Atlas of Small Animal Ultrasonography

Atlas of Small Animal Ultrasonography

Dominique Penninck

Marc-André d'Anjou

Illustrations by Beth Mellor

Blackwell Publishing

Dominique Penninck, DVM, PhD, is a Professor of Diagnostic Imaging in the Department of Clinical Sciences, Cummings School of Veterinary Medicine, Tufts University.

Marc-André d'Anjou, DVM, is an Assistant Professor of Diagnostic Imaging, Department of Clinical Sciences, Faculté de Médecine, Vétérinaire, Université de Montréal.

Blackwell Publishing Professional
2121 State Avenue, Ames, Iowa 50014, USA

Orders: 1-800-862-6657
Office: 1-515-292-0140
Fax: 1-515-292-3348
Web site: www.blackwellprofessional.com

Blackwell Publishing Ltd
9600 Garsington Road, Oxford OX4 2DQ, UK
Tel.: +44 (0)1865 776868

Blackwell Publishing Asia
550 Swanston Street, Carlton, Victoria 3053, Australia
Tel.: +61 (0)3 8359 1011

First edition, 2008

Library of Congress Cataloging-in-Publication Data

Atlas of small animal ultrasonography/[edited by] Dominique Penninck, Marc-André d'Anjou.–1st ed.
p. ; cm.
Includes bibliographical references and index.
ISBN 978-0-8138-2800-8 (alk. paper)
1. Veterinary ultrasonography–Atlases. I. Penninck, Dominique. II. d'Anjou, Marc-André.
[DNLM: 1. Ultrasonography–veterinary–Atlases. 2. Veterinary Medicine–methods–Atlases. SF 772.58 A881 2008]

SF772.58A85 2008
636.089'607543–dc22

2007013146

The last digit is the print number: 9 8 7 6

Dedication

To my children, Anaïs and Loïc for their loving support, continuous encouragement and . . . patience!

To Marianne Spehl, an inspiring mentor and friend.

In memory of my father, Albert Penninck, and my nephew, Vincent Dupierreux.

Dominique Penninck

To Annabelle, Olivier, and Héloïse, for their constant love, comprehension, and energizing presence.

To all participants in our veterinary community that allow us to advance in pure mutualism.

In memory of my brother Charles.

Marc-André d'Anjou

Contents

Contributors

Donald Brown, DVM, PhD, DACVIM Cardiology
Associate Professor Cardiology
Department of Clinical Sciences
Tufts Cummings School of Veterinary Medicine
200 Westborough Road
North Grafton, MA 01536, USA

Nancy R. Cox, DVM, MS, PhD
Scientist, Scott-Ritchey Research Center and
Associate Professor, Department of Pathobiology
College of Veterinary Medicine
Auburn University
Auburn, AL 35849, USA

Marc-André d'Anjou, DMV, DACVR
Assistant Professor, Diagnostic Imaging
Department of Clinical Sciences
Faculty of Veterinary Medicine
University of Montreal
3200 Sicotte
Saint-Hyacinthe Quebec, Canada J2S 7C6

Hugues Gaillot, DMV
Imagerie Médicale Vétérinaire de Paris 15
10, 12 rue Robert de Flers
75015 Paris, France

John Graham, MVB, MSc, DVR, MRCVS, DACVR, DECVDI
Affiliated Veterinary Specialists,
9905 South US Highway 17-92
Maitland, FL 32751, USA

Silke Hecht, Dr.med.vet., DACVR, DECVDI
Assistant Professor of Radiology
Department of Small Animal Clinical Sciences
University of Tennessee College of Veterinary Medicine
Knoxville, TN 37996, USA

Judith A. Hudson, DVM, PhD, DACVR
Professor of Diagnostic Imaging
Department of Clinical Sciences
College of Veterinary Medicine
Auburn University
Auburn, AL 35849, USA

Martin Kramer, Dr.med.vet., PhD, DECVDI
Professor
Department of Veterinary Clinical Sciences
Clinic for Small Animals
Justus-Liebig University–Giessen
Frankfurter Str. 108
35392 Giessen, Germany

Dominique Penninck, DVM, PhD, DACVR, DECVDI
Professor Diagnostic Imaging
Department of Clinical Sciences
Tufts Cummings School of Veterinary Medicine
200 Westborough Road
North Grafton, MA 01536, USA

Kathy Spaulding, DVM, DACVR
Clinical Professor Radiology
Large Animal Clinical Sciences
College of Veterinary Medicine and Biomedical Sciences
Texas A&M University
4475 TAMU
College Station, TX 77843-4475, USA

James Sutherland-Smith, BVSc, DACVR
Assistant Professor, Diagnostic Imaging
Department of Clinical Sciences
Tufts Cummings School of Veterinary Medicine
200 Westborough Road
North Grafton, MA 01536, USA

Erik Wisner, DVM, DACVR
Professor of Diagnostic Imaging
Department of Surgical and Radiological Sciences
School of Veterinary Medicine, University of California
1 Shields Avenue
Davis, CA 95616, USA

Allison Zwingenberger, DVM, DACVR, DECVDI
Assistant Professor of Diagnostic Imaging
Department of Surgical and Radiological Sciences
School of Veterinary Medicine, University of California
1 Shields Avenue
Davis, CA 95616, USA

Preface

Since the start of veterinary ultrasonography in the late 1970s, many technological changes have transformed this diagnostic modality. Research and publications have enabled all sonographers to increase their level of expertise significantly. Today, ultrasonography is an integral part of the diagnostic approach in academic institutions, as well as in private practice.

The main goal of this book is to provide its readers with a vast collection of high-quality sonographic images and illustrations addressing the normal anatomy and common disorders of most body parts in small animals. These images were carefully selected or created for their teaching capability.

The choice of contributors reflects some of the international expertise available today.

We hope that this atlas will be a reference source for veterinary students, interns, and residents, as well as for radiologists, internists, and surgeons eager to learn and excel in this modality.

Acknowledgments

We are pleased to acknowledge the "behind the scenes" contributions of many colleagues, technicians, students, and residents, past and present, who helped in gathering the necessary image collections to assemble this atlas. Special thanks to those at Tufts University Cummings School of Veterinary Medicine and at the Faculty of Veterinary Medicine, University of Montreal.

We express our deep gratitude also to the contributors for sharing their expertise and passion and to the publishing team at Blackwell who assisted us with this project.

Finally, we thank the many pets that patiently participated in these studies, enabling us to learn and teach with their images.

Special thanks to Beth Mellor, who produced most of the illustrations. Her artistic talent has greatly enhanced the mission of this book.

Atlas of Small Animal Ultrasonography

CHAPTER ONE

Nervous System

SECTION 1

Brain

Judith Hudson and Nancy Cox

Scanning Technique

The brain of most small animals can be imaged adequately with a high-frequency transducer (7.5–10 MHz) to provide the best resolution. The use of a lower-frequency transducer (3–5 MHz) may also be necessary in large dogs or in dogs with thick bone. Although sector scanners, linear array transducers, and curvilinear array transducers all can be used, sector scanners and curvilinear array transducers provide better visualization of peripheral structures. A small footprint is also helpful.

Sedation is usually not necessary. Most small animals can be imaged while wrapped in a warm towel and held gently in the sonographer's lap. Fur can usually be parted for the acoustic gel to be applied. In some individuals with a thick hair coat, clipping may improve the quality of the images.

In young puppies, the bregmatic fontanel can be used as an acoustic window to the brain up to approximately 1 month of age (Hudson et al. 1991). In some individuals, particularly in toy-breed dogs, the bregmatic fontanels may persist into adult life. A kitten's brain can be imaged through the fontanel up to about 5 months of age although accessibility decreases over time (Jäderlund et al. 2003). Unless the fontanel or defect is very large, the tip of the transducer must be held relatively stationary; the transducer can slide only a short distance. The brain is imaged by using a "windshield wiper" technique, with the tip of the probe acting as a pivot point to scan from rostral to caudal and back to obtain transverse images and from side to side to obtain longitudinal images. Because the probe is usually angled to view rostral and caudal structures, most images are made in oblique rather than perpendicular planes (Figure 1.1). Therefore, it should be remembered that, in rostral transverse images, ventral structures seen are actually located rostrally to dorsal structures in the image whereas, in the caudal transverse images, the ventral structures are located caudally to dorsal structures seen in the image.

In absence of a fontanel, a lower-frequency transducer (e.g., 5 MHz) can be used to penetrate the skull, enabling partial visualization of the brain. Penetration of the temporal bone can be used for this purpose in some small dogs in which the brain cannot be otherwise imaged (Figure 1.2A).

Visualization of caudal structures of the brain can be achieved by imaging at the foramen magnum (Figure 1.2B).

Craniotomy sites, and defects caused by trauma or disease, can be used in imaging the brain. Prenatal neurosonography is common in human medicine but is seldom used in animals. The brain of unborn puppies and kittens can be evaluated in utero, however. Prenatal sonographic diagnosis of hydranencephaly has been reported (Cruz et al. 2003). Based on findings in human patients, ultrasound images of the brain of puppies and kittens in late gestation in utero should enable the detection of other major defects in brain development, such as anencephalies, encephaloceles, and meningogoceles.

Normal Sonographic Anatomy of the Brain

In Dogs

Transverse Images

The sonographic anatomy of the brain of normal dogs has been described (Hudson et al. 1989) (Figure 1.3). The longitudinal fissure and splenial sulci form a hyperechoic umbrella-like structure that can be used as a landmark to locate the midline of the brain. This is particularly useful when a natural or created defect in the skull is located asymmetrically. The cingulate

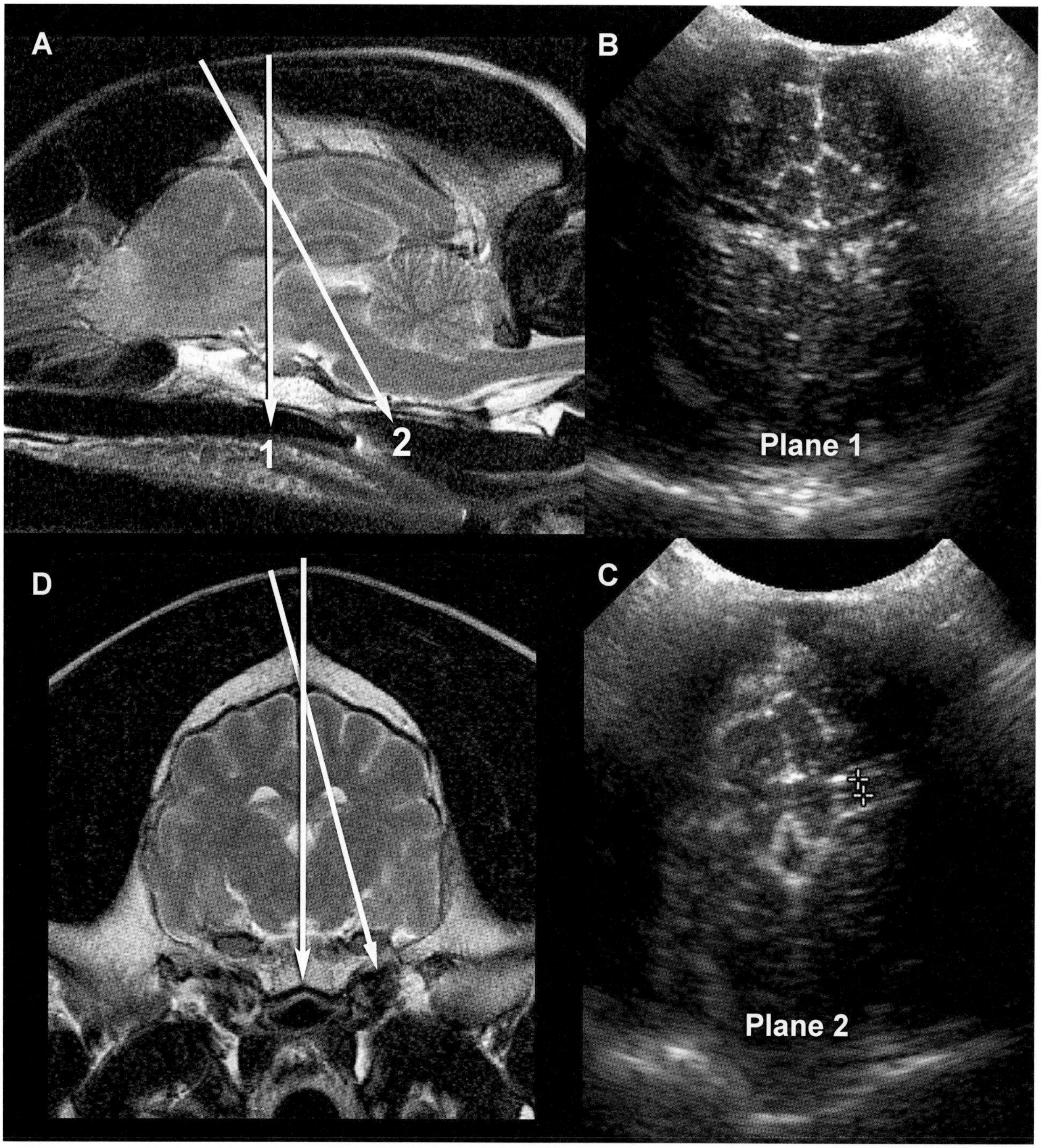

Figure 1.1. Normal brain in a dog and ultrasound beams resulting in planes 1 and 2. **A:** Sagittal magnetic resonance image of the brain of a normal golden retriever illustrating how the ultrasound beam (planes 1 and 2 represented by the arrows) passes through the brain when the beam is placed over the fontanel to obtain transverse sonograms. **B:** Plane 1 shows the ultrasound beam angled perpendicular to the long axis of the brain to image the rostral horns of the lateral ventricles. **C:** Plane 2 shows the ultrasound beam angled caudally to image the third ventricle and mesencephalon. **D:** Transverse magnetic resonance image of the brain of a normal dog showing the axis of an ultrasound beam over the fontanel to obtain midline and parasagittal sonograms (arrows).

Figure 1.2. **A: Hydrocephalus.** Transverse magnetic resonance image of a dog with hydrocephalus showing the axis of an ultrasound beam to obtain parasagittal images (arrows and corresponding planes 1 and 2). Plane 1 shows the beam angled laterally to obtain a parasagittal image. Plane 2 shows the axis of the beam to image the brain through the temporal bone. 3, third ventricle; CN, caudate nucleus; LLV, left lateral ventricle; and T, thalamus. **B: Foramen magnum window.** Sagittal magnetic resonance image of a cat showing the axis of the ultrasound beam (arrow) for imaging of the brain through the foramen magnum. The plane of the ultrasound beam passes through the cerebellum and midbrain. A sonogram of a normal cat made through the foramen magnum is on the bottom right. A histological image made in a similar plane is on the bottom left. M, midbrain; and V, vermis.

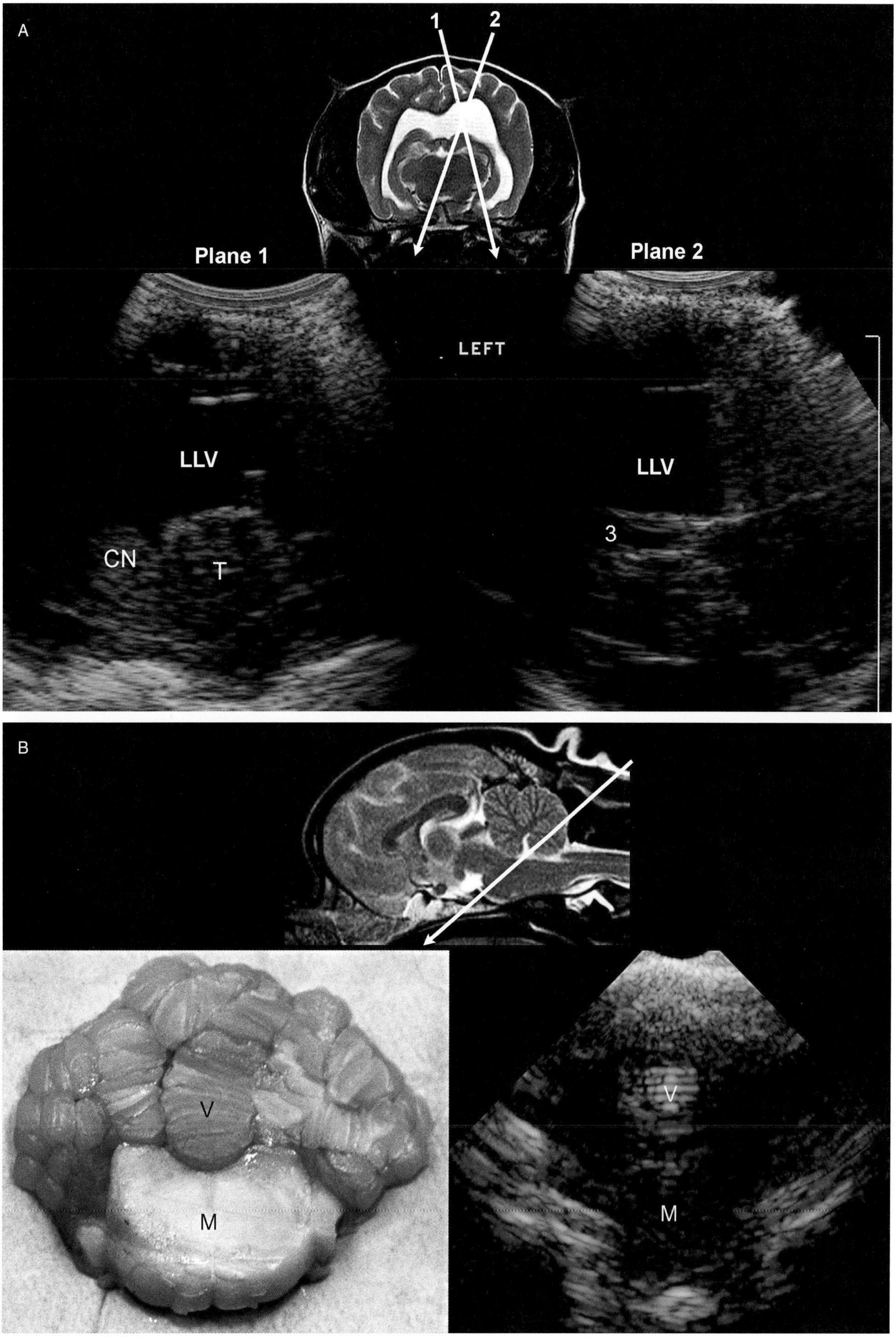

Figure 1.2

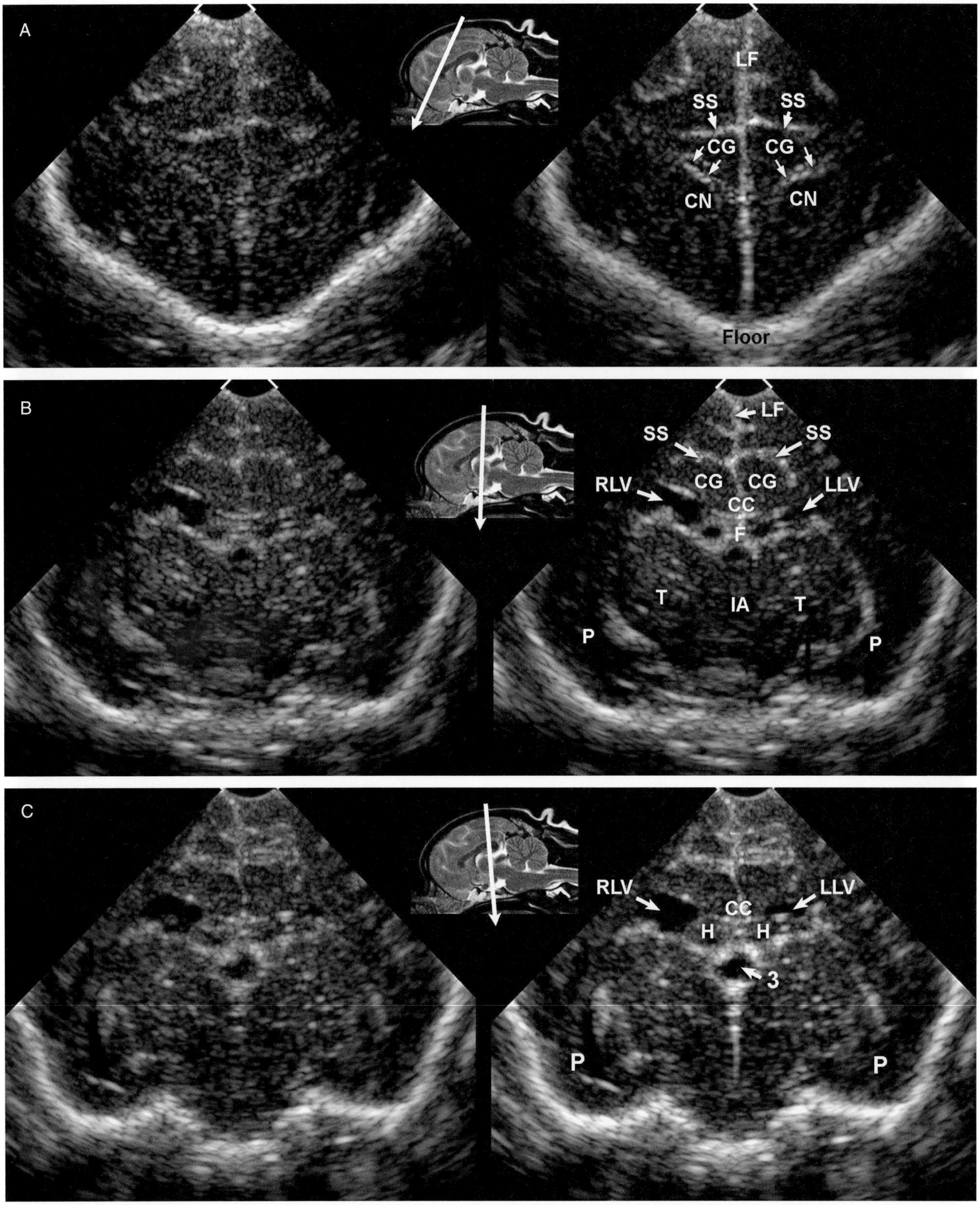

Figure 1.3. Transverse sonograms of the brain of a 1-month-old Yorkshire terrier. The ventricles are asymmetrical but within normal limits. **A:** Rostral sonogram. **B:** Sonogram at the level of the interthalamic adhesion. **C:** Sonogram at the level of the third ventricle. **D:** Sonogram with the ultrasound beam angled caudally to image the mesencephalon. **E:** Sonogram with the ultrasound beam angled caudally to image the cerebellum. 3, third ventricle; CC, corpus callosum; CG, cingulate gyrus; CN, caudate nucleus; F, fornix; H, hippocampus; IA, interthalamic adhesion; LF, longitudinal fissure; LLV, left lateral ventricle; M, mesencephalon; P, pyriform lobe; Po, pons; RLV, right lateral ventricle; SS, splenial sulcus; Su, subarachnoid space; T, thalamus; and V, vermis.

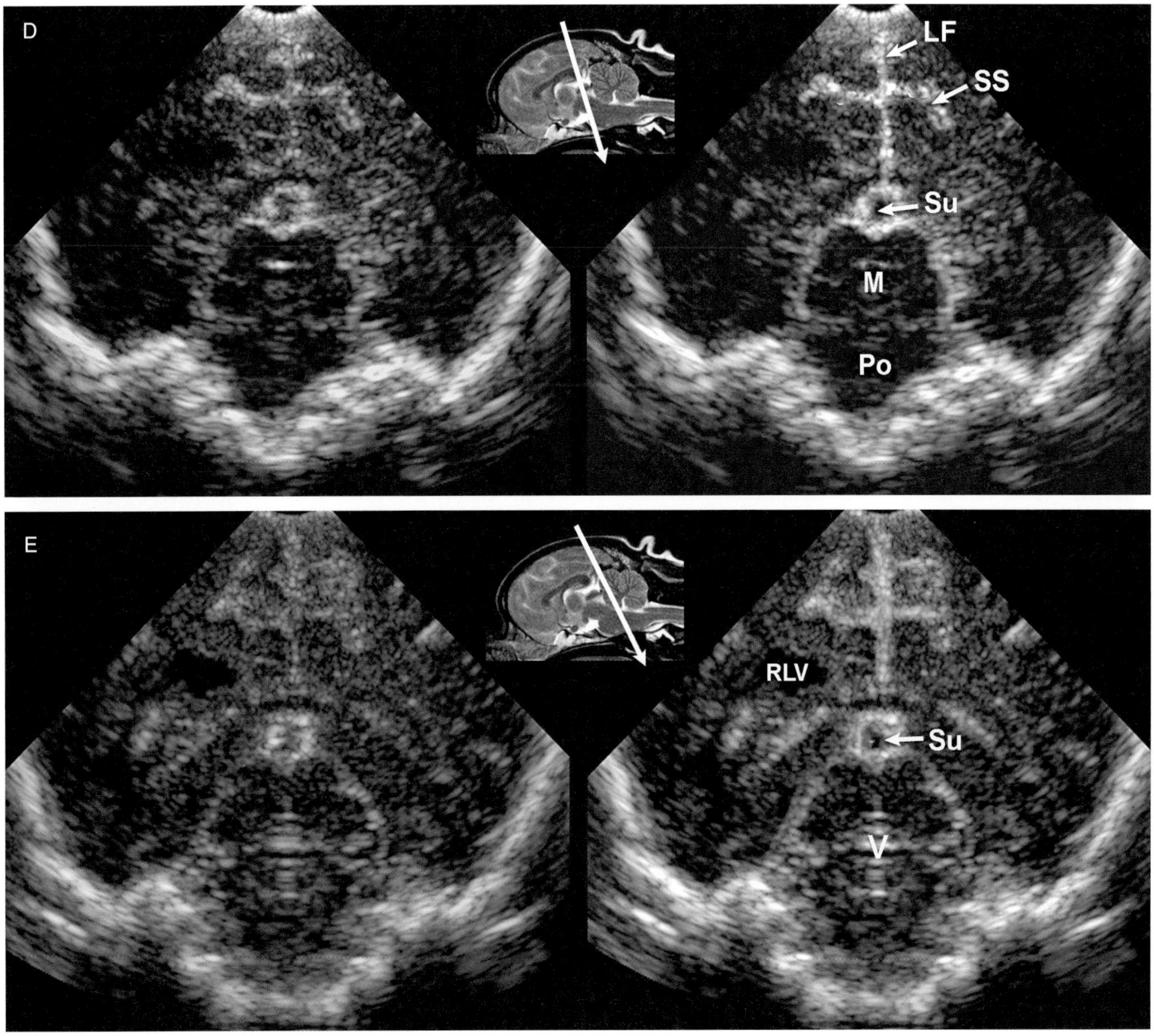

Figure 1.3. *Continued*

gyrus is found deep to each splenial sulcus. Rostrally, the caudate nuclei are recognizable as hyperechoic curved structures. The lateral ventricles are located medial to the caudate nuclei and vary greatly in size according to the breed, age, and individual. Asymmetry is common. Cerebrospinal fluid (CSF) is anechoic and may cause the lateral ventricles to appear as small anechoic slits in some individuals.

As the beam is swept slightly more caudally, the rostral fornix comes into view. Choroid plexus is hyperechoic while it lies on the floor of the central portion of the lateral ventricle and the roof of the temporal horn. It may be difficult to distinguish between the caudate nucleus and the adjacent choroid plexus in the lateral ventricle, so only a single hyperechoic focus might be seen on each side of the midline in some dogs. If there is sufficient CSF, the lateral ventricle can be seen.

In older puppies and adult dogs, alternating hyperechoic and hypoechoic lines represent the callosal sulcus, corpus callosum, and fornix. Comparison with histological samples suggests that the most superficial hyperechoic layer is the callosal sulcus, which contains vessels that pulsate. The corpus callosum is comprised of a hypoechoic surface with a deeper hyperechoic border. The fornix is hypoechoic. In the first few days of life, these structures may appear only as a single hyperechoic region. Detail improves as myelination progresses after birth. Most of the brain is uniformly hypoechoic, but the pyriform lobes are visible because of hyperechoic meninges dorsal to each lobe.

When the probe is tilted to sweep the ultrasound beam caudally, the dorsal portion of each hippocampus appears as a hypoechoic structure close to the midline. Dorsolateral to each of these structures, a hyperechoic area represents choroid plexus in each lateral ventricle. Another hyperechoic area is seen in the midline ventral to the level of the dorsal portions of the hippocampi. Depending on the angle of ultrasound section, this hyperechoic area may represent choroid plexus in the dorsal portion of the third ventricle or pia mater that is located more caudally in the adjacent subarachnoid space. Vessels and trabeculae in the subarachnoid space may create a complex of echoes that outline the mesencephalon and cause it to appear as a dome-shaped hypoechoic structure. The petrous temporal bones will create irregular hyperechoic echoes on the floor of the cranium on each side of the midline deep to the hypoechoic pyriform lobes.

More caudally, the osseous tentorium is a hyperechoic structure shaped like an inverted V. In older animals, this structure often prevents visualization of the caudal brain, but the medulla and cerebellum can be imaged in neonatal animals. The medulla is hypoechoic. The vermis of the cerebellum is represented by a stack of hyperechoic lines seen in the midline. Each lateral cerebellar hemisphere is located more laterally as a hypoechoic structure.

Parasagittal Images

Longitudinal images made near the midline are true sagittal images, but when the probe is moved past the edge of the fontanel, the probe must be angled to enable the beam to reach the lateral margins of the brain. The floor of the cranium appears curved in images showing the lateral portions of the brain, whereas the floor of the cranium is more irregular in images made near the midline (midsagittal images). As the probe is angled laterally, structures that are anatomically closer to the midline appear in the near field of the ultrasound image, whereas more lateral structures are seen in the far field (Figure 1.4).

The interthalamic adhesion and, more caudally, the mesencephalon can be seen in midsagittal images as hypoechoic structures surrounded by echoes created mainly by choroid plexus in the third ventricle and meninges and in vessels in the subarachnoid space. In some areas, the third ventricle will appear anechoic or hypoechoic because of the presence of CSF. The osseous tentorium is incompletely ossified in neonates, enabling visualization of hyperechoic echoes created by the vermis in the posttentorial area of the brain. More superficially, the callosal sulcus is seen as a hyperechoic line. The corpus callosum has an appearance similar to that seen in transverse images. It is hypoechoic, with a deep hyperechoic interface.

When the probe is angled to obtain a lateral parasagittal image, the subarachnoid space and third ventricle are no longer seen; the thalamus and lateral ventricle are now visible on the imaged side. The thalamus appears as a hypoechoic structure outlined by hyperechoic choroid plexus in the lateral ventricle. Areas of the lateral ventricle with sufficient CSF may appear anechoic or hypoechoic. The caudate nucleus is imaged rostral to the thalamus as a hypoechoic structure with increased echogenicity superficially. This structure is more apparent in older dogs than in neonates. The thalamocaudate groove is seen between the thalamus and caudate nucleus. This groove is more apparent in older dogs, but in neonates a hyperechoic clump of choroid plexus is often seen in the lateral ventricle in this region. Care should be taken not to mistake this normal appearance for intraventricular hemorrhage that is also hyperechoic. In lateral parasagittal images, the splenial sulcus is seen in addition to the callosal sulcus and corpus callosum and appears as an undulating hyperechoic line. The cingulate gyrus shows as a hypoechoic structure deep to the splenial sulcus.

In Cats

The feline brain can be evaluated by using transverse and longitudinal sonographic planes (Figures 1.5 and 1.6).

The lateral ventricles are slitlike in kittens. In some normal magnetic resonance images of the adult feline brain (Hudson et al. 1995), the lateral ventricles cannot be discerned. Using ultrasound, measurement of lateral ventricles is also more problematic in cats than in dogs because landmarks such as the thalamocaudate groove and the interthalamic adhesion are less recognizable (Jäderlund et al. 2003). In the study by Jäderlund and colleagues, the most reliable and repeatable measurements were obtained by measuring the central portion of the lateral ventricle in parasagittal views angled 5°–10° from the midline. In these images, the dorsal and ventral walls of each lateral ventricle were parallel to each other, but the walls on each side were perpendicular to the ultrasound beam (Figure 1.6). The caudal portion of each lateral ventricle was larger than the more rostral portions, which provided clear

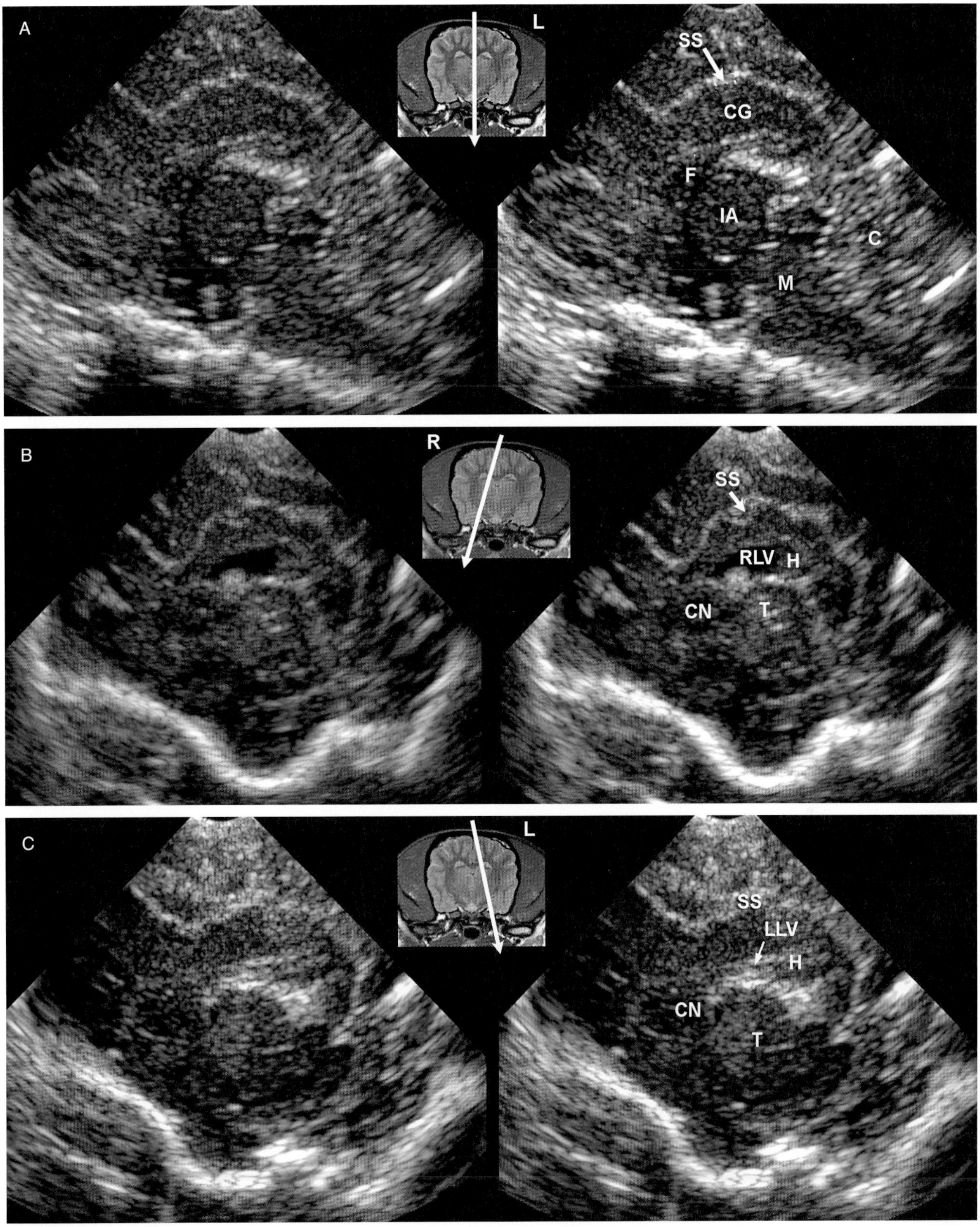

Figure 1.4. Sagittal to parasagittal sonograms of the brain of a normal 1-month-old Yorkshire terrier. **A:** Midline sagittal sonogram. **B:** Parasagittal sonogram with the ultrasound beam angled laterally to image the right lateral ventricle. **C:** Parasagittal sonogram with the ultrasound beam angled laterally to image the left lateral ventricle. C, cerebellum; CG, cingulate gyrus; CN, caudate nucleus; F, fornix; H, hippocampus; IA, interthalamic adhesion; L, left; M, mesencephalon; R, right; RLV, right lateral ventricle; SS, splenial sulcus; and T, thalamus.

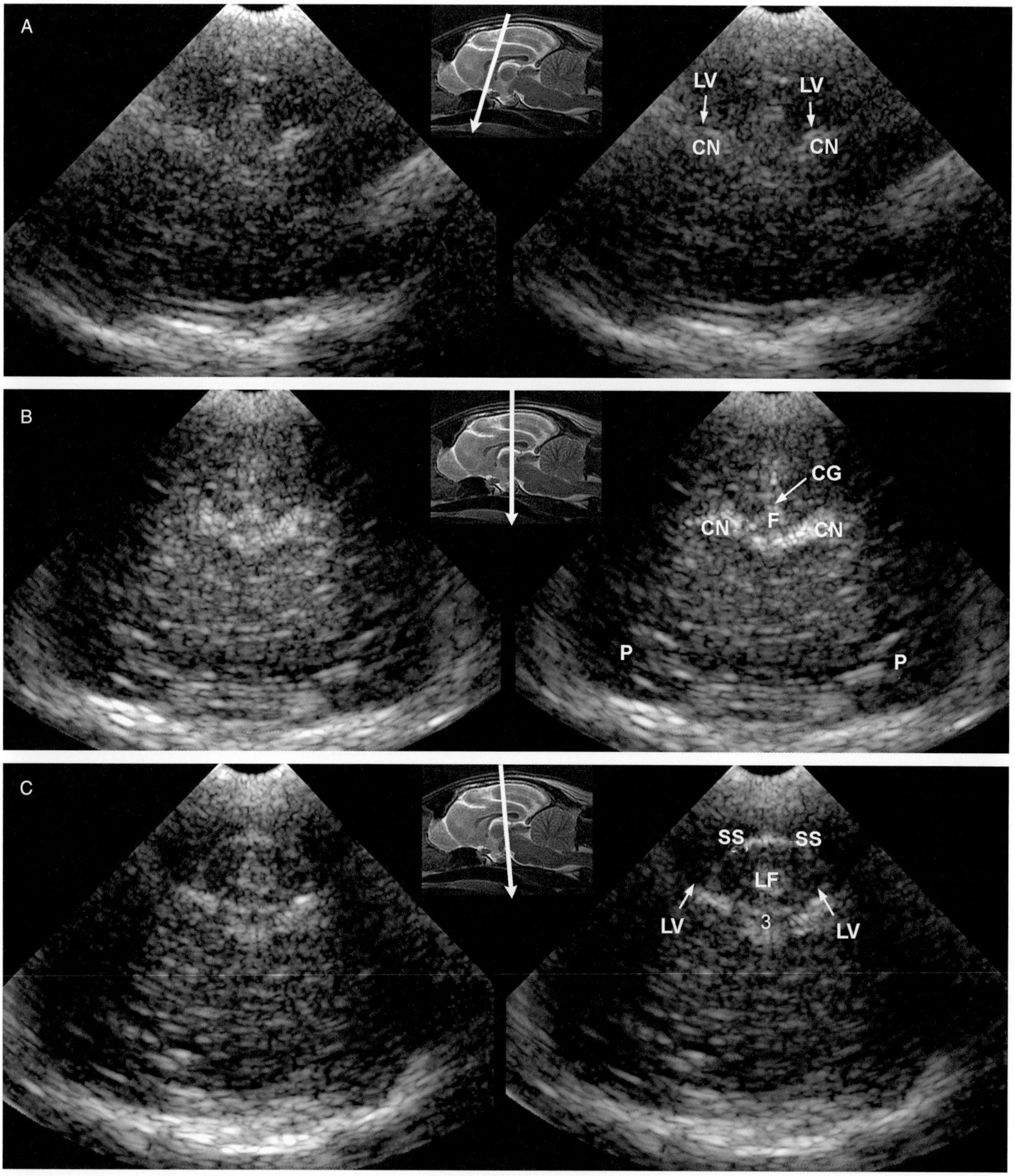

Figure 1.5. Transverse sonograms of the brain of a normal 1-week-old kitten. The ventricles in a kitten are slitlike and much smaller than those of a puppy. **A:** Rostral sonogram showing the caudate nuclei and lateral ventricles (arrows). **B:** Sonogram with the ultrasound beam perpendicular to the brain. **C:** Sonogram at the level of the third ventricle. **D:** Sonogram at the level of the mesencephalon. **E:** Sonogram with the probe angled caudally to image the cerebellum. The vermis appears as a series of stacked linear echoes. 3, third ventricle; CC, corpus callosum; CG, cingulate gyrus; CN, caudate nucleus (plus the choroid plexus in the lateral ventricle); F, fornix; LF, longitudinal fissure; LV, lateral ventricle; M, mesencephalon; P, pyriform lobe; SS, splenial sulcus; and V, vermis.

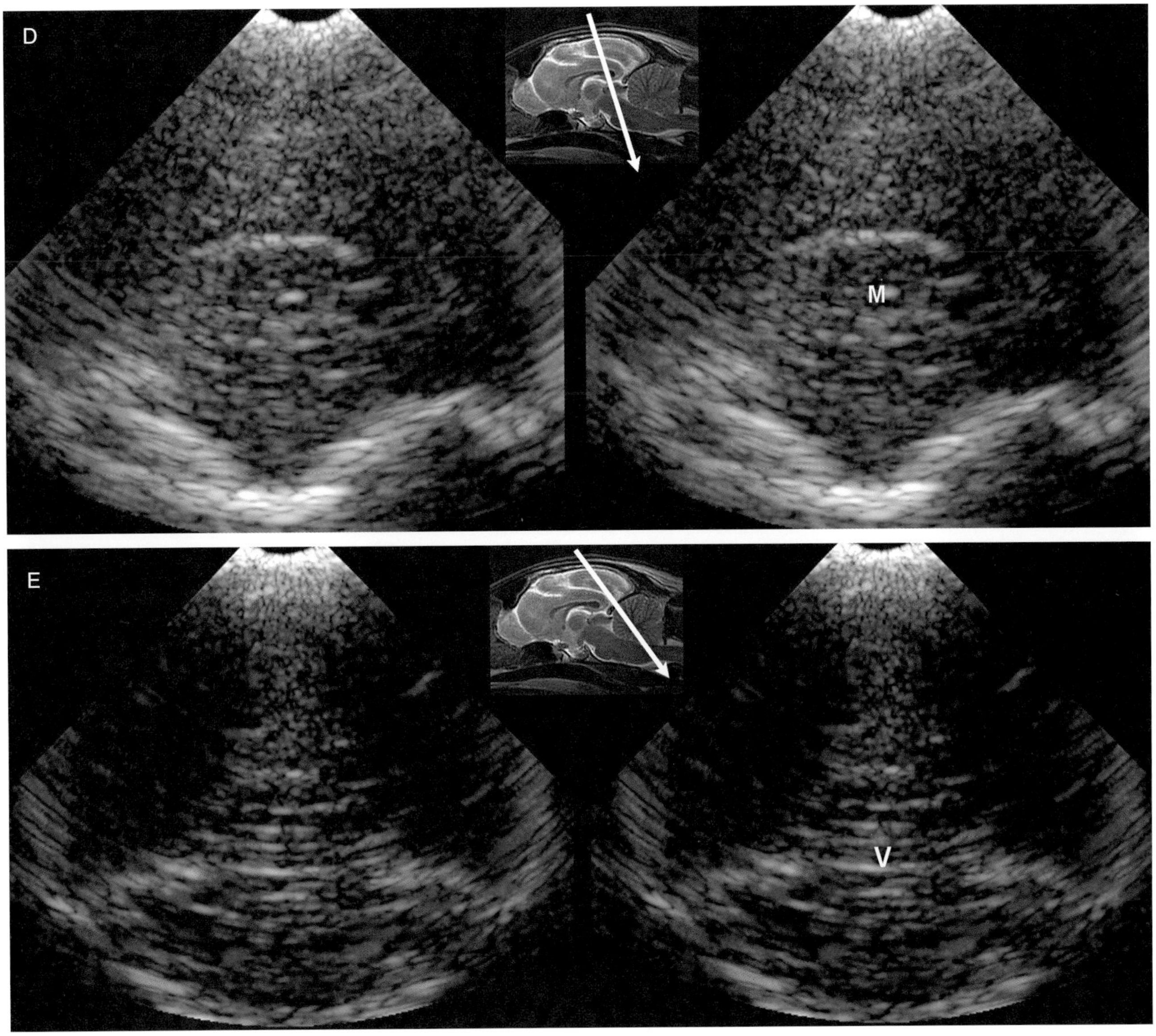

Figure 1.5. *Continued*

visualization in parasagittal scans. Curving of the occipital horn made accurate measurement difficult, however. Difficulty was also experienced when measuring the lateral ventricles in transverse images. Measurement was recommended at the junction of the sella turcica and the cranial fossa to provide a landmark for greater repeatability, but the ventricular walls were at a slightly oblique angle to the beam in transverse images at this level.

Brain Vasculature

In dogs, the internal carotid artery enters the cranial vault and divides into the rostral cerebral artery, the middle cerebral artery, and the caudal communicating artery (Schaller 1992) (Figure 1.7).

The rostral cerebral artery runs rostrally and dorsally and then curves caudally along the medial aspect of the hemisphere. The artery anastomoses with a branch of the caudal communicating artery that supplies the caudomedial portion of the cerebrum. The middle cerebral artery sends central branches that enter the midportion of the brain. A lateral branch supplies the surface of the brain. In the area of the spine, the vertebral arteries unite to form the basilar artery, which enters the brain caudally and divides into the right and left caudal communicating arteries. Each caudal communicating artery connects the basilar artery with the ipsilateral internal carotid artery.

Cats differ from dogs in that the terminal extracranial portion of the internal carotid artery is regressed (Figure 1.8).

In cats and dogs, the ascending pharyngeal artery arises from the external carotid artery and runs rostrally to anastomose with the internal carotid artery, but, in cats, the ascending pharyngeal artery is a major source of blood to the brain.

Color flow Doppler imaging can be used to image the cerebral arteries, particularly the rostral cerebral artery and the central branch of the middle cerebral artery. Velocities in these vessels can be measured by switching the sonographic mode to pulsed-wave or continuous-wave Doppler imaging. The most accurate measurements are made from sagittal images because the sonographer can ensure that the *Doppler angle* (the angle between the path of the ultrasound beam and the direction of flow) is as close to zero as possible. Velocities are likely to be underestimated when made

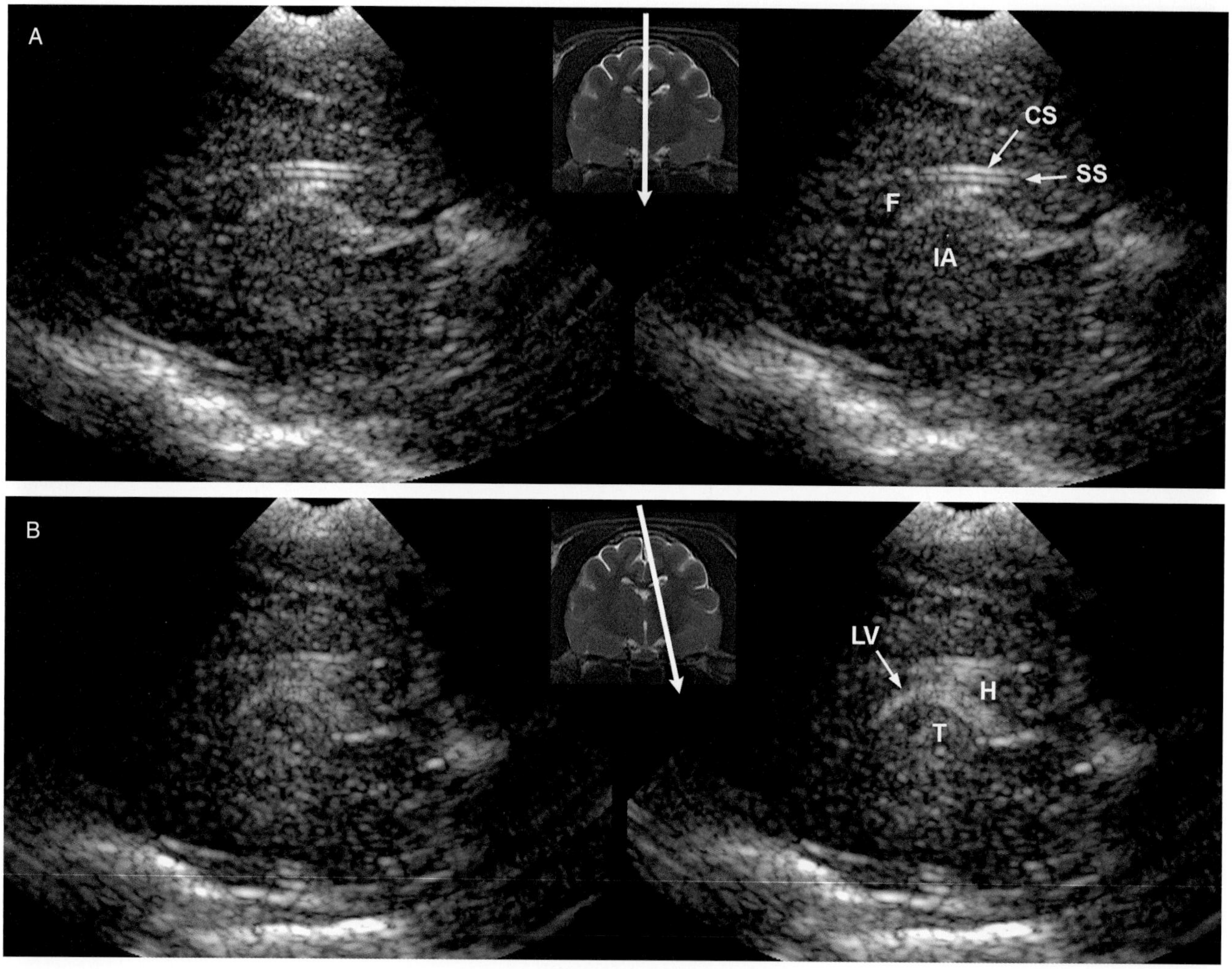

Figure 1.6. Sagittal to parasagittal sonograms of the brain of a normal 1-week-old kitten. **A:** Midline sagittal sonogram. **B:** Parasagittal sonogram with the beam angled lateral to the midline. CS, callosal sulcus; F, fornix; H, hippocampus; IA, interthalamic adhesion; LV, lateral ventricle; SS, splenial sulcus; and T, thalamus. The arrow in the magnetic resonance image insert shows sagittal and parasagittal planes corresponding to the sonograms.

Figure 1.7. Sonograms with color Doppler imaging to show the vasculature of the brain of a normal dog. **A:** Parasagittal sonogram showing the branches of the internal carotid artery. **B:** Parasagittal sonogram of the brain showing placement of the pulsed Doppler cursors on the rostral cerebral artery. **C:** Transverse sonogram of the rostral brain showing the dorsal portion of the rostral cerebral artery (R). The electronic cursors have been placed to measure velocity and calculate the resistance index from the Doppler waveform. Arrows indicate the location of the lateral ventricles. ACC, branch of the rostral cerebral artery (artery along the corpus callosum); CB, callosal branches; ICA, internal carotid artery; MCA, middle branch of the middle cerebral artery; and RCA, rostral cerebral artery.

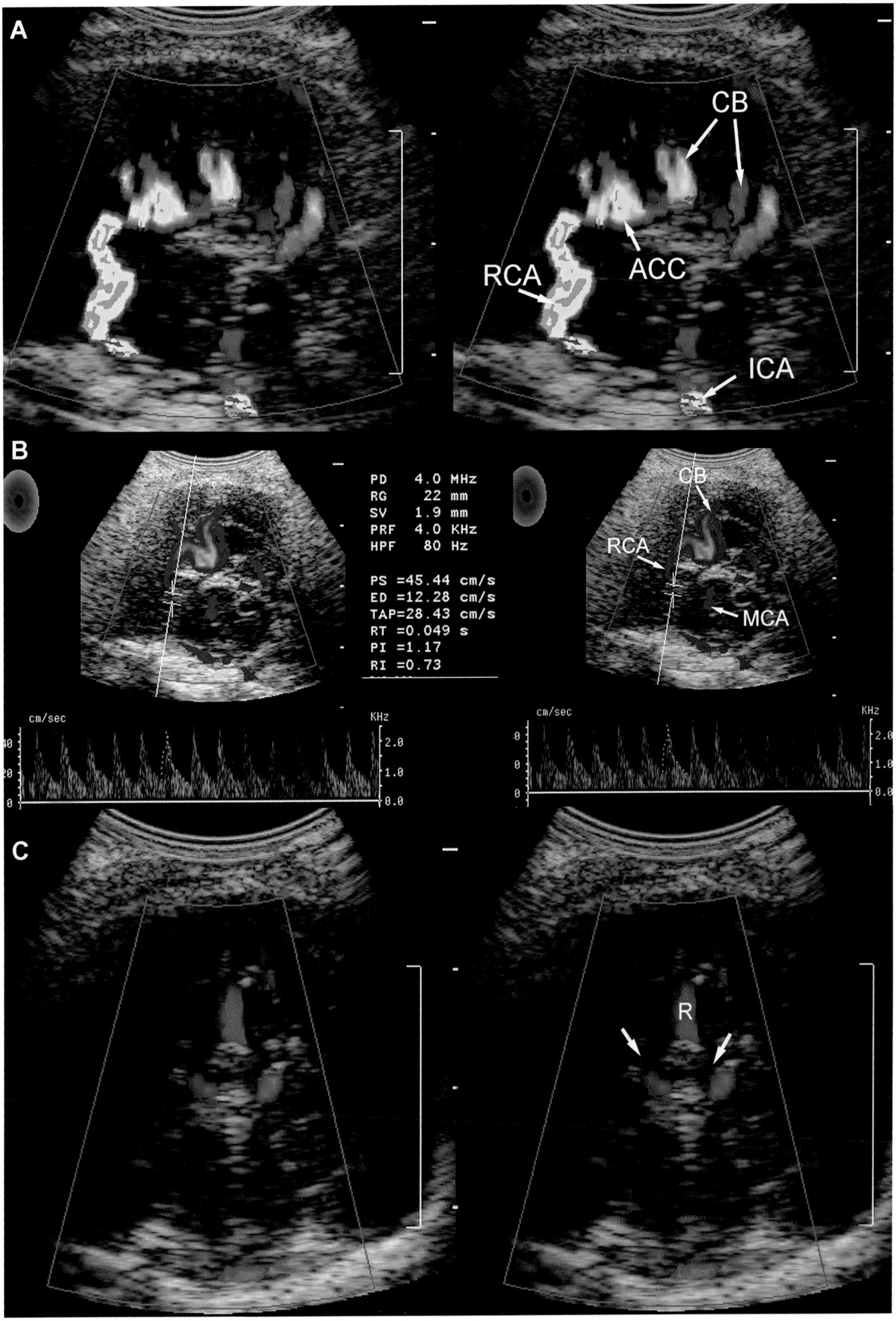
A
CB
ACC
RCA
ICA
B
PD 4.0 MHz
RG 22 mm
SV 1.9 mm
PRF 4.0 KHz
HPF 80 Hz
PS =45.44 cm/s
ED =12.28 cm/s
TAP=28.43 cm/s
RT =0.049 s
PI =1.17
RI =0.73
CB
RCA
MCA
cm/sec
KHz
C
R

Figure 1.7

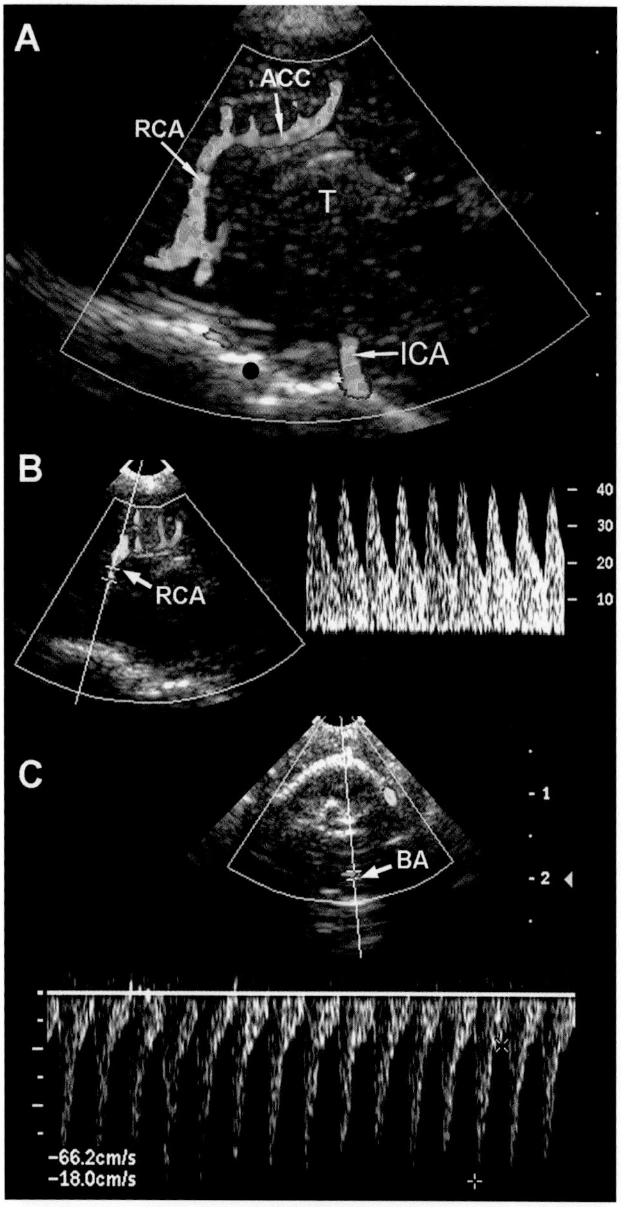

Figure 1.8. Sonograms made using color Doppler imaging to show the vasculature of the brain of a normal cat. **A:** Parasagittal sonogram showing the branches of the internal carotid artery. **B:** Parasagittal sonogram of the feline brain showing placement of the pulsed Doppler cursors on the rostral cerebral artery. A normal waveform is shown. **C:** Sonogram of the caudal aspect of the brain made through the foramen magnum showing the pulsed Doppler cursor placed on basilar artery. The resistance index can be calculated from the peak systolic and diastolic velocities. The ascending pharyngeal artery anastomoses with the internal carotid artery becoming a major source of blood to the brain. A portion of the extracranial internal carotid artery is not patent. ACC, branch of the rostral cerebral artery (artery along the corpus callosum); BA, basilar artery; ICA, internal carotid artery; RCA, rostral cerebral artery; and T, thalamus.

from transverse images, because the Doppler angle cannot be accurately measured. Nevertheless, in some cases, transverse images must be made because the sonographic window is too small and the probe too large to enable sonographers to tilt the probe adequately to obtain parasagittal images of the rostral brain. Although the Doppler cursor is best placed using the color flow Doppler image as a guide, pulsations can be seen on gray-scale images, and the Doppler cursor can be placed on these pulsations to obtain velocity measurements (Hudson et al. 1997).

Evaluation of vessels may be helpful when the brain is injured or is damaged by disease. Color flow Doppler imaging can be used to identify overcirculated or undercirculated areas. The resistance index (RI) is calculated as the following ratio:

$$(\text{systolic velocity} - \text{diastolic velocity}) / \text{diastolic velocity}$$

High RI may be associated with a poor prognosis in some disease processes (Saito et al. 2003).

Sonography of Brain Disorders

The most common application of neurosonography of the brain is to measure ventricular size when diagnosing hydrocephalus. Other applications include evaluation of animals with traumatic cranial defects for evidence of hemorrhage or infection, intraoperative or postoperative examination of brain neoplasms, and imaging of masses associated with bony lysis. Additionally, ultrasound can be used to guide biopsy or fine-needle aspiration of brain lesions or to guide injection of substances into the brain.

Hydrocephalus

Hydrocephalus can be congenital or acquired. The disorder is common in toy-breed dogs, which may have persistent fontanels (Figure 1.9).

It should not be assumed that a dog has hydrocephalus merely because there is a persistent fontanel. Not all toy-breed dogs with a persistent fontanel have hydrocephalus, and, conversely, toy-breed dogs can have hydrocephalus without having a persistent fontanel. In some toy-breed or small breed dogs without a persistent fontanel, the temporal bone is thin enough to allow transcranial imaging. In addition, limited imaging of the caudal fossa can be achieved using the foramen magnum. Because the fontanel ossifies in many larger dogs, other imaging modalities may be

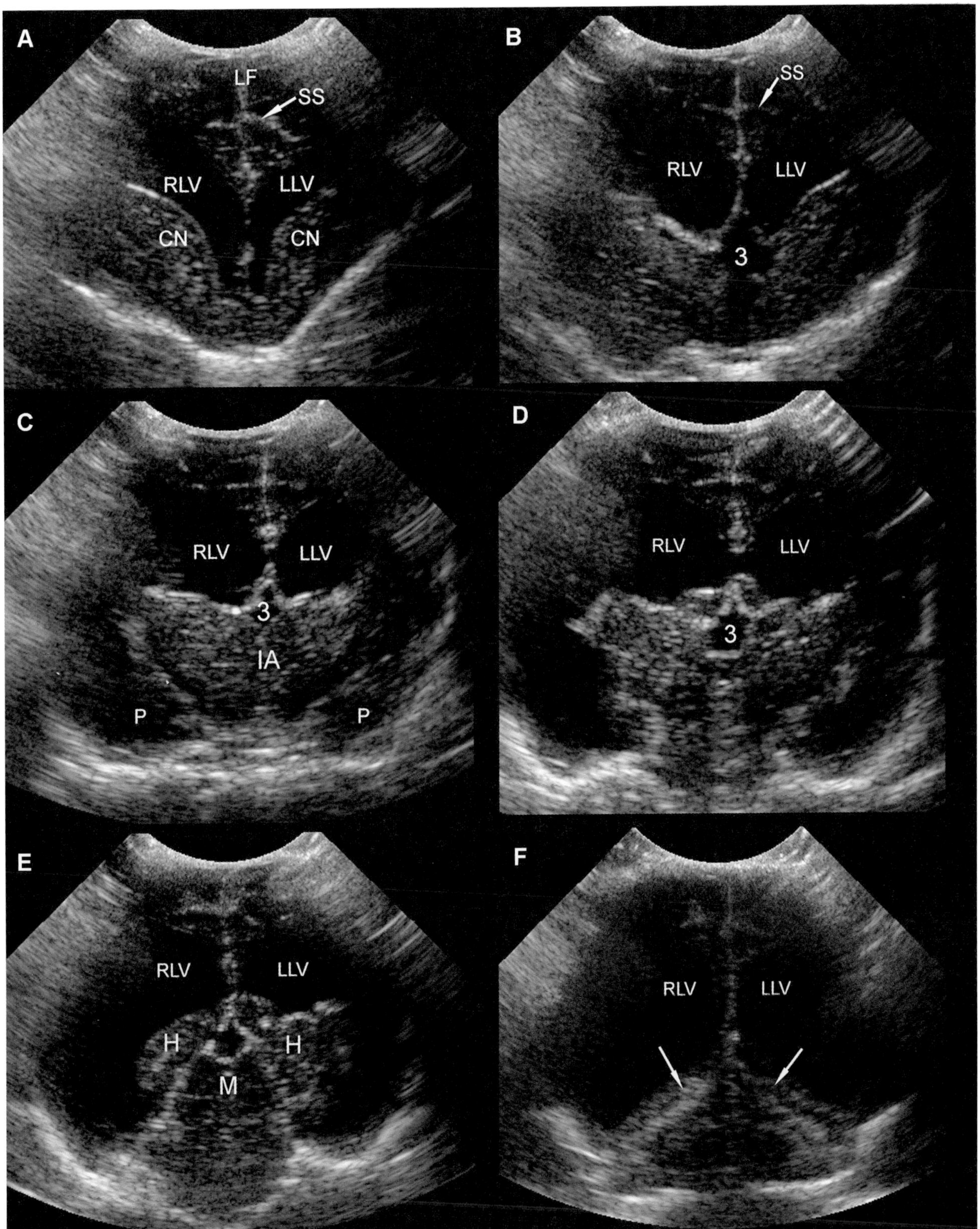

Figure 1.9. Sonograms of a 1-year-old Chihuahua with severe ventriculomegaly. **A:** Rostral sonogram showing the caudate nuclei and lateral ventricles. **B:** Sonogram made at the level of the rostral portion of the third ventricle. **C:** Sonogram made at the level of the thalami. **D:** Sonogram made at the level of the pituitary gland. Notice the irregularity of the floor of the cranium at this level. **E:** Sonogram made with the ultrasound beam pointed caudally to display mesencephalon. **F:** Sonogram showing the osseous tentorium (arrows). 3, third ventricle; CN, caudate nuclei; H, hippocampus; IA, interthalamic adhesion; LF, longitudinal fissure; LLV, left lateral ventricle; M, mesencephalon; P, pyriform lobe; RLV, right lateral ventricle; and SS, splenial sulcus on the left side.

necessary to examine the brain for hydrocephalus in these dogs after the first few weeks of life.

Acquired hydrocephalus can be caused by obstruction at various locations in the ventricular system. Neoplasia, hemorrhage (including intraventricular hemorrhage in the perinatal period), and infection are among the possible causes of obstruction. Location of the obstruction dictates the pattern of dilation of the ventricular system; therefore, a finding of asymmetrical dilation recognizable via ultrasound images can assist in determining the focus of the obstruction. Interference with absorption of CSF from the subarachnoid space into the venous system can cause nonobstructive hydrocephalus. Ex vacuo hydrocephalus is caused by the atrophy or failure of the brain to develop (Ettinger and Feldman 2005).

Several methods have been proposed for evaluating enlarged lateral ventricles on sonograms (Figure 1.10 and Table 1.1). The degree of ventriculomegaly ranges from the ventricles being only slightly enlarged to ventricles occupying most of the brain. Midline structures between the lateral ventricles are intact in some animals, but the lateral ventricles become confluent in others (Figure 1.11).

Several studies using ultrasonography or magnetic resonance imaging (MRI) have shown that the severity of clinical signs is not directly related to the degree of ventriculomegaly, and ventriculomegaly can be seen in neurologically normal dogs (De Haan et al. 1994; Vullo et al. 1997). A study using MRI to compare ventricular volume in Yorkshire terriers to that in German shepherds indicated that percentage of ventricle area to hemispheric area was significantly greater in the Yorkshire terriers, but the range of ventricle area for neurologically normal Yorkshire terriers overlapped that of neurologically abnormal Yorkshire terriers (Estave-Ratsch et al. 2001). Ventriculomegaly should not be equated with clinically significant hydrocephalus (Hudson et al. 1990; Spaulding and Sharp 1990; Ettinger and Feldman 2005). Breed differences and severity of clinical signs should be considered. Measurement of blood flow in the basilar artery might help to identify animals in which enlarged ventricles are significant or are likely to become clinically significant (Saito et al. 2003). In one study, RI at the basilar artery was higher in dogs with clinical hydrocephalus or other brain disease compared with normal dogs or dogs with asymptomatic hydrocephalus. Additionally,

Table 1.1.
Guidelines for measurements of the ventricular system as currently available in the literature

Parameter	How Measured	Normal	Ventriculomegaly
Hudson et al. (1990)			
Lateral ventricular height: transverse	Measure the dorsoventral dimension of the lateral ventricle with the probe perpendicular at or caudal to the interthalamic adhesion	0.04–0.35 cm Mean, 0.15 cm	>0.35 cm
Cerebral mantle thickness: transverse	Measure the thickness of brain tissue dorsal to each lateral ventricle	1.63–1.91 cm	Often decreased; may be very thin
Ventricle-hemisphere ratio (measured on transverse images)	Ratio of the lateral ventricular height to the width of the ipsilateral hemisphere	Mean, 0.19	>0.19
Ventricle-mantle ratio (measured on transverse images)	Ratio of the lateral ventricular height to the thickness of the cerebral mantle	Mean, 0.25	>0.25
Lateral ventricular height: sagittal	Measure the dorsoventral dimension of the lateral ventricle with the probe perpendicular at the thalamocaudate sulcus	Mean, 0.14 cm	
Spaulding and Sharp (1990)			
Dorsoventral dimension of lateral ventricle	Measure the dorsoventral dimension of the lateral ventricle at the level of the pituitary fossa	NA	NA
Dorsoventral percentage	Ratio of the dorsoventral dimension of the lateral ventricle to the dorsoventral dimension of the brain	0–14%	15%–25% → moderate ventriculomegaly >25% → severe ventriculomegaly

NA, not applicable.

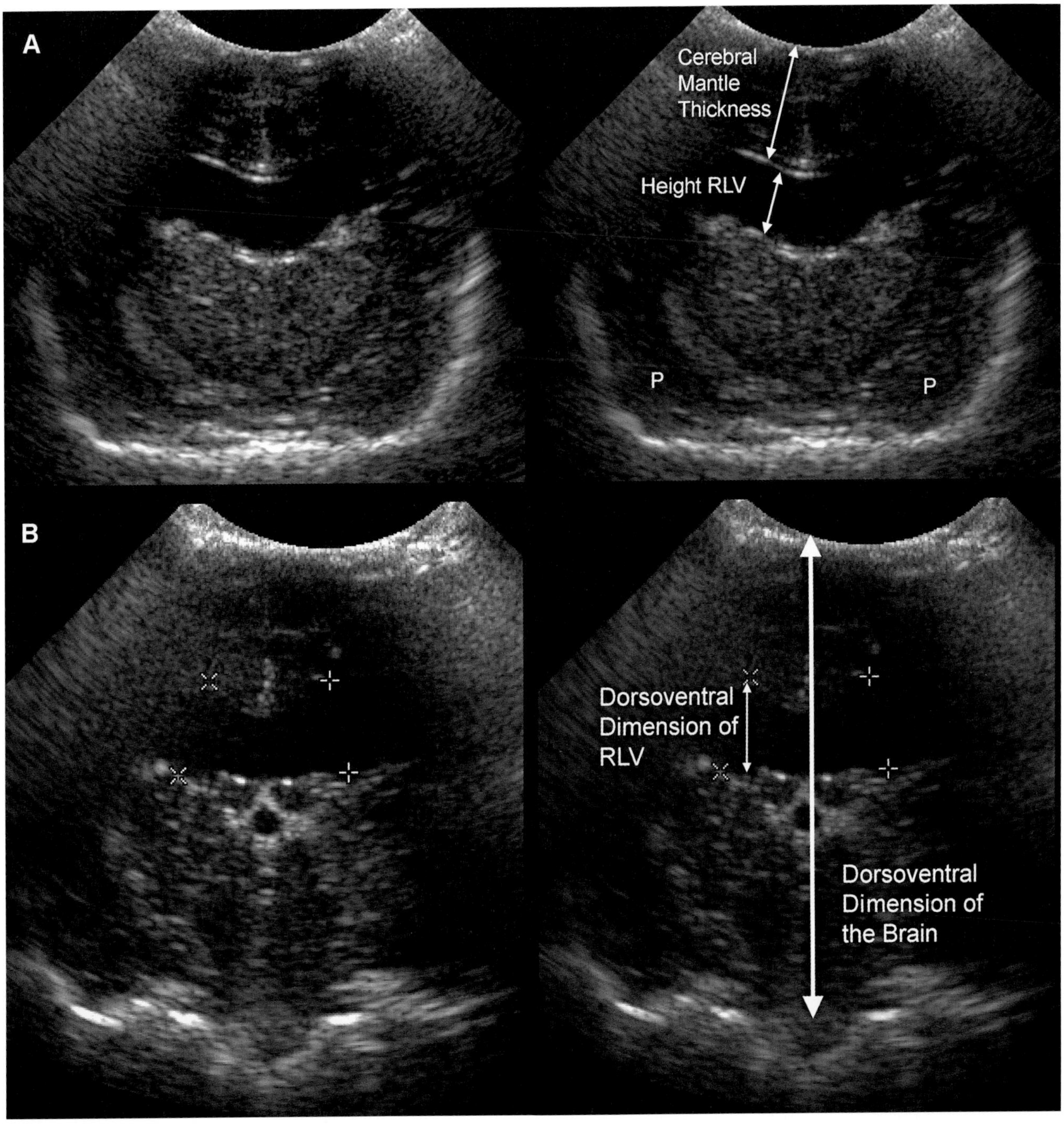

Figure 1.10. Measurement of the lateral ventricles in a 3-month-old Chihuahua. **A:** Transverse sonogram at the level of the interthalamic adhesion showing measurement using the method of Hudson et al. (1990) The lateral ventricular height can be compared with the cerebral mantle thickness (the thickness of the parenchyma dorsal to the lateral ventricle) to obtain the ventricle-mantle ratio. **B:** Transverse sonogram at the level of the pituitary gland showing measurement by using the method of Spaulding and Sharp (1990). Another method of measurement calculates the dorsoventral measurement of the lateral ventricle as a percentage of the dorsoventral measurement of the brain. RLV, right lateral ventricle.

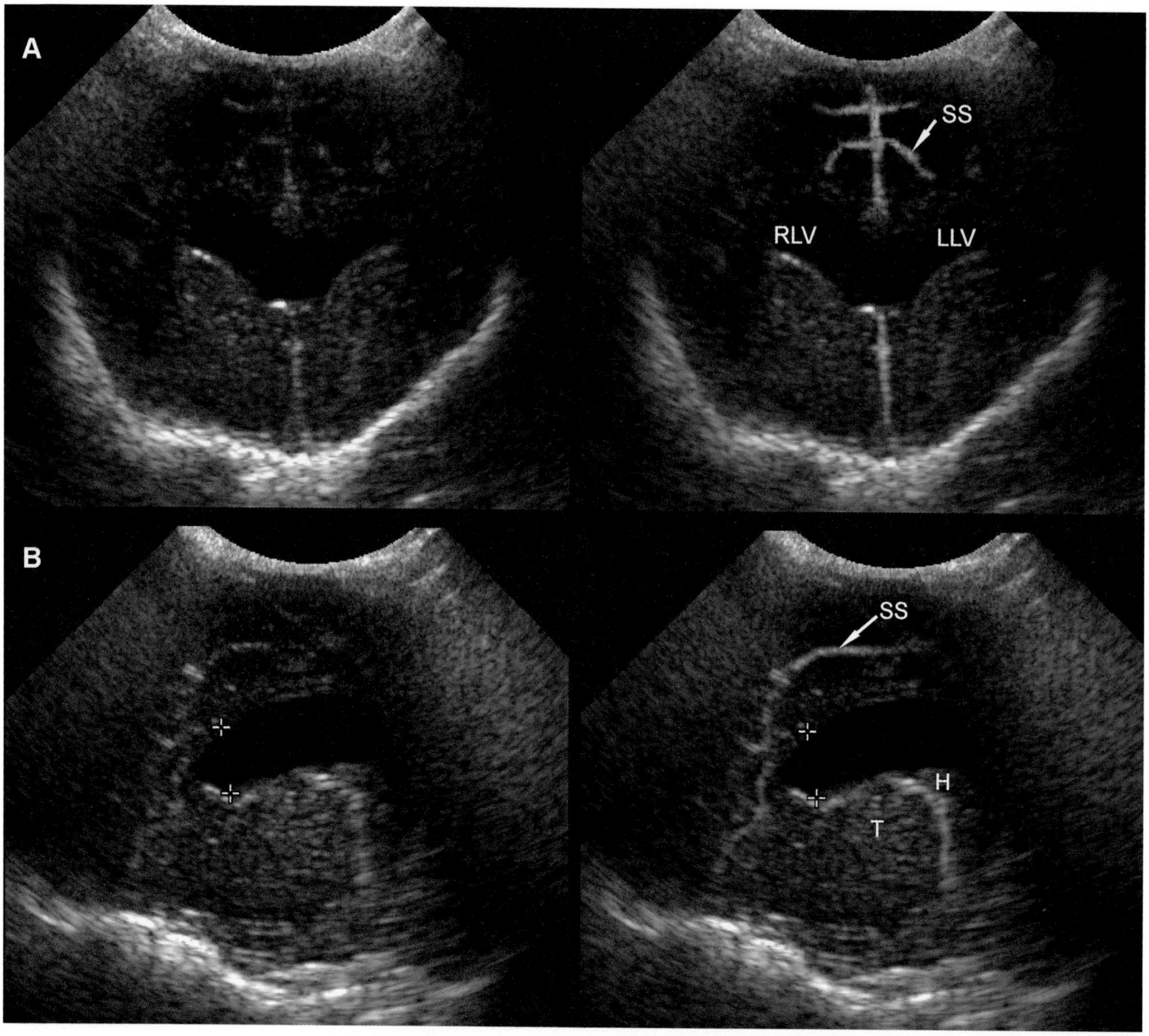

Figure 1.11. Variability in expansion of the ventricular system in hydrocephalus. Additional images from the brain of the 3-month-old Chihuahua shown in Figure 1.10 indicate that the temporal horns are minimally affected, but there is a confluence of the rostral horns. The third ventricle is not enlarged. Sonograms of another Chihuahua in Figure 1.9 show that ventriculomegaly involves the temporal horns, as well as rostral horns and central parts, and there is enlargement of the third ventricle in that dog. Midline structures remain mainly intact, however. **A:** Rostral transverse sonogram. **B:** Parasagittal sonogram. H, hippocampus; LLV, left lateral ventricle; RLV, right lateral ventricle; SS, splenial sulcus; and T, thalamus.

asymptomatic dogs with severe ventriculomegaly and high RI later developed clinical signs, although the use of high RI by itself did not identify asymptomatic dogs that were likely to become symptomatic (Saito et al. 2003).

It may also be useful to evaluate the amount of brain tissue spared by the dilated ventricles. Animals with very little brain tissue commonly have severe neurological deficits, although that is not always true (Figure 1.12).

The suggested methods of measurement are not always useful (Table 1.1). Some animals may have minimal enlargement in the described planes for measurement but have greatly enlarged ventricles in other areas, such as the caudal part of the central horn and the temporal horn. The third or fourth ventricles may

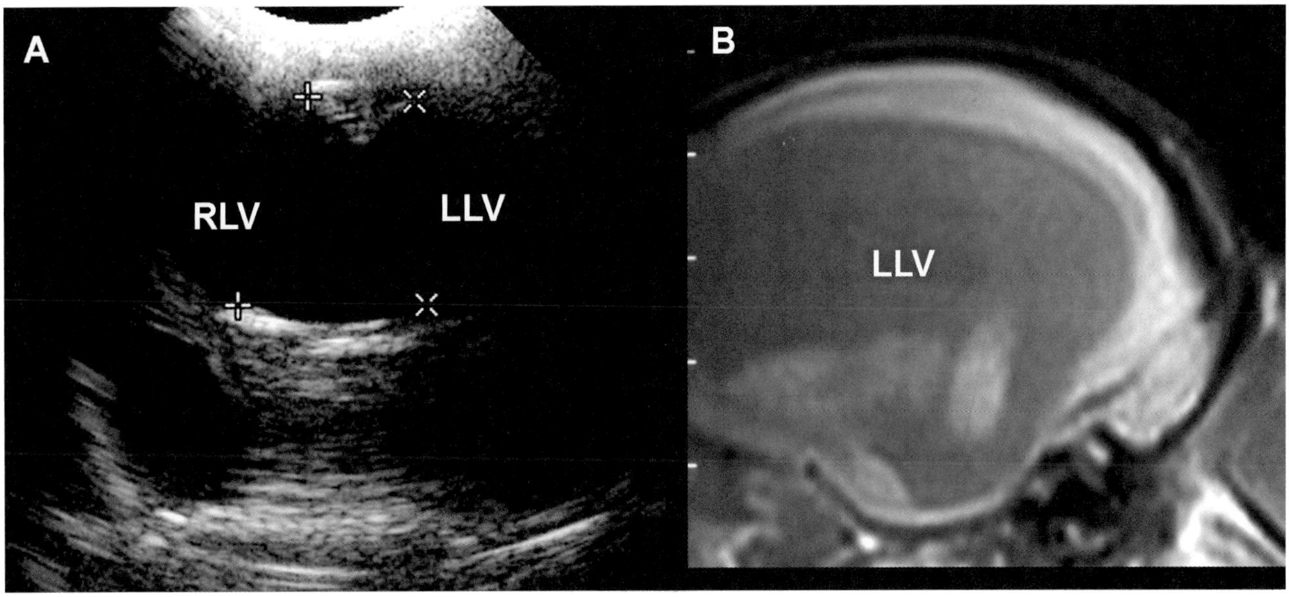

Figure 1.12. Incidental ventriculomegaly. Sonogram and magnetic resonance image (MRI) of the brain of a 10-year-old Maltese with severe but incidental ventriculomegaly. The ventriculomegaly was noted during spinal MR imaging performed to evaluate intervertebral disc herniation in the cervical region. The dog was not showing clinical evidence of brain abnormalities. **A:** Transverse sonogram showing massive ventriculomegaly involving the right and left lateral ventricles (RLV and LLV, respectively). **B:** Parasagittal MRI showing a severely dilated left lateral ventricle (LLV).

also be enlarged. Sonographers should be careful to record these findings, as well as any other abnormalities, including additional anomalies or masses that may be related to the ventriculomegaly.

Neoplasia

In most animals with brain neoplasia, MRI or computed tomography is used to make the initial diagnosis because the thick bone of the cranium precludes diagnosis with ultrasonography. Ultrasonography is more likely to be used either intraoperatively or postoperatively, although a window might provided by a persistent fontanel or by bone lysis associated with a neoplasm (Figure 1.13).

Most neoplasms in people and animals are hyperechoic to the adjacent normal brain.

Ultrasonography can assist in defining the borders of a mass intraoperatively so that most or all of the abnormal tissue can be removed. The vessels associated with a mass or other lesion can also be evaluated. Ultrasound-guided biopsy can be performed if the nature of a lesion is questionable. This enables preliminary diagnosis to establish the neoplastic or nonneoplastic nature of the lesion and establish a prognosis and selection of treatment. If a cranial defect remains following surgical intervention, ultrasonography can be used to follow the patient postoperatively to determine response to therapy.

Infectious Lesions

In rare instances, a brain abscess or granulomatous mass might occur in either a very young animal or an older animal with a persistent fontanel or other cranial defect (Klopp et al. 2000). Abscessation can appear as a cavitary and hypoechoic lesion containing swirling cellular material compressing the surrounding brain parenchyma (Figure 1.14).

In case of organized granuloma, a well-marginated hyperechoic lesion can be detected. Thus, a granulomatous mass should be considered as a differential diagnosis for neoplasia when a hyperechoic mass is seen on ultrasonography (Figure 1.15).

Traumatic Hemorrhage

Ultrasonography is used to examine the brain of animals with traumatic cranial defect to determine whether hemorrhage has occurred. Comatose or

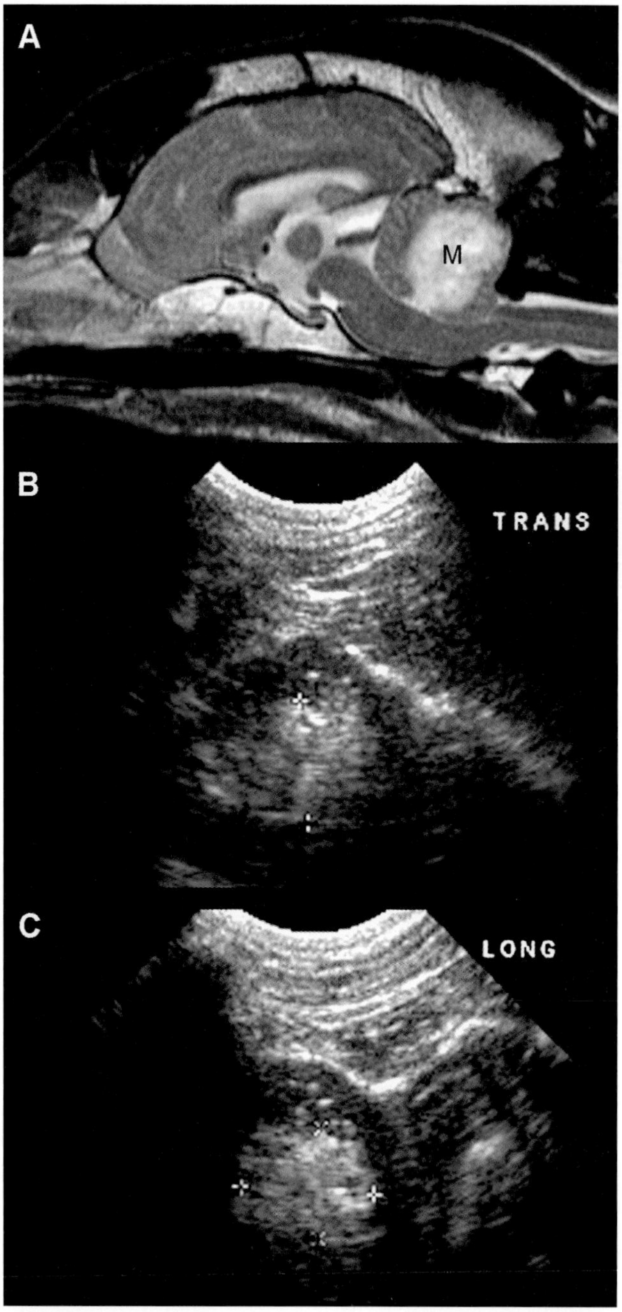

Figure 1.13. Astrocytoma in the cerebellum of an 8-year-old terrier. **A:** Magnetic resonance image shows a hyperintense mass (M) in the cerebellum. A craniotomy was done to enable an intraoperative ultrasound-guided biopsy of the mass. **B:** Transverse (trans) sonogram showing the hyperechoic mass (between the cursors) in the cerebellum. **C:** Parasagittal (long) sonogram showing the cerebellar mass. Images courtesy of D. Penninck and S. Hecht.

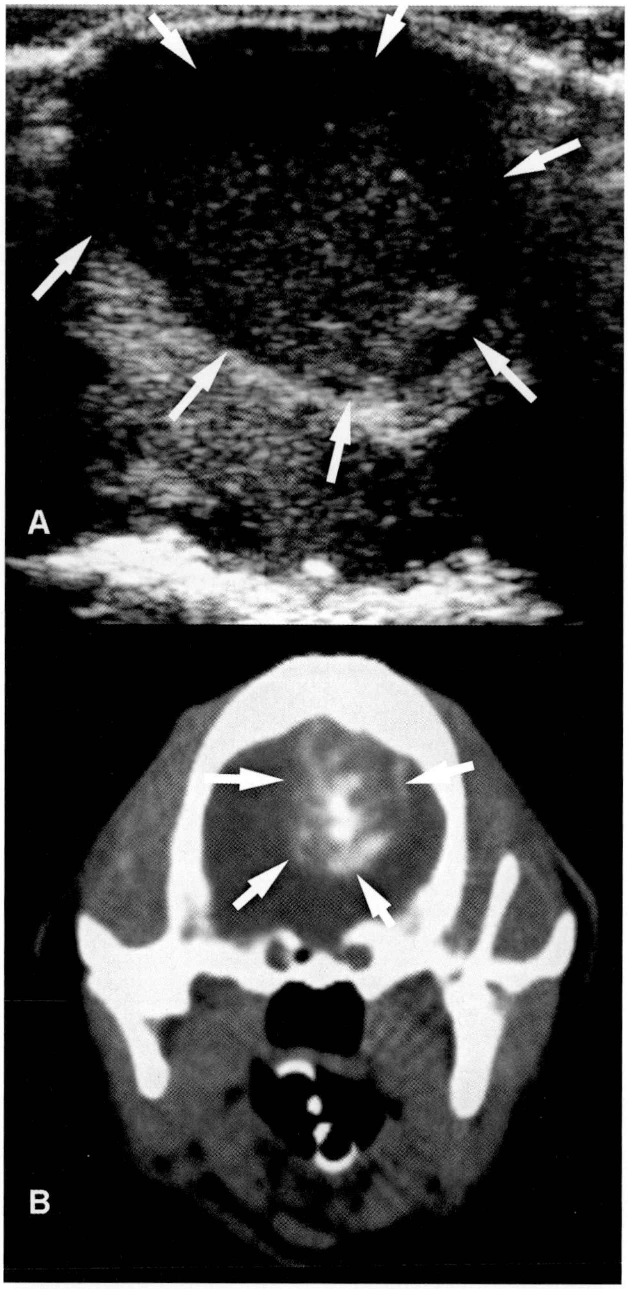

Figure 1.14. Abscess in the cerebrum of a kitten. The kitten had ventrolateral strabismus and soft-tissue swelling on its head. An abscess was diagnosed and drained via a palpable fontanel. **A:** Transverse ultrasonographic plane showing a large pocket of cellular fluid within the cerebrum (arrows). **B:** Transverse postcontrast computed tomography, on which a large, heterogeneous, contrast-enhancing mass lesion is observed (arrows).

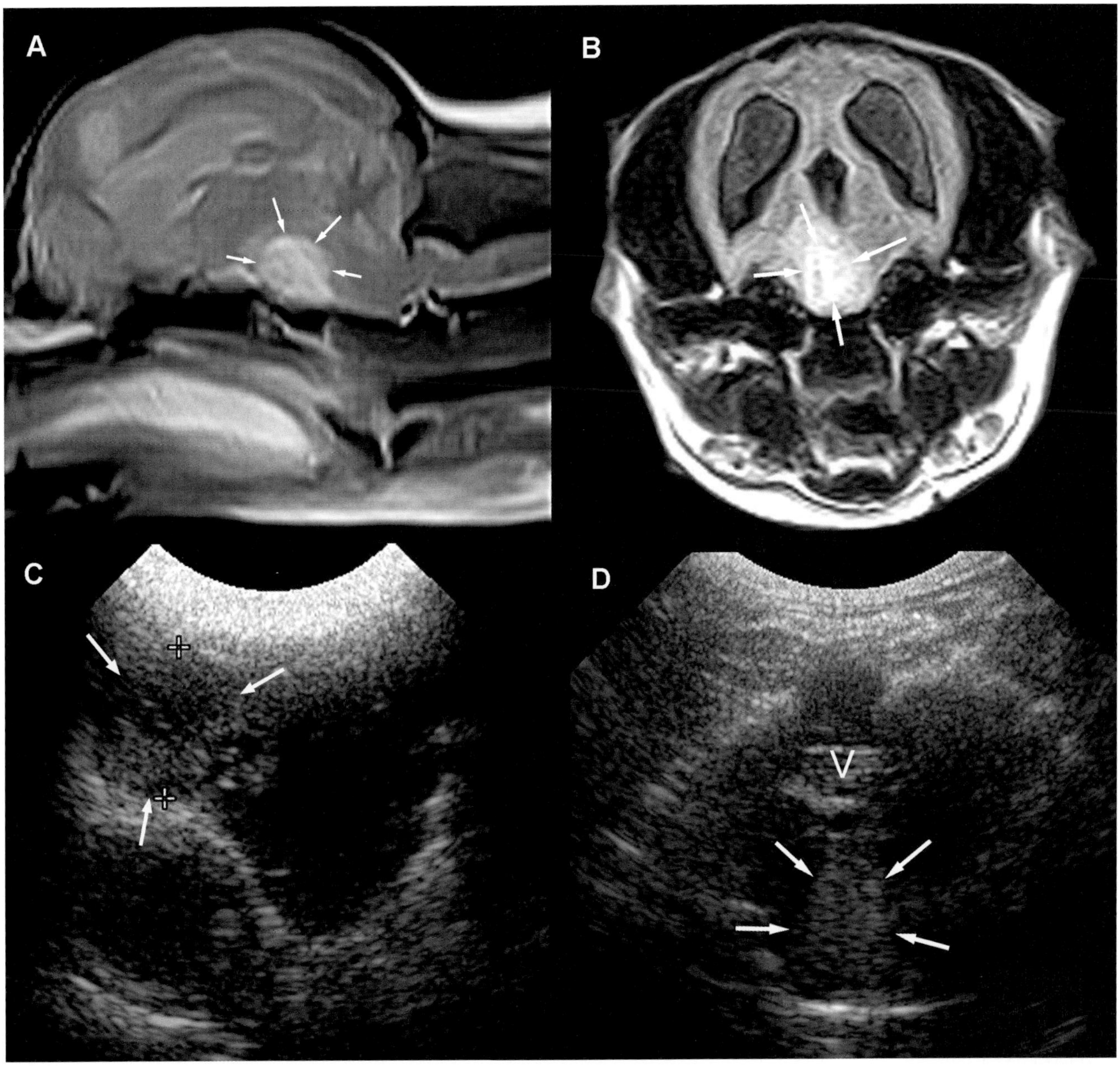

Figure 1.15. Granulomatous meningoencephalitis in a 5-year-old Yorkshire terrier. A mass was identified in the brain stem and subsequently biopsied. The mass could be seen with ultrasonography performed at the foramen magnum although ventriculomegaly was not apparent from that location. **A:** Sagittal T1-weighted magnetic resonance image after intravenous administration of gadolinium showing a hyperintense lesion in the rostral brain stem (arrows). **B:** Transverse T2-weighted magnetic resonance image showing a hyperintense lesion in the brain stem to the right of the midline (arrows). The lateral and third ventricles are dilated. **C:** Sagittal sonographic image obtained through the foramen magnum. Cursors have been placed to measure the mass (arrows). **D:** Transverse sonographic image obtained through the foramen magnum. In the brain stem is a hyperechoic mass (arrows) just ventral to the cerebellar vermis (V).

semicomatose animals can be evaluated for evidence of active hemorrhage requiring surgical intervention if a suitable sonographic window is available (Figure 1.16).

Bleeding into the brain is usually seen immediately as a hypoechoic area, but erythrocyte aggregation causes a lesion to become hyperechoic. As the clot breaks down, anechoic or hypoechoic areas may be seen (Figure 1.17).

Serial sonograms enable continuing evaluation of patients without anesthesia and with little stress to the patients. Recheck ultrasonographic evaluation is

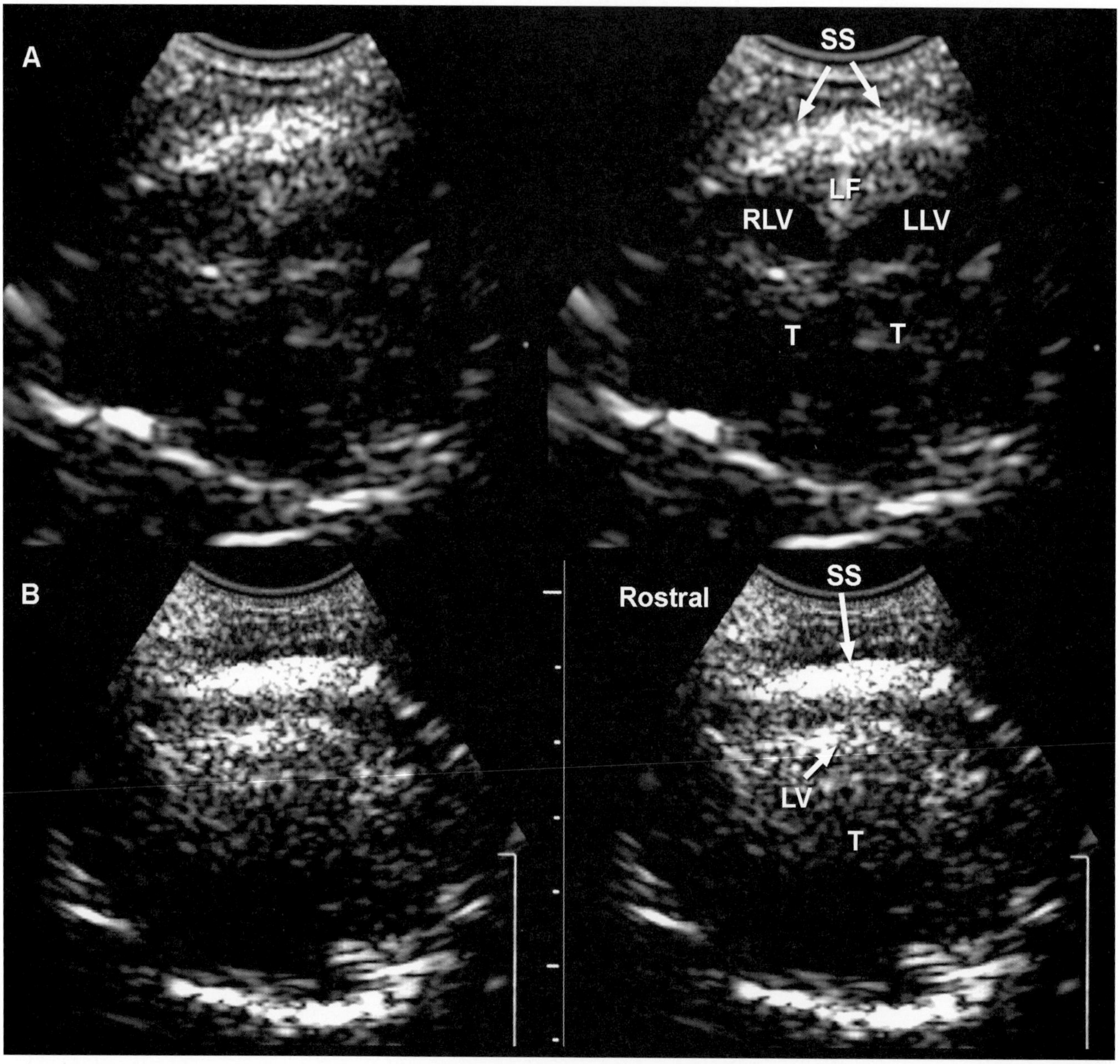

Figure 1.16. Sonograms of the brain of a puppy hit by a car and comatose. On these transverse **(A)** and parasagittal **(B)** sonograms, there is thickening of the splenial sulci (SS) suggesting localized hemorrhage. Other areas of the brain appear normal, and the patient recovered uneventfully. LF, longitudinal fissure; LV, choroid plexus in the lateral ventricle; LLV, area of the left lateral ventricle; RLV, area of the right lateral ventricle; SS, splenial sulcus; and T, thalamus.

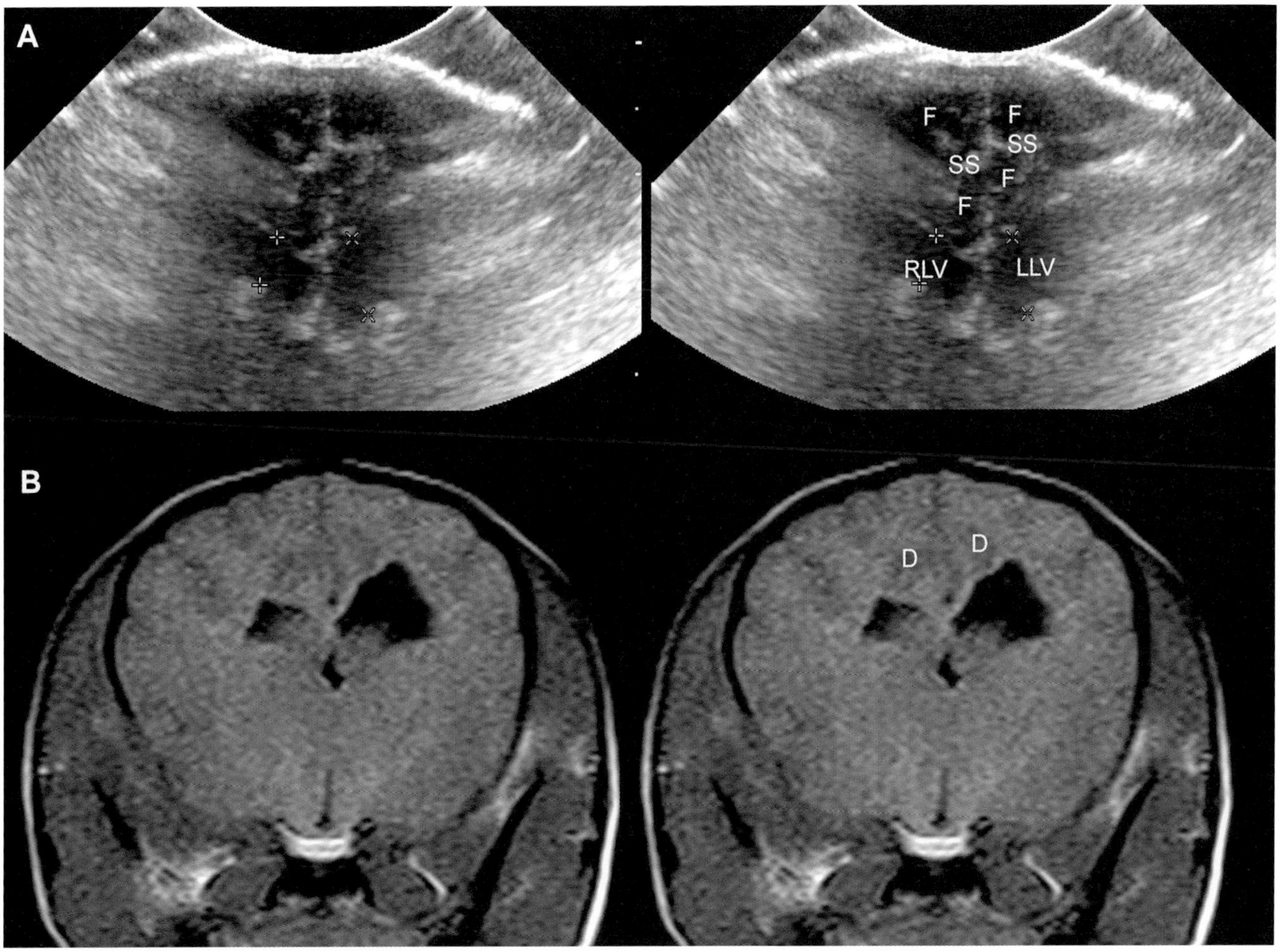

Figure 1.17. Head trauma in a 4-year-old Chihuahua. **A:** Transverse sonogram of the brain after head trauma and subsequent seizures. The dog was in lateral recumbency and was minimally responsive. A collection of fluid (F) surrounds the splenial sulcus (SS) on each side. The right splenial sulcus is displaced ventrally. The right lateral ventricle (RLV) and left lateral ventricle (LLV) are mildly dilated. **B:** T1-weighted magnetic resonance image showing decreased signal intensity (D) in the region of the splenial sulci.

warranted especially when patients have changed mentation.

Cystic Lesions

Cystic lesions can be produced by infectious disease or neoplasia or may have no apparent cause (Cruz et al. 2003) (Figure 1.18).

Choroid plexus cysts, intracranial arachnoid cysts, and epidermoid and dermoid cysts associated with the fourth ventricle, quadrigeminal cistern, or cerebellopontine angle have been reported. Arachnoid cysts are seen most commonly in the quadrigeminal cistern, where they appear as a well-defined anechoic mass between the caudal aspect of the cerebral hemispheres. The midbrain will be found ventral to the cyst, and the cerebellum will be caudal (Saito et al. 2001). Congenital cysts secondary to abnormal development or destruction of brain parenchyma, such as in Dandy-Walker syndrome and porencephaly or hydranencephaly, can also occur. Hydranencephaly is diagnosed when the cerebral hemispheres are absent or almost completely absent (Cruz et al. 2003).

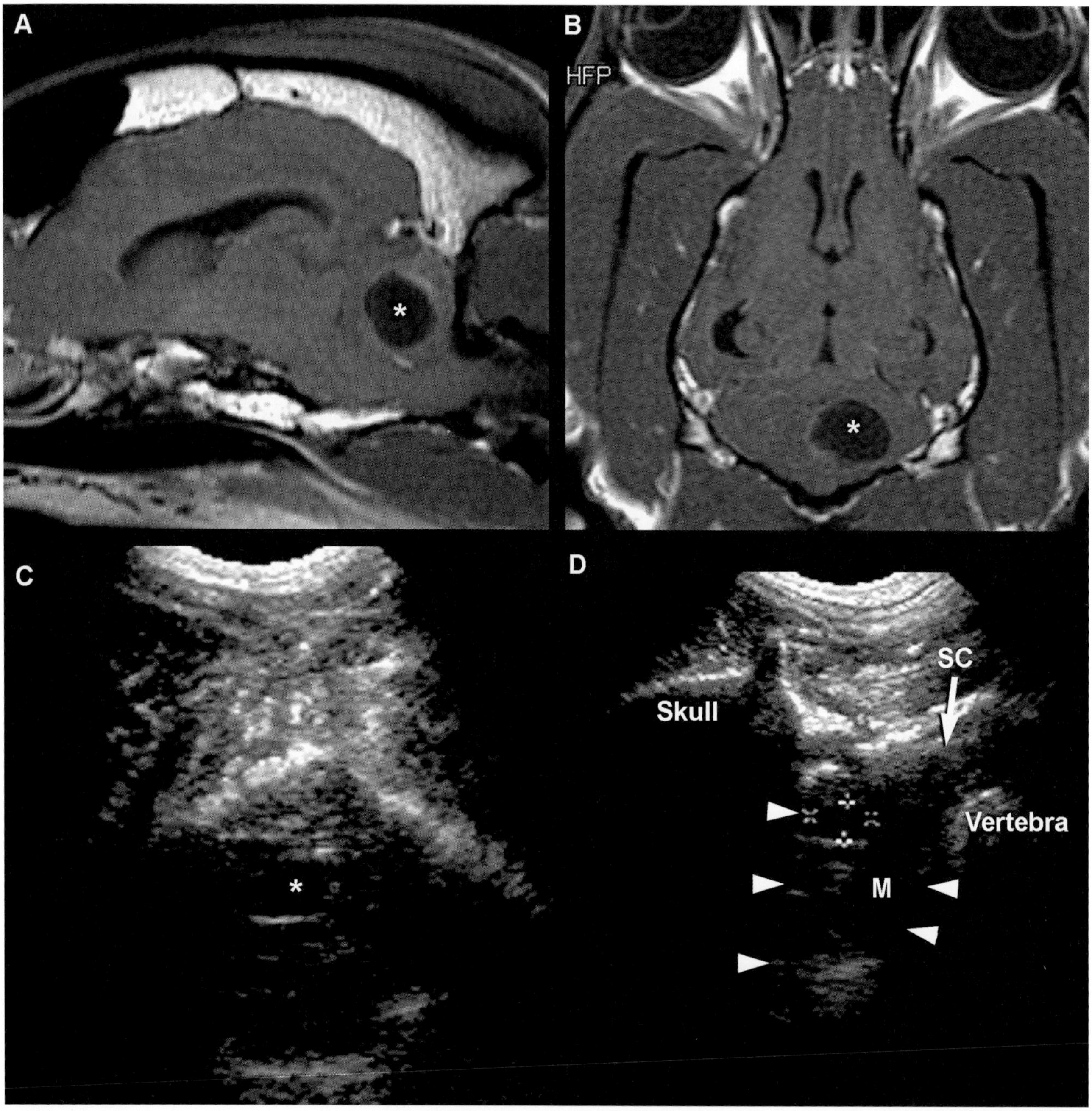

Figure 1.18. Cyst in the cerebellum of an 8-year-old terrier. The cyst was drained surgically, but an astrocytoma was later diagnosed at the site (as seen in Figure 1.13). **A and B:** Sagittal and dorsal postcontrast T1-weighted images of the brain on which a well-defined, hypointense cystlike lesion is identified (*). **C:** Transverse sonogram of the cerebellum imaged from the foramen magnum on which the cyst appears as a well-defined, oval, anechoic lesion (*). **D:** Longitudinal sonogram of the cyst. The bone of the skull and vertebral column prevents visualization of portions of the brain and spine, but the part of the brain (arrowheads) can be seen through the foramen magnum. A portion of the spinal cord (SC) can also be observed as it joins the medulla oblongata (M) rostrally. Cursors have been placed to measure the cyst in the cerebellum. Images courtesy of D. Penninck and S. Hecht. **E and F: Sonograms of a 1-year-old Chihuahua with hydrocephalus and a quadrigeminal cyst.** **E:** Sagittal sonogram showing the quadrigeminal cyst (Q) and confluence of the dilated lateral ventricles (LV). **F:** Transverse sonogram. LLV, left lateral ventricle; M, midbrain; and RLV, right lateral ventricle. Images courtesy of B. Poteet, Gulf Coast Veterinary Specialists, Houston.

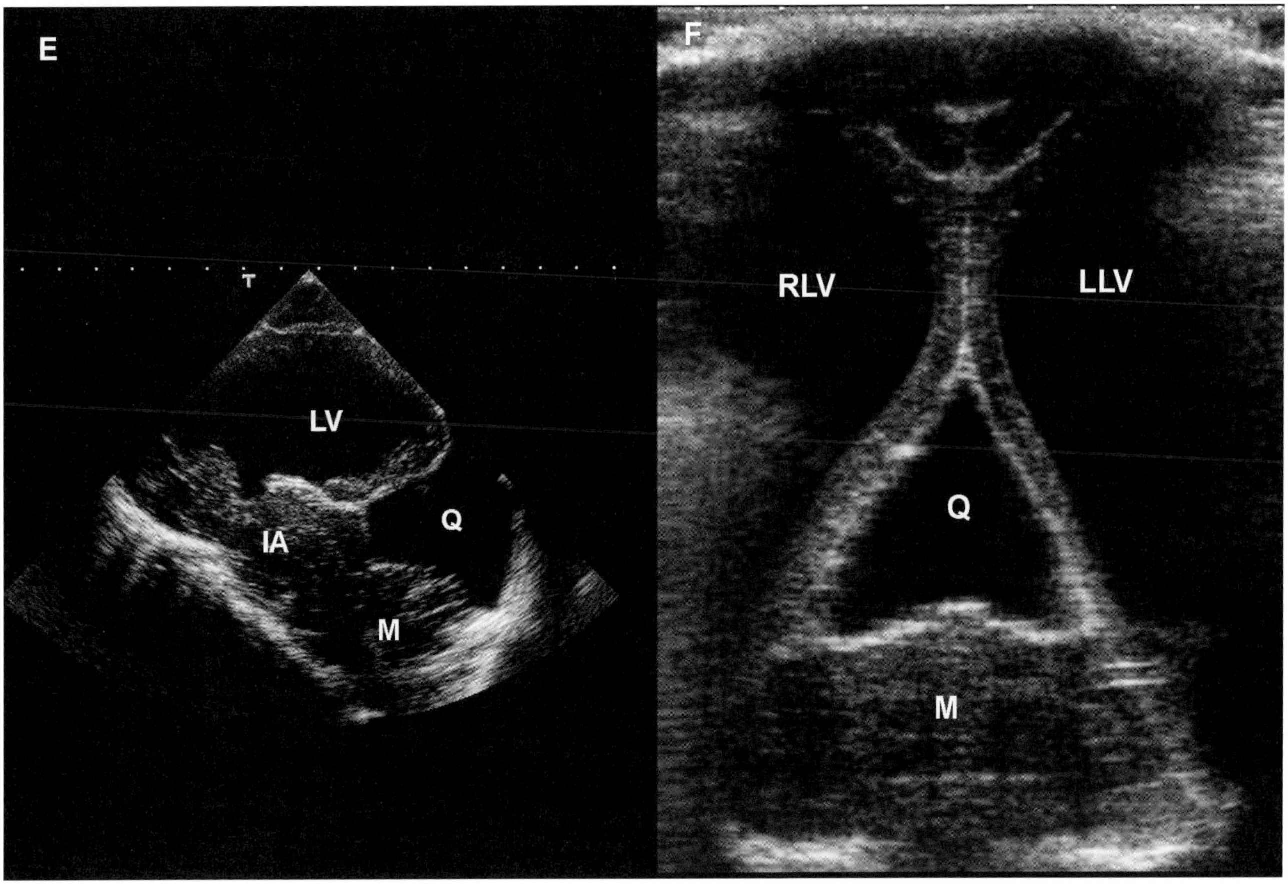

Figure 1.18. *Continued*

Congenital Disease

Agenesis of the Corpus Callosum

Agenesis of the corpus callosum has been reported uncommonly in dogs (Spaulding and Sharp 1990). In people, sonographic findings include lateral separation of the rostral horns and bodies of the lateral ventricles, elevation and variable dilation of the third ventricle, and dilation of the occipital horns. The bundles of Probst cause concavity of the medial wall of the lateral ventricles. In dogs, enlargement and dorsal displacement of the third ventricle can be seen (Figure 1.19).

Chiari-like Malformations

Chiari-like malformations are conditions in which there is variable pathology, such as malformation of the craniovertebral junction, cerebellar dysplasia, and elongation or displacement of portions of the cerebellum (Figure 1.20).

Herniation of the cerebellum can obstruct CSF flow, causing hydrocephalus and syringomyelia (Ettinger and Feldman 2005). Chiari type I malformations have been reported to occur in the Cavalier King Charles breed, with anomalies of the first cervical vertebra and skull, and in Maltese dogs (Kirberger et al. 1997). In some dogs, these conditions can be diagnosed by using the foramen magnum to provide an acoustic window in evaluating the cerebellum, fourth ventricle, spinal cord, and central canal.

Dandy-Walker–like Syndrome

A condition resembling Dandy-Walker syndrome of children has been reported in a Boston terrier (Nourreddine et al. 2004). The puppy exhibited ataxia, rolling, and intention tremors. Sonographic findings can include hypoplasia of the cerebellar vermis, confluence of the lateral ventricles, enlargement of the third and lateral ventricles, and cystic lesions within the cerebellum. A fluid accumulation seen between the

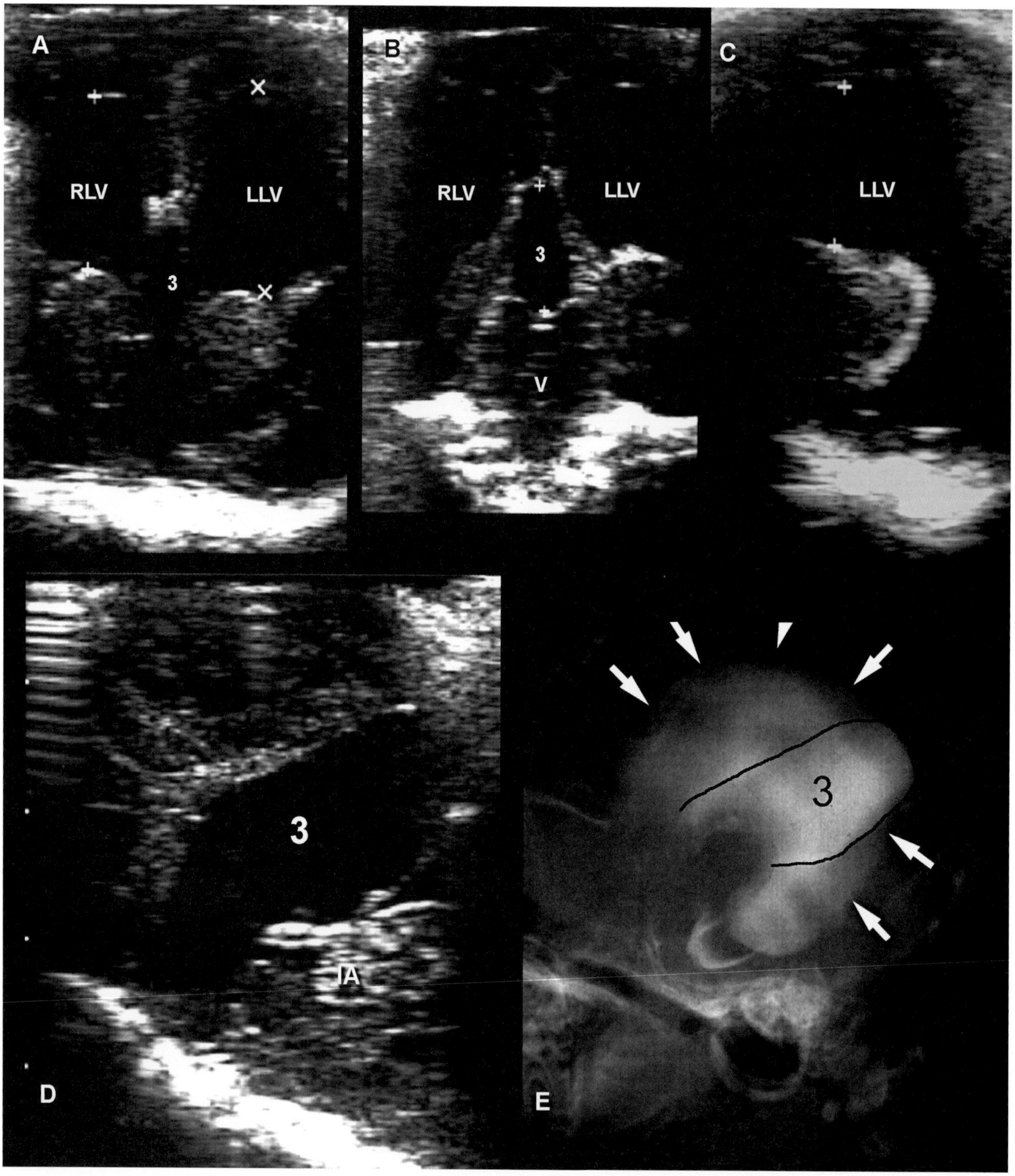

Figure 1.19. Agenesis of the corpus callosum and hydrocephalus. Images of the brain of a young puppy with severe neurological deficits. The right and left lateral ventricles are greatly dilated. The third ventricle is enlarged and displaced dorsally. **A:** Rostral transverse sonogram showing marked dilation of the lateral ventricle. **B:** Transverse sonogram angled caudally to image the vermis of the cerebellum. The third ventricle is enlarged and displaced dorsally. **C:** Parasagittal sonogram with the ultrasound beam angled laterally to image the enlarged left lateral ventricle. **D:** Sagittal sonogram showing marked enlargement and dorsal displacement of the third ventricle. **E:** Radiograph of the brain after ventriculography was performed using an iodinated contrast medium. The lateral ventricles (arrows) are greatly dilated. The third ventricle (outlined in black) is greatly dilated and displaced dorsally. 3, third ventricle; IA, interthalamic adhesion; LLV, left lateral ventricle; RLV, right lateral ventricle; and V, vermis.

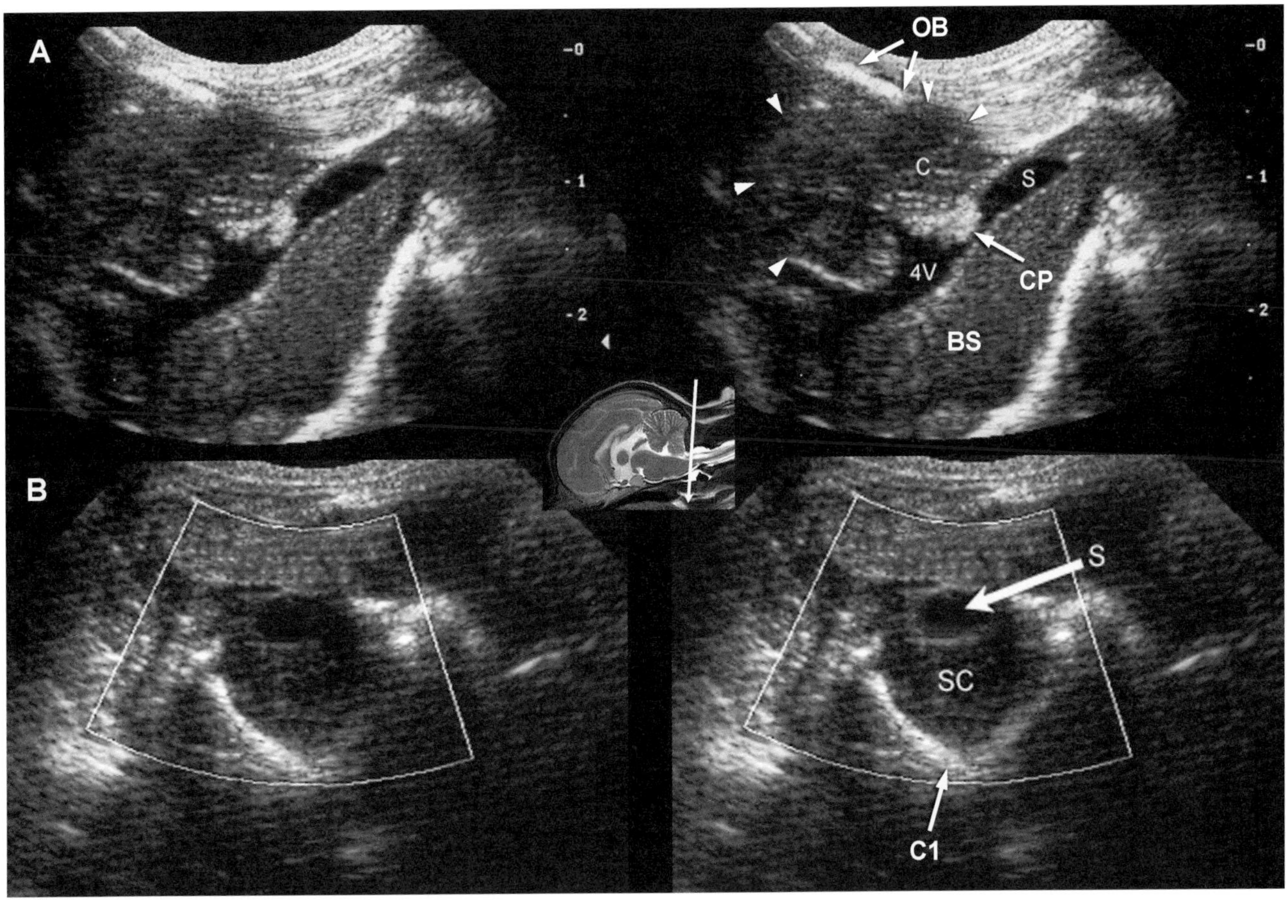

Figure 1.20. Chiari-like malformation. Sagittal **(A)** and transverse **(B)** sonographic images obtained through a large foramen magnum in a dog with occipital dysplasia. The cerebellum (C, arrowheads) protrudes into the foramen, below the occipital bone (OB). A tubular anechoic fluid collection is observed along the middorsal portion of the cranial cervical spinal cord (SC), consistent with syringomyelia (S). The fourth ventricle (4V) is also dilated. Malformation of the skull enables better visualization of the brain than usual (compare with Figure 1.18). BS, brain stem; and CP, choroid plexus of the fourth ventricle. Images courtesy of M. A. d'Anjou.

lateral ventricles and the cerebellum was determined to be a cyst associated with the fourth ventricle.

Hypoplasia

Cerebrocortical hypoplasia has been reported to be caused by loss or abnormal proliferation and/or migration of cortical neurons because of specific inherited abnormalities, toxins, in utero infections, or vascular insults. In some cases, lack of development shown as decreased detail of the brain echotexture might be apparent with ultrasonography either through a persistent fontanel or by viewing the brain through the foramen magnum (Figure 1.21).

Cerebellar hypoplasia, which is reduced size of the cerebellum because of abnormal development, can be caused by viral infections such as panleukopenia (feline parvovirus) in cats, toxins or other environmental influences, or genetic abnormalities, or the cause may be unknown.

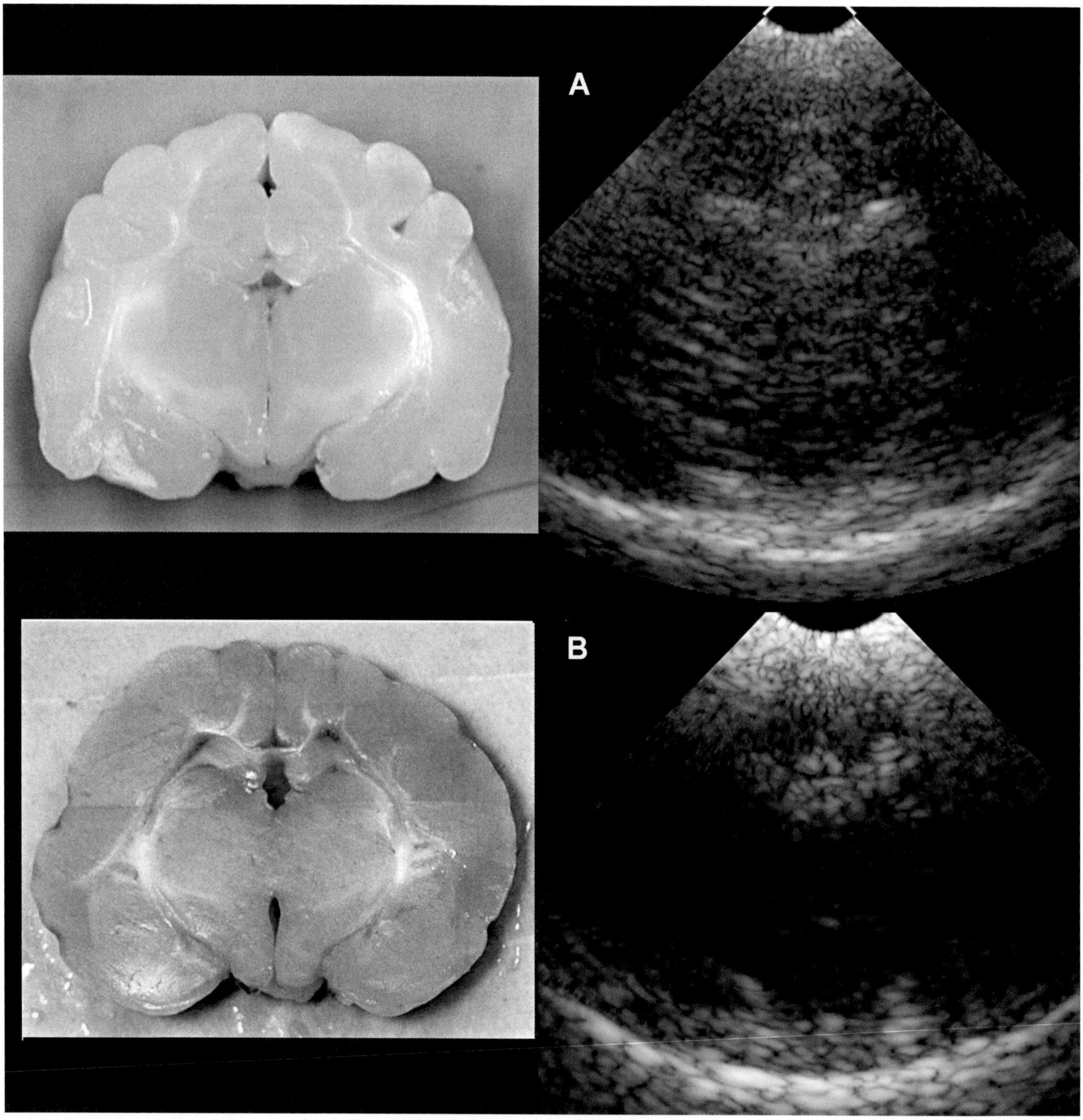

Figure 1.21. Sonograms of a normal kitten and a kitten with abnormal brain development. **A:** Sonogram of a normal 1-week-old kitten next to the gross transverse section from a normal 1-month-old kitten. **B:** Sonogram of an 8-week-old kitten with severe neurological deficits caused by cerebrocortical dysplasia and abnormal myelinization. The sonogram shows a lack of detail compared with the normal kitten. The cause of this lack of detail is unknown. A gross transverse section from the kitten is seen on the left. Note the decreased visualization of white matter tracks and decreased depth of sulci.

Figure 1.22. Cystic cerebellar lesion in a dog. **A:** Sagittal T2-weighted spin echo magnetic resonance image showing a well-defined, hyperintense cystic lesion in the cerebellum. **B:** Intraoperative sonogram shows an anechoic circular lesion (cyst) with some hypoechoic material around the margins. Fluid has been placed at the surgical site to enable imaging. **C:** Intraoperative sonogram showing the brain after drainage of the cyst. The arrow indicates the area of the lesion after suction. Images courtesy of D. Penninck and S. Hecht.

Interventional Procedures

When the brain is examined intraoperatively, the probe head should be coated with sterile acoustic gel and enclosed in sterilized material, such as a surgical glove or sterilized plastic wrap. Sterile probe sleeves are available commercially. Some of these extend for some distance along the probe cord to ensure sterility. Alternatively, the cord can be wrapped in sterile elastic bandaging material so that asepsis can be more easily maintained. Sterile physiological saline placed at the surgical site prevents drying of the tissues and achieves an acoustic match between the probe and the brain.

Ultrasound can be used intraoperatively to guide needle placement for drainage of cystic lesions or during debulking of brain masses to ensure complete removal of a mass and to localize vessels and minimize hemorrhage (Figures 1.22 and 1.23).

Lesions with uncertain etiology can be biopsied using ultrasound to guide placement of the biopsy needle. Ultrasound can also guide insertion of tubes for treatment of obstructive hydrocephalus or needles for injection of drugs or chemotherapeutic agents into the lesion. Postoperative sonography can be used to evaluate the surgical site (Figure 1.24).

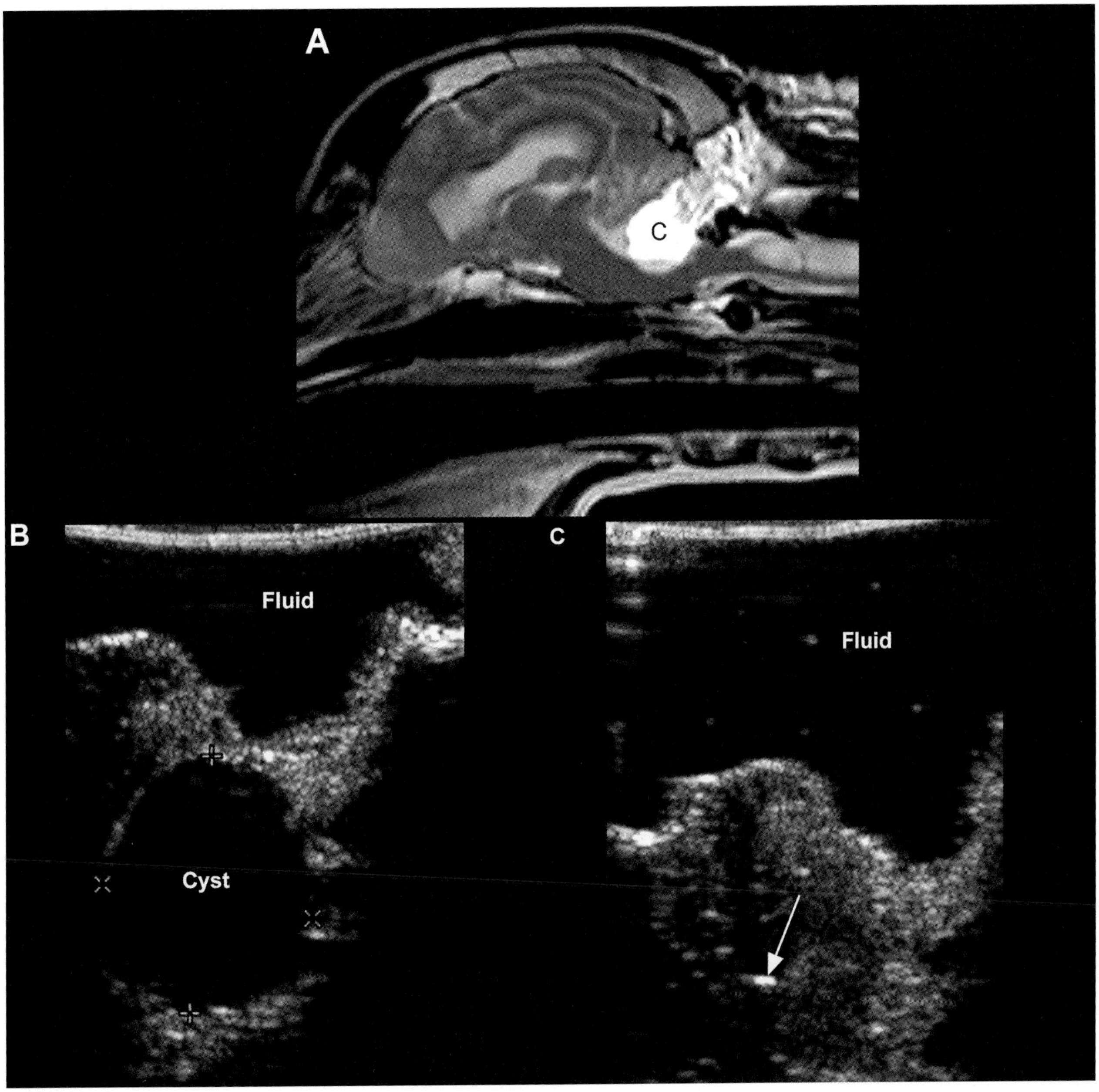

Figure 1.22

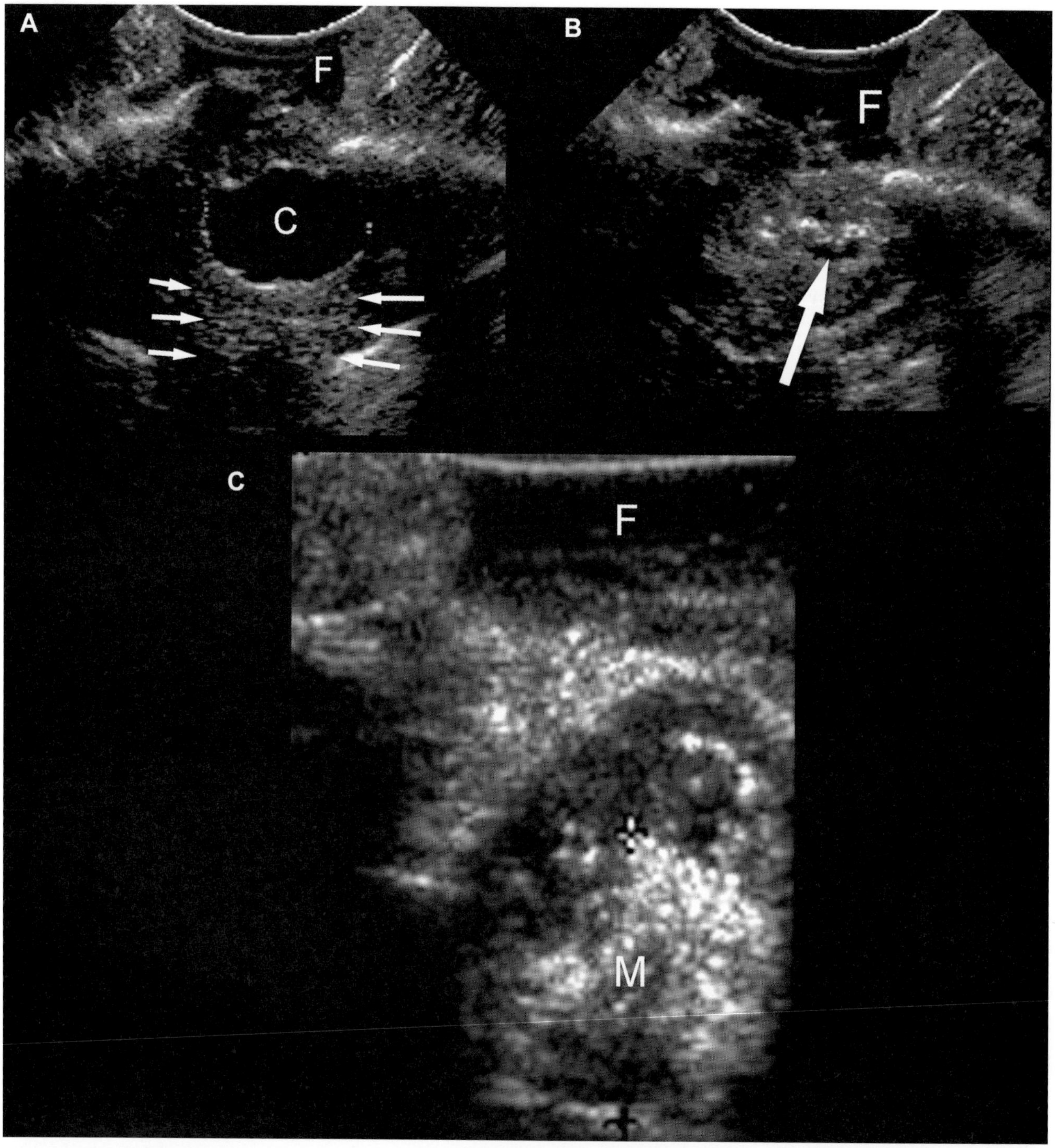

Figure 1.23. Cerebellar astrocytoma. **A:** Transverse sonogram of the brain of the 8-year-old terrier in Figures 1.13 and 1.18. This dog had a cerebellar cyst. When intraoperative ultrasonography was performed, the cyst (C) was a well-defined anechoic lesion with mild distal enhancement (arrows). Fluid (F) can be seen at the surgical site. **B:** After drainage, only a small amount of fluid remains, as is evidenced by a small anechoic area (arrow). **C:** Subsequently, clinical signs recurred. Magnetic resonance images and sonograms revealed that a mass was in the area of the previously imaged cyst. Intraoperative ultrasonography was used to measure the mass (M) prior to debulking. Histopathology revealed that the mass was an astrocytoma. Images courtesy of D. Penninck and S. Hecht.

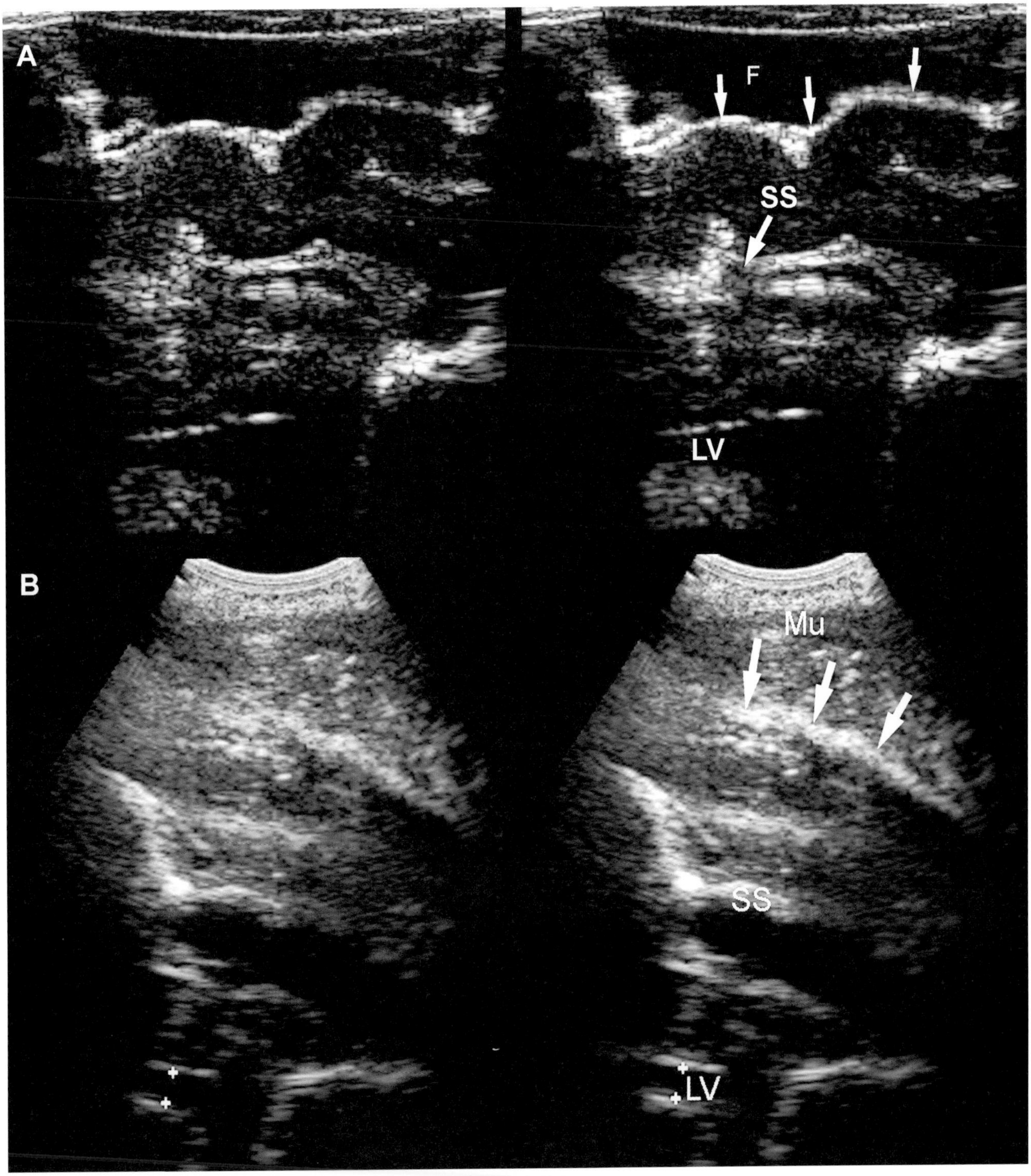

Figure 1.24. Seizuring dog with hyperintense focus in the cerebral cortex on magnetic resonance imaging. **A: Intraoperative parasagittal sonogram.** No mass lesions are visible, and biopsy findings suggested previous trauma. **B: Postoperative parasagittal sonogram** made by imaging through the intact skin and muscle over the craniotomy site. There is considerable facial swelling after surgery. Ultrasonography was performed to check for a possible dural fistula. No dural cyst was seen, and the lateral ventricles were normal. The dog recovered uneventfully. Arrows indicate the surface of the brain. F, fluid at the surgical site; LV, lateral ventricle; Mu, muscle under the craniotomy site; and SS, splenial sulcus.

References

Cruz R, Alvarado MS, Sandoval JE, Vilchez E (2003) Prenatal sonographic diagnosis of fetal death and hydranencephaly in two Chihuahua fetuses. Vet Radiol Ultrasound 44:589–592.

De Haan CE, Kraft SL, Gavin PR, Wendling LR, Griebenow ML (1994) Normal variation in size of the lateral ventricles of the Labrador retriever dog as assessed by magnetic resonance imaging. Vet Radiol Ultrasound 35:83–86.

Estave-Ratsch B, Kneissl S, Gabler C (2001) Comparative evaluation of the ventricles in the Yorkshire Terrier and the German Shepherd dog using low-field MRI. Vet Radiol Ultrasound 42:410–413.

Ettinger SJ, Feldman EC (2005) Primary Brain Diseases. In: Ettinger SJ, ed. Textbook of Veterinary Internal Medicine, 6th edition. Philadelphia: WB Saunders, pp 820–835.

Hudson JA, Buxton DF, Cox NR, Finn-Bodner ST, Simpson ST, Wright JC, Wallace SS, Mitro A (1997) Color flow Doppler imaging and Doppler spectral analysis of the brain of neonatal dogs. Vet Radiol Ultrasound 38:313–322.

Hudson JA, Cartee RE, Simpson ST, Buxton DF (1989) Ultrasonographic anatomy of the canine brain. Vet Radiol 30:13–21.

Hudson LC, Cauzinille L, Kornegay JN, Tompkins MB (1995) Magnetic resonance imaging of the normal feline brain. Vet Radiol Ultrasound 36:267–275.

Hudson JA, Simpson ST, Buxton DF, Cartee RE, Steiss JE (1990) Ultrasonographic diagnosis of canine hydrocephalus. Vet Radiol 31:50–58.

Hudson JA, Simpson ST, Cox NR, Buxton DF (1991) Ultrasonographic examination of the normal canine neonatal brain. Vet Radiol 32:50–59.

Jäderlund KH, Hansson K, Berg A-L, Sjöström A, Narfström K (2003) Cerebral ventricular size in developing normal kittens measured by ultrasonography. Vet Radiol Ultrasound 44:581–588.

Kirberger RM, Jacobson LS, Davies JV, Engela J (1997) Hydromyelia in the dog. Vet Radiol Ultrasound 38:30–38.

Klopp LS, Hathcock JT, Sorjonen DC (2000) Magnetic resonance imaging features of brain stem abscessation in two cats. Vet Radiol Ultrasound 41:300–307.

Nourreddine C, Harder R, Olby NJ, Spaulding K, Brown T (2004) Ultrasonographic appearance of Dandy Walker–like syndrome in a Boston terrier. Vet Radiol Ultrasound 45: 336–339.

Saito M, Olby NJ, Spaulding K (2001) Identification of arachnoid cysts in the quadrigeminal cistern using ultrasonography. Vet Radiol Ultrasound 42:435–439.

Saito M, Olby NJ, Spaulding K, Munana K, Sharp NJH (2003) Relationship among basilar artery resistance index, degree of ventriculomegaly, and clinical signs in hydrocephalic dogs. Vet Radiol Ultrasound 44:667–694.

Schaller O (1992) Illustrated Veterinary Anatomical Nomenclature. Stuttgart, Germany: Enke.

Spaulding KA, Sharp NJH (1990) Ultrasonographic imaging of the lateral cerebral ventricles in the dog. Vet Radiol 31:59–64.

Vullo T, Korenman E, Manzo RP, Gomez DG, Deck MDF, Cahill PT (1997) Diagnosis of cerebral ventriculomegaly in normal adult beagles using quantitative MRI. Vet Radiol Ultrasound 38:277–281.

SECTION 2

Spine

Judith Hudson and Martin Kramer

Scanning Technique

Because of acoustic shadowing created by bone, ultrasonography of the spinal cord can usually be performed only during or following surgical laminectomy, corpectomy, or foraminotomy (Nakayama 1993; Gallagher et al. 1995) (Figures 1.25 and 1.26).

The cervical spinal cord can be partially visible through the foramen magnum and between the atlas and axis while the neck is fully flexed (Figure 1.27). In addition, windows through ventral slot surgery or surgical sites involving the caudal portion of the brain enable partial evaluation of the cranial cervical spine (Figures 1.27 and 1.28).

A portion of the lumbar spinal cord can be seen through the intervertebral disc space either with a dorsolateral approach through the lumbar musculature or from the ventral aspect when performing abdominal ultrasonography (Figures 1.29 and 1.30). Using a ventral transabdominal approach, the spinal cord can only be assessed at the disc space. Intervertebral disc calcification and bridging spondylosis deformans can significantly limit its visibility.

The spinal cord is small and superficial, making a high-frequency transducer (usually 7.5–12 MHz) the optimal choice. Transducers with a small footprint are preferred to better fit the narrow surgical sites. Perhaps the most common use of spinal cord ultrasonography is intraoperatively to evaluate whether all disc material has been removed from the spinal canal during a laminectomy or cervical ventral slot surgery. Other intraoperative applications include evaluation of the cord because of trauma, suspected neoplasia, developmental abnormalities, and infection. For intraoperative applications, the probe must be placed in a long, sterile, plastic cover, and sterile acoustic gel must be used. Postoperatively, the spinal cord can be monitored if a remaining defect in the vertebra provides a sonographic window. Vertebral bone lysis because of neoplasia or infection can also provide an acoustic window for the spinal cord. Additionally, the spinal cord may be visible perinatally because of incomplete vertebral ossification.

Normal Sonographic Anatomy of the Spine

The spinal cord is relatively hypoechoic, the meninges are hyperechoic, and the cerebrospinal fluid (CSF) is anechoic (Figure 1.31). The more superficial bright line represents the dura mater and arachnoid together, whereas the deeper line represents the pia mater (Finn-Bodner et al. 1995). Anechoic CSF separates these two hyperechoic lines. Centrally, one or two lines are present at the location of the central canal. Deep to the central canal, two more hyperechoic lines represent the meninges. The surface of the bone deep to the spinal cord and meninges appears as a thick hyperechoic line. Absorption of sound prevents imaging of structures deep to the bone.

Transverse images can be obtained if the available probe has a small footprint. In these images, the spinal cord is hypoechoic with a circular or oval shape, whereas the central canal appears as a central hyperechoic dot (Finn-Bodner et al. 1995).

The spinal cord is supplied by ventral and dorsal branches of spinal arteries that originate from vertebral, thoracic vertebral, and lumbar arteries. The ventral branches unite to form the ventral spinal artery, from which a central branch supplies the central portion of the spinal cord. Both ventral and dorsal branches supply the spinal cord from the periphery. Examination of intraparenchymal branches with Doppler ultrasound has been described (Hudson et al. 1995).

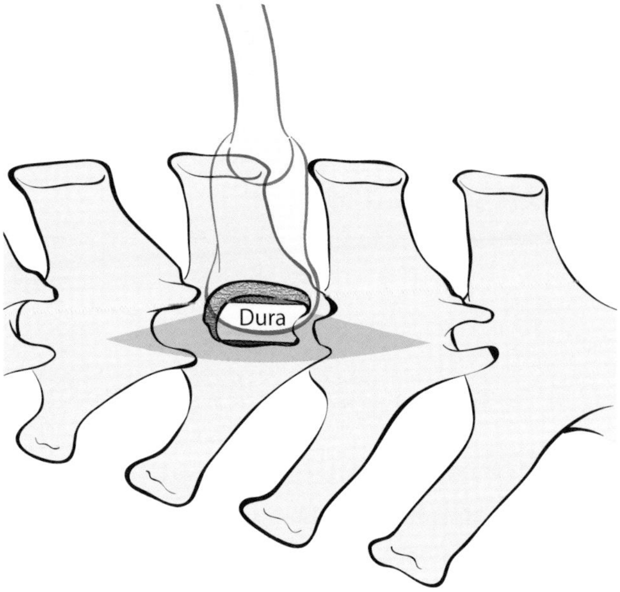

Figure 1.25. Position of probe. Illustration of a hemilaminectomy site of a dog with a sectorial probe positioned at the surgical site to evaluate the spinal cord.

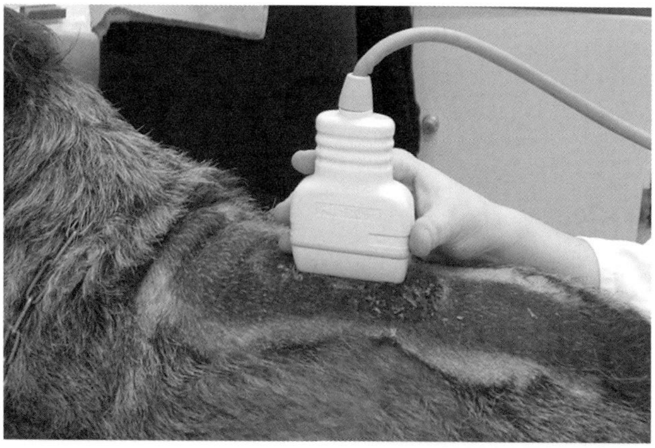

Figure 1.26. Position of probe in a longitudinal plane on the thoracolumbar spine in a dog with recent back surgery. Both longitudinal and transverse images should be obtained.

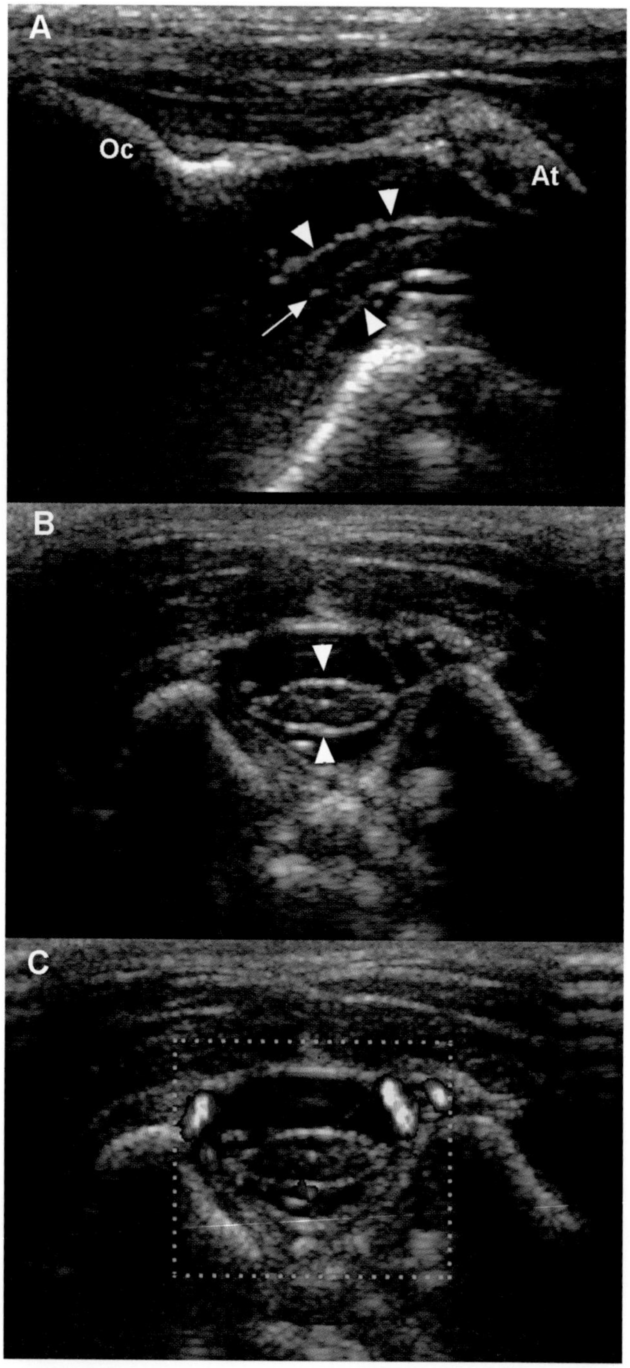

Figure 1.27. Normal canine cranial cervical spine. Longitudinal **(A)** and transverse **(B)** sonograms obtained at the atlanto-occipital junction. **C:** Power Doppler mode of the neighboring vessels at the same location. Arrowheads outline the cranial portion of the cervical spine. The arrow points to the central canal. At, lamina of the atlas; and Oc, occipital bone.

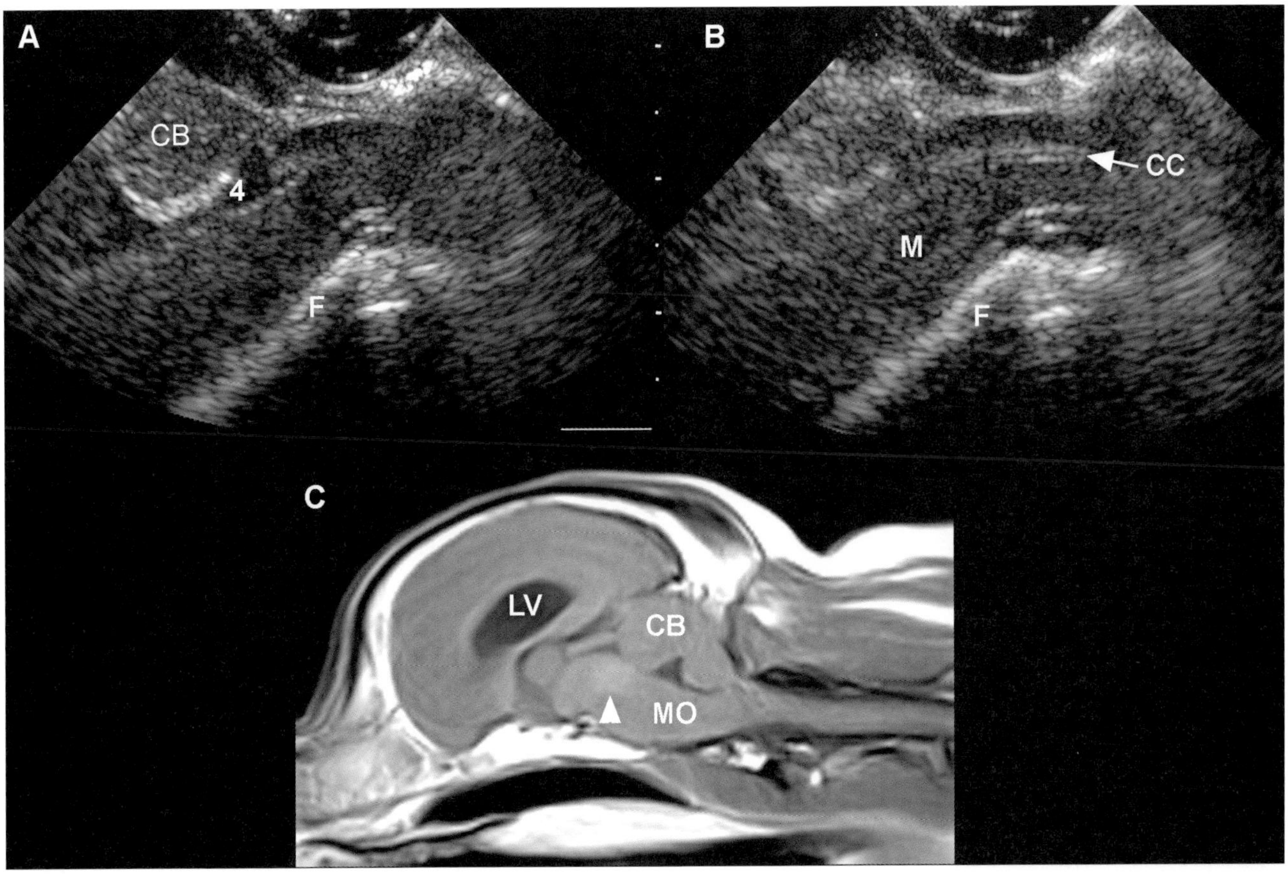

Figure 1.28. Sonograms of a Boston terrier undergoing brain surgery. The brain mass caused herniation of the cerebellum (CB). A craniotomy has been performed and an incision made through the dura mater. **A:** Longitudinal sonogram showing the fourth ventricle (4) and spinal cord. CC, central canal of the spinal cord; and F, floor of the cranium. **B:** Longitudinal sonogram made with the transducer moved slightly to the midline, making the central canal more visible. CC, central canal; F, floor of the cranium; and M, medulla oblongata. **C:** Sagittal magnetic resonance image of the brain and the spinal cord. The arrowhead points to the brain-stem mass. CB, cerebellum; LV, lateral ventricle; and MO, medulla oblongata.

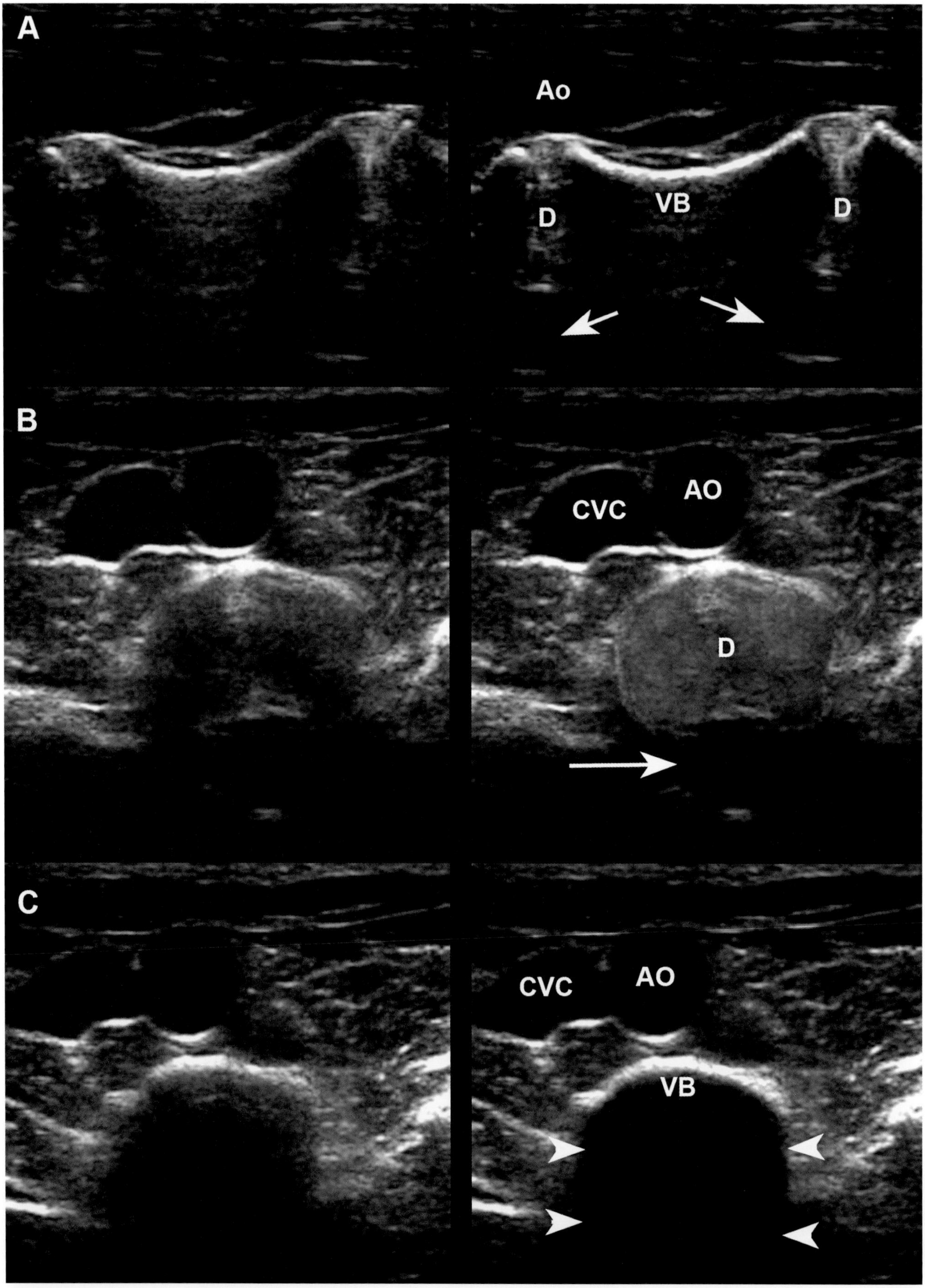

Figure 1.29

Figure 1.29. Ventral sonographic anatomy of the lumbar spine. **A:** Longitudinal sonogram and corresponding labeled schematic image, obtained via a transabdominal approach, of the caudal lumbar spine of an adult beagle. The vertebral body (VB) has a distinct curvilinear shape. In normal dogs, the intact disc (D) can be an acoustic window to see part of the cord (arrows). **B:** Transverse sonogram and corresponding labeled schematic image at the level a disc. The spinal cord is observed dorsally (arrow). **C:** Transverse sonogram and corresponding labeled schematic image at the level of the caudal aspect of the vertebral body. The arrowheads point to the shadowing associated with the vertebral body. AO, aorta; and CVC, caudal vena cava. Images courtesy of D. Penninck.

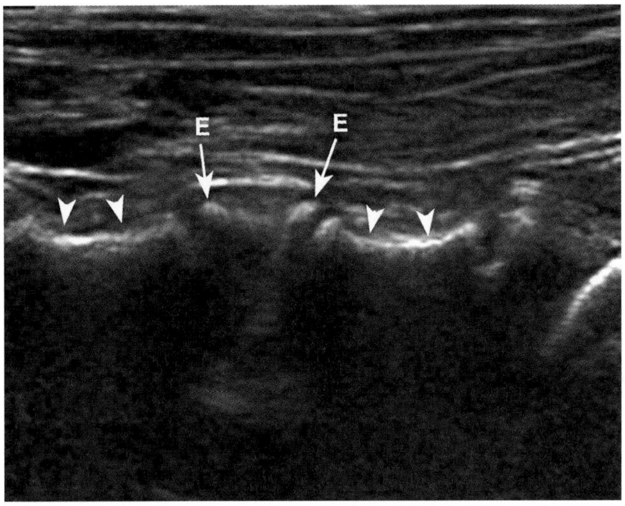

Figure 1.30. Normal lumbar spine of a 3-month-old Samoyed dog. Sagittal sonogram of the caudal lumbar spine in a puppy. Arrowheads point to vertebral bodies. E, vertebral end plates. Image courtesy of D. Penninck.

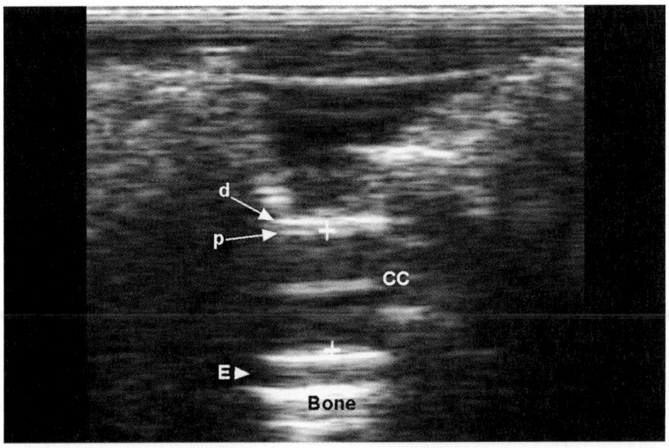

Figure 1.31. Longitudinal sonograms of a normal canine spinal cord during surgery. The spinal cord (between the cursors) is relatively hypoechoic, and the meninges are hyperechoic and outline the anechoic cerebrospinal fluid. CC, central canal; d, dura mater and arachnoid mater; E, epidural space; and p, pia mater. The bone interface is hyperechoic and hyperattenuating, limiting evaluation of any structure deeper to it.

Sonography of Spinal Disorders

Disc Herniation

Disc material is hyperechoic to the spinal cord parenchyma and therefore easily identified (Hudson et al. 1998). Herniated disc material may appear as amorphous, bright material with irregular margins (Figure 1.32). During surgery, sonography may assist the surgeon in assessing complete removal of disc fragments. Acute compressive lesions tend to increase focally the spinal diameter and obliterate the central canal (Figure 1.33). In situ hemostatic gel or foam can mimic the presence of disc material (Figure 1.34).

Some authors have reported oscillations in the spinal cord that they attributed to pulsations in arterial branches and suggested that there might be a relationship between the absence of oscillations and poor outcome in some animals (Nakayama 1993). The significance of the lack of oscillations remains controversial.

Hemorrhage

In research studies evaluating the efficacy of various drugs for the treatment of spinal cord trauma, ultrasonography was performed to document the appearance of hemorrhage (Finn-Bodner et al. 1995). Hemorrhage appeared as a hyperechoic region that obscured visualization of the linear echoes normally associated with the spinal cord (Figure 1.35). Traumatic hematomas in the vertebral canal are amorphous, inhomogeneous, and irregularly marginated (Jones et al. 1996; Rault et al. 2004; Tanaka et al. 2006) (Figure 1.36).

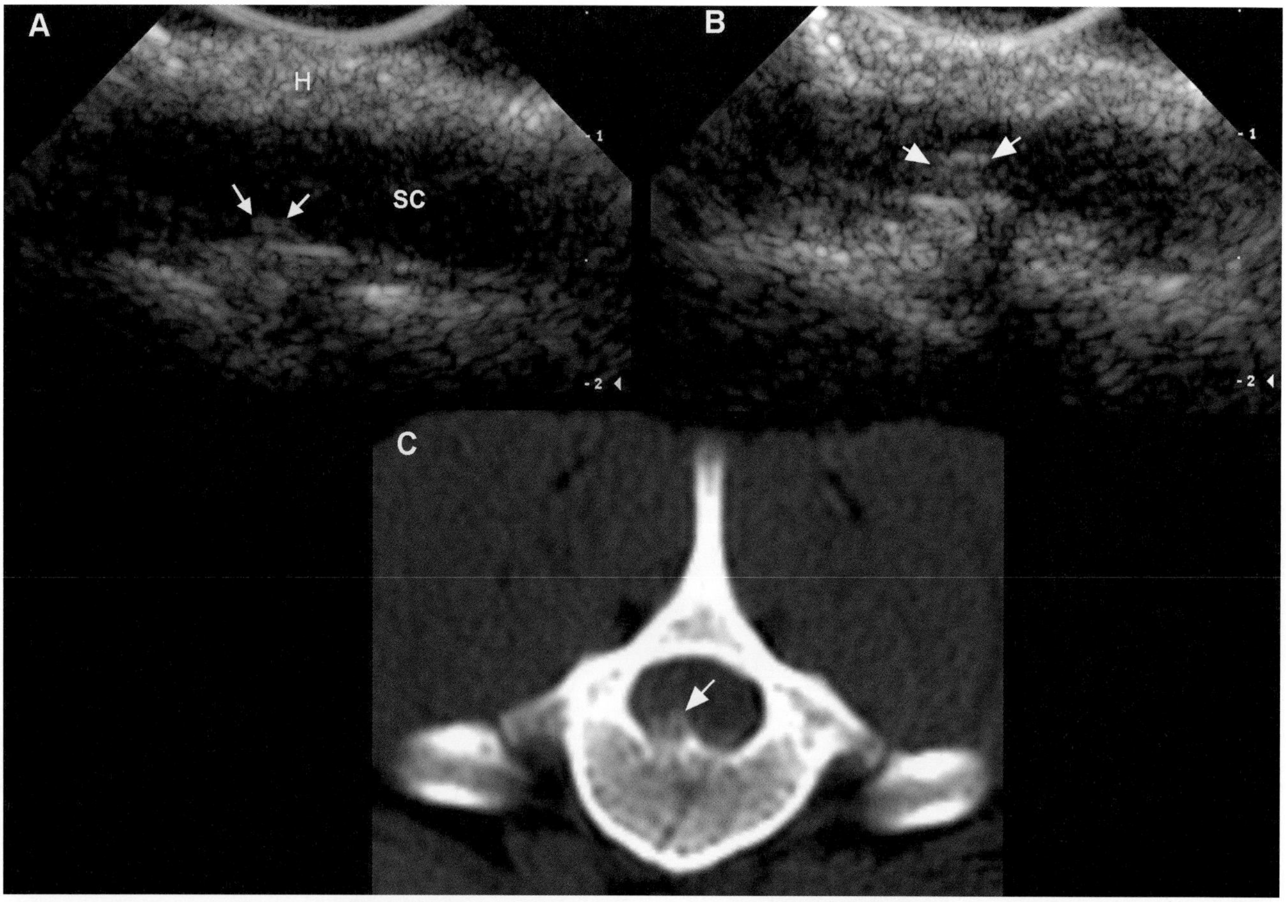

Figure 1.32. Images of a dog with intervertebral disc herniation. **A:** Longitudinal sonogram made near the midline. A small amount of hyperechoic disc material (arrows) is seen deep to the hypoechoic spinal cord (SC). Some hemorrhage (H) shows as a hyperechoic region superficial to the spinal cord. **B:** A larger amount of disc material (arrows) is apparent in this longitudinal sonogram made more laterally. **C:** Computed tomographic image of the spinal cord of the same dog showing the hyperdense disc material (arrow) on the right side of the midline.

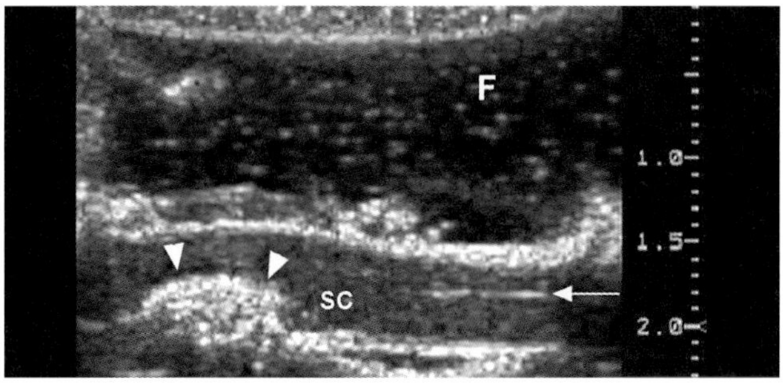

Figure 1.33. Compressive herniated disc material in the vertebral canal of a dog. The hyperechoic disc material (arrowheads) has irregular margins and compresses the spinal cord (SC). Part of the visible central canal (arrow) is seen away from the lesion. F, fluid at the surgical site.

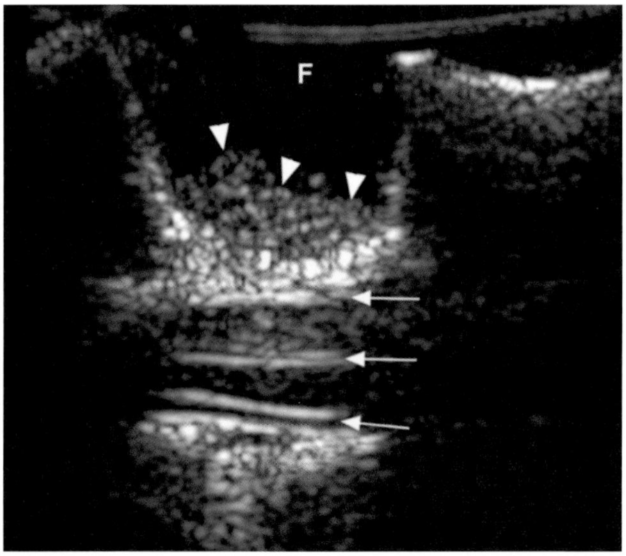

Figure 1.34. Successfully removed disc material in a dog. Compressive disc material was removed at the C4-5 intervertebral disc space. The subarachnoid spaces and central canal (arrows) are normal; there is no evidence of cord compression. The echogenic structure (arrowheads) seen dorsal to the spinal cord represents hemostatic foam in situ and should not be confused with disc material. F, fluid at surgery site. Image courtesy of D. Penninck.

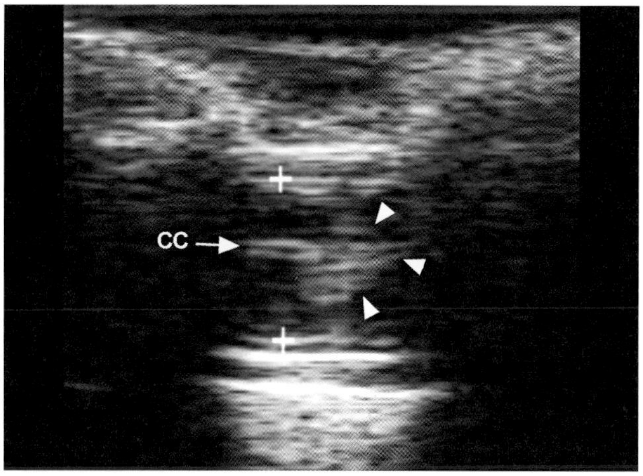

Figure 1.35. Sonogram of a traumatized spinal cord in a dog. Spinal cord hemorrhage appears as a hyperechoic region (arrowheads) obscuring the linear echoes normally seen in the spinal cord. CC, central canal.

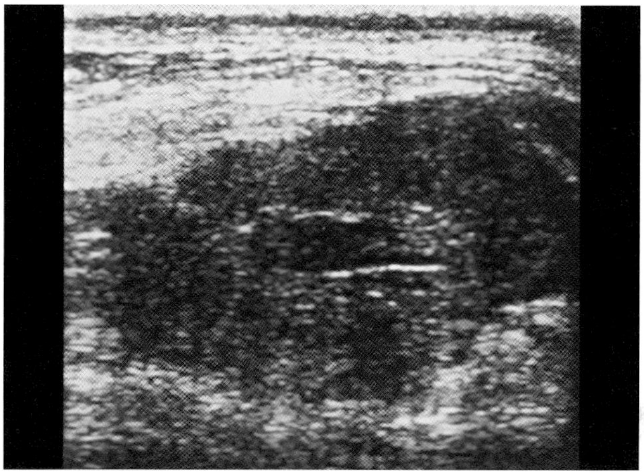

Figure 1.36. Hematoma in a dog, 2 days after lumbar hemilaminectomy. On this sagittal sonogram, the irregular, inhomogeneous, echotexture lesion represents a hematoma.

Neoplasia

The appearance of neoplasia is nonspecific and varies in echogenicity and uniformity (McConnell et al. 2003; Tanaka et al. 2006) (Figures 1.37 and 1.38). Tumors may arise from the vertebrae or soft tissues of the spinal canal, such as the meninges or spinal cord. The exact location or origin and nature of the lesion cannot be diagnosed solely on the ultrasonographic appearance. Tumors arising from neurological tissue may appear in unexpected locations such as the kidney (Figure 1.39). Multinodal or metastatic neoplasms, such as multiple myeloma and disseminated histiocytic sarcoma, can affect multiple vertebral segments and other body regions such as the abdomen, requiring complete body imaging in most cases. Serial ultrasound examinations may also help to evaluate progression of neoplastic disease or response to chemotherapy.

Cystic Lesions

Spinal arachnoid or intradural cysts have been reported as cystlike lesions in the subarachnoid space of dogs and cats (Galloway et al. 1999). These are not lined

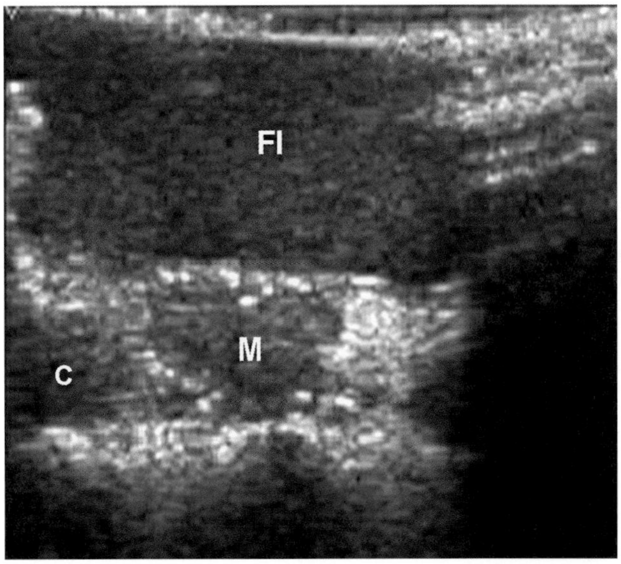

Figure 1.37. Intramedullary tumor (sarcoma) in a dog. On this longitudinal sonogram obtained after dorsal laminectomy, an irregularly marginated mass (M) is noted in the spinal canal (c). Fl, fluid at the surgery site.

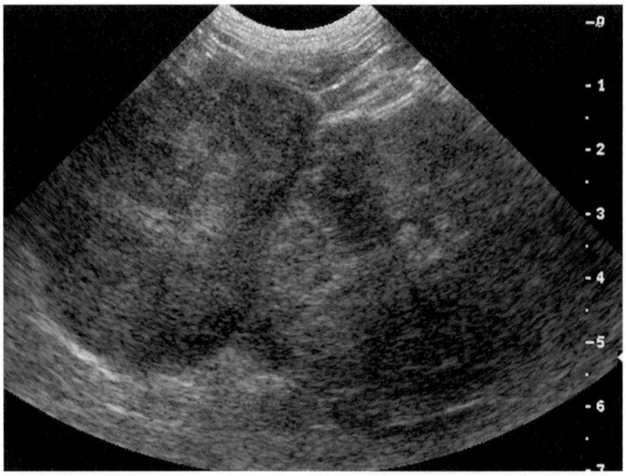

Figure 1.39. Neuroblastoma in the kidney of a cat. The large mass deforms the contours of the kidney and is heterogeneous, with both hypoechoic and hyperechoic areas intermingled. Only a small portion of the kidney was recognizable as renal tissue (not shown).

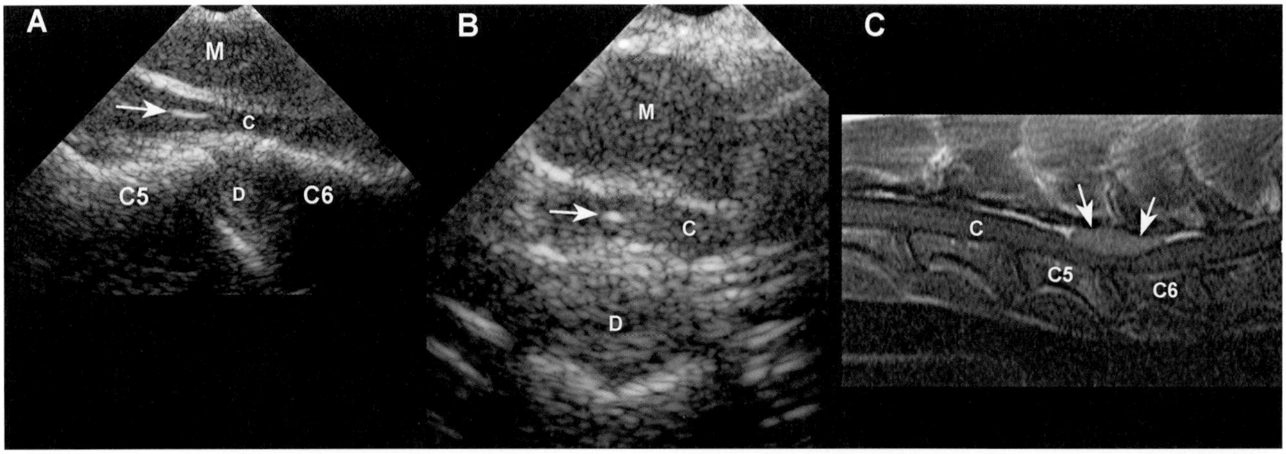

Figure 1.38. Intradural extramedullary mass (M) in an American foxhound with a 2-month history of chronic progressive tetraparesis. A dorsal laminectomy was performed at C5-6. **A:** Longitudinal sonogram at the laminectomy site showing a hypoechoic mass (M) compressing and flattening the spinal cord (C). The central canal (arrow) cannot be visualized where compression is greatest on this plane. **B:** Transverse sonogram at C5-6. The spinal cord is flattened and displaced laterally although the central canal is visible (arrow) on this image. A small amount of hemorrhage appears bright and can be seen on the ventral surface of the mass. D, intervertebral disc at C5-6. **C:** Sagittal magnetic resonance image showing the mass (arrows) dorsal to the spinal cord (C) at C5-6. C5, body of the fifth cervical vertebra; and C6, body of the sixth cervical vertebra.

with a secreting epithelium and therefore not considered as true cysts.

The fluid contents may be anechoic to isoechoic to the spinal cord (Galloway et al. 1999). The lesions can appear septated with irregular hyperechoic lines. An irregular and thickened dura may be present. The central canal may or may not be recognized, and the compressed spinal cord may be increased in echogenicity. The line thought to represent the pia in normal animals is not always visible (Galloway et al. 1999). After drainage of arachnoid or intradural cysts, the spinal cord can be monitored for recurrence by using the surgical site as an acoustic window (Hudson et al. 1998).

Syringomyelia

Dilation of the central canal with an ependymal lining (*hydromyelia*) and cavitation within the spinal cord lacking an ependymal lining (*syrinx*), a combined condition known as *syringomyelia*, can occur secondary to numerous conditions (Rusbridge et al. 2006). Syringomyelia has been mainly described in relation to Chiari type I–like malformation syndrome in Cavalier King Charles spaniels and other small breeds of dogs. Other processes such as trauma, neoplasia, intracranial epidermoid cysts, and arachnoiditis can lead to this condition (Kirberger et al. 1997; MacKillop et al. 2006; Rusbridge et al. 2006) (Figure 1.40).

In all cases, syringomyelia is thought to occur as a consequence of altered CSF dynamics (Rusbridge et al. 2006). Concurrent myelomalacia might also be found, with a tendency to increase the spinal cord echogenicity with an obliteration of the central canal (Figure 1.41).

Meningocele

Tethering of the spinal cord with an associated meningocele, extramedullary intradural cyst, and lipoma was sonographically evaluated in a Manx-type cat (Plummer et al. 1993). The lipoma appeared as a hyperechoic region located within a hypoechoic tract representing the meningocele. A hyperechoic linear structure located within the meningocele was believed to be the filum terminale, although this could not be confirmed on histology.

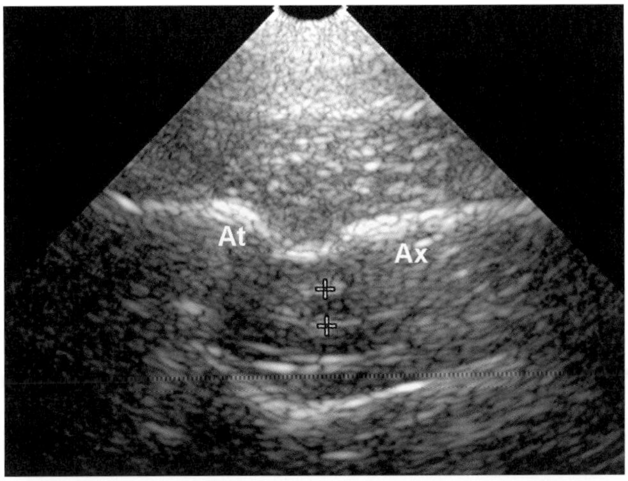

Figure 1.40. Syringomyelia in a Cavalier King Charles spaniel with Chiari type I–like malformation syndrome. Longitudinal image obtained at the level of the atlantoaxial junction. The dilated central canal (between the cursors) measures 2.5 mm in diameter. At, atlas; and Ax, axis.

Vertebral and Perivertebral Changes

Many changes—such as malformation (spina bifida), spondylosis, spondylarthrosis, or articular facet osteoarthrosis, osteomyelitis, discospondylitis, fracture, and tumor—can affect the shape and echogenicity of the vertebral and perivertebral structures.

Ventral spondylosis bridges two vertebral bodies along the ventral longitudinal ligament and appears as a hyperechoic bridge associated with acoustic shadowing. The disc at that space cannot be visualized.

Spondylarthrosis or articular facet osteoarthrosis is visible as hyperechoic, irregularly lined surfaces over the joint space and is associated with acoustic shadowing (Figure 1.42).

In discospondylitis, a ventral approach to the affected disc enables visualization of a partial or complete loss of the fiber organization of the discs. The vertebral hyperechoic contours become irregular and may be interrupted by the presence of hypoechoic or anechoic lytic foci. A hypoechoic area of swelling is

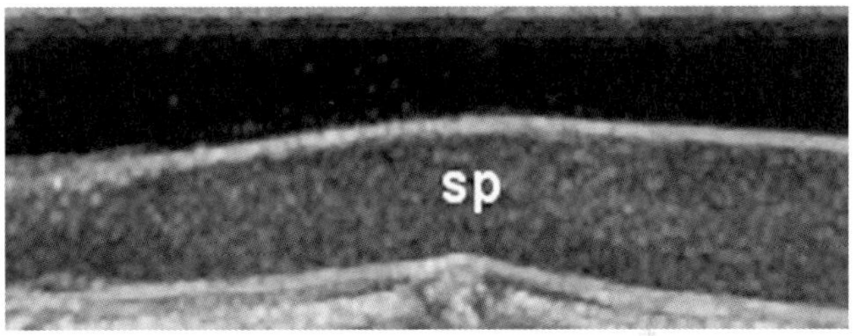

Figure 1.41. Myelomalacia in a dog. Sagittal sonogram of a segment of spine (sp) after laminectomy and durotomy. The cord is uniformly mildly echogenic, and the central canal is not visible. Anechoic fluid is noted in the near field, placed to serve as an acoustic window.

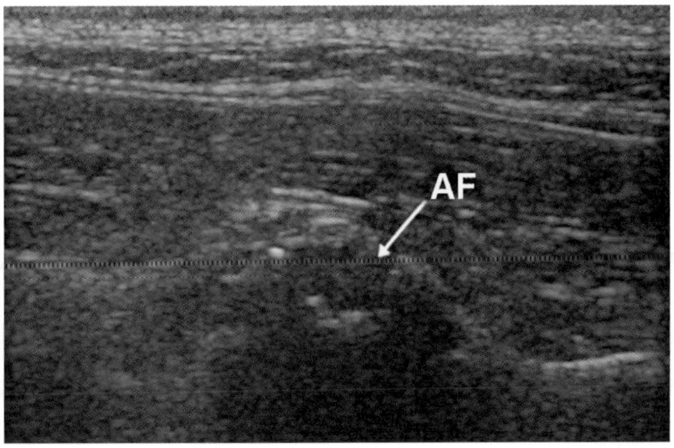

Figure 1.42. Articular facet osteoarthrosis in a dog. Sagittal sonogram of a segment of spine with an irregular hyperechoic surface at the level of the articular facets (AF).

often seen laterally and ventrally to the disc space. The surrounding fat or muscles may also be affected. Ultrasound-guided fine-needle aspirates of the affected discs can be done (Rault et al. 2004; Packer et al. 2005).

A sublumbar abscess appears as a hypoechoic to anechoic, inhomogeneous to homogeneous area with irregular and ill-defined margins. Neighboring organs may be affected. In some cases, a foreign body can be identified within the abscess. Foreign material often appears as hyperechoic with or without acoustic shadowing (Figure 1.43) (Packer et al. 2005).

Primary bony tumors or metastases are visible as irregular and inhomogeneous areas destroying the hyperechoic bony structure (Figure 1.44). The involved soft tissue usually appears more hypoechoic than normal, with irregular borders.

Fractures of the vertebral bodies can be visualized as interruptions of the continuous hyperechoic line of the surface of the bone. In acute cases, an inhomogeneous, mixed echotexture hematoma can be seen at the fracture site.

Postoperative seromas can be observed at the incision sites. They often are regularly marginated and

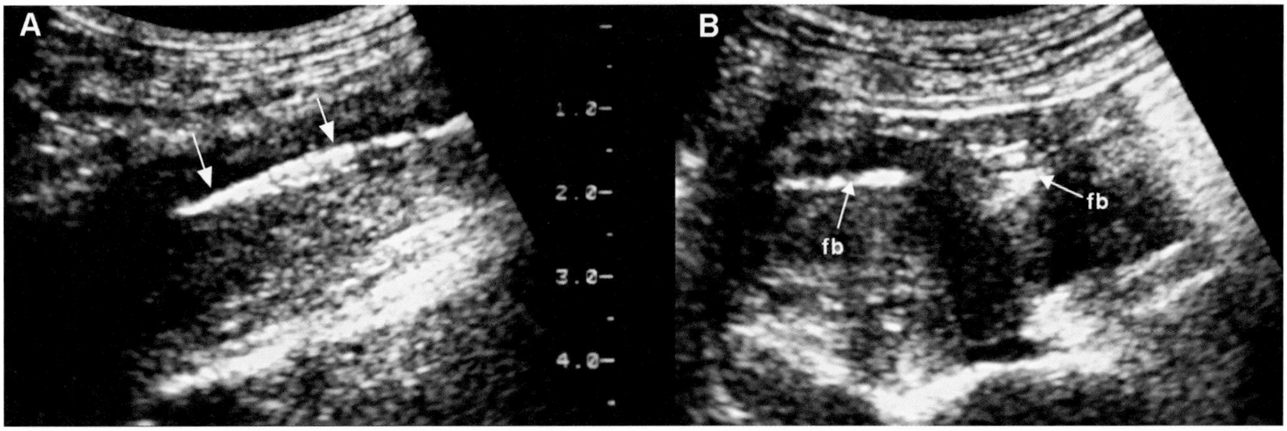

Figure 1.43. Sublumbar abscess with foreign bodies (wooden sticks) in a dog. Sagittal **(A)** and transverse **(B)** sonograms of the swollen, inhomogeneous, and mostly hypoechoic sublumbar region. The wooden sticks appear as hyperechoic linear interfaces (fb and arrows). In the far field, the surface of the adjacent vertebral bodies is irregular, most likely because of periostitis.

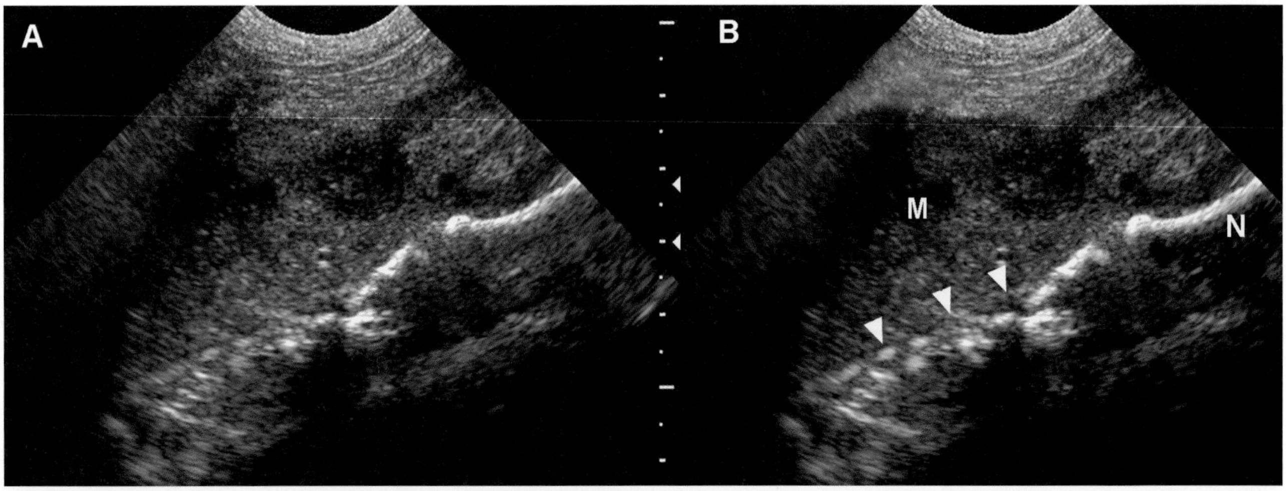

Figure 1.44. Vertebral osteosarcoma in a dog. Sagittal sonogram **(A)** and schematic labeled image **(B)**. The ventral cortical surface of this lumbar vertebral body is moderately irregular and interrupted (arrowheads). An inhomogeneous and mostly hypoechoic soft-tissue mass (M) extends along the ventral aspect of the vertebra. N, normal adjacent vertebra. Image courtesy of D. Penninck.

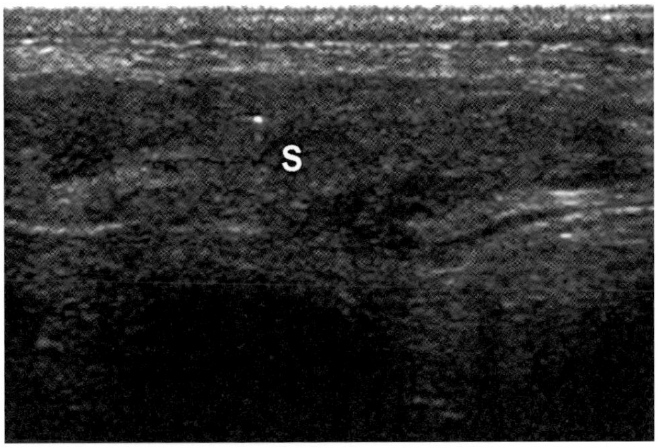

Figure 1.45. Seroma at a recent hemilaminectomy site in a dog. Sagittal sonogram of a hypoechoic and inhomogeneous lesion with irregular margins, representing a superficial seroma (S) at the surgical site.

hypoechoic to anechoic, with or without thin linear hyperechoic septa (Figure 1.45).

Interventional Procedures

Intraoperative ultrasonography can be useful in determining whether herniated disc material remains in the vertebral canal or foramina (Nakayama 1993). The use of spinal ultrasonography has also been described during dorsal laminectomy in dogs with caudal cervical vertebral instability and malformation to ensure that the spinal cord has been adequately decompressed (Nanai et al. 2006). Sonography can also be useful for evaluating cystic lesions after drainage to ensure that fluid has not recurred (Hudson et al. 1998). As in other locations, ultrasound-guided aspirates or tissue-core biopsies of focal lesions can be done if a satisfactory acoustic window is available.

References

Finn-Bodner ST, Hudson JA, Coates JR, et al. (1995) Ultrasonographic anatomy of the normal canine spinal cord and correlation with histopathology after induced spinal cord trauma. Vet Radiol Ultrasound 36:39–48.

Gallagher JG, Penninck D, Boudriaux RJ, Schelling SH (1995) Ultrasonography of the brain and vertebral canal in dogs and cats: 15 cases (1988–1993). J Am Vet Med Assoc 207:1320–1324.

Galloway AM, Curtis NC, Sommerlad SF, Watt PR (1999) Correlative imaging findings in seven dogs and one cat with spinal arachnoid cysts. Vet Radiol Ultrasound 40:445–452.

Hudson JA, Finn-Bodner ST, Coates JR, et al. (1995) Color Doppler imaging and Doppler spectral analysis in the spinal cord of normal dogs. Vet Radiol Ultrasound 36:542–547.

Hudson JA, Finn-Bodner ST, Steiss JE (1998) Neurosonography. Vet Clin North Am Small Animal Pract 28:943–971.

Jones JC, Hudson JA, Sorjonen DC, et al. (1996) Effects of experimental nerve root compression on arterial blood flow velocity in the seventh lumbar spinal ganglion of the dog: Measurement using intraoperative Doppler ultrasonography. Vet Radiol Ultrasound 37:133–140.

Kirberger RM, Jacobson LS, Davies JV, Engela J (1997) Hydromyelia in the dog. Vet Radiol Ultrasound 38:30–38.

MacKillop E, Schatzberg SJ, de Lahunta A (2006) Intracranial epidermoid cyst and syringohydromyelia in a dog. Vet Radiol Ultrasound 47:339–344.

McConnell JF, Garosi LS, Dennis R, Smith KC (2003) Imaging of spinal nephroblastoma in a dog. Vet Radiol Ultrasound 44:537–541.

Nakayama M (1993) Intraoperative spinal ultrasonography in dogs: Normal findings and case-history reports. Vet Radiol Ultrasound 34:264–268.

Nanai B, Lyman R, Bichsel P (2006) Intraoperative use of ultrasonography during continuous dorsal laminectomy in tow dogs with caudal cervical vertebral instability and malformation ("Wobbler syndrome"). Vet Surg 35:465–469.

Packer RA, Coates JR, Cook CR, Lattimer JC, O'Brien DP (2005) Sublumbar abscess and discospondylitis in a cat. Vet Radiol Ultrasound 46:396–399.

Plummer SB, Bunch SE, Khoo LH, Spaulding KA, Kornegay JN (1993) Tethered spinal cord and an intradural lipoma associated with a meningocele in a Manx-type cat. J Am Vet Med Assoc 203:1159–1161.

Rault DN, Besso JG, Ruel Y, et al. (2004) Ultrasonography of discospondylitis: Seven dogs and three cats. In: Annual Scientific Conference of the European Association of Veterinary Diagnostic Imaging, September 8–11, Ghent, Belgium, p 151.

Rusbridge C, Greitz D, Iskandar BJ (2006) Syringomyelia: Current concepts in pathogenesis, diagnosis, and treatment. J Vet Intern Med 20:469–479.

Tanaka H, Nakayama M, Takase K (2006) Intraoperative spinal ultrasonography in two dogs with spinal disease. Vet Radiol Ultrasound 47:99–102.

SECTION 3

Peripheral Nerves

Martin Kramer and Judith Hudson

Scanning Technique

Because of their small size and superficial location, peripheral nerves are preferably scanned with high-frequency (>10 MHz) linear transducers. If needed, a stand-off pad can be used to place the nerve into the focal zone. Color flow Doppler imaging can be useful in differentiating vessels from nerves. Imaging in multiple planes and following structures distally can also be helpful. In addition, nerves are not compliant to pressure, unlike vessels, and moving a limb can help in differentiating a tendon from a nerve.

The region of the brachial plexus can be scanned with lower-frequency probes, depending on the size of the dog. The patient is placed in lateral recumbency with the affected limb up. The plexus is assessed with the limb fully extended and abducted. The axilla is examined with the probe positioned craniocaudally (perpendicular to the limb axis).

Normal Sonographic Anatomy of Peripheral Nerves

In longitudinal section, nerves appear as tubular hypoechoic structures with linear echogenic walls (Hudson et al. 1996). The midportion of the nerve is mainly hypoechoic, with small dispersed hyperechoic internal echoes (Figure 1.46). The walls of nerves are brighter and better defined than vessels walls; vascular walls are less distinct. In transverse section, nerves are circular or oval hypoechoic structures.

The brachial plexus can also be evaluated. In the axilla, the largest structures are the axillary vessels (arteries and veins), which appear tubular and anechoic, with smooth hyperechoic walls (Figure 1.47). By means of Doppler ultrasonography, veins can be distinguished from arteries by their Doppler signature, larger size, and lack of visible pulsation. They can be more easily compressed than the arteries. Normal nerves are small (2–3 mm) linear hypoechoic structures outlined by bright walls.

The axillary lymph nodes located adjacent to the vessels are smooth ovoid, homogeneous, and echogenic structures. Sometimes the hilar fat can be seen as a hyperechoic line in the center of the parenchyma.

Sonographic Features of Peripheral Nerve Disorders

Rupture

Rupture or transection of nerves can occur associated with fractures, sharp-object penetration, or other injuries. Research has shown that nerve degenerates rapidly after transection. Wallerian degeneration in the distal segment causes a breakdown of myelinization that is more severe in the more distal portion. The proximal stump undergoes traumatic degeneration and is more likely to be visualized. After injury, loss of visualization of the distal segment strongly suggests rupture. It is important, however, to remember that nerves often dive into or between muscular and tendinous structures. Knowledge of anatomy is necessary to ensure that the nerve is transected and has not altered course.

Serial examination can be useful to determine if there is any evidence of repair after injury. In some animals, a neuroma may form at the site of transection, often appearing as a hypoechoic bulb on ultrasonography. Regeneration has been described as irregular regrowth with or without neuroma formation.

Demyelinization Without Rupture

Demyelinization also can occur after trauma or inflammation that is not severe enough to cause transection.

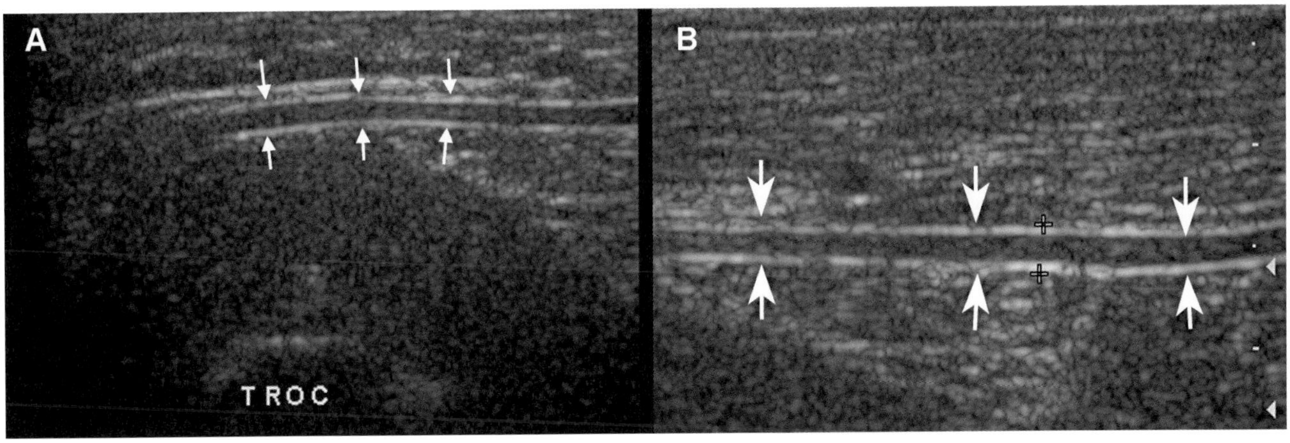

Figure 1.46. Longitudinal sonograms of a normal sciatic nerve in a dog. A normal nerve is a tubular, poorly echogenic structure with small hyperechoic internal echoes, outlined by linear hyperechoic walls. **A:** Proximal portion of the nerve (arrows) near the greater trochanter (troc). **B:** Normal sciatic nerve in the midfemoral region showing sharp linear echogenic walls (arrows). The nerve measures 2.5 mm in diameter.

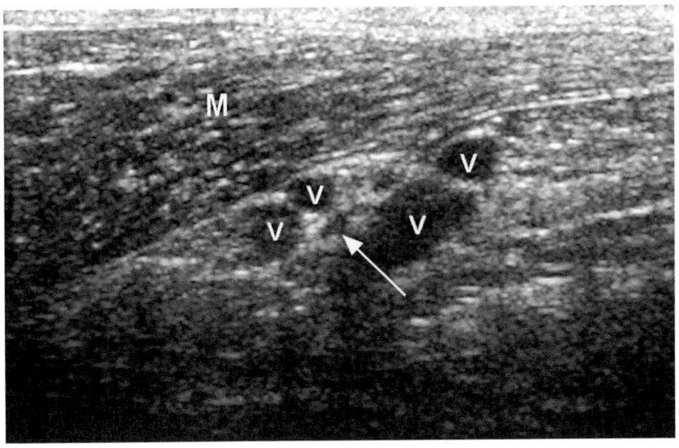

Figure 1.47. Normal brachial plexus in a dog. The brachial plexus (arrow) is present between the round anechoic vascular structures (v). The nerves are poorly echogenic and slightly inhomogeneous. M, adjacent muscle.

In such cases, the nerve is poorly visualized distal to the site of injury. Comparison with the nerve on the healthy contralateral side is helpful (Figure 1.48).

Compression

Nerve compression can be caused by local masses such as neoplasms or hematomas, by incorrectly applied external bandaging, or by compartmental syndrome. Carpal tunnel syndrome in people causes swelling of the median nerve that can be imaged external to the carpal tunnel. Ultrasonography can be useful in determining whether compression has caused demyelinization or other abnormalities in the affected nerve.

Neoplasia

Peripheral nerve sheath tumors in the brachial plexus of dogs were described as hypoechoic tubular structures (Rose et al. 2005) or as fusiform masses exhibiting mixed echogenicity (Platt et al. 1999) (Figures 1.49 and 1.50). These tumors can occur in unusual locations such as the thorax (Essman et al. 2002).

Other Disorders of the Brachial Plexus

In acute partial or complete avulsions of the brachial plexus, a hypoechoic to anechoic, inhomogeneous, and irregularly demarcated area is seen in the axillary region. This area represents the hematoma. Torn nerve tissue can usually not be seen sonographically.

Tumors of the brachial plexus can usually be visualized by ultrasonography if they exceed 5 mm. These masses appear round to oval, vary in echogenicity from hyperechoic to anechoic areas (Figure 1.51), and can be inhomogeneous.

Metastases to the axillary lymph nodes in the area of the brachial plexus can also be identified. Affected lymph nodes are typically rounded, moderately to severely enlarged, and mildly to moderately inhomogeneous. The hilar fat usually disappears. A definitive diagnosis can be obtained by ultrasound-guided needle biopsy.

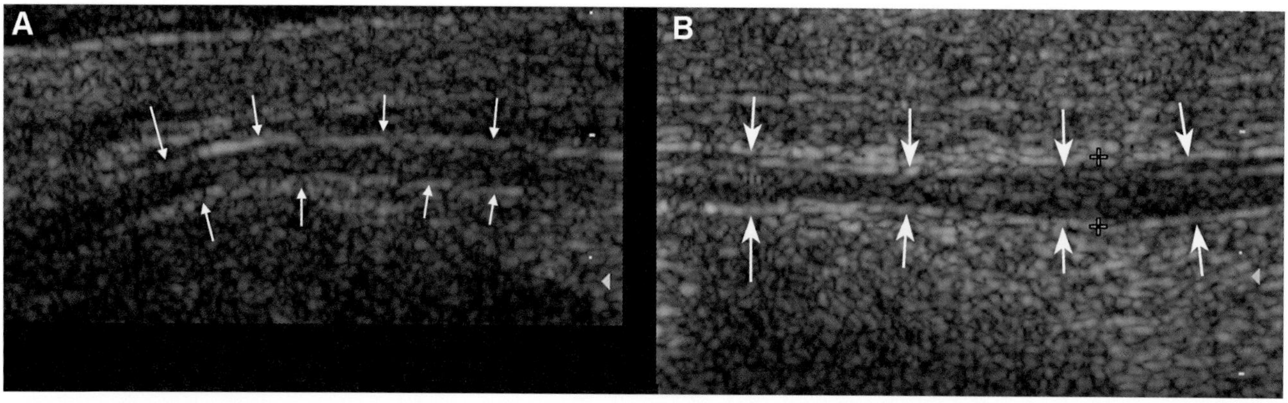

Figure 1.48. Sonogram of the right sciatic nerve in a dog with neurological deficits. Compare these images with those of the left sciatic nerve of the same dog shown in Figure 1.1. **A:** Sciatic nerve (arrows) near the greater trochanter. **B:** Sciatic nerve near the midfemoral region (arrows). The nerve has a variable diameter and irregular interrupted walls (arrows). The nerve is swollen in the midfemoral region and measures 2.9 mm.

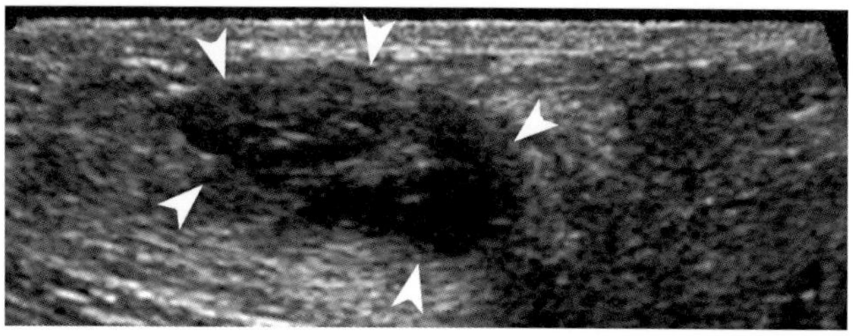

Figure 1.49. Median nerve sarcoma in a dog. A 20-mm-long by 5-mm wide, mostly hypoechoic lesion (arrowheads) is distal and medial to the elbow joint, along the path of the median nerve.

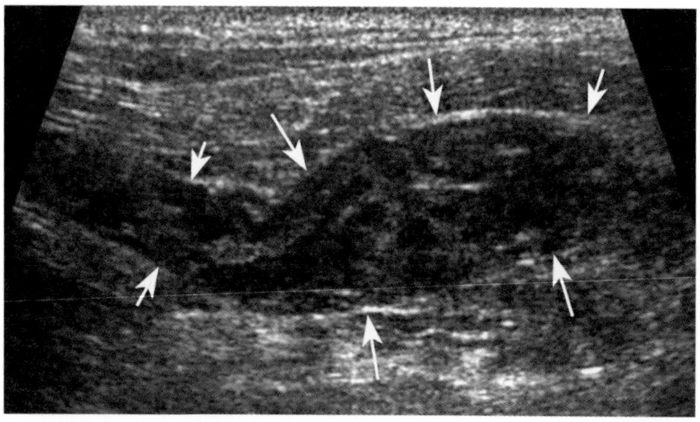

Figure 1.50. Radial nerve sheath tumor. A large (5 cm long) mass (arrows) is on the cranial aspect of the left elbow in a 5-year-old Labrador retriever with lameness and forelimb muscle atrophy. The elongated mass is well defined and inhomogeneously hypoechoic. Image courtesy of K. Spaulding.

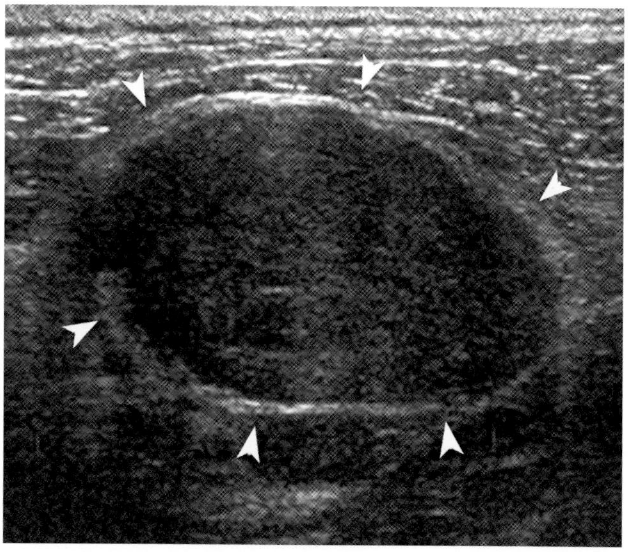

Figure 1.51. Brachial plexus tumor. A large (2 cm long by 1 cm wide), well defined, oval and poorly echogenic mass (arrowheads) is in the axillary region of this Bernese mountain dog that presented with lameness. A histiocytic sarcoma was identified.

Interventional Procedures

Ultrasonography can be used to guide fine-needle aspirations or biopsies, or to locate nerve endings prior to surgical repair. Following anastomosis, ultrasonography can be used to monitor the nerves and determine whether healing is occurring. Sonography could also be useful in the resection of masses associated with nerves.

References

Essman SC, Hoover JP, Bahr RJ, Ritchey JW, Watson C (2002) An intrathoracic malignant peripheral nerve sheath tumor in a dog. Vet Radiol Ultrasound 43:255–259.

Hudson JA, Steiss JE, Braund KG, Toivio-Kinnucan M (1996) Ultrasonography of peripheral nerves during wallerian degeneration and regeneration following transection. Vet Radiol Ultrasound 37:302–312.

Platt SR, Graham J, Chrisman CL, et al. (1999) Magnetic resonance imaging and ultrasonography in the diagnosis of a malignant peripheral nerve sheath tumor in a dog. Vet Radiol Ultrasound 40:367–371.

Rose S, Long C, Knipe M, Hornof B (2005) Ultrasonographic evaluation of brachial plexus tumors in five dogs. Vet Radiol Ultrasound 46:514–517.

CHAPTER TWO

EYE AND ORBIT

Kathy Spaulding

PREPARATION AND SCANNING TECHNIQUE

There are three primary methods for imaging the globe: directly on the cornea, through the eyelid, or imaging through a water bath over the globe.

Imaging with the transducer applied directly on the cornea, which is the method most frequently used, produces the highest-quality images (Figure 2.1).

Artifacts and image degradation occur when imaging through the eyelid. The technique of imaging through the closed lid is recommended if there is a deep corneal ulcer, recent severe globe trauma, or recent ocular surgery. Using a water bath helps to image the near field (anterior chamber). However, a water bath is cumbersome to hold in position and not often used or needed with current ultrasound equipment. The recently available high-resolution transducers either have a water bath attached to the transducer or do not require a water bath to image the superficial structures of the globe.

The examination is generally performed with the dogs awake. For the safety of the imager and the patient, mild sedation of an unruly patient may be advised if manual restraint is inadequate to securely position it. If the animal is heavily sedated or anesthetized, then the globe tends to rotate ventrally. The angle of the incident beam through the eye is then affected. With a transducer covering the surface of the globe, seeing the direction of gaze of the globe may be difficult (Figure 2.2).

This is important when localizing a lesion within the globe. A topical anesthetic is applied at a dose of 1–2 drops to the cornea 2–5 min prior to the examination.

Different acoustic coupling gels can be used. A sterile, water-soluble lubricating acoustic gel approved for the eye is recommended. It is important that the gel does not contain preservatives or perfumes. At the end of the examination, the gel should be flushed from the eye with approved sterile eyewash.

High-frequency transducers are selected depending on the equipment available and the region of the eye and orbit to be imaged. The highest resolution available is recommended. Transducers with a range from 7.5- to 50-MHz range are used to image the globe and orbit. The 25- to 50-MHz transducers are generally ocular specific because they are designed for optimally imaging the near-field structures within the globe. They are excellent for resolution of the cornea, anterior chamber, iris, ciliary body, and lens. The vitreous body and the retrobulbar area are often best imaged with the 7.5- to 13-MHz transducers. A linear transducer provides optimum imaging of the near-field structures, but manipulating a sector or convex probe with a small footprint may be easier.

The patient's eyelids are manually held open by the restrainer while the head is secured (Hager et al. 1987; Dziezyc et al. 1988). Large-breed dogs are often more difficult to image because they may squint or retract the globe into the orbit and thus limit access to the eye. The globes of brachiocephalic breeds are generally more accessible.

Geometrically speaking, the globe is nearly a sphere. It is important to identify the direction of the beam; that is, where it enters the globe and the corresponding location on the opposite side of it. The globe should be imaged in sagittal, dorsal, and transverse planes (Figures 2.3–2.8). Selected oblique planes are used to delineate a lesion better. The entire globe is systematically scanned with a fanning motion. The globe is scanned from one side to the other in each sagittal and dorsal plane and from rostrally to caudally in a transverse plane. Access to the posterior section of the globe is often more difficult in patients with a retracted globe. The zygomatic salivary gland, located ventrally to the globe, can be imaged with the probe placed ventrolaterally to the zygomatic arch (Figure 2.9). Doppler imaging or standardized A-mode scanning may provide additional vascular and measurement information.

Appropriate positional markers identifying the location of the transducer relative to the globe are documented on the image and changed with new positions. The probe position marker is usually placed on the image to identify the nasal (medial) aspect for a horizontal plane and superior (dorsal) for a vertical plane (Figures 2.3 and 2.5).

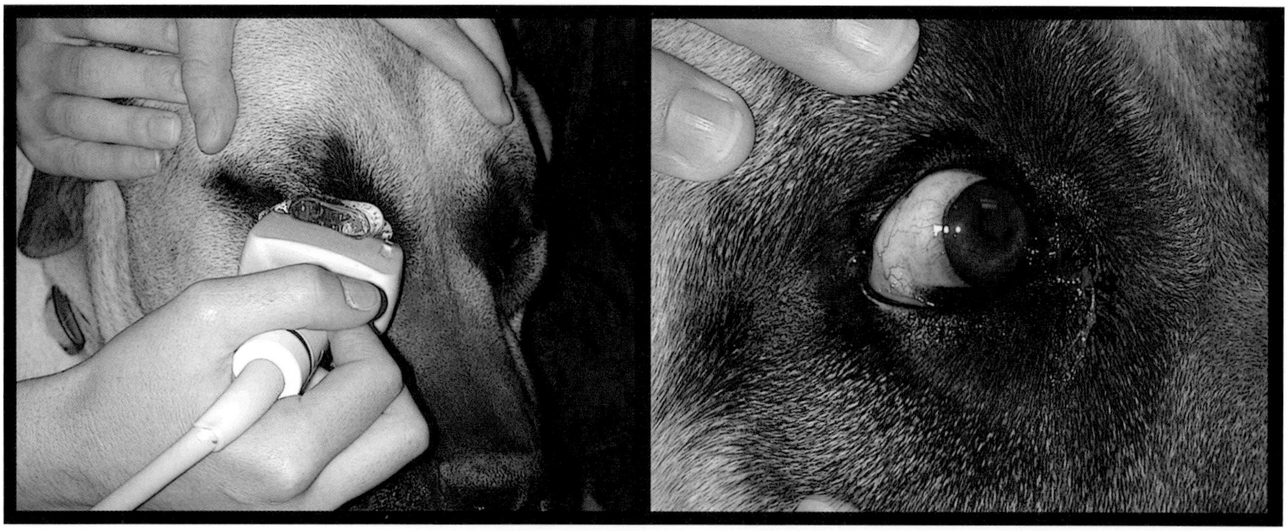

Figure 2.1. Probe placement. Images can be made either through the eyelid **(left)** or directly on the cornea. Imaging directly on the cornea produces the best images. This requires digitally retracting the eyelids **(right)**.

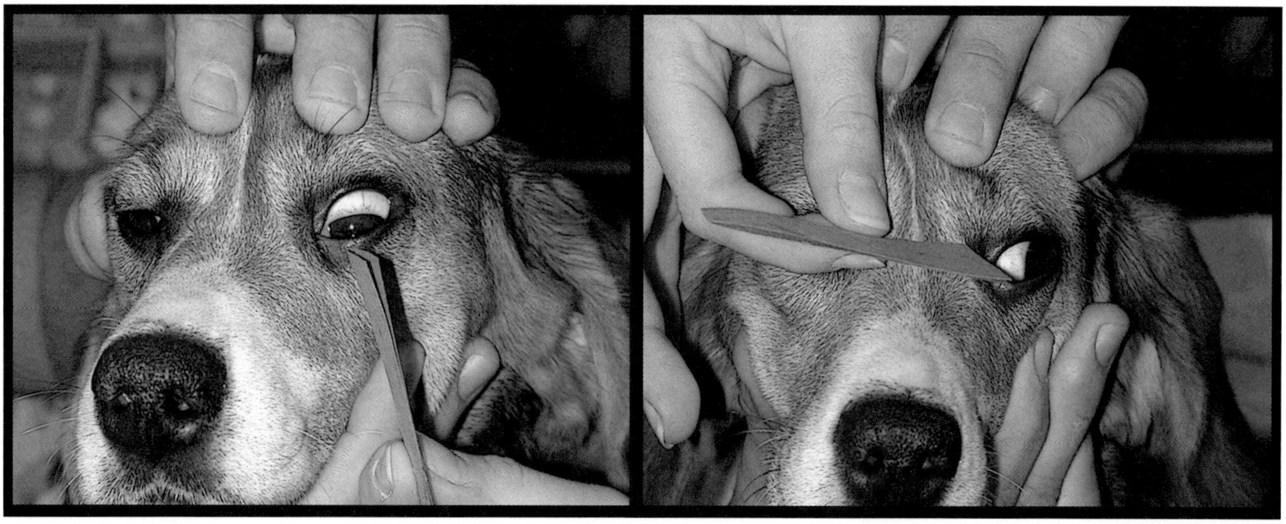

Figure 2.2. Directions of the gaze. The direction of the gaze influences the globe section displayed. Control of the direction of the gaze is limited. When the transducer is placed over the globe, the direction of the gaze is often obscured. This can lead to erroneous location of a lesion within the eye.

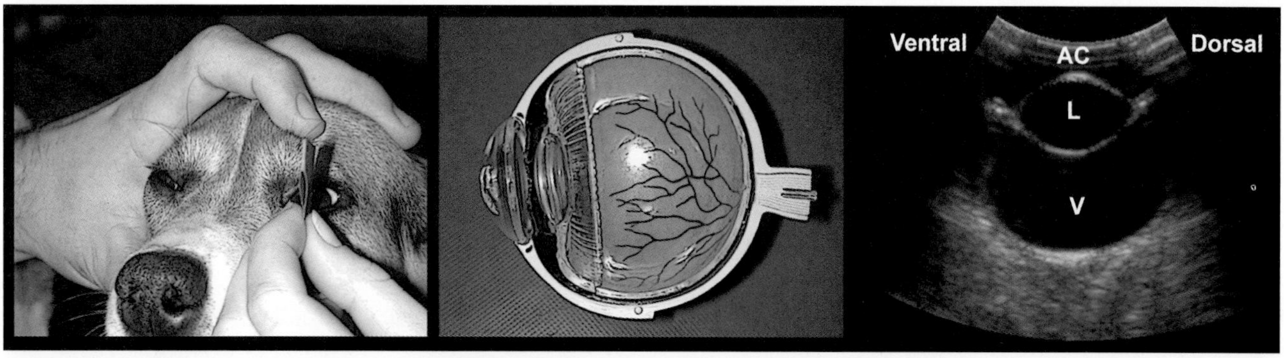

Figure 2.3. Sagittal plane. A sagittal plane through the eye divides it into right and left halves. The near field of the image is on the cornea and anterior chamber. The far field represents the vitreous and retina. The dorsal part is by convention placed on the left of the image. AC, anterior chamber; L, lens; and V, vitreous body.

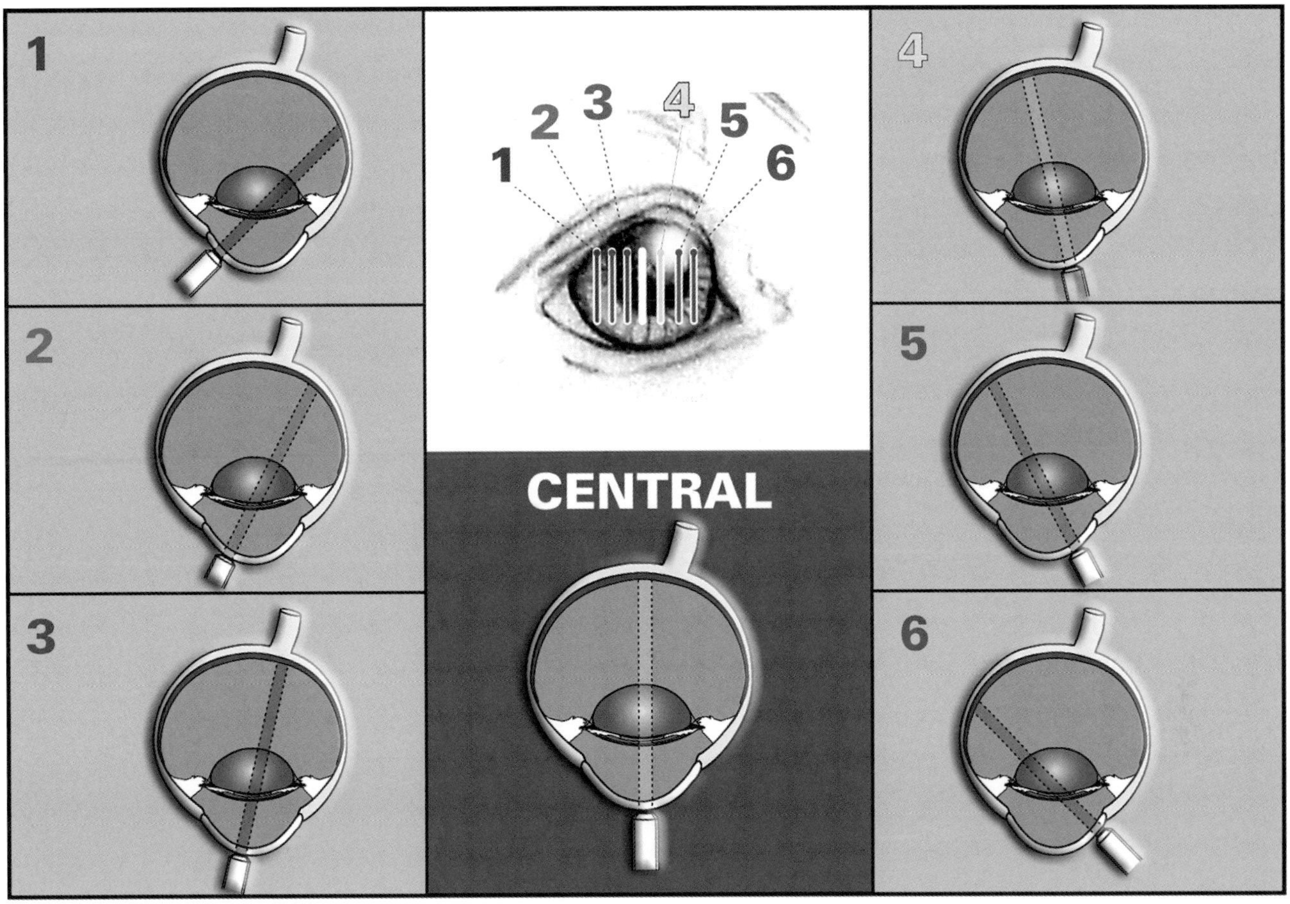

Figure 2.4. Array of sagittal images. The central image represents the sagittal view through the globe with equal divisions into right and left halves. The globe is then scanned from one side to the other to obtain a complete view of the entire globe (planes 1–6). When imaging from one side of the eye, the opposite side of the far side of the globe is displayed.

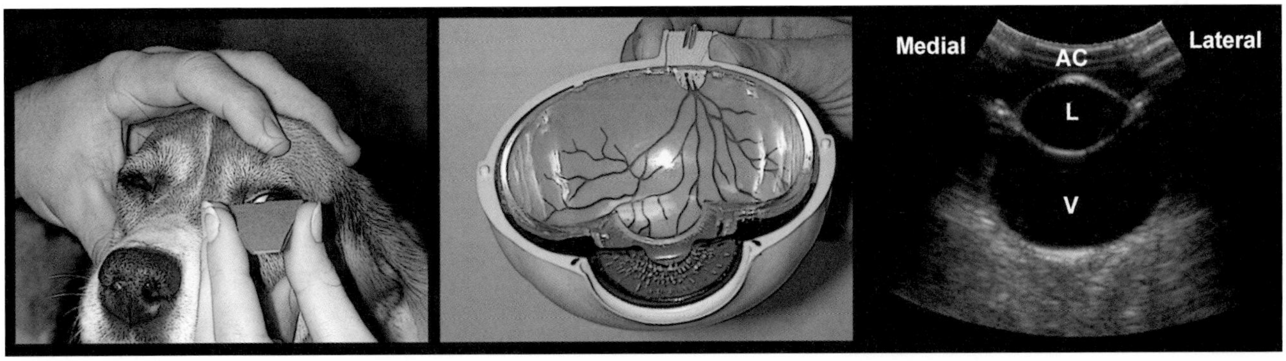

Figure 2.5. Dorsal plane. A dorsal plane divides the globe into dorsal and ventral halves. The image should be displayed such that the right side of the image represents the medial (nasal) side of the eye. AC, anterior chamber; L, lens; and V, vitreous body.

The directional terms used with reference to the globe are anterior and posterior (rostral to caudal), superior and inferior (dorsal to ventral), and medial and lateral (nasal to temporal). The planes and axis of the globe can be thought of in similar terms as those of the longitudinal and latitudinal directions of the earth. The central axis of the eye is an imaginary line from the center of the cornea (anterior pole) to the posterior center of the sclera (posterior pole) (Figure 2.10).

This is analogous to the axis of the earth between the north and south poles. The degrees around the

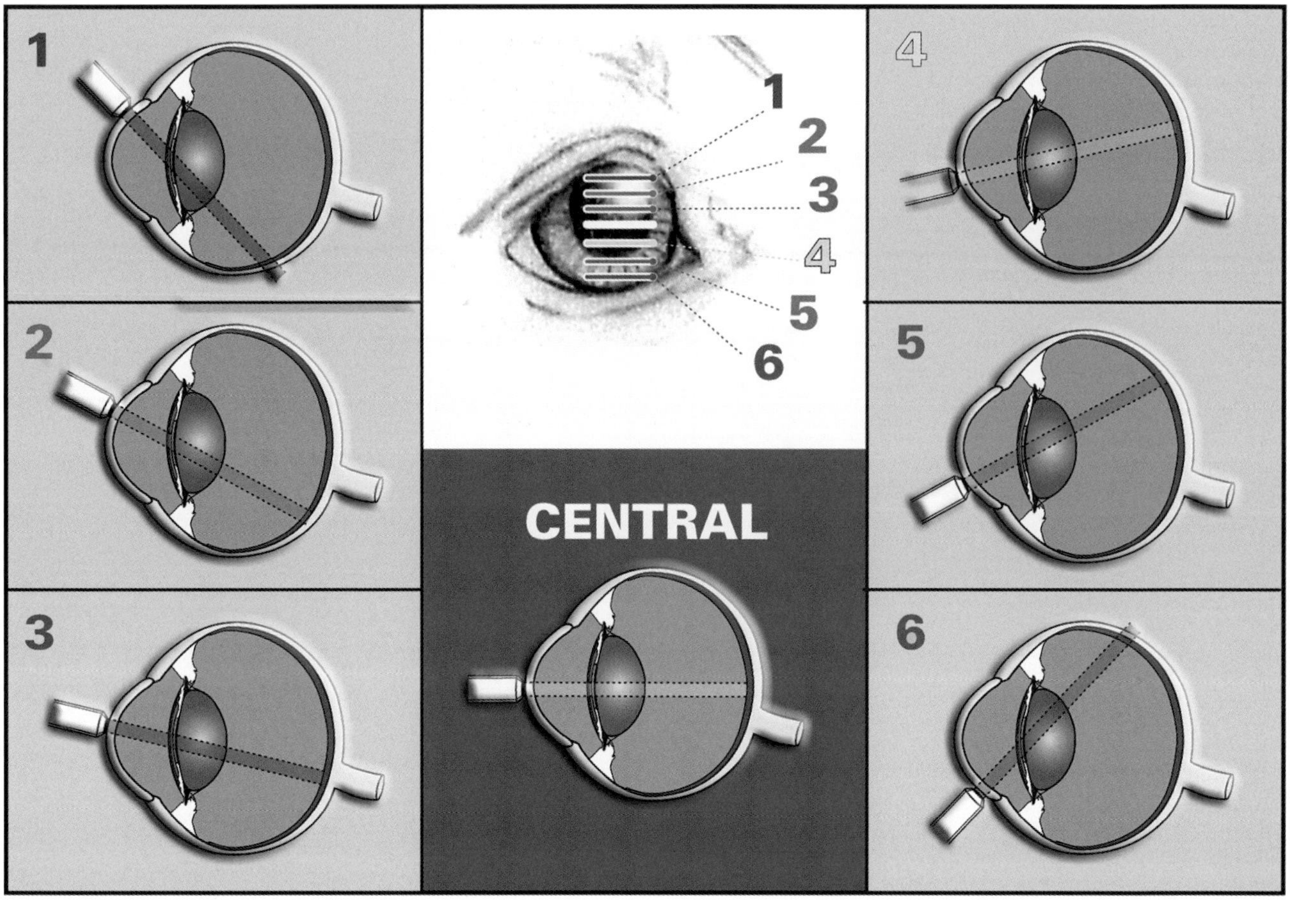

Figure 2.6. Array of dorsal planes. The central image represents the dorsal plane through the globe with equal divisions into dorsal and ventral halves. The globe is then scanned from dorsal to ventral to include the entire globe (planes 1–6).

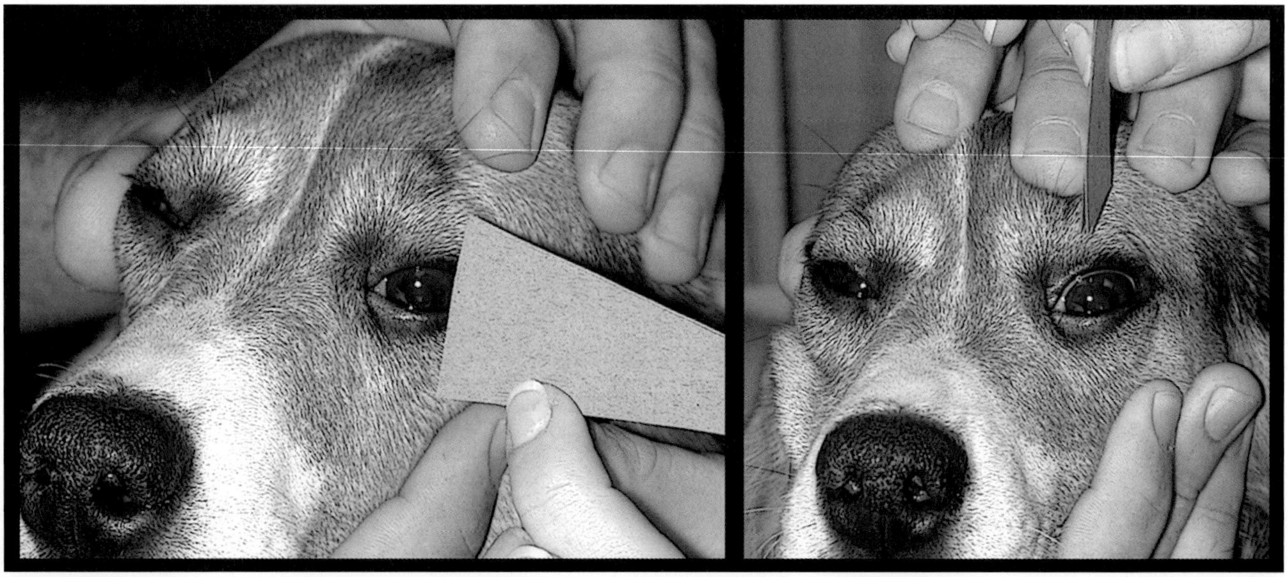

Figure 2.7. Transverse plane. A transverse image of the globe can be achieved by placing the transducer at the limbus and scanning across the globe. Radial views of the globe can be achieved by moving the transducer around the globe.

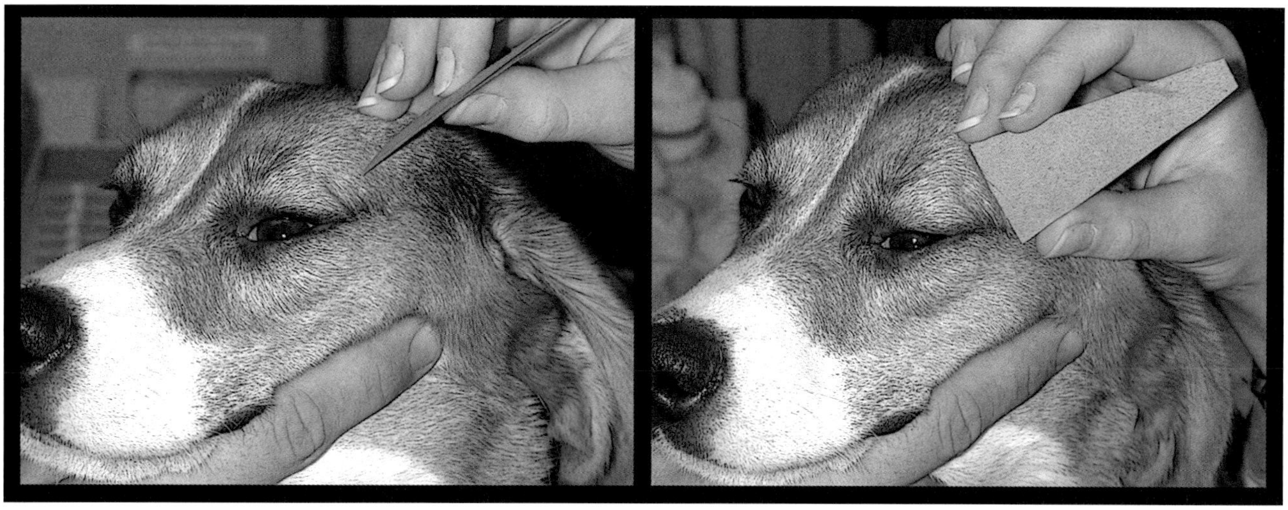

Figure 2.8. Retro-orbital scanning. Both longitudinal **(left)** and transverse **(right)** images should be made of the retro-orbital region to include the orbital cone. This is achieved by placing the transducer caudal to the eye and dorsal to the zygomatic arch.

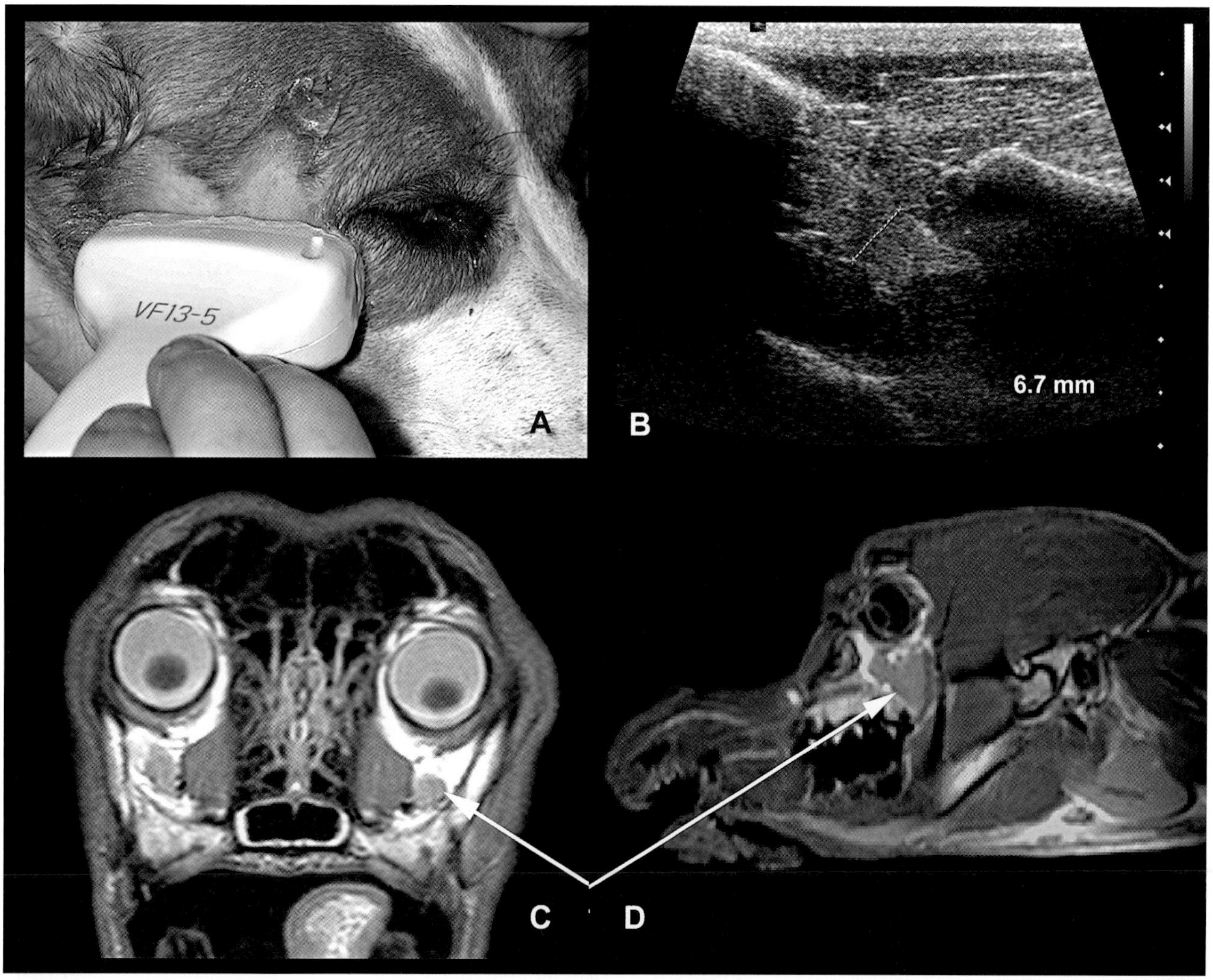

Figure 2.9. Zygomatic gland scanning. **A:** Images of the zygomatic salivary gland are obtained by placing the transducer ventral to the zygomatic arch and caudoventral to the globe. **B:** The zygomatic salivary gland is identified as a well-defined echogenic tissue (between the cursors) with a thin capsule located deep to the zygomatic arch depicted by the hyperechoic shadowing bone. **C:** Corresponding transverse magnetic resonance image. The zygomatic gland is identified by the arrows ventral to the globe. **D:** Corresponding parasagittal magnetic resonance image.

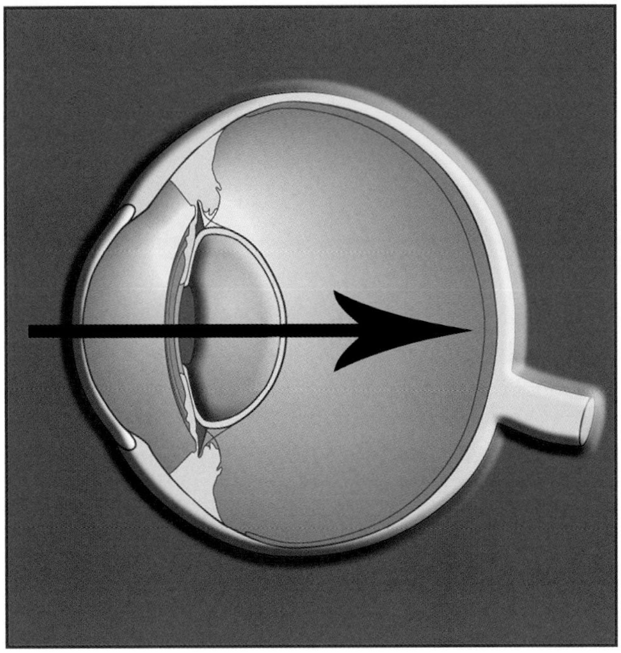

Figure 2.10. Central axis of the globe. This central line (arrow) is the pivotal line through the center of the globe. This is the central reference point. Two planes perpendicular and intersecting this reference point are the equatorial and the meridional planes. Localization of a lesion on a round globe without specific landmarks is achieved by using these planes and the positions around the clock.

globe in each plane can be thought of in terms of the hours on the face of a clock. Using the central axis as a central reference point, there are two primary perpendicular planes: The equatorial (transverse) and the meridional (longitudinal) planes are perpendicular to each other.

Ultrasonographic Anatomy of the Normal Eye

Ultrasound imaging of the orbit primarily consists of the globe (eyeball or bulbus oculi) and ocular adnexa, including the tissues within the periorbital cone in the retro-orbital area (optic nerve, extrinsic ocular muscles, vessels, fat, and surface of adjacent orbital bone) and the soft tissues and glands (lacrimal gland and zygomatic salivary gland) around the globe.

The globe is composed of two chambers (the anterior and the posterior) and the vitreal body (Figure 2.11). The globe contains the uveal tract (vascular tract), which consists anteriorly of the iris and ciliary body and posteriorly of the choroid. A single lens is secured between the anterior part of the eye and the

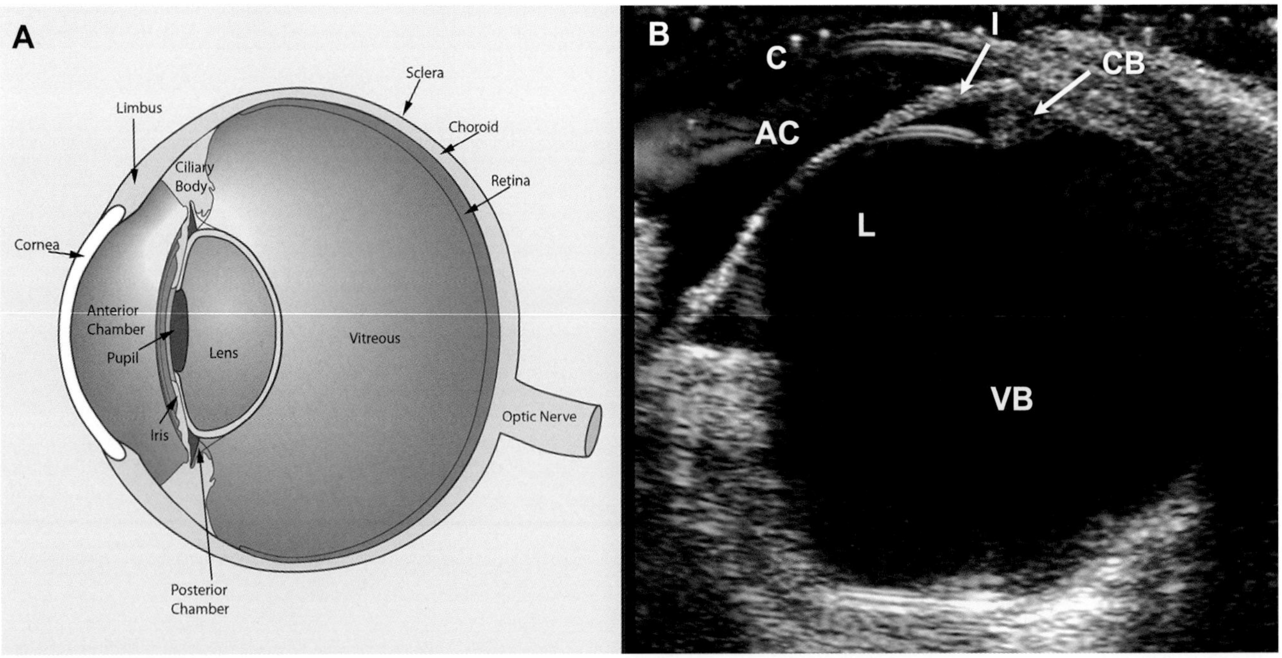

Figure 2.11. Normal ocular globe. **A:** The globe contains the anterior chamber, the posterior chamber, and the vitreous body. **B:** The three chambers are identified on this ultrasound image. Each chamber contains anechoic fluid. The anterior chamber (AC) is bordered by the cornea (C) anteriorly and the iris (I) posteriorly. The posterior chamber is a small area located posterior to the iris and anterior to the ciliary body (CB) and the lens (L). The vitreous body (VB) is bounded posteriorly and peripherally by the retina and anteriorly by the lens and ciliary body (CB).

vitreous body. The retina represents the innermost of the three layers of the globe wall in the posterior segment.

In the normal young eye, the three cavities (anterior chamber, posterior chamber, and vitreous body) have an anechoic appearance, with few reflectors present (Figure 2.11). It is best evaluated with a frequency of 25 MHz or greater. The thickness of the cornea and various parts of the eye has been recorded in different species (Schiffer et al. 1982; Cottrill et al. 1989; Boroffka et al. 2006).

Depending on the probe frequency, the cornea presents as a single or double parallel echogenic line with an anechoic center (Figure 2.12). The first highly reflective line is the corneal surface. The stroma is low reflective, with a second highly reflective line at the endothelium or Descemet's membrane.

The corneoscleral junction (limbus) is defined by the transition between the lowly reflective cornea and highly reflective sclera. The sclera is imaged as a highly reflective structure compared with the cornea. The sclera can usually be differentiated from overlying episclera and underlying ciliary body and retina (Figure 2.13).

The anterior chamber can be difficult to image because of its compressibility, size, and location in the near field. The anterior chamber is delineated by the cornea, the iris, and the central anterior lens capsule.

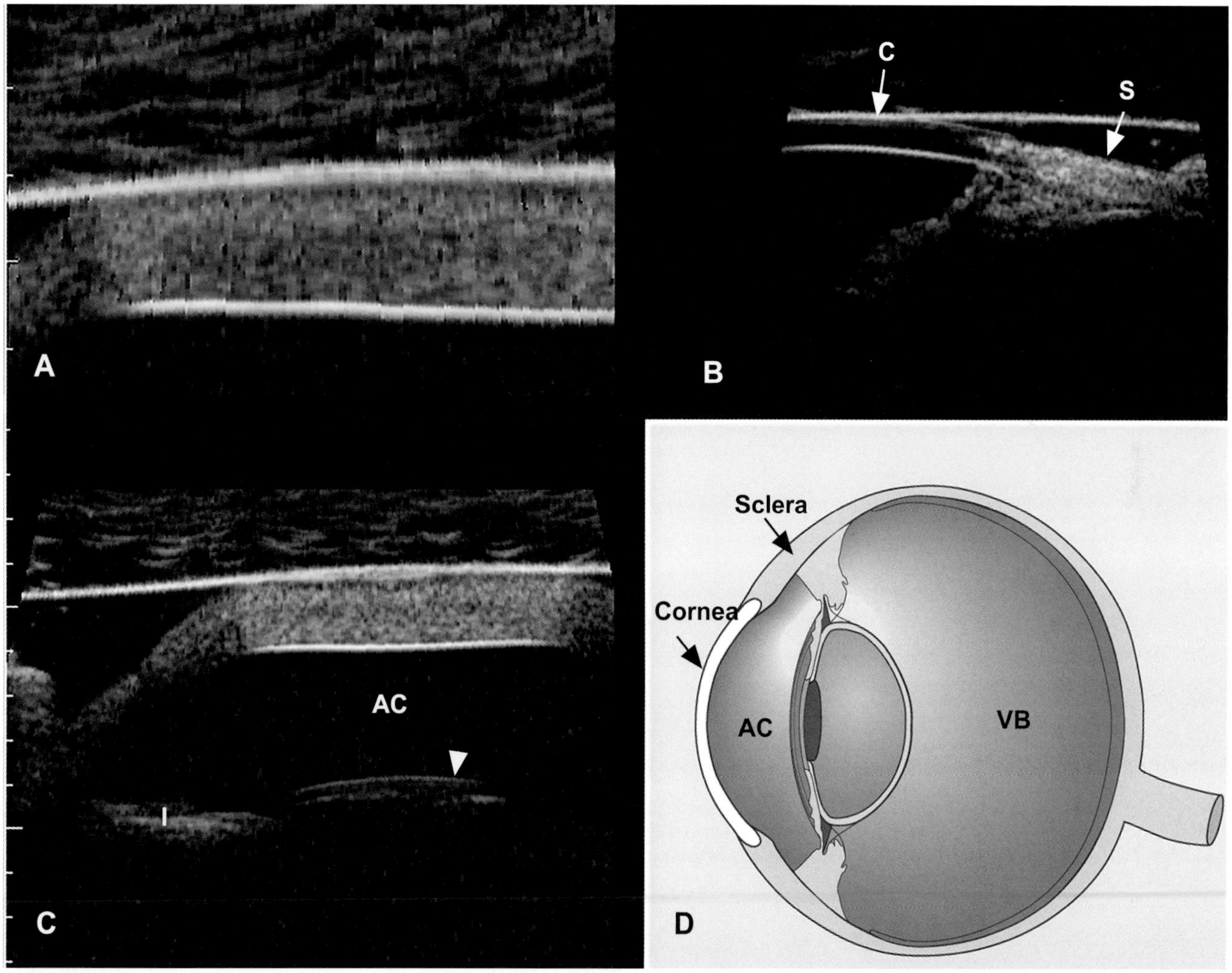

Figure 2.12. Normal cornea. The cornea is best seen with a 25- to 50-MHz transducer. The cornea has two parallel lines with an anechoic to mildly echogenic center. **A:** High-resolution sonogram of the cornea. **B:** The junction is imaged with a 25-MHz transducer. The corneal-scleral junction is defined by the transition between the two parallel lines with an anechoic to echogenic center representing the cornea (C) and the wider, more uniform, echo distribution of the highly reflective sclera (S). **C:** The corneal-scleral junction, anterior chamber (AC), anterior lens capsule (arrowhead), and part of the iris (I). The cornea surface is slightly flattened by the standoff. **D:** Schematic representation of these structures. VB, vitreous body.

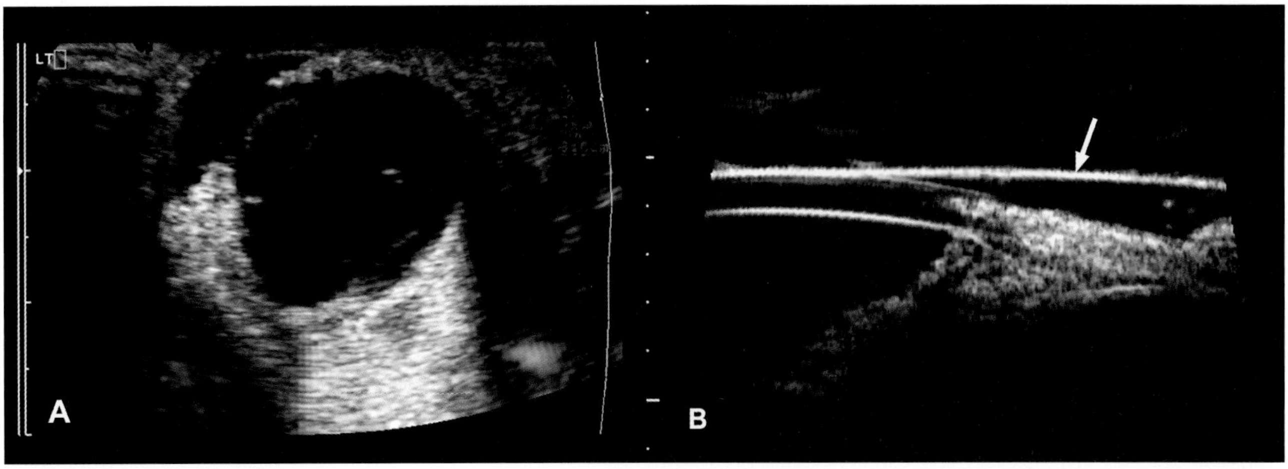

Figure 2.13. Corneal-scleral junction. **A:** The corneal-scleral junction cannot be adequately evaluated with a 7.5-MHz transducer. **B:** High-resolution sonogram of the corneal-scleral junction. The bright superficial straight line (arrow) represents the standoff interface.

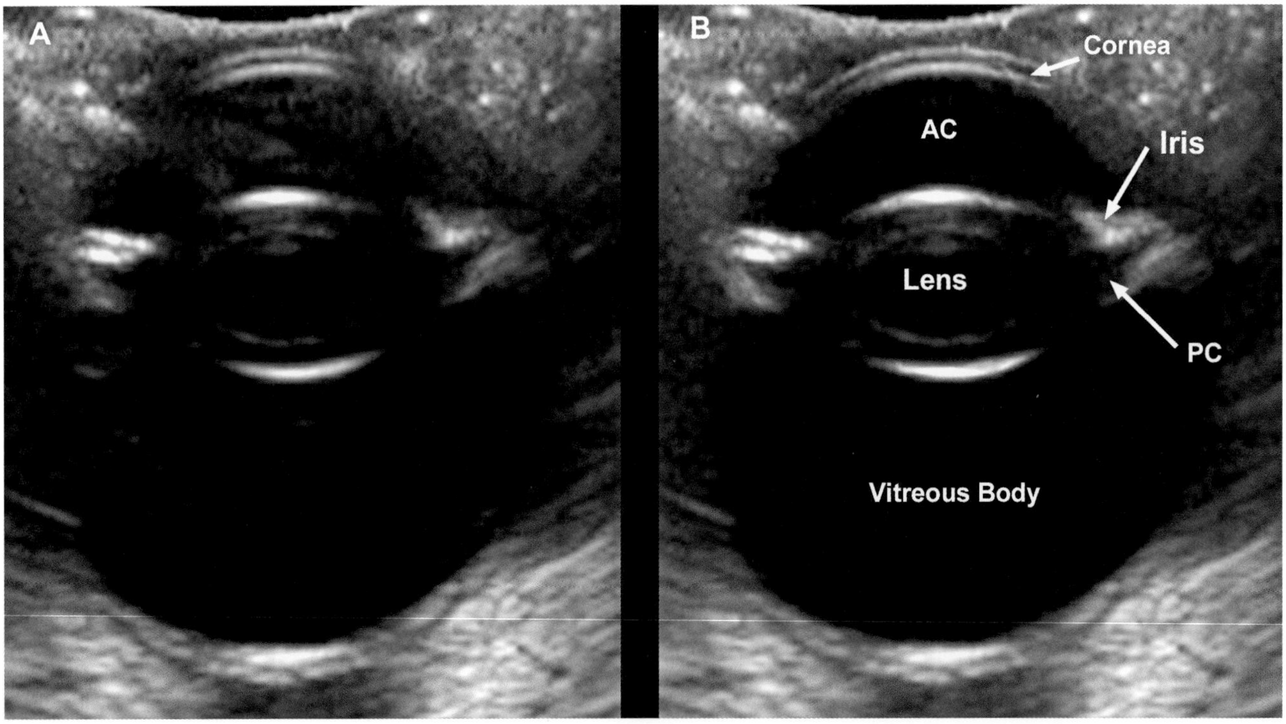

Figure 2.14. Sagittal plane of a normal globe. The anterior chamber, the vitreous body, and the internal contents of the lens are anechoic. **A:** Longitudinal sonogram of a canine eye. **B:** Modified and labeled image. AC, anterior chamber; and PC, posterior chamber. Note the nucleus sclerosis affecting the lens. Image courtesy of D. Penninck.

It is distended with noncellular anechoic aqueous humor (Figure 2.14).

The normally shallow posterior chamber, which is located between the iris and the peripheral lens, contains aqueous humor that is produced by the ciliary body and flows from the posterior chamber to the anterior chamber through the pupil.

The uvea, which represents the vascular layer of the globe, is composed posteriorly by the choroid, whereas the anterior uvea is composed by the ciliary body and the iris (Figures 2.15 and 2.16).

The iris is a dynamic, muscular, contractile diaphragm with a central opening (the pupil). The size of the pupil, which can vary rapidly in diameter

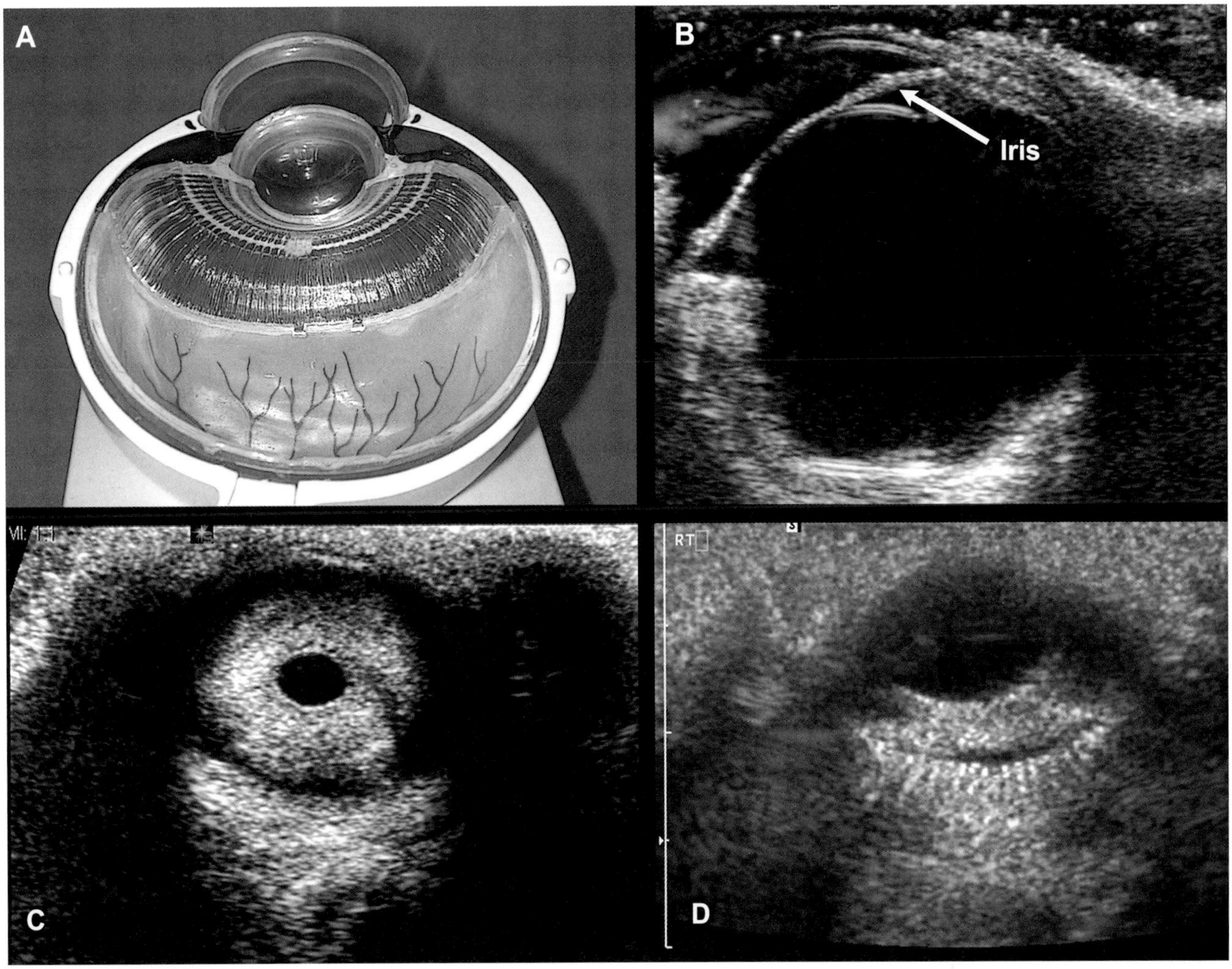

Figure 2.15. Normal iris and ciliary bodies. **A:** Plastic model of the iris and ciliary body, which are part of the uveal system. **B:** The iris (I) is seen on the anterior surface of the lens and anterior to the ciliary body. **C:** The iris encircles the pupil and controls the pupil size as seen on a transverse imaging plane. **D:** The iris is in close apposition to the ciliary body as seen around the periphery of the iris.

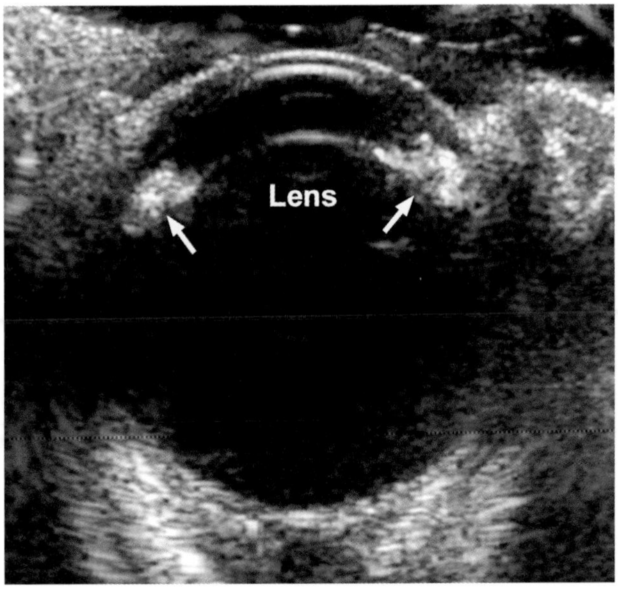

Figure 2.16. Normal ciliary bodies. The ciliary body with the zonules to connect to the lens is seen as the hyperechoic structures (arrows) at the equator (periphery) of the lens. This is a frequent area of primary ocular neoplasia. With contraction of the muscle fibers in the ciliary body, the zonules assist in adjusting the shape of the lens.

(Figure 2.17), allows varying amounts of light to penetrate to the retina on the posterior surface of the globe. The muscles in the iris control the pupil size. The pupil appears as a circular void in the iris. When the pupil is constricted or when the beam is off axis, the iris may be mistaken for the anterior surface of the lens. The iris, which is the anatomical demarcation between the anterior and posterior chambers, is contiguous at the equatorial plane in the periphery of the globe to the ciliary body. The ciliary body is highly vascular and at the junction with the choroid forms the ora serrata. The aqueous humor is produced by the ciliary epithelium, which lies on the surface of the ciliary process. The ciliary body contains muscle fibers that regulate the shape of the lens. The lens is supported at the equator by the suspensory ligaments (zonular fibers). The zonules are seen as striations that attach to the lens contour. The iris, ciliary body, and zonules are often best imaged from a transverse or oblique view.

The lens is composed of a capsule, anterior epithelium, lens fibers, and nucleus. The capsule is like an envelope that encases the lens. The lens fibers that make up the majority of the lens are positioned in layers with the cortex forming the outer layer of the

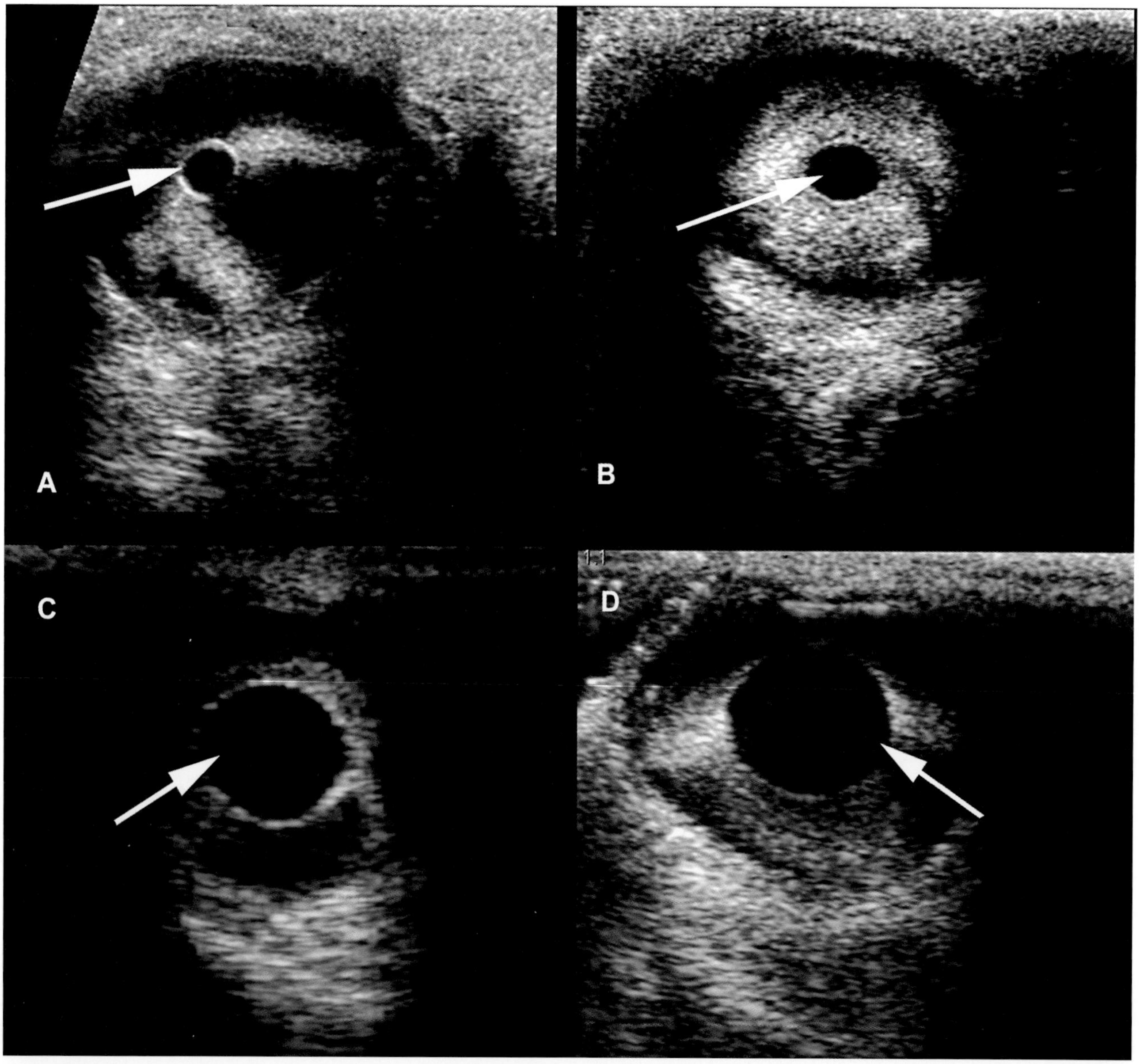

Figure 2.17. Normal pupil. The pupil size is dynamic and is controlled by the contraction of the iris. **A–D:** These images represent four varying sizes of the pupil (arrows) as imaged from a transverse plane.

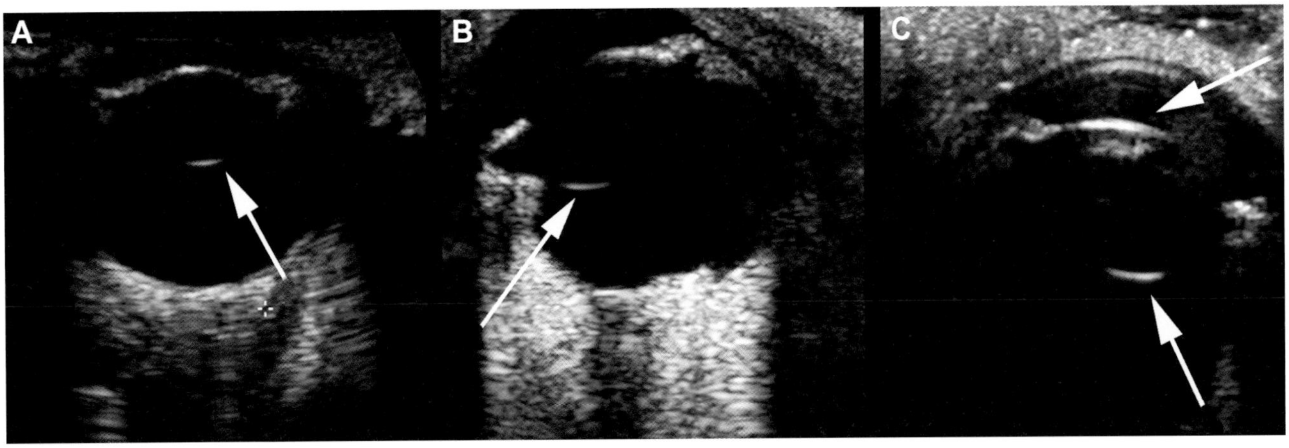

Figure 2.18. Normal lens. When the sound beam interacts with the surface of the lens, there is a change in acoustic impedance and a strong reflection is produced. This is seen as a thin curvilinear hyperechoic line on both the anterior and posterior surfaces of the normal lens. The position changes depending on the angle at which the incident beam hits the lens, which is often useful in identifying the margin of the lens. This is seen only at the perpendicular angle with the lens and not around the entire curve of the lens. **A–C:** In the three images, note the change in position of the specular reflection (arrows) as the angle through the globe is changed.

lens and the nucleus located in the center. The lens is primarily supported in place by the zonular ligaments at the equator. The vitreous body contributes to maintain the lens position posteriorly.

The internal appearance of the normal lens is anechoic. Curvilinear hyperechoic interfaces appear at the anterior and posterior margins of the lens, as the result of specular reflection, when scanned perpendicularly. This reflection is caused by the acoustic impedance difference between the fluid in the anterior chamber and the sound interacting with the surface of the lens (Figure 2.18). The peripheral curved margins of the normal lens are not seen. The surface of the lens is smooth and slightly convex. The size of the lens varies with the species. The anterior surface of the lens can be difficult to separate from the iris unless the pupil is dilated. The normal nucleus has the same appearance as the cortex of the lens. The lens can produce artifacts as the sound is accelerated through it, and because of its shape, the sound may be refracted. This is manifested in the posterior chamber and the posterior wall as Baum's bumps with an abnormal shape to the globe (Figure 2.19).

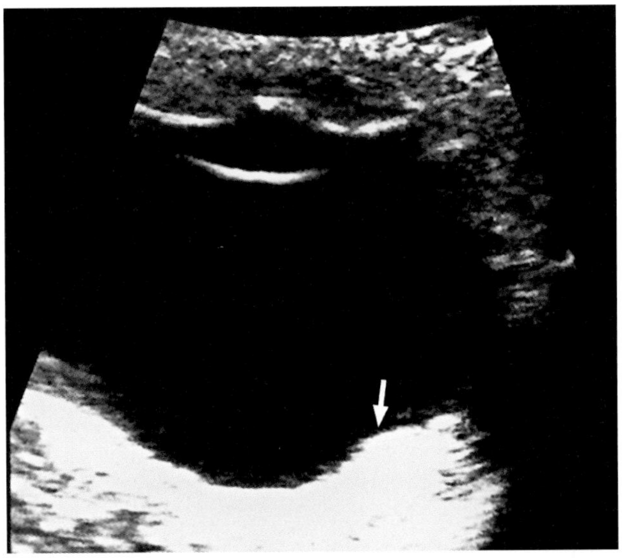

Figure 2.19. Braum's bump artifact. This may produce an abnormal shape to the posterior wall of the globe. This occurs because of refraction of the sound as the sound goes through the lens. The bent or refracted sound may then be reflected from a more anterior and closer part of the globe. The echoes are then displayed at a wrong position and appear to be "bumps" (arrow) on the posterior surface of the globe. When the sound goes through the center of the lens, refraction does not occur, and the posterior wall is not foreshortened.

Posterior to the lens and extending to the posterior aspect of the globe is the vitreal body, which fills the vitreous cavity. This vitreous body is a thick, acellular, gelatinous structure composed of 98% water, mucopolysaccharides, and hyaluronic acid. The vitreous cavity is bounded by the lens zonules and posterior capsule anteriorly and retina posteriorly (Figure 2.20). The vitreous body attaches primarily at the region of the optic disc (vitreous base) and at the ora serrata and forms the hyaloid fossa, a fibrillar dense indentation, to adapt the posterior surface of the lens. The vitreous body is densely packed at the posterior surface of the lens except at the posterior pole of the lens, where it encircles the attachment of the hyaloid canal (Cloquet's

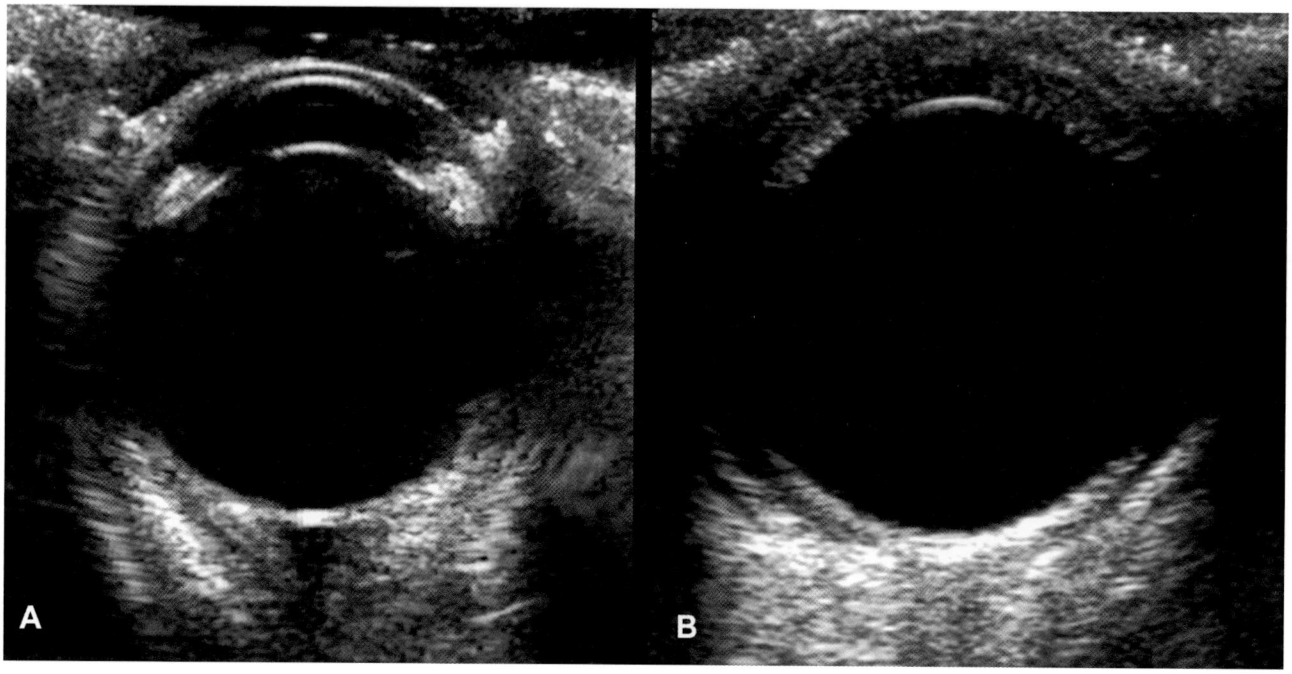

Figure 2.20. Normal vitreous body and cavity. The vitreal body is a thick, acellular, round, gelatinous mass that is normally anechoic and is located in the vitreous cavity. It is bounded by the retina, choroid, and sclera posteriorly and the ciliary body and posterior surface of the lens anteriorly. It is attached primarily at the optic disc and on the posterior surface of the lens. **A:** Sagittal plane **B:** Transverse-oblique.

or central canal) (Figure 2.21). This canal extends from the posterior surface of the lens through the vitreous body to the optic disc on the posterior surface of the globe. This potential space in the vitreous body contains the hyaloid artery in an embryonic eye (Figure 2.22). Remnants of this vessel may be present in adults. The posterior surface of the vitreal body, located in close proximity to the retina, does not have a true membrane but is referred to as the posterior hyaloid membrane.

The posterior wall of the globe is formed by a thin, hyperechoic, smooth layer that represents the combined layers of the sclera, choroid, and retina. There is not clear demarcation between the three layers in the normal globe. The retina is the most anterior, and the sclera forms the posterior layer. The retina extends from the optic nerve to the ora serrata located just posteriorly to the ciliary body. Located slightly ventrally and medially in the posterior wall of the globe in dogs and cats is the optic disc. The optic nerve courses in a straight or undulating course from the posterior surface of the globe at the optic disc into the periorbita of the retrobulbar region to the optic canal in the skull (Figure 2.23).

The retrobulbar space (periorbital cone), which includes the extrinsic ocular muscles, the optic nerve,

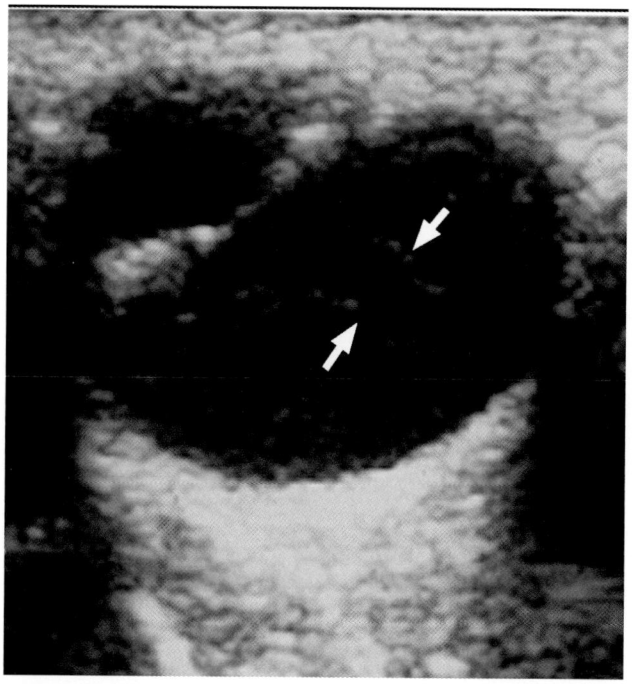

Figure 2.21. Hyaloid canal. This may be seen as faint membranes extending from the posterior surface of the lens to the optic disc. When vitreal degeneration occurs, this area may be more evident (between the arrows). On this dorsal plane, faint echoes representing mild vitreal degeneration are present, but the canal is echo free.

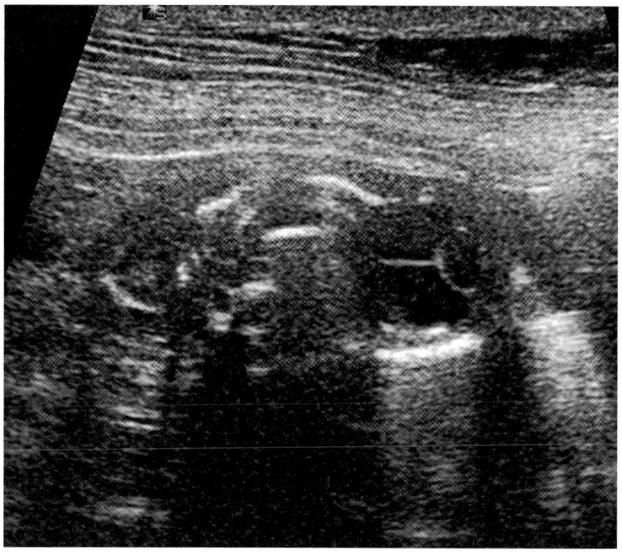

Figure 2.22. Fetal eye. This is the globe of an approximately 54-day-old fetus. Note the straight line from the posterior surface of the lens to the posterior surface of the globe. This is a patent hyaloid vessel supplying nutrition to the lens. This vessel typically is not present after birth.

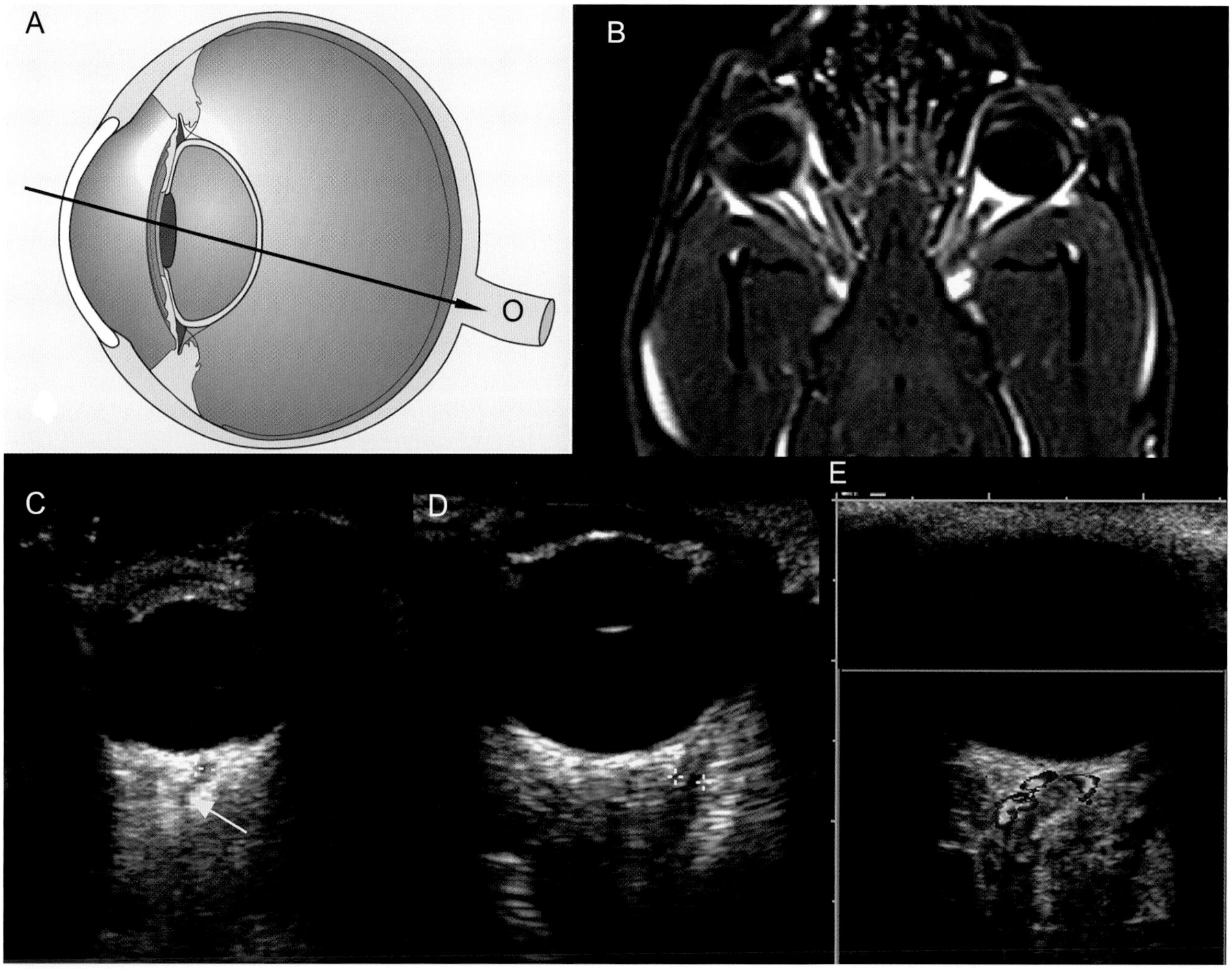

Figure 2.23. Normal optic disc and nerve. The optic disc and nerve in dogs and cats are located slightly ventrally and medially on the posterior wall of the globe. **A:** The angle of the beam often is from a slightly anterior dorsal to posterior ventral direction (arrow). O, section of the optic nerve. **B:** The magnetic resonance image displays the optic nerve in the center and the extraocular muscles at the periphery. **C:** The optic nerve is seen as a hypoechoic, often undulating, linear structure (arrow) coursing from the posterior wall of the globe into the retro-orbital region. It is hypoechoic relative to the surrounding fat. **D:** The hypoechoic muscles may appear similar in size and echogenicity but attach primarily to the periphery of the globe, and their position will help to distinguish them from the optic nerve. The optic nerve is usually less than 3 mm wide (between the cursors). **E:** Color Doppler of ocular vessels along the optic nerve.

arteries and veins, and periorbital fat, can also be evaluated (Figure 2.8). The frontal bone, which forms the medial wall of the orbit, appears as a hyperechoic interface associated with shadowing. The extraocular orbital muscles are hypoechoic linear structures that attach to the globe. The optic nerve is a thin, linear, hypoechoic structure outlined by adjacent hyperechoic fat. The lobular lacrimal gland, which is on the lateral (temporal) side of the orbit, and the zygomatic salivary gland, which is ventral and caudal to the globe and ventral to the orbital cone, can also be imaged (Figure 2.9). This approach may be used to aspirate tissue from a mass located posterior to the globe.

Sonography of Ocular and Orbital Abnormalities

Cornea and Anterior Chamber

The size, echogenicity, and appearance of the layers of the cornea may change with corneal disease, because of inflammation, degeneration, neoplasia, trauma, or specific corneal disorders, such as bullous keratopathy that occurs with diseases affecting the endothelial cells of the posterior corneal surface (Figure 2.24). Their degeneration does not any longer regulate the amount of intrastromal fluid, leading to bullae formation and possible corneal ulcers. Limbal infiltration caused by neoplasia or granulation tissue may be identified as focal thickening of the cornea or sclera. Determining the depth and involvement of the mass is helpful because the prognosis is more guarded if a limbal mass extends beyond the sclera to the ciliary body (Figure 2.25). Scleral thickening may support scleritis or episcleritis.

The cornea and the sclera merge at the limbus or corneoscleral junction and form the iridocorneal angle with the iris. In small animals, this angle represents the most relevant site for aqueous humor outflow. Any primary or secondary change in the angle may interfere with normal flow of the aqueous humor and cause glaucoma. An enlarged anterior chamber may be associated with glaucoma, aphakia, or posterior lens dislocation (Figure 2.26). A small chamber size may be associated with an anteriorly subluxated lens, with trauma, with tumor, or with compression by the transducer (Figure 2.27).

Cells and fibrin debris within the aqueous humor often present as echogenic foci that are moved along by ocular motion (Figure 2.28). Mass can be free or attached to iris, lens, or cornea (Figure 2.29). The presence of vascular flow within a mass is often helpful in determining whether the mass is a blood clot or tumor and may assist in determining the tissue of origin.

Uveitis is an inflammation of the uveal tract (Sapienza et al. 2000; Van der Woerdt 2000). When involving the anterior uvea, it is referred to as iritis and iridocyclitis. If the inflammation involves the posterior part of the uveal tract, it is classified as choroiditis. Often the inflammatory process involves the retina and is then referred to as chorioretinitis. The primary abnormalities associated with the uveal tract include cysts, neoplasia, and inflammation. Iridociliary cysts present as singular or multiple (Deehr and Dubielzig 1998; Spiess et al. 1998). The cysts are thin walled and have no internal reflectivity. Cysts may form on the iris

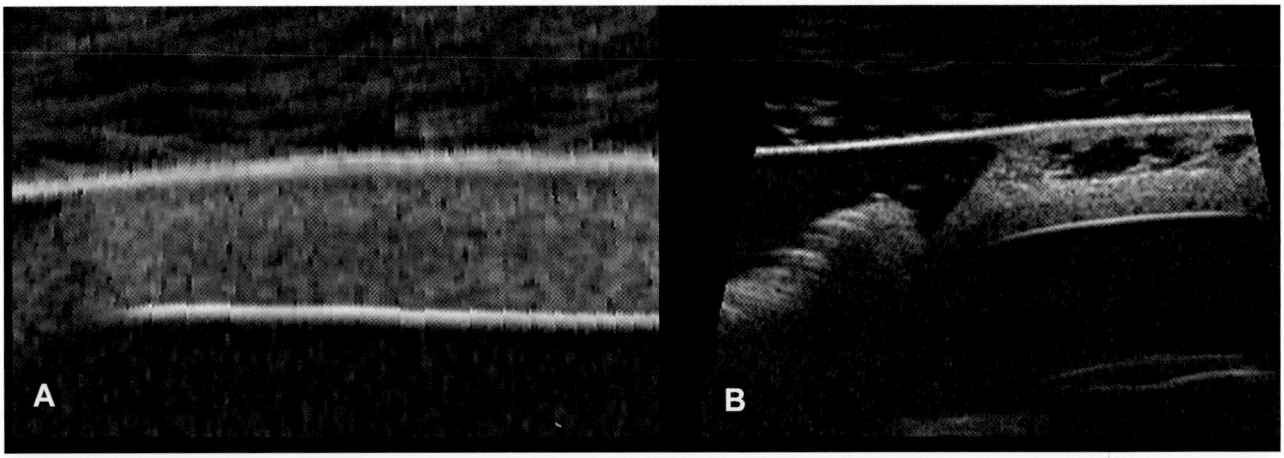

Figure 2.24. Bullous keratopathy. The cornea can be seen with a 10-MHz transducer, but more diseases are being evaluated with 25-MHz (or above) transducers. **A:** The normal cornea. **B:** Bullous keratopathy. Note the cystic areas within the abnormal cornea.

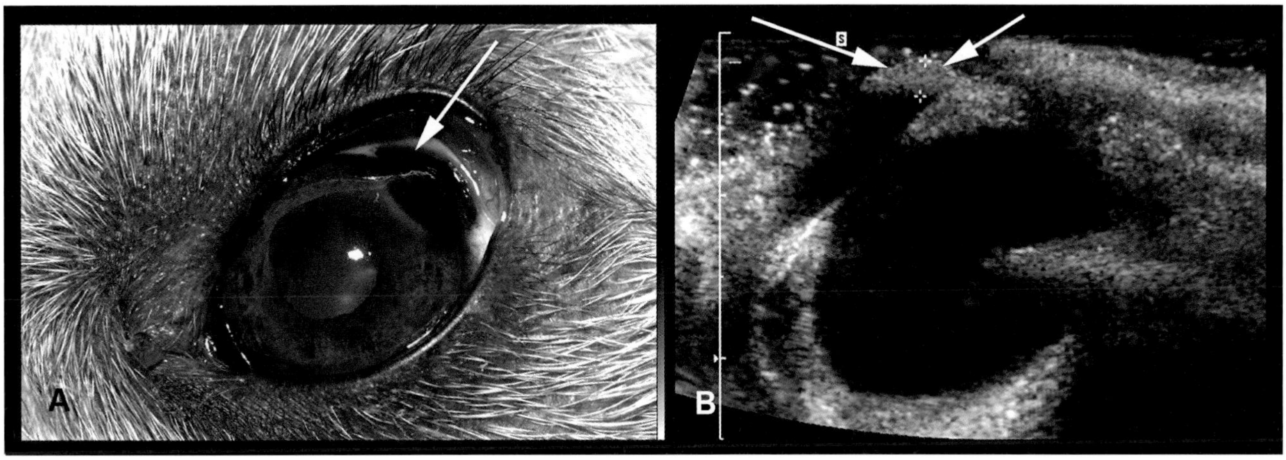

Figure 2.25. Limbal tumor. **A:** Photograph of a canine limbal melanoma (arrow). **B:** The arrows depict the echogenic mass, which appears to communicate with the adjacent ciliary body. The ciliary body is thickened, and local infiltration is suspected.

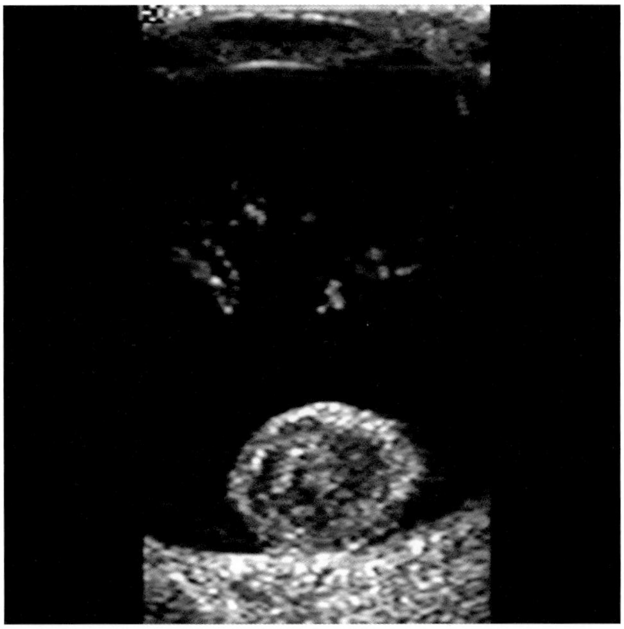

Figure 2.26. Posterior lens luxation. The echogenic lens (cataract) is in the posterior portion of the vitreous body, near the optic disc. Irregular curvilinear structures are seen near the posterior lens capsule. Image courtesy of D. Penninck.

or ciliary body and extend into either the anterior or posterior chamber or vitreous body. They may occur in any breed, but golden retrievers, Great Danes, Rottweilers, or Labrador retrievers are predisposed. The cysts, which are usually congenital, may be free floating or attached to the ciliary body, posterior iris, or cornea. Their finding may be incidental, but iridociliary cysts can also cause uveitis or glaucoma (Figure 2.30).

Tumors of the iris and ciliary body may present as focal masses or a diffuse infiltrative process. The most common intraocular tumor in dogs is melanoma and is most often associated with the anterior uvea. It is important to distinguish limbal melanomas from uveal tract melanomas in dogs because the treatments differ. The ciliary body is also commonly affected by other tumors, such as lymphoma, adenoma, adenocarcinoma, and medulloepithelioma or metastasis.

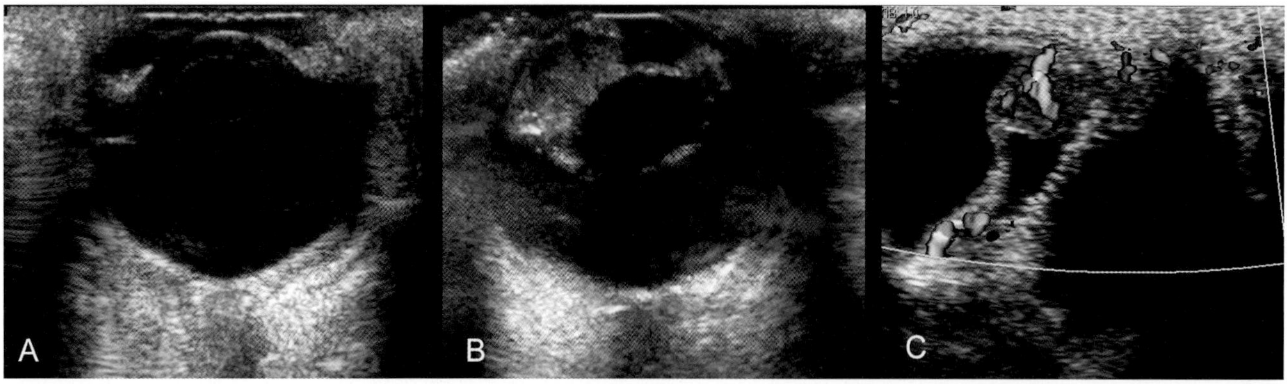

Figure 2.27. Anterior chamber changes. **A:** The anterior chamber normally contains anechoic fluid. The chamber can be compressed by transducer mild pressure, which hampers evaluation of this chamber. **B:** Ciliary body tumor with local extension into the anterior chamber. The mass is an anaplastic, malignant, round-cell tumor with invasion into the iris, sclera, and cornea. It was poorly differentiated, and a malignant melanoma was suspected. **C:** There is a focal thickening of the iris caused by the presence of a melanoma (arrows). There is blood flow within the mass. The anterior chamber is enlarged because of glaucoma.

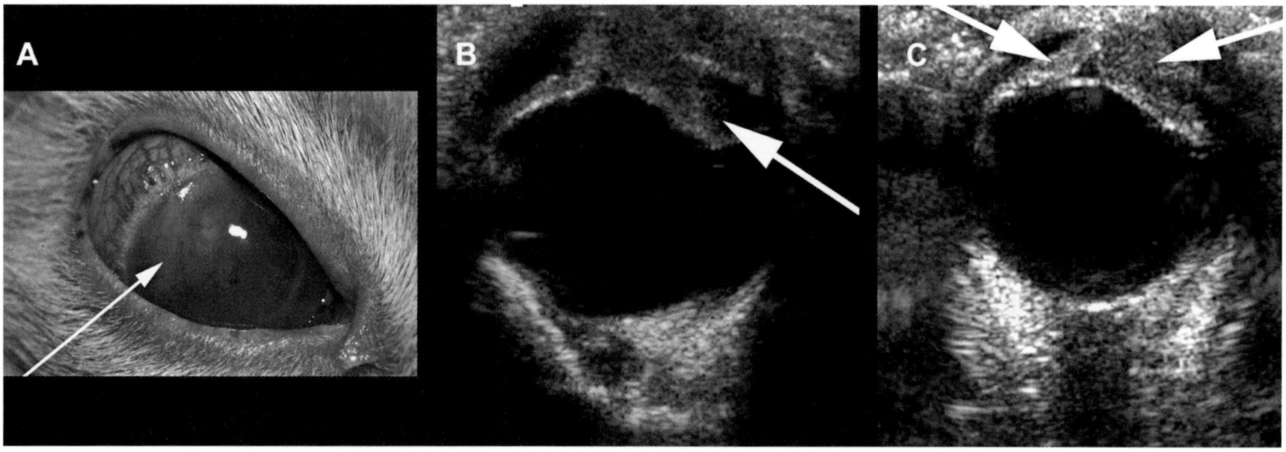

Figure 2.28. Iridal lymphoma. **A:** Photograph of a thickened iris and focal infiltrate (arrow) in the anterior chamber. **B and C:** The echogenic mass has invaded the anterior chamber (arrow) and is in continuity with the iris (arrows).

Lens

Abnormalities of the lens include cataracts (cortical or nuclear), liquefaction of the cortex, intumescence (swelling) of the lens, rupture of the anterior or posterior capsule, posterior lenticonus, retrolenticular membrane, subluxation, or dislocation.

Cataracts are degenerative changes in the lens (Gelatt and MacKay 2005). A cataract produces increased echoes in various locations within an anechoic lens. The echogenicity, shape, and size of the lens may change with the type of cataract and its duration. The changes within a cataractous lens produce acoustic inhomogeneities.

The most commonly used ways to classify cataractous changes are based on topography or stage of maturation. Although both can be used clinically by slit lamp examination, a classification that describes the topographical location of the lens degeneration seems more appropriate when imaging is used. According to their location within the lens, cataracts will be addressed as capsular, cortical (anterior, posterior, or equatorial) or nuclear (the core of the lens). The classification based on the stage of progression of

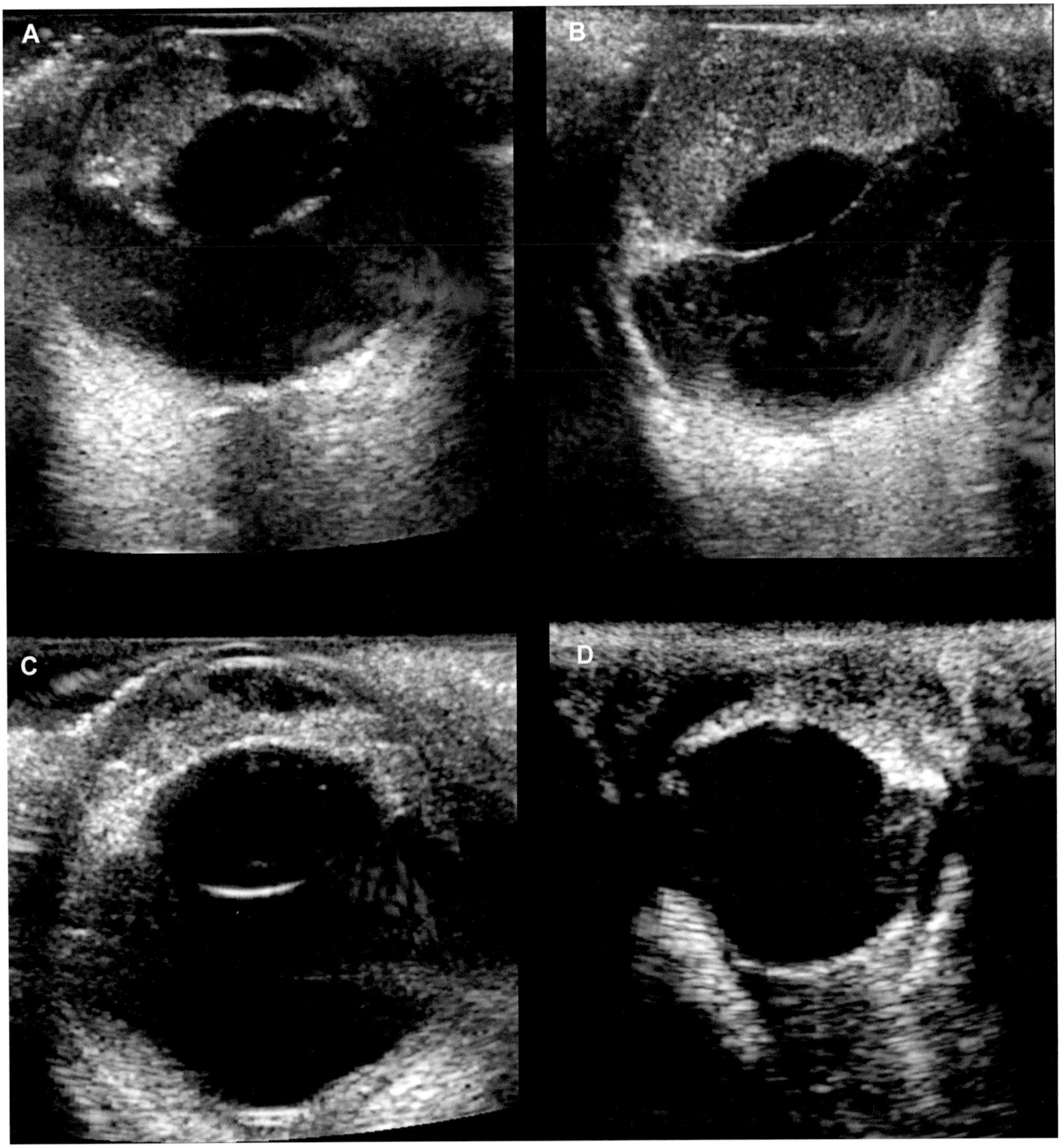

Figure 2.29. Anterior chamber masses. **A:** Ciliary body tumor with local extension into the anterior chamber. The mass is an anaplastic, malignant, round-cell tumor with invasion into the iris, sclera, and cornea. It was poorly differentiated, and a malignant melanoma was suspected. A large echogenic mass is in the anterior chamber, which is distended, consistent with a malignant melanoma arising from the iris. **B:** The anterior chamber is enlarged and diffusely filled with echogenic cellular contents. This was an epithelial adenoma arising from the iridociliary body. **C:** The iris is thickened and has poorly defined irregular margins because of an infiltrative lymphoma. **D:** The iris is diffusely thickened especially on the left side. This is a malignant histiocytosis involving the iris and the ciliary body.

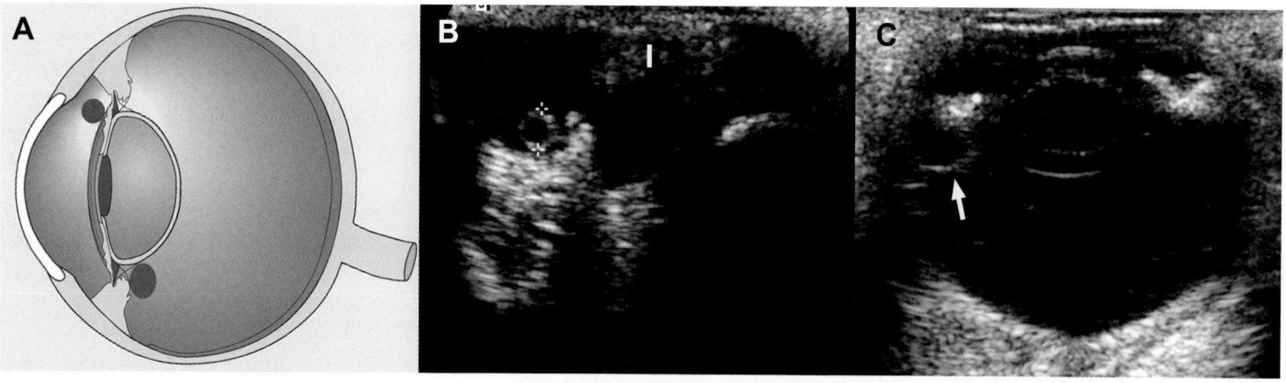

Figure 2.30. Iridociliary cysts. They may be identified within the anterior or posterior chambers. **A:** The most common locations are shown in this illustration. There may be one or multiple cysts. **B:** There is one cyst (between the cursors) in the anterior chamber of this Jack Russell terrier. The iris (I) is irregular and thickened because of anterior uveitis. **C:** There is a large single cyst (arrow) on the posterior surface of the ciliary body at the medial (nasal) aspect of the eye.

the cataract is clinical and includes incipient, immature and mature cataract with <10%, 10-100% partial opacity, 100% complete opacity respectively. These stages maintain the lens volume (it may be slightly increased in diabetic mature hyperosmotic cataracts). Hypermature and Morgagnian cataracts are later stages with cortical reabsorption. In these stages the lens thickness is reduced and the capsules appear wrinkled; these changes can be assessed ultrasonographically. Resorption can be detected as a decrease in the anteroposterior thickness of the lens. In a cortical cataract, the anterior and/or posterior cortices become echogenic, and the entire capsule may be apparent and not just the region of the specular reflection. The cortical sutures may become echogenic and be identified especially from a transverse plane (Figures 2.31 and 2.32). A nucleus that becomes echogenic is referred to as a nuclear cataract. The changes might progress to involve the entire lens. (Figure 2.33) A morgagnian cataract, which occurs when the content of the lens becomes liquefied, with the nucleus becoming free and mobile within the lens, is identified when the nucleus is not within the center of the lens (Figure 2.34). A markedly calcified cataractous lens has an increased sound velocity, which can result in an artifactually shortened globe. The amount of refraction through the lens may vary and cause an abnormal shape to the globe. An intumescent lens, which is associated with imbibition of fluid, is manifested as a thick, echogenic lens caused by an osmotic gradient difference as seen in early cataracts or in diabetes mellitus (Figure 2.35). Hypermature cataracts are often thin because the lens protein has liquefied and absorbed (Figure 2.36). This shrunken lens has fibrotic changes of the capsule and may pull on the zonules, which dislocates the lens. In one clinical study comparing lens morphometry in normal and cataractous lenses, diabetic cataracts had an increased axial thickness (Beam et al. 1999). Mature cataracts had a trend toward increased axial thickness, whereas immature cataracts demonstrated a trend toward reduced thickness (Williams 2004).

Posterior lenticonus is a developmental anomaly of the lens with localized cone-shaped protrusion of the axial portion of its posterior surfaces. The lens may have an isolated protrusion of the posterior thin capsule. The posterior capsule may appear irregular or wrinkled. This may be seen in association with a retrolenticular membrane and a persistent hyperplastic primary vitreous (Figure 2.37). A posterior capsule cataract and irregularity are important to recognize prior to surgery because they can lead to surgical complications when removal of the lens is attempted.

The lens rupture may be associated with anterior uveitis, fibrin or granulation tissue proliferation, or adherence to the pupil. The rupture may occur anteriorly, posteriorly, or peripherally. Equatorial ruptures are more common in diabetic patients (Figure 2.38). A posterior lenticonus has an eventration on the posterior surface, but the lens is still contained.

Lenticular nodular proliferations, also called lenticular fibroxanthomatous nodules, occur when the lens ruptures. The lens capsule and lens epithelium have undergone fibrous metaplasia, which is associated with trauma and a rupture of the lens (Figure 2.39).

A dislocated lens is identified by its abnormal position. Subluxation occurs when the zonule partially ruptures, and the lens is tilted from its normal position

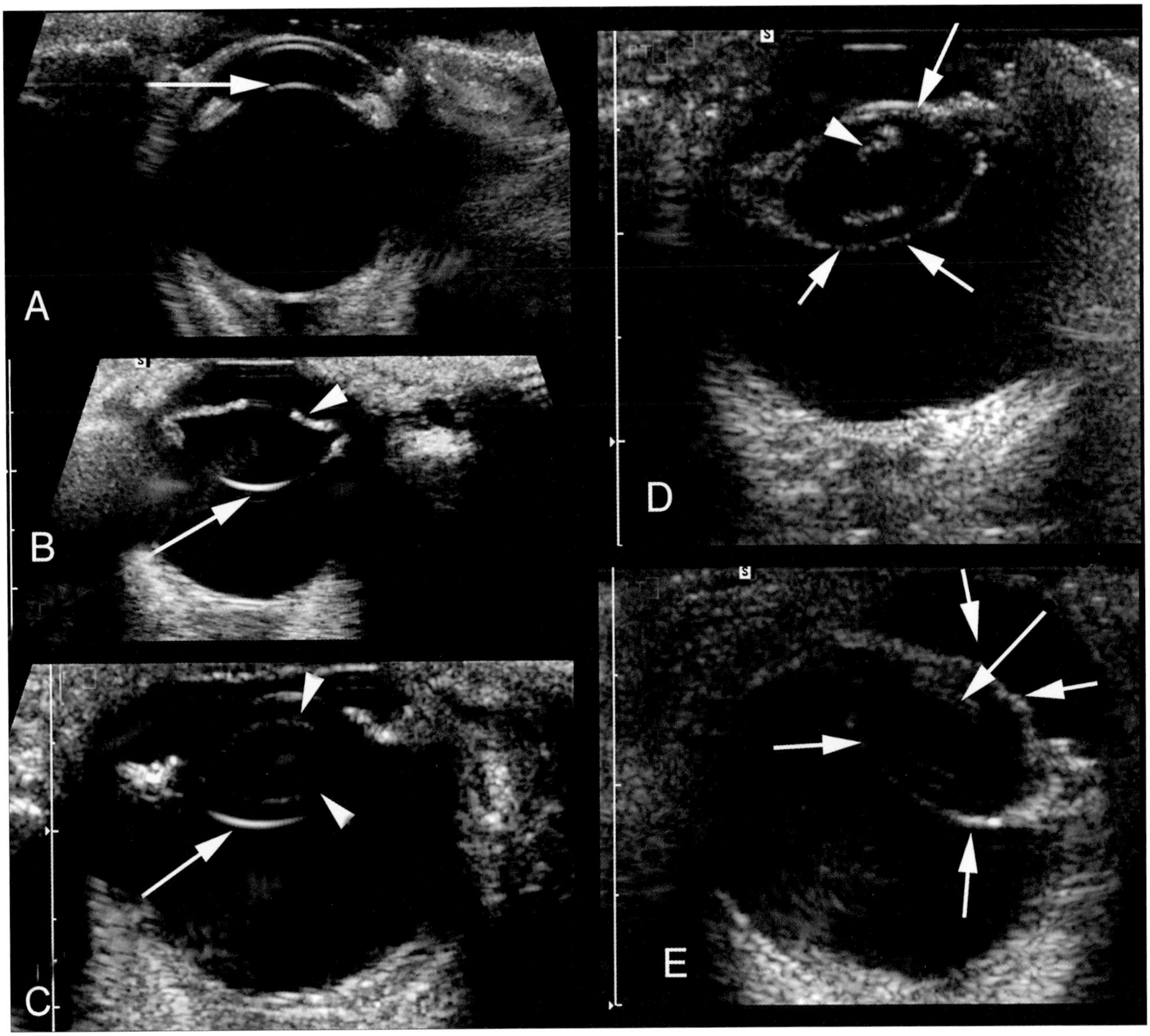

Figure 2.31. Cortical cataracts and other conditions mimicking cataracts. **A:** The normal hyperechoic curvilinear specular reflection (arrow) is perpendicular to the incident sound beam. **B:** The iris (arrowhead) is on the anterior surface of the lens, the pupil is in the center, and the curvilinear specular reflection is on the posterior surface of the lens (arrow). **C:** The lens has thin hyperechoic lines (arrowheads), indicating early cataract changes. The strong hyperechoic curvilinear line (arrow) is the posterior specular reflection at the surface of the lens. This helps to identify the position within the lens of the cataract. This is more likely on the surface of the nucleus. **D:** The lens has a thin hyperechoic line (arrows) around the lens consistent with a cortical cataract. The thicker hyperechoic focal areas (arrowhead) in the lens represent incomplete cataractous involvement of the sutures of the cortex of the lens. **E:** The surface of the lens has a hyperechoic rim (short arrows) around it that represents cortical cataracts (long arrow). The anterior part of the cortex is thickened and hyperechoic.

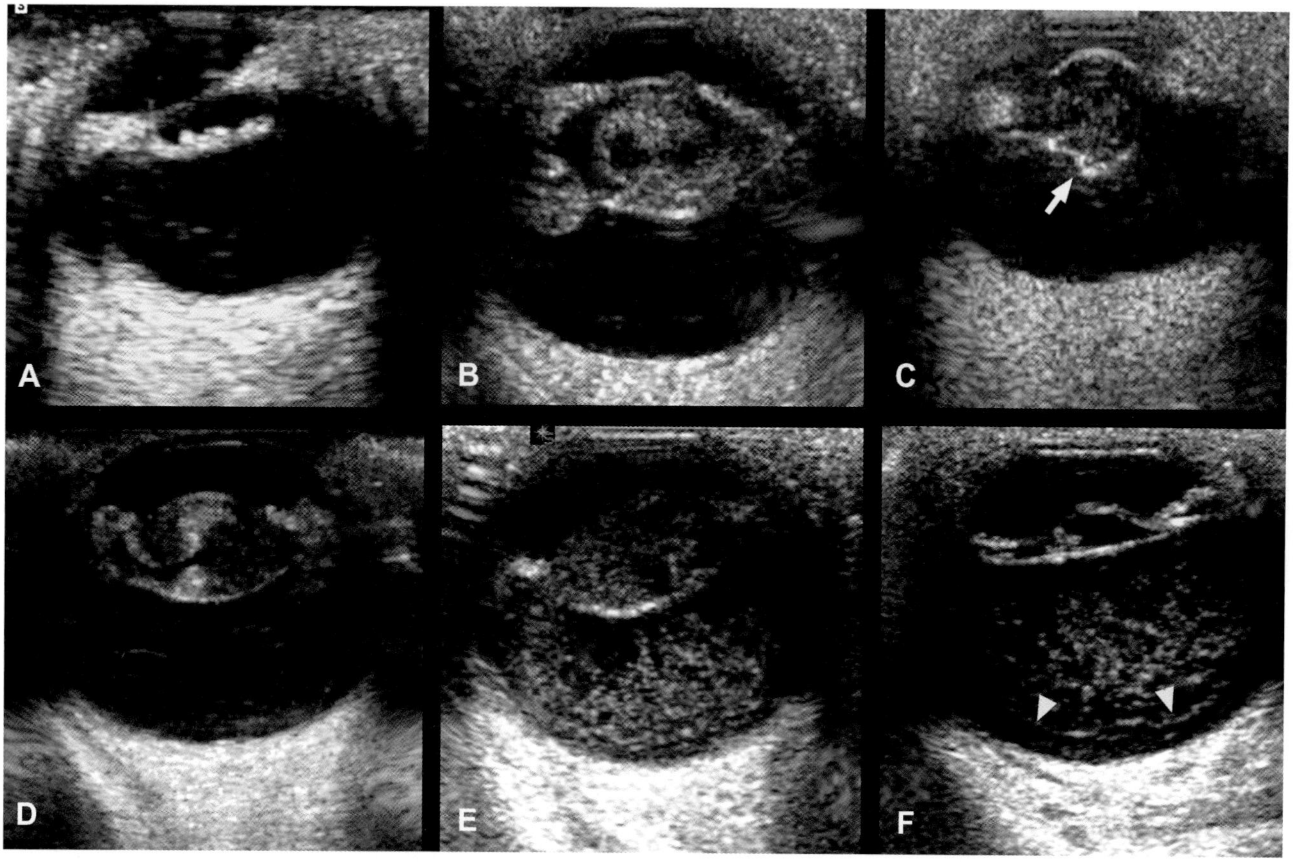

Figure 2.32. Various stages of cataract. **A:** An irregular hyperechoic posterior cataract is present. Noticing this change is important when a lens is being extracted, because the change may lead to complications. **B:** A large amount of nuclear cataract is present. **C:** An irregularity (arrow) is noted on the posterior surface of the cataractous lens. This may be caused by posterior rupture or, in this case, by a retained primary vitreous. **D:** Asymmetric but nearly complete nuclear cataract is present. **E:** The entire lens is echogenic, consistent with a complete cataract. Echoes within the vitreous are consistent with degenerative changes. **F:** Note that the lens is much smaller than normal. The margins of the lens are hyperechoic. This is a supermature cataract with resorption of lens contents. These changes are responsible for traction on the retina and can cause retinal detachment. Note the retraction of the vitreal body (arrowheads) and the echoes in the vitreous, consistent with degenerative changes.

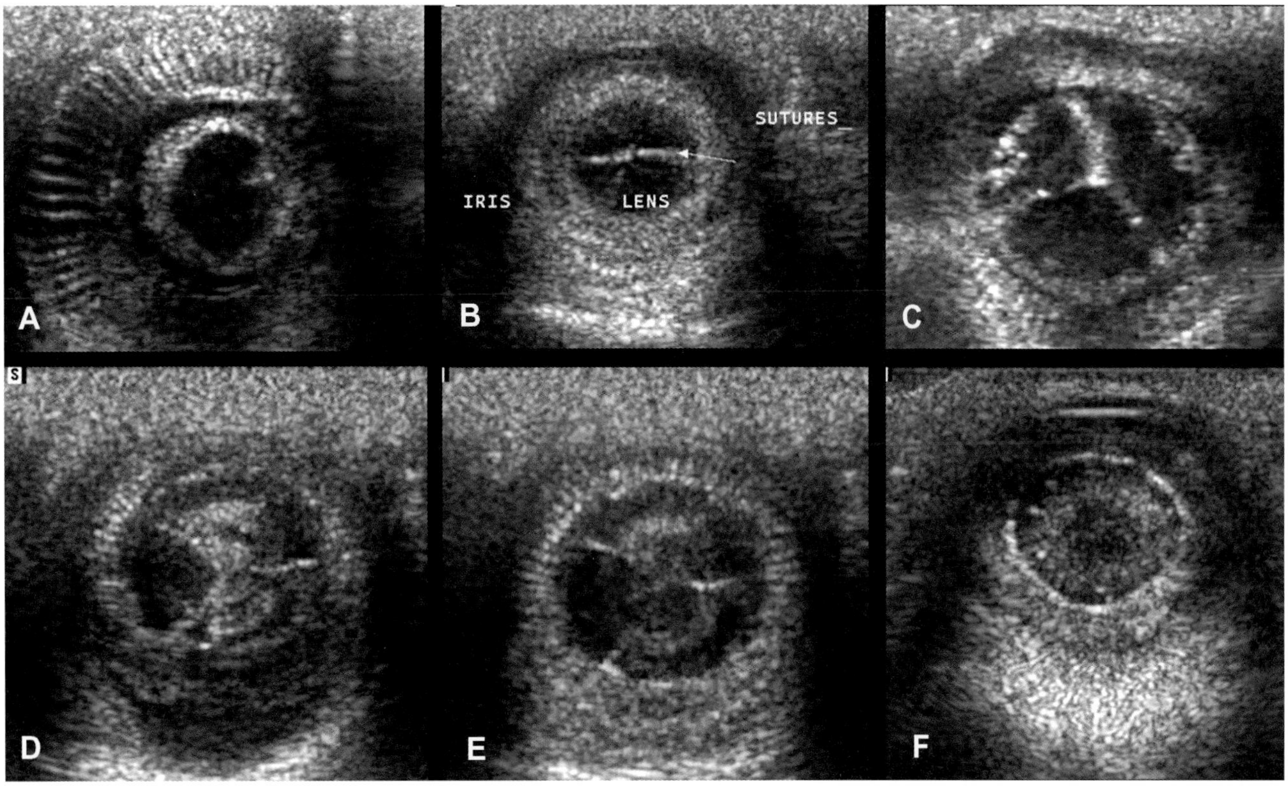

Figure 2.33. Cataracts involving the sutures of the lens. The involvement becomes more extensive from **A** to **F**. All are transverse images of the lens. With the first image, the involvement is cortical, and by **F** there is complete cortical and nuclear involvement with progression of disease and type of involvement. Notice the iris surrounding the lens in each image.

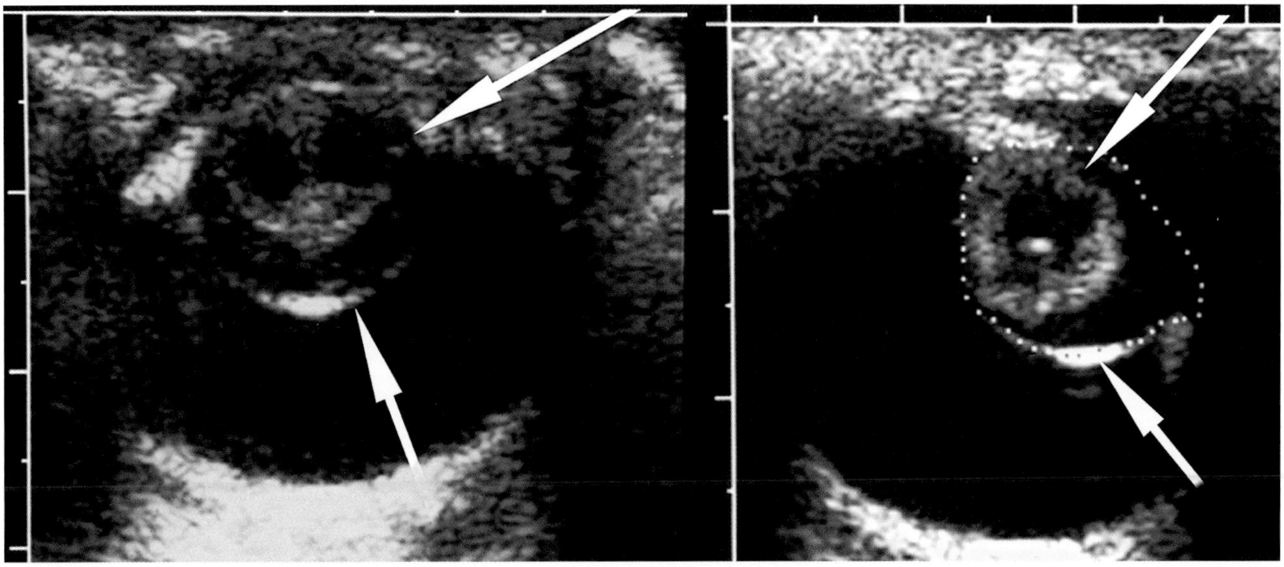

Figure 2.34. Morgagnian cataract. The contents of the lens has liquefied (arrows). The cataractous nucleus is mobile within the lens and may change in position. The lens is often smaller than normal because the lens contents has been resorbed.

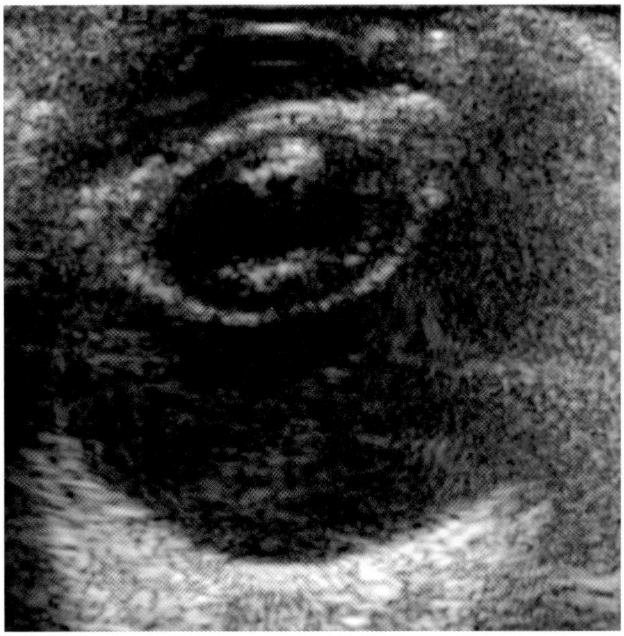

Figure 2.35. Swollen lens. This is often caused by the imbibition of fluid because of the osmotic gradient difference of fluid within the lens. It may be seen with various disorders but is often associated with diabetes mellitus.

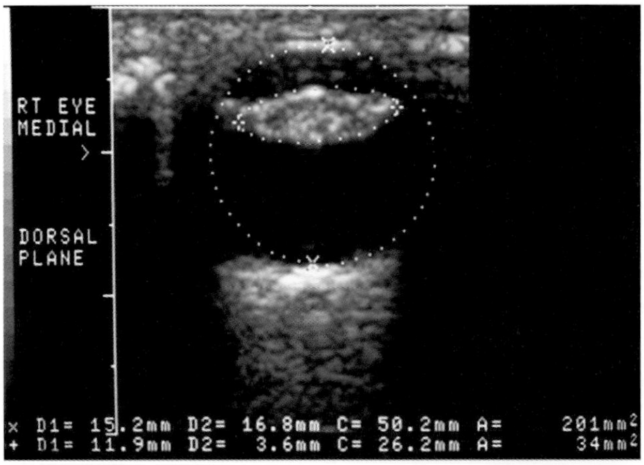

Figure 2.36. Supermature cataract. The lens is entirely hyperechoic and is smaller than normal. The lens protein has liquefied and been absorbed. Traction on the retina by the shrunken lens may lead to retinal detachment.

but still behind the iris and in front of the patellar fossa of the vitreous. Luxation occurs when the zonules at the peripheral ligamentous attachments totally rupture, and the lens is displaced anteriorly to the iris or posteriorly into the vitreal cavity. A luxated lens is often cataractous, especially if it has been luxated for any duration of time because of nutrition loss. Lens dislocation may occur secondary to trauma, space-occupying masses, glaucoma, or hereditary predisposition (Figure 2.40).

Vitreous and Retina

Clinical conditions with sonographically visible vitreal changes include changes in the shape of the globe, vitreous opacities (such as asteroid hyalosis, synchysis scintillans, vitreous hemorrhage, and uveitis), posterior vitreous detachment, persistence and hyperplasia of the primary vitreous or remnant of the hyaloid artery, retinal detachment, or presence of a foreign body or a mass.

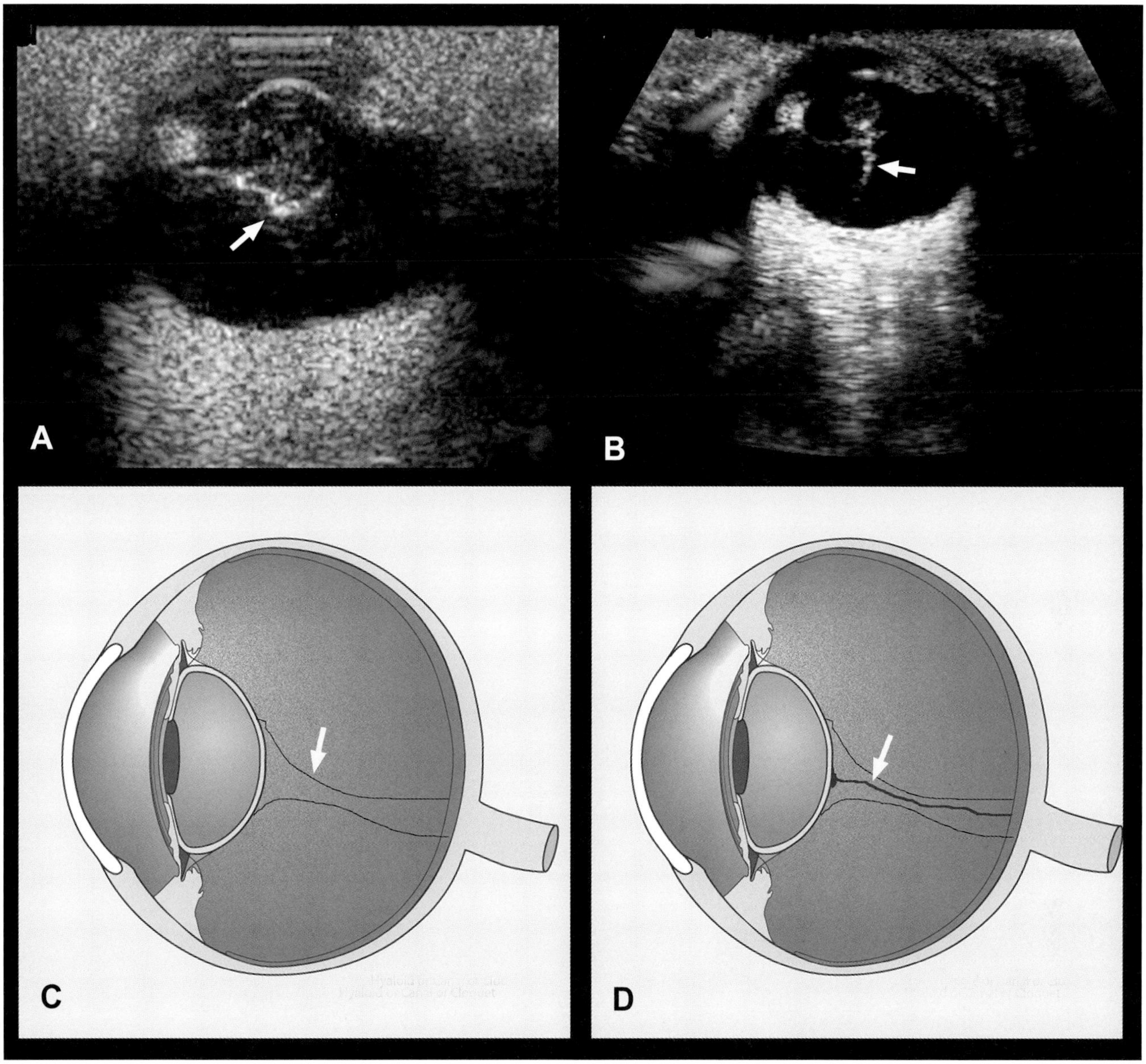

Figure 2.37. Posterior lenticonus. This is a developmental anomaly of the lens with localized cone-shaped protrusion of the axial portion of the anterior or posterior surfaces. The lens may have an isolated protrusion of the thinned capsule lined by a single layer of epithelium. **A:** The posterior capsule may appear irregular (arrow) or wrinkled. **B:** A remnant of the hyaloid vessel is noted as a linear hyperechoic line (arrow) extending from the posterior surface of the lens. **C:** The hyaloid canal (arrow) is depicted as the central canal. **D:** Persistent vessels (arrow) may be found extending from the posterior surface of the lens to the optic disc within the canal.

The globe shape may be altered by developmental anomalies, trauma, glaucoma, an internal mass, or by pressure from an extraocular mass (Figures 2.41 and 2.42). Microphthalmos (reduction in eye volume) may be caused by developmental defects or may be acquired (phthisis bulbi) secondary to chronic wasting diseases (uveitis or end-stage glaucoma) or trauma. Buphthalmos (an enlarged globe) instead may be associated with coloboma (an absence or defect of ocular tissue), a mass, or chronic glaucoma.

Echogenic foci or debris within the vitreous can have several causes. They appear as dotlike reflectors within the normally anechoic vitreous body (Figure 2.43). Membranes may be imaged and appear as hyperechoic lines within the vitreous. These reflectors are more common in eyes that have sustained trauma or

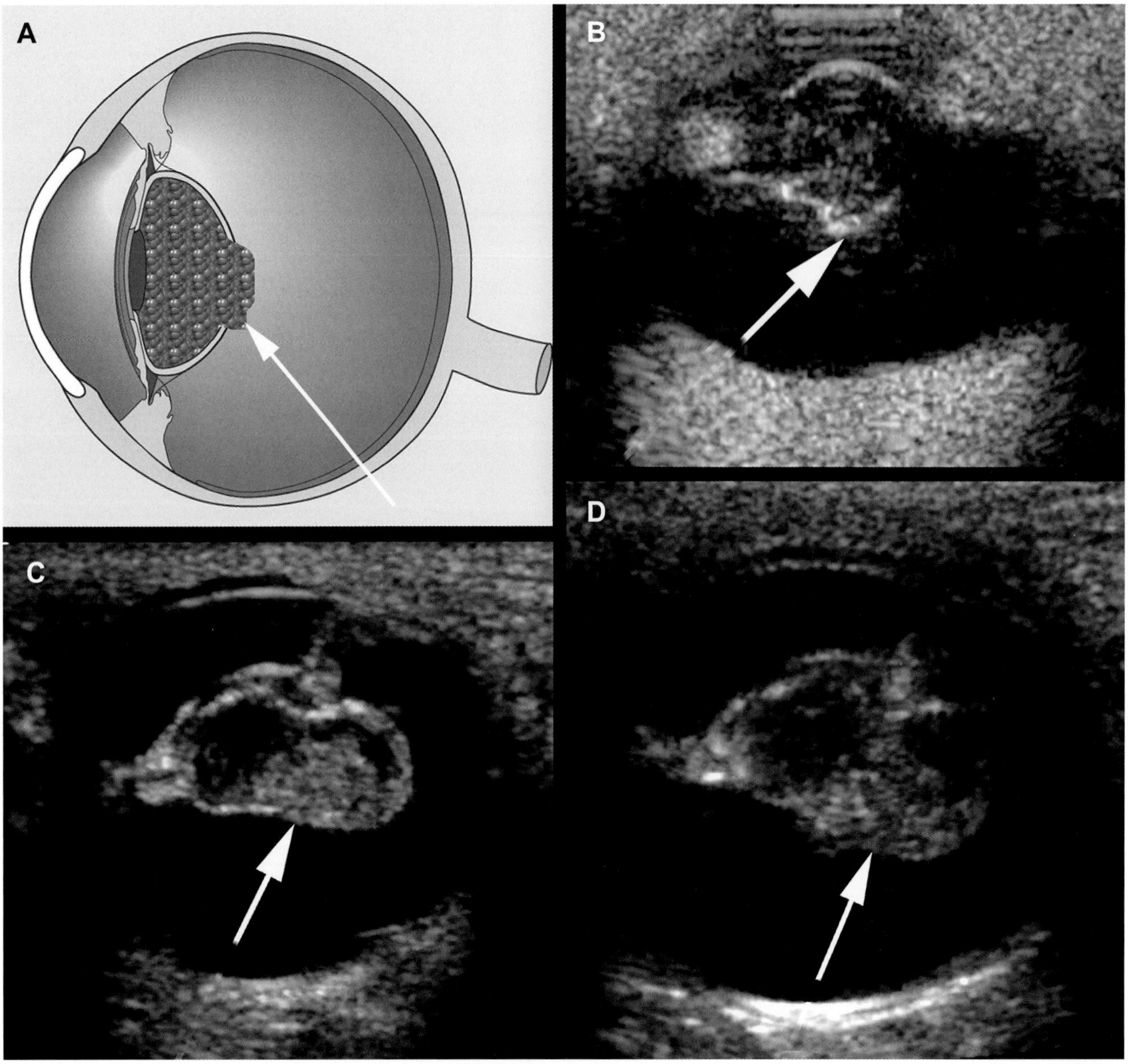

Figure 2.38. Posterior rupture of the lens. **A:** Schematic drawing of a rupture of posterior lens capsule (arrow). **B–D:** Examples of irregular posterior lens capsules (arrows)

disease and are often pronounced in myopic or senile vitreous.

Degenerative changes are common and become more common as one ages. They include asteroid hyalosis, synchysis scintillans, vitreal degeneration, and posterior vitreal detachment. Asteroid hyalosis is caused by calcium containing lipids suspended in the vitreous framework. These small foci of 0.03- to 0.1-mm calcium-lipid complexes are discrete pinpoint reflectors. A few may be present or a large number may be dispersed throughout the vitreous (Figure 2.44). In synchysis scintillans, the cholesterol crystals are not suspended. They sink to the bottom of the liquefied vitreous body. This is often seen in eyes with end-stage disease. Vitreal degeneration is often identified in dogs with cataracts. In one study, vitreal degeneration was seen in 55%, 89%, and 100% of dogs with immature, mature, and hypermature cataracts, respectively (Dietrich et al. 1995).

A detached vitreous may appear as a linear or curvilinear convex echo in the posterior aspect of the vitreous cavity. High gain may be useful to assist in

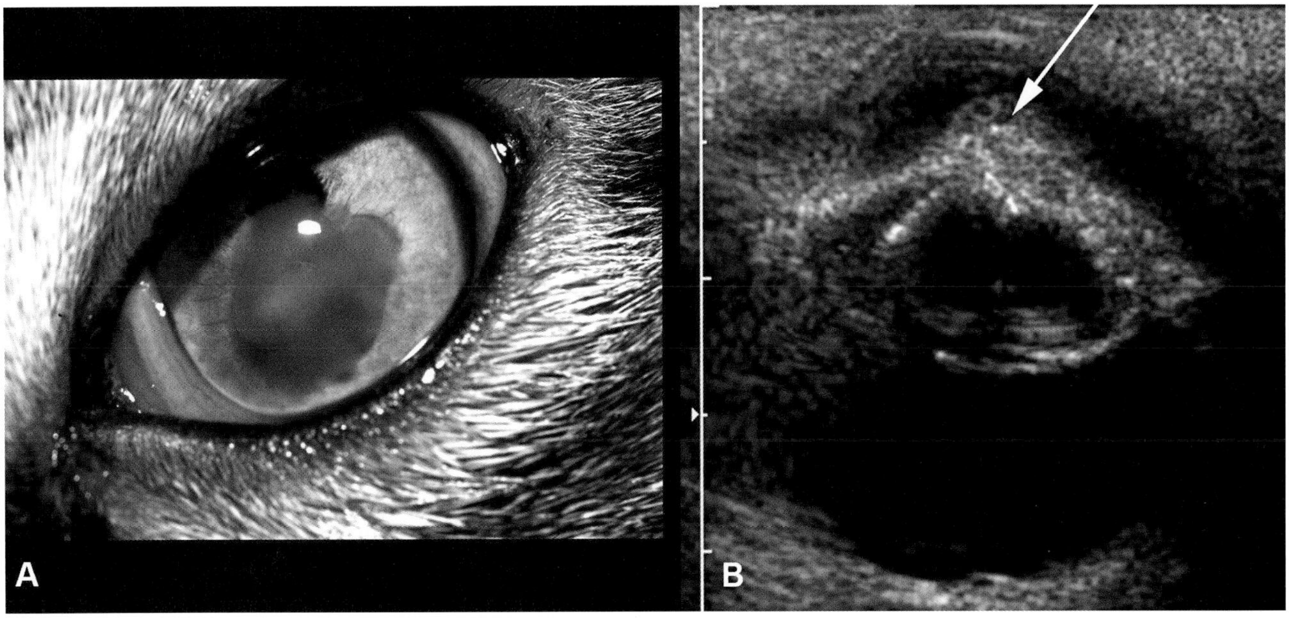

Figure 2.39. Anterior rupture of the lens in a cat. **A:** Photograph of the affected eye. **B:** Granulation tissue has formed (arrow). When the lens of a cat is damaged, the incidence of malignant transformation increases.

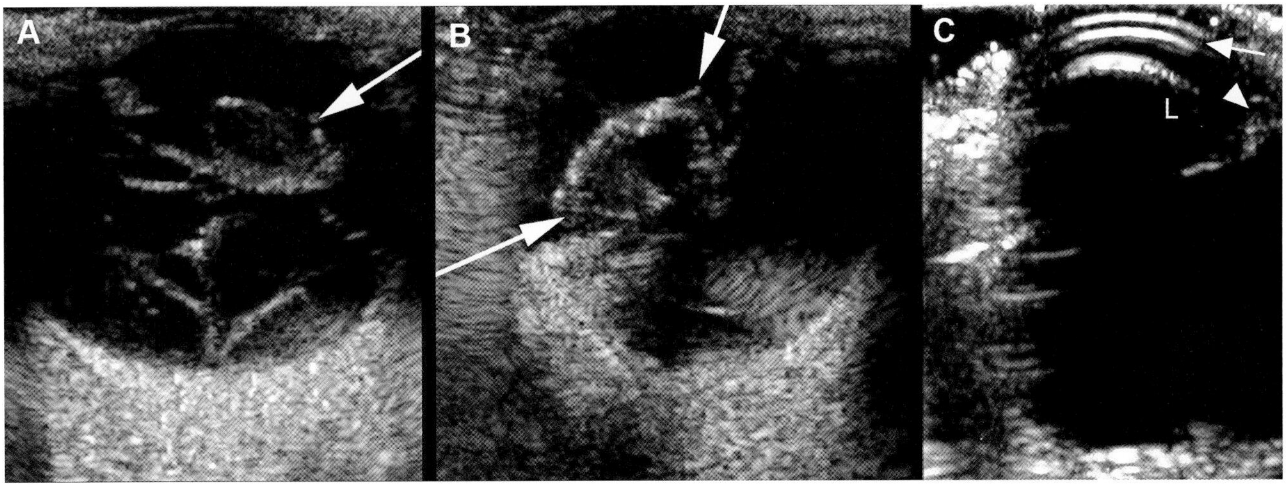

Figure 2.40. Anterior luxation of the lens. Note that the lens is not longer in the center of the ciliary body and posterior to the iris. **A:** Multiple membranes in the vitreous represent retinal detachments and possible fibrin tags (arrow). **B:** Echogenic material is present in the anterior chamber secondary to a uveitis because of the luxated lens (arrows). Both lenses are cataractous. A cataract can be a sequela of lens luxation caused by loss of nutrients. **C:** Another case of anterior lens luxation. The lens (L) is clearly displaced within the anterior chamber, anteriorly to the ciliary bodies (arrowhead). The two hyperechoic curved lines (arrow) represent the cornea. Image C courtesy of D. Penninck.

imaging this subtle change. The detached vitreous body is characterized by multicurved lines with varying reflectivity. Anechoic fluid may accumulate between the retracted vitreal body and the retina (Figure 2.45).

Echoes within the vitreous may be caused by inflammation, infection, or hemorrhage. Hemorrhage into the vitreous may produce a multitude of echoes within the anechoic vitreous cavity, varies in appearance, and often depends on the duration, severity, and the location of the bleed. Acute hemorrhage may not be evident for several days or until a clot forms. Hemorrhage may be seen as diffuse pointlike multiple echoes. The posterior hyaloid artery may bleed into the vitreous

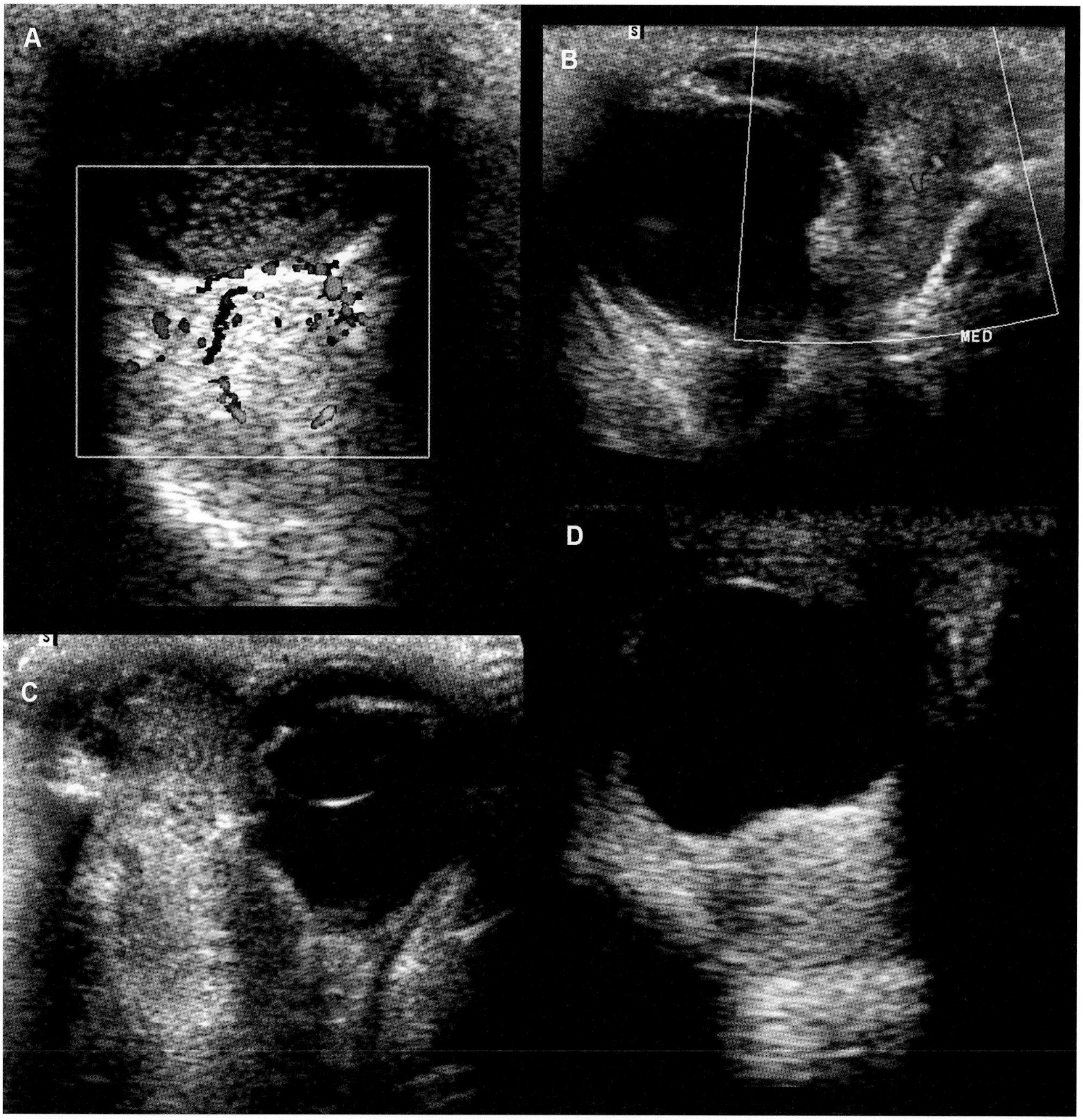

Figure 2.41. Changes in globe shape. **A:** A mass (undifferentiated mesenchymal tumor) posterior to the globe displaces the vessels and indents the posterior surface of the globe. **B:** Limbal mass (melanoma) with extension into the ciliary body. The entire globe is displaced and distorted by the mass. MED, medial. **C:** Mass medial to the globe. The mass, which is a lacrimal adenocarcinoma, distorts the normal round shape of the globe. **D:** A rounded mass (nasal cavity adenocarcinoma) posterior to the globe indents and distorts the vitreous cavity and the contour of the globe.

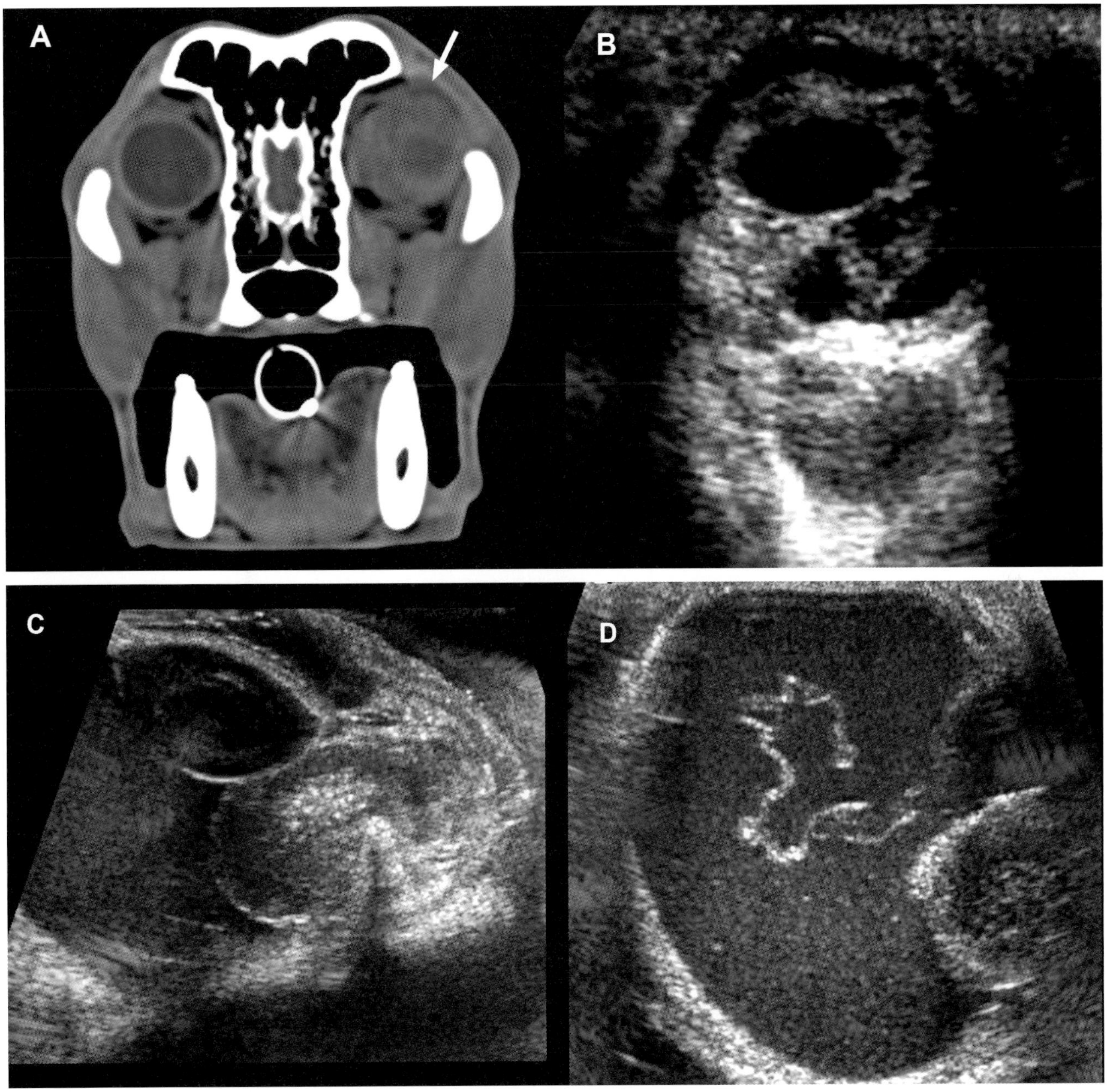

Figure 2.42. Eye trauma. **A and B:** Corresponding computed tomographic **(A)** and sonographic **(B)** images of a dog with marked disruption of the globe (arrow) caused by impact trauma from a golf ball. **C and D:** Rupture of the globe secondary to a kick to the eye. The globe has been lacerated and ruptured as supported by its irregular contour. Note the echogenic hemorrhagic contents with fibrin tags floating in the vitreous body.

especially in young animals. Erythrocytes often precipitate onto a preexisting vitreous strand, acquired membrane, or the posterior hyaloid membrane, and this may lead to an increase in densification of the membranes and an increase in the acoustic reflectivity (Figure 2.46). Fibrous strands may develop secondary to clot formation. These strands may cause tractional retinal detachment when they contract. The vitreal membranes are typically lower in intensity when compared with detached retinal membranes. Blood within the vitreous framework typically is absorbed more slowly (Zeiss and Dubielzig 2004). Bleeding into the vitreous may present as a mass that mimics a tumor. Similar sonographic changes are present in inflammatory and hemorrhagic vitreous changes (Figure 2.47).

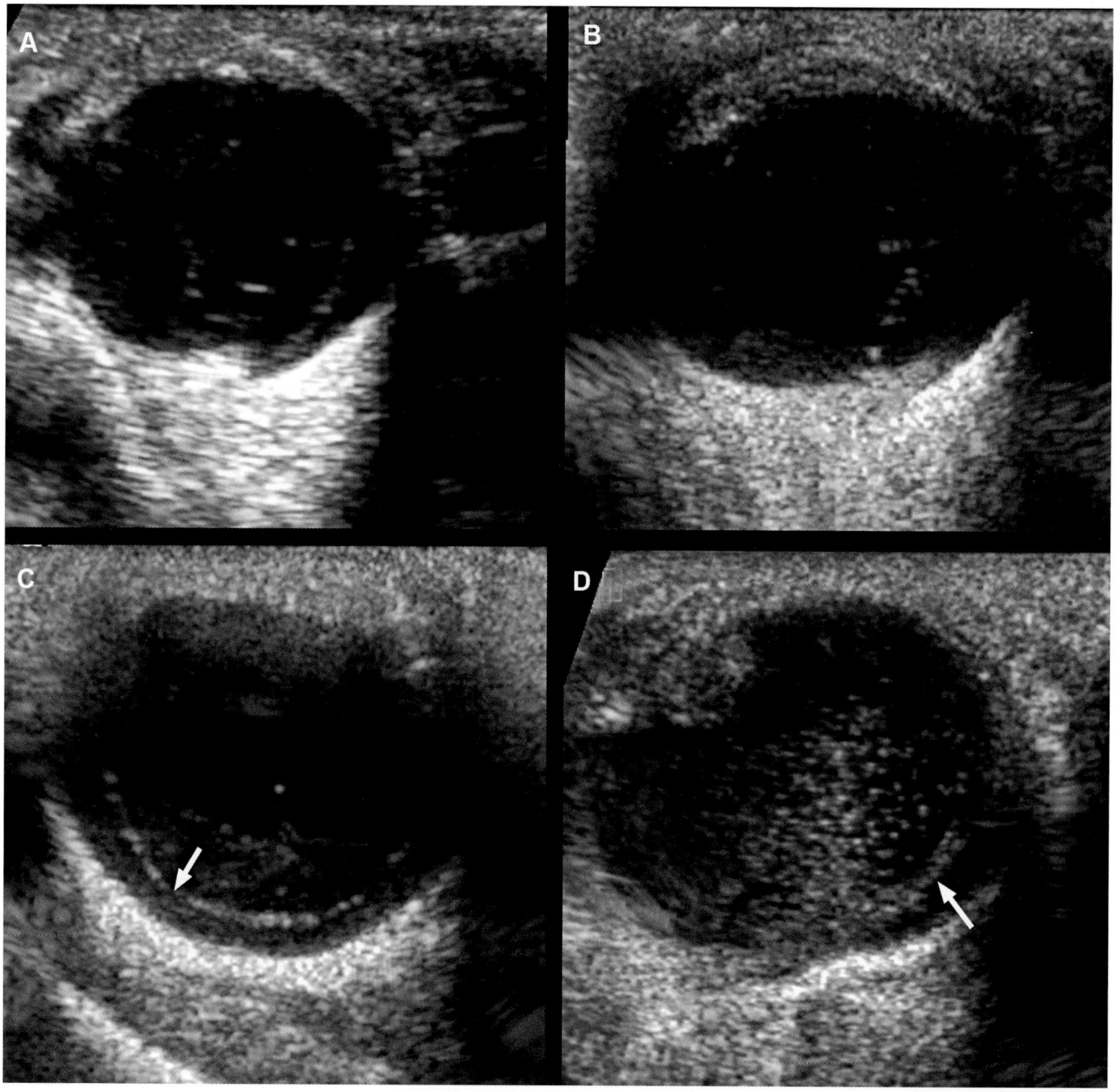

Figure 2.43. Vitreal foci and membranes. **A and B:** Within the vitreous are several faint echogenic foci and membranes. **C and D:** The posterior margin of the retracted vitreal body is seen along the inner part of the orbital wall (arrows). Small, pinpoint, hyperechoic foci are in the vitreous body in **D**, consistent with asteroid hyalosis. When present, the membranes may be confused with retinal detachment.

Endophthalmitis, which is an inflammatory process involving the internal structures of the eye, may appear identical to diffuse vitreal hemorrhage. There may be small pointlike hyperechoic lesions that demonstrate movement within the globe after the eye moves. It has a tendency to organize faster than hemorrhage and often produces vitreal membranes. The echoes may be located within the vitreous or have echoes between the detached retina and the choroid (chorioretinitis) (Figures 2.48 and 2.49).

Persistent and hyperplastic primary vitreous is a congenital condition (Bayon et al. 2001; Gemensky-Metzler and Wilkie 2004; Grahn et al. 2004). The primary vitreous (hyaloid artery and posterior tunica vasculosa lentis) incompletely regresses after birth. Severe forms include microphthalmia, cataract

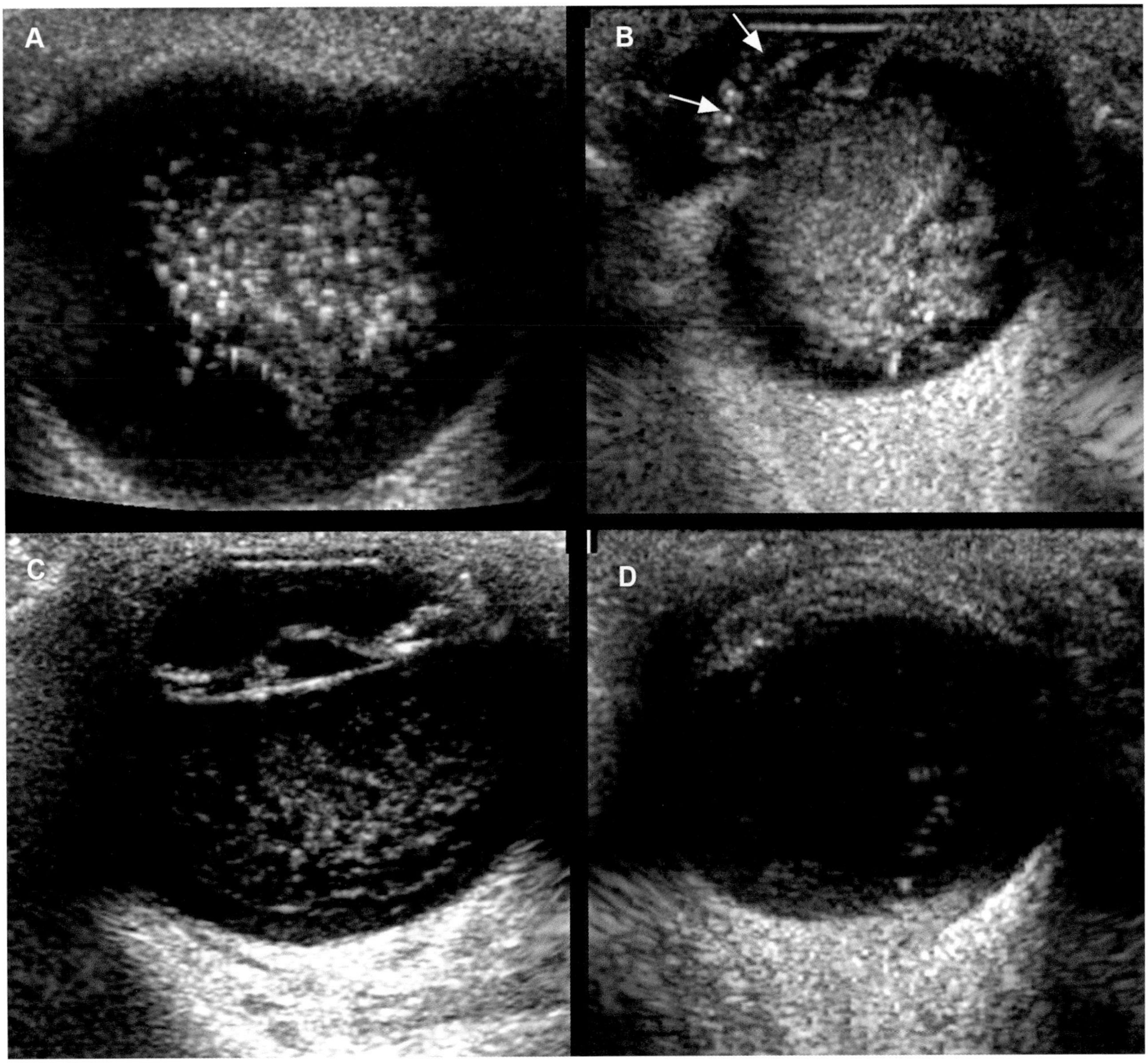

Figure 2.44. Degenerative changes in the vitreous. **A:** Pinpoint hyperechoic foci with faint small comet tails caused by asteroid hyalosis. **B:** Anterior luxated lens (arrows) and suspected hemorrhage in the vitreous body. An anechoic area is around the periphery of the vitreous, likely because of resorption. **C:** Retraction of the vitreal body, a supermature cataract, and asteroid hyalosis. **D:** Faint membranes within the vitreous, most consistent with fibrin tags.

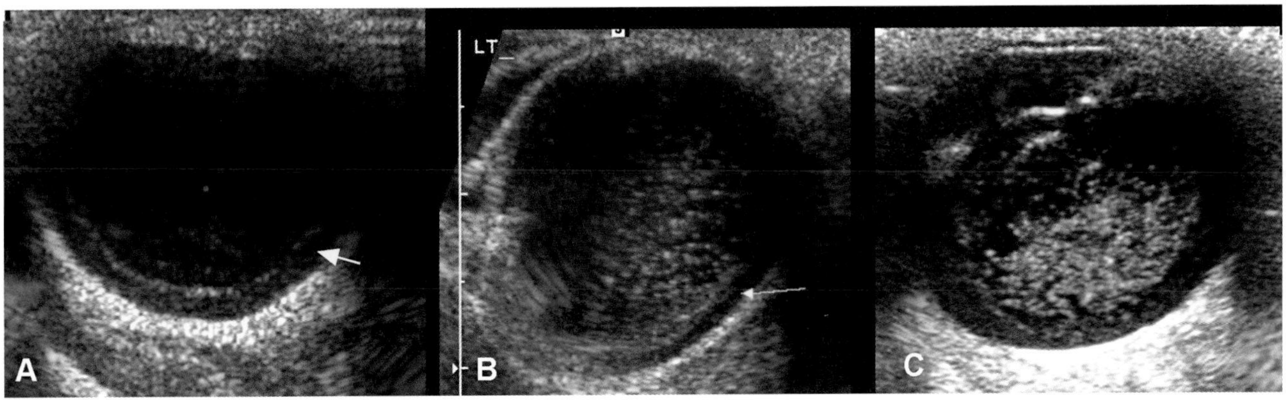

Figure 2.45. Vitreal retraction. **A–C:** There is a progressive liquefaction and separation of the posterior vitreous from the retinal membrane. A faint, hyperechoic, curvilinear area around the periphery of the vitreal body may identify the vitreal margin. The region between the vitreal body and the retina is often anechoic (arrows). LT, left.

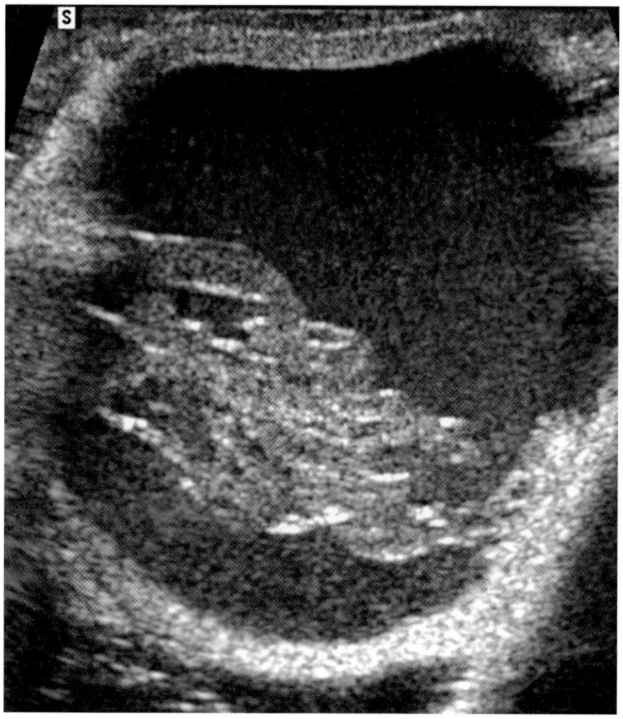

Figure 2.46. Post-traumatic hemorrhage. The vitreous contains mobile low-level echoes. The membranes are fibrin tags. Retinal detachment is also present but not clearly seen on this plane.

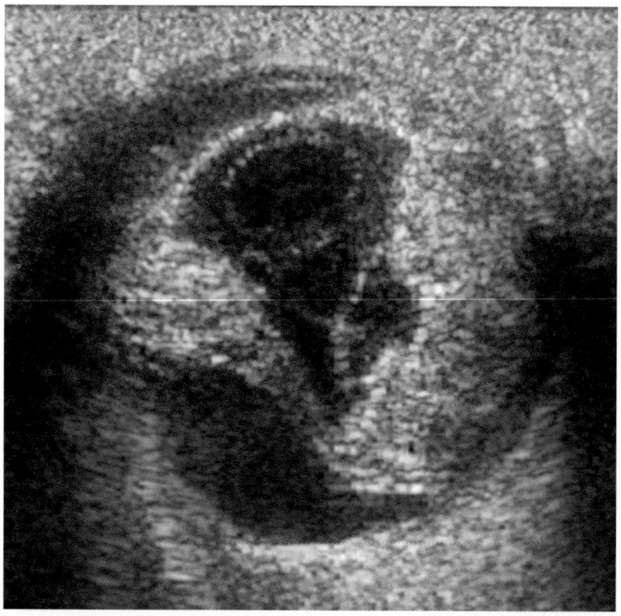

Figure 2.47. Ciliary body tumor. The large echogenic mass originating from the temporal side of the ciliary body has caused retinal detachment and hemorrhage in the vitreous. It is difficult to separate the mass from the hemorrhage on the image. Blood flow may be useful in determining the extent of involvement.

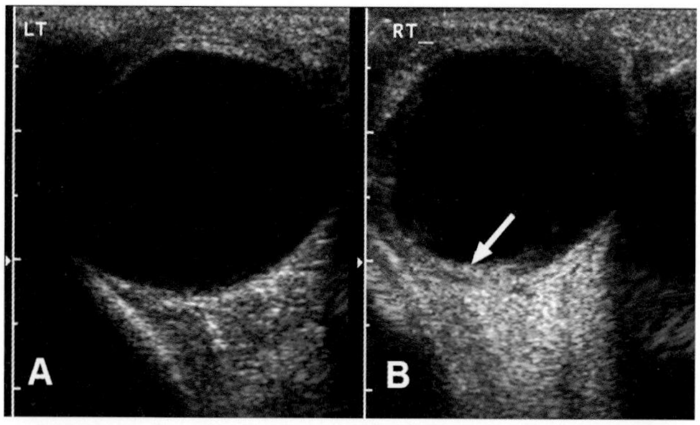

Figure 2.48. Chorioretinitis. **A:** Normal retina for comparison. LT, left eye. **B:** Thickening and mild irregularity of the surface of the retina is noted (arrow). This is consistent with a chorioretinitis in this patient. RT, right eye.

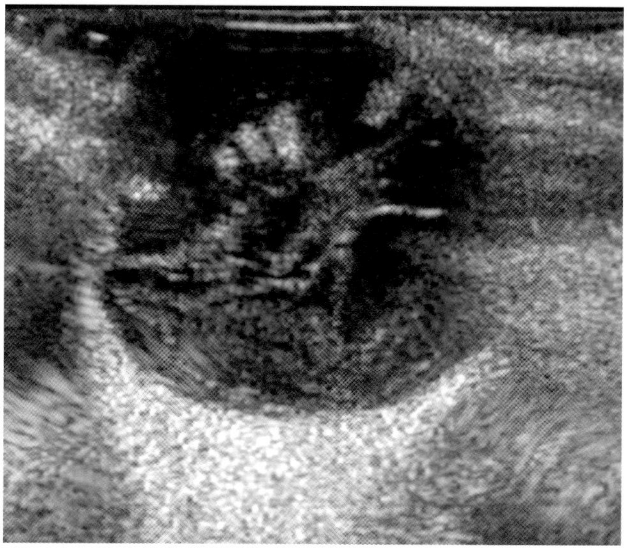

Figure 2.49. Endophthalmitis. Note the numerous membranes and cellular contents in the vitreous. This appearance can be similar to hemorrhage. The membranes usually move in random directions and not usually as hyperechoic as the retina detached membrane. Retinal detachments may occur in conjunction with this process.

formation, and a connective-tissue strand (retrolenticular fibrovascular tissue) between the posterior surface of lens and the area of optic nerve head. A funnel-shaped retrolenticular mass with a thin echogenic stalk emerging from the lens and coursing to the optic disc may be seen. The axial length of the globe may be shortened. The strand between the surface of the lens and the area of the optic nerve head may contain patent hyaloid vessels (Figure 2.50).

A retinal detachment is a commonly encountered abnormality that can be sonographically diagnosed. The retina normally adheres firmly to the optic nerve

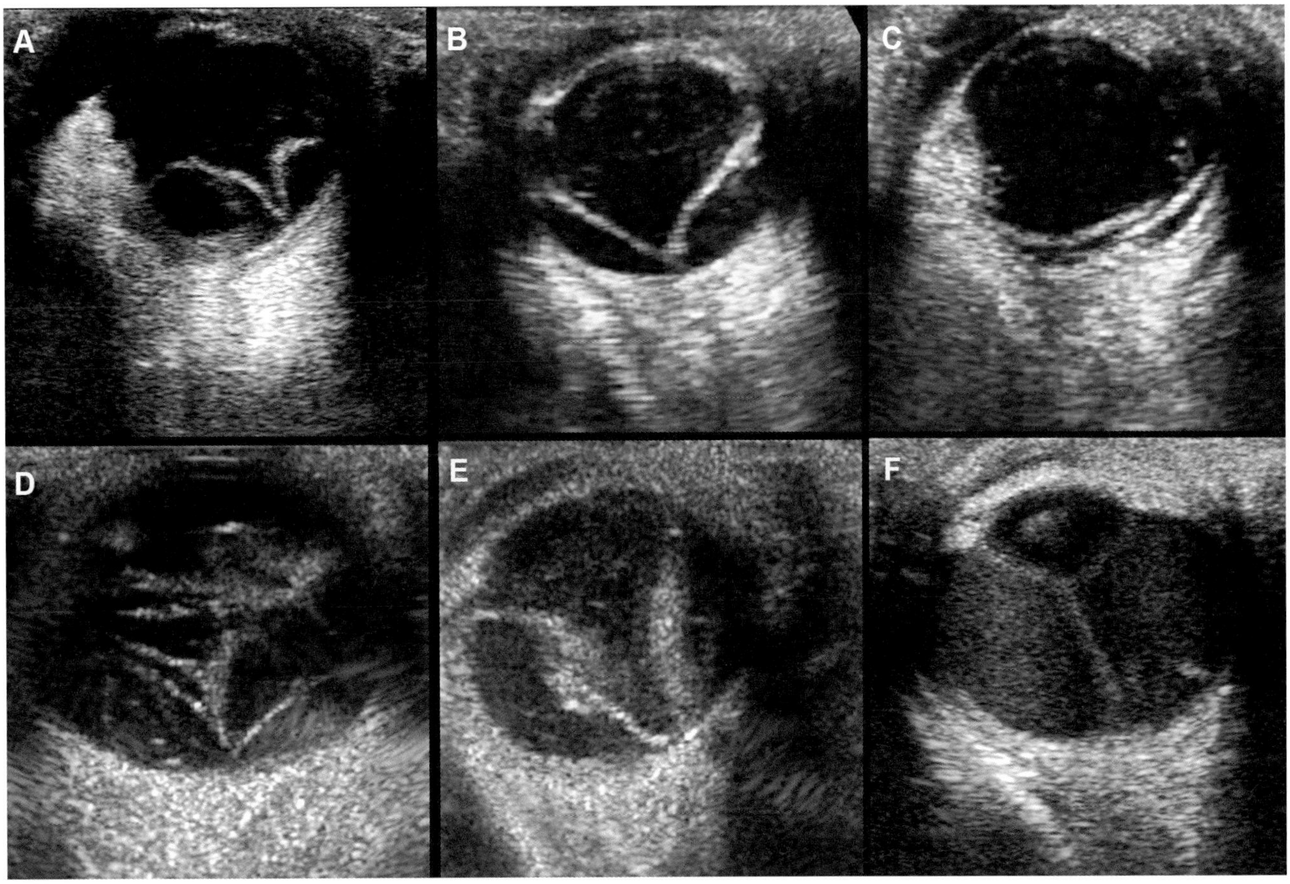

Figure 2.50. Retinal detachments. **A:** Classic example of the retinal membranes coursing from their attachment at the optic disc. **B:** Complete detached retinal membranes from the optic disc to the orra serrata. **C:** Flat retinal detachment. **D:** Retinal detachment with numerous other membranes making the diagnosis more challenging. **E:** Posterior to the detached retinal membranes, there is echogenic material representing pus from a *Prototheca* infection. **F:** Chronic complete retinal detachment. Note the retinal membrane course directly from the optic disc to the posterior surface of the lens. Echogenic contents are posterior to the retinal membrane because of blastomycosis.

head posteriorly and to the ora serrata anteriorly. With a retinal detachment, the retinal layers will remain attached at these two points but may be separated from the adjacent choroid by fluid anywhere between them. The detachment may occur focally or along the entire surface between these two points. The different types of retinal detachments include the rhegmatogenous (tear), the mechanical (traction), the serous or inflammatory infiltrate located between the choroid and the retina. A complete retinal detachment has been referred to as a "morning glory" sign (Figure 2.51). In a sagittal plane, the detachment looks like an isosceles triangle that is open toward the anterior segment. The retina in an acute detachment is usually thin and highly echogenic. With time, the membrane becomes thicker, more fixed, and less mobile, and the membrane moves to the center of the vitreous to form a funnel-shaped configuration.

A vitreal membrane and a detached taunt retina have a similar appearance. Attachment to the optic disc must be demonstrated. The retinal membrane is typically thicker and more echogenic. Incomplete retinal detachment may also occur in various locations (Figure 2.52). Hypermature cataracts have a higher incidence of retinal detachments because of traction and tearing caused by the shrinking lens. Trauma, inflammation, tumors, or systemic hypertension may also cause a detachment. Identification of a retinal detachment can be difficult if different membranes are in the vitreous complicated by strands and floating opacities. Vitreal degeneration and detachment occur as the hyaloid body shrinks. A potential space is produced between the vitreous and the retina, which is considered an incidental degenerative change in older patients. Adhesions may form between the vitreal body and the retina and lead to focal retinal detach-

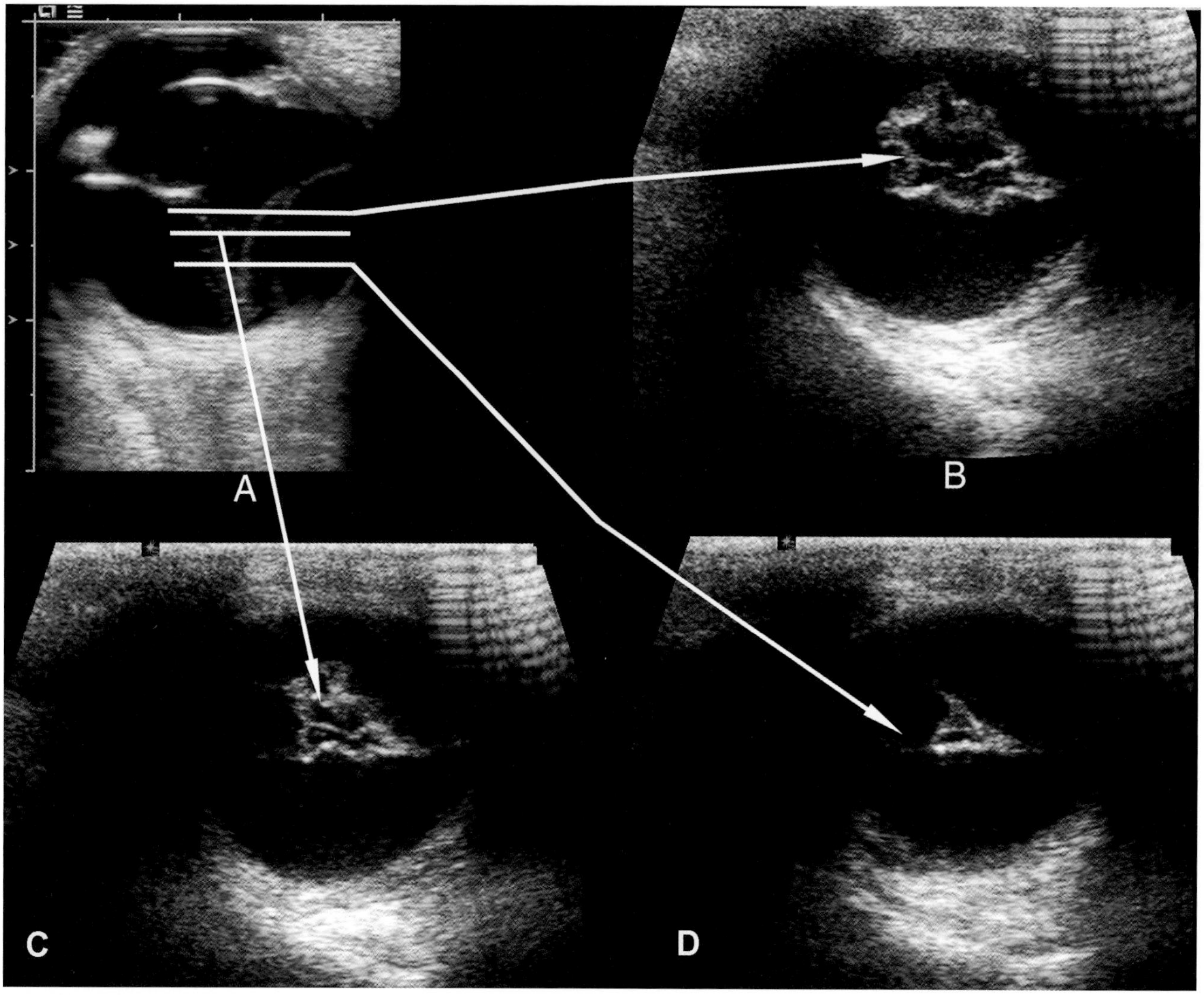

Figure 2.51. Retinal detachment, different planes (parallel lines). **A:** Longitudinal sonogram of a detached retina. **B–D:** Transverse images showing the detached retina as an isosceles triangle, depending on where the slice was taken through the membrane (see corresponding lines from **A**). The detached membrane can then appear as a three-dimensional parachute.

ments. The adhesions and membranes may be confused with a retinal membrane. Blood flow within the membrane is consistent with a retinal detachment. A chorioretinitis may cause an exudate to accumulate between the retina and the choroid. Echogenic material is identified in the subretinal area, and the retina is separated from the choroid, leading to this diagnosis.

Intraocular Foreign Bodies

The appearance of intraocular foreign bodies varies depending on the type and shape of foreign material present and their location. Metal has a typical comet ring–down artifact with a hyperechoic surface to the reflector. Wooden foreign material might be associated with shadowing (Figure 2.53). The sound impedance within the foreign body, the foreign body's and surface characteristics, and its direction relative to the incident beam will help in locating the foreign body and in identifying the type of material present. A hypoechoic tract around the foreign body may assist in locating a foreign body.

Some normal structures in the eye can mimic a foreign body. These include specular reflection from the lens and the shadowing bone forming the orbit.

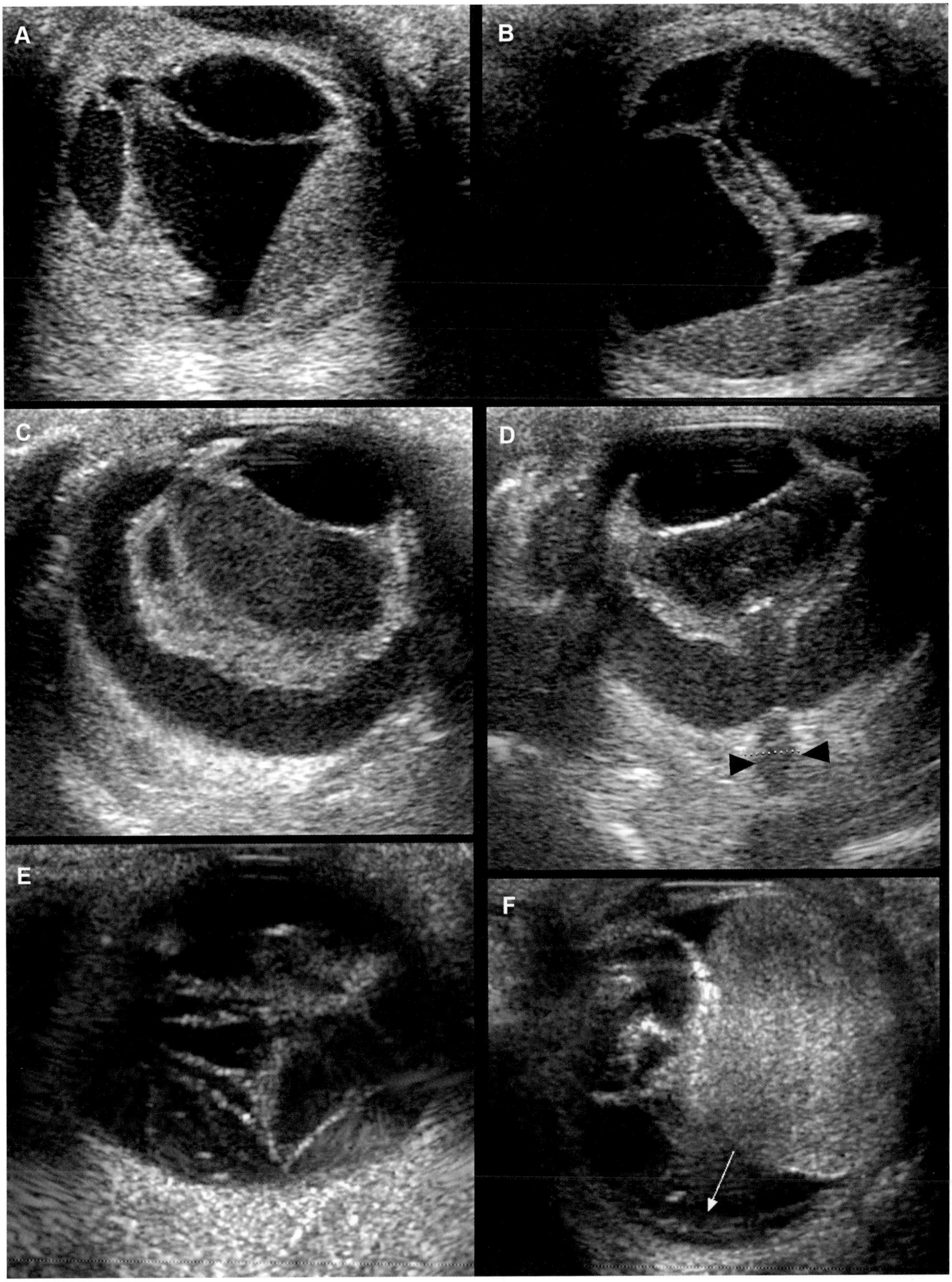

Figure 2.52. Complicated retinal detachments. **A:** Chorioretinitis with secondary retinal detachments caused by blastomycosis. **B:** Note the very echogenic contents posterior to the retinal membrane of the same dog. The cellular contents are mobile and move with gravity. **C:** Retinal detachment secondary to chorioretinitis and neuritis from an unknown organism. Note the echogenic material posterior to the thickened retinal membrane. **D:** Note also that the optic nerve is thickened (arrowheads) (same dog as in **C**). **E:** Traumatic lens luxation with hemorrhage and retinal detachment that is difficult to distinguish from the fibrin membranes. **F:** Large ciliary body tumor. A flat retinal detachment (arrow) is secondary to tearing of the retina by the mass. Note the displacement of the lens by the mass.

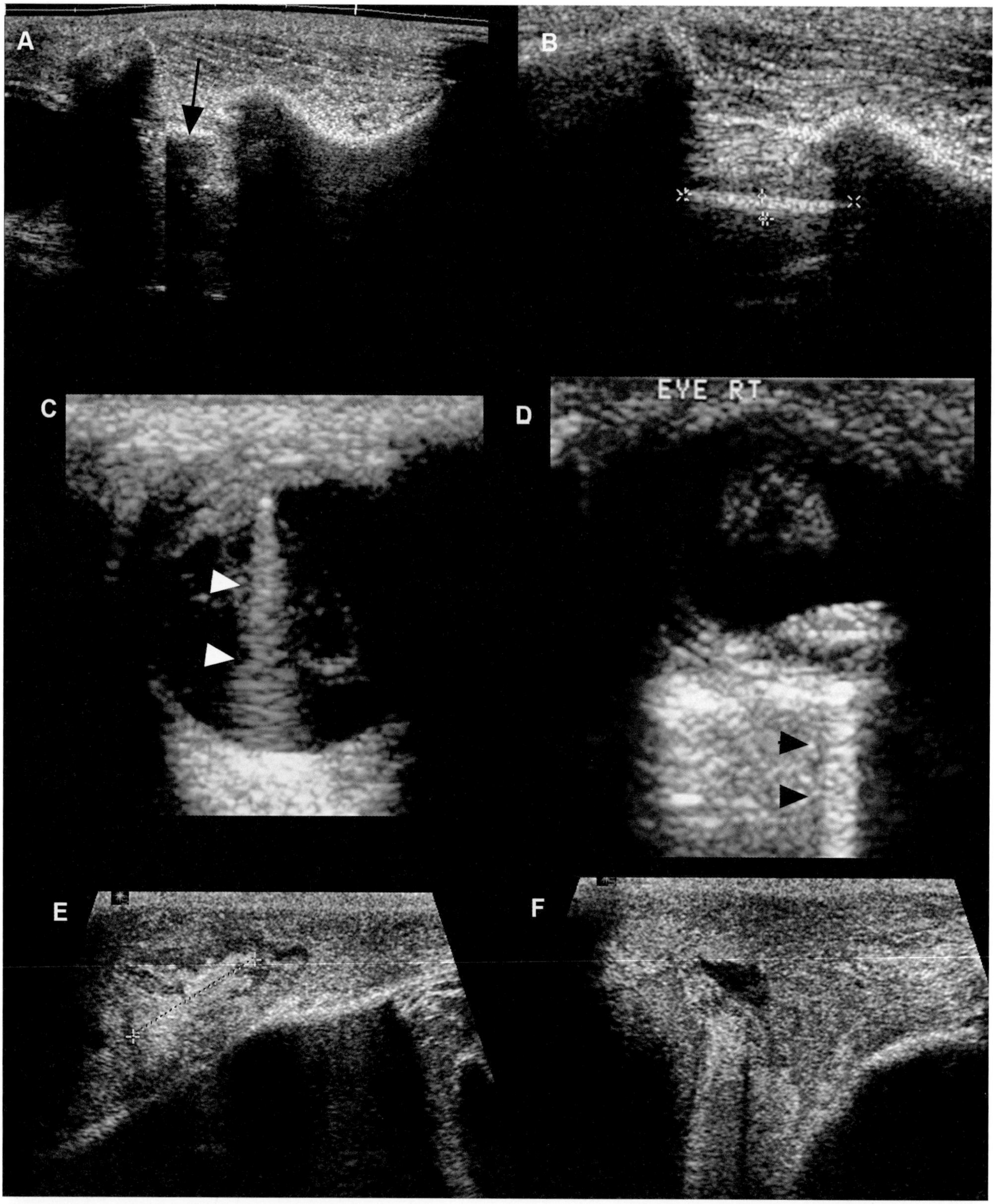

Figure 2.53. Foreign bodies. **A and B: Wooden stick.** A hyperechoic line (arrow) associated with shadowing is present between the margins of the zygomatic bone. The globe is to the left of the image. The wooden foreign body is between the cursors in **B**. **C and D: Pellet-gun metallic foreign bodies** (BBs) with associated comet-tail artifact (arrowheads). The BB appears within the globe in **D**. RT, right eye. **E and F: Short linear foreign object.** Soft-tissue swelling is adjacent and ventral to the globe. A mixed echogenic and anechoic area is around the foreign object, consistent with purulent material in the fistular tract around.

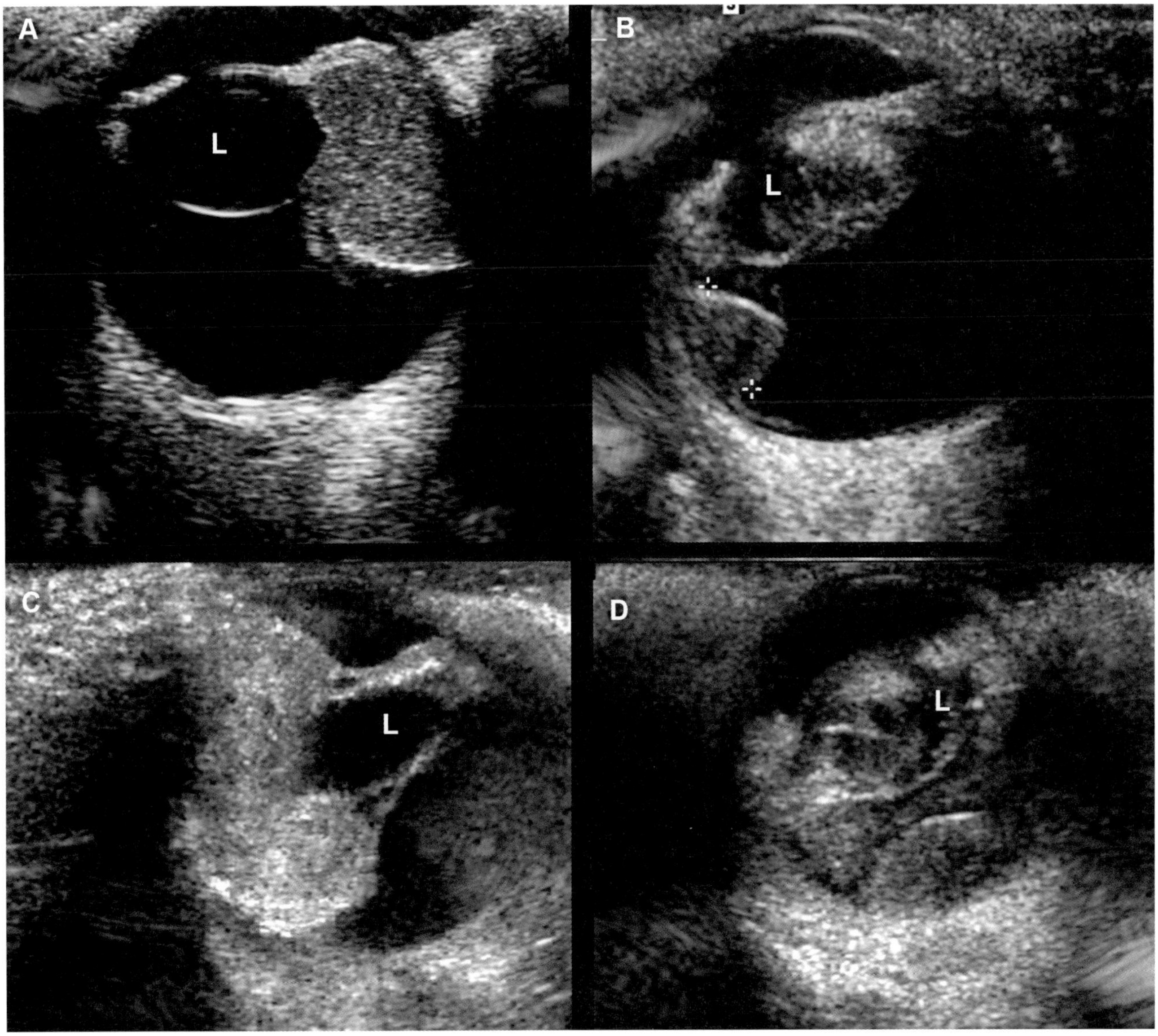

Figure 2.54. Ciliary body tumors. **A–D:** Different size, extension, and echogenicity of ciliary body masses. L, lens. Final diagnosis: melanoma **(A)**, limbal melanoma **(B)**, ciliary body carcinoma **(C)**, and melanoma **(D)**.

Intraocular Neoplasia

Ocular tumors are usually echogenic. Ultrasound may be used to locate the lesion and assess the degree of involvement. Masses (unlike blood clots) are vascularized, often have a broad base, and the attachment to the wall or the tissue of origin can be identified. Extraocular masses may have intraocular extensions. Ocular neoplasia may be primary, multicentric, or metastatic. Tumors of the melanocytic origin are the most common primary intraocular neoplasms in cats and dogs. Diffuse iridal melanomas (cats), epibulbar melanocytoma anterior uveal melanocytoma, choroidal melanocytoma, malignant ocular melanoma, trauma-associated sarcoma (cats), iridociliary epithelial tumor (Dubielzig et al. 1989), medulloepithelioma, and plasmacytoma have been reported as primary ocular neoplasms. Metastatic tumors reported include lymphoma, squamous cell carcinoma, adenocarcinoma (often mammary or pulmonary), oral melanoma, and hemangiosarcoma (Dubielzig 2002). Tumoral masses may be difficult to distinguish from blood clots or a granuloma (Figure 2.54). Lymphoma may have very echogenic thickening of the iris and ciliary

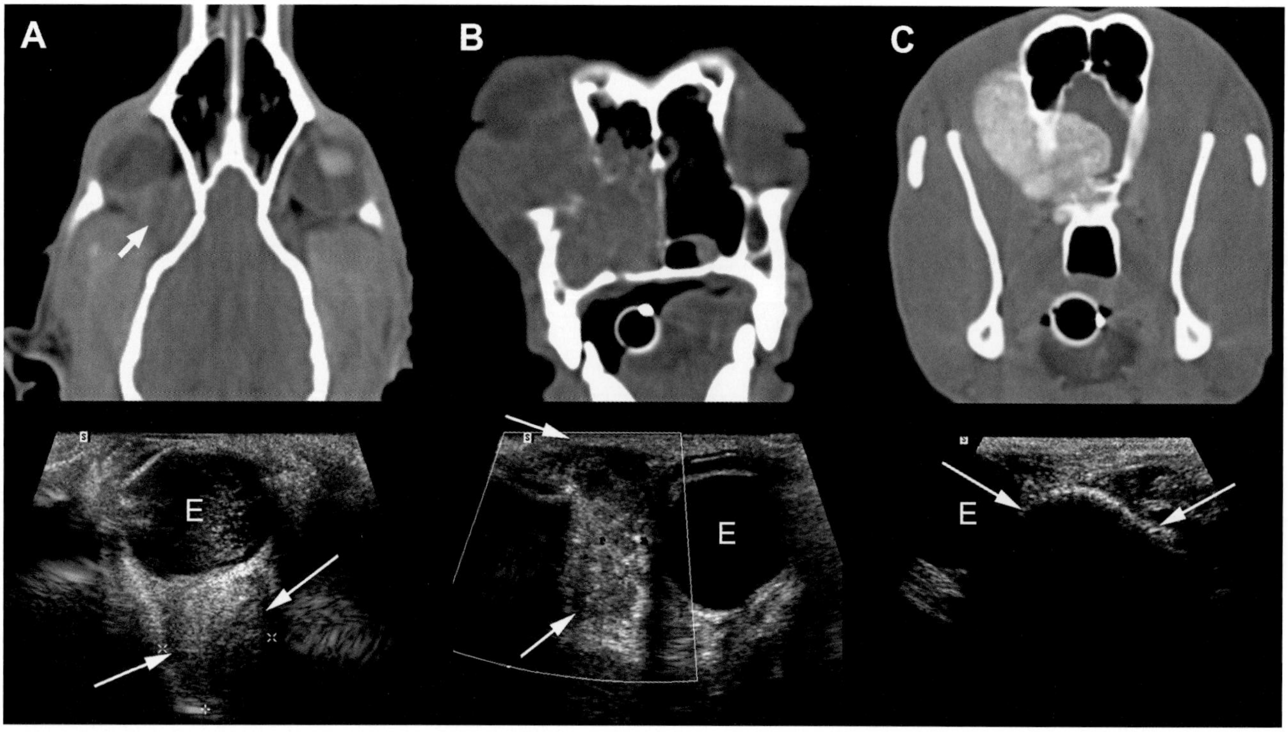

Figure 2.55. Periocular tumors and secondary displacement of the globe. The corresponding computed tomographic image is displayed at the **top** of each case. **A:** Undifferentiated mesenchymal tumor (arrows) located posterior to the globe and displacing it anteriorly. **B:** Nasal adenocarcinoma with extensive lysis of the bony orbit and extension into the periorbital tissues. The globe is displaced laterally and dorsally (arrows). **C:** Osteosarcoma involving the skull, with secondary ocular involvement. Note the hyperechoic and shadowing structure (arrows) displacing the globe. E, ocular globe.

body, echoes in the anterior and posterior chambers, and thickening of the choroid, with possible retinal detachment.

Retrobulbar Disease

The bone surrounding the ocular cone limits the sonographic evaluation of orbital lesions. Abnormalities include blunting of the posterior aspect of the globe; diffuse, increased echogenicity of the retrobulbar space, with failure to delineate the optic nerve; a discrete, hypoechoic mass in the retrobulbar space; and a discrete, highly echogenic mass deforming the posterior aspect of the globe (Morgan 1989; Attali-Soussay et al. 2001). Retrobulbar malignancies present as hyperechoic or hypoechoic changes with various degrees of deformity of the posterior aspect of the globe (Figure 2.55). The appearance of inflammatory changes varies from a diffuse hyperechoic to a discrete hypoechoic mass with possible blunting of the posterior aspect of the globe. Diffuse, non-deforming lesions often are most compatible with retrobulbar cellulitis, but the margins may be sharp and discrete or diffuse and ill-defined.

Tumors involving the tissues around the eye include nasal tumors, primary benign or malignant bone tumors, oral melanomas, squamous cell carcinomas, hemangiosarcomas. These tumors may invade the orbital space. The adjacent bone may be destroyed and have an irregular appearance.

Additional periorbital tissues that may affect the globe include the lacrimal gland and the zygomatic gland (Giudice et al. 2005). Either inflammation or neoplasia may affect the size, shape, and echogenicity of the different periorbital glands. Enlargement or a mass from the affected glands can produce a mass effect that displaces the globe (Figures 2.56–2.61).

The optic nerve is a curvilinear, hypoechoic structure coursing from the posterior surface of the globe into the orbital cone. Abnormalities of the nerve include neuritis (Figure 2.62) with diffuse enlargement or neoplasia with either focal or diffuse enlargement (Figure 2.63). Tumors of the optic nerve include meningioma, neurofibroma, astrocytoma, and lymphoma.

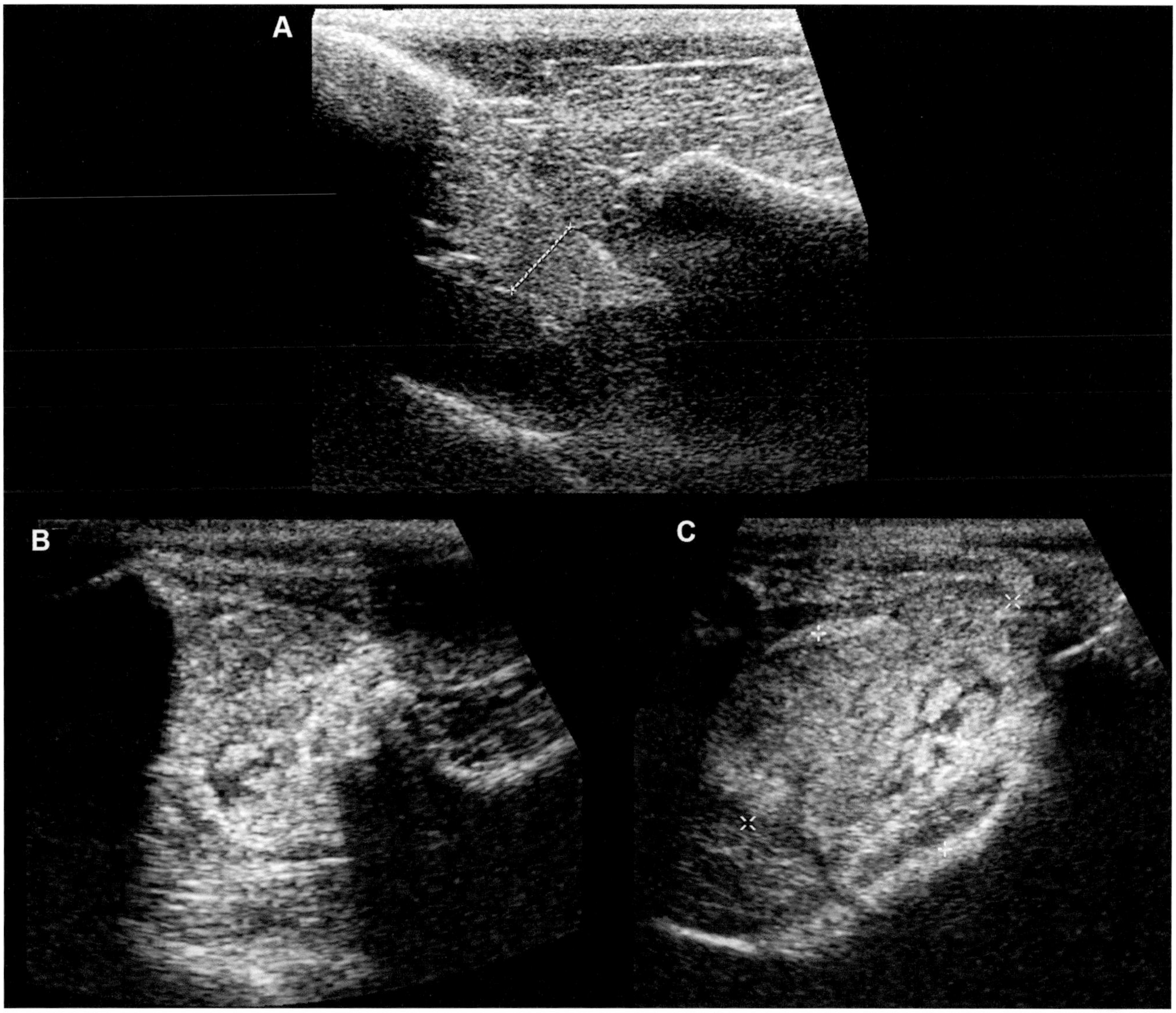

Figure 2.56. Inflamed zygomatic gland. **A:** Normal appearance of the zygomatic gland. **B and C:** Enlarged zygomatic salivary gland from inflammation.

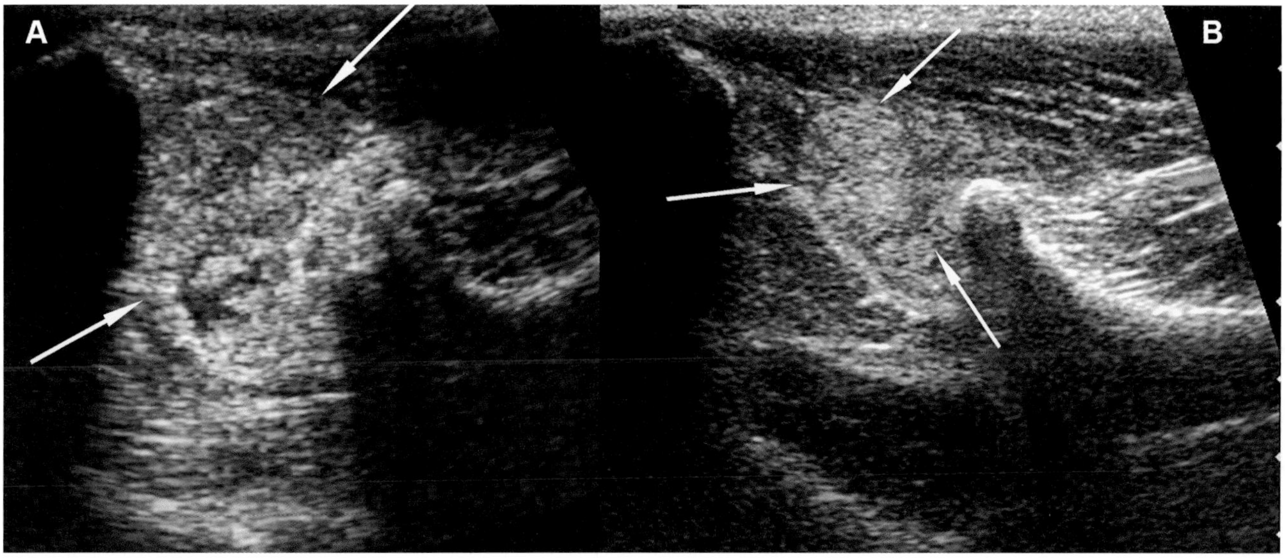

Figure 2.57. Chronic myositis. **A and B:** The masseter muscle (arrows) is hyperechoic and has disrupted fibers. The muscle size is reduced. This is caused by fibrosis secondary to chronic myositis.

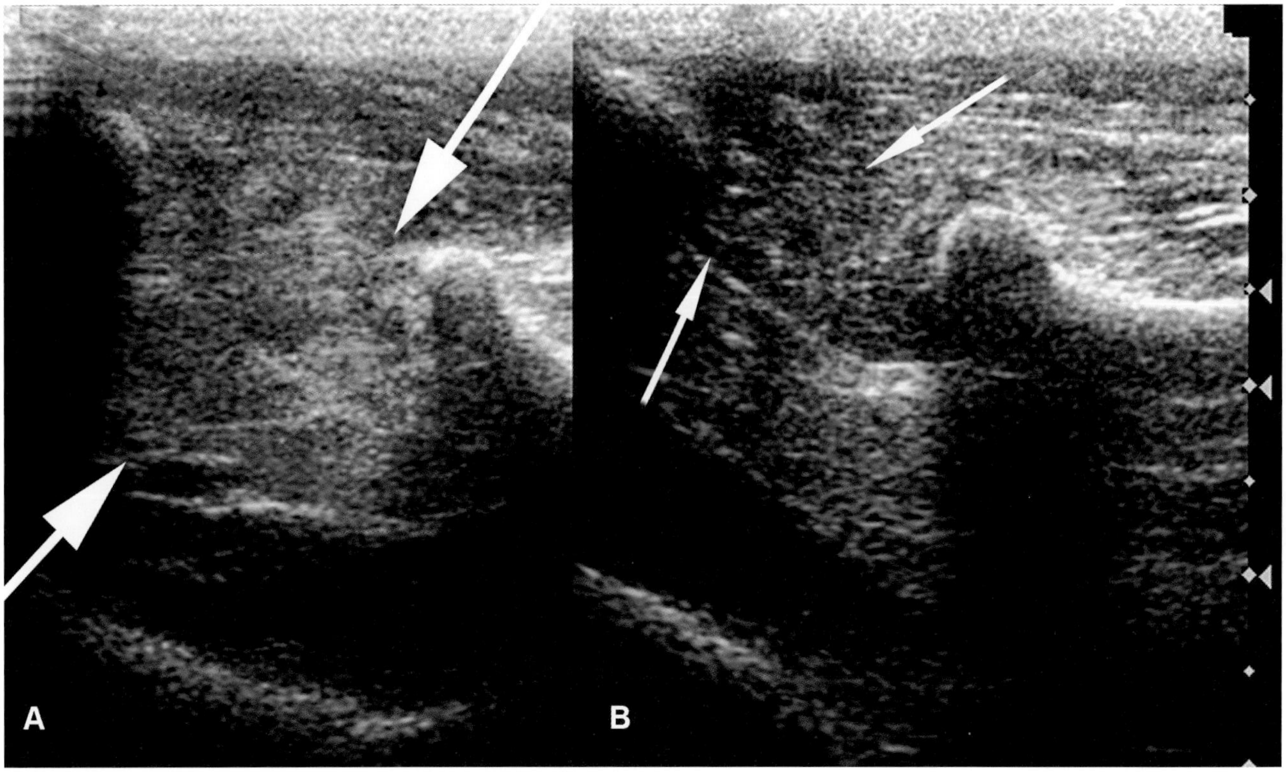

Figure 2.58. Temporalis myositis. **A:** The temporalis muscle (arrows) is markedly thickened secondary to acute myositis. **B:** Normal temporalis muscle (arrows) for comparison.

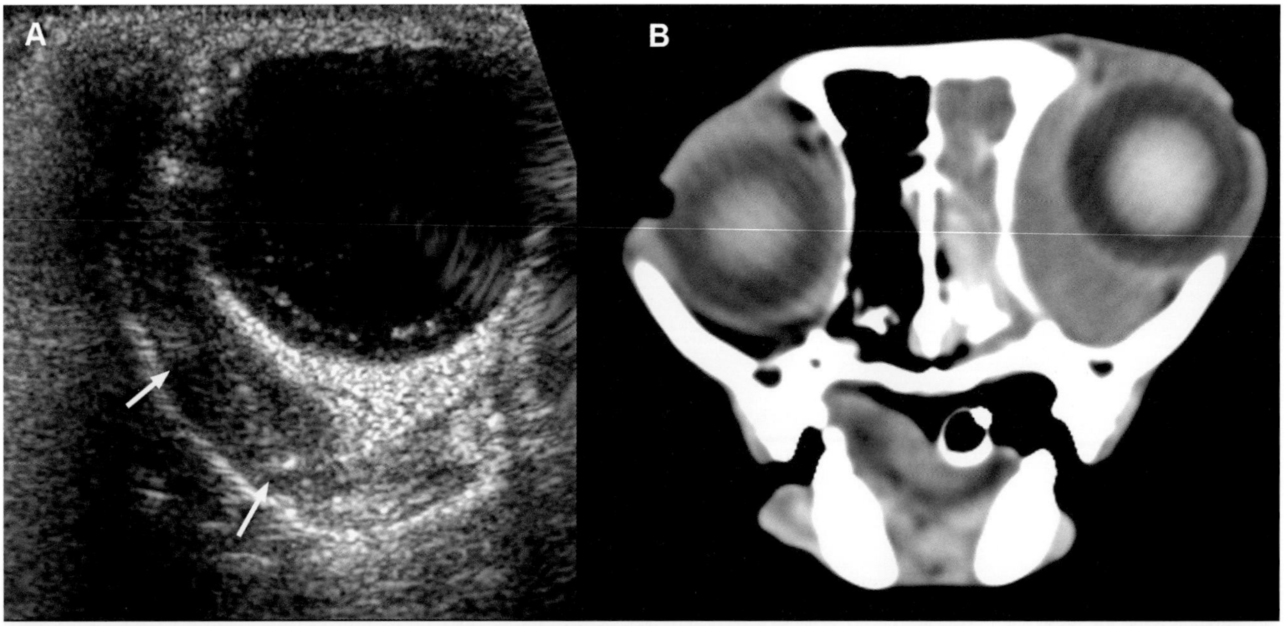

Figure 2.59. Lacrimal gland adenocarcinoma. **A:** Echogenic soft-tissue infiltrate is present on the medial aspect of the left globe (arrows). **B:** Corresponding transverse computed tomographic image showing the lateral displacement of the globe by the infiltrate.

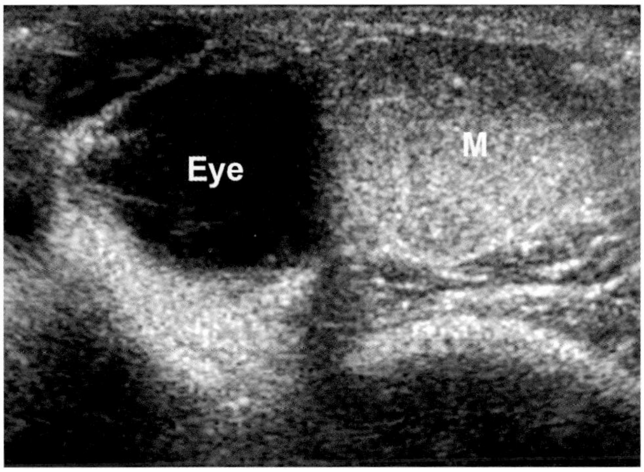

Figure 2.60. Lacrimal gland adenoma. A homogeneous echogenic mass (M) is lateral to and displacing the globe.

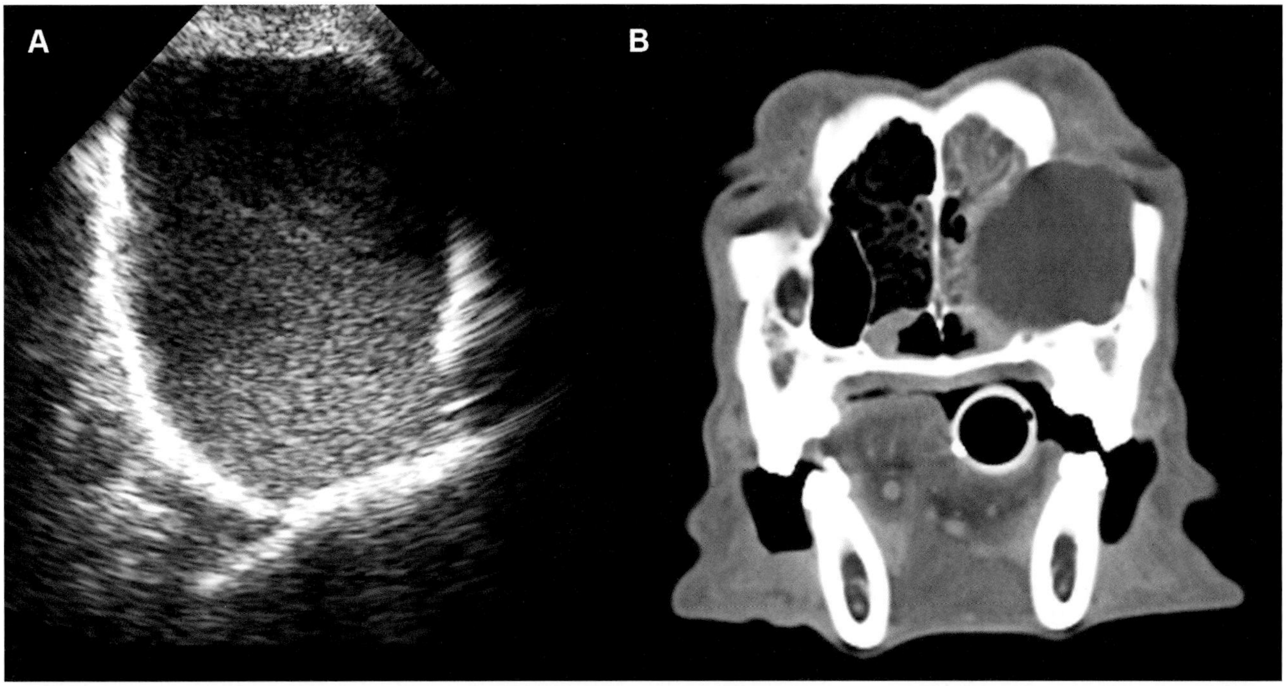

Figure 2.61. Maxillary cyst. **A:** The cyst is filled with mobile echogenic contents, creating pressure necrosis on the orbit, and displaces the globe. Ultrasound was used to aspirate the fluid contents. **B:** Corresponding transverse computed tomographic image of the large lesion.

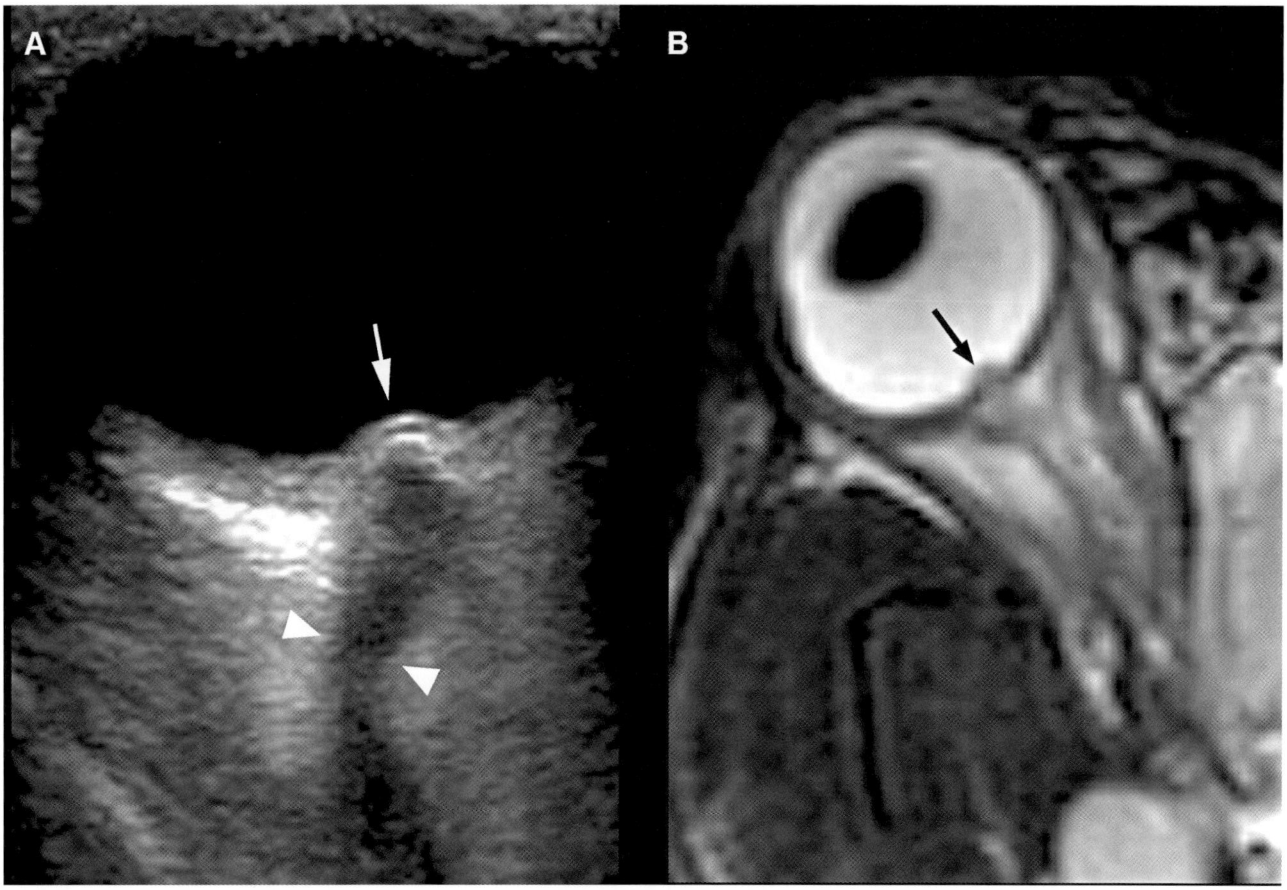

Figure 2.62. Optic neuritis. An indentation (arrows) into the globe at the optic disc is seen in both the ultrasound **(A)** and the magnetic resonance **(B)** images. The optic nerve (arrowheads) is thickened. Image courtesy of D. Penninck.

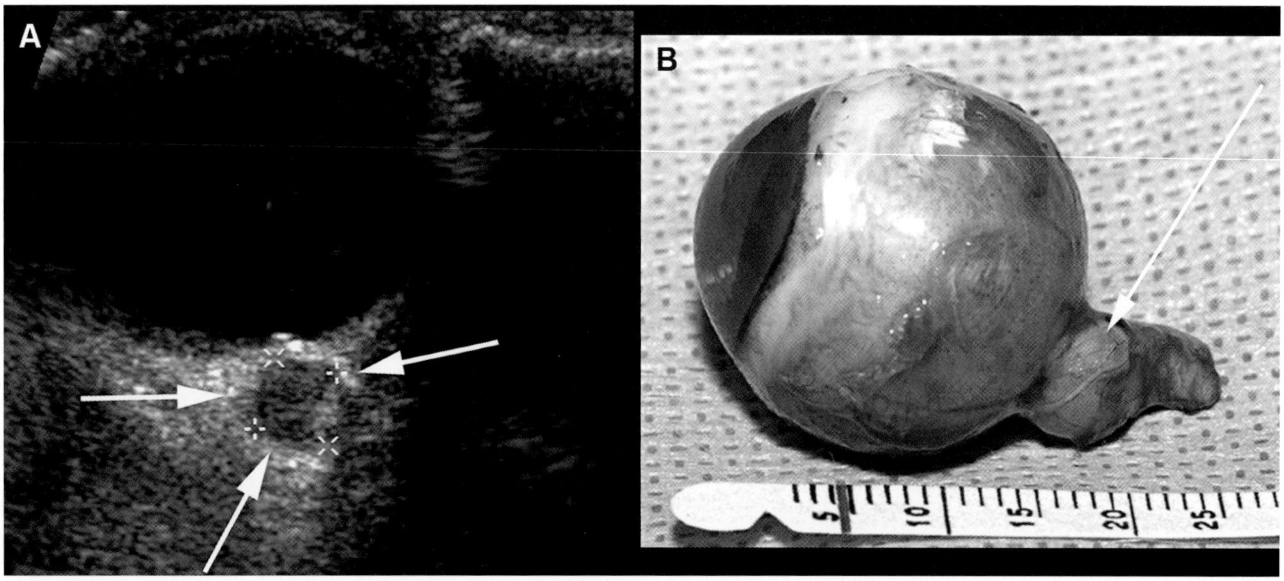

Figure 2.63. Optic nerve meningioma. Focal thickening of the optic nerve is seen in the ultrasound image (arrows) **(A)**, as well as on the specimen (arrow) **(B)**.

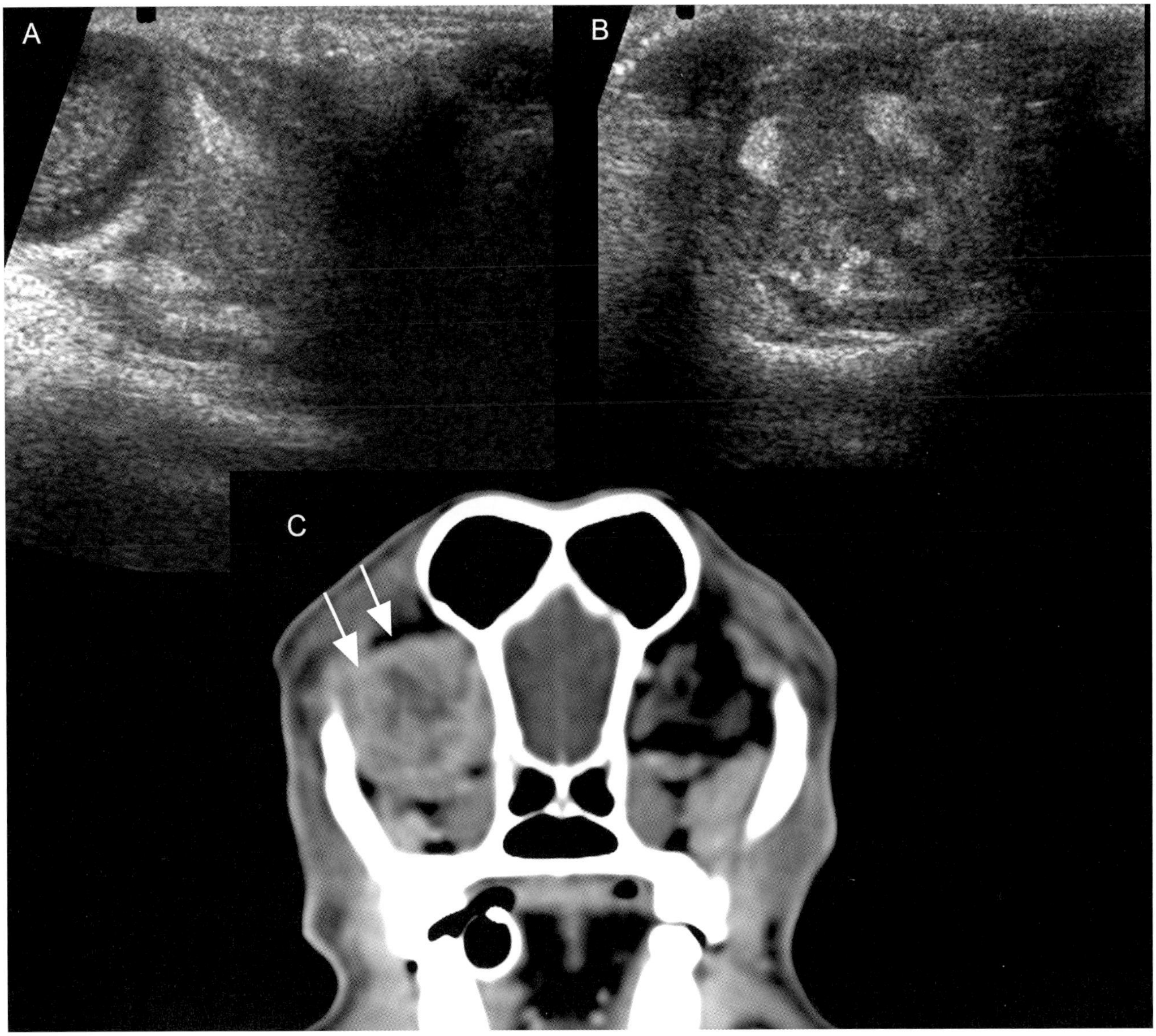

Figure 2.64. Polymyositis of the extraocular muscles. **A:** Longitudinal image of thickened extraocular muscles within the orbital cone. **B:** Transverse to oblique view of the same area. **C:** Corresponding transverse computed tomographic image. The arrows point to the thickened muscles.

Extraocular muscles include the four rectus muscles (dorsal, medial, ventral, and lateral), retractor bulbi muscle, and dorsal and ventral oblique muscles. Normally the muscles attach in the equatorial zone of the globe and form a cone whose apex is at the posterior orbital bony wall. The muscles run around the optic nerve and are hypoechoic, being surrounded by hyperechoic fat. Diseases affecting these muscles include an immune-mediated myositis (Allgoewer et al. 2000) that results in enlarged and hypoechoic muscles in the acute phase. Muscular fibrosis is the outcome in chronic cases. Neoplasia is possible but less common (Figure 2.64).

Interventional Procedures

Ultrasound-guided fine-needle aspiration of masses in the periorbital and retro-orbital region can be performed. This technique enables visualization of the mass and the needle placement into the lesion. The angle in which the needle is placed relative to the direction of the transducer is vital in order to position the tip of the needle accurately. Aspiration in the retro-orbital region with ultrasound guidance is helpful in avoiding vital structures such as the optic nerve, the globe, and the vessels. It is also helpful in placing the

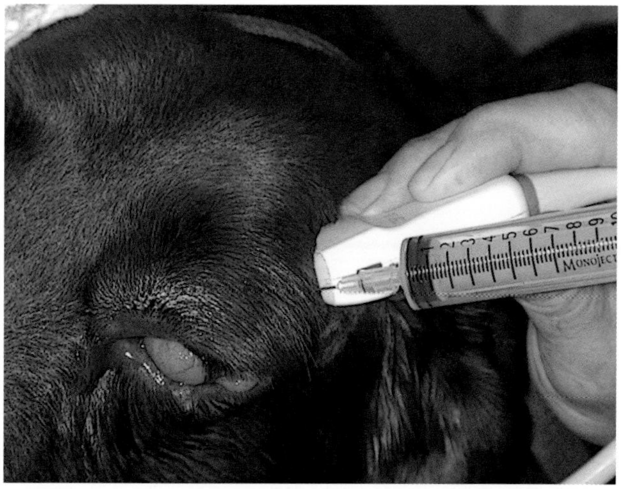

Figure 2.65. Ultrasound-guided freehand aspirate of a retro-orbital mass. The needle attached to a syringe is placed into the retrobulbar lesion.

needle within the mass or infiltrate to acquire appropriate cells for cytology, or to drain the abscess cavity (Figure 2.65).

References

Allgoewer I, Blair M, Basher T, Davidson M, et al. (2000) Extraocular muscle myositis and restrictive strabismus in 10 dogs. Vet Ophthalmol 3:21–26.

Attali-Soussay K, Jegou J, Clerc B (2001) Retrobulbar tumors in dogs and cats: 25 cases. Vet Ophthalmol 4:19–27.

Bayon A, Tovar MC, Fernandez del Palacio MJ, Agut A (2001) Ocular complications of persistent hyperplastic primary vitreous in three dogs. Vet Ophthalmol 4:35–40.

Beam A, Correa M, Davidson M (1999) A retrospective-cohort study on the development of cataracts in dogs with diabetes mellitus: 200 cases. Vet Ophthalmol 2:169–172.

Boroffka SA, Voorhour G, Verbruggen AM, Teske E (2006) Intraobserver and interobserver repeatability of ocular biometric measurements obtained by means of B-mode ultrasonography in dogs. Am J Vet Res 67:1743–1749.

Cottrill N, Banks WJ, Pechman RD (1989) Ultrasonographic and biometric evaluation of the eye and orbit of dogs. Am J Vet Res 50:898–903.

Deehr AJ, Dubielzig RR (1998) A histopathological study of iridociliary cysts and glaucoma in golden retrievers. Vet Ophthalmol 1:153–158.

Dietrich U, Kostlin R, Tassani M (1995) Ultrasonographic examination of the eyes of dogs with cataracts [Abstract]. Vet Radiol Ultrasound 36:436.

Dubielzig RR (2002) Tumors of the eye. In: Meuten D, ed. Tumors in Domestic Animals, 4th edition. Ames, IA: Blackwell, pp 739–754.

Dubielzig RR, Steinberg H, Garvin H, Deehr AJ, Fischer B (1998) Iridociliary epithelial tumors in 100 dogs and 17 cats: A morphological study. Vet Ophthalmol 1:223–231.

Dziezyc J, Hager DA (1988) Ocular ultrasonography in veterinary medicine. Semin Vet Med Surg (Small Anim) 3:1–9.

Gelatt K, MacKay E (2005) Prevalence of primary breed-related cataracts in the dog in North America. Vet Ophthalmol 8:101–111.

Gemensky-Metzler A, Wilkie DA (2004) Surgical management and histologic and immunohistochemical features of a cataract and retrolental plaque secondary to persistent hyperplastic tunica vasculosa lentis/persistent hyperplastic primary vitreous (PHTVL/PHPV) in a bloodhound puppy. Vet Ophthalmol 7:369–375.

Giudice C, Marco R, Mirko R, Luca M, Giorgio C (2005) Zygomatic gland adenoma in a dog: Histochemical and immunohistochemical evaluation. Vet Ophthalmol 8: 13–16.

Grahn BH, Storey ES, McMillan C (2004) Inherited retinal dysplasia and persistent hyperplastic primary vitreous in Miniature Schnauzer dogs. Vet Ophthalmol 7:151–158.

Hager DA, Dziezyc J, Millchamp NJ (1987) Two-dimensional real-time ocular ultrasonography in the dog: Technique and normal anatomy. Vet Radiol 28:60–65.

Morgan RV (1989) Ultrasonography of retrobulbar diseases of the dog and cat. J Am Anim Hosp Assoc 25:393–399.

Sapienza JS, Simo FJ, Prades-Sapienza A (2000) Golden retriever uveitis: 75 cases (1994–1999). Vet Ophthalmol 3:214–246.

Schiffer SP, Rantanen NW, Leary GA, Bryan GM (1982) Biometric study of the canine eye, using A-mode ultrasonography. Am J Vet Res 43:826–830.

Spiess BM, Bolliger JO, Guscetti F, Haessig M, Lackner PA, Ruehli MB (1998) Multiple ciliary body cysts and secondary glaucoma in the Great Dane: A report of nine cases. Vet Ophthalmol 1:41–45.

Van der Woerdt A (2000) Lens-induced uveitis. Vet Ophthalmol 3:227–234.

Williams DL (2004) Lens morphometry determined by B-mode ultrasonography of the normal and cataractous canine lens. Vet Ophthalmol 7:91–95.

Zeiss CJ, Dubielzig RR (2004) A morphologic study of intravitreal membranes associated with intraocular hemorrhage in the dog. Vet Ophthalmol 7:239–243.

CHAPTER THREE

Neck

Allison Zwingenberger and Erik Wisner

Scanning Technique

Because the ventral cervical region is anatomically complex, ultrasound is uniquely suited to evaluating cervical organs and tissues that are not readily characterized on survey or contrast radiographs. In addition to defining gross anatomy of the neck, high-resolution ultrasound can also be used to examine very small structures such as the thyroid and parathyroid glands. High-frequency (8- to 15-MHz) linear transducers and curvilinear transducers provide the best images of small structures and those with complex internal architecture. Tissue harmonic imaging is also available on some newer machines, which can further improve image resolution by decreasing artifacts.

For ultrasonography of most structures, the animal is positioned in dorsal recumbency with the area of interest clipped (Figure 3.1A). Because many of the organs in the neck are symmetrically paired, it is useful to clip both sides in order to compare them. Positioning the patient so that the neck is as straight as possible is important to locate anatomical landmarks reliably and to compare one side of the neck accurately with the other. For imaging the tympanic bullae, positioning the patient in sternal recumbency (Figure 3.1B) or seated with the head held straight and extended is preferred. Any structure can be investigated while the animal is in lateral recumbency (Figure 3.1C) according to operator preference or for dyspneic animals, with the caveat that anatomy may appear somewhat distorted and comparisons to the contralateral neck will be impaired.

Although the ultrasound beam cannot penetrate air within hollow structures such as the tympanic bullae, trachea, and larynx, the interface between air and adjacent soft tissues can still be evaluated for regularity of contours and physiological motion as exemplified by examination of the vocal folds.

In addition to two dimensional B-mode imaging, color flow Doppler, power Doppler, and pulsed-wave Doppler imaging can be used to evaluate vascularity of organs, vessels, and tissues. Flow characteristics of large vessels such as the common carotid artery and jugular vein can be determined with color and pulsed-wave Doppler.

Normal Sonographic Anatomy

There are a few anatomical landmarks that are useful for locating cervical structures of clinical interest. The ventral margin of the mandible appears as a smooth, hyperechoic interface surrounded by skeletal muscle. Structures surrounding it include the parotid and mandibular salivary glands, the external ear canal, and the tympanic bulla caudally. The parotid salivary gland is caudal to the external ear canal, and the tympanic bulla is medial to the canal.

The mandibular salivary gland is a marker for the origin of the external jugular vein, the bifurcation of the common carotid artery, and the medial retropharyngeal lymph node.

The larynx is located on the ventral midline, and the paired hyperechoic arytenoid cartilages are landmarks for the vocal folds. Structures located near the larynx from cranial to caudal include the parotid salivary gland, mandibular salivary gland, medial retropharyngeal lymph node, mandibular lymph nodes, maxillary and linguofacial veins, and internal and external carotid arteries.

The trachea is on ventral midline and commonly used as a fixed midline anatomical landmark when the thyroid and parathyroid glands are imaged and is used to define the caudal aspect of the larynx.

The jugular vein and common carotid artery are easily located and can serve as landmarks for identifying the thyroid and parathyroid glands.

Bullae

The external ear canal and tympanic bulla are best imaged with a curvilinear transducer of medium frequency (5–8 MHz) with a small footprint. The contact area for imaging these structures is small, and

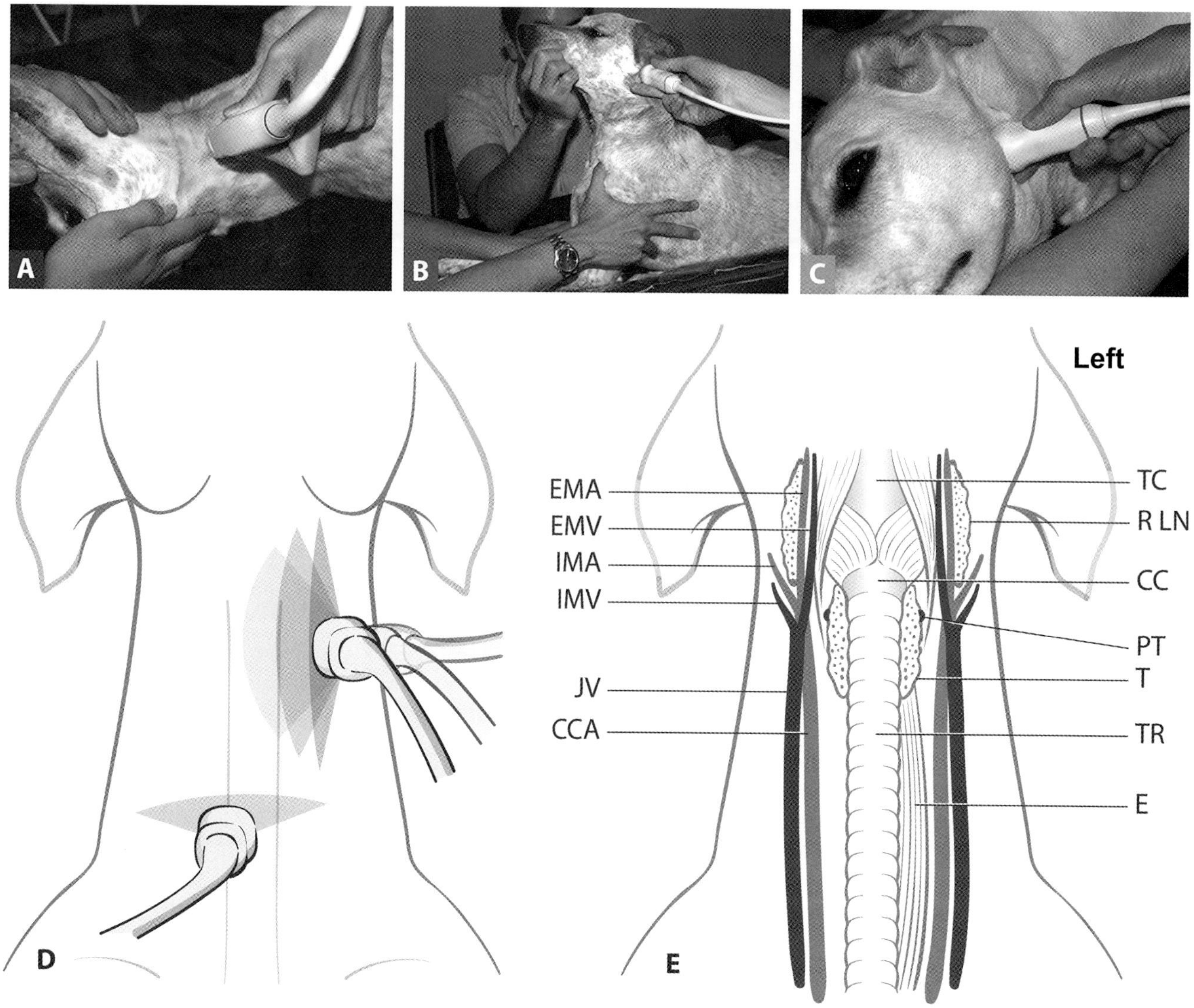

Figure 3.1. Images of positioning for the ultrasound probe on the neck of a dog. **A:** Dorsal recumbency is convenient for imaging most of the structures of the neck. It enables comparison of bilaterally symmetrical structures, and it is easy to maintain true sagittal and transverse orientation. **B:** Sternal positioning for ultrasonography of the tympanic bulla. **C:** Lateral recumbency is an alternate position for investigating the structures of the neck. **D:** Schematic representation of probe positioning and corresponding scan planes on the neck. **E:** Schematic main anatomical structures evaluated with ultrasound. CC, cricoid cartilage; CCA, common carotid artery; E, esophagus; EMA, external maxillary artery; EMV, external maxillary vein; IMA, internal maxillary artery; IMV, internal maxillary vein; JV, jugular vein; PT, parathyroid gland; RLN, retropharyngeal lymph node; T, thyroid gland; TC, thyroid cartilage; and TR, trachea.

a higher-frequency linear transducer is often too large to position evenly on the skin. In addition, the bone of the tympanic bulla absorbs the ultrasound beam, and higher frequencies may not penetrate the bullae wall adequately to generate an image of the lumen.

The external ear canal and bulla are imaged from both a lateral approach and a ventral approach (Figure 3.1B and C) with the patient in sternal, seated, or lateral recumbency (Dickie et al. 2003). From a lateral position with the transducer oriented in a dorsal plane, the cross section of the vertical external ear canal is visible as a curvilinear hyperechoic line filled with air producing reverberation artifact. In a transverse plane with respect to the head, the external ear canal appears in longitudinal orientation. The ear canal lies just caudal to the zygomatic arch, with the masseter muscle lateral to the arch and the sternocephalicus muscle caudal to it. The horizontal portion of the ear canal is imaged from a ventral position either in longitudinal or in transverse orientation (Figure 3.2). From the

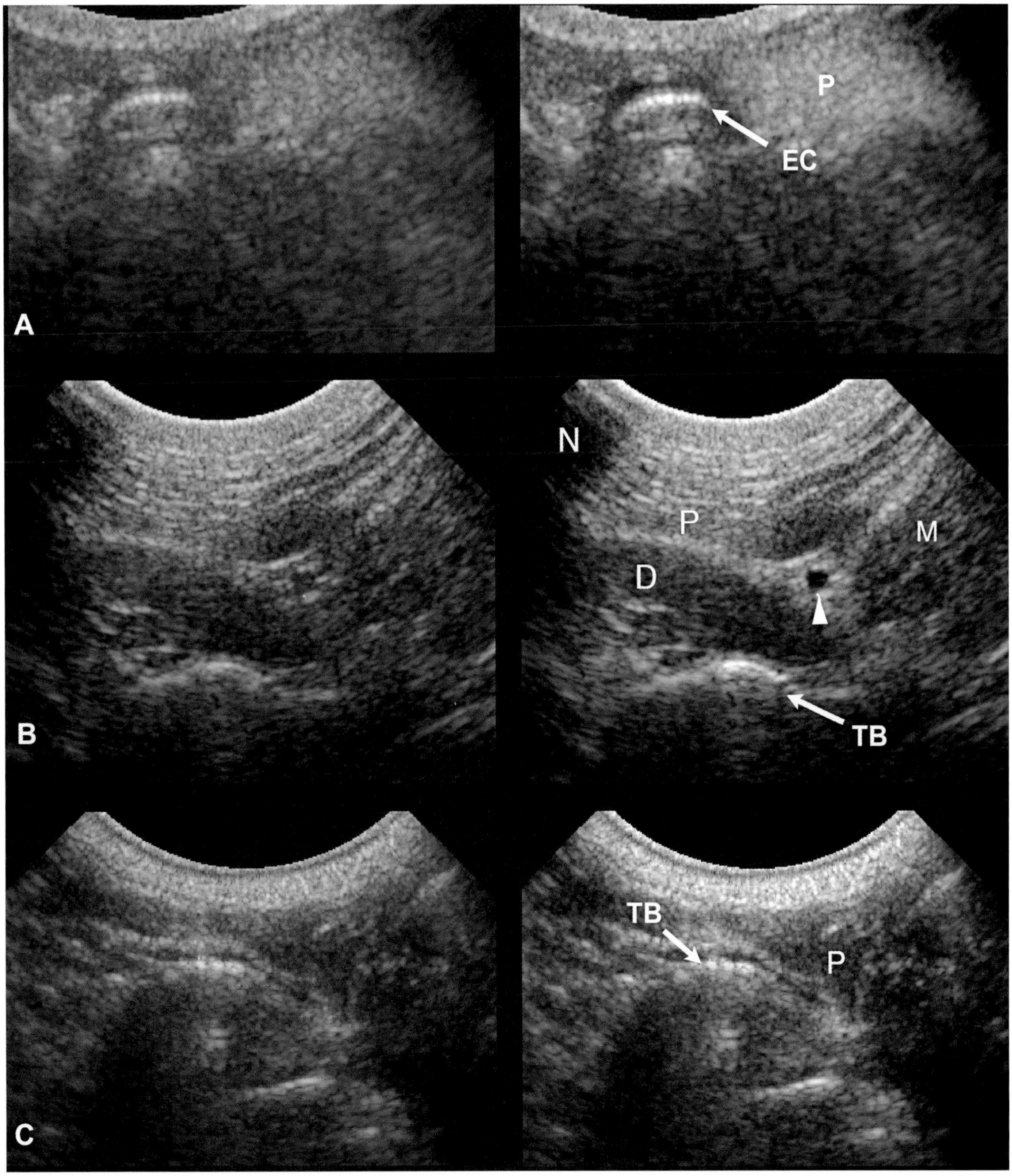

Figure 3.2. Normal external ear canal and tympanic bulla of a dog. **A and B:** Ultrasonographic and schematic images obtained from the ventral approach to the external ear canal and tympanic bulla. Cranial is to the left of the images. A: Beginning with the transducer positioned just caudal to the zygomatic arch, slide the transducer ventrally and then rotate to a vertical (sagittal with respect to the head) orientation. The external ear canal (EC) is visible as a curved, bright, soft-tissue–air interface with reverberation and acoustic shadowing in the far field. The parotid salivary gland (P) is a triangular, hyperechoic structure caudal and superficial to the external ear canal. **B:** Moving medially from the external ear canal, the tympanic bulla (TB) is visible as a semicircular hyperechoic line. The far wall is not visible because of acoustic shadowing and reverberation. The mandible is superficial cranially (N) and is seen as acoustic shadowing. The digastricus muscle (D), mandibular salivary gland (M), and parotid salivary gland (P) are in the near field. The maxillary artery (arrowhead) is caudal to the bulla. **C:** Ultrasonographic and schematic images of the tympanic bulla in a cat. When imaged from a lateral approach (dorsal orientation with respect to the head), the tympanic bulla (TB) is located more superficially. The parotid salivary gland (P) is hypoechoic and located superficially and caudally to the bulla.

longitudinal position, the transducer can be rotated slightly to view the tympanic bulla and external ear canal in the same image.

The middle ear is imaged from the lateral and ventral positions. The lateral position is just ventral to the external ear canal, with the transducer positioned between the zygomatic arch and the wing of the atlas and directed medially in a dorsal plane. In this window, the parotid salivary gland is hypoechoic to the surrounding tissue and superficial to the tympanic bulla. The bulla itself is curvilinear, with internal gas associated with acoustic shadowing. The maxillary artery can be identified with Doppler ultrasound caudally and laterally to the tympanic bulla at the junction of the external ear canal and the bulla.

From the ventral approach, the mandibular salivary gland is visible in the near field, with the digastricus muscle imposed between it and the tympanic bulla (Figure 3.2). Mandibular lymph nodes may appear as hypoechoic structures at the caudal aspect of the bulla.

The tympanic bulla is composed of thin bone and is filled with air. The normal bulla wall appears as an echogenic curved line, and the air within it causes reverberation artifact and dirty shadowing deep to the bone margin. The bone is thin enough that the ultrasound beam penetrates it, and therefore within the bulla cavity the presence of soft tissue or fluid caused by a middle-ear disorder can be identified.

Salivary Glands

The mandibular salivary gland is easily visible caudal to the ramus of the mandible, and between the linguofacial and maxillary veins as they join to form the jugular vein (Figure 3.3). A portion of the sublingual salivary gland shares the capsule of the rostral portion of the mandibular salivary gland, but may not be distinguished as a separate entity. The parotid salivary gland is oriented vertically lateral to the external ear canal and dorsally and superficially to the mandibular salivary gland (Figure 3.2A).

In the parasagittal imaging plane, the mandibular salivary gland is caudal to the more hypoechoic digastricus muscle, with the medial retropharyngeal lymph node medial to it (Figure 3.4A). To image the mandibular salivary gland in a sagittal orientation, the transducer can be rotated slightly from the parasagittal plane relative to the head and neck. It is well defined and triangular or round, with a hyperechoic capsule

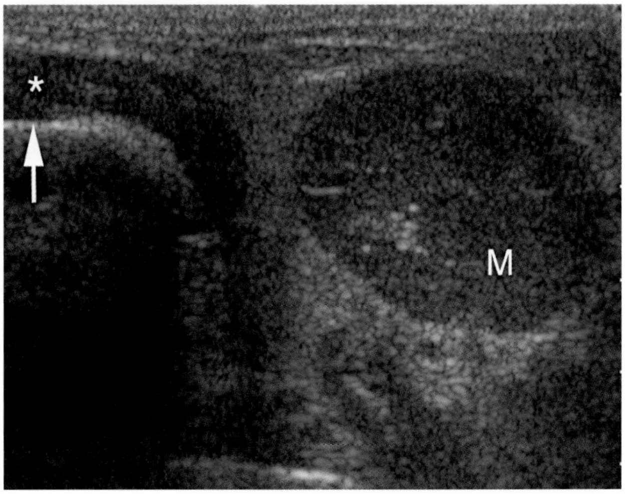

Figure 3.3. Normal mandibulary salivary gland in a dog. Parasagittal image taken with the transducer rotated slightly medially. Cranial is to the left of the image. The mandibular salivary gland (M) has a striated echotexture with a central linear echo. The digastricus muscle (asterisk) is the hypoechoic band overlying the mandible (arrow), which appears as a hyperechoic line with distal acoustic shadowing.

Figure 3.4. Images of the carotid artery and jugular vein of a normal dog. **A:** Sagittal image of the internal carotid artery (IC) and external carotid artery (EC) as they join to form the common carotid artery (CC). The mandibular salivary gland (M) is lateral to the origin of the common carotid artery and appears as a hypoechoic, lobular structure in the near field. The medial retropharyngeal lymph node (R) is between the mandibular salivary gland and the common carotid artery. The maxillary vein (MV) is caudal to the mandibular salivary gland. The common carotid artery has a distinct hyperechoic wall (arrowhead). **B:** At the caudal edge of the mandibular salivary gland, the maxillary vein (MV) and linguofacial vein (L) join to form the jugular vein (not shown). **C:** Sagittal image of the common carotid artery (CC) in the midcervical region. The artery has a thicker, more hyperechoic wall (arrow) compared with the jugular vein. **D:** The jugular vein (J), which is in the jugular furrow, has a much thinner wall than the common carotid artery and is easily compressed. **E:** Longitudinal image of the jugular vein by using color Doppler. Light transducer pressure must be used to avoid compressing the vessel. The color signal changes from blue to red as the blood flow passes perpendicular to the ultrasound beam. **F:** Pulsed-wave Doppler imaging of the jugular vein produces a smooth, laminar, low-velocity signal. **G:** Pulsed-wave Doppler of the carotid artery has distinct pulsatile flow with higher velocity. Note the characteristic arterial systolic peaks (arrow). The velocities are lower than actual velocities because no angle correction can be used.

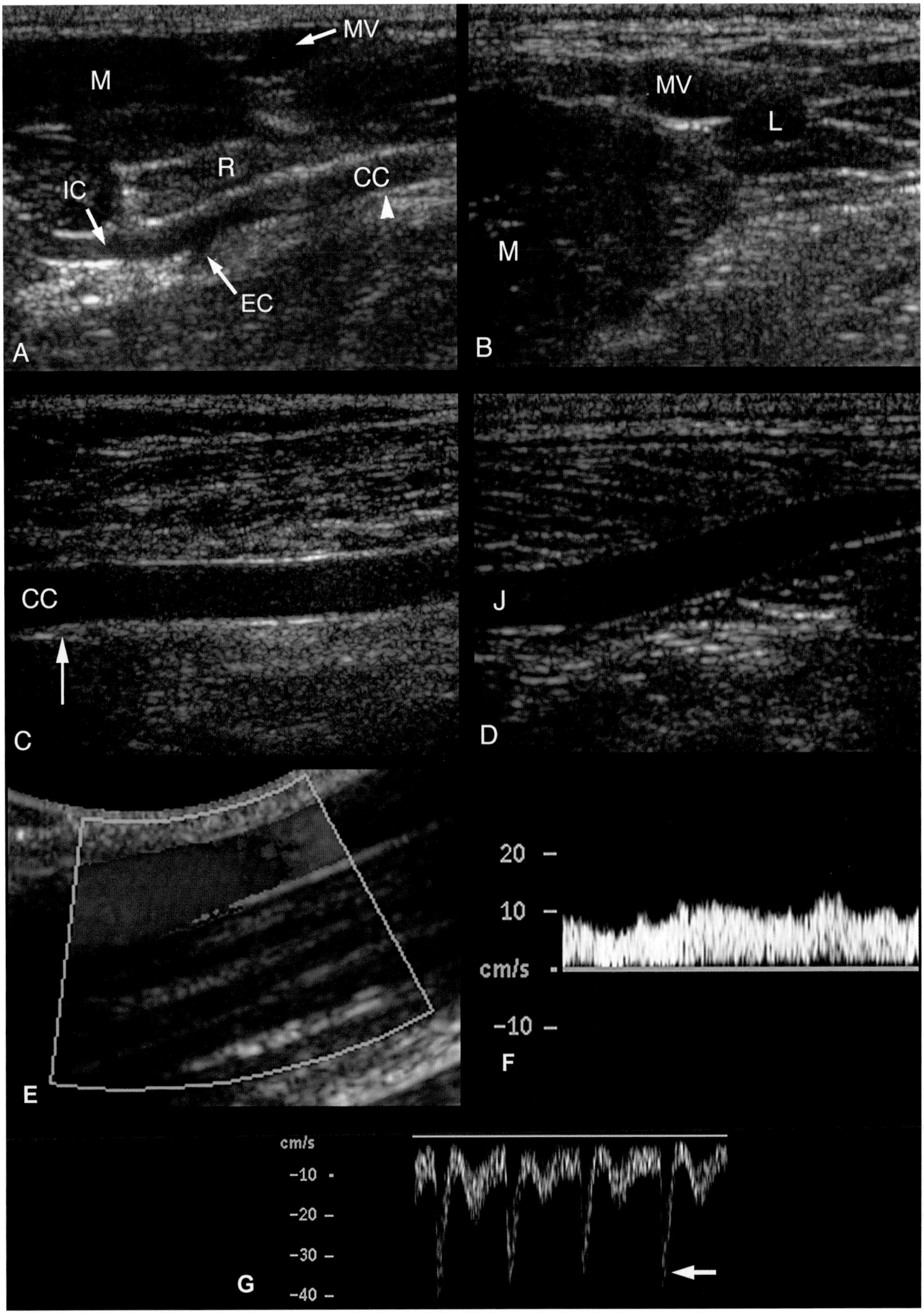

Figure 3.4.

and linear echogenic streaks within finely textured hypoechoic parenchyma (Figure 3.3).

Moving dorsally from the mandibular salivary gland by using a dorsal plane, the parotid salivary gland appears as a less-distinct, heterogeneous, and poorly marginated structure lateral or caudal to the curvilinear external ear canal.

Vessels and Nerves

The major neck vessels that can be seen with ultrasound are the jugular veins and their primary tributaries and the common carotid arteries and their major branches (Wisner et al. 1991). Other vessels, such as thyroid arteries and veins, are smaller and seen inconsistently. All of these structures are imaged in transverse or sagittal plane. Some may be seen from ventral midline, whereas others may be seen better with the transducer positioned lateral to midline. For the vascular structures and thyroid glands, the sagittal plane is obtained by orienting the transducer in a cranial to caudal direction and rotating the imaging plane 30°–45° medially.

The external jugular vein (Figure 3.4D and E) lies superficially within the jugular furrow. Cranially, the maxillary and linguofacial veins join to form the external jugular vein at the caudal aspect of the mandibular salivary gland (Figure 3.4B). The jugular vein is easily compressed, so very little transducer pressure should be used to image it. The transducer should be placed in the jugular furrow in a sagittal orientation and angled 45° toward midline. The wall of the jugular vein is thin, and the lumen is anechoic. With color Doppler or pulsed-wave Doppler ultrasound, a smooth, laminar flow is seen (Figure 3.4F). This is sometimes difficult to demonstrate because the Doppler signal is weakest when the vessel lies at nearly 90° to the beam. Slight angulation of the transducer in a caudal direction, as well as angle correction controls, will improve the Doppler image. Weak pulsatile flow referred from the carotid artery will be seen occasionally.

The common carotid artery is located in close association and parallel to the trachea. The artery has a thick, hyperechoic wall and anechoic lumen (Figure 3.4A and C), with a pulsatile Doppler waveform (Figure 3.4G). Each artery is located at the dorsolateral margin of the trachea, and the sternohyoid and sternothyroid muscles are located ventromedially to them. The sternocephalicus muscle lies between the common carotid artery and the more superficial jugular vein. The common carotid artery branches into the internal and external carotid arteries medial to the mandibular salivary gland. The external carotid artery continues in a straight line from the common carotid artery, whereas the internal carotid artery is slightly smaller in diameter and travels medially at a 30° angle (Figure 3.4A). The carotid bulb, a focal dilatation of the arterial lumen at the origin of the internal carotid artery, can be seen occasionally.

Using a high-frequency transducer (8–12 MHz), the vagosympathetic trunk is near the internal jugular vein and dorsal to the common carotid artery within the carotid sheath. In transverse orientation, the carotid sheath appears hyperechoic and encompasses the common carotid artery, vagosympathetic trunk, and internal jugular vein. The vagosympathetic trunk is dorsal to the common carotid artery and appears hypoechoic. It can be seen from the laryngeal region to the thoracic inlet, and no visible vascular structures are within it. The vagosympathetic trunk is approximately 1.2 ± 0.4 mm in diameter, which varies with the weight of the animal (Reese et al. 2001).

Lymph Nodes

Mandibular lymph nodes are small, oval or kidney-shaped structures located medially and caudally to the mandibular salivary glands and clustered around the jugular vein. These nodes are usually mildly hypoechoic to surrounding fat, although they can be isoechoic. There are usually 2–3 lymph nodes on each side. The medial and lateral retropharyngeal lymph nodes are dorsal to the pharynx and medial to the mandibular salivary gland (Figure 3.3). The medial retropharyngeal lymph node is larger than most other cervical lymph nodes and can be more than 0.5 cm in diameter and 2–4 cm long. The cranial portion of these nodes is typically wider than the caudal part, which is more fusiform. These occasionally appear as two to three closely associated nodes. Mandibular, retropharyngeal, and cranial cervical lymph nodes can be seen in normal dogs, depending on the size of the lymph nodes and the transducer frequency. The nodes are usually well defined, oval, and less than 0.5 cm in diameter. The superficial cervical lymph nodes, located in the lateroventral aspect of the caudal neck, are often paired and significantly larger than those in the cranial cervical region. These nodes can be found superficially in the prescapular region and slightly dorsal to the jugular furrow.

Tongue

The tongue is attached to the paired mylohyoid and geniohyoid muscles that are attached to the ramus of the mandible and the hyoid apparatus. The mylohyoid originates from the medial side of the mandible, and the geniohyoid from the ramus of the mandible. Both muscles attach to the basihyoid bone caudally. The tongue is hyperechoic to the supporting musculature (Figure 3.5).

Larynx

Just caudal to the tongue, the thyroid and cricoid cartilages have echogenic surfaces and produce acoustic shadowing in the far field. In sagittal orientation, the epiglottis is a short echogenic line parallel to the transducer surface and dorsal to the cranial portion of the thyroid cartilage. Its motion during swallowing assists its identification.

In transverse section, the arytenoid cartilages appear as a pair of echogenic lines oriented parallel to the transducer and within the thyroid cartilage near the lateral walls (Figure 3.6). Between the arytenoid cartilages and the true vocal folds are hypoechoic bands medial to the wall of the thyroid cartilage. These

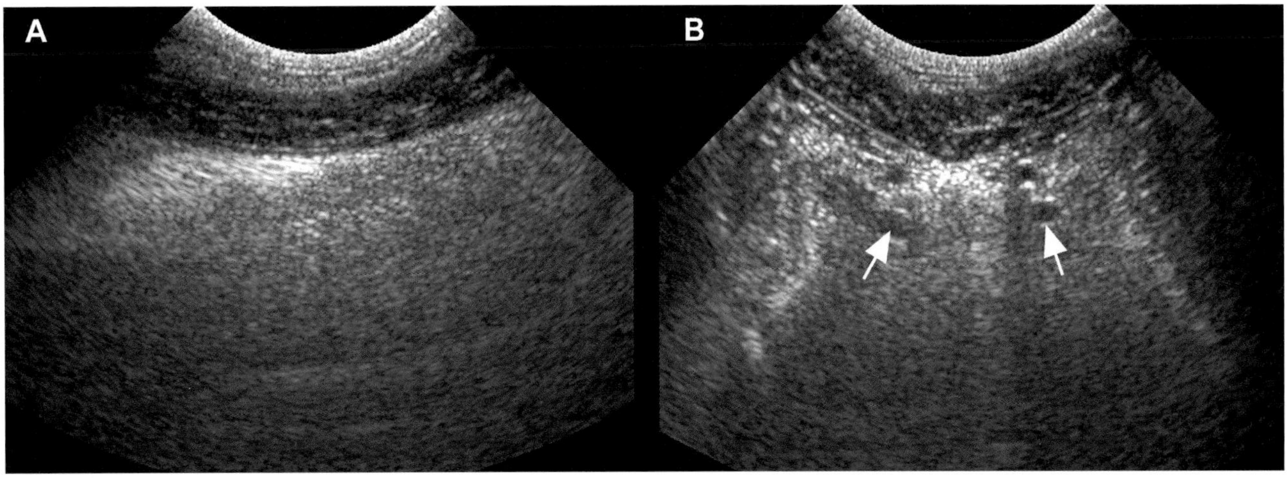

Figure 3.5. Transverse and parasagittal images of the canine tongue. **A:** The muscle of the tongue is hyperechoic to the more ventral geniohyoid and mylohyoid muscles. In parasagittal orientation, the fibers have a diagonal pattern. **B:** In transverse orientation, the round hypoechoic structures (arrows) represent the lingual and sublingual veins. The lingual muscles have a butterfly shape.

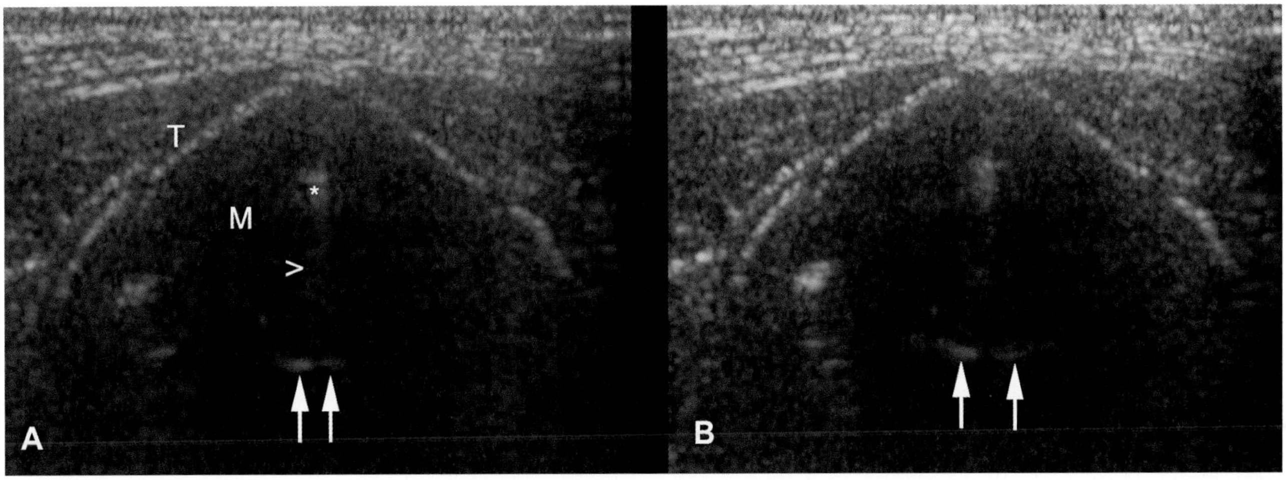

Figure 3.6. Normal larynx in a dog. **A:** Transverse image of the larynx taken through the thyroid cartilage at **expiration**. Ventral is at the top of the image, and the right side is on the left. The thyroid cartilage is visible as a hyperechoic V-shaped line (T). The rima glottis is the air-filled space (asterisk) between the hyperechoic vocal ligaments (>). Dorsal to the vocal ligaments, the cuneiform processes of the arytenoid cartilages appear as hyperechoic dots (arrows). The vocal muscles (M) are hypoechoic and fill the space between the ligaments and the thyroid cartilage on either side. **B:** Transverse image of the canine larynx taken during **inspiration**. The cuneiform processes move in abduction in inspiration and in adduction in expiration (compare with **A**).

represent the insertion of the aryepiglottic fold from the epiglottis on the ventral portion of the cuneiform process of the arytenoid cartilage and are called the false vocal folds.

Orienting the transducer transversely ventral to the thyroid cartilage shows the moving vocal folds. The transducer is then moved caudally to the junction of the thyroid and cricoid cartilages and directed cranially toward the vocal folds, which are attached to the vocal process of the arytenoid cartilage dorsally and the thyroid cartilage ventrally. The vocal folds consist of the vocal ligaments located craniomedially, and the vocal muscle continues laterally and caudally from it to join with the larynx. The vocal ligaments appear as vertical hyperechoic bands in the central larynx that contact each other in the ventral portion of the thyroid cartilage. The vocal processes of the arytenoid cartilage are hyperechoic lines that join with the vocal ligaments dorsally. The air-filled space between the vocal folds is the rima glottis. Mineralization of the laryngeal cartilages may hinder viewing of the vocal folds through the thyroid cartilages.

Normal motion of the vocal folds is abduction during inspiration and adduction during expiration. The cuneiform and vocal processes of the arytenoid cartilages also move in this manner. The motion may be more apparent when an animal is panting. Motion should be evaluated for symmetry, and overall motion is minimal in normal dogs.

Thyroid and Parathyroid Glands

The left and right thyroid lobes lie between the common carotid artery and the trachea and are often positioned at slightly different levels craniocaudally. To locate the thyroids, place the transducer in a transverse plane centered on the trachea just caudal to the larynx and move it caudally until triangular structures are seen between the trachea and carotid (Figure 3.7). Each thyroid may also be located separately by sliding the probe lateral to the trachea and by following the correspondent common carotid artery on cross section, which serves as an important landmark. Once a thyroid is located, rotate the transducer 90° to a sagittal plane, keeping the thyroid in the middle of the screen. This motion can be challenging because the thyroid gland is thin. The transducer may need to be angled medially from the jugular furrow to get the best sagittal plane (Figure 3.8A).

The thyroid is fusiform or ellipsoid in sagittal section, and round, oval, or triangular in transverse section. Thyroid glands in dogs are isoechoic to surrounding tissue, though a small percentage can be hypoechoic or hyperechoic. The glands are uniformly echogenic, though occasionally they have hyperechoic or hypoechoic foci or are diffusely mottled. Small vessels may sometimes be seen as anechoic structures coursing through the thyroid tissue, which can be confirmed with Doppler ultrasound. Both canine and feline thyroids can be imaged by using a 10- to 13-MHz transducer for best resolution. Cats may also occasionally have ectopic thyroid tissue located in the caudal cervical region or cranial mediastinum.

Thyroid volume can be estimated by measuring the length, width, and height of the gland, and using the formula $\pi/6$ (length × width × height) to calculate volume. The thyroid gland volume is correlated with body weight and body surface area more than with breed. There is more intraobserver variability in measuring the length of the glands because they taper caudally and the distal limit may be difficult to define (Table 3.1).

On average, there are four parathyroid glands located in each thyroid lobe, with two in each cranial and caudal pole. However, there is significant normal individual variation in both parathyroid numbers and distribution. Normal parathyroid glands are usually well margined, hypoechoic to anechoic, and less than 2 mm in diameter and 3.3 mm long (Reusch et al. 2000; Wisner et al. 2002) (Figure 3.8). All parathyroid glands are not always visible in normal dogs.

Trachea and Esophagus

Both structures contain air that causes reverberation artifacts and acoustic shadowing. However, their near walls (ventral and lateral) can be examined using ultrasound. The trachea has a hyperechoic, round to oval wall and travels in a sagittal plane. In a longitudinal view, the tracheal rings are visible (Figure 3.9A). In transverse view, in the midportion of the neck, the near wall is curved and echogenic, with distal acoustic shadowing obscuring the lumen (Figure 3.9B).

The esophagus is also sagittally oriented, but varies in position from dorsal to the trachea caudal to the larynx, to left of the trachea at the thoracic inlet. The lumen of the esophagus has a star shape in transverse orientation and contains a small amount of gas and mucus. In sagittal orientation, the muscularis layer is visible as a hypoechoic band superficially, and gas or fluid may be seen in the lumen (Figure 3.10A). If imaged obliquely, the folds of the mucosal surface appear as parallel hyperechoic bands (Figure 3.10B). The esophagus can be seen medial to the left common carotid artery and left thyroid gland.

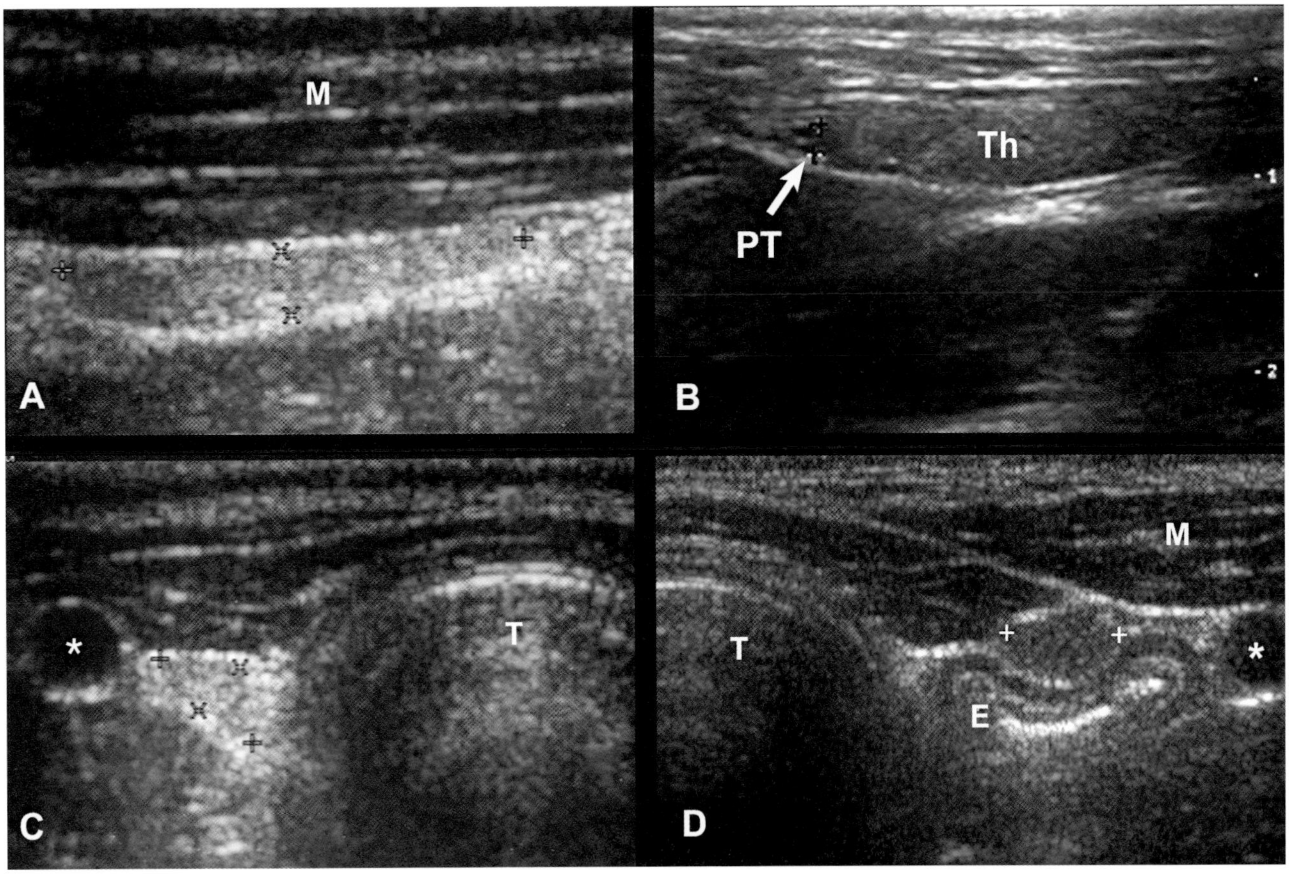

Figure 3.7. Normal thyroid glands in a dog. Sagittal **(A and B)** and transverse **(C and D)** images of normal thyroid glands. **A:** In sagittal orientation, the thyroid (cursors) is fusiform to elliptical and isoechoic or hyperechoic to the surrounding musculature (M). **B:** The normal cranial parathyroid gland (PT, between the cursors) is at the cranial extremity of the thyroid gland (Th). Image courtesy of D. Penninck. **C: Right thyroid gland.** In the transverse orientation, the thyroid is triangular and lies between the trachea (T) and common carotid artery (asterisk). **D: Left thyroid gland in another dog.** In transverse orientation, the left thyroid (between the cursors) is ventral or lateral to the esophagus (E), dorsal to the ventral musculature (M), and also between the trachea (T) and common carotid artery (asterisk).

Table 3.1.
Measurements of normal structures in the neck

Structure	Width/Diameter (mm)	Length (mm)	Height (mm)	Volume (mm^3)
Vagosympathetic trunk	1.2 ± 0.4			
Medial retropharyngeal lymph node	5	20–40		
Mandibular lymph node	<5			
Thyroid, feline (single lobe)				66–103
Left		20.5 (18.9–22.1)	3.3 (2.5–4.1)	89 (66–112)
Right		20.3 (18.7–21.9)	3.0 (2.4–3.6)	80 (61–99)
Cats (total volume)				124–215
Thyroid, canine				
Beagles	5.3 (3.3–7.3)	24.5 (20.4–28.5)	5.3 (3.3–7.3)	380
Akitas				63–1912
Golden retrievers				315–1580
Toy and miniature poodles				128–713
Parathyroid	<2	3.3 (2.0–4.6)		

Combined data from Wisner et al. (1991 and 1994), Reusch et al. (2000), Reese and Ruppert (2001), Taeymans et al. (2005), and Bromel et al. (2005).

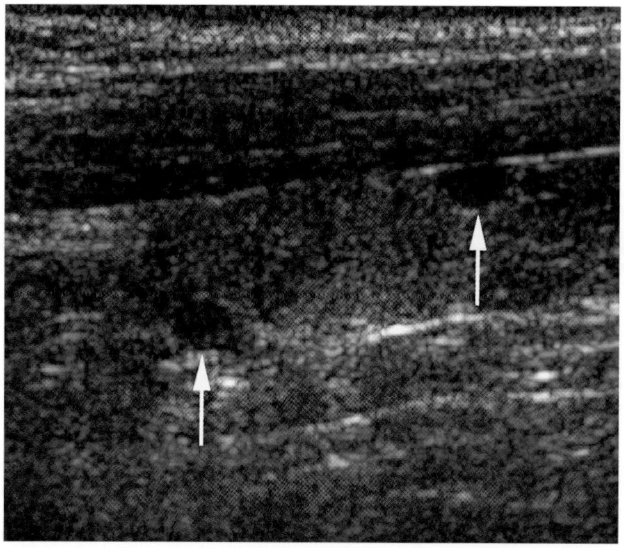

Figure 3.8. Normal parathyroid glands in a dog. Sagittal image of a normal thyroid. Two small, round, hypoechoic parathyroid glands (arrows) are visible in the cranial and caudal aspects of the thyroid lobe.

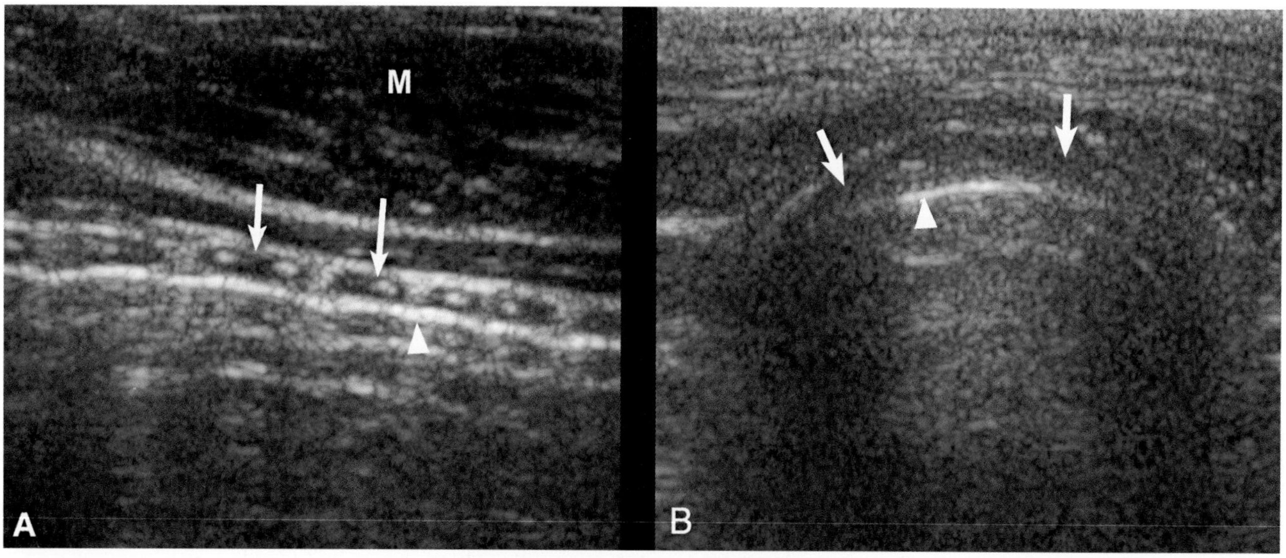

Figure 3.9. Normal trachea in a dog. **A: Sagittal plane.** The tracheal rings are visible in the sagittal plane as rectangular, hypoechoic structures (arrows) with central hyperechoic dots, dorsal to the hyperechoic air column (arrowhead). The air-tissue interface causes reverberation artifact in the far field, which appears as equally spaced and progressively less echogenic lines parallel to the original air interface. The hypoechoic ventral muscles (M) of the neck are in the near field. **B: Transverse plane.** The cartilage ring is visible as a curved hypoechoic band (arrows) with a thin, superficial, hyperechoic interface. The tracheal ring-air interface is hyperechoic (arrowhead). The tracheal lumen cannot be evaluated because of the presence of reverberation and shadowing.

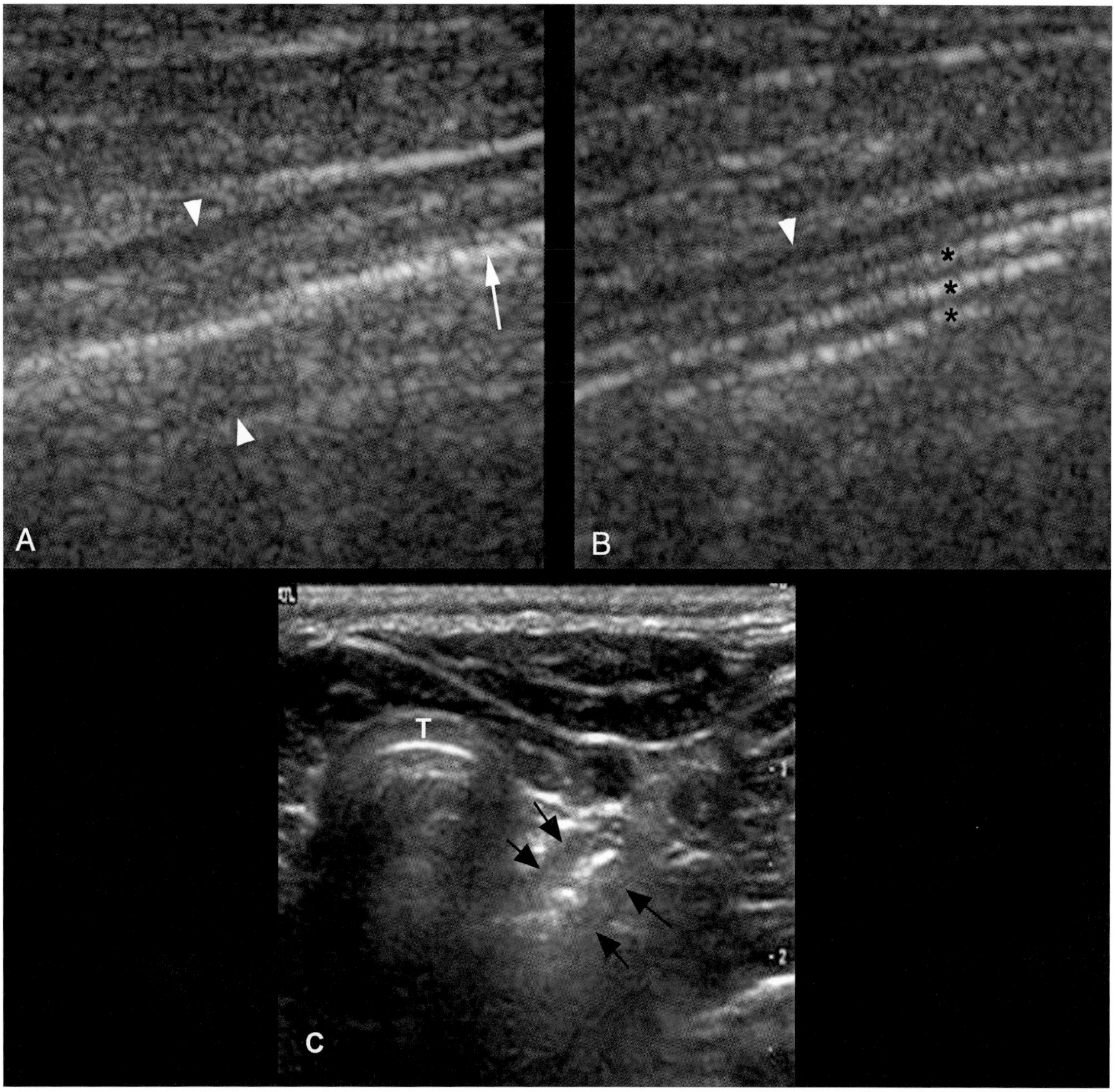

Figure 3.10. Normal esophagus of a dog. Cranial is to the left of the image. **A:** The muscularis layer is seen as a hypoechoic line (arrowheads) in the near and far fields. The small amount of mucus or gas in the lumen causes a hyperechoic appearance (arrow). **B:** If the esophagus is imaged at an oblique angle, the mucosal folds appear as multiple parallel hyperechoic lines (asterisk) deep to the mucosa (arrowhead). **C:** Transverse sonogram of the esophagus (arrows) in a normal dog. The presence of gas in the lumen prevents optimal visualization of the wall. T, trachea. Image courtesy of D. Penninck.

Sonographic Features of Neck Disorders

Bulla

Middle-ear disease is often characterized by the presence of fluid in the tympanic bulla. Fluid in the bulla appears hypoechoic, replacing the normal gas shadows. The transmission of the ultrasound beam through the fluid also renders the far wall of the bulla visible (Figure 3.11). If air and gas are present in the bulla, a dependent scanning position may be the most sensitive. Fluid can also be found incidentally as a transient bulla effusion rather than as a result of inflammatory or obstructive disease, so its presence should be correlated with clinical signs of middle-ear disease.

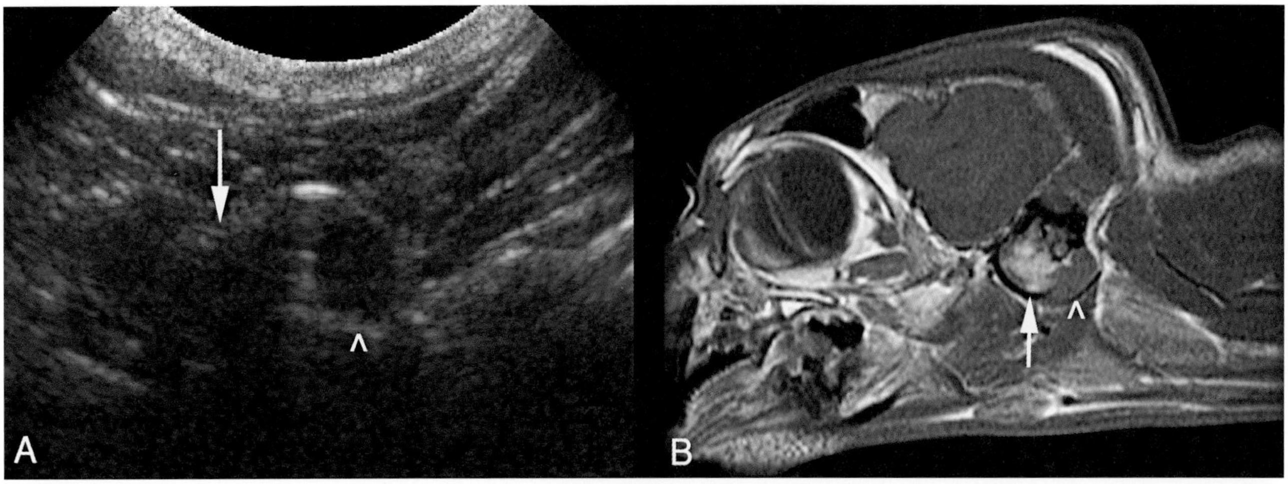

Figure 3.11. Otitis media in a cat. **A:** Sagittal image of the tympanic bulla. The sonogram is taken from the ventral position, with cranial to the left of the image. The ventromedial compartment of the bulla is filled with anechoic fluid, and the near wall is seen more clearly. The far wall (>) is also visible because the fluid has transmitted the ultrasound. The dorsolateral compartment (arrow) appears hypoechoic, and there is no reverberation artifact, suggesting soft-tissue content. **B:** Magnetic resonance T1-weighted postcontrast sagittal image of the tympanic bulla. The magnetic resonance image confirms the presence of fluid in the ventromedial compartment (>) and contrast-enhancing soft tissue in the dorsolateral compartment (arrow) of the tympanic bulla.

Tumors and inflammatory polyps cause soft-tissue filling of the bulla on computed tomographic and magnetic resonance images, but has not been reported with ultrasound imaging. Bulla thickness irregularity or alteration may indicate more severe ear disease such as neoplasia, osteomyelitis, or craniomandibular osteopathy.

Experimentally, a fluid-filled external ear canal improves the visualization of canal size and cartilage thickness. The tympanic membrane cannot be seen directly; however, if the ear canal is fluid filled and the bulla is air filled, the membrane is likely intact. If the membrane is ruptured, the bulla is also fluid filled.

Salivary Glands

Disorders that affect the salivary glands include true cyst, mucocele, sialolith, sialitis (Figure 3.12), sialocele (Figure 3.13), salivary duct cyst (Figure 3.14), and neoplasia.

Most of these conditions are rare in dogs and cats. Localization of the lesion is based on the anatomical site and surrounding landmarks. Common findings in inflammatory or obstructive disease include enlargement of the gland and/or salivary ducts and edema in the surrounding tissues. Cystic lesions, nodular lesions, and enlarged salivary glands can be aspirated to determine their origin.

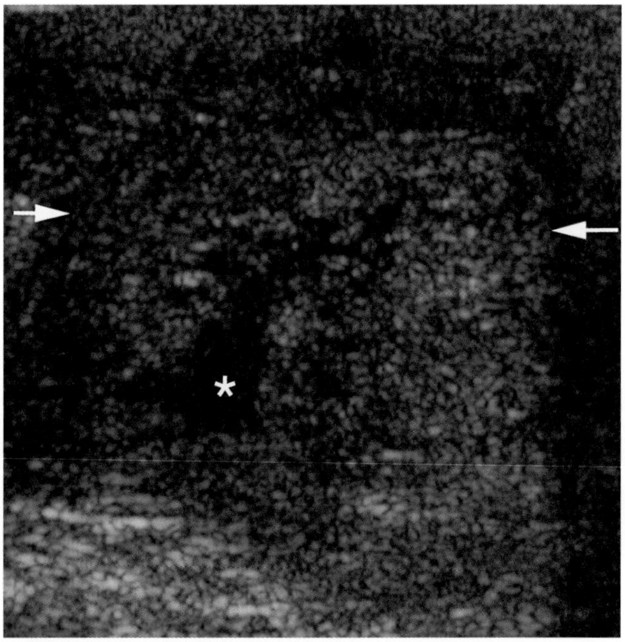

Figure 3.12. Lymphoplasmacytic sialoadenitis in a dog. On this sagittal image, the right mandibular gland is rounded, hypoechoic, and enlarged (arrows), and the salivary ducts are dilated (asterisk).

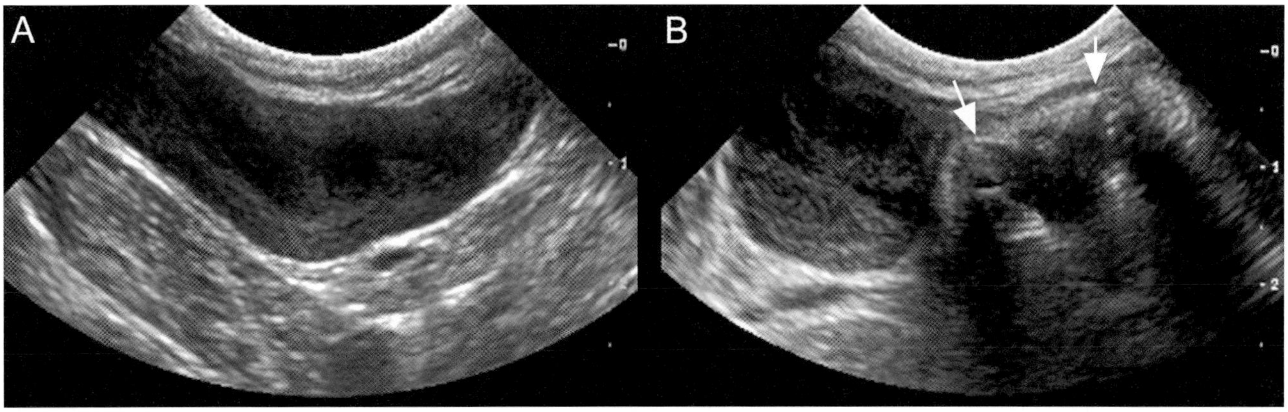

Figure 3.13. Sialocele in a 13-year-old Jack Russell terrier. **A:** A dilated mandibular and sublingual duct system is present. **B:** Transverse sonogram of the dilated duct filled with poorly echogenic fluid. The larynx (arrows) is near the dilated duct. A fine-needle aspirate confirmed the presence of saliva. Images courtesy of D. Penninck.

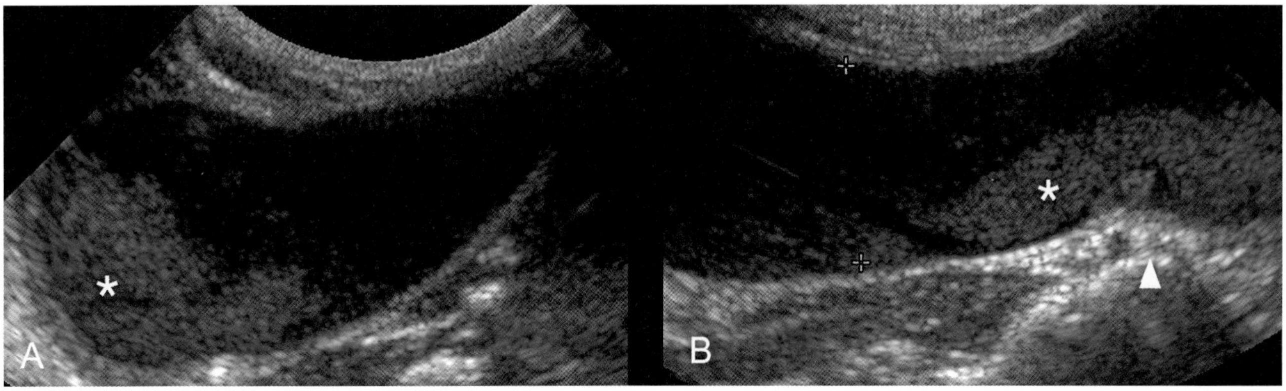

Figure 3.14. Salivary duct cyst in a cat. On these transverse **(A)** and sagittal **(B)** images, a well-demarcated fluid filled structure is ventral and lateral to the mandible (arrowhead). The cyst contains hyperechoic sedimenting debris (asterisk).

Vessels

Abnormalities involving the carotid artery and jugular veins may include thrombosis in hypercoagulable animals (e.g., hyperadrenocorticism and protein-losing nephropathy) and may be a complication of catheter placement. The acute thrombus may be anechoic and is recognized only by a flow void in the color Doppler signal. More chronically, the thrombus becomes more echogenic and visible in B-mode imaging. Stenosis of these vessels can occur as a complication of surgery, trauma, or invasive neoplasia. Stenosis appears as a narrowing of the vessel lumen, with increased velocity or turbulent flow.

Carotid-body tumors are rare neuroendocrine tumors that arise from the pressure sensors in the carotid artery. Older brachycephalic breeds may be predisposed to developing chemodectomas. Chronic hypoxia and overstimulation of the carotid bodies caused by brachycephalic syndrome may contribute to the increased prevalence of disease in these breeds. Other neuroendocrine tumors, such as thyroid tumors, may occur in conjunction with chemodectomas. On ultrasound examination, these tumors are located at the bifurcation of the common carotid artery into the internal and external carotid arteries. Tumors may surround the common carotid artery and its branches and are generally highly vascular. They are hypoechoic to surrounding tissues, lobulated, and well marginated (Wisner et al. 1994; Fife et al. 2003) (Figure 3.15). Fine-needle aspirates should be performed with caution, considering the vascularity and proximity of major vessels.

Any invasive tumor, such as thyroid carcinoma, can cause local distortion of vasculature. Invasion of the common carotid artery can cause erosion of the

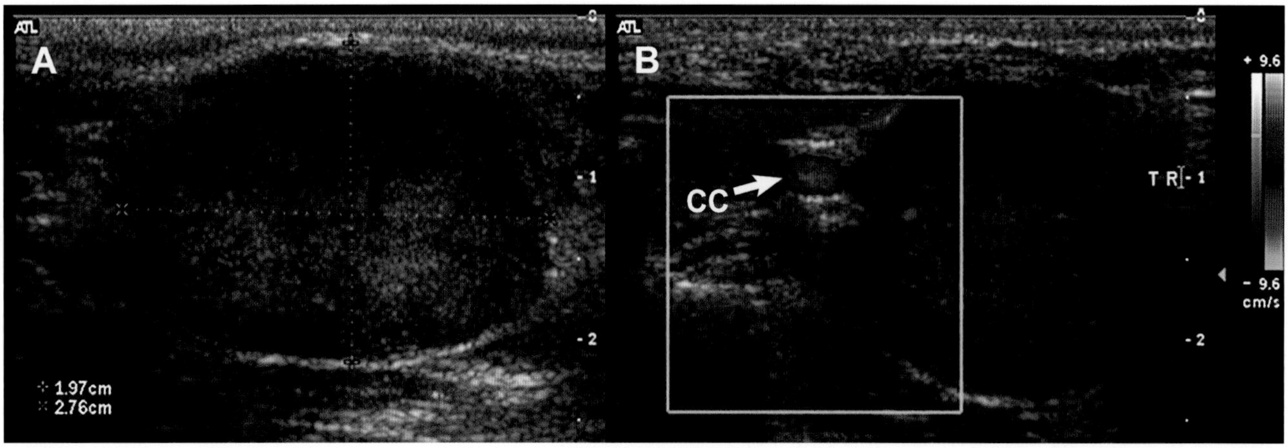

Figure 3.15. Chemodectoma in a 12-year-old dog. Sagittal B-mode **(A)** and transverse color Doppler **(B)** ultrasound images of a mass found in the neck. A smooth, well-circumscribed, hypoechoic mass is noted at the medial aspect of the right common carotid artery (CC). Initially the mass was suspected to originate from the thyroid gland. At surgery, the thyroid glands were normal. Images courtesy of M.A. d'Anjou.

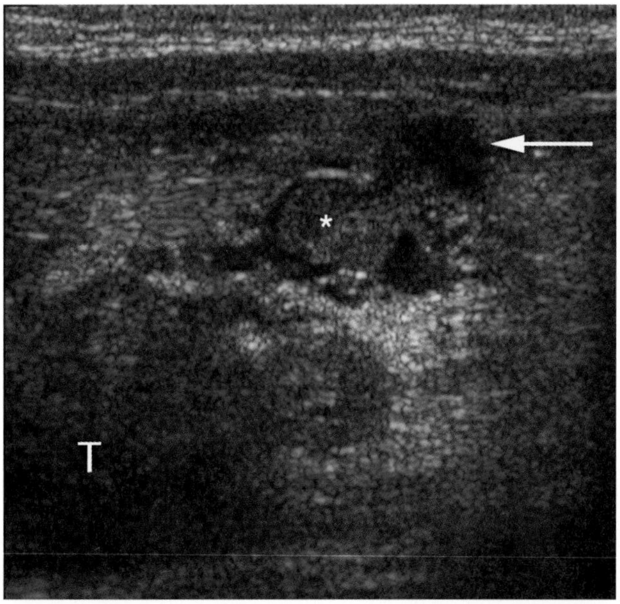

Figure 3.16. Venous invasion and thrombosis in a dog. Transverse image of the thyroid with thyroid carcinoma. A large, ill-defined, hypoechoic mass (T) has replaced the thyroid gland. The mass had invaded the thyroid vein, with a tumor thrombus occupying most of the lumen (asterisk). The tumor thrombus continued into the jugular vein (arrow).

wall and massive hemorrhage (Slensky et al. 2003). Local vessels may be infiltrated by the neoplasia (Figure 3.16), recruited into the tumor, compressed, or thrombosed. Other small vessels may also distend to supply the mass. Tumors of the caudal neck and thoracic inlet may also invade local vessels or cause thrombosis. If the cranial vena cava is thrombosed, distended, or occluded, veins may be seen more cranially. Obstruction of venous flow may also cause subcutaneous edema of the head and neck.

Arteriovenous fistula in association with a recurrent thyroid carcinoma has been reported in the neck (Wisner et al. 1994). These abnormal connections between the arterial system and the venous system often have multiple tortuous vessels with arterial flow characteristics. The local veins may be distended, and left heart failure can occur.

Cervical masses such as lymphoma and thyroid carcinoma may also involve the vagosympathetic trunk, causing Horner's syndrome (Melian et al. 1996) and laryngeal paralysis (Schaer et al. 1979). There is also a single report of a neoplastic mass originating from the vagus nerve (Ruppert et al. 2000).

Lymph Nodes and Soft Tissues

Enlarged mandibular, retropharyngeal, or cervical lymph nodes may be caused by local inflammation, tumoral infiltration, or regional metastatic disease. Tumors of the mouth often metastasize to the mandibular lymph nodes. Lymph nodes affected by inflammatory disease (Figure 3.17) or neoplastic disease are enlarged, rounded, and hypoechoic. The margins of the lymph nodes can be indistinct if there is local inflammation.

Cavitation can also occur in reactive nodes because of abscessation and in metastatic nodes because of

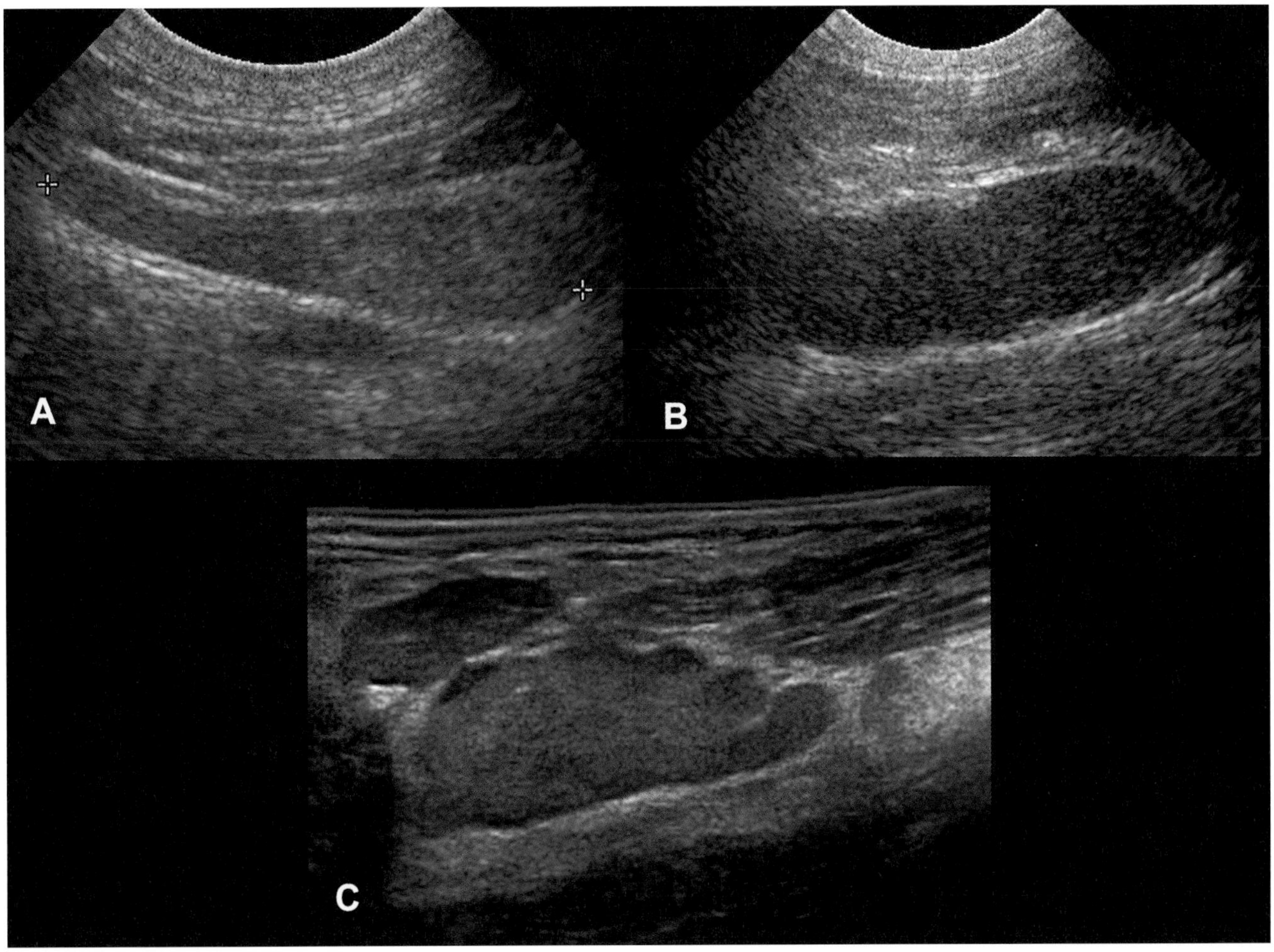

Figure 3.17. Mandibular lymphadenopathy in a dog. **A:** Sagittal image of the normal left mandibular lymph node (cursors). It is oval and is slightly hypoechoic to the surrounding tissues. **B:** The right mandibular lymph node is reactive. It is hypoechoic and rounded compared with the left, with a margin that is homogeneous in echotexture and slightly irregular. **C:** Sagittal image of enlarged mandibular lymph nodes with pyogranulomatous lymphadenitis and cellulitis. The lymph nodes are slightly inhomogeneous and have irregular contours. Image C courtesy of D. Penninck.

hemorrhage and necrosis. Metastatic lymph nodes can also be hypoechoic or heterogeneous without enlargement. They tend to become rounder and thicker from their normal oval or elongated shape. Reactive and metastatic lymph nodes appear very similar, and fine-needle aspiration is generally needed for a diagnosis.

Lymphoma causes generalized peripheral lymphadenopathy in dogs, but rarely in cats. Affected lymph nodes of the head and neck are enlarged and hypoechoic. The nodes may have indistinct margins and disrupted internal architecture. In dogs with lymphoma, the cervical and mandibular lymph nodes enlarge to a lesser degree than the retropharyngeal lymph nodes (Figure 3.18A). These hypoechoic lymph nodes may also have distal acoustic enhancement and be surrounded by slightly hyperechoic tissue (Figure 3.18B). The distal enhancement can cause the nodes to be confused with anechoic cysts.

Other cervical masses that are nonlymphoid, thyroid, or parathyroid in origin, such as lipomas, hemangiosarcomas, fibrosarcomas, hematomas, and abscesses. Masses in the neck can appear solid, cystic, or complex (Gooding et al. 1977). Neoplastic masses are usually solid or complex, and hematomas are complex or cystic. Acutely, hematomas appear as hypoechoic masses with a hypoechoic center. With time, septations can develop, echogenicity increases, and a capsule may form (Wisner et al. 2002). Hematomas should become smaller with time. Lipomas are usually well marginated, are elliptical, and are striated and

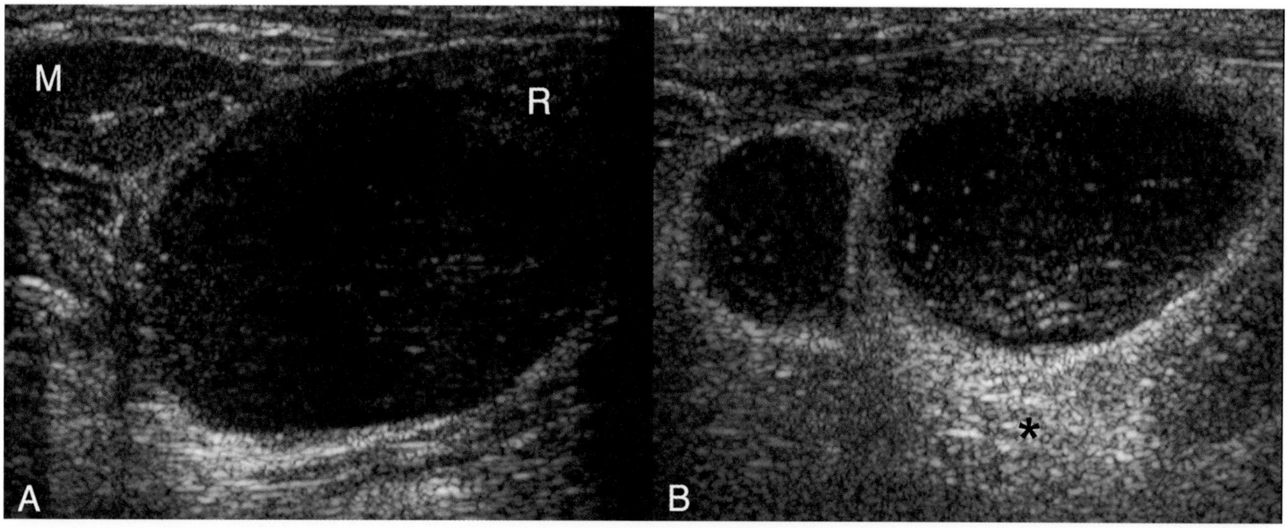

Figure 3.18. Sonograms of the neck of a dog with lymphoma. Cranial is to the left of the image. **A:** The medial retropharyngeal lymph node (R) is markedly enlarged, rounded, and hypoechoic. It is medial to the normal mandibular salivary gland (M) and many times its size. **B:** The paired superficial cervical lymph nodes are also markedly enlarged and are not normally seen. They are rounded, with a hypoechoic, speckled echotexture. There is also distal acoustic enhancement deep to the lymph nodes (asterisk). The tissues surrounding the lymph nodes are hyperechoic, indicating inflammation or edema.

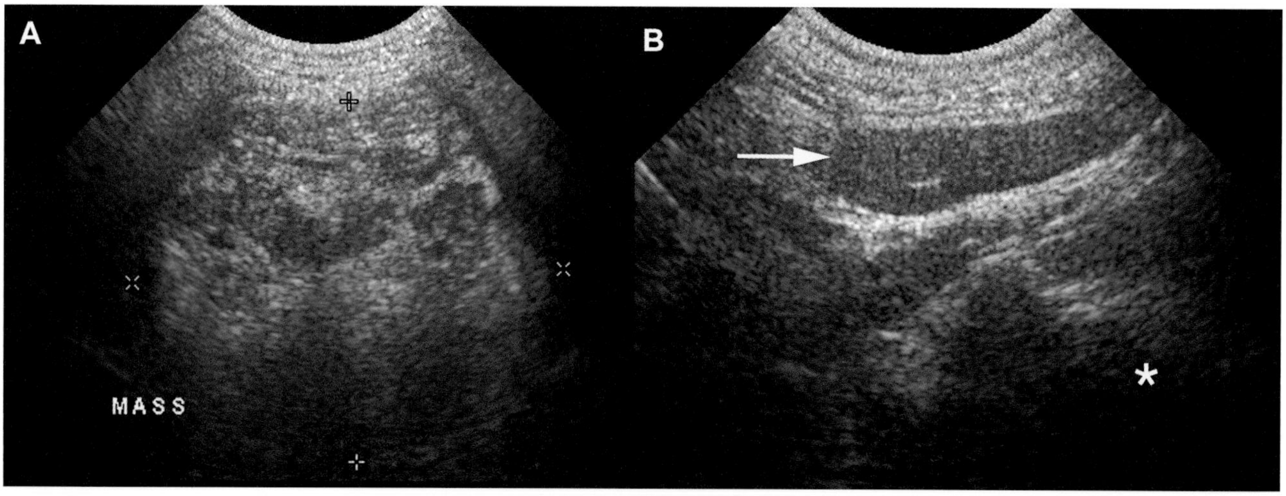

Figure 3.19. Intermandibular cellulitis in a dog. **A:** Transverse image taken between the mandibles from a ventral position. A large, heterogeneous mass is in the soft tissues of the neck (cursors). The margin is hypoechoic, which suggests edema, and the mass is attenuating, with decreased signal in the far field. **B:** In this more cranial image, an enlarged, hypoechoic reactive lymph node (arrow) is superficial to the mass (asterisk).

hyperechoic to surrounding musculature. However, lipomas can be infiltrative and poorly defined. Interfascial planes or muscles can be infiltrated.

Penetrating wounds from the skin or esophagus, with or without foreign bodies, may cause diffuse or localized cellulitis of the soft tissues of the neck (Figures 3.19–3.22). Edema can be seen dissecting between fascial planes or within the subcutaneous fat as anechoic or hypoechoic areas separated by thin hyperechoic septa (Figure 3.20C). Inflamed fatty tissues are often thickened, hyperechoic, and hyperattenuating (Figure 3.20D). Abscesses are often septated, with a thick wall and echogenic fluid contents (Figure 3.22). Cystic lesions are rare and usually thyroid or branchial in origin (Wisner et al. 2002). Foreign bodies can be challenging to identify. Their detection is greatly influenced by the their acoustic characteristics and by their size, location, and shape (Figure 3.21).

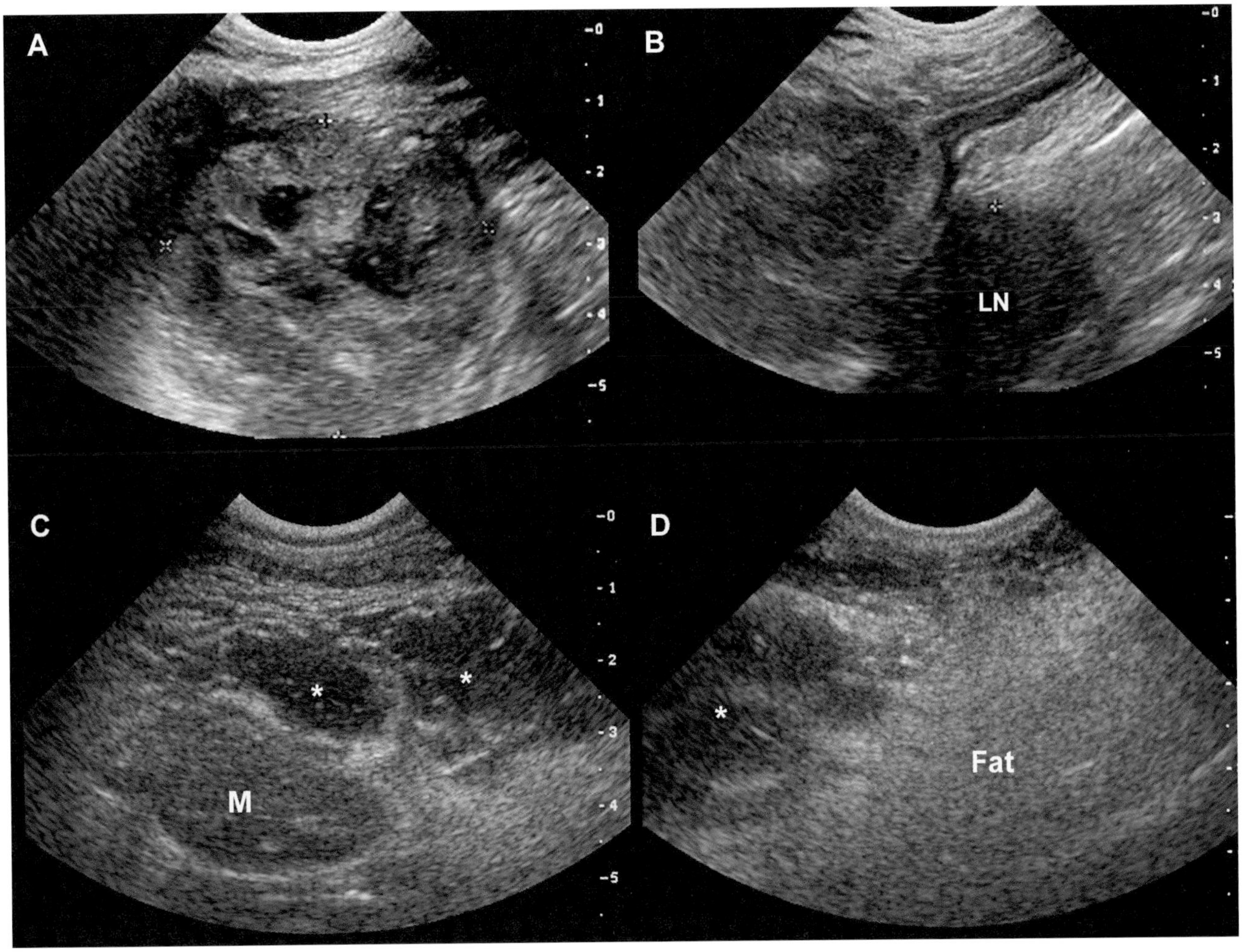

Figure 3.20. Septic suppurative cellulitis and abscess formation in two dogs. **A and B:** Sagittal images of the cranioventral neck in an 11-year-old Irish setter, on which a multicavitated mass measuring about 4.5 × 6 cm is caudoventral to the larynx. A local lymph node is enlarged and hypoechoic (LN). Images courtesy of D. Penninck. **C and D:** Sagittal images obtained in another large-breed dog with a history of neck pain and swelling and inappetance. The subcutaneous fat is swollen and presents several hypoechoic, septated cavities (*) located caudal to one of the mandibular (M) salivary glands. The neighboring fat is hyperechoic and hyperattenuating. The presence of serohemorrhagic fluid and pus was confirmed by fine-needle aspirations. Images courtesy of M.A. d'Anjou.

Larynx

Neoplasia (Figure 3.23), trauma (Figure 3.24), inflammation (Figure 3.25), and cysts can affect the larynx and paralaryngeal structures. The most common neoplasia of the larynx in cats is lymphoma, and in dogs is malignant epithelial neoplasia (Carlisle et al. 1991). These tumors can appear as masses in the laryngeal wall and may also distort or obliterate the normal laryngeal structures. Lymphoma in cats appears as a well-circumscribed, hypoechoic or mixed echogenic mass arising from the ventral or lateral larynx. The mass may narrow the lumen of the larynx or displace the larynx to the side. Squamous cell carcinoma may appear more destructive and occurs in the ventral larynx, as well as on the vocal cords. Laryngeal cysts have been reported infrequently in dogs and cats and may originate from the epiglottis, laryngeal wall, or paralaryngeal tissues. They are seen as anechoic masses distorting the rima glottides.

Laryngeal paralysis, which is a neuropathy of the recurrent laryngeal nerve, causes unilateral or bilateral paralysis of the vocal folds. Ultrasound can be used to evaluate the motion of the vocal folds and cuneiform cartilages to diagnose the condition. The criterion for diagnosing laryngeal paralysis is reduced or asymmetrical motion of the vocal folds. This appears as lack of abduction of the cuneiform cartilages and vocal folds during inspiration on one or both sides

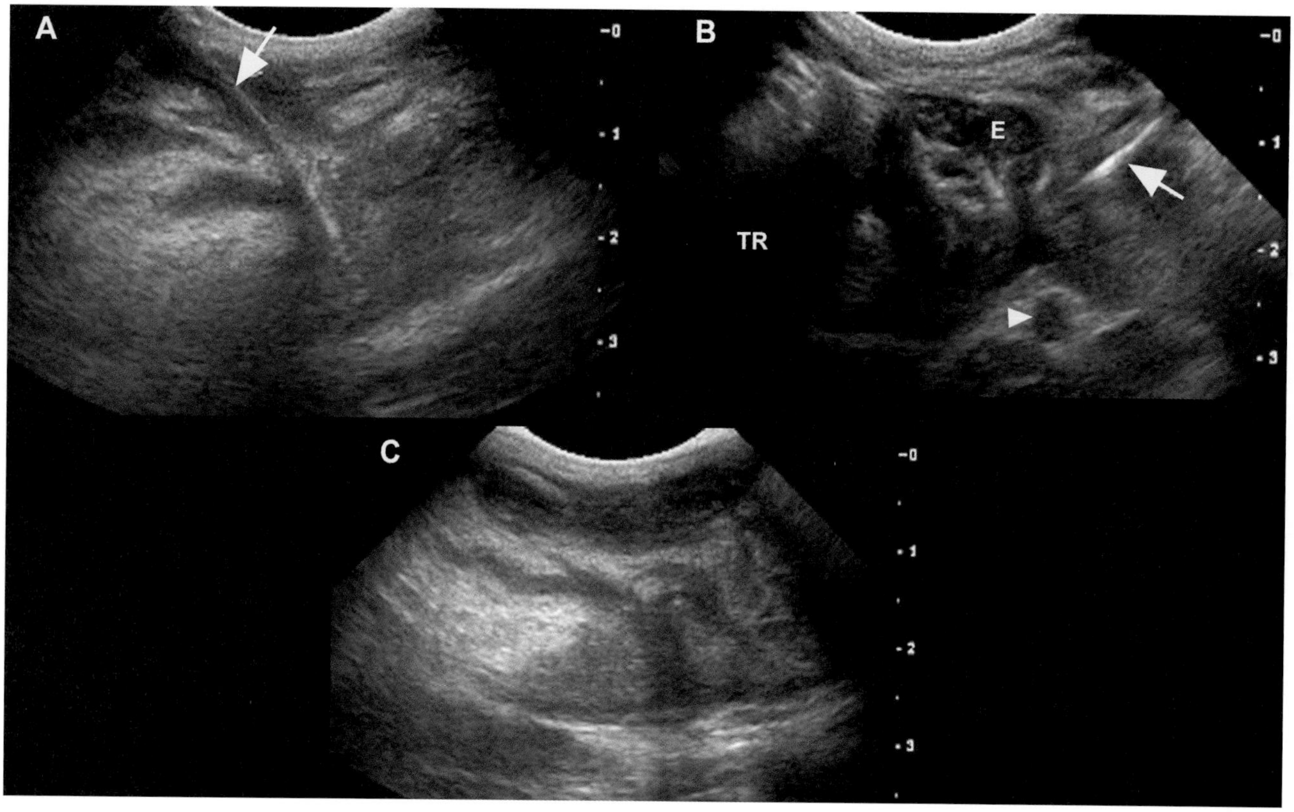

Figure 3.21. Sewing needle and associated cellulitis in a dog. **A:** The needle (arrow) appears as a discrete hyperechoic line surrounded by a poorly marginated hypoechoic area representing extensive cellulitis and edema. **B:** The needle tip (arrow) is close to the esophagus (E) and the carotid artery (arrowhead). TR, trachea. **C:** Hypoechoic arborization through the superficial and deep cervical soft tissue is noted and is often seen in abscess formation, dissecting cellulitis, and edema. Images courtesy of D. Penninck.

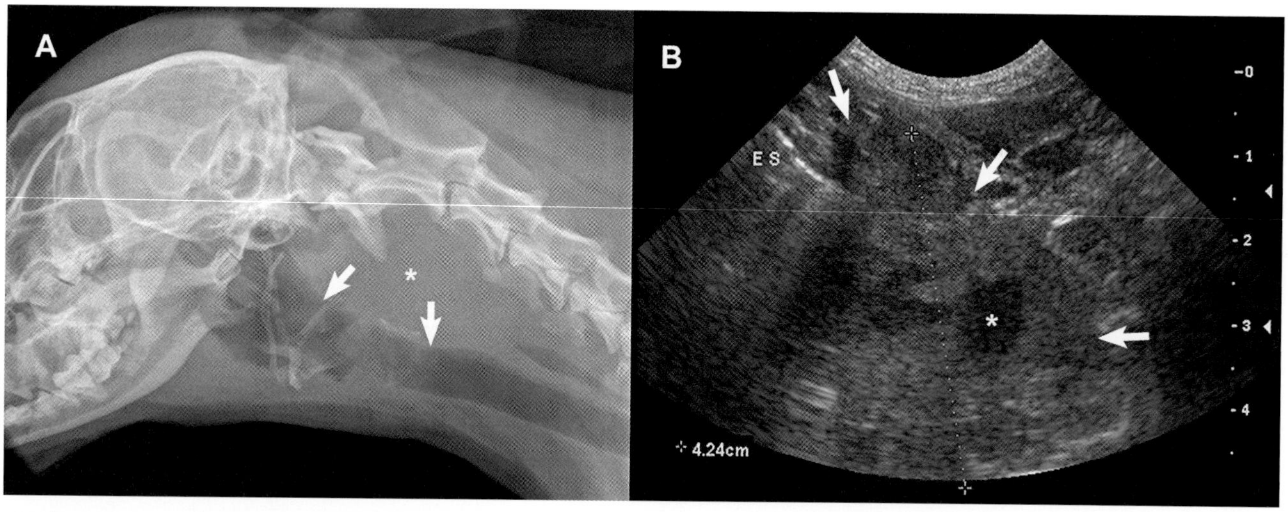

Figure 3.22. Retropharyngeal abscess in a dog. **A:** Lateral oblique radiograph of the head and neck of a dog with a history of difficulties in swallowing and of neck pain. A soft-tissue mass effect (asterisk) is in the retropharyngeal region, causing ventral displacement of the nasopharynx, larynx, and trachea (arrows). **B:** Transverse sonogram in the region of the mass. A large, irregular, moderately echogenic mass (arrows) is lateral and caudal to the esophagus (ES). This mass has a thick wall encircling an irregular cavity filled with echogenic fluid. Fine-needle aspirations and surgical biopsies confirmed the presence of a sterile, pyogranulomatous abscess of uncertain origin. Images courtesy of M.A. d'Anjou.

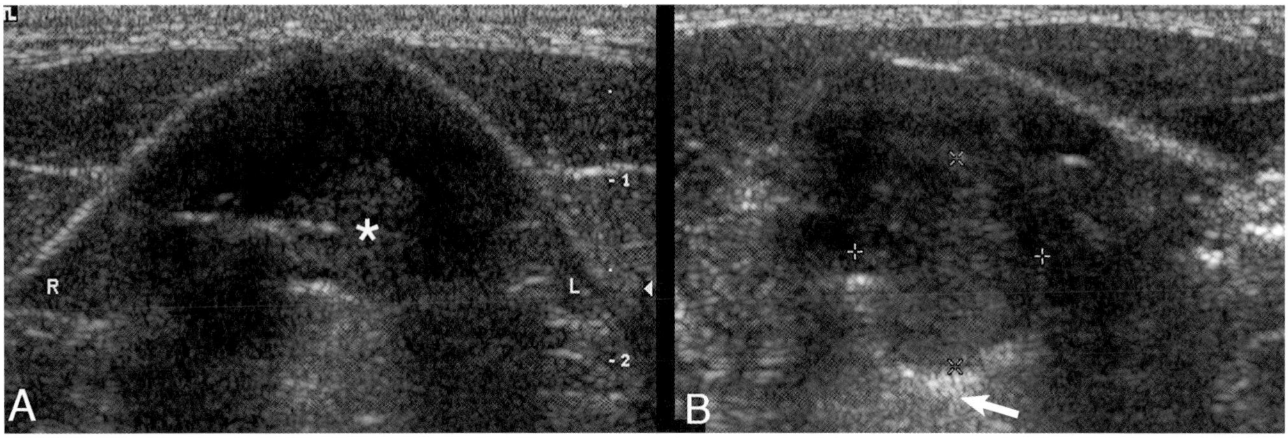

Figure 3.23. Laryngeal melanoma in a dog. **A:** Transverse image of the larynx through the thyroid cartilage. An ill-defined soft tissue mass (asterisk) is within the left side of the lumen of the larynx. **B:** In left sagittal orientation, the mass is better delineated originating from the left laryngeal wall (cursors). Cranial is to the left side of the image. Hyperechoic reverberating artifact caused by the soft-tissue–air interface is in the far field (arrow).

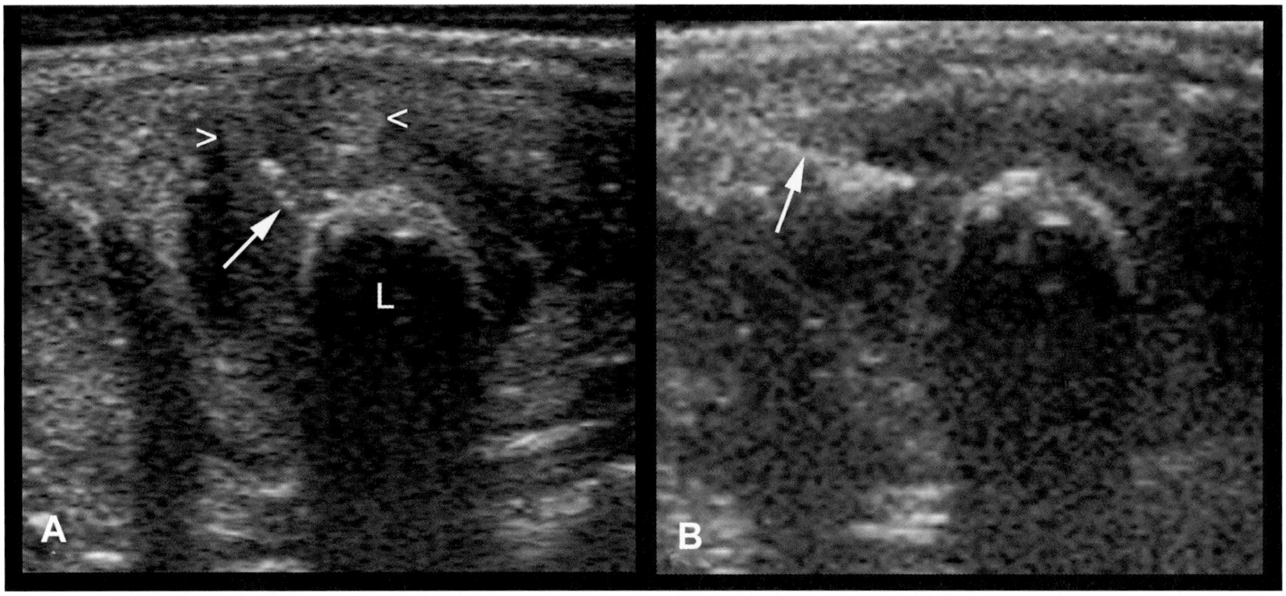

Figure 3.24. Penetrating laryngeal foreign body in a dog. **A:** On this transverse image, the air-filled larynx is visible as an anechoic acoustic shadowing artifact (L). There is a hyperechoic linear structure (arrow) exiting the larynx at a ventrolateral oblique angle. The tissues surrounding this foreign body are distorted (between the carets). **B:** The foreign body (arrow) can be followed from the larynx to the right ventral neck.

(Figure 3.26). Approximately 50% of dogs with laryngeal paralysis have abnormal dorsal and ventral movement of the arytenoid cartilages that is caused by the unaffected contraction of the cricothyroid muscle (Rudorf et al. 2001). Signs of severe upper-airway obstruction include collapse of the pharynx during inspiration, paradoxical movement of the vocal folds (blowing laterally during expiration), and caudal displacement of the whole larynx.

Laryngeal paralysis and vocal cord thickening have been reported in cats. Vocal cord thickening can be caused by inflammation, edema, or neoplasia. The anatomy and motion of the cuneiform cartilage are similar to those of dogs, but the smaller size of the feline larynx may cause incomplete visibility of the vocal folds.

Thyroid Glands

Hyperthyroidism caused by functional thyroid adenoma or adenomatous hyperplasia is very common in older cats (Mooney 2002). This can manifest as a

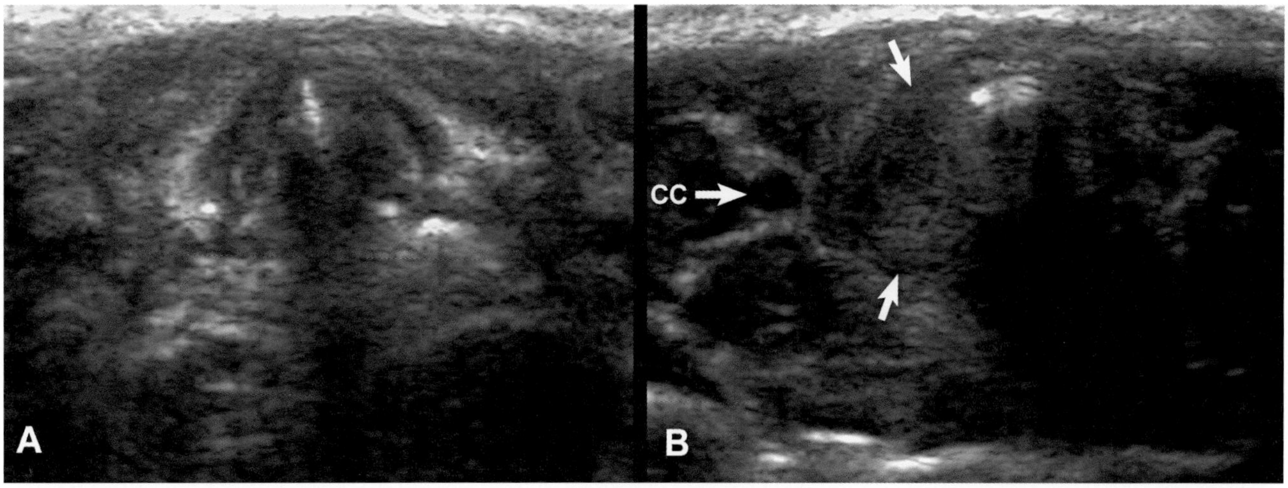

Figure 3.25. Lymphofollicular laryngitis in a cat. **A:** Transverse image of the larynx with the right side on the left of the image. The vocal folds appear normal at this level. **B:** Just caudal to the vocal folds is a lobulated, hypoechoic mass (arrows) involving the right side of the larynx and trachea. CC points to the common carotid artery.

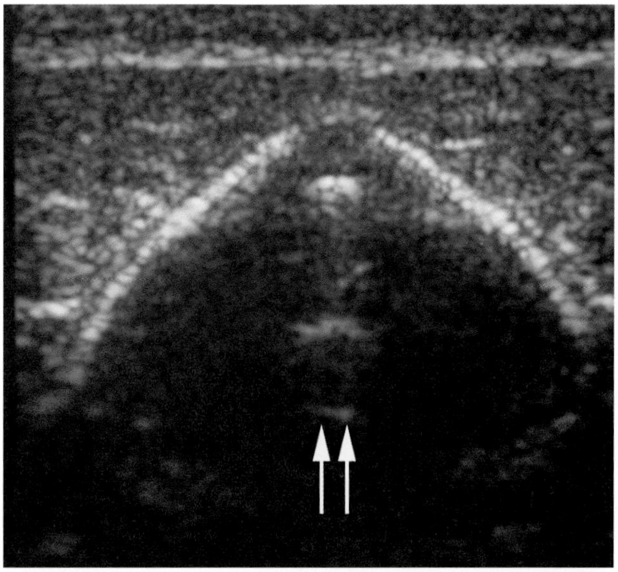

Figure 3.26. Laryngeal paralysis in a dog. The cuneiform processes of the arytenoid cartilage (arrows) fail to abduct during inspiration.

discrete nodule within the thyroid gland or as diffuse thyroid enlargement. Ultrasound can be used to measure the volume of the thyroid glands to detect enlargement. Although this is not a functional test as is nuclear scintigraphy, enlarged glands are indicative of thyroid disease. Both thyroid lobes are affected in 70% of cats (Mooney 2002).

Hyperplastic thyroid glands are hypoechoic or isoechoic to surrounding tissue and hypoechoic to normal thyroids. In thyroid adenomas, the glands can be focally or diffusely affected, often with a lobular margin and tubular shape (Figure 3.27B).

Thyroid glands occasionally contain cysts with distal acoustic enhancement. These cysts can be confused with normal parathyroid glands, which can also appear hypoechoic or anechoic. The cyst may be irregular in shape, but its margin should be visible in both planes. Thyroid and parathyroid neoplasia, such as thyroid cystadenoma and parathyroid adenocarcinoma, can also appear cystic (Phillips et al. 2003) (Figure 3.27A and C). Thyroid glands that cannot be identified on ultrasound are rarely hyperfunctioning, so cats with unilateral thyroid hyperplasia may only have one visible lobe.

Dogs are more often affected by hypothyroidism. On ultrasound examination in one study, hypothyroid lobes were more rounded on transverse imaging rather than their normal triangular shape (Reese et al. 2005). However, a further study of normal dogs revealed many with a similar transverse shape, making the earlier observation nonspecific. Hypothyroid lobes are also hypoechoic and smaller than normal lobes (Figure 3.28). They may be heterogeneous in echotexture and have an irregularly shaped capsule (Bromel et al. 2005).

Thyroid carcinoma is a rare but aggressive neoplasia that affects dogs and cats. It often presents at an advanced stage, with the mass involving a large area of the ventral cervical region and distorting local anatomy. This may make localizing the origin of the mass to the thyroid difficult. On ultrasound examination, the mass appears heterogeneous and hypoechoic to normal thyroid tissue, with good to poor margination (Figure 3.29). The trachea and esophagus may be displaced ventrally and laterally, and the enlarging

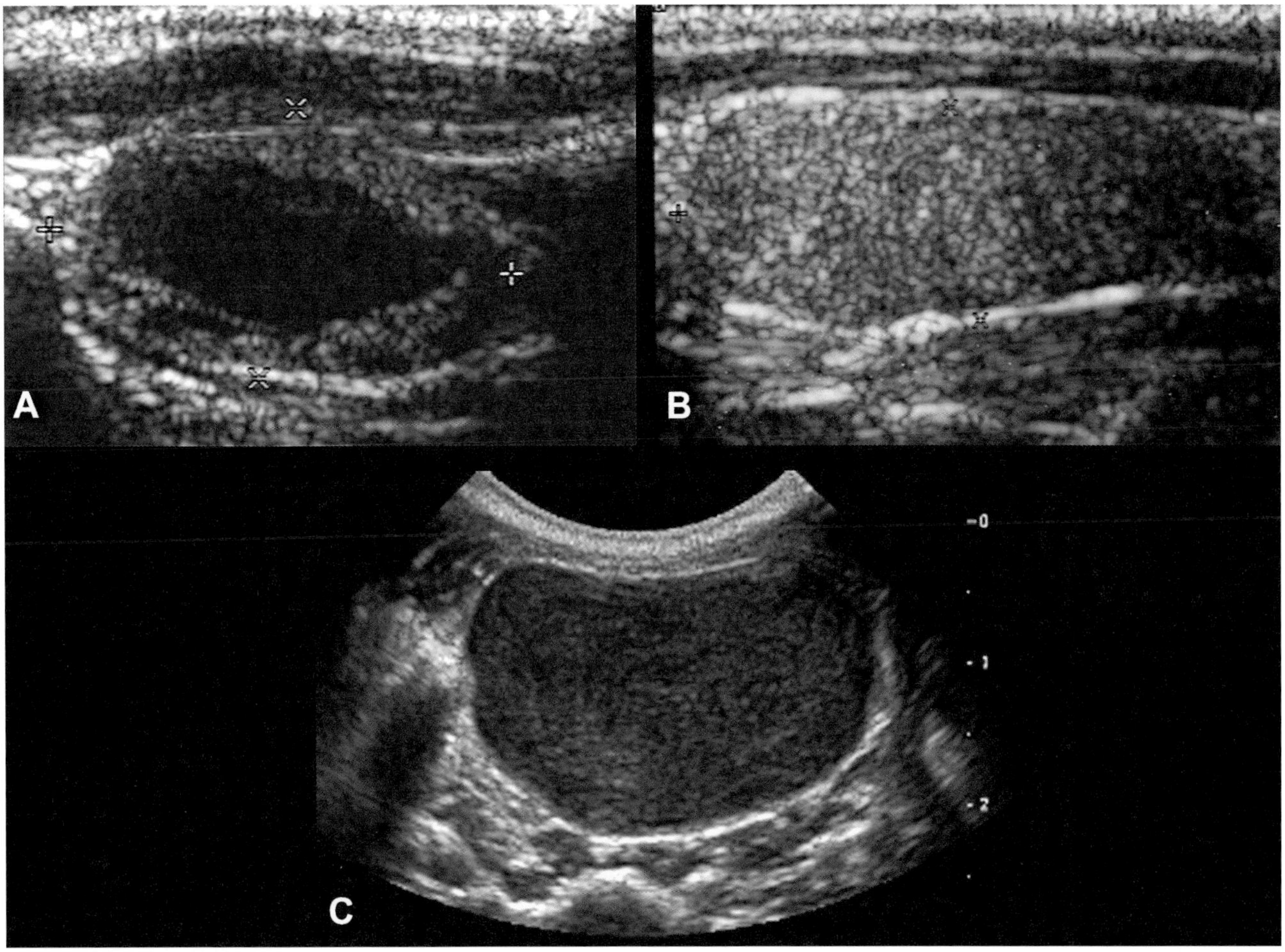

Figure 3.27. Thyroid adenoma in cats. **A:** Transverse image of the right thyroid with a cystic thyroid adenoma. The thyroid lobe is outlined by cursors, and the center is filled with anechoic fluid. **B:** Sagittal image of the right thyroid with thyroid adenoma. The thyroid lobe is outlined by cursors. The gland is enlarged and rounded, with an irregular border, and is isoechoic to surrounding tissue. **C:** Sagittal image of a thyroid cystic adenoma in a 16-year-old Burmese cat. The lesion is primarily cystic but filled with echogenic fluid mimicking a solid mass. Image C courtesy of D. Penninck.

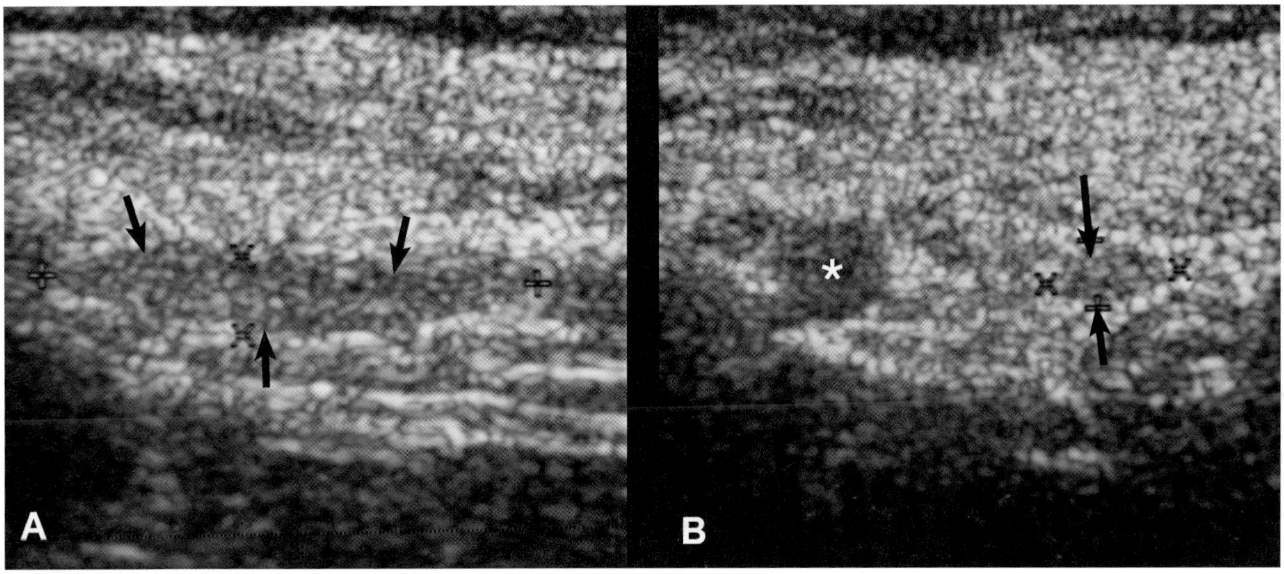

Figure 3.28. Right thyroid lobe of a dog with hypothyroidism. Sagittal **(A)** and transverse **(B)** images of the small thyroid lobe outlined by cursors and arrows. It is poorly marginated and slightly hypoechoic to the surrounding tissue (arrows). * points to the common carotid artery.

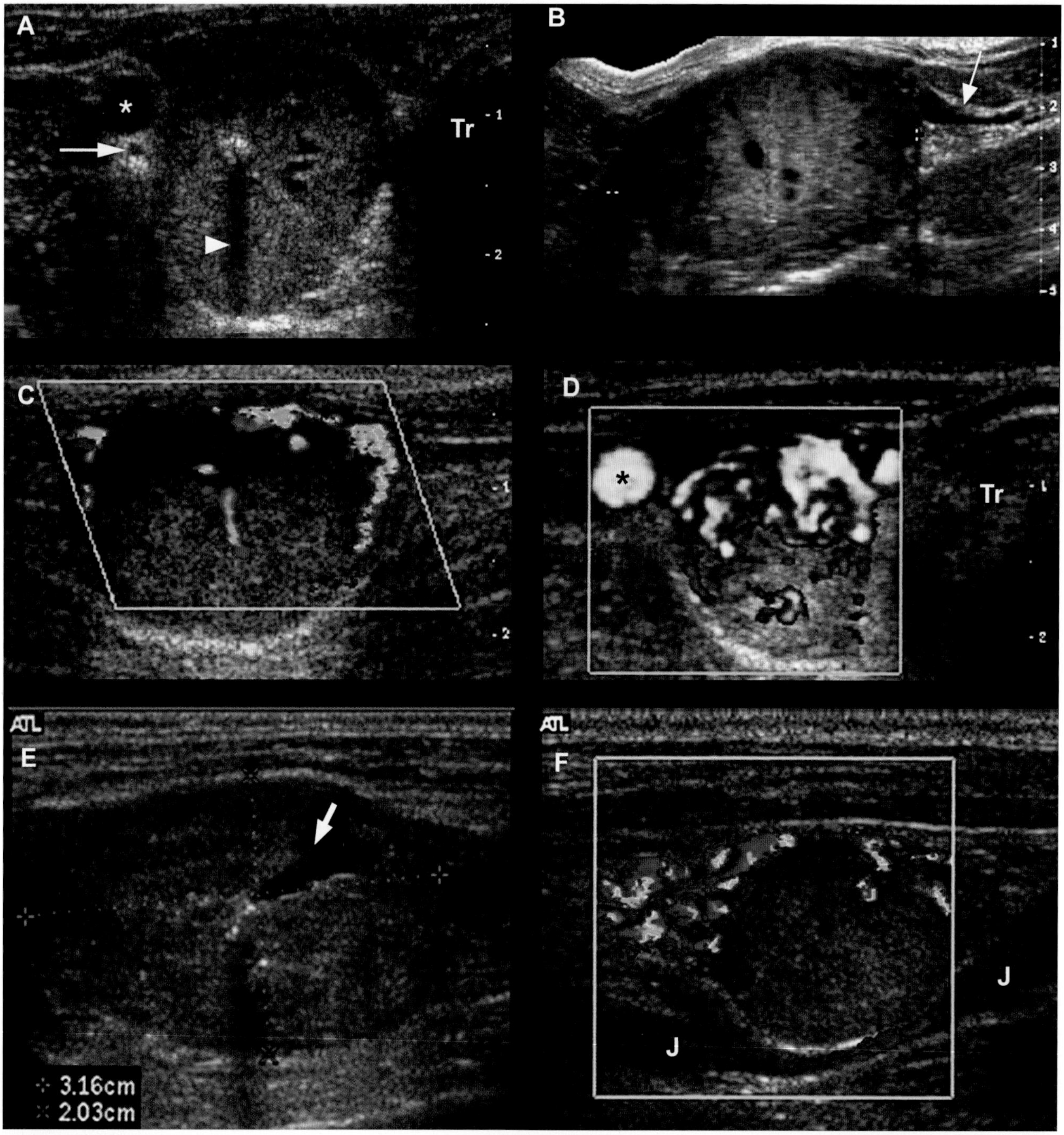

Figure 3.29. Thyroid carcinoma in dogs. **A:** Transverse image of the left thyroid gland. The large, hypoechoic thyroid carcinoma is displacing the common carotid artery (asterisk) laterally. The trachea (Tr) is visible on the medial side of the mass. Foci of mineralization are within the mass, causing acoustic shadowing (arrowhead). The vagosympathetic trunk (arrow) is dorsal to the common carotid artery. **B:** Panoramic view of a large thyroid carcinoma (over 5 cm long) deviating the carotid (arrow) laterally. The mass is inhomogeneous and multicavitated. Image courtesy of D. Penninck. **C:** Color Doppler of the thyroid carcinoma presented in **B**. Prominent vessels are at the ventral periphery of the mass. **D:** Power Doppler of another thyroid carcinoma, which is highly vascularized. The mass is between the common carotid artery (asterisk) and the trachea (Tr). Image courtesy of D. Penninck. **E and F:** Sagittal B-mode and color Doppler images of another thyroid carcinoma. The mass contains discrete, hyperechoic mineral foci and a fluid cavitation (arrow). Prominent vessels are noted at the ventral periphery, and the external jugular vein (J) is displaced and compressed, but not invaded. Images E and F courtesy of M.A. d'Anjou.

mass can cause upper-airway obstruction. The local vasculature and esophagus can be compressed or invaded by thyroid carcinoma (Figures 3.16 and 3.29F). Mineralization of the mass can be observed as hyperechoic foci with distal acoustic shadowing (Figure 3.29A and E), and metastasis to local lymph nodes is common.

Parathyroid Glands

Dogs with hypercalcemia may have primary or secondary parathyroid disease, and ultrasonography often helps to differentiate between them (Reusch et al. 2000). Primary hyperparathyroidism is caused by hyperplasia, adenoma, or less commonly, adenocarcinoma and presents as a single parathyroid nodule. Secondary hyperparathyroidism is caused by parathyroid hyperplasia secondary to renal disease or nutritional deficiencies, and often more than one parathyroid gland is visible.

Parathyroid nodules are hypoechoic to anechoic and often have distal acoustic enhancement. They tend to be well circumscribed and are round or oval (Figure 3.30). Parathyroid nodules that are greater than 4 mm in diameter are more likely to be parathyroid adenomas or carcinomas, whereas those less than 4 mm in diameter are more often primary hyperplastic, or secondary to chronic renal disease or hypercalcemia of malignancy (Wisner et al. 1997). Parathyroid neoplasia tends to involve one gland, though a second nodule has been reported in a case of adenoma (Wisner et al. 1997). Cats rarely have parathyroid adenoma.

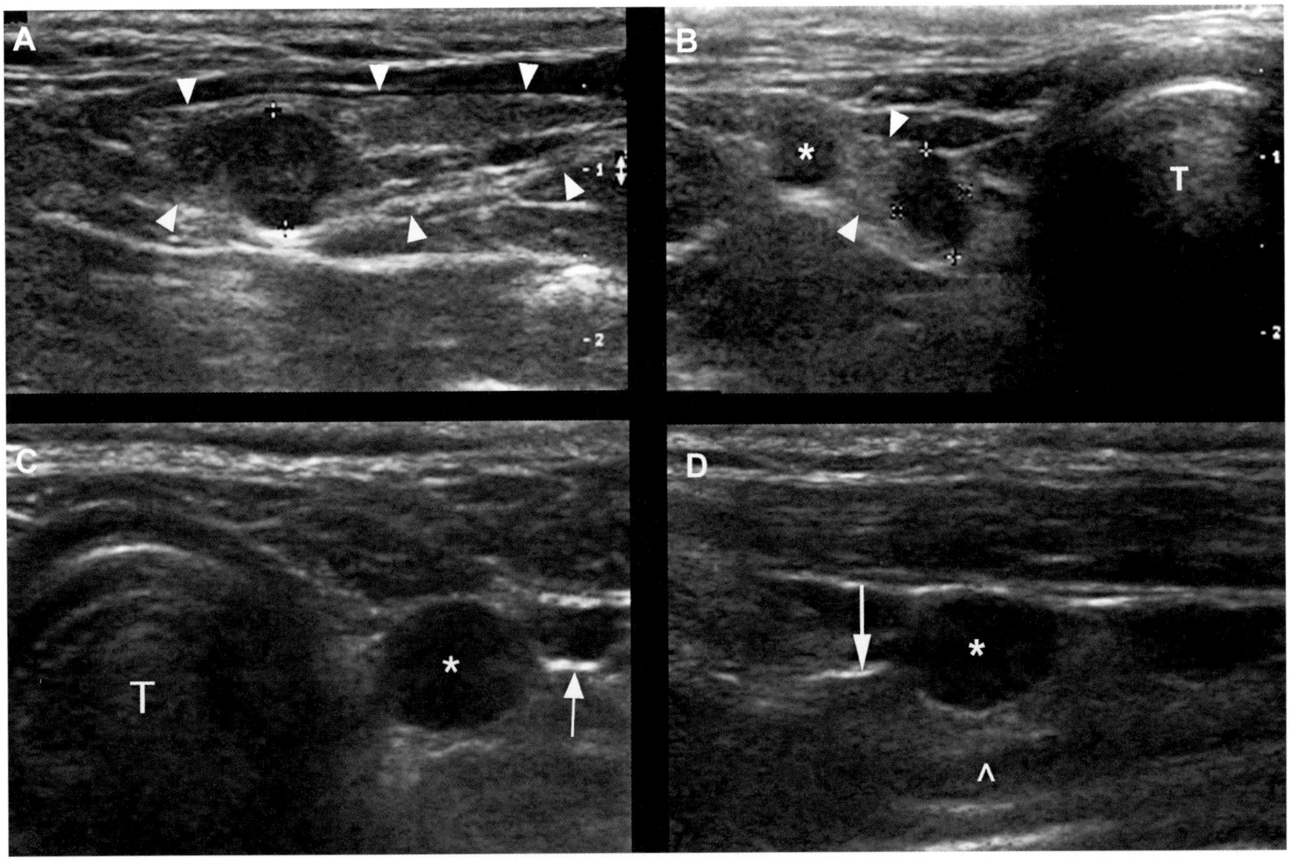

Figure 3.30. Parathyroid chief cell adenoma in dogs. **A:** Sagittal image of the right thyroid (arrowheads) and parathyroid glands of a 10-year-old English setter. A discrete hypoechoic nodule (between the cursors) measuring 7 mm in diameter is present cranially. Image courtesy of D. Penninck. **B:** Transverse image of the right thyroid (arrowheads) and parathyroid glands of a 10-year-old Siberian husky. A discrete hypoechoic nodule (between the cursors) measuring 8 × 4 mm is deforming the medial contour of the thyroid gland. The diagnosis is parathyroid chief cell adenoma. The adjacent common carotid artery (asterisk) seen on cross section should not be confused with a parathyroid nodule. T, trachea. Image courtesy of D. Penninck. **C:** Transverse image of the left parathyroid of a dog with parathyroid carcinoma. A round, hypoechoic nodule (asterisk) is between the trachea (T) and the common carotid artery (arrow) in the left neck. **D:** In sagittal orientation, the nodule protrudes from the cranioventral aspect (arrow) of the thyroid gland. The dorsal border of the thyroid gland is marked with the caret.

In acute renal failure, parathyroid length (median, 2.7 mm) is similar to that in normal dogs (median, 3.3 mm). In dogs with chronic renal failure, however, the parathyroid glands are longer (median, 5.7 mm) (Reusch et al. 2000). This may help to differentiate between acute and chronic renal failure, although there is likely to be some overlap between the two groups.

Trachea

In dogs with tracheal collapse, the hyperechoic air column just caudal to the cricoid cartilage appears oval and flattened (Rudorf et al. 1997). This may be associated with tracheal collapse in the thoracic inlet, as well. The dorsal tracheal membrane is not visible directly, but this alteration in shape of the air column is indicative of invagination. The flattening of the air column may worsen slightly with the head in an extended position. Other tracheal lesions such as masses, trauma, or edema may occasionally be seen (Figure 3.31).

Esophagus

Ultrasonography can be used to identify mass lesions in the cervical esophagus to monitor correct placement of an endotracheal tube or to confirm megaesophagus (Wisner et al. 2002). Other lesions, such as thickening, can also be detected (Figures 3.32 and 3.33).

Intraluminal esophageal ultrasound has also been used to investigate lesions such as enlarged lymph nodes and mediastinal masses in the thorax (Gaschen et al. 2003).

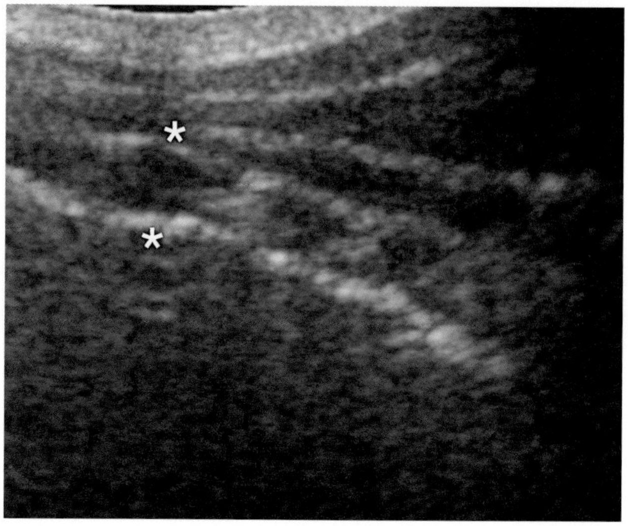

Figure 3.31. Tracheal edema in a dog. Sagittal image of the trachea of a dog with postanesthetic regurgitation and aspiration causing tracheal edema. Cranial is to the left of the image. The tracheal wall is mildly thickened and irregular in the caudal portion of the neck. The asterisks outline a hypoechoic tracheal cartilage ring.

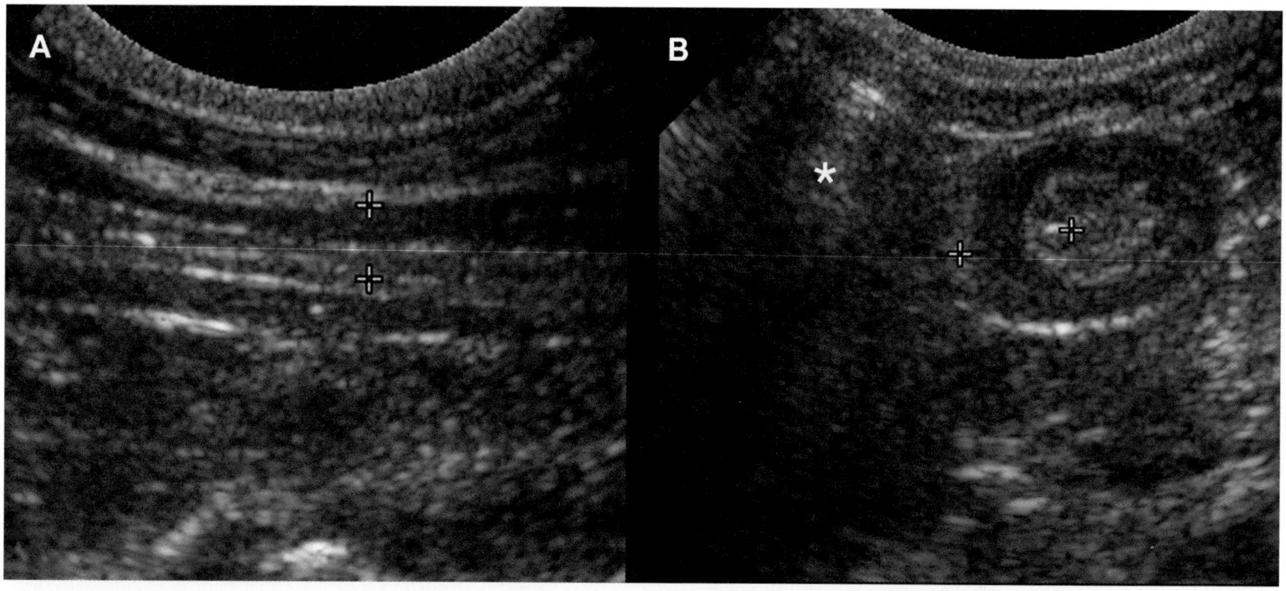

Figure 3.32. Esophagus of a dog with esophageal fibrosis and muscular hypertrophy. **A:** Cranial is on the left of the image. In the sagittal orientation, the lumen of the esophagus is indicated by the far-field cursor and the serosal surface by the near-field cursor. The muscularis layer is hypoechoic, and the entire esophageal wall is thickened. **B:** Transverse image of the esophagus. The trachea (asterisk) is visible on the left side of the image, to the right of the esophagus. Images were taken with a curvilinear 5- to 8-MHz transducer.

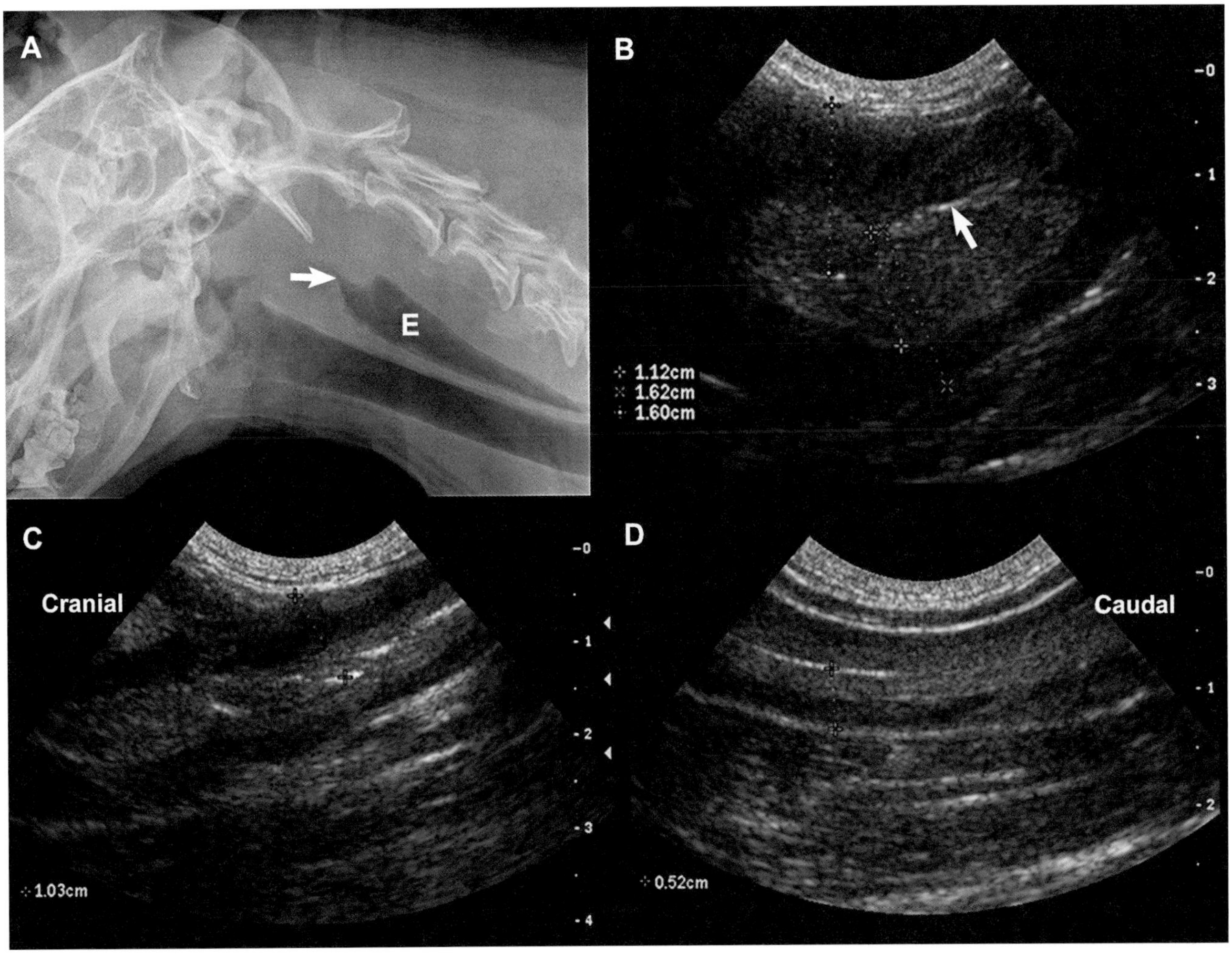

Figure 3.33. Idiopathic esophageal hypertrophy in a dog. **A:** Lateral radiograph of the cranial neck in a dog with chronic swallowing disorder. The esophagus (E) is abnormally dilated with air, and a soft-tissue mass–like projection is noted within its cranial lumen (arrow), caudal to the cricopharyngeal muscle. **B–D:** Transverse **(B)** and sagittal **(C and D)** sonograms of the diffusely and markedly thickened esophagus, involving especially the muscular layer. The mucosa is hyperechoic and confluent with the submucosa. Cranial and caudal portions of the esophagus are represented in **C** and **D**, respectively. The arrow points to the collapsed lumen. Mucosal and muscular hyperplasia and hypertrophy, as well as nonspecific inflammation, were diagnosed by means of ultrasound-guided biopsies. There was no evidence of a neoplastic process. Images courtesy of M.A. d'Anjou.

Special Procedures

Tissue samples of neck lesions are most often obtained by using a fine-needle aspirate, though tissue-core biopsies of larger lesions are possible using ultrasound guidance (Figure 3.34). However, because of the high vascularity of some organs and masses such as those of thyroid origin, and the presence of large arteries and veins often adjacent to cervical lesions, particular care should be taken when either fine-needle aspiration or tissue-core biopsy is attempted.

Vessels of masses and tissues can be identified with color and power Doppler imaging to gauge vascularity, to map vessels prior to fine-needle aspiration or biopsy, and to determine operability of a mass lesion.

Feline hyperthyroidism has been treated using both heat ablation and percutaneous ethanol ablation (Wells et al. 2001; Mallery et al. 2003) (Figure 3.35). Complications from both of these procedures include Horner's syndrome and laryngeal paralysis. Heat ablation obtained better results than ethanol ablation, with a mean euthyroid period of 4 months. The longest euthyroid period with ethanol ablation was 27 weeks, with a higher complication rate. Neither of these methods is as effective as the surgical, medical, or radiotherapeutic methods currently in use.

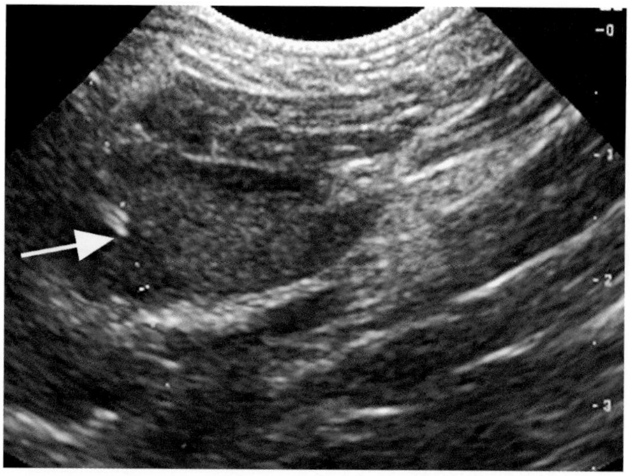

Figure 3.34. Fine-needle aspiration of an enlarged mandibular lymph node in a dog. The final diagnosis is pyogranulomatous lymphadenitis (the same dog as in Figure 3.17C). Image courtesy of D. Penninck.

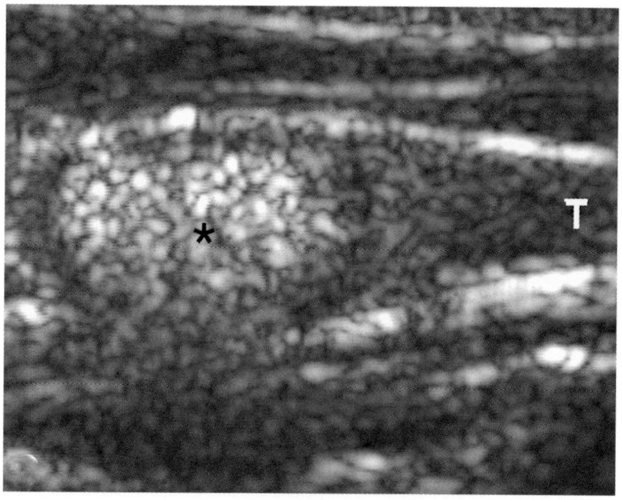

Figure 3.35. Intralesional ultrasound-guided injection in a dog. Sagittal image of a thyroid gland during ablation with intralesional injection of ethanol. The ethanol accumulation is a round, hyperechoic area (asterisk) within the thyroid gland (T). The needle originates from the left superficial aspect of the image, and the tip is at the asterisk.

Ablation of thyroid carcinoma by using injection of pure medical ethanol has been reported (Wisner et al. 2002). The target volume of injection is approximately half of the tumor volume, although the amount injected depends on the tumor characteristics. Complications include inadvertent injection or diffusion of ethanol to the local blood vessels or vagosympathetic trunk and recurrent laryngeal nerve.

References

Bromel C, Pollard RE, Kass PH, Samii VF, Davidson AP, Nelson RW (2005) Ultrasonographic evaluation of the thyroid gland in healthy, hypothyroid, and euthyroid golden retrievers with nonthyroidal illness. J Vet Intern Med 19:499–506.

Carlisle CH, Biery DN, Thrall DE (1991) Tracheal and laryngeal tumors in the dog and cat: Literature review and 13 additional patients. Vet Radiol 32:229–235.

Dickie AM, Doust R, Cromarty L, Johnson VS, Sullivan M, Boyd JS (2003) Ultrasound imaging of the canine tympanic bulla. Res Vet Sci 75:121–126.

Fife W, Mattoon J, Drost WT, Groppe D, Wellman M (2003) Imaging features of a presumed carotid body tumor in a dog. Vet Radiol Ultrasound 44:322–325.

Gaschen L, Kircher P, Hoffmann G, et al. (2003) Endoscopic ultrasonography for the diagnosis of intrathoracic lesions in two dogs. Vet Radiol Ultrasound 44:292–299.

Gooding GA, Herzog KA, Laing FC, McDonald EJ Jr (1977) Ultrasonographic assessment of neck masses. J Clin Ultrasound 5:248–252.

Mallery KF, Pollard RE, Nelson RW, Hornof WJ, Feldman EC (2003) Percutaneous ultrasound-guided radiofrequency heat ablation for treatment of hyperthyroidism in cats. J Am Vet Med Assoc 223:1602–1607.

Melian C, Morales M, Espinosa de los Monteros A, Peterson ME (1996) Horner's syndrome associated with a functional thyroid carcinoma in a dog. J Small Anim Pract 37:591–593.

Mooney CT (2002) Pathogenesis of feline hyperthyroidism. J Feline Med Surg 4:167–169.

Phillips DE, Radlinsky MG, Fischer JR, Biller DS (2003) Cystic thyroid and parathyroid lesions in cats. J Am Anim Hosp Assoc 39:349–54.

Reese S, Breyer U, Deeg C, Kraft W, Kaspers B (2005) Thyroid sonography as an effective tool to discriminate between euthyroid sick and hypothyroid dogs. J Vet Intern Med 19:491–498.

Reese S, Ruppert C (2001) Ultrasonographic imaging of the vagosympathetic trunk in the dog. Vet Radiol Ultrasound 42:272–275.

Reusch CE, Tomsa K, Zimmer C, et al. (2000) Ultrasonography of the parathyroid glands as an aid in differentiation of acute and chronic renal failure in dogs. J Am Vet Med Assoc 217:1849–1852.

Rudorf H, Barr FJ, Lane JG (2001) The role of ultrasound in the assessment of laryngeal paralysis in the dog. Vet Radiol Ultrasound 42:338–343.

Rudorf H, Herrtage ME, White RA (1997) Use of ultrasonography in the diagnosis of tracheal collapse. J Small Anim Pract 38:513–518.

Ruppert C, Hartmann K, Fischer A, Hirschberger J, Hafner A, Schmidt P (2000) Cervical neoplasia originating from the vagus nerve in a dog. J Small Anim Pract 41:119–122.

Schaer M, Zaki FA, Harvey HJ, O'Reilly WH (1979) Laryngeal hemiplegia due to neoplasia of the vagus nerve in a cat. J Am Vet Med Assoc 174:513–515.

Slensky KA, Volk SW, Schwarz T, Duda L, Mauldin EA, Silverstein D (2003) Acute severe hemorrhage secondary to arterial invasion in a dog with thyroid carcinoma. J Am Vet Med Assoc 223:649–653.

Taymans O, Duchateau L, Schreurs E, Kramer M, Daminet S, Saunders JH (2005) Intra- and interobserver variability of ultrasonographic measurements of the thyroid gland in healthy beagles. Vet Radiol Ultrasound 46:139–142.

Wells AL, Long CD, Hornof WJ, et al. (2001) Use of percutaneous ethanol injection for treatment of bilateral hyperplastic thyroid nodules in cats. J Am Vet Med Assoc 218:1293–127.

Wisner ER, Mattoon JS, Nyland TG (2002) Neck. In: Nyland TG, ed. Small Animal Diagnostic Ultrasound. Philadelphia: WB Saunders, pp 285–304.

Wisner ER, Mattoon JS, Nyland TG, Baker TW (1991) Normal ultrasonographic anatomy of the canine neck. Vet Radiol Ultrasound 32:185–190.

Wisner ER, Nyland TG, Mattoon JS (1994) Ultrasonographic examination of cervical masses in the dog and cat. Vet Radiol Ultrasound 35:310–315.

Wisner ER, Penninck D, Biller DS, Feldman EC, Drake C, Nyland TG (1997) High-resolution parathyroid sonography. Vet Radiol Ultrasound 38:462–466.

CHAPTER FOUR

Thorax

Silke Hecht

Preparation and Scanning Technique

In a normal animal, evaluation of intrathoracic structures is hampered by the interposition of aerated lung tissue. However, collapsed or consolidated lung, thoracic masses, or pleural effusion can provide a suitable acoustic window. Thoracic radiography should always precede thoracic ultrasonography to confirm the presence of a lesion, identify a suitable acoustic window, and rule out entities, such as severe pneumothorax, which preclude an ultrasonographic examination (Tidwell 1998). Since pleural effusion may facilitate the examination of intrathoracic structures, thoracocentesis should be postponed until the ultrasonographic examination has been performed, unless the patient has respiratory compromise.

To optimize image quality, hair should be clipped in the region to be scanned, and acoustic gel should be applied. An intercostal approach is most commonly used and involves examination of the thoracic structures by positioning the transducer on the chest wall between adjacent ribs (Figure 4.1A and B). Animals are generally positioned in lateral recumbency, although scanning in sternal recumbency or while a patient is standing may be considered in compromised patients or for an initial screening. A thoracic inlet approach can sometimes help in visualizing cranial thoracic lesions (Figure 4.1C).

A subcostal (transhepatic) approach may be used to assess caudal mediastinal or caudal pulmonary lesions. The examination technique is similar to that used for evaluation of the liver. The animal is positioned in dorsal or lateral recumbency, and the transducer is aimed cranially under the rib cage.

Some examiners prefer imaging the dependent portion of the thorax by using a cardiac table. This approach optimizes the acoustic window, because pleural fluid accumulates in the dependent portion of the thorax, and the pulmonary structures in the near field contain less air because of positional atelectasis. However, ultrasound-guided interventional procedures are difficult to perform using this approach, and the field of view is limited to the size of the table window and the ability to position the area of interest over the opening.

Usually, a sector transducer or a curvilinear or microconvex sonographic probe with a small footprint should be selected when using an intercostal window, although a linear probe may also be used. The optimal frequency depends on the size of the animal and the location of the lesion. For the examination of the cranial mediastinum in large dogs, a 5-MHz transducer may be used, whereas examination of small superficial pulmonary lesions necessitates the use of a higher-frequency transducer (7.5 or 10.0 MHz). A standoff pad may improve image quality during the evaluation of thoracic wall lesions. For a transhepatic or thoracic inlet approach, sector or curvilinear transducers are most commonly used.

The examination is performed in at least two planes, depending on the nature, size, and location of the lesion.

Normal Sonographic Anatomy

Intercostal Approach

The soft tissues of the thoracic wall (skin, subcutaneous fat, and muscle) appear as layered tissues of alternating echogenicity in the near field (Figure 4.2). The parietal pleura is rarely recognized as a discrete structure, but may be differentiated from the visceral pleura in real time by the sliding motion of the lung during respiration. The ribs appear as smoothly marginated, curvilinear, hyperechoic structures with distal acoustic shadowing (Figure 4.2). The lung interface is seen as an echogenic linear band with distal reverberation artifacts and dirty shadowing. The pulmonary parenchyma deep to the lung surface cannot be evaluated in normal animals because of these artifacts (Figure 4.2).

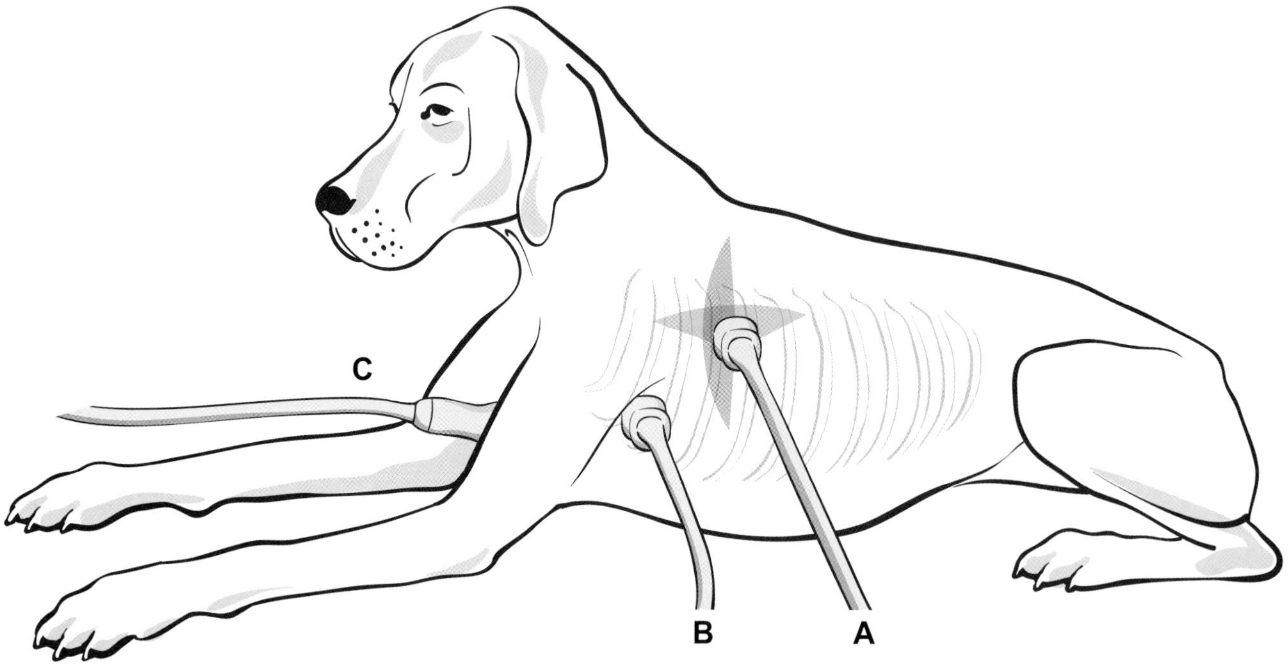

Figure 4.1. Ultrasonographic examination of the thorax. The patient can be examined while it is standing or in sternal, lateral, or dorsal recumbency. **A and B: Intercostal approach.** The transducer is placed on the thoracic wall in the area of interest; for example, at the level of a pulmonary lesion suspected radiographically **(A)**. To better evaluate the cranial mediastinum **(B)**, the thoracic limbs are pulled forward. The transducer is placed on the thoracic wall caudal to the elbows and dorsal to the sternum. Transverse and dorsal or sagittal planes can be used. **C: Thoracic inlet approach** to evaluate the most cranial aspect of the thoracic cavity. The transducer is placed midline on the caudal neck and aimed caudally into the thorax. An initial dorsal plane view is useful to identify the trachea, esophagus, and great vessels. Sagittal and oblique views are obtained subsequently.

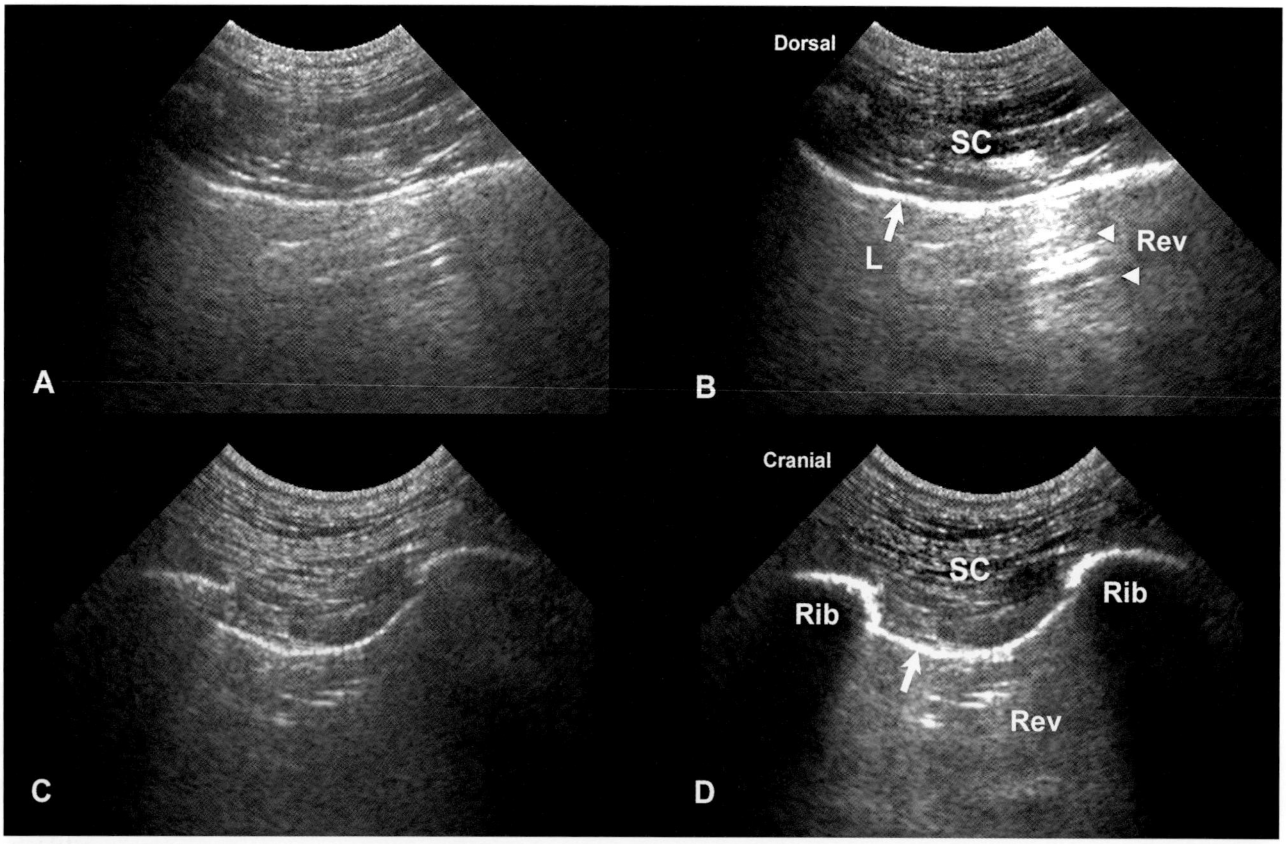

Figure 4.2.

Evaluation of the normal cranial and caudal mediastinum by means of an intercostal approach is often hampered by interposition of aerated lung. However, cranial mediastinal vessels may be visualized as tubular anechoic structures that show flow on Doppler examination (Figure 4.3).

The thymus may be visible in young animals. Care must be taken not to confuse abundant mediastinal fat with intrathoracic mass lesions. Normal cranial mediastinal or sternal lymph nodes are usually not visible.

Transhepatic (Subcostal) Approach

The diaphragm-lung interface appears as a curvilinear, strongly hyperechoic structure in the far field cranial to the liver (Figure 4.4). The diaphragm cannot be distinguished from the adjacent hyperechoic lung interface, except in cases of pleural effusion or consolidation of the caudal lung lobes. The caudal thoracic esophagus is occasionally seen traversing the diaphragm (see Figure 8.3). Using this approach, the examiner has to be aware of the commonly observed mirror artifact (see Figure 6.4).

Thoracic Inlet Approach

By using a thoracic inlet approach, mediastinal fat, cranial thoracic trachea, and esophagus are usually seen (Figure 4.5). Cranial mediastinal vessels may be visible.

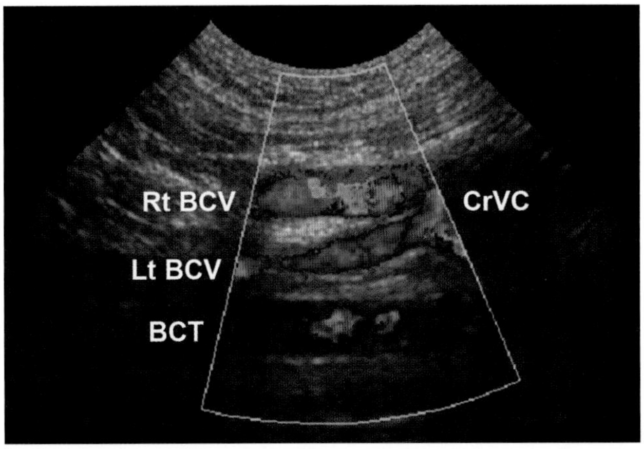

Figure 4.3. Normal cranial mediastinum in a dog when using a right intercostal approach (dorsal plane) and color Doppler. The cranial mediastinal vessels are clearly visible. The confluence of the brachiocephalic veins to form the cranial vena cava is observed. BCT, brachiocephalic trunk; CrVC, cranial vena cava; Lt BCV, Left brachiocephalic vein; and Rt BCV, right brachiocephalic vein.

Figure 4.2. Normal thoracic wall when using an intercostal approach. Transverse **(A and B)** and longitudinal **(C and D)** ultrasonographic and schematic images. The subcutaneous tissues (SC), which include muscle, fat, and fascial planes, are recognized as multiple alternating hypoechoic and hyperechoic layers in the near field. The lung surface (L, arrows) appears as a smooth, strongly hyperechoic line. Distal to the lung surface are dirty shadowing and reverberation artifacts (Rev) that prevent evaluation of the normal air-filled lung. The normal ribs are visible as strongly hyperechoic curvilinear structures (Rib), with clean distal shadowing in the far field.

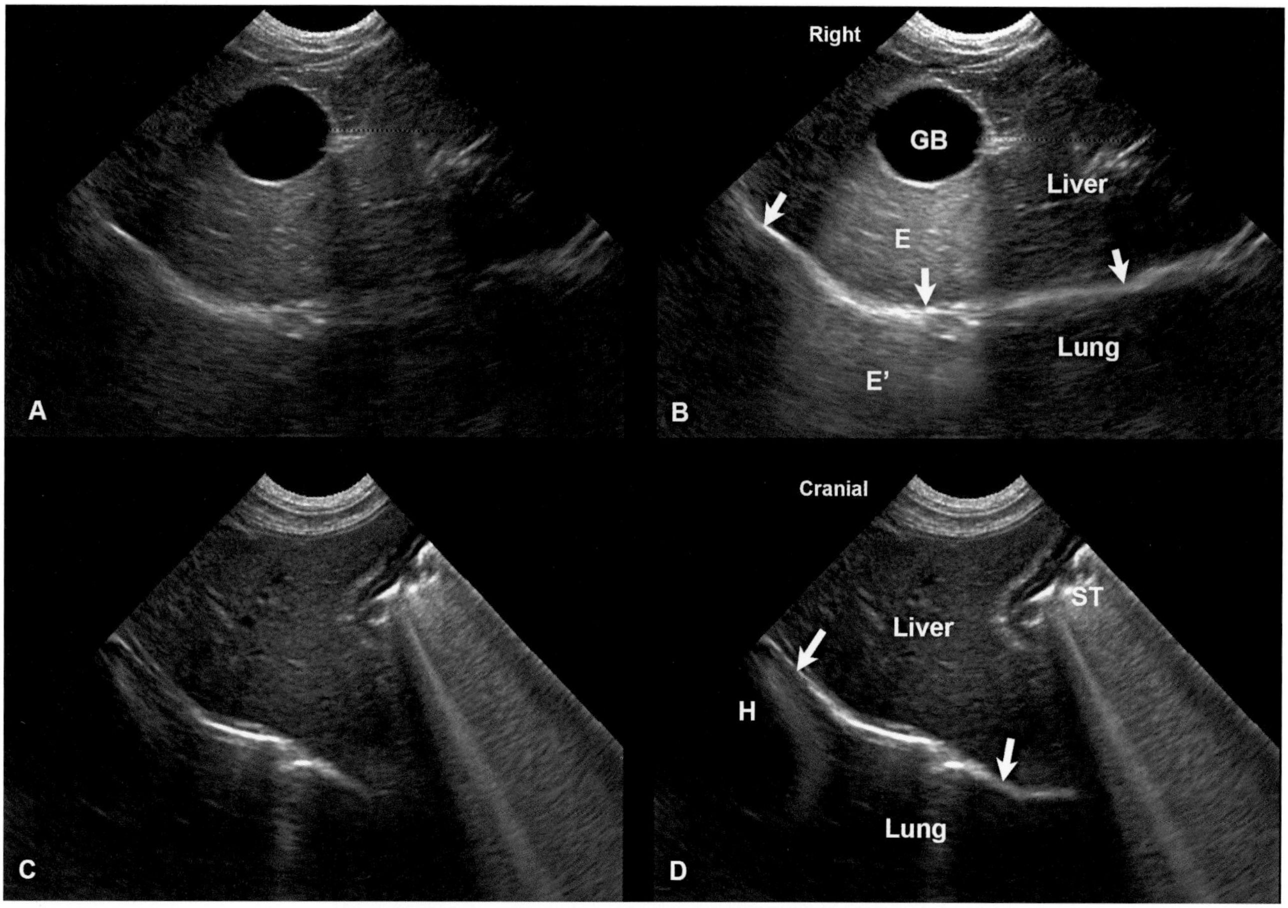

Figure 4.4. Normal caudal thorax in a dog when using a transhepatic (subcostal) approach. Transverse **(A and B)** and sagittal **(C and D)** ultrasonographic and schematic images. The diaphragm-lung interface (arrows) appears as a curvilinear hyperechoic line cranial to the liver. A mirror image of the hyperechoic acoustic enhancement (E) deep to the gallbladder (GB) is in the lung region (E′). H, heart; and ST, stomach.

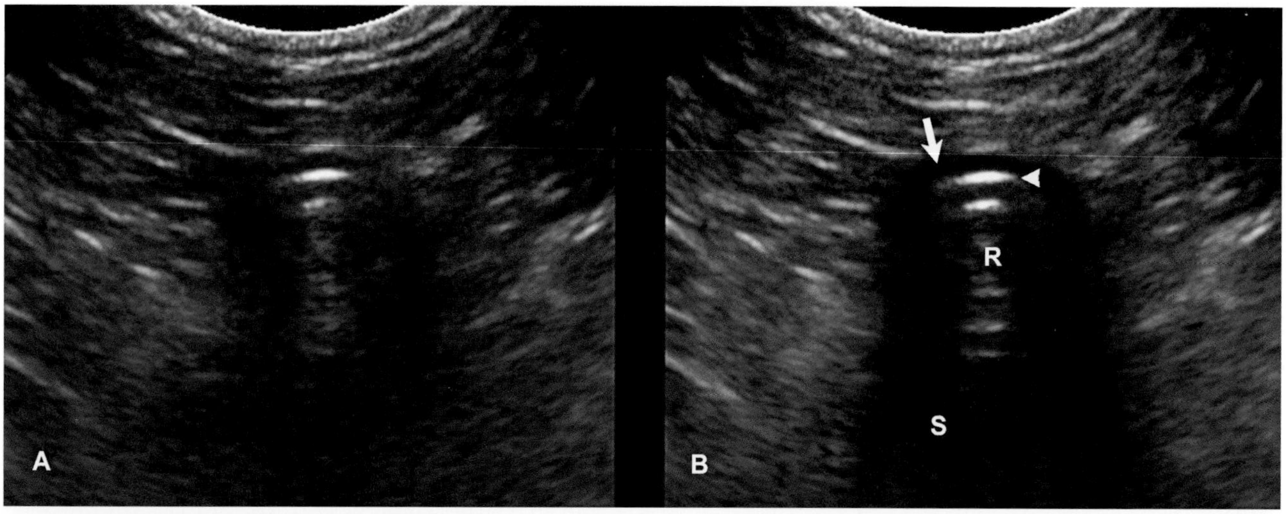

Figure 4.5. Normal cranial thorax in a dog when using a thoracic inlet approach. Transverse to dorsal ultrasonographic **(A)** and schematic **(B)** images. The transducer is positioned midline and aimed caudally. The ventral tracheal wall is visible as a hypoechoic crescent (arrow). The adjacent hyperechoic crescent (arrowhead) represents the interface between tracheal wall and intraluminal gas. A combination of acoustic shadowing (S) and reverberation (R) is visible in the far field.

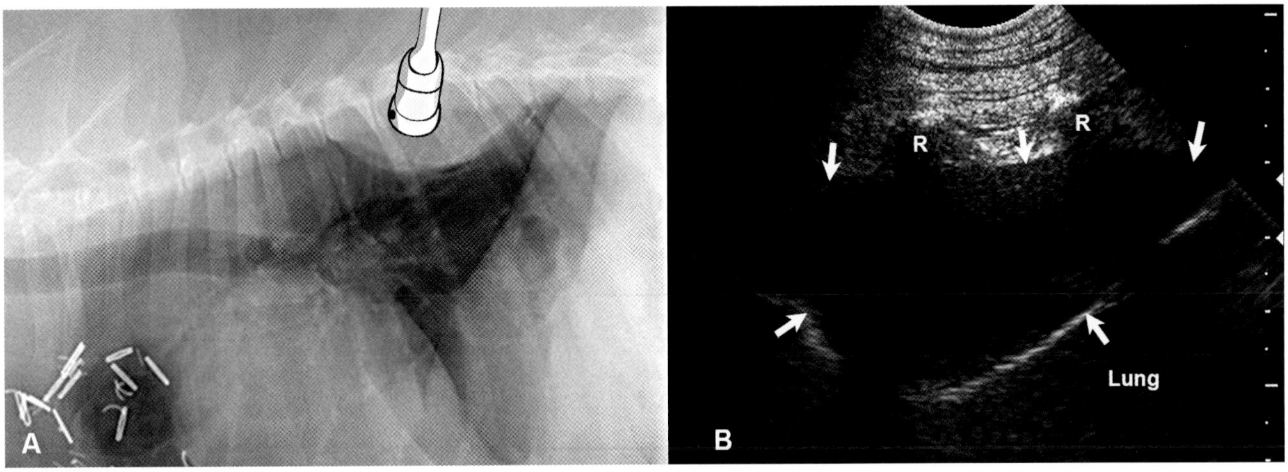

Figure 4.6. Extrapleural mass (metastatic thymoma) in a 7-year-old elkhound. **A:** On this right lateral radiograph is a fusiform mass lesion associated with the caudal dorsal thorax (under the sonographic probe). This mass is in broad-based contact with the dorsal thoracic wall (*extrapleural sign*). Metallic hemoclips associated with the cranial ventral thorax are consistent with previous removal of a cranial mediastinal mass (thymoma). **B:** The mass, which is visualized by using a left dorsal intercostal approach, appears as a homogeneously hypoechoic mass lesion (arrows) forming an obtuse angle with the adjacent thoracic wall. The hyperechoic interface of the normal lung is visible in the far field, as well as acoustic shadows associated with ribs (R).

Sonographic Features of Thoracic Disorders

Lesions of the Thoracic Wall

Thoracic wall lesions include neoplasms, inflammatory lesions, and trauma. Ultrasound allows assessment of the extent and margination of a lesion, bone involvement (such as in rib neoplasms or trauma), echotexture (solid and/or fluid filled), invasion of adjacent structures, and presence of foreign material or gas (e.g., in abscesses). A thoracic wall mass is convex, in broad-based contact with the chest wall, and displaces the normal lung interface (*extrapleural sign*). In contrast to most mass lesions originating from the pulmonary parenchyma, the angle between the extrapleural mass and the adjacent thoracic wall is obtuse (Figure 4.6). Additionally, the dynamic visualization of lung motion underneath thoracic wall lesions enables their extrapulmonary origin to be confirmed. In contrast to pulmonary masses, thoracic wall mass lesions are static or move with the chest wall during respiration.

Masses originating from ribs or sternum are most commonly neoplastic in etiology (e.g., chondrosarcoma or osteosarcoma). These masses cause irregular disruption of the smooth contour of the affected bone and are accompanied by an intrathoracic and extrathoracic mass lesion of variable size and echogenicity (Figures 4.7 and 4.8).

Benign or malignant neoplastic processes, such as infiltrative lipomas or soft-tissue sarcomas, may also invade the thoracic wall (Figure 4.9). Metastatic disease may also involve one or several of these bones, causing variable alteration in their normal hyperechoic, shadowing surface. The osseous proliferation and/or lysis encountered in aggressive bone lesions are typically irregular and poorly defined when compared with benign processes, such as chronic rib fractures.

Inflammatory lesions affecting the thoracic wall include cellulitis, abscesses, and granulomas. Ultrasound enables identification of fluid pockets and differentiation of well-circumscribed processes from infiltrative processes. Ultrasonography has been proven to be more accurate than fistulography in the detection of foreign material in animals with chronic draining tracts or abscesses (Armbrust et al. 2003). Depending on their size and composition, foreign bodies are usually hyperechoic to the surrounding soft tissues and often cast an acoustic shadow (Figure 4.10).

In cases of thoracic trauma, ultrasonography can be used as an alternative to radiography in the diagnosis of rib fractures. Findings include discontinuity of cortical alignment (Figure 4.11), as well as edge shadowing and reverberation artifacts arising from the margin of the displaced rib segment (Hurley et al. 2004). However, based on the literature on human patients, ultrasonography does not significantly increase the detection rate of rib fractures, may be uncomfortable for a patient, and is more time-consuming than radiography.

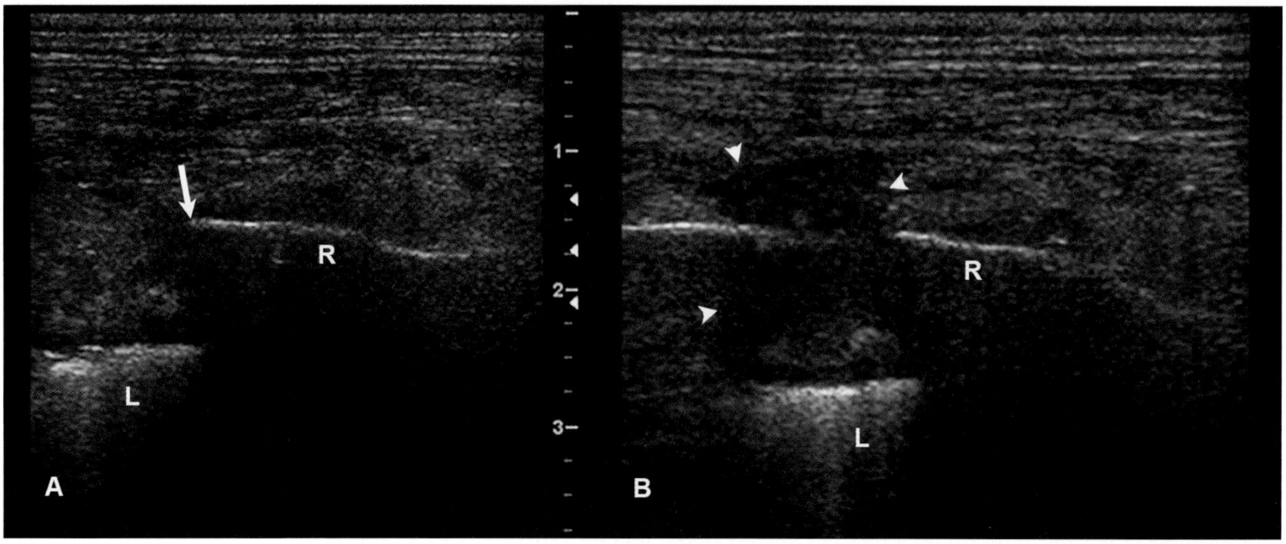

Figure 4.11. Rib fracture in a dog. Ultrasonographic images obtained in a transverse plane in respect to the thoracic cavity, which corresponds to the long axis of the rib. Images **A** and **B** were obtained at different levels of the rib fracture. There is disruption of the smooth hyperechoic contour of the rib (R), with displacement of the fracture fragments (arrow). Material of inhomogeneous soft-tissue echogenicity is noted at the fracture site (arrowheads), consistent with a hematoma. The lung (L) surface is focally visible beyond the fracture site. Images courtesy of M. Kramer.

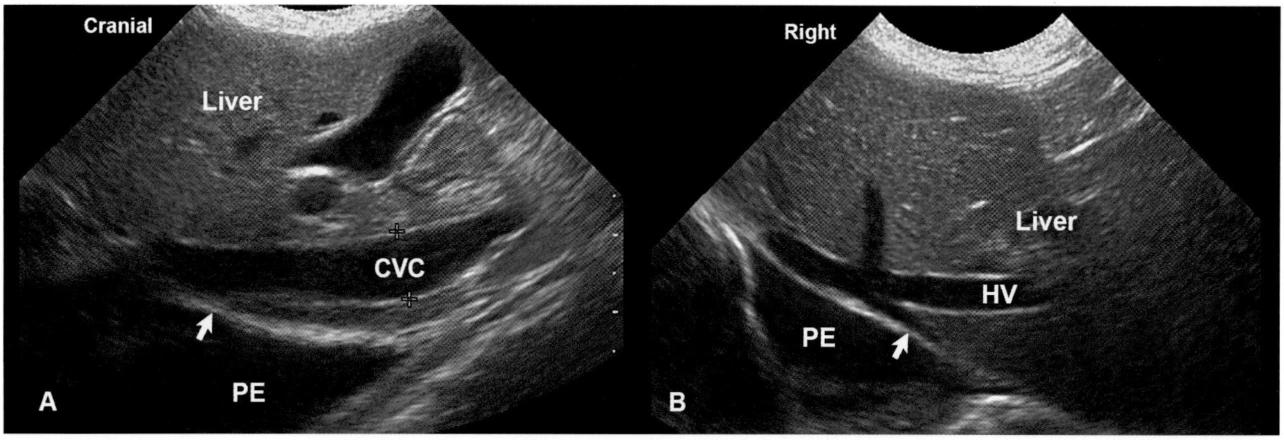

Figure 4.12. Congestive heart failure in a dyspneic cat. Sagittal **(A)** and parasagittal oblique **(B)** subcostal images of the caudal thorax. There is anechoic pleural effusion (PE) cranial to the diaphragm (arrows), and distension of caudal vena cava (CVC) and hepatic veins (HV).

effusion are generally hypoechoic or anechoic (Figures 4.12 and 4.13). Exudates, malignant pleural effusions, or hemorrhages are usually echogenic (Figures 4.14 and 4.15).

Free fluid may be differentiated from trapped fluid pockets by scanning the patient in different recumbent positions. Although free fluid accumulates in the dependent portion of the thorax, trapped fluid is not influenced by gravity and remains in the same region of the pleural space.

Chronic pleural effusion causes echogenic strands to develop within the pleural space, consistent with pleural adhesions or fibrinous bands (Figure 4.16).

Pleural Lesions

The pleural cavity can be affected by inflammation (pleuritis), neoplasia (carcinomatosis, mesothelioma, and metastatic disease), and loss of integrity subsequent to trauma. The detection of smaller pleural

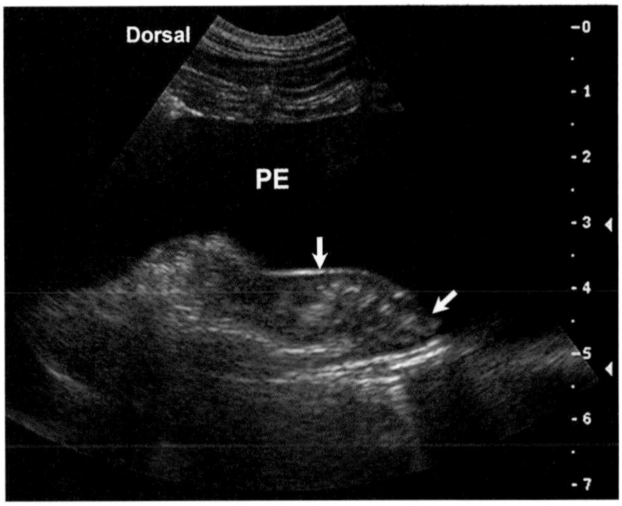

Figure 4.13. Transverse image in a cat with severe chylothorax. A large volume of anechoic pleural effusion (PE) is visible, delineating a collapsed lung lobe (arrows). Image courtesy of M.A. d'Anjou.

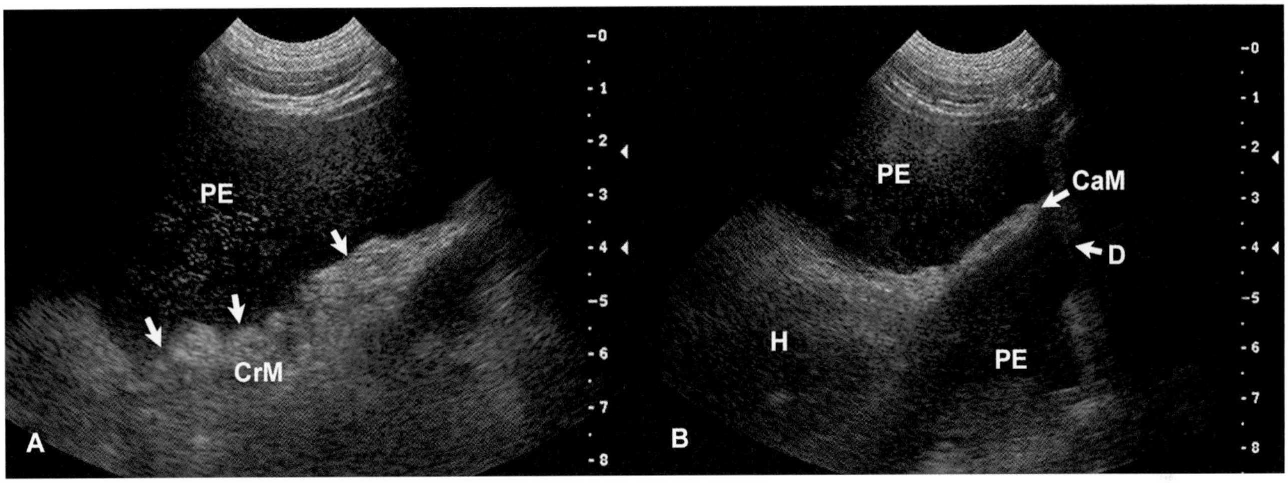

Figure 4.14. Severe pleural effusion in a dyspneic dog. Oblique intercostal sonographic images of the cranial **(A)** and caudal **(B)** thorax. A large volume of echogenic effusion (PE) is in both pleural spaces, on each side of the caudal mediastinum (CaM). In **A**, the border of the cranial mediastinum (CrM) is irregular and hyperechoic (arrows). The diaphragm (D) is visualized, as well as the liver just caudal to it. Carcinomatosis secondary to metastatic disease was diagnosed at necropsy. Images courtesy of M.A. d'Anjou.

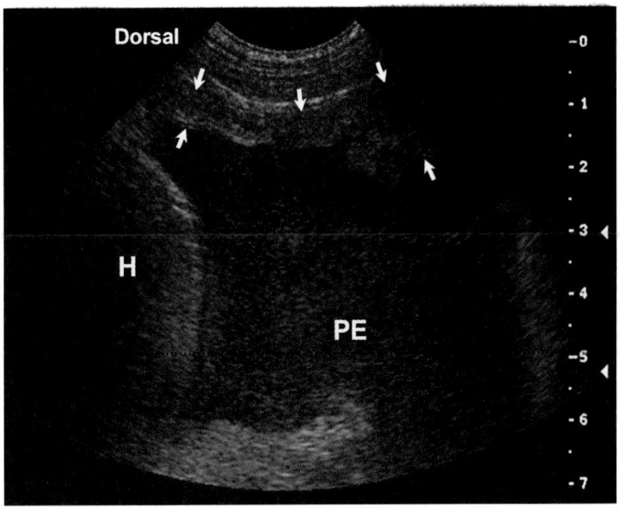

Figure 4.15. Chronic chylothorax and pleuritis in a 10-year-old mixed-breed dog. Severe, echogenic pleural effusion (PE) is seen when using a left intercostal approach caudal to the heart (H). Irregular thickening of the parietal pleural is observed (arrows). Image courtesy of M.A. d'Anjou.

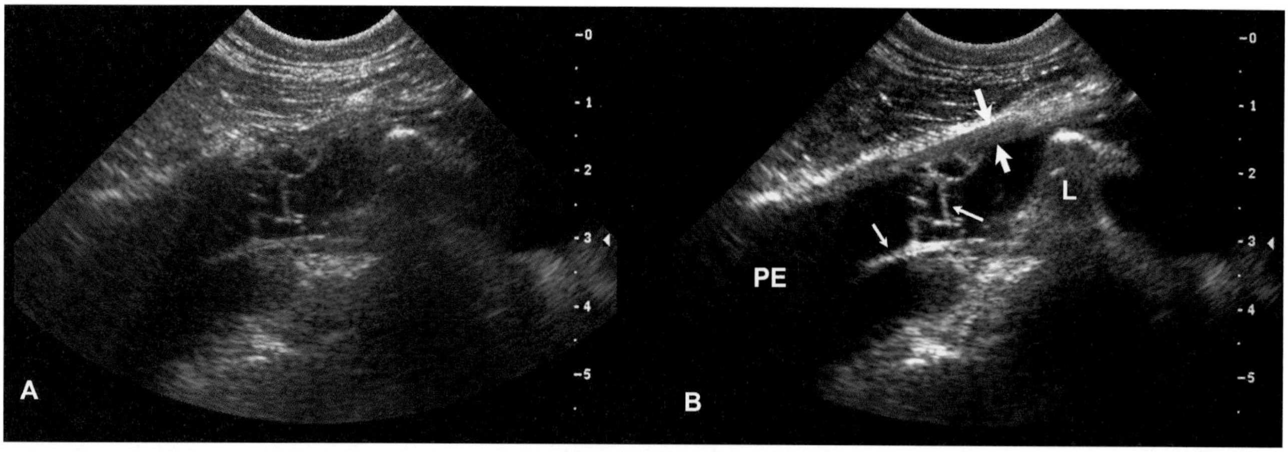

Figure 4.16. Chronic pleuritis in a 2-year-old cat. Ultrasonographic **(A)** and schematic **(B)** transverse images on which anechoic pleural fluid (PE) is associated with lung atelectasis (L). Hyperechoic linear strands (thin arrows) are visible within the fluid, consistent with pleural adhesions or fibrin strands and indicative of chronicity. The visceral pleura is also thickened (wide arrows).

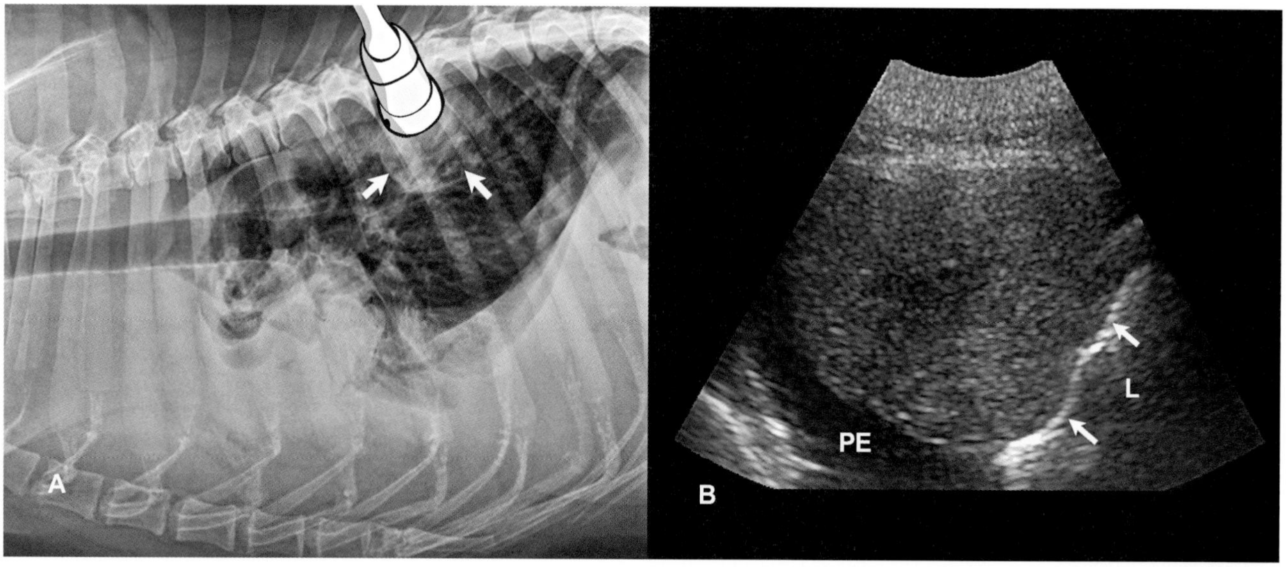

Figure 4.17. Pleural carcinomatosis and cranial mediastinal mass in a 9-year-old dog. **A:** Left lateral radiograph of the thorax. Moderate pleural effusion, as well as a cranial mediastinum mass, cause dorsal displacement of the trachea and lungs. A round soft-tissue opacity is associated with the dorsal thorax bordering the thoracic spine (arrows). **B:** Intercostal ultrasonographic image of the dorsal thoracic mass. The mass is seen arising from the pleura and is separate from the hyperechoic lung interface (L, arrows) in the far field. Pleural effusion (PE) is also present. Fine-needle aspirates of the cranial mediastinal and pleural lesions were consistent with carcinoma.

nodules and masses on radiographs is commonly hampered by the presence of pleural effusion. Additionally, radiographic distinction between pleural and pulmonary masses may be challenging. On ultrasonographic examination, pleural disease manifests as thickening, irregularity, or mass lesions of variable echogenicity associated with the pleura. Lesions arising from the parietal pleura are readily recognized, especially in the presence of pleural effusion (Figures 4.15–4.18). Even in the absence of pleural effusion, differentiation between pulmonary and parietal pleural lesions is usually possible based on real-time ultrasonography. Whereas a pulmonary mass moves with respiration, a mass arising from the parietal pleura remains stationary in comparison with the sliding lung (Mattoon and Nyland 1995).

Nodules or masses arising from the visceral pleura cannot be easily distinguished from lesions originating from the pulmonary parenchyma (Figure 4.19).

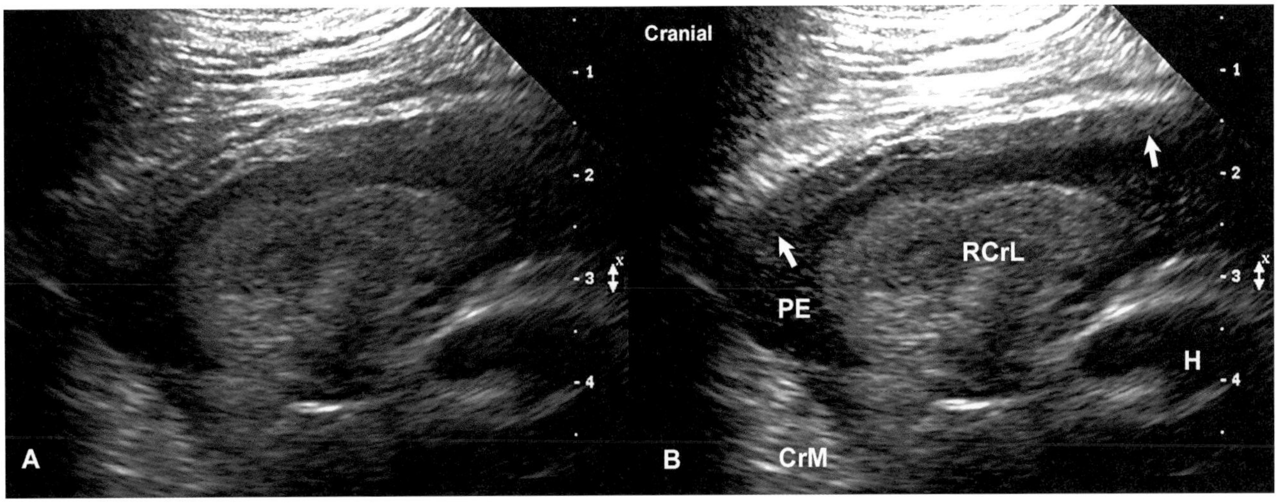

Figure 4.18. Pleural carcinomatosis and pulmonary carcinoma in a 10-year-old cat. Intercostal approach. On these dorsal ultrasonographic **(A)** and schematic **(B)** images, the right cranial lung lobe (RCrL) is rounded, irregular, and has assumed soft-tissue echogenicity because of replacement of normally air-filled parenchyma by neoplastic cells. Echogenic fluid separates the lung lobe from the parietal pleura (PE). The parietal pleura (arrows) is thickened, slightly irregular, and unusually hypoechoic. CrM, cranial mediastinum; and H, heart.

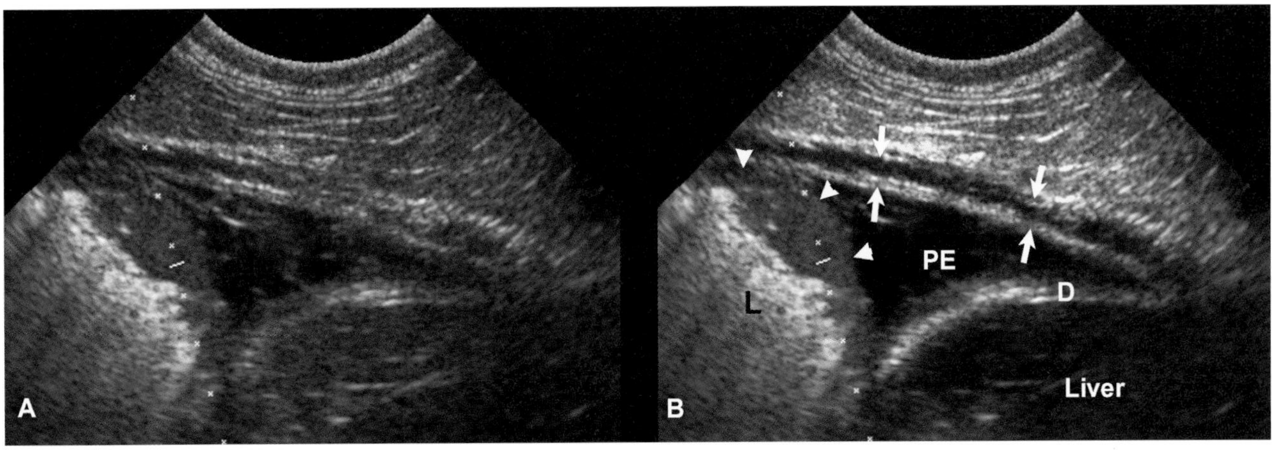

Figure 4.19. Chronic pleuritis in a 2-year-old cat (the same patient as in Figure 4.16). Ultrasonographic **(A)** and schematic **(B)** images obtained by using a left caudodorsal intercostal approach. The superficial parietal pleura (arrows) is irregularly thickened, irregular, and hypoechoic. The visceral pleura of the left caudal lung lobe is also markedly thickened (arrowheads). Pleural effusion (PE) separates the lung lobe from the diaphragm (D). The visceral pleural lesion cannot be differentiated from a primary pulmonary lesion by means of ultrasonography.

Pneumothorax

Although radiography remains the imaging modality of choice to diagnose air within the pleural space, ultrasonographic assessment of the pleural space should always be performed after interventional procedures, and the examiner should be aware of the ultrasonographic appearance of pneumothorax. Free air within the pleural space may create similar reverberation artifacts as normal lung (see Figures 4.20 and 4.41). However, the classic *gliding sign* of the lung against the parietal pleura is not observed. In cases of concurrent pleural effusion, a gas-fluid interface may be visualized.

Abnormalities of the Mediastinum

Ultrasound facilitates differentiation of entities, such as accumulation of fat, fluid, or true mediastinal

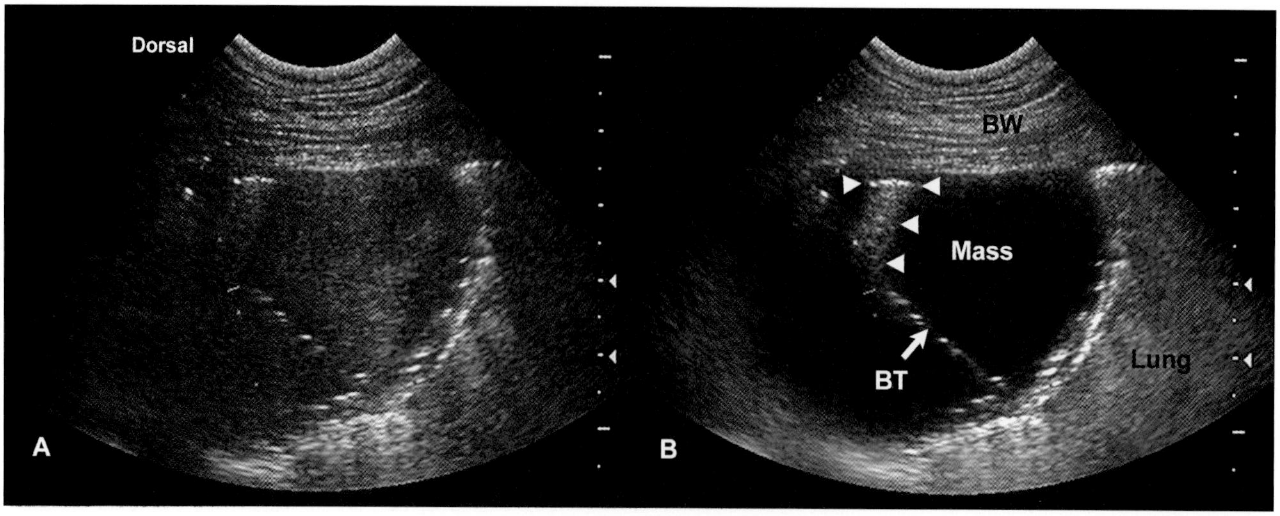

Figure 4.20. Mild pneumothorax after biopsy of a pulmonary mass in a dog. A linear hyperechogenicity with distal reverberation artifacts (arrowheads) is in the near field superficial to the mass. The biopsy tract (BT) is characterized by a line of punctate hyperechogenicities through the mass. BW, body wall.

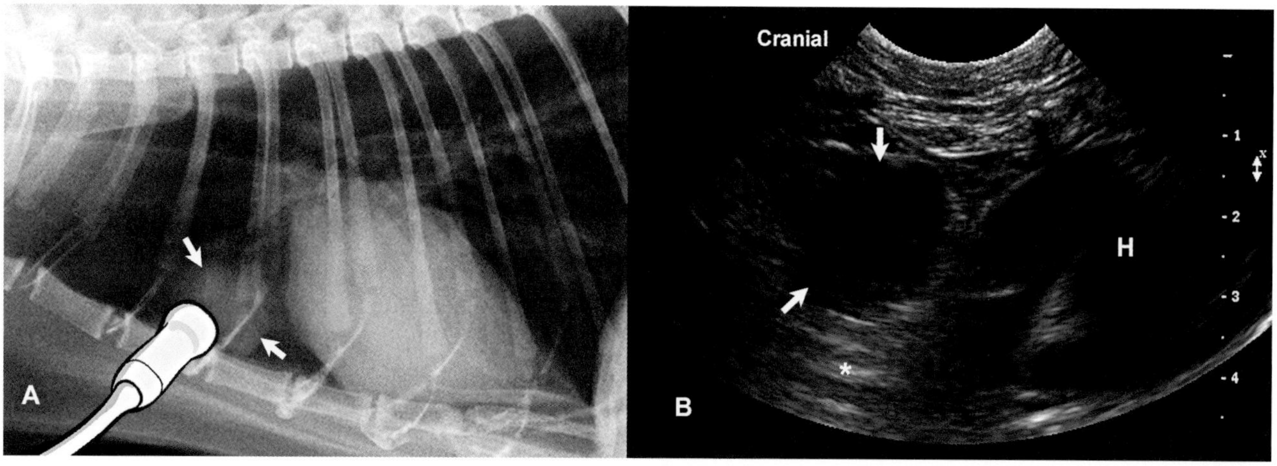

Figure 4.21. Cranial mediastinal cyst in a 9-year-old cat. **A:** Lateral thoracic radiograph demonstrating an ovoid area of increased opacity immediately cranial to the heart (arrows). **B:** Ultrasonographic image obtained by using an intercostal approach immediately dorsal to the sternum at the level of the fourth intercostal space. Cranial to the heart (H) is a round anechoic structure with distal enhancement (*), consistent with the presence of a cranial mediastinal cyst.

masses, which cause cranial mediastinal widening on radiographs. Additionally, it enables identification of a cranial mediastinal mass in the presence of pleural effusion, facilitates characterization of cranial mediastinal mass lesions (cystic in contrast to solid), and is helpful in the identification of a window suitable for interventional procedures.

Mediastinal Mass Lesions

These are most commonly found in the cranioventral mediastinum and are often accompanied by pleural effusion (Reichle and Wisner 2000). Their visualization depends on their location, size, and the presence of a suitable acoustic window. Differential diagnoses for cranial mediastinal masses include cysts, enlarged lymph nodes, neoplasms (e.g., lymphoma or thymoma), inflammatory lesions (abscesses or granulomas), and hematomas. An accumulation of fat may occasionally appear masslike and has the potential for a false-positive diagnosis of a mediastinal mass (Konde and Spaulding 1991).

Cranial mediastinal cysts are an occasional incidental finding in cats (Zekas and Adams 2002). They are usually well circumscribed, thin walled, and filled with anechoic fluid (Figure 4.21).

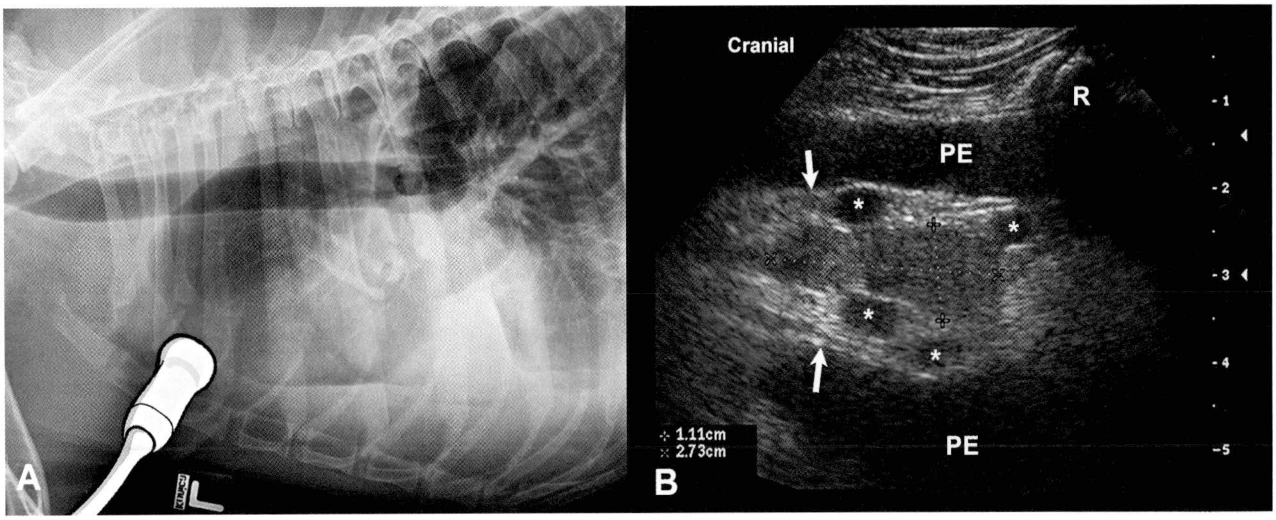

Figure 4.22. Reactive sternal lymph node in a dog with chylothorax. **A:** Lateral thoracic radiograph showing significant pleural effusion that mask mediastinal structures such as the cardiac silhouette. Lung lobes are retracted from the body wall. **B:** Ultrasonographic image at the right second intercostal space immediately dorsal to the sternum. Hypoechoic effusion is on both sides of the cranial mediastinum (arrows). A mildly enlarged sternal lymph node (cursors) is surrounded with hyperechogenic fat and cross-sectional views of hypoechoic vessels (*). A curved hyperechoic interface casting strong shadowing, consistent with a rib, is in the near field (R). PE, pleural effusion. Images courtesy of M.A. d'Anjou.

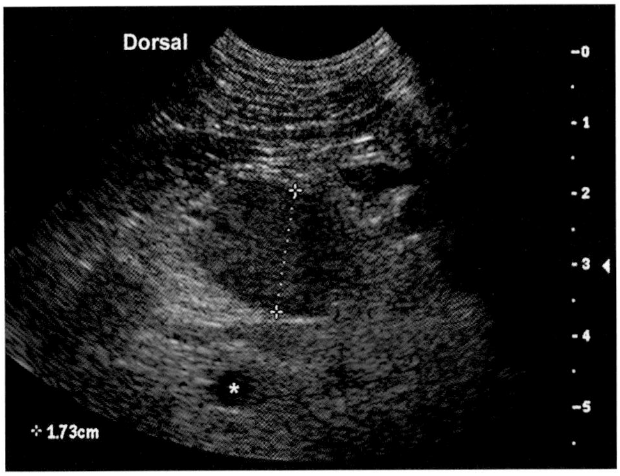

Figure 4.23. Metastatic sternal lymph node in a dog with splenic hemangiosarcoma and hemoabdomen. Transverse ultrasonographic image of an enlarged sternal lymph node (cursors) via an intercostal approach dorsal to the sternum at the level of the second intercostal space. The enlarged lymph node appears as a round hypoechoic nodule surrounded by echogenic fat, and adjacent to cross-sectional anechoic vessels (*). The final histopathologic diagnosis is metastatic hemangiosarcoma. Image courtesy of M.A. d'Anjou.

Enlarged sternal lymph nodes are recognized as rounded nodules or masses of variable size, margination, echotexture, and echogenicity immediately dorsal to the sternum (Figures 4.22–4.24). As the peritoneal cavity is partly drained by these nodes, ultrasonographic examination of the abdomen for underlying disease processes may be warranted in affected patients. Although reactive lymph nodes tend to be smaller than neoplastic or granulomatous lesions, ultrasonographic differentiation of these entities, and differentiation of an enlarged lymph node from cranial mediastinal mass lesions of other etiology, may not be possible.

Masses of inflammatory or neoplastic etiology may appear rounded or lobulated, solid, or cystic, homogeneous, or inhomogeneous (Figures 4.25–4.32). Larger aggressive lesions may infiltrate the surrounding structures, hampering determination of their origin. Lymphoma is most commonly associated with the presence of markedly enlarged and variably homogeneous, hypoechoic lymph nodes or mass(es) in the cranial mediastinum. Thymomas have a tendency to appear cystic (Tidwell 1998). However, cranial mediastinal masses cannot be differentiated based on their ultrasonographic appearance, and histopathology or cytology is needed to assess the nature of the lesion.

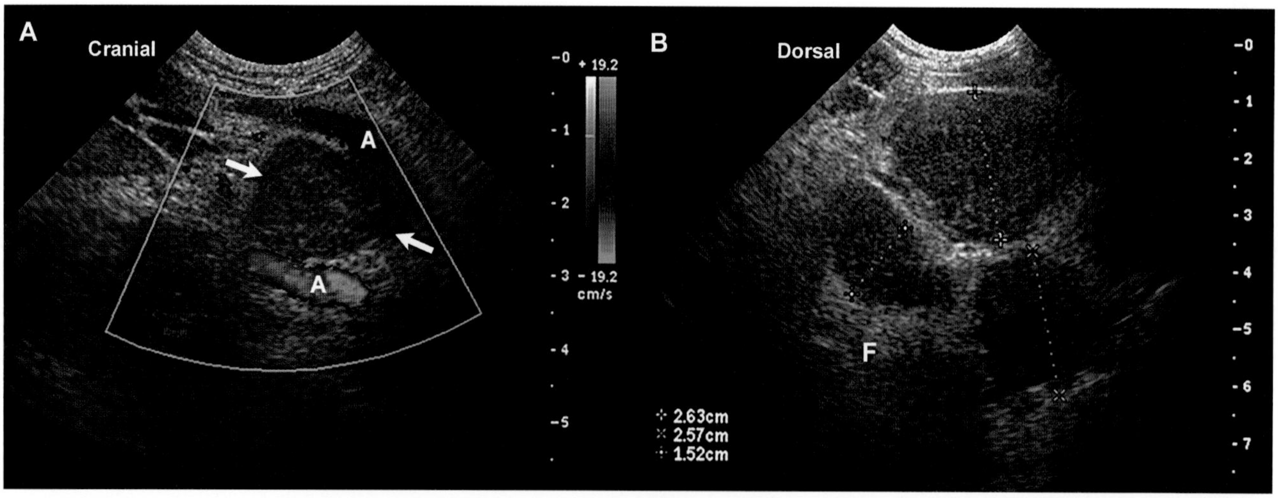

Figure 4.24. Disseminated histiocytic sarcoma in a 5-year-old Bernese mountain dog. Sagittal B-mode **(A)** and transverse color Doppler **(B)** intercostal sonographic images of the cranioventral thorax. A cranial mediastinal mass was suspected on radiographs. Multiple well-defined, hypoechoic nodules and masses (arrows and cursors) are surrounded by mediastinal hyperechoic fat (F) and arteries (A). Images courtesy of M.A. d'Anjou.

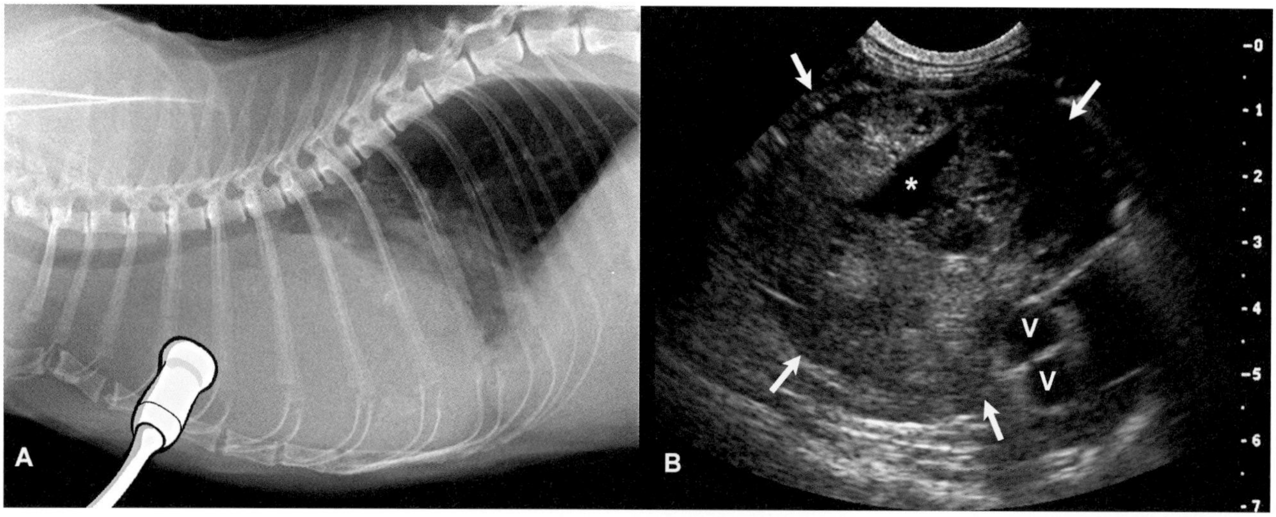

Figure 4.25. Thymoma in a 12-year-old cat. **A:** Lateral thoracic radiograph demonstrating a large cranial mediastinal mass (arrow) causing dorsal displacement of the trachea and silhouetting with the cardiac silhouette. **B:** Ultrasonographic image obtained through a right cranial intercostal approach. A large cranial mediastinal mass lesion (arrows) is of mixed echogenicity, with several anechoic (cystic or cavitated) areas (*). Cranial mediastinal vessels (V) are seen in the far field as anechoic circular structures on cross section. Thymoma was diagnosed based on ultrasonographically obtained biopsy samples.

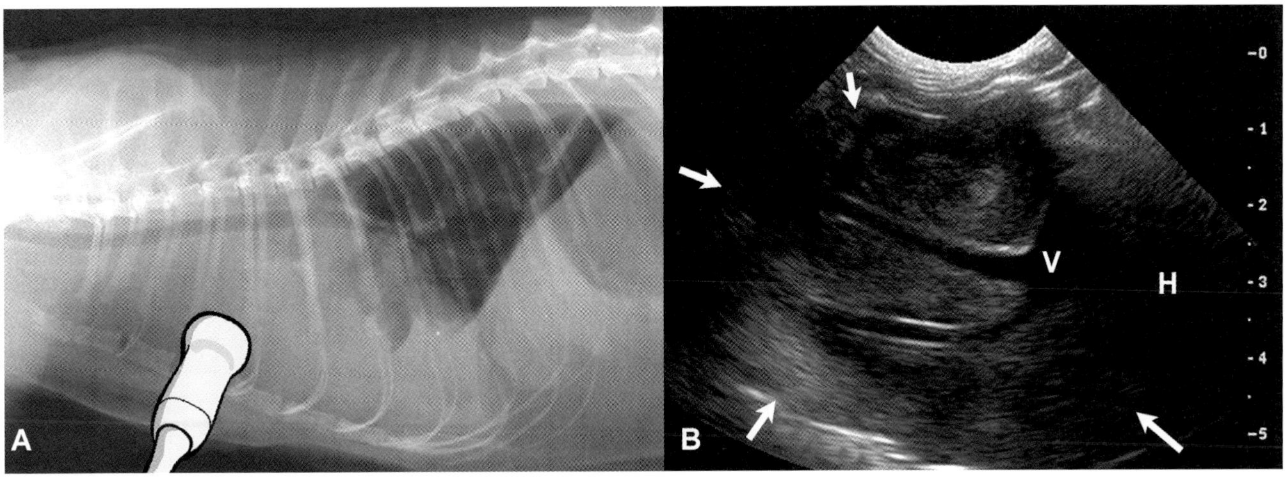

Figure 4.26. Lymphoma in a 4-year-old cat. **A:** In the lateral thoracic radiograph is a large cranial mediastinal mass silhouetting with the heart and displacing the trachea dorsally. Pleural effusion is also present, as indicated by scalloped fluid tissue opacity associated with the ventral thorax, pleural fissure lines, and retraction of the caudodorsal lung lobes from the thoracic wall and diaphragm. **B:** Longitudinal sonogram via an intercostal approach. A large homogeneous mass (arrows) is associated with the cranial mediastinum and in contact with the heart (H). Large vessels are visible within this mass as anechoic tubular structures with strongly hyperechoic vessel walls (V). Lymphoma was diagnosed based on histopathology.

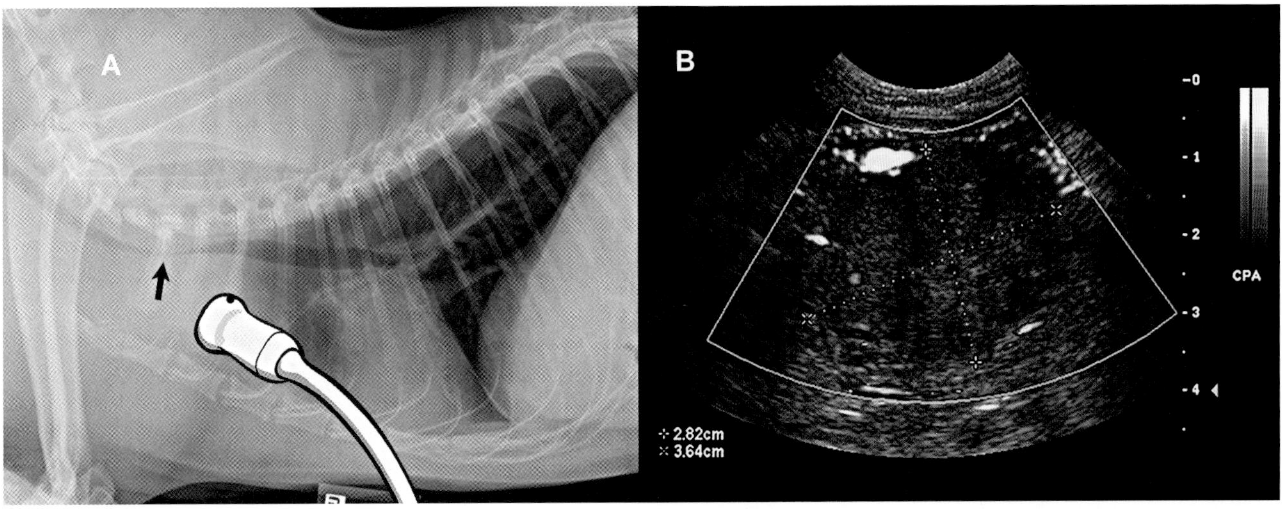

Figure 4.27. Granulomatous lymphadenopathy in a cat. **A:** On the lateral thoracic radiograph is a large, ill-defined, cranial mediastinal mass displacing and compressing the trachea (arrow). Severe swelling was also apparent throughout the neck. **B:** Transverse sonogram via an intercostal approach. A large heterogeneous mass (cursors) is associated with the cranial mediastinum. Increased vascularity is noted at the periphery of the mass by using power Doppler. Cryptococcosis was diagnosed based on ultrasound-guided fine-needle aspiration. Images courtesy of M.A. d'Anjou.

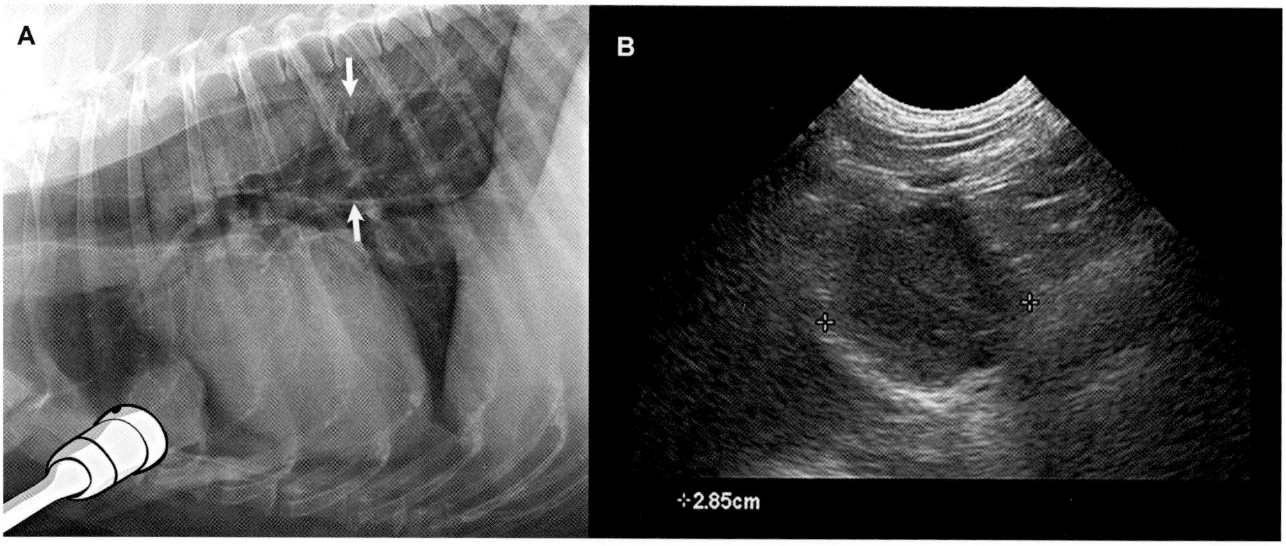

Figure 4.28. Thymoma in a 10-year-old golden retriever. **A:** On the lateral radiograph of the thorax is a well-circumscribed, round, soft-tissue opacity associated with the cranial mediastinum immediately cranial to the cardiac silhouette. The esophagus (arrows) is gas distended, consistent with megaesophagus. **B:** Transverse sonogram via a right intercostal approach immediately dorsal to the sternum. The mass (cursors) appears as a homogeneous, round, hypoechoic structure. Thymoma was diagnosed based on histopathology.

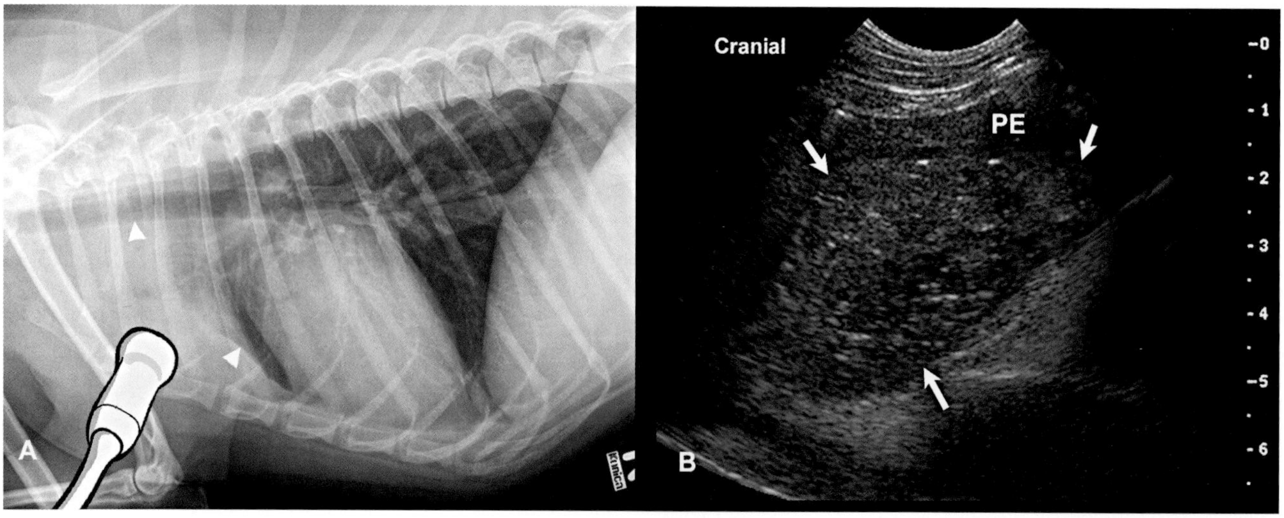

Figure 4.29. Cranial mediastinal lymphoma in a 7-year-old Labrador retriever. **A:** Lateral thoracic radiograph of a large soft-tissue opacity in the cranial mediastinum. The opacity is displacing the trachea and cranial lung ventral margin dorsally (arrowheads). **B:** Corresponding ultrasonographic image by using a dorsal oblique plane through a right intercostal window. A well-defined hypoechoic mass with hyperechoic speckles is in the cranial mediastinum (arrows). A small amount of anechoic pleural effusion (PE) is also observed around the mass. Images courtesy of M.A. d'Anjou.

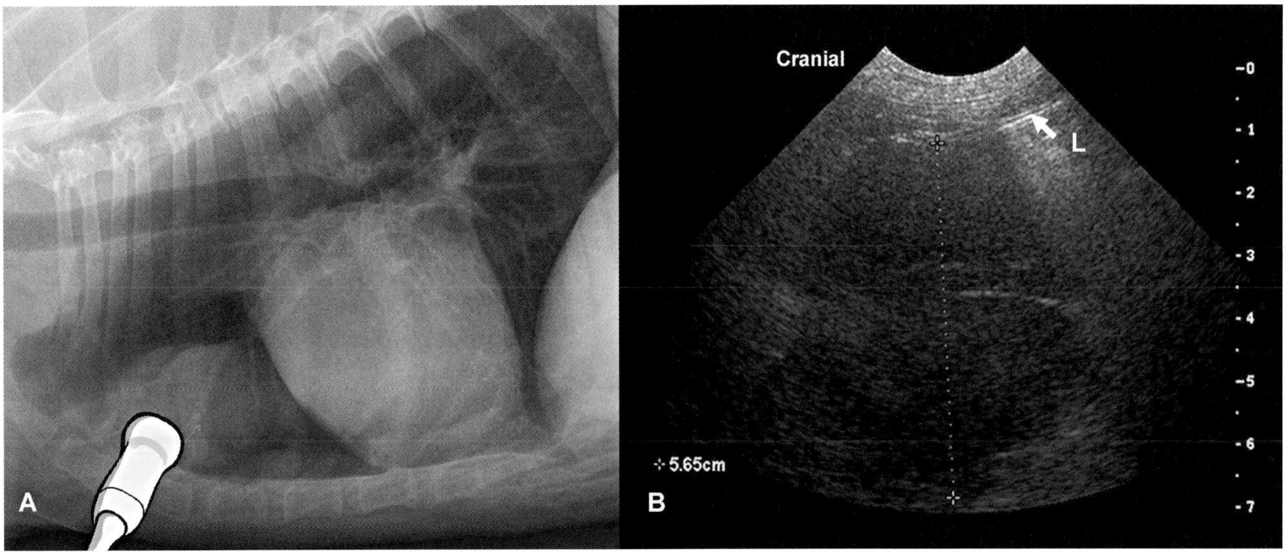

Figure 4.30. Cranial mediastinal mass in an 11-year-old large, mixed-breed dog. **A:** On this lateral thoracic radiograph, a well-circumscribed, round, soft-tissue opacity in the cranial thorax is suspected to originate from the mediastinum on the ventrodorsal radiograph (not shown). **B:** Using a right parasternal intercostal approach, a lobulated hypoechoic mass is noted. Fine-needle aspiration was performed, and a mast cell tumor was diagnosed cytologically. The displaced lung interface (L) and associated reverberation artifacts are in the near field. Images courtesy of M.A. d'Anjou.

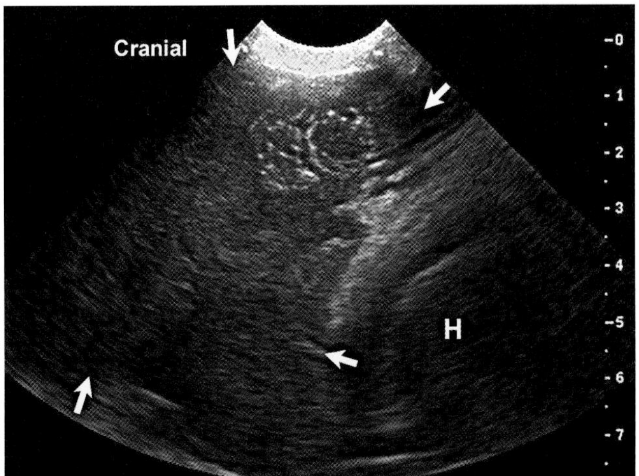

Figure 4.31. Cranial mediastinal lymphoma in a 1-year-old Lhasa apso. Dorsal sonogram via a right intercostal approach. A large, ill-defined mass lesion (arrows) is cranial to the heart (H). The lesion is mainly hypoechoic, with hyperechoic foci in the near field.

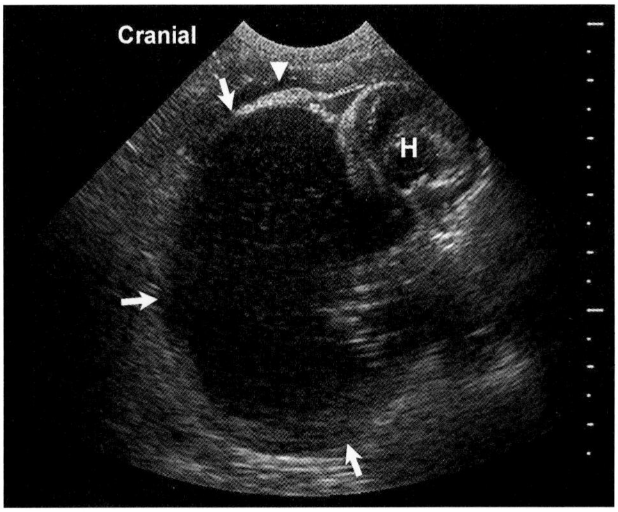

Figure 4.32. Cranial mediastinal mass in a domestic long-hair cat. The examination is performed by using a right intercostal approach. A large mass, mixed in echogenicity, with a large, hypoechoic cavitary component (arrows) is cranial to the heart (H). A small amount of pleural effusion is in the near field (arrowhead). The histopathologic diagnosis was adenocarcinoma.

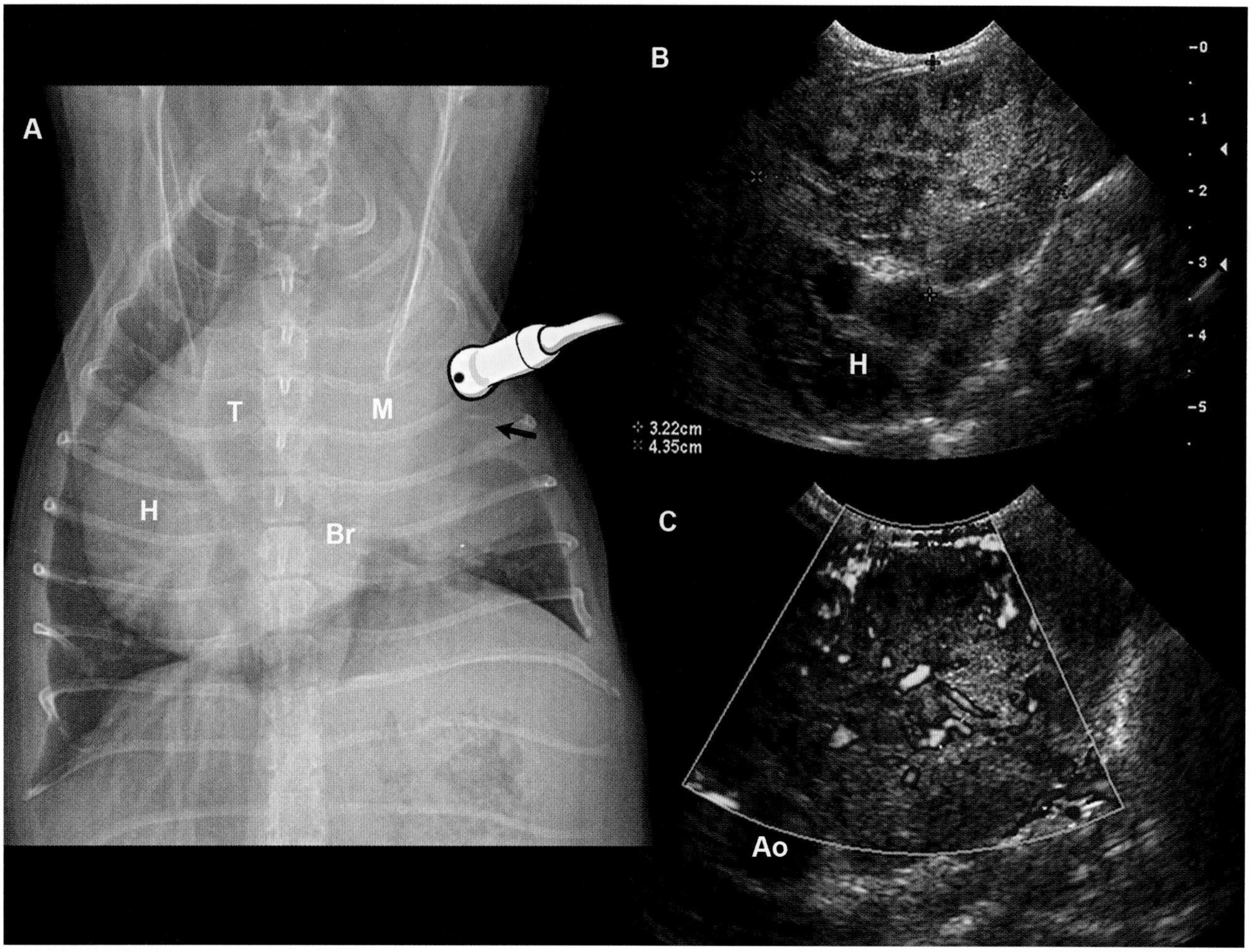

Figure 4.33. Heart base tumor in a small-breed dog. **A:** Ventrodorsal thoracic radiograph in which a soft-tissue opacity associated with a mass effect (M) is in the left cranial hemithorax. The trachea (T) and cardiac silhouette (H) are displaced to the right, and the main left bronchus (Br) is partially compressed. An alveolar pattern is in the caudal portion of the left cranial lobe (arrow). **B:** B-mode sonogram obtained by using a transverse intercostal approach (as shown in **A**). A well-defined solid mass (cursors), mixed in echogenicity, in the near field is displacing the heart (H). **C:** When power Doppler is used, this mass appears hypervascularized. The aorta (Ao) is in the far field, adjacent to the mass. A neuroendocrine tumor was highly suspected on cytological specimens obtained with fine-needle aspiration. Images courtesy of M.A. d'Anjou.

Other Mediastinal Lesions

Radiography (including contrast procedures) and thoracic computed tomography remain the imaging modalities of choice for the diagnosis of lesions associated with the dorsal mediastinum, trachea, and esophagus. Transesophageal ultrasonography may also be of great value when available. Heart base tumors may be visualized through the heart or by using an intercostal approach, if large enough (Figure 4.33). Esophageal dilation and mass lesions (neoplasms, foreign bodies, or granulomas) may occasionally be visualized via a thoracic inlet or transhepatic approach, depending on their location and size (Figure 4.34).

Ultrasonography has been described as an alternative to fluoroscopy in the diagnosis of tracheal collapse (Rudorf et al. 1997). Additionally, it may prove useful in distinguishing between tracheal collapse and other causes of tracheal narrowing such as tracheal wall thickening or compressive mass lesions (Figure 4.35). The ultrasonographic examination is performed using a thoracic inlet approach and is limited to the cervical and cranial thoracic trachea.

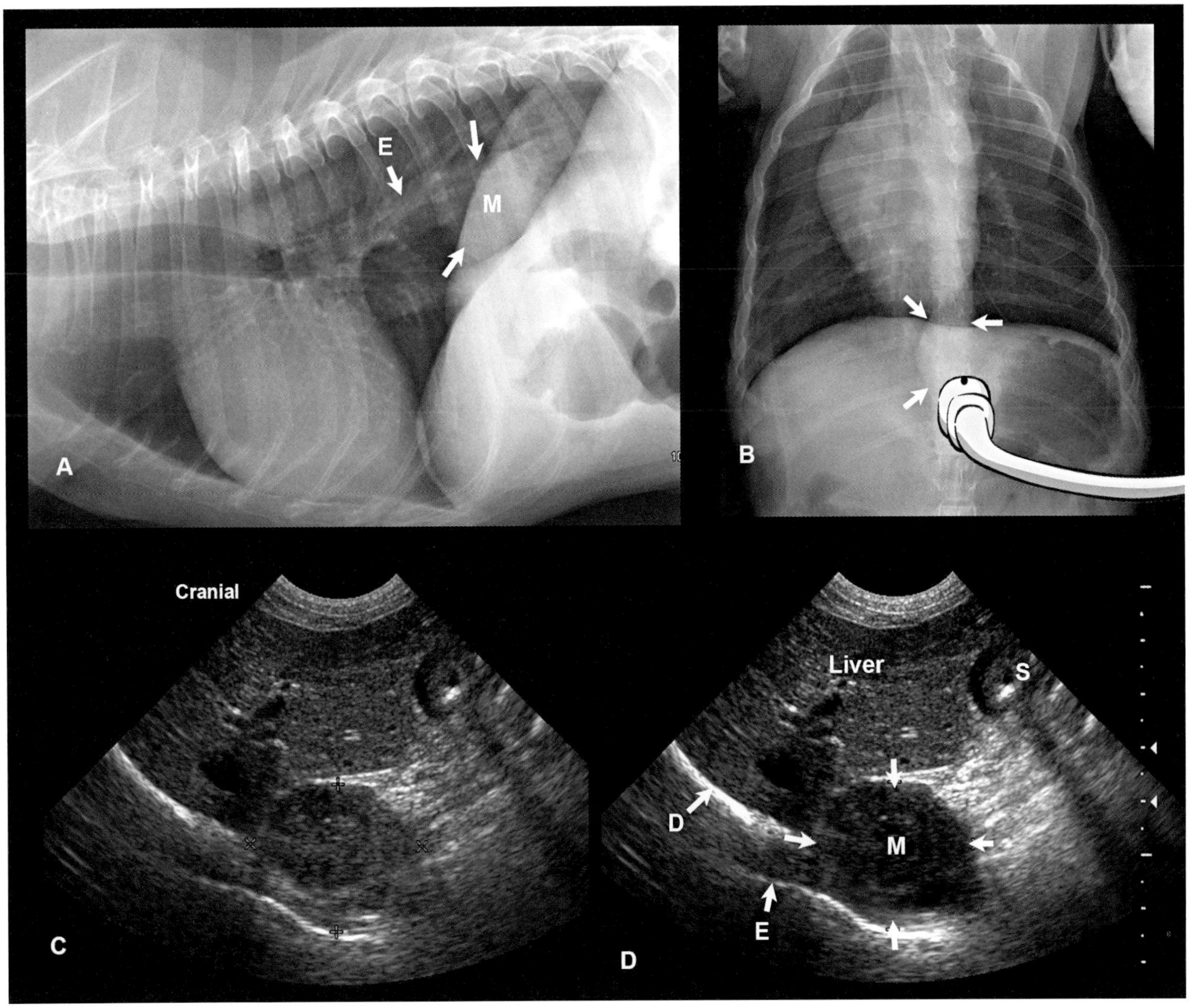

Figure 4.34. Esophageal mass in a 14-year-old Welsh corgi. **A and B:** Thoracic radiographs reveal a homogeneous, soft-tissue opacity (M, arrows) associated with the caudal mediastinum, in the caudal region of the esophagus (E), summating with the diaphragm. The position of the ultrasound transducer is shown in **B**. **C and D:** Ultrasonographic and schematic images obtained with a ventral transhepatic approach (sagittal plane). At the level of the esophageal hiatus, the mass (M, arrows) is associated with the esophagus (E). Liver and stomach (S) are visible in the near field, and the lung-diaphragm interface (D) manifests as a curvilinear, strongly hyperechoic structure bordering the esophageal mass.

Pulmonary Disorders

The ability to assess pulmonary lesions depends on the location and size of the lesion, as well as the presence of a suitable acoustic window. Normally aerated lung, and lesions surrounded by normally aerated lung, cannot be evaluated ultrasonographically. However, when fluid or cells replace the air within alveoli and/or airways, or if a lung lobe collapses, evaluation of the affected lung becomes possible. Pulmonary abnormalities commonly detected and investigated by means of ultrasonography are atelectasis, consolidation, and pulmonary mass lesions. The presence of pleural effusion facilitates the evaluation of lobar size, shape, and contour. A comparative illustration of the ultrasonographic appearance of different pulmonary disorders is shown in Figure 4.36. Although tendencies in ultrasonographic appearance exist for some of the processes, fine-needle aspirations or biopsies are required in most instances to confirm the diagnosis.

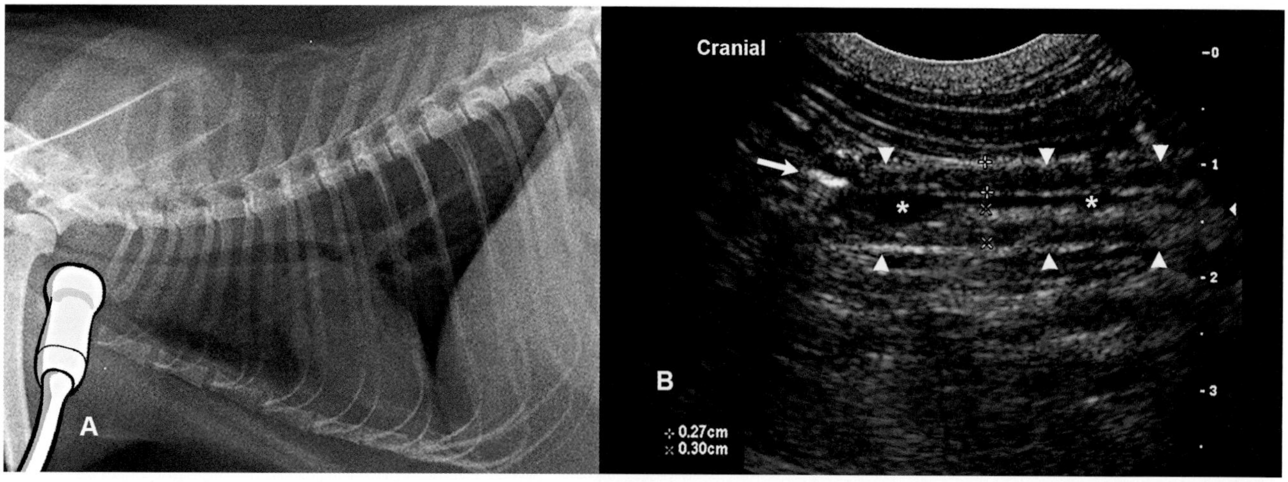

Figure 4.35. Tracheal wall thickening caused by eosinophilic airway disease in a 4-year-old cat. **A:** The lateral thoracic radiograph shows extensive narrowing of the cranial thoracic trachea. **B:** An ultrasonographic examination of the trachea (arrowheads) is performed by using a thoracic inlet approach. The tracheal wall (cursors) is thickened (0.3 cm) and hypoechoic. Anechoic material, consistent with mucus, is present within the severely narrowed tracheal lumen (*). A gas bubble is present more cranially, appearing as a reverberating hyperechoic focus in the nondependent portion of the lumen (arrow).

Atelectasis

Atelectasis (pulmonary collapse) may occur secondary to increased pressure within the pleural space (pneumothorax or pleural effusion) and may be a sequela to bronchial obstruction or a result of decreased pulmonary compliance and inability of the lung to inflate properly. Ultrasonographic assessment of atelectatic lung is easy in cases of concurrent pleural effusion, but impossible in cases of pneumothorax. Affected lung lobes appear as small, smoothly marginated, triangular structures that are commonly surrounded by pleural fluid (Figure 4.13). The echogenicity of atelectatic lung depends on the amount of residual air within the airspaces and may range from uniformly hypoechoic to strongly hyperechoic. Linear and speckled hyperechoic foci, indicating residual air within bronchi and alveoli, as well as bronchial walls, are often seen. Additionally, vessels can usually be visualized, particularly by means of color or power Doppler. Completely collapsed lung lobes tend to be similar in echogenicity and echotexture to liver lobes. In cases of obstructive atelectasis, ultrasonography may prove useful in identification of the obstructive lesion (e.g., mass).

Consolidation

When fluid or cells uniformly infiltrate the pulmonary air spaces, the lung often becomes hypoechoic and assumes an echotexture similar to liver (*hepatized lung*) (Schwarz and Tidwell 1999). The affected lung lobe typically retains its normal shape and volume (Figures 4.36–4.38 and 4.41). Air-filled bronchi appear as hyperechoic *air bronchograms* radiating from the hilus, which are commonly associated with reverberation artifacts or dirty shadowing. Residual air within alveoli also remains hyperechoic (Figure 4.38). If the bronchial lumen is filled with secretions or cellular debris, *fluid bronchograms* develop, which resemble vessels but can be distinguished by means of color or power Doppler by their lack of flow (Figure 4.39). Although pulmonary consolidation is most commonly associated with pneumonia, it may also be encountered in lung contusion, lobe torsion (d'Anjou et al. 2005), and infiltrative pulmonary neoplasia (Figures 4.39–4.41). Dispersed, hyperechoic, and reverberating foci, indicating vesicular emphysema, are commonly observed in the central portion of a twisted lung lobe (Figures 4.39 and 4.40), and lobes infiltrated with neoplasia are often heterogeneous and deformed. Additionally, concurrent pleural effusion is expected in cases of lung-lobe torsion and in some cases of pulmonary neoplasia, as opposed to pneumonia. Color or power Doppler can prove useful in confirming the lack of flow in a twisted lobe. However, ultrasonographic differentiation of these entities, which may coexist in the same lobe, may not be possible.

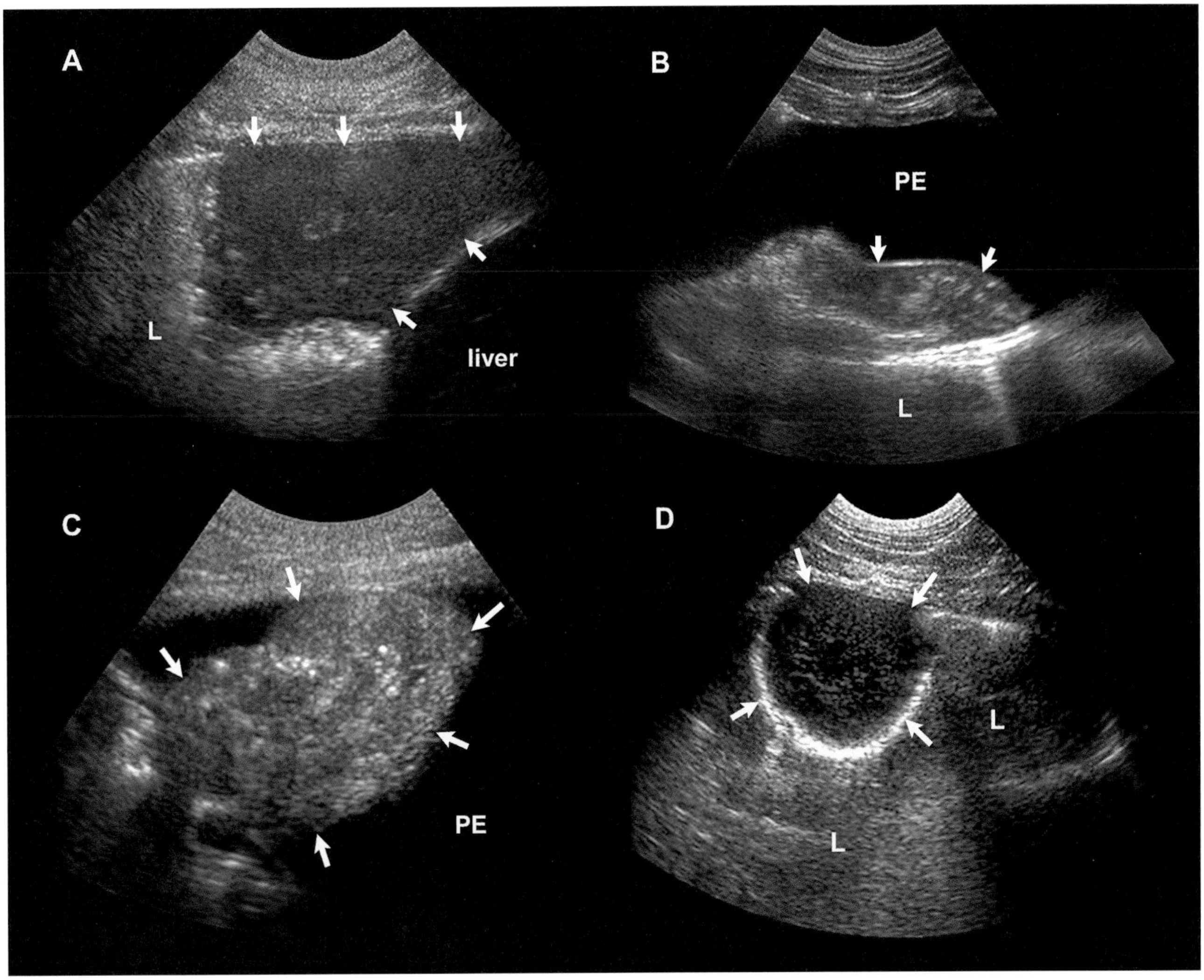

Figure 4.36. Schematic ultrasound images of pulmonary abnormalities. **A: Consolidation.** Normal pulmonary parenchyma is filled with fluid or replaced with inflammatory or neoplastic infiltrates. The affected portion (arrows) is hypoechoic when compared with the normally aerated, hyperechoic lung portion (L). The lung lobe retains its normal size, shape, and contour. **B: Atelectasis.** The lung is collapsed because of pleural effusion (PE). The affected lung lobe is significantly reduced in volume (arrows). Occasional hyperechoic foci within the collapsed lung lobe are consistent with a small amount of residual air. The reverberating interface of the contralateral air-filled lung is seen in the far field. **C: Pulmonary mass lesion.** With increasing size, pulmonary mass lesions cause loss of the normal shape and margination of a lung lobe, with distortion of the pulmonary border and the normal triangular form of a lung lobe (arrows). These changes are enhanced if pleural effusion is present (PE). The echogenicity of pulmonary mass lesions is variable. **D: Pulmonary nodule.** Lung nodules are typically spherical and well demarcated from the peripheral aerated lung (arrows). These nodules can only be detected if they are in contact with the thoracic wall. L, aerated lung.

Pulmonary Masses and Nodules

Although pulmonary masses in small animals are most commonly neoplastic in etiology, benign lesions such as abscesses, cysts, hematomas, or granulomas may also be encountered. In the absence of pleural effusion, pulmonary masses can be evaluated ultrasonographically only if located at the periphery of the lung field and if a suitable acoustic window is present.

Pulmonary neoplasms usually appear hypoechoic or mixed echogenic and solid. They cause focal disruption of the reflective lung surface and commonly form an acute angle with the thoracic wall

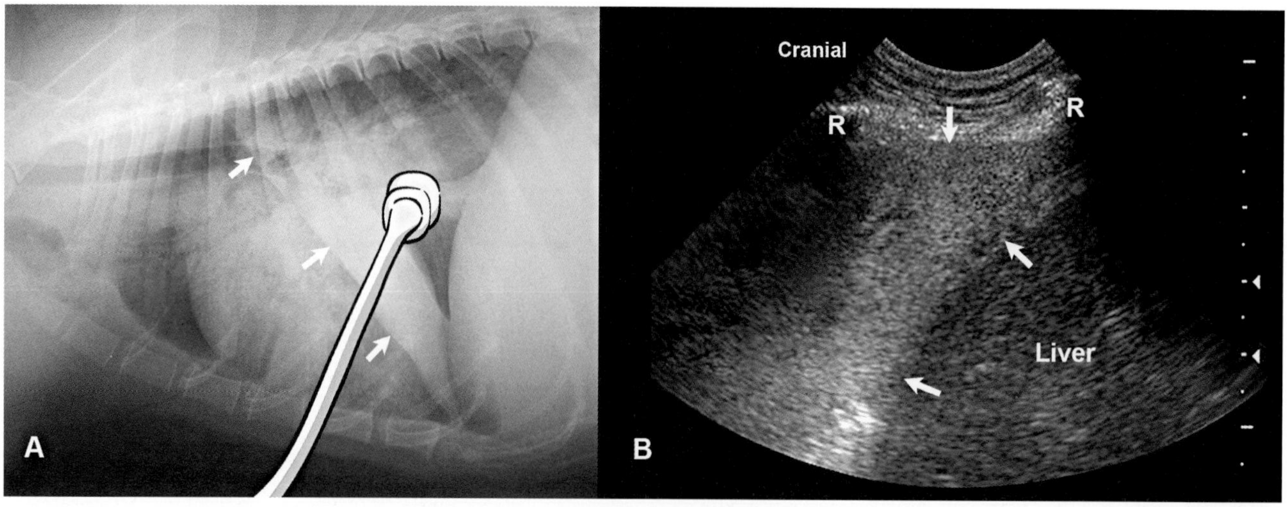

Figure 4.37. Acute suppurative pneumonia with hemorrhage in a 10-year-old Labrador retriever. **A:** The right lateral radiograph of the thorax shows an alveolar pattern in the left caudal lung lobe and a clear border between the left cranial and caudal lung lobe (lobar margination [arrows]). There is also a mixed alveolar pattern and an interstitial pattern in the left cranial lung lobe. **B:** The ultrasonographic examination is performed in a dorsal plane by using a left caudal dorsal intercostal approach. The left caudal lung lobe is homogeneously echogenic (arrows) and is hyperechoic to the hepatic parenchyma seen caudal to the diaphragm. Acoustic shadows related to superficial ribs (R) are present.

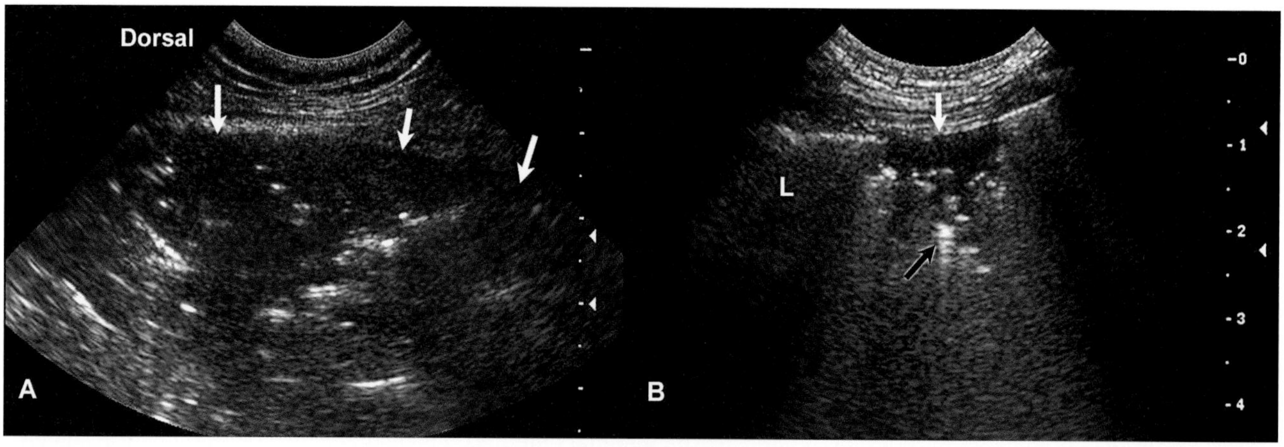

Figure 4.38. Aspiration pneumonia in two dogs. Both examinations are performed with a right intercostal approach. **A:** The right middle lung lobe (arrows) is homogeneous and mostly hypoechoic, with a few hyperechoic foci representing gas inclusions. The lung lobe retains its normal triangular shape and size. There is no evidence of pleural effusion. **B:** Focal pneumonia (white arrow) involving the right middle lobe, which appears as an irregular, hypoechoic region with gas speckles associated with comet-tail artifacts (black arrow). Deeper foci of pneumonia cannot be visualized because of overlying aerated lung (L). Image B courtesy of M.A. d'Anjou.

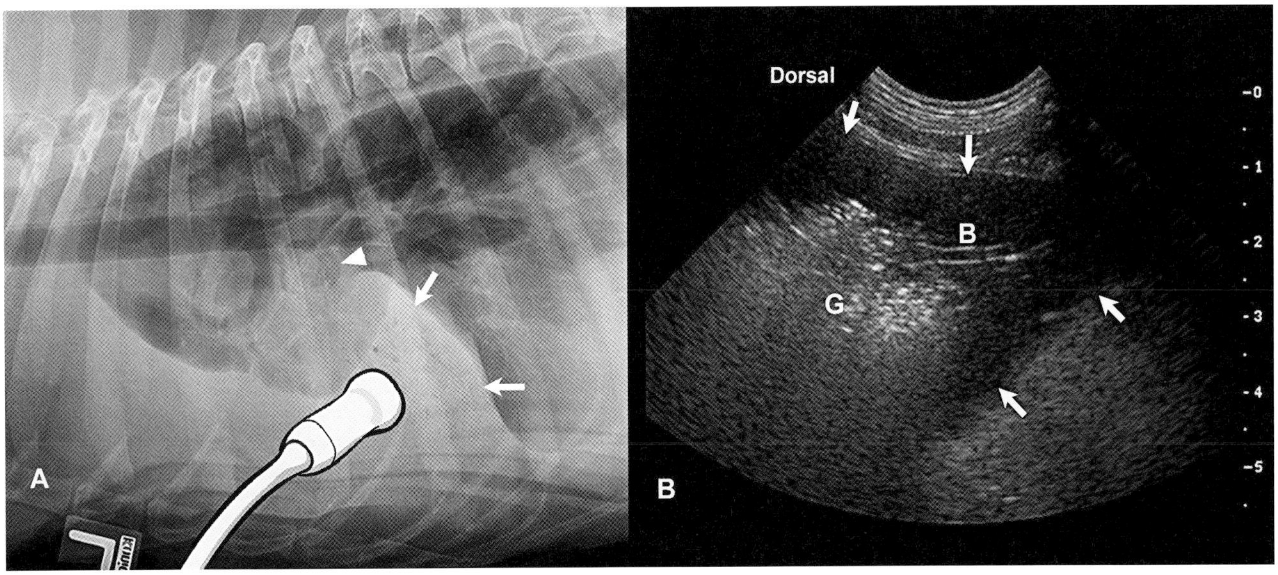

Figure 4.39. Torsion of the right middle lung lobe in a 5-year-old mixed large-breed dog. **A:** On the lateral thoracic radiograph, marked pleural effusion is noted, as well as right middle lung lobe opacification and enlargement (arrows). The main bronchus is interrupted (arrowhead), and punctate and linear gas lucencies are observed in the consolidated lobe. **B:** The ultrasound examination is performed by using a right intercostal approach at the level of the sixth intercostal space. The peripheral portion of the lung lobe is hypoechoic, and dispersed and hyperechoic foci are in the central portion, in association with reverberation artifacts, consistent with gas (G). This pattern is commonly encountered with lung-lobe torsion. A fluid-filled bronchus (fluid bronchogram) appears in the apex of this lobe (B). Images courtesy of M.A. d'Anjou.

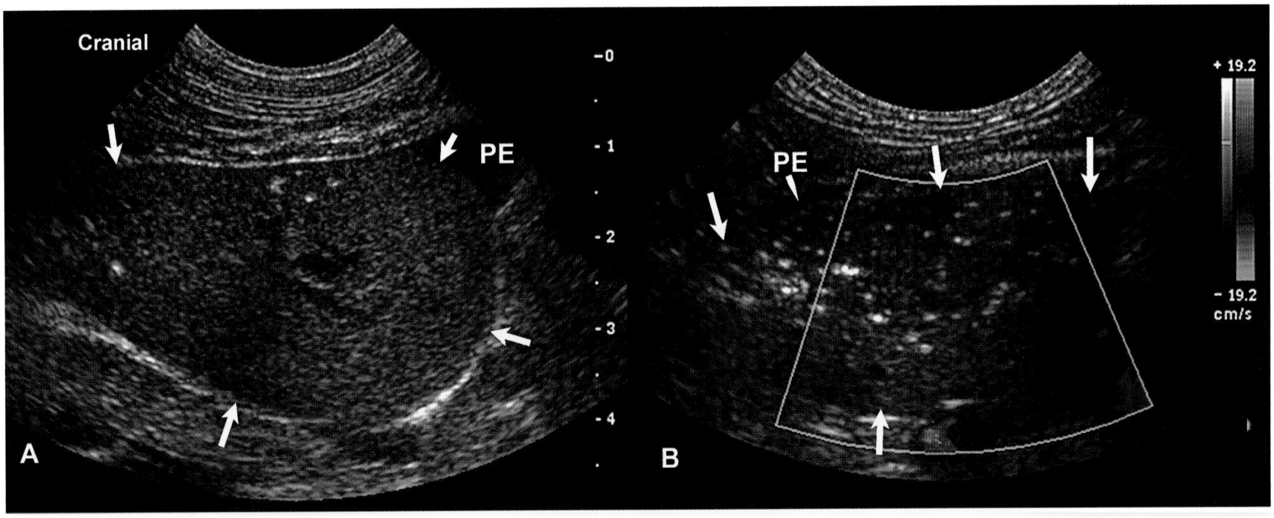

Figure 4.40. Lung-lobe torsion in a small-breed dog. **A and B:** Ultrasonographic images of different portions of the right cranial lung lobe, which appears "hepatized" and enlarged (arrows). The lobe is diffusely mildly echogenic and presents dispersed hyperechoic foci that were consistent with gas. When color Doppler is used **(B)**, there is no evidence of any vascular flow. A small volume of hypoechoic pleural effusion (PE) is also apparent around the lobe. Images courtesy of M.A. d'Anjou.

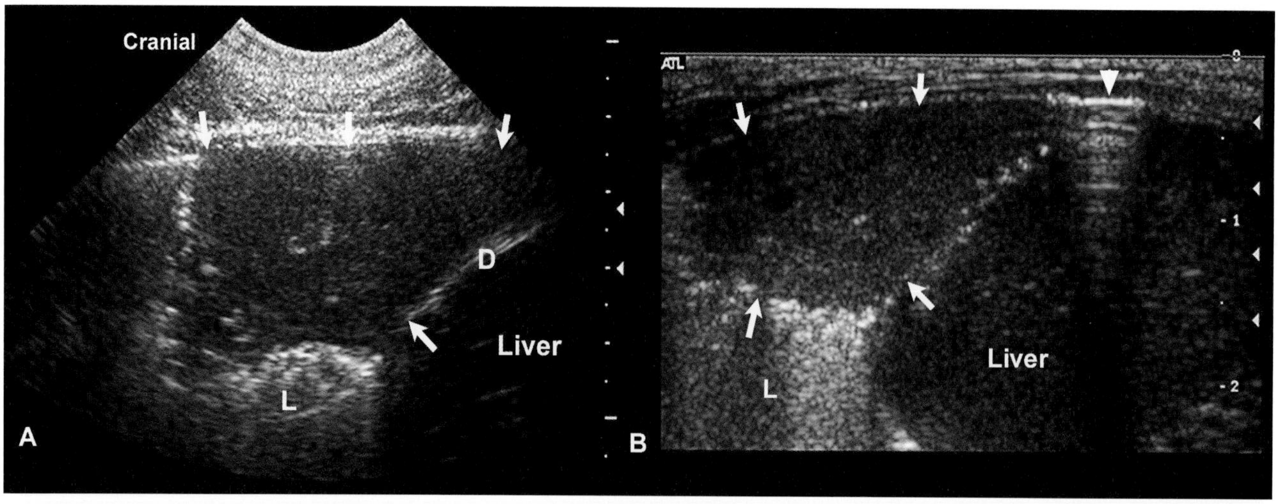

Figure 4.41. Uniform lung consolidation in two dogs. **A:** Bronchoalveolar carcinoma in a 15-year-old mixed-breed dog. Dorsal sonogram by using a right intercostal approach. The tip of the right caudal lung lobe (arrows) is uniformly hypoechoic and has retained its normal triangular shape. The abnormal portion of this lobe is in contact with the diaphragm (D). The normal lung portion, which remains aerated, is seen in the far field (L). **B:** Traumatic lung contusion in another dog in which the affected portion of the right caudal lobe (arrows) is uniformly moderately echogenic. Additionally, a short linear hyperechogenicity is in the caudolateral portion of the pleural space (arrowhead), in association with a comet-tail artifact, consistent with mild pneumothorax. L, normal aerated lung. Image B courtesy of M.A. d'Anjou.

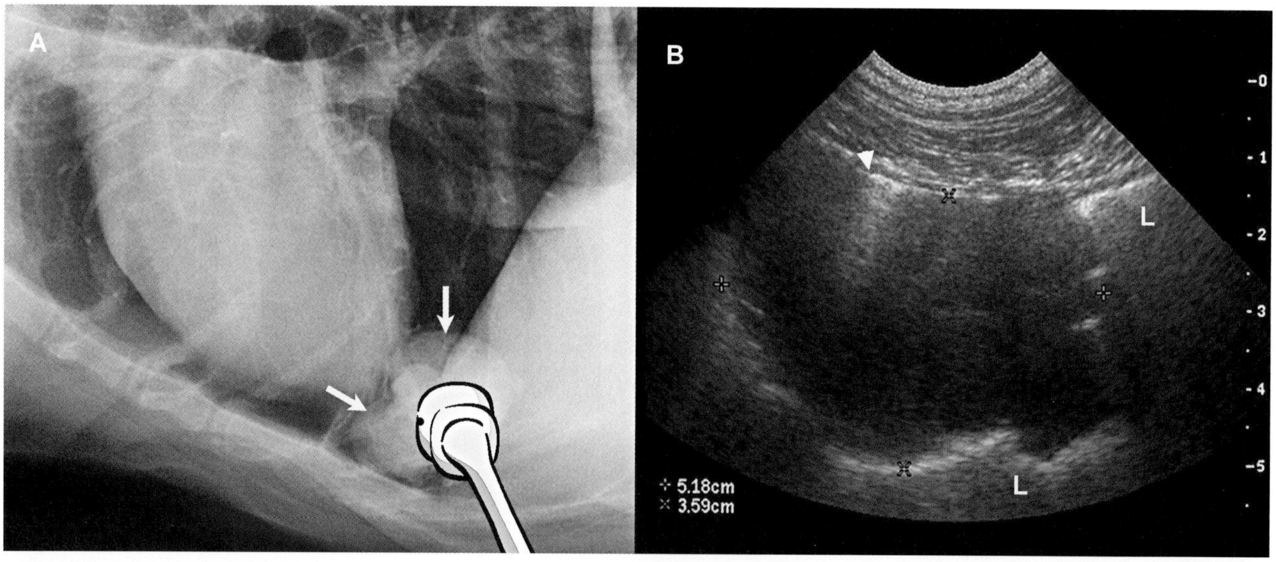

Figure 4.42. Disseminated histiocytic sarcoma in a 6-year-old Bernese mountain dog. **A:** On the left lateral radiograph of the thorax is an approximately 5-cm soft-tissue mass in the caudal ventral thorax, summating with the diaphragm (arrows). **B:** The ultrasonographic examination of the caudal ventral thorax was performed by using an intercostal approach immediately dorsal to the sternum. The mass (cursors) is irregular, homogeneous, hypoechoic, and associated with the ventral aspect of the right caudal lung lobe. The peripheral border is strongly hyperechoic and associated with reverberation artifacts, consistent with aerated portion of the lung lobe (L). On real-time examination, it was seen to be sliding with respiration. A reverberating artifact originating from the pleural space and consistent with free air is also observed in the near field (arrowhead).

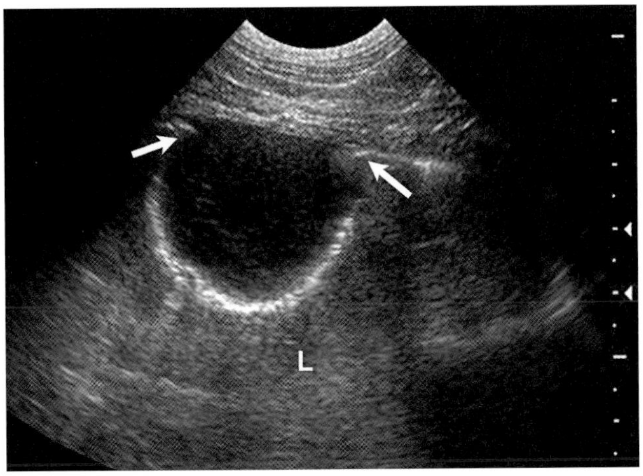

Figure 4.43. Pulmonary carcinoma in an 8-year-old Labrador retriever. The examination was performed by using an intercostal approach. The pulmonary mass is well circumscribed, almost anechoic, forms an acute angle with the thoracic wall (arrows), and is surrounded by normally aerated lung parenchyma (L).

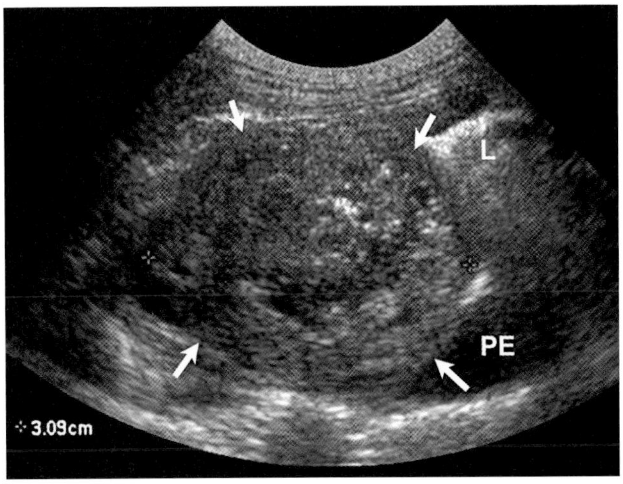

Figure 4.44. Pulmonary carcinoma in a 12-year-old cat. The examination is performed by using an intercostal approach. A 3-cm mixed echogenic mass (arrows) associated with the pulmonary parenchyma distorts the normal lung margins. The adjacent normal lung is characterized by a hyperreflective interface (L). A small amount of pleural effusion (PE) is present.

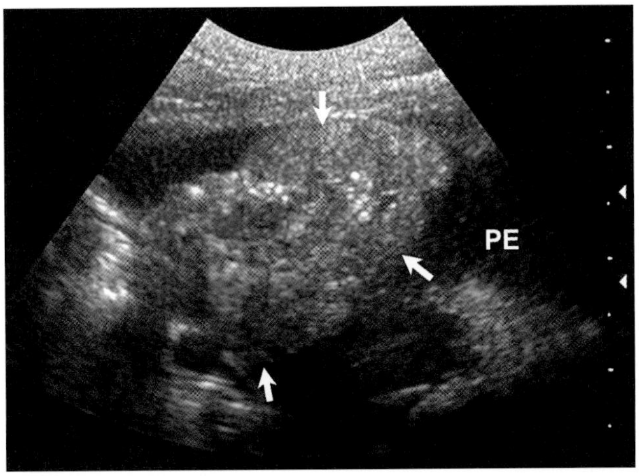

Figure 4.45. Pulmonary carcinoma in a 9-year-old cat. The examination is performed by using a right intercostal approach. A mixed echogenic mass associated with the right lung (suspected right middle lung lobe) distorts the normal lung margins. Concurrent pleural effusion (PE) is noted, delineating the irregular contours of the lung lesion.

(Figures 4.42 and 4.43). Lung masses or nodules are easily identified as pulmonary in origin when they move with the rest of the lung during respiration. However, this feature is not observed in cases of pleural adhesions. In contrast to atelectasis or consolidation, pulmonary mass lesions frequently cause distortion of the normal contour of the affected lung lobe (Figures 4.44 and 4.45). Central tumor necrosis can vary in appearance and may lead to confusion with a pulmonary abscess, particularly when hypoechoic or anechoic. Air cavities and dystrophic mineralization, appearing as hyperechoic foci with or without rever-

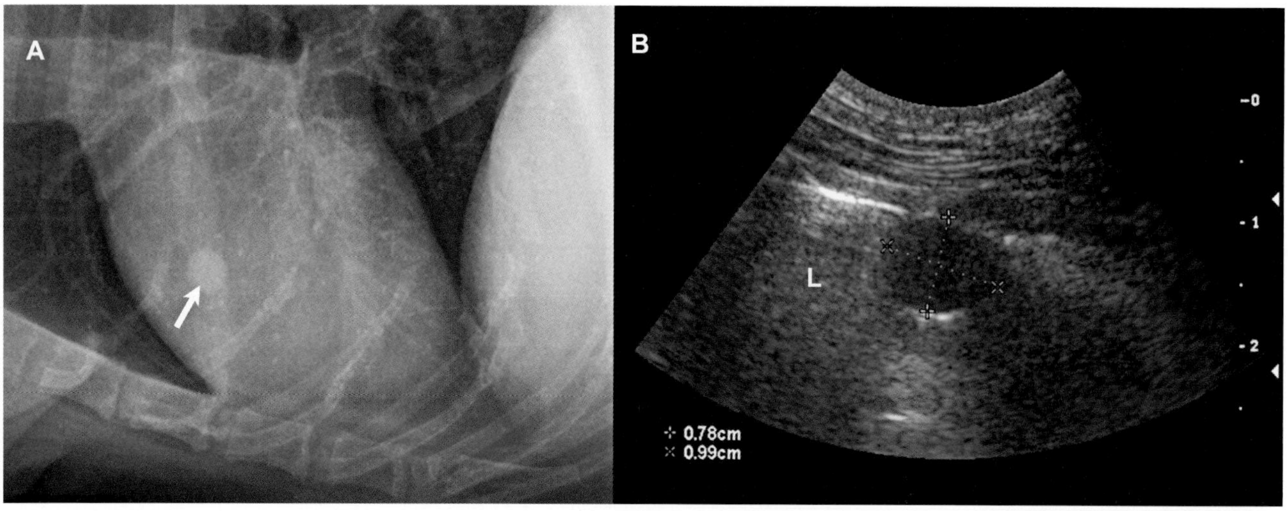

Figure 4.46. Pulmonary nodule in a Dalmatian with a history of weight loss. **A:** A small, round, soft-tissue opacity is observed on this left lateral thoracic radiograph in the right hemithorax (arrow). **B:** Using a left intercostal approach, a spherical hypoechoic nodule was observed at the superficial aspect of the lung (L). Fine-needle aspiration by using ultrasound guidance revealed a metastatic sarcoma. An abdominal fibrosarcoma was identified. Images courtesy of M.A. d'Anjou.

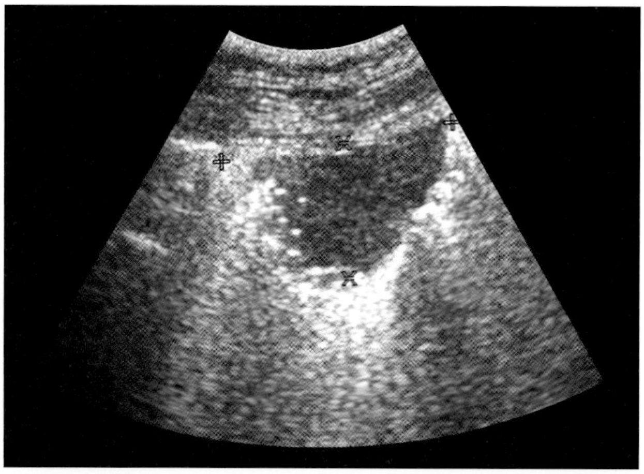

Figure 4.47. Fungal granuloma (blastomycosis) in a dog. A small, superficial, homogeneous, hypoechoic mass (cursors) is associated with the pulmonary parenchyma.

berating and shadowing artifacts, are often seen in primary lung tumors.

Pulmonary metastases may be recognized as peripherally distributed, round, hypoechoic nodules moving with the aerated lung (Figure 4.46). Larger metastases may show similar ultrasonographic features as primary pulmonary neoplasms. However, these lesions may also resemble benign mass lesions such as granulomas and chronic hematomas, necessitating cytological or histological analysis for a definitive diagnosis (Figure 4.47).

Pulmonary cysts, acute hematomas, and abscesses can be fluid filled. Cysts are usually thin walled and contain anechoic fluid. Abscesses and hematomas have

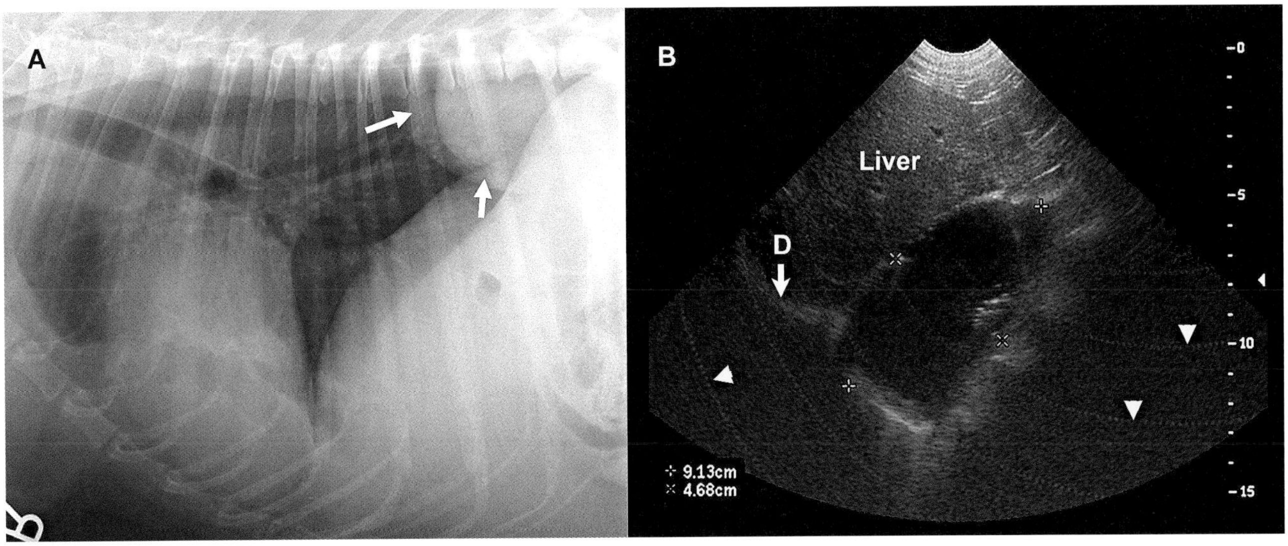

Figure 4.48. Pulmonary abscess in a 5-year-old collie. **A:** On the lateral thoracic radiograph is a large, well-circumscribed, homogeneous mass lesion associated with the caudal dorsal lung fields immediately cranial to the diaphragm (arrows). **B:** The ultrasonographic examination is performed by using a transhepatic approach (dorsal plane). The abscess (cursors) is seen immediately cranial to the diaphragm (D). It is anechoic and surrounded by a thin, hyperechoic rim. The concentric dotted lines (arrowheads) represent an artifact likely caused by electrical interference.

variable wall thickness and margination, and the echogenicity of their contents may range from anechoic to echogenic (Figures 4.48–4.50). Abscessing pneumonia may also cause lobar enlargement and marked heterogeneity, mimicking neoplasia and necrosis. Furthermore, these processes can coexist.

Diaphragmatic Disorders

Hernia

Although challenging, ultrasonography represents an important diagnostic tool in the investigation of traumatic diaphragmatic hernias (i.e., ruptures), true (congenital) diaphragmatic hernias, and congenital peritoneo-pericardial diaphragmatic hernias (PPDH) (Spattini et al. 2003).

The ultrasonographic characteristics of a diaphragmatic hernia or rupture are an irregular or asymmetrical cranial aspect of the liver and the presence of abdominal viscera in the thorax (Figures 4.51–4.55).

If an ultrasonographic examination is performed to confirm or exclude a diaphragmatic hernia, the examiner has to be aware of common artifacts occurring at the level of the diaphragm. If the animal has ascites, refraction of the beam at the liver surface may cause the diaphragm to appear discontinuous. The commonly seen mirror-image artifact might be mistaken for a herniation of liver into the thorax (see Figure 6.4). Adhesions between liver and lung in cases of chronic diaphragmatic rupture might resemble the appearance of an intact diaphragm and lead to a false-negative result on the ultrasonographic examination. Diaphragmatic, pulmonary, or pleural mass lesions may also lead to misinterpretation by mimicking abdominal contents in the thoracic cavity (Spattini et al. 2003)

The ultrasonographic diagnosis of a PPDH is usually straightforward if abdominal organs (e.g., liver or intestine) are present within the pericardial sac (Figures 4.54 and 4.55).

Other Diaphragmatic Disorders

Other disorders of the diaphragm are extremely rare. Benign or malignant mass lesions are occasionally encountered (Figure 4.56).

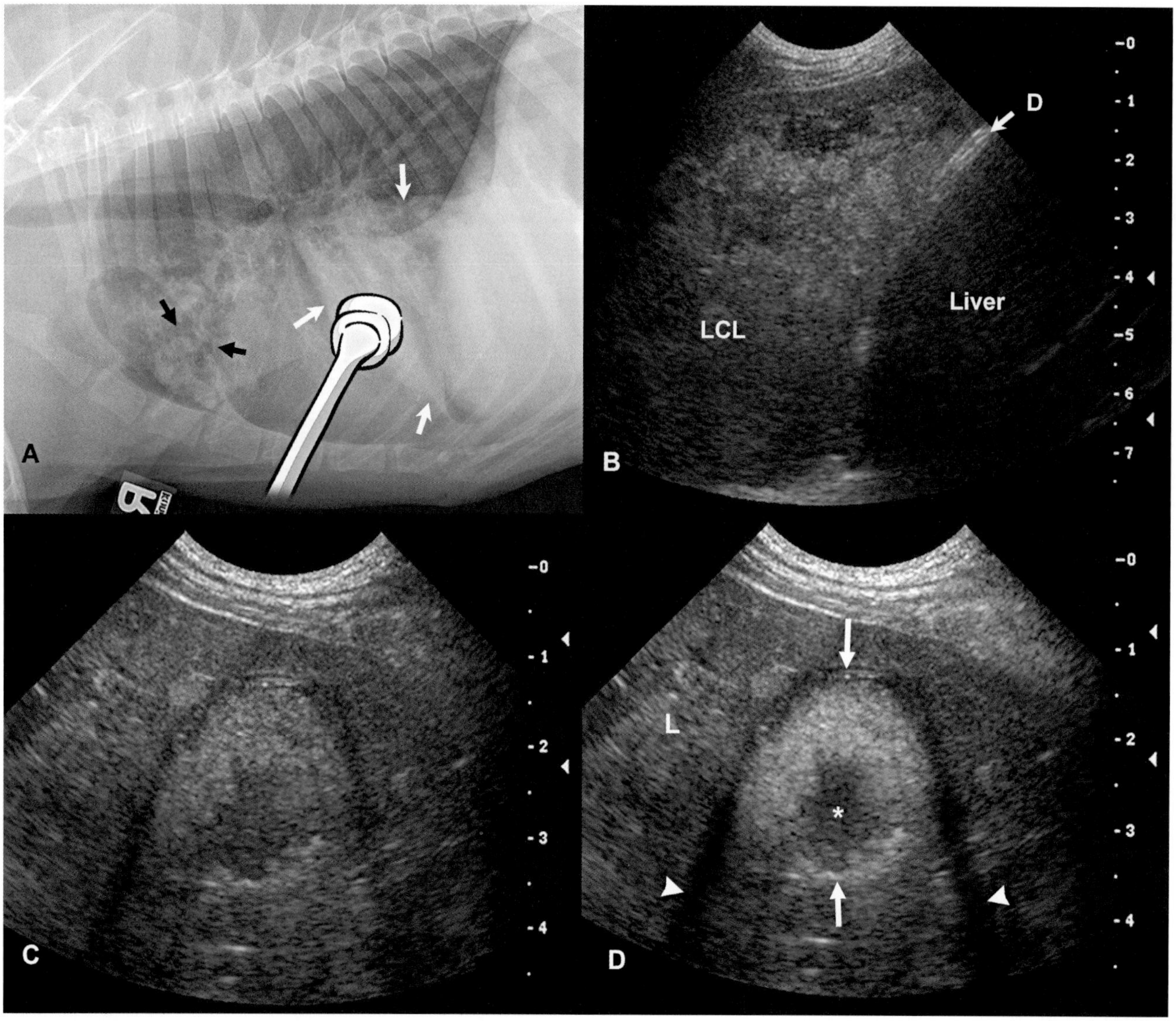

Figure 4.49. Chronic pyogranulomatous pneumonia in a large-breed dog. **A:** A soft-tissue opacity is in the caudoventral lung field on the right lateral radiograph (white arrows). An alveolar pattern is also apparent in the cranioventral lung field, as well as irregular, air-filled, dilated bronchi consistent with bronchiectasis (black arrows). **B:** On this ultrasonographic image obtained through the left sixth intercostal space, a large portion of the left caudal lung lobe (LCL) in contact with the diaphragm (D) is heterogeneous, moderately echogenic, and enlarged. **C and D:** Sonographic and schematic images. In a portion of this lung lobe (L) is a spherical hyperechoic mass (arrows) with an irregular hypoechoic center (*). A thin hypoechoic rim is at the periphery of this mass, as well as edge-shadowing artifacts (arrowheads). Fine-needle aspiration confirmed the presence of a pyogranuloma. Images courtesy of M.A. d'Anjou.

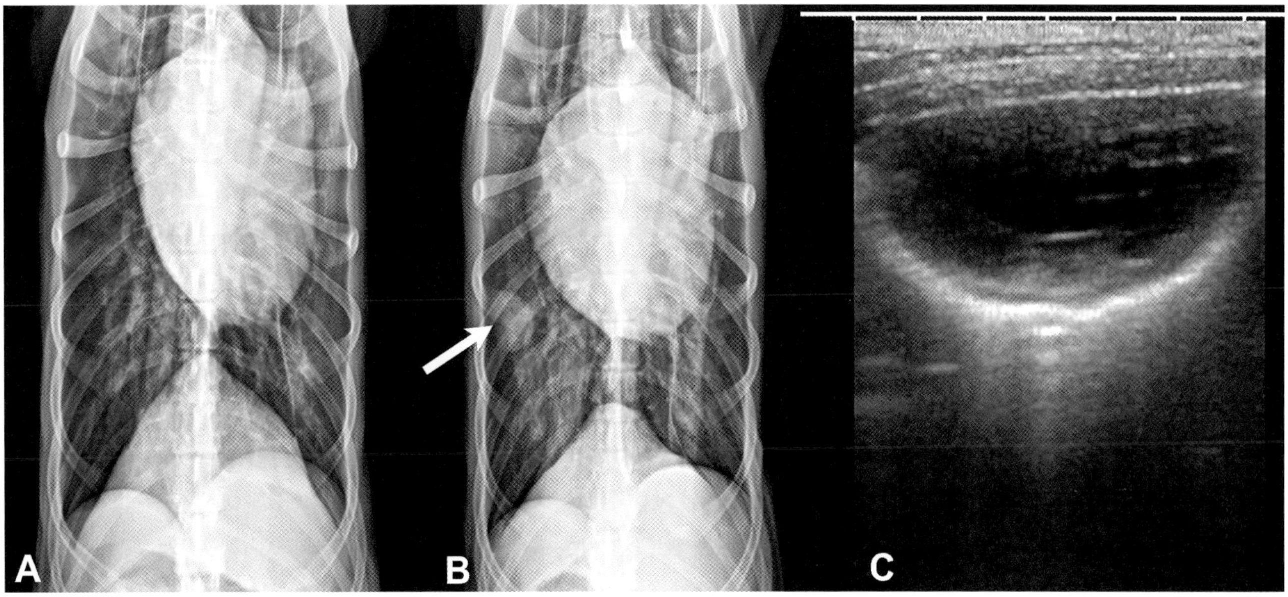

Figure 4.50. Traumatic pulmonary hematoma in a 9-year-old Scottish deerhound. Radiographs and sonogram of the lung after bronchoalveolar lavage. **A:** The ventrodorsal radiograph, at the time of presentation, reveals a generalized unstructured interstitial pattern. No other abnormality is detected at this time. A bronchoalveolar lavage was then performed. **B:** Recheck radiographs 6 days later show a homogeneous 3-cm mass lesion associated with the right lung at the level of the sixth rib (arrow). **C:** The ultrasonographic examination was performed by using a linear probe with a transverse intercostal approach. An anechoic, well-circumscribed lesion of 3-cm diameter is associated with the lung. Aspiration yielded blood, consistent with a hematoma.

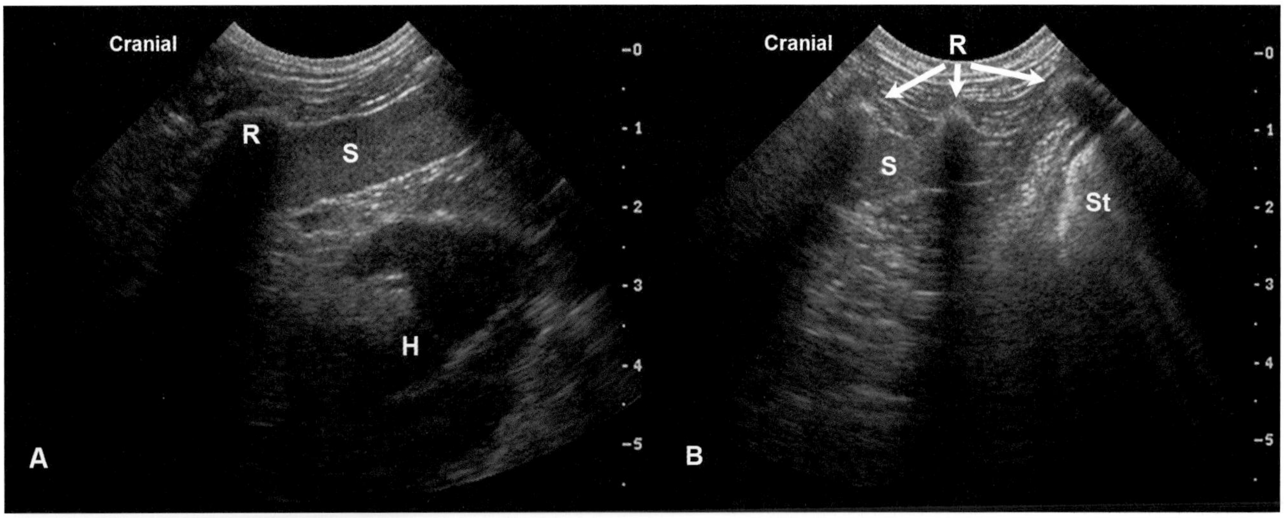

Figure 4.51. Diaphragmatic rupture in a 5-year-old cat. Longitudinal sonogram via a left intercostal approach. Images of the midthorax **(A)** and the caudal thorax **(B)**. The spleen (S) is displaced within the thoracic cavity, lateral to the heart (H). The stomach (St) is also displaced cranial to the liver. The ribs (R) in the near field are characterized by strong acoustic shadows (arrowheads). Images courtesy of M.A. d'Anjou.

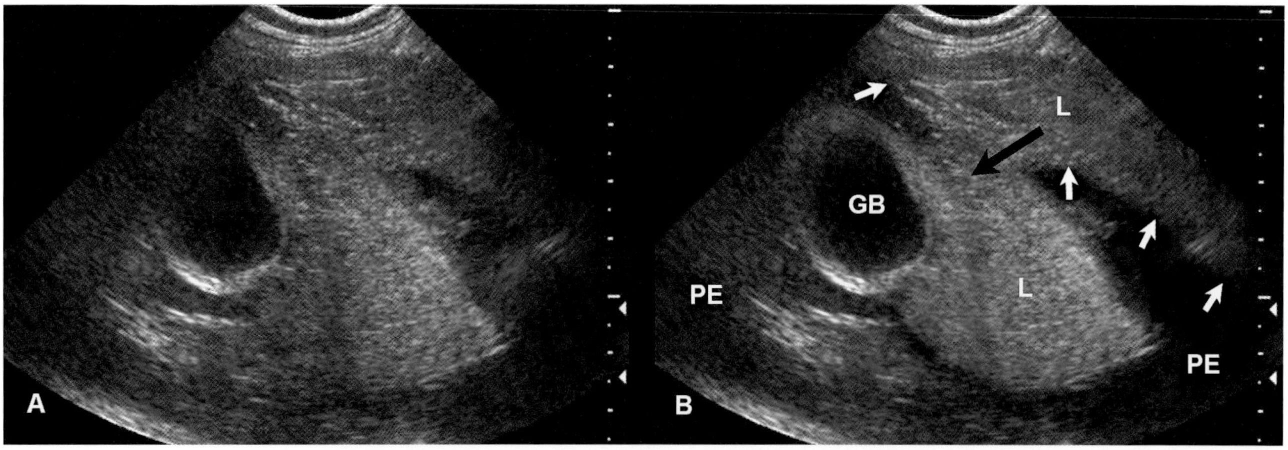

Figure 4.52. Diaphragmatic rupture in a 3-year-old mixed-breed dog. Ultrasonographic **(A)** and schematic **(B)** images of the caudal thorax obtained by using an intercostal approach. The margin of the diaphragm (arrows) is disrupted, and part of the liver (L) and the gallbladder (GB) are herniated into the thoracic cavity (black arrow). In the far field is echogenic pleural effusion (PE), consistent with hemorrhage.

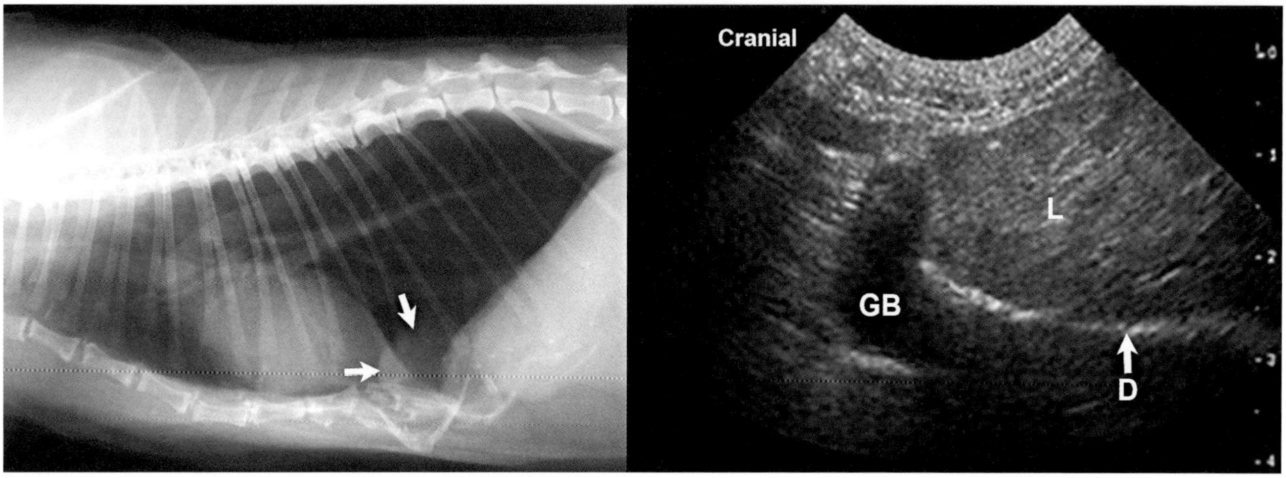

Figure 4.53. Herniation of the gallbladder in a cat. **A:** On the lateral thoracic radiograph, a well-circumscribed, round opacity (arrows) is between the diaphragm and cardiac silhouette. **B:** The ultrasonographic examination is performed by using a right ventral intercostal approach. The diaphragm (D) is the strongly hyperechoic curvilinear structure in the far field. The diaphragm is discontinuous in the near field, with herniation of the gall bladder (GB) into the thoracic cavity.

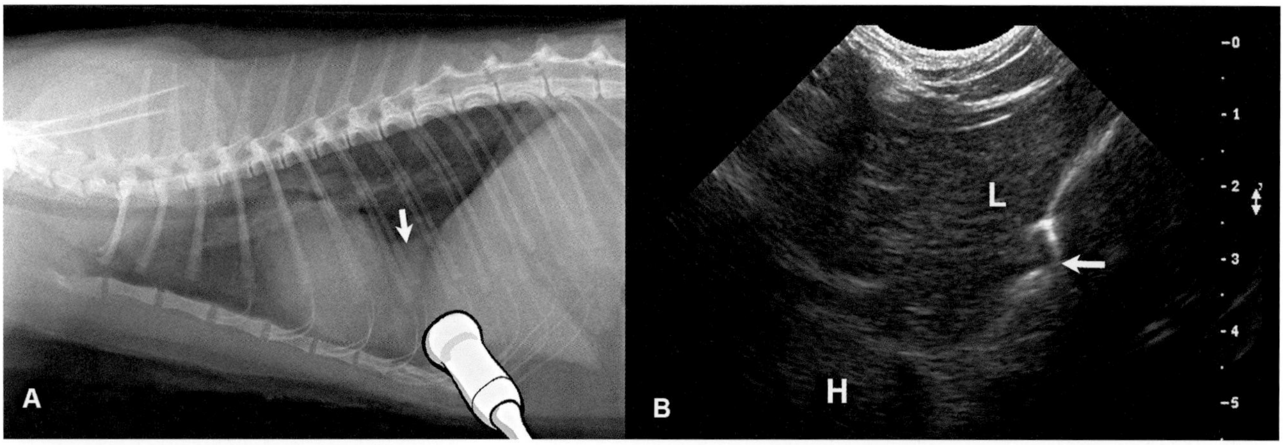

Figure 4.54. Peritoneo-pericardial diaphragmatic hernia in a 2-year-old cat. **A:** The lateral thoracic radiograph reveals loss of the ventral part of the diaphragmatic silhouette and silhouetting of abdominal and peritoneal contents. A "mesothelial remnant" sign is ventral to the caudal vena cava (arrow). The cardiac silhouette is enlarged. **B:** The ultrasonographic examination was performed by using an intercostal approach. There is discontinuity of the diaphragm (arrow), and hepatic parenchyma (L) is visible in the near field close to, and displacing, the heart (H).

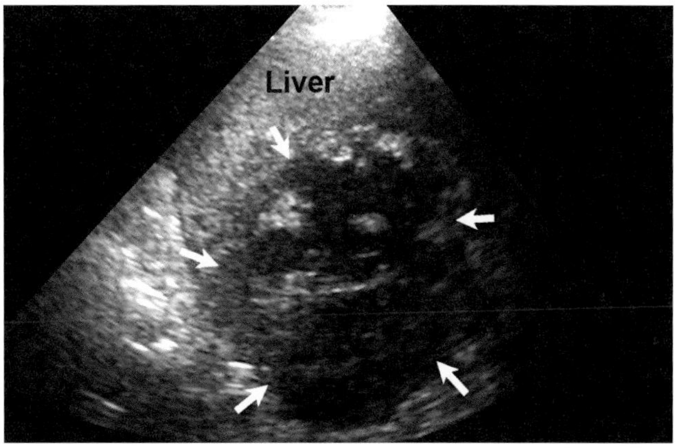

Figure 4.55. Peritoneo-pericardial diaphragmatic hernia in an 8-year-old Rhodesian ridgeback. The examination is performed via a right intercostal approach. Normal hepatic parenchyma is visible in the near field. There is a 9-cm mixed echogenic hepatic mass within the pericardial sac (arrows). Histopathologic examination of the herniated liver lobe revealed hepatocellular atrophy and hepatic dysplasia caused by compression and circulatory compromise. There was no evidence of neoplasia.

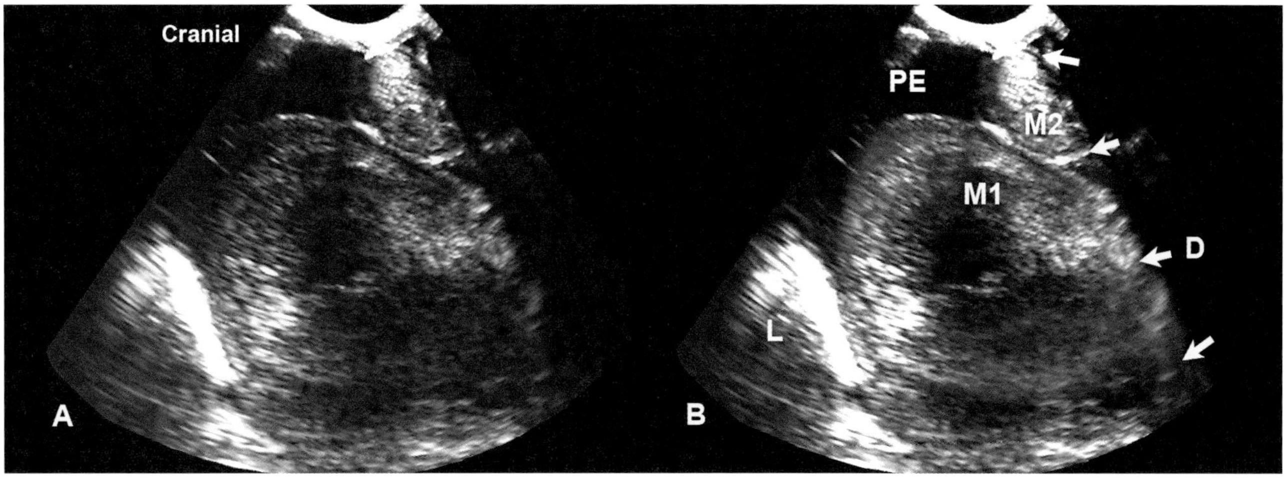

Figure 4.56. Diaphragmatic rhabdomyosarcoma in a 4-month-old cat. Ultrasonographic **(A)** and schematic **(B)** images obtained with an intercostal approach. Two mixed echogenic mass lesions (M1 and M2) are arising from the diaphragm (D, arrows). The larger mass measures more than 6 cm in maximum diameter, and the smaller mass measures 2.5 cm. The lung is displaced cranially (L), and anechoic pleural effusion is in the near field (PE), as well as anechoic peritoneal effusion caudal to the diaphragm.

Interventional Procedures

Ultrasound is very useful to aid diagnostic or therapeutic thoracocentesis, especially if only a small volume of pleural effusion is present (Figure 4.57). Additionally, fine-needle aspiration or biopsies of thoracic mass lesions are commonly performed. These procedures are safe and have a high diagnostic yield (Wood et al. 1998) (Figure 4.58). Although an intercostal approach is most commonly used, a thoracic inlet approach and even a transdiaphragmatic approach may be chosen. Patient preparation (sedation with or without anesthesia, sterile preparation) is routinely performed. Depending on the size and location of the lesion, 20- to 22-gauge injection or spinal needles are used for fine-needle aspiration, and 16- to 18-gauge biopsy needles are used to obtain core biopsy samples. Fine-needle aspiration can be performed freehand, with an extension tube or directly attached to a 5- to 10-mL syringe, enabling, with practice, faster and safer interventions. Biopsy samples can also be obtained freehand or by using a biopsy guide.

To facilitate fine-needle aspiration or biopsy of pulmonary lesions, it might be necessary to induce

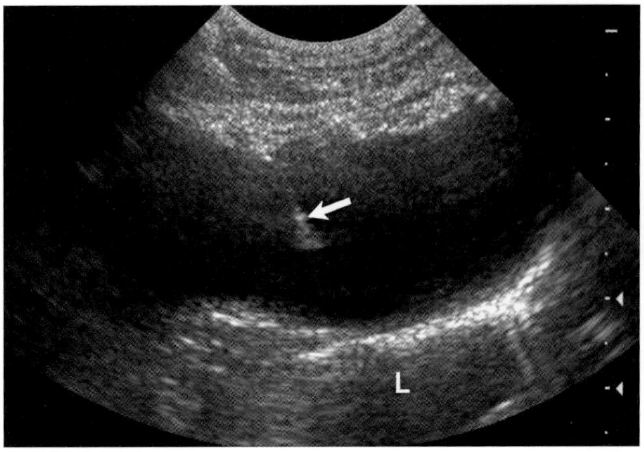

Figure 4.57. Ultrasound-guided thoracocentesis in a cat with pleural effusion. The needle is traversing the thoracic wall, and the needle tip, which appears as a hyperechoic line (arrow), is within the pleural space. The aerated lung (L) is partially retracted medially.

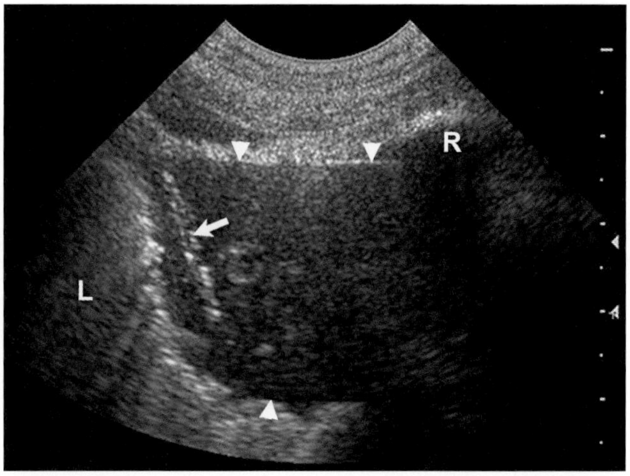

Figure 4.58. Biopsy of a pulmonary mass (bronchoalveolar carcinoma) in a dog. Two closely aligned needle tracts are visible as hyperechoic lines (arrow) in the periphery of the mass (arrowheads) adjacent to the aerated portion of the lung (L). There is no evidence of pneumothorax. The hyperechoic superficial margin of a rib (R), associated with acoustic shadowing, is in the near field.

respiratory standstill for the duration of the procedure, warranting endotracheal intubation of the patient. In addition to hemorrhage, which is a potential sequela to any biopsy, fine-needle aspiration or biopsy of pulmonary lesions might also cause pneumothorax. However, severe complications necessitating therapeutic intervention are rare.

References

Armbrust LJ, Biller DS, Radlinsky MG, Hoskinson JJ (2003) Ultrasonographic diagnosis of foreign bodies associated with chronic draining tracts and abscesses in dogs. Vet Radiol Ultrasound 44:66–70.

d'Anjou MA, Tidwell AS, Hecht S (2005) Radiographic diagnosis of lung lobe torsion. Vet Radiol Ultrasound 46:478–484.

Hurley ME, Keye GD, Hamilton S (2004) Is ultrasound really helpful in the detection of rib fractures? Injury 35: 562–566.

Konde LJ, Spaulding K (1991) Sonographic evaluation of the cranial mediastinum in small animals. Vet Radiol 32:178–184.

Mattoon JS, Nyland TG (1995) Thorax. In: Nyland TG, Mattoon JS, eds. Small Animal Diagnostic Ultrasound. Philadelphia: WB Saunders, pp 325–353.

Reichle JK, Wisner ER (2000) Non-cardiac thoracic ultrasound in 75 feline and canine patients. Vet Radiol Ultrasound 41:154–162.

Rudorf H, Herrtage ME, White RA (1997) Use of ultrasonography in the diagnosis of tracheal collapse. J Small Anim Pract 38:513–518.

Schwarz LA, Tidwell AS (1999) Alternative imaging of the lung. Clin Tech Small Anim Pract 14:187–206.

Spattini G, Rossi F, Vignoli M, Lamb CR (2003) Use of ultrasound to diagnose diaphragmatic rupture in dogs and cats. Vet Radiol Ultrasound 44:226–230.

Tidwell AS (1998) Ultrasonography of the thorax (excluding the heart). Vet Clin North Am Small Anim Pract 28: 993–1015.

Wood EF, O'Brien RT, Young KM (1998) Ultrasound-guided fine-needle aspiration of focal parenchymal lesions of the lung in dogs and cats. J Vet Intern Med 12:338–342.

Zekas LJ, Adams WM (2002) Cranial mediastinal cysts in nine cats. Vet Radiol Ultrasound 43:413–418.

CHAPTER FIVE

Heart

Donald Brown and Hugues Gaillot

Echocardiographic Technique

Instrumentation

Echocardiographic methods differ from abdominal techniques in that transducer placement is confined to limited windows of access between the ribs and aerated lung. This limitation imposes the need for a small transducer footprint. Echocardiographic examinations are then best performed using sector or curvilinear scanning transducers, preferably with phased-array technology. Echocardiography also requires greater temporal resolution. Maximal temporal resolution is obtained by decreasing field depth and minimizing the sector angle (sector width). The ultimate in temporal resolution is obtained by using motion-mode echocardiography (M-mode). Numerous dedicated abbreviations and conventions are used in this chapter and are listed in Table 5.1.

Suggested guidelines for transducer frequencies include 8–12MHz for cats and similarly sized dogs, 4–8MHz for dogs in the 5- to 40-kg range, and 2–4MHz for large dogs (>40kg). When performing an echocardiogram, a concurrent electrocardiogram may be valuable or essential, depending on the goals of the study.

Preparation of Patients

Patients are positioned in lateral recumbency, with the transducer applied to the patient from below with the aid of a table with cutouts designed for this purpose (Figure 5.1). Acoustic transmission is facilitated either by clipping the hair over the point of transducer application or by fully saturating the fur with ultrasound coupling gel.

Two-dimensional Echocardiography

Cardiac image orientation and transducer placement are referenced with respect to the heart itself (Henry et al. 1980; Thomas 1984; Bonagura et al. 1985; O'Grady et al. 1986; Thomas et al. 1993). The central left ventricular (LV) axis can be conceptualized as an imaginary line that extends between the cardiac apex and base in the center of the LV lumen. When the transducer is oriented such that the scan plane includes or is parallel to this axis, a *long-axis image* is obtained. If the scan plane is perpendicular to this axis, a *short-axis image* is obtained (Figure 5.1).

Because of impedance mismatching and ultrasound attenuation imposed by the ribs and air-filled lungs, transthoracic echocardiography is limited to relatively small windows of access. These surround the heart on both the right and left sides of the ventral thorax, i.e., next to the sternum (*parasternal*). The size of these access windows depends on individual thoracic conformation and may be increased by pulmonary underinflation (e.g., secondary to pleural effusion or atelectasis) and decreased by overinflation as may occur with many cardiopulmonary diseases. Additional access can be gained from the subcostal (*subxiphoid*) position, imaging the heart through the liver and caudal mediastinum; limited views of the aortic arch may be available from the thoracic inlet (*suprasternal* transducer position), as well.

Right Parasternal Views

Usually there are two or more rib spaces available for right parasternal (RPS) views, including a cranial location, corresponding typically to the fourth intercostal space, and a more caudal location at the fifth (Figure 5.2).

For images suitable for LV quantification, the transducer is positioned within the selected rib space so that the central beam of the transducer is perpendicular to the LV long axis at the tips of the mitral valve leaflets. A short-axis image is obtained by twisting the transducer so that the LV cross section is as close to circular as possible. Angulation in the base-apex direction yields a series of RPS short-axis views, depending on the transection level (Figure 5.2).

Long-axis images are obtained from the RPS position by applying a 90° counterclockwise transducer

Table 5.1.
Abbreviations and conventions used throughout this chapter

Anatomical designations	
AML	Anterior mitral valve leaflet
Ao	Aorta or aortic
AV	Aortic valve
CaVC	Caudal vena cava
CrVC	Cranial vena cava
CT	Chordae tendinae
IVS	Intraventricular septum
LA	Left atrium or left atrial
LAA	Left atrial appendage
LPA	Left main pulmonary artery
LV	Left ventricle or left ventricular
LVOT	Left ventricular outflow tract
LVW	Left ventricular wall
MV	Mitral valve
P	Pericardium
PM	Papillary muscle
PML	Posterior mitral valve leaflet
PT	Pulmonary trunk
PV	Pulmonic valve
RA	Right atrium or right atrial
RAA	Right atrial appendage
RPA	Right main pulmonary artery
RV	Right ventricle or right ventricular
RVOT	Right ventricular outflow tract
RVW	Right ventricular wall
TV	Tricuspid valve
Echocardiographic modality	
CFD	Color flow Doppler
CWD	Continuous-wave Doppler
M-mode	Motion mode
PWD	Pulsed-wave Doppler
TD	Tissue Doppler
TDI	Tissue Doppler imaging
2DE	Two-dimensional echocardiography
Transducer position and orientation	
Ap	Apex
Bs	Base
Ca	Caudal
Cr	Cranial
LAp	Left apical
LPS	Left parasternal
LAx	Long-axis (orientation)
RPS	Right parasternal (position)
SAx	Short-axis (orientation)
Diseases and conditions	
AI	Aortic insufficiency
CDVD	Chronic degenerative valve disease
DCM	Dilated cardiomyopathy
HCM	Hypertrophic cardiomyopathy
LCHF	Left-sided congestive heart failure
MR	Mitral regurgitation
PI	Pulmonic insufficiency
RCHF	Right-sided congestive heart failure
TR	Tricuspid regurgitation

twist, relative to the short-axis orientation, and fanning so that the LV central axis lies within the scan plane; a four-chamber view results (Figure 5.3). From this view, slight cranial angulation and clockwise twisting brings the LV outflow tract and aorta into view.

Left Apical Views

Left apical position (LAp) images are best obtained with the patient in left lateral recumbency, with the transducer applied to the left ventral thorax from below (Figure 5.4). A true apical view results when the transducer is placed at an extreme ventral and caudal location, approaching a subcostal position. The transducer is angled cranially so that the central ultrasound beam is pointed toward the heart base along the LV central axis. The true apical view may be technically challenging, so a more cranial transducer position may be suitable but results in a foreshortened LV view that is unsuitable for ventricular quantification.

Cranial angulation of the transducer from the LAp four-chamber position brings the aortic root into the scan plane and enables visualization of the aortic valve. This scan plane constitutes the *apical five-chamber* image and often is suitable for aortic flow-velocity quantification. However the subcostal transducer location typically is better aligned for maximal velocity measurements in dogs (Abbott and MacLean 2003).

From the apical four-chamber view, a 90° clockwise twist yields the apical two-chamber view including the left ventricle and atrium in the near and far fields, respectively.

Left Parasternal Views

Left parasternal position (LPS) views of the heart, also called left cranial views, are obtained preferably with the patient in left lateral recumbency. The transducer is positioned so that it is cranial to the heart, at the fourth to fifth intercostal space, and approximately at the level of the costal-chondral junction in the dorsal-ventral direction.

Baseline left cranial long-axis images are obtained with the scan plane oriented parallel to the ascending aorta, twisting so as to include a longitudinal view of this structure (Figure 5.5). Portions of the left ventricle and atrium, mitral valve, and right ventricular (RV) outflow tract may be visible from this position. The view is particularly useful for evaluation of heart base tumors and the RV outflow tract.

With dorsal and slightly caudal angulation of the transducer, the scan plane encounters the left atrium

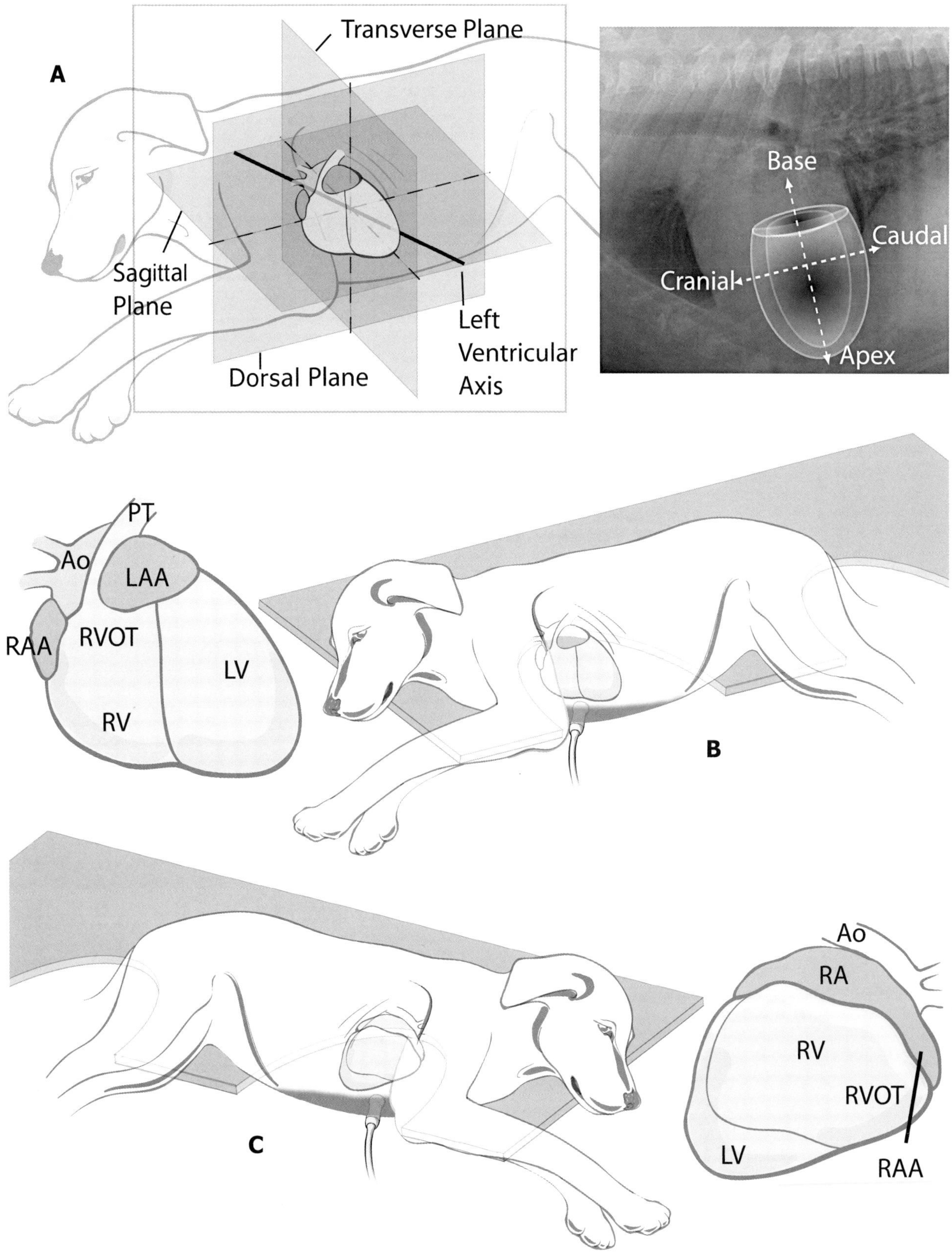

Figure 5.1. Echocardiographic orientation and anatomy. **A:** A prevailing coordinate system is defined in terms of the LV axis for the individual's heart. The terms *base* and *apex* are specific to the heart and do not usually correspond precisely with *dorsal* and *ventral* directions referenced with respect to the animal. Similarly, the *cranial-caudal* axis of the heart is perpendicular to the *base-apex* axis and does not coincide precisely with the anatomical definitions. **B and C:** The transducer is most commonly applied to recumbent patients from below with the aid of a specially designed table. *For the definition of abbreviations in the figures in this chapter, see Table 5.1.*

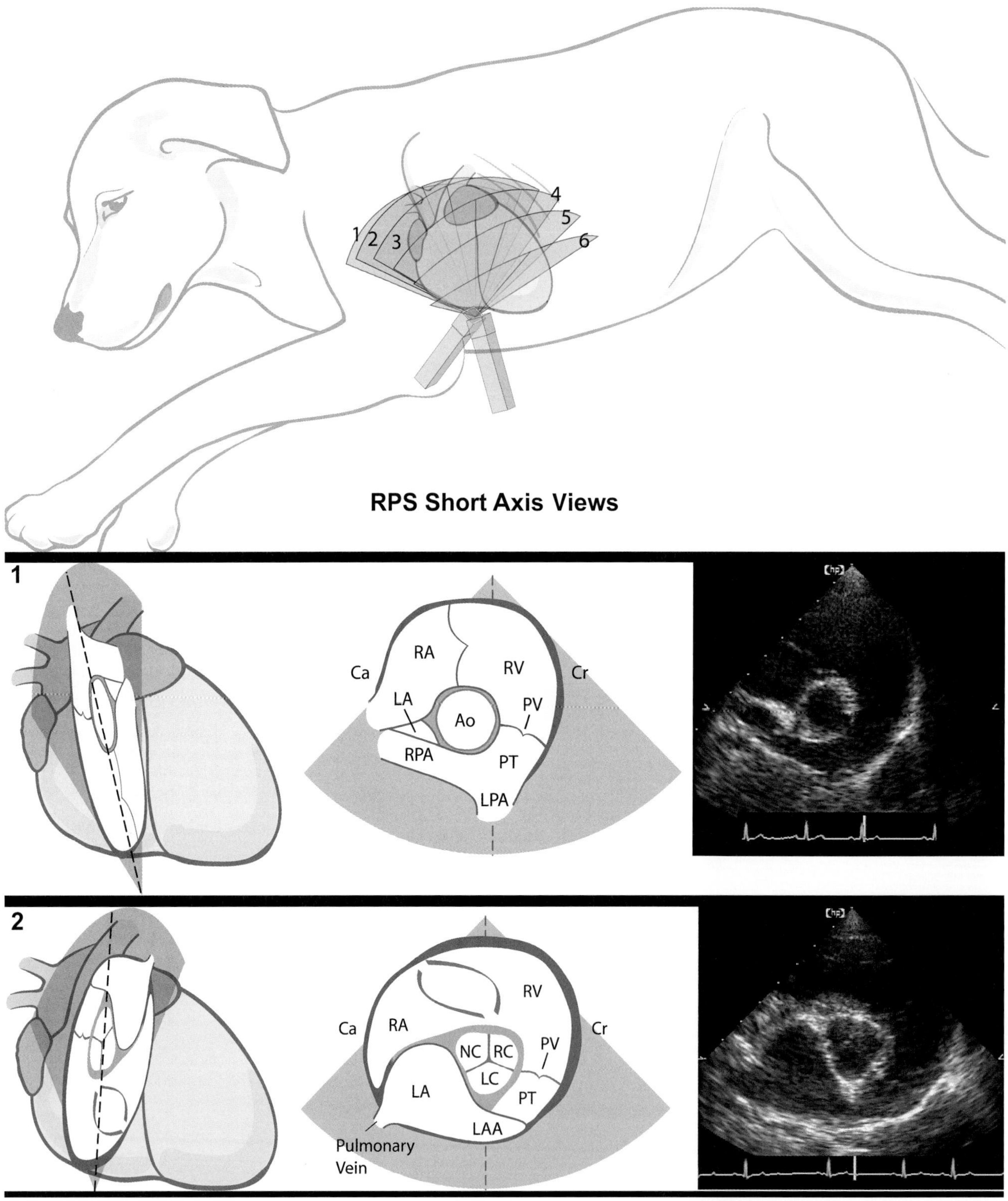

Figure 5.2. RPS SAx scanning technique. For RPS SAx views, the transducer is positioned so that the scan plane slices perpendicularly to the LV central axis at the level of the CT. Numbers 1–6 refer to the scan plane orientation and image obtained. Slice 6 is not shown on subsequent images. **1:** Slice 1 at the PT level. **2:** Slice 2 at the Ao root level. The right coronary (RC), left coronary (LC), and noncoronary (NC) cusps of the Ao valve may be visible. **3:** Slice 3 at the mitral level. The mitral leaflets are widely separated while blood flows between the leaflets into the LV chamber. **4:** Slice 4 at the chordal level. **5:** Slice 5 at the LV level. P, pericardium.

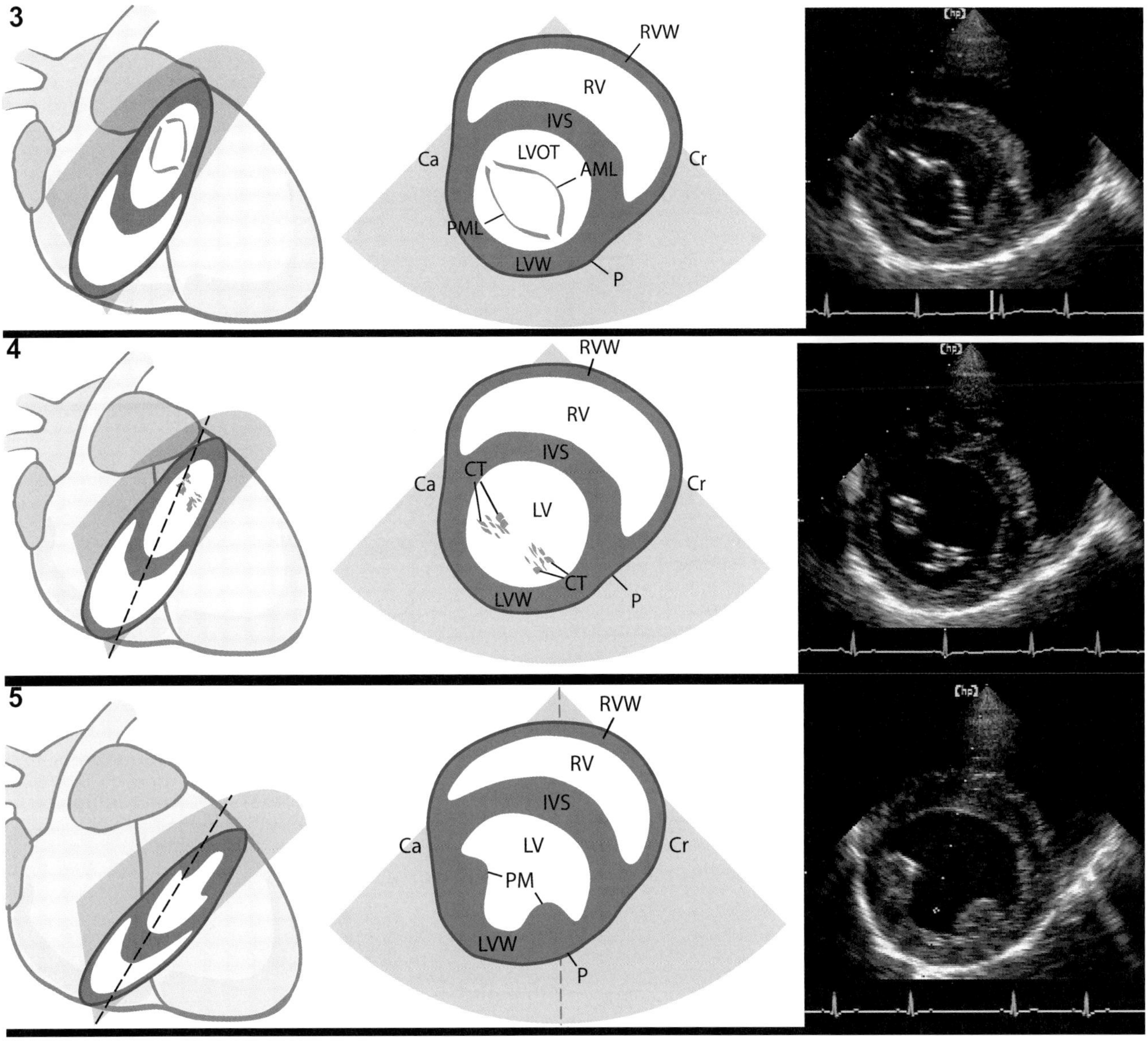

Figure 5.2. *Continued*

and ventricle, RV outflow tract, and pulmonary trunk; the pulmonary bifurcation typically can be visualized.

Relative to the initial LV outflow tract position, ventral and slightly cranial angulation causes the scan plane to transect the right atrium, right atrial (RA) appendage, tricuspid valve, and RV inflow. The RA appendage can be closely inspected from this vantage point for evidence of neoplasia.

From the initial LPS view of the LV outflow tract, a clockwise twist results in a scan plane that slices the aortic root transversely (Figure 5.6). Fanning the transducer in a cranial-dorsal direction produces a range of images for optimal viewing of the right atrium and RV inflow tract, RV inflow and outflow tracts, and pulmonary trunk. The latter enables visualization of the pulmonary bifurcation, ascending aorta, and structures associated with the heart base.

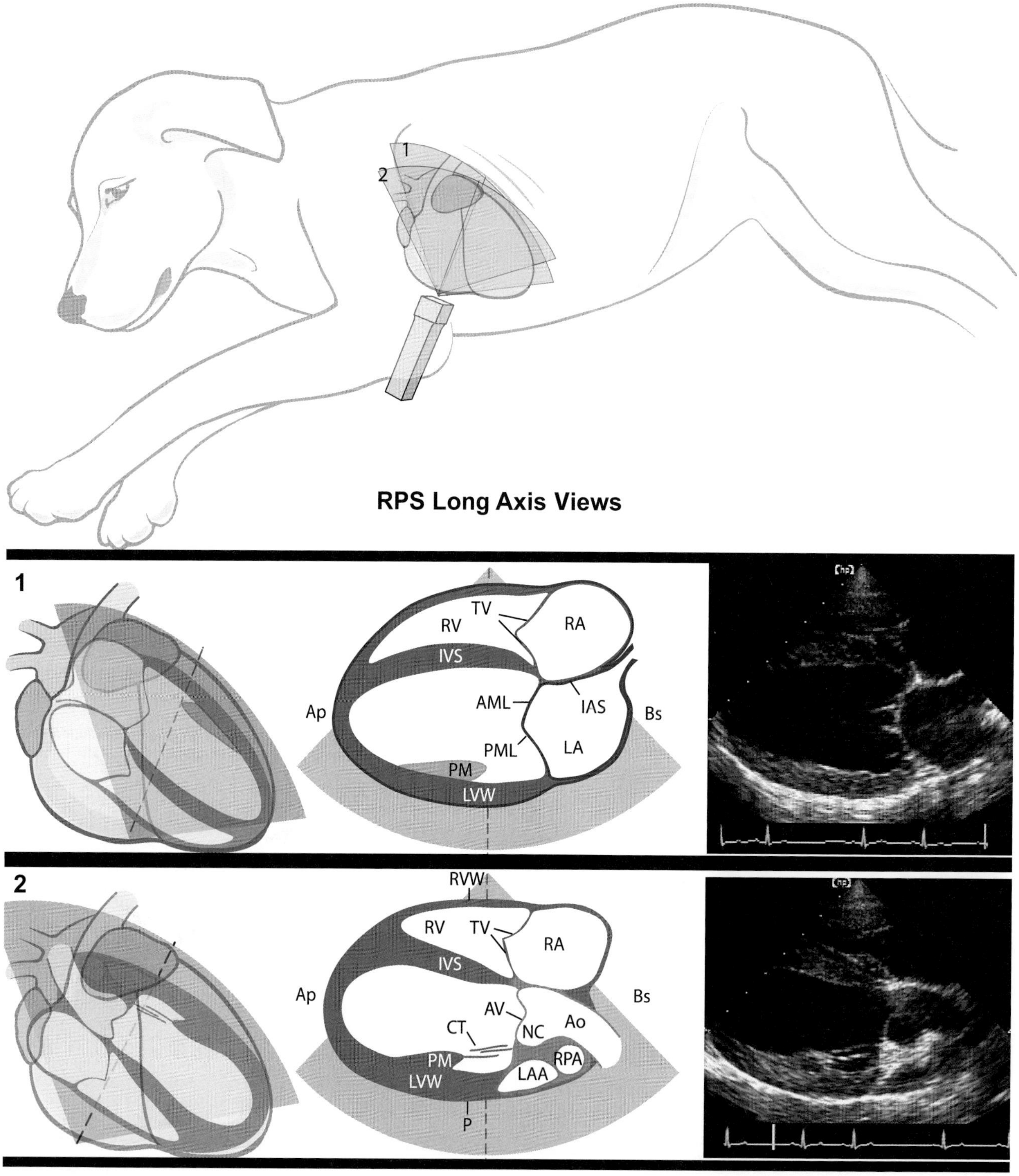

Figure 5.3. RPS LAx scanning technique. For RPS LAx views, the transducer is positioned so that the scan plane contains, or is parallel to, the LV central axis. **1:** Slice 1 with a four-chamber view. **2:** Slice 2 with an LVOT view. NC is the noncoronary portion of the Ao sinus of Valsalva. IAS, interatrial septum.

Figure 5.4. LAp scanning technique. The transducer is positioned at the left apex of the heart. Cranial angulation brings the heart into the scan plane. **1:** LAp four-chamber view. **2:** LAp five-chamber view. **3:** LAp two-chamber view. IAS, interatrial septum.

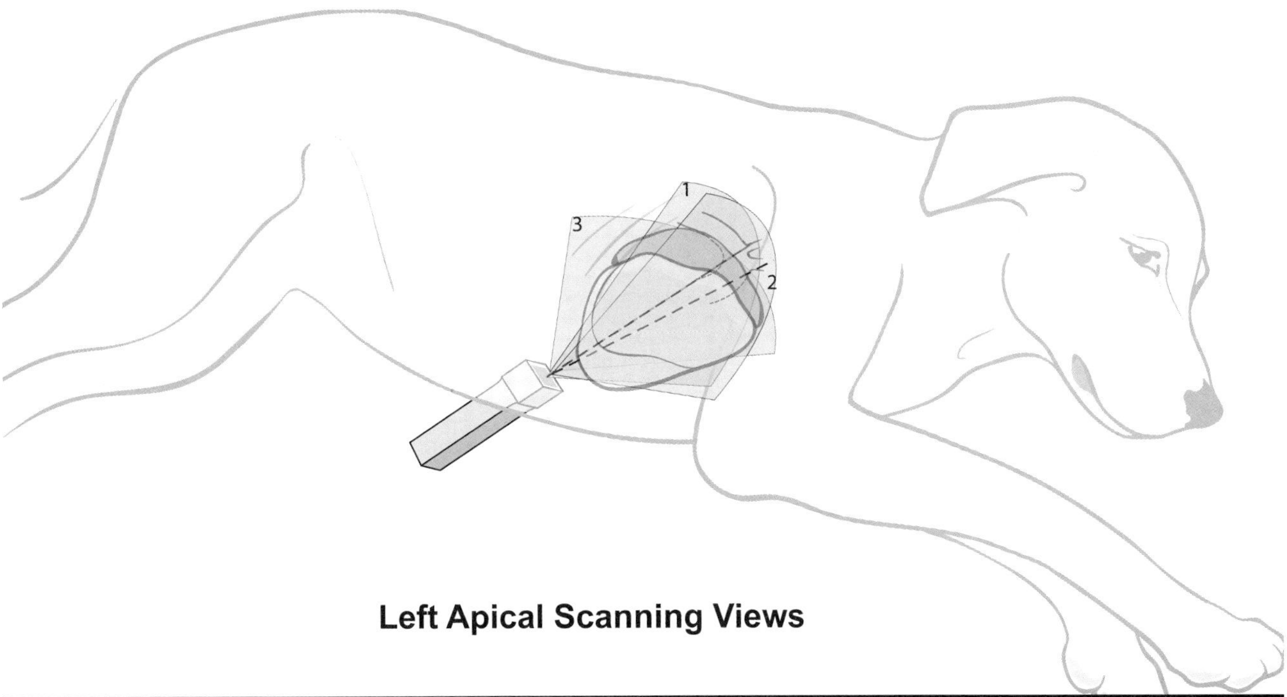

Left Apical Scanning Views

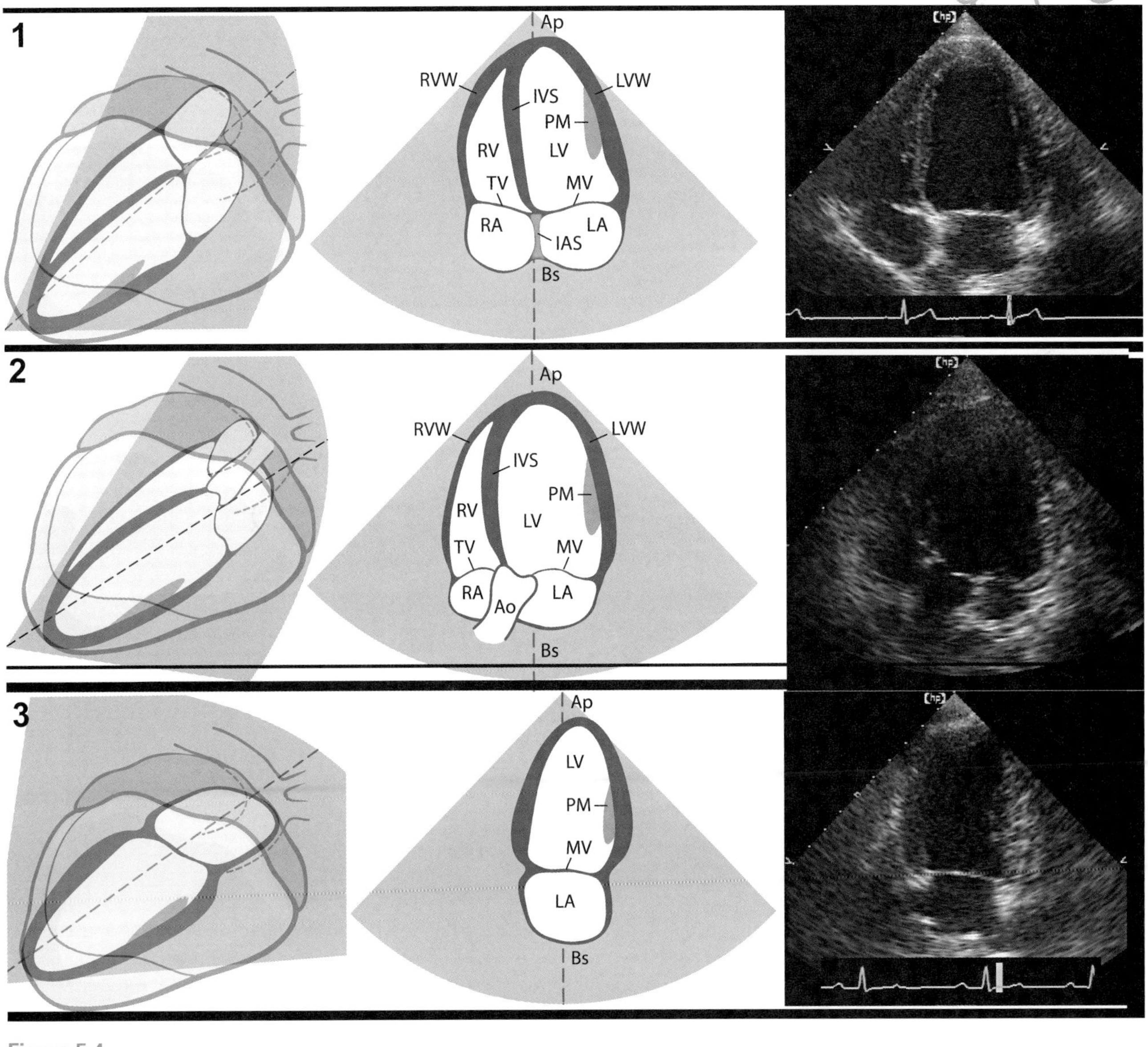

Figure 5.4.

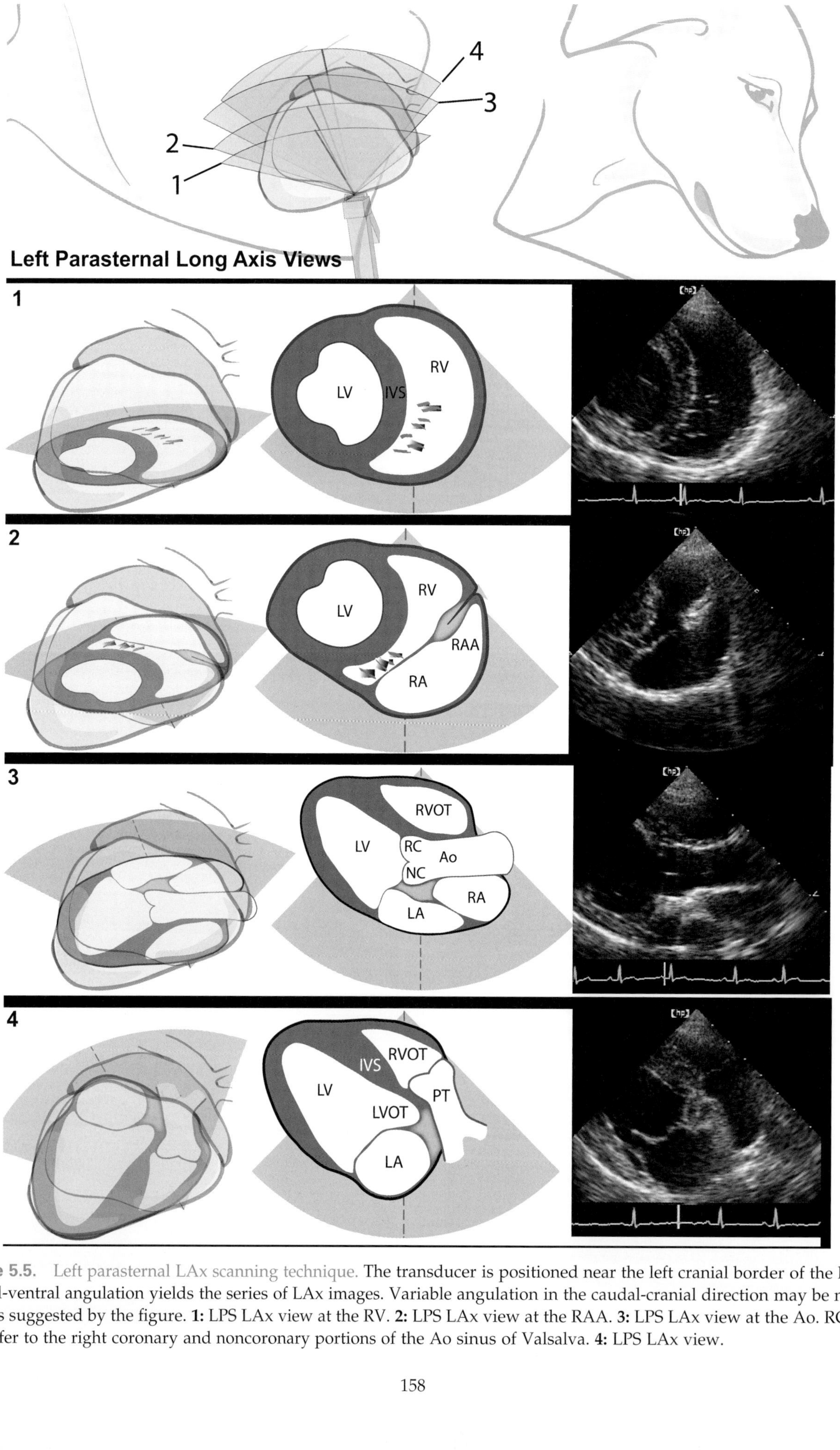

Figure 5.5. Left parasternal LAx scanning technique. The transducer is positioned near the left cranial border of the heart. Dorsal-ventral angulation yields the series of LAx images. Variable angulation in the caudal-cranial direction may be necessary as suggested by the figure. **1:** LPS LAx view at the RV. **2:** LPS LAx view at the RAA. **3:** LPS LAx view at the Ao. RC and NC refer to the right coronary and noncoronary portions of the Ao sinus of Valsalva. **4:** LPS LAx view.

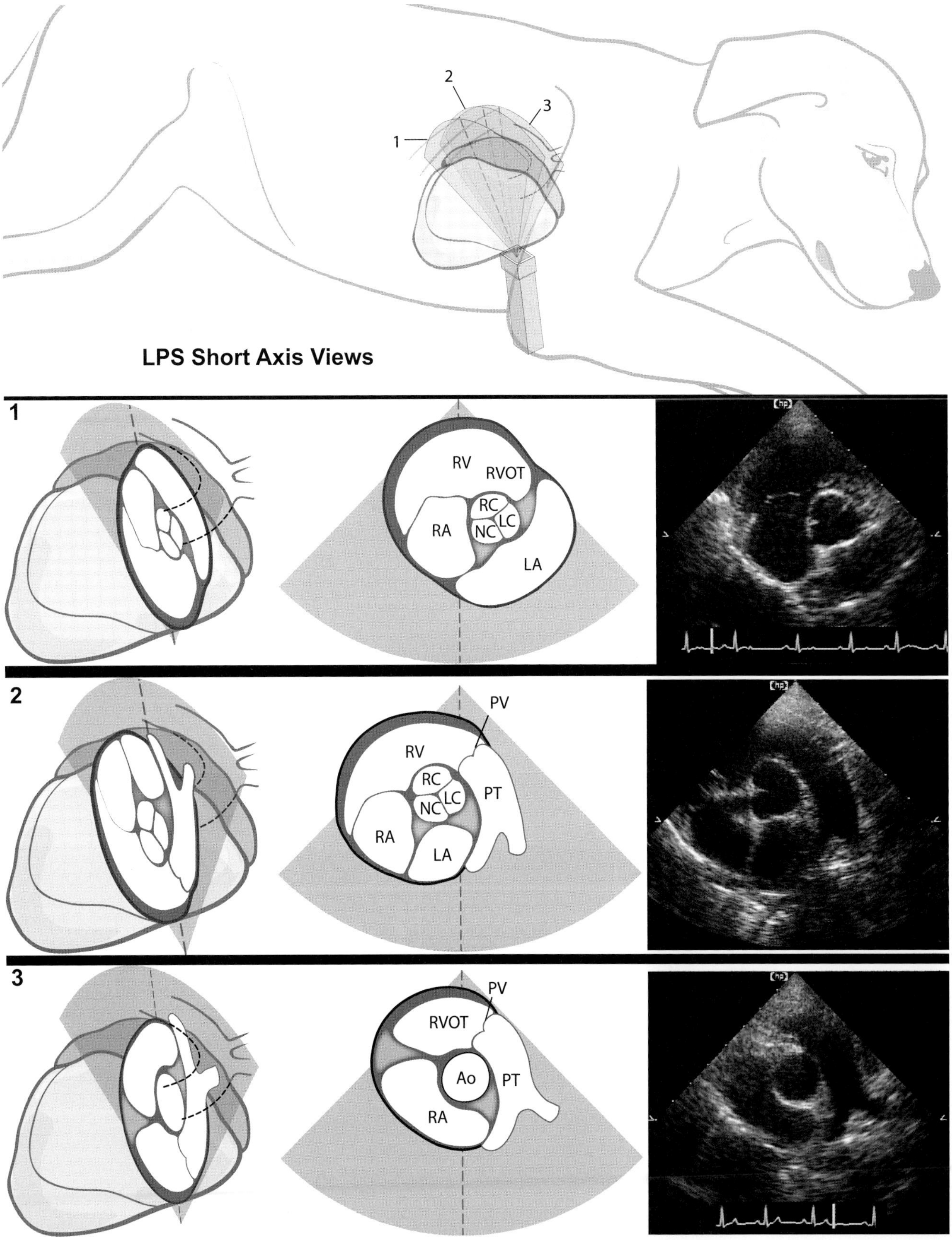

Figure 5.6. Left parasternal SAx scanning technique. The transducer is positioned near the left cranial border of the heart. Cranial-caudal yields the series of SAx images. Variable angulation in the dorsal-ventral direction may be necessary as suggested by the figure. **1:** LPS SAx view at the RV inflow tract. The right coronary (RC), left coronary (LC), and noncoronary (NC) cusps of the Ao valve may be visible. **2:** LPS SAx view at the inflow-outflow. Both the inflow and outflow tracts of the right heart may be visible with subtle angulation and twist adjustments. The right coronary (RC), left coronary (LC), and noncoronary (NC) cusps of the Ao valve may be visible. **3:** LPS SAx view at the PT. PV, pulmonary vein.

Subcostal and Suprasternal Views

The suprasternal view necessitates transducer positioning at the thoracic inlet with the scan plane oriented parallel to the patient's sagittal plane. This view is best for imaging the aortic arch and valuable, consequently, for quantification of aortic insufficiency. The subcostal view is obtained, with the patient in lateral recumbency, by positioning the transducer at the xiphoid process and pressing into the abdomen while pointing the transducer almost directly cranially (Figure 5.7). The twist is adjusted to be approximately parallel to the sagittal plane. For Doppler aortic velocity recordings, the transducer is fanned to include the aortic root.

Motion-mode Echocardiography (M-mode)

The majority of M-mode dimensional recordings are made from the RPS transducer position (Bonagura 1983; Bonagura et al. 1985). One of the principal applications of M-mode is for the recording of time-dependent short-axis dimensions of the heart, and this dictates a specific external transducer location that is determined by the cardiac anatomy (Figures 5.8–5.12).

Doppler Echocardiography

Doppler echocardiography uses the Doppler principal to determine the velocity of moving blood or tissue

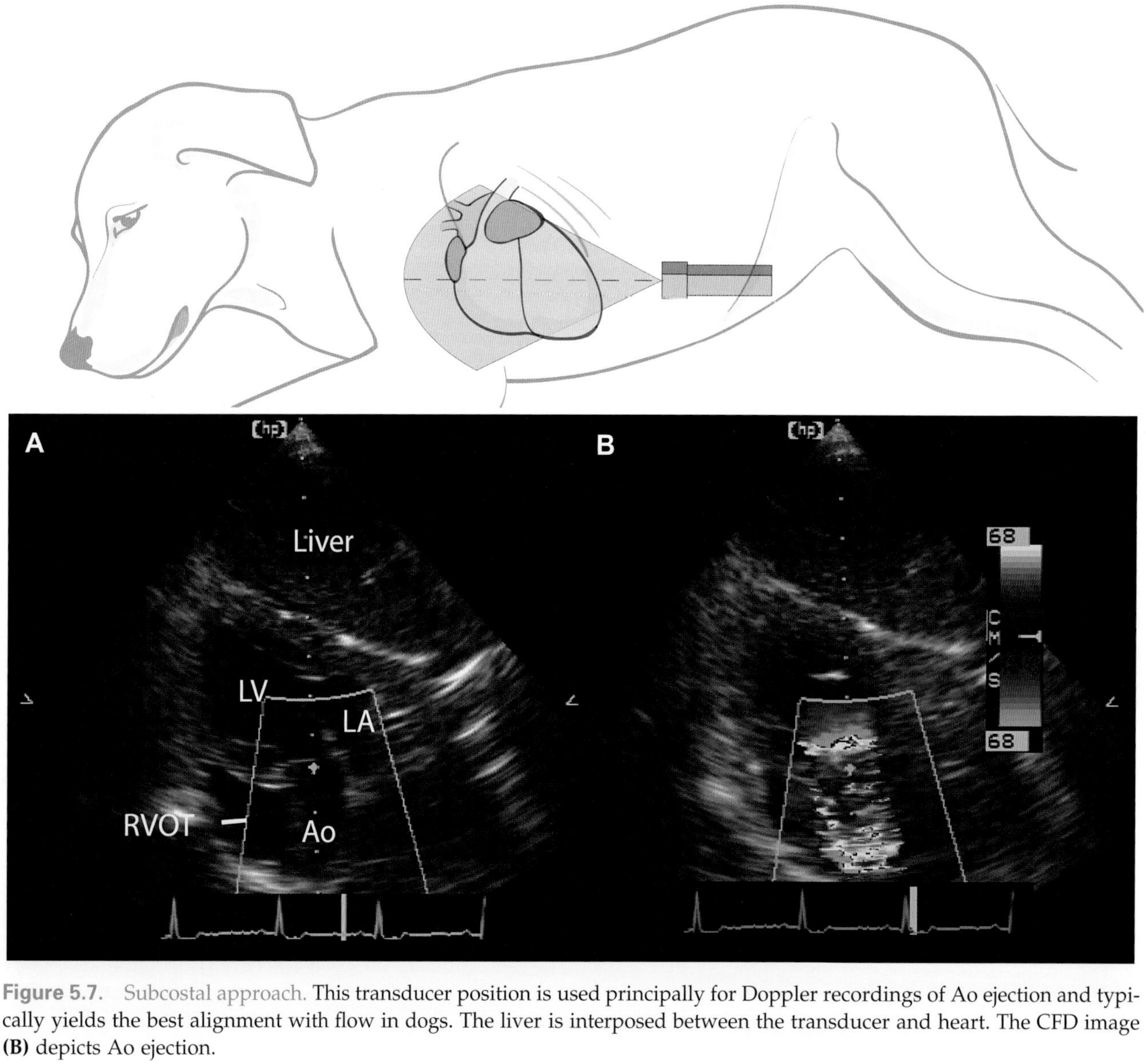

Figure 5.7. Subcostal approach. This transducer position is used principally for Doppler recordings of Ao ejection and typically yields the best alignment with flow in dogs. The liver is interposed between the transducer and heart. The CFD image **(B)** depicts Ao ejection.

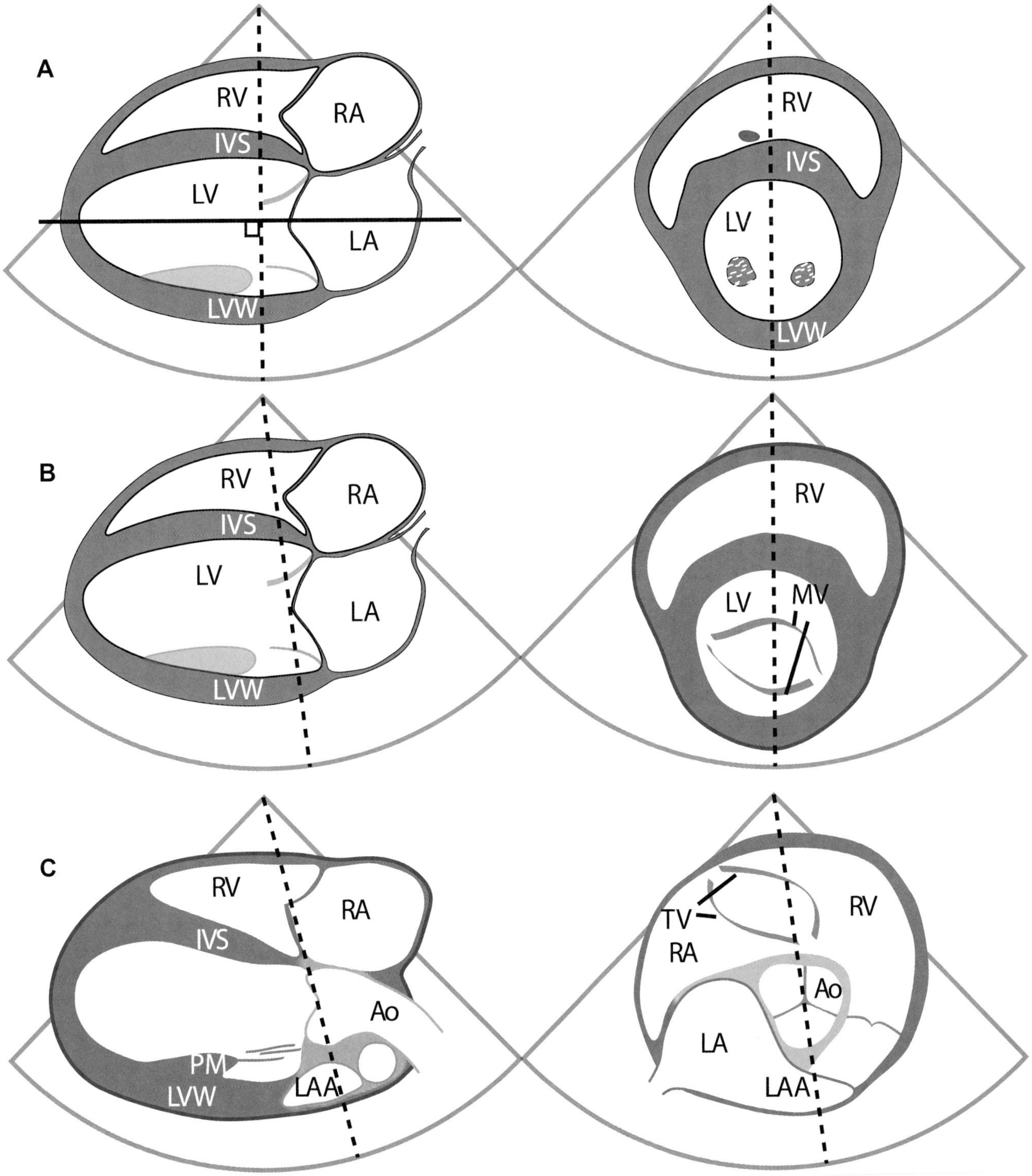

Figure 5.8. M-mode scan-line orientation. 2DE is used to position the transducer and orient the scan line throughout M-mode recordings as shown. Orientations are depicted for LV **(A)**, MV **(B)**, and Ao-LA **(C)** recordings.

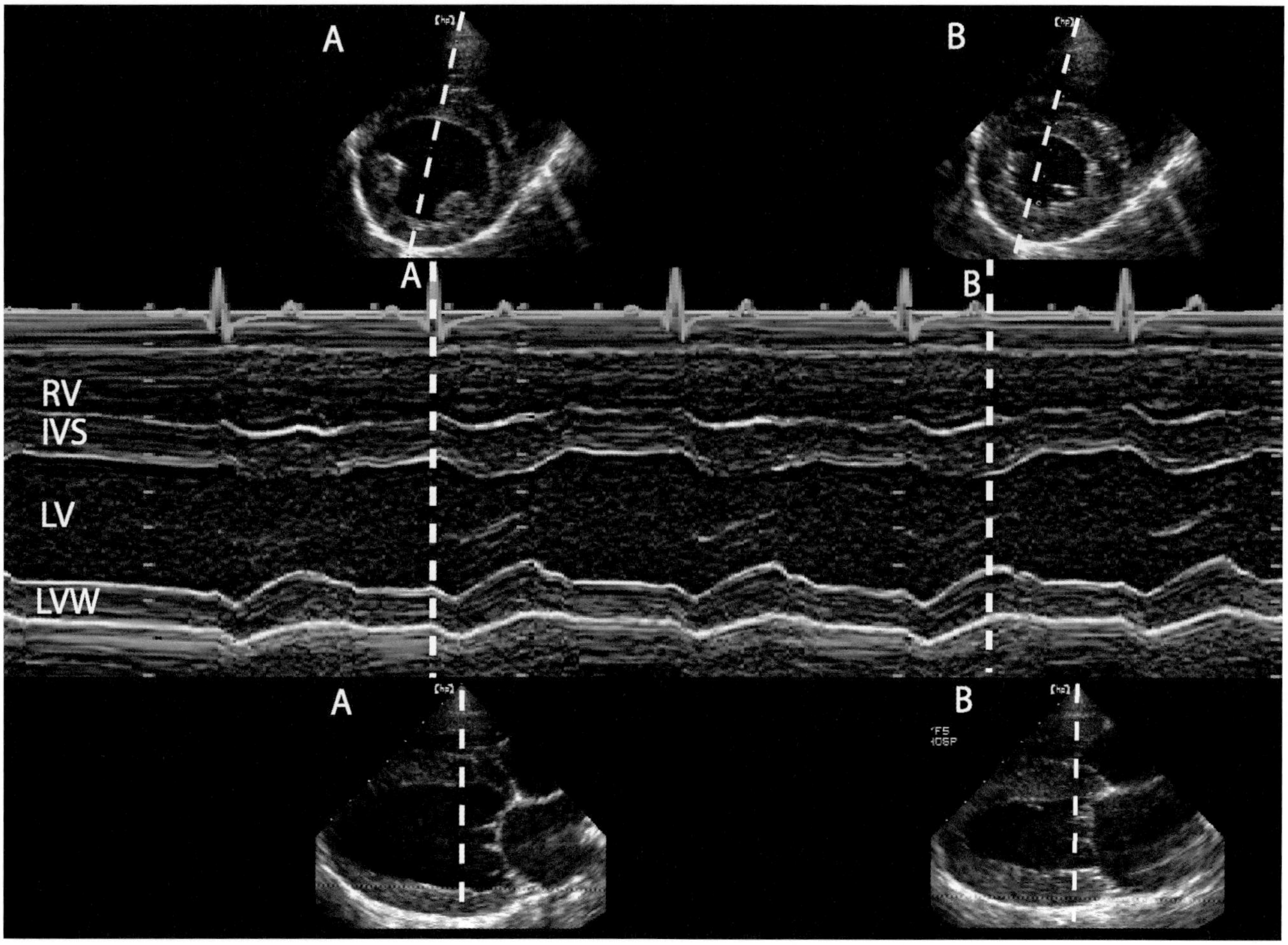

Figure 5.9. M-mode at the LV level. The M-mode recording (middle tier) is generated from the selected scan line shone in the RPS SAx (top tier) and LAx (bottom tier) images. Time marker A is at end diastole coinciding with the onset of the QRS complex of the electrocardiogram. Time marker B is at end systole, which coincides with the minimum LV dimension near the end of the electrocardiographic T wave.

(Darke 1992; Kirberger et al. 1992; Bonagura and Miller 1998; Bonagura et al. 1998). With *pulsed-wave Doppler* (PWD), the round-trip time of the ultrasound pulse is used to determine the tissue depth at which the velocity occurs; the maximum depth dictates a specific pulse-repetition frequency. In turn, repetitive pulsation of the ultrasound is directly responsible for the aliasing phenomenon whereby measured velocity is observed to occur at an alias velocity. The alias velocity may be a gross misrepresentation of actual velocity (Figure 5.13). In contrast to PWD, ultrasound is emitted continuously in the *continuous-wave Doppler* modality, which does not suffer from the velocity ambiguity of PWD. There is no practical limit to the velocity magnitude that can be measured with continuous-wave Doppler (CWD). However, this mode does not enable determination of the tissue depth from which the measured velocities arise, so the anatomical location of velocities must be inferred or determined using other means (e.g., PWD).

Color flow Doppler (CFD) is a pulsed-wave modality in which velocity characteristics are encoded to a color display, via a user selected mapping, and overlaid onto the real-time 2DE image. This enables the ultrasonographer to visualize directly the source of velocities within the heart and great vessels within the anatomical framework of the image. Being a pulsed-wave modality, CFD is subject to velocity measurement ambiguity caused by aliasing (Figure 5.14). PWD and CFD are better suited for differentiation between laminar and turbulent flow patterns than is CWD.

Aortic flow velocity is recorded from the subcostal or LAp transducer position for velocity quantification. The normal aortic ejection signal peaks early in the

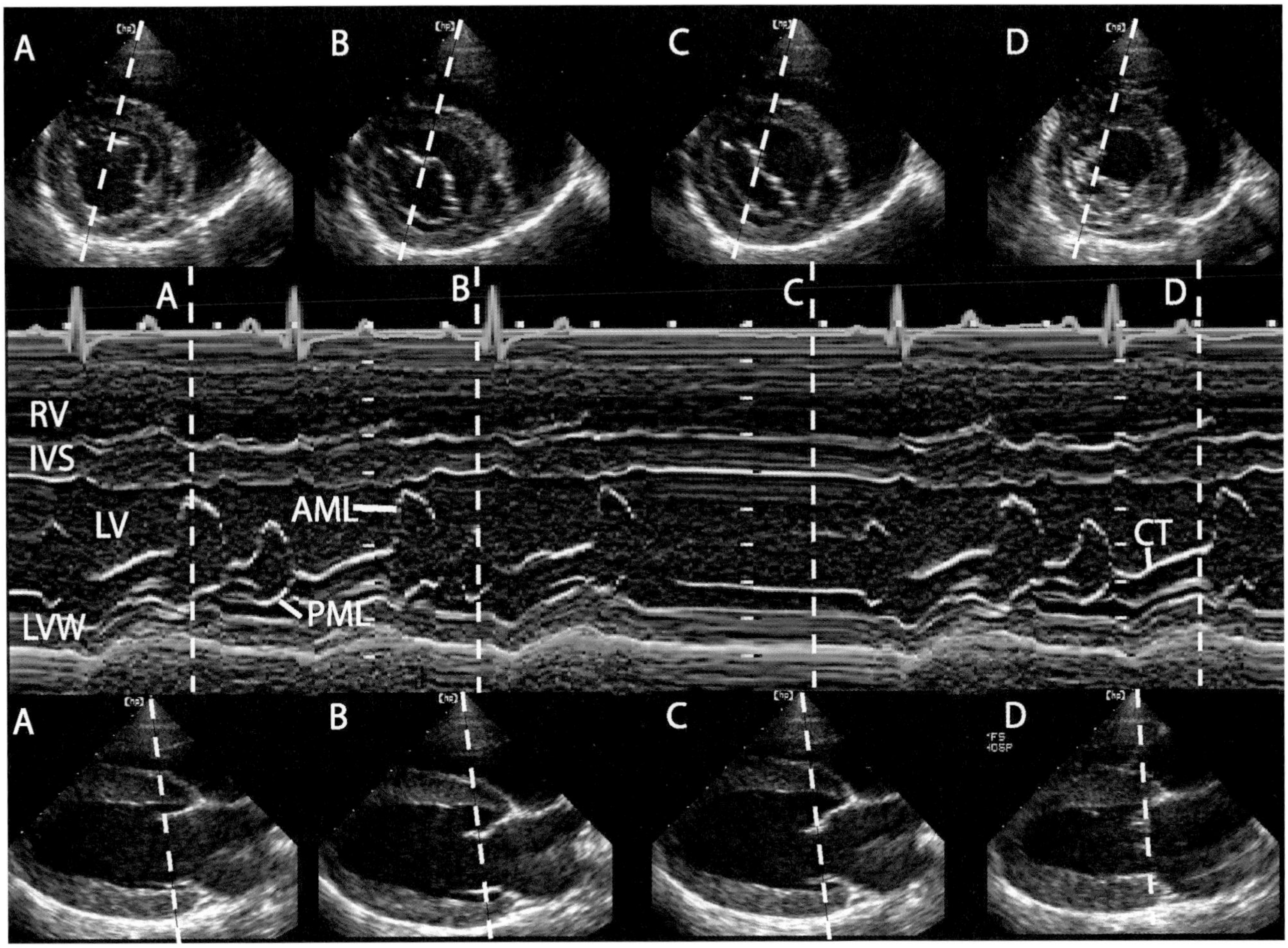

Figure 5.10. M-mode at the MV level. The M-mode recording (middle tier) is generated from the selected scan line shone in the RPS SAx (top tier) and LAx (bottom tier) images. The two primary mitral leaflets are separated from each other during diastole and apposed during systole. Time marker A is at early diastole, and marker B is at late diastole immediately after the P wave of the electrocardiogram. Marker C is at a prolonged diastasis, i.e., middiastole, and D is at end systole.

ejection cycle and may impart a daggerlike shape to the velocity envelope (Figure 5.15). By comparison, pulmonary ejection from the same individual exhibits a later peak velocity with a lower maximal value, and a longer duration of ejection (Figure 5.16). Pulmonic ejection recordings may be obtained from either the RPS or LPS transducer positions, and it may be appropriate to attempt both if quantification of maximal velocity is desired. It is normal for the pulmonic valve to exhibit a small amount of insufficiency (see Figure 5.18).

Mitral and tricuspid inflow velocities are usually recorded from the LAp position to best align the ultrasound beam with the direction of inflow (Figure 5.15). PWD recordings are made by placing the sample volume near the tips of the open mitral or tricuspid leaflets to include maximal velocities. Like their M-mode counterparts, velocity signals exhibit phasic changes that reflect the physiology of ventricular filling. The tricuspid inflow-velocity signal is similar to the mitral but normally exhibits diminished velocity magnitude in comparison, in part because of greater effective orifice area for the tricuspid valve. Recording of tricuspid inflow is facilitated by placing the transducer one or more rib spaces farther cranially as compared with the optimal position for mitral recordings.

Examples of normal CFD recordings are shown in Figures 5.17 and 5.18.

Tissue Doppler Recordings

Tissue Doppler recordings are employed to quantify the velocity of motion of cardiac tissue directly. The

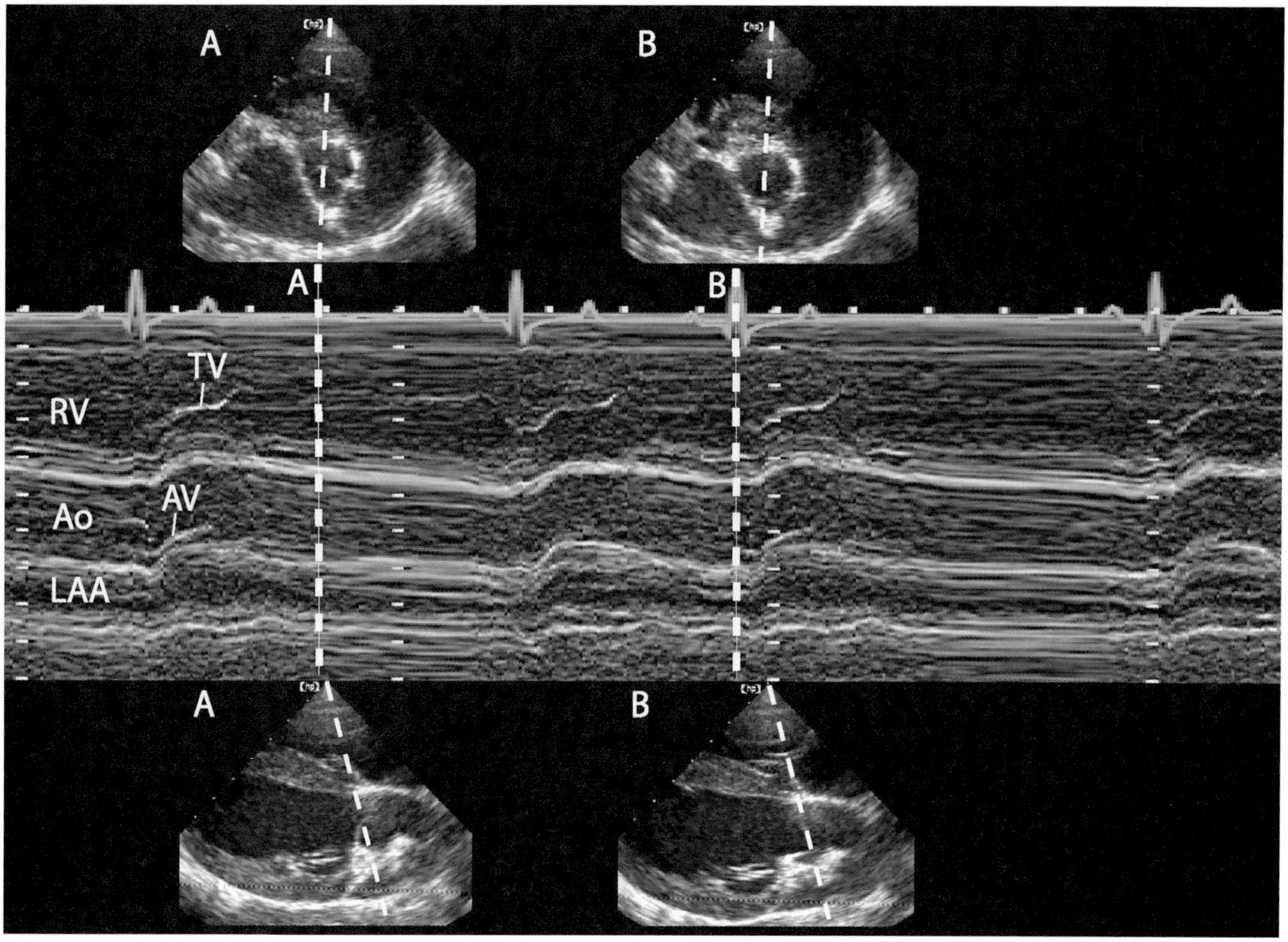

Figure 5.11. M-mode at the Ao root level. The M-mode recording (middle tier) is generated from the selected scan line shone in the RPS SAx (top tier) and LAx (bottom tier) images. Because of the orientation of the scan line, only the left coronary cusp is typically visible during systole in the dog. Time marker A is at middiastole, and the AV is shown closed during this phase. Time marker B coincides with systole, and the left coronary cusp is visible near the far-field Ao wall.

most common use of tissue Doppler in cardiology is to record the longitudinal (base-apex) velocity of the mitral annulus from the LAp four-chamber position. Velocity recordings may be obtained from either the septal or lateral mitral annulus, adjusting transducer position so that annular motion of the chosen site is directed along the Doppler scan line to the extent possible (Figure 5.19).

Echocardiographic Measurements and Indices

Besides direct visual observation, structural and functional evaluation of the heart may entail echocardiographic measurements of linear dimensions, areas, time intervals, or velocities, and calculation of performance indices from these raw data. To characterize and quantify the heart echocardiographically, the ultrasonographer must possess a detailed understanding of cardiovascular physiology, pathophysiology, and the sources of variation for observations (Table 5.2).

Measurement and Index Normalization

A basic, but troublesome, aspect of veterinary cardiology has been to interpret raw measurements for the range of body-size and breed variations encountered, particularly for dogs. Although no entirely satisfactory approach has been determined, a common feature of many well-normalized indices is that they derive from a ratio of two measurements with the same physical units. Echocardiographic ratio indices have long been used in cardiology, with examples dating from the beginning of the technique. Left atrial (LA) size, for example, may be expressed in terms of aortic

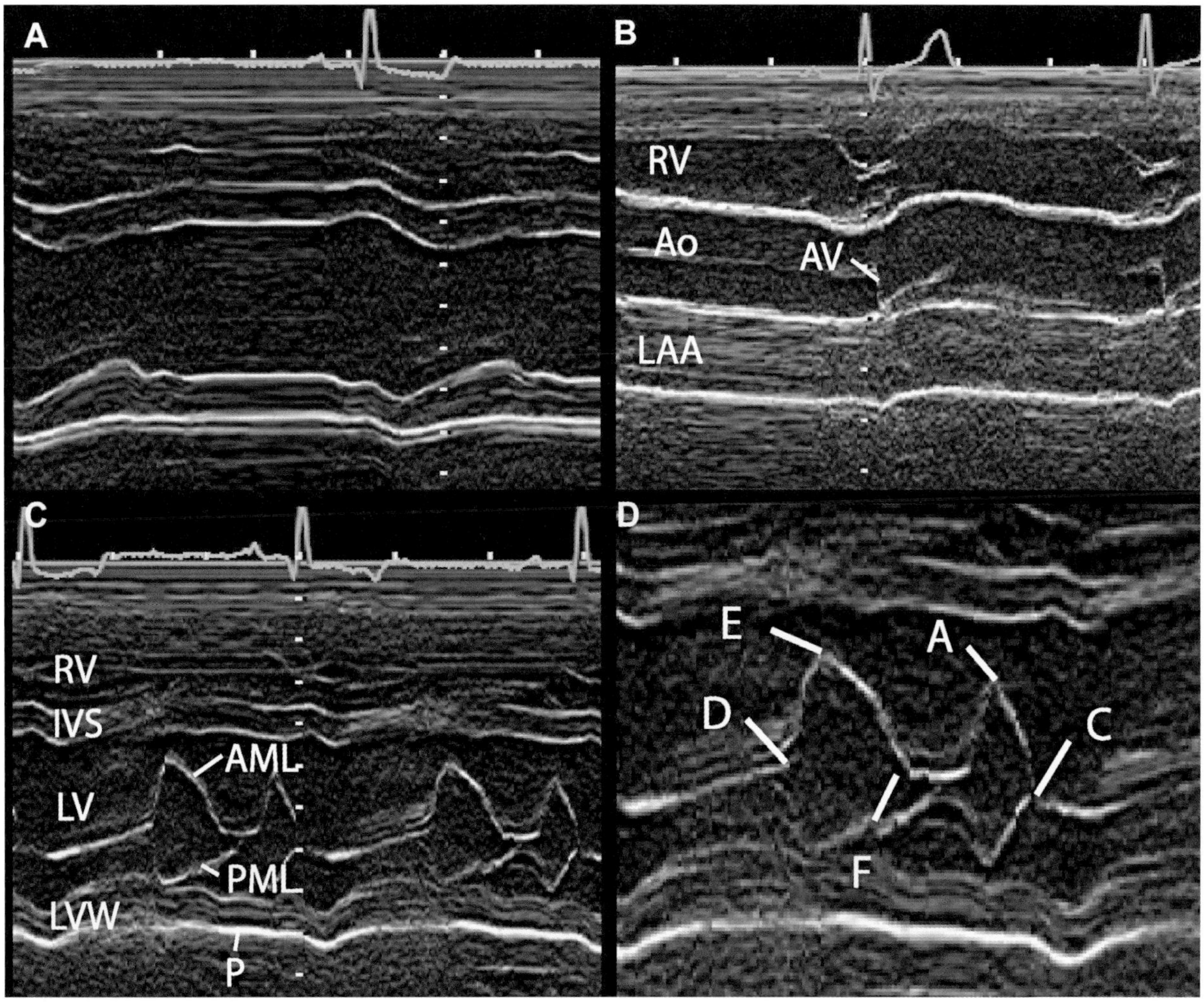

Figure 5.12. M-mode recordings. **A:** This recording is made at the LV level corresponding to the scan-line orientation shown in Figure 5.8A. Epicardial and endocardial surfaces of the IVS and LVW are well delineated throughout the recording, which is necessary for measurement accuracy. **B:** This Ao root recording corresponds to the orientation in Figure 5.8C. The AV is visible. **C:** This recording is at the MV level (Figure 5.8B). **D:** Depicted are letter designations A–F of MV motion.

Table 5.2.
Sources of echocardiographic variation

Image acquisition	**Genetic variation**
Observer technique	Body size
Instrument settings	Species variation
Measurement from images	Breed variation
Observer technique	Individual variation
Hemodynamic variation (short term)	**Pathophysiology**
Autonomic balance	Disease consequences
Preload	Cardiovascular remodeling
Afterload	**Interpretive methods**
Contractility	Observer experience
Heart rate	Statistical methods
Drugs	Spectrum of normal
Environmental variation (long term)	Data availability
Nutrition	
Athletic training level	
Drugs	

Expertise as an echocardiographer necessitates an extensive understanding of these factors and interrelationships.

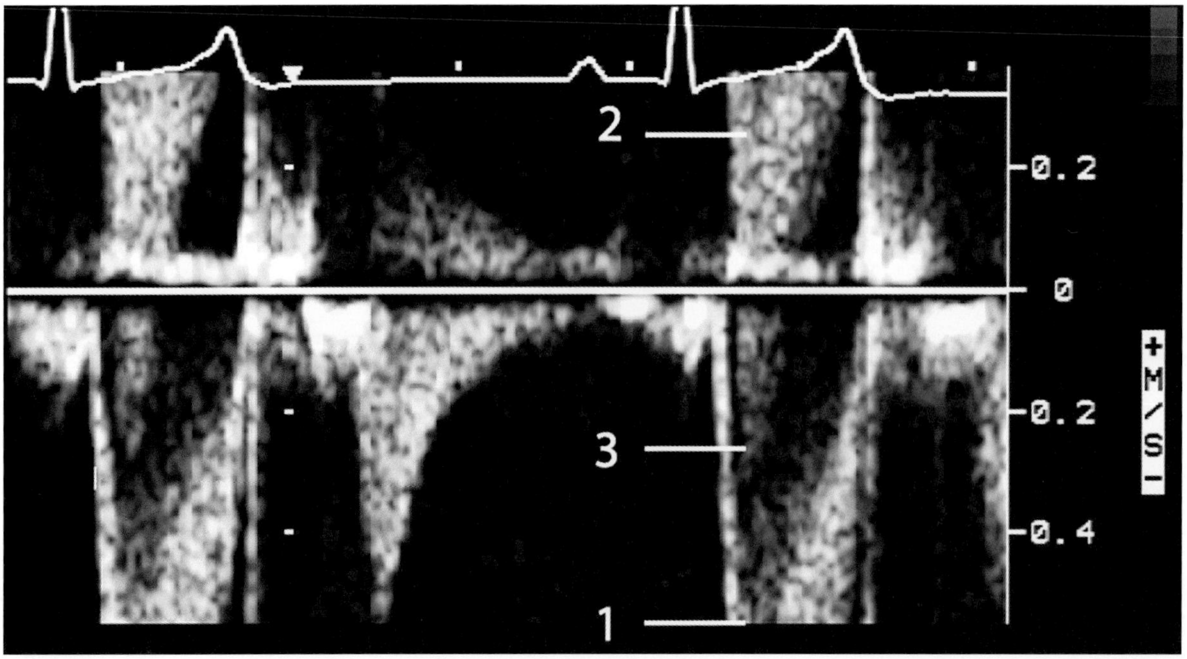

Figure 5.13. Spectral PWD aliasing. Spectral Doppler recordings represent velocity along the *y*-axis, corresponding to Doppler shift frequency, and time along the *x*-axis. In this example of Ao ejection, flow is directed away from the transducer, and velocity in this direction is depicted below the baseline. The velocity reaches the alias velocity (Nyquist limit) at position 1 and further increases causing the signal to wrap around to the positive side of the velocity scale (position 2). Velocity continues to increase, actually passing the zero baseline to the peak velocity indicated at position 3.

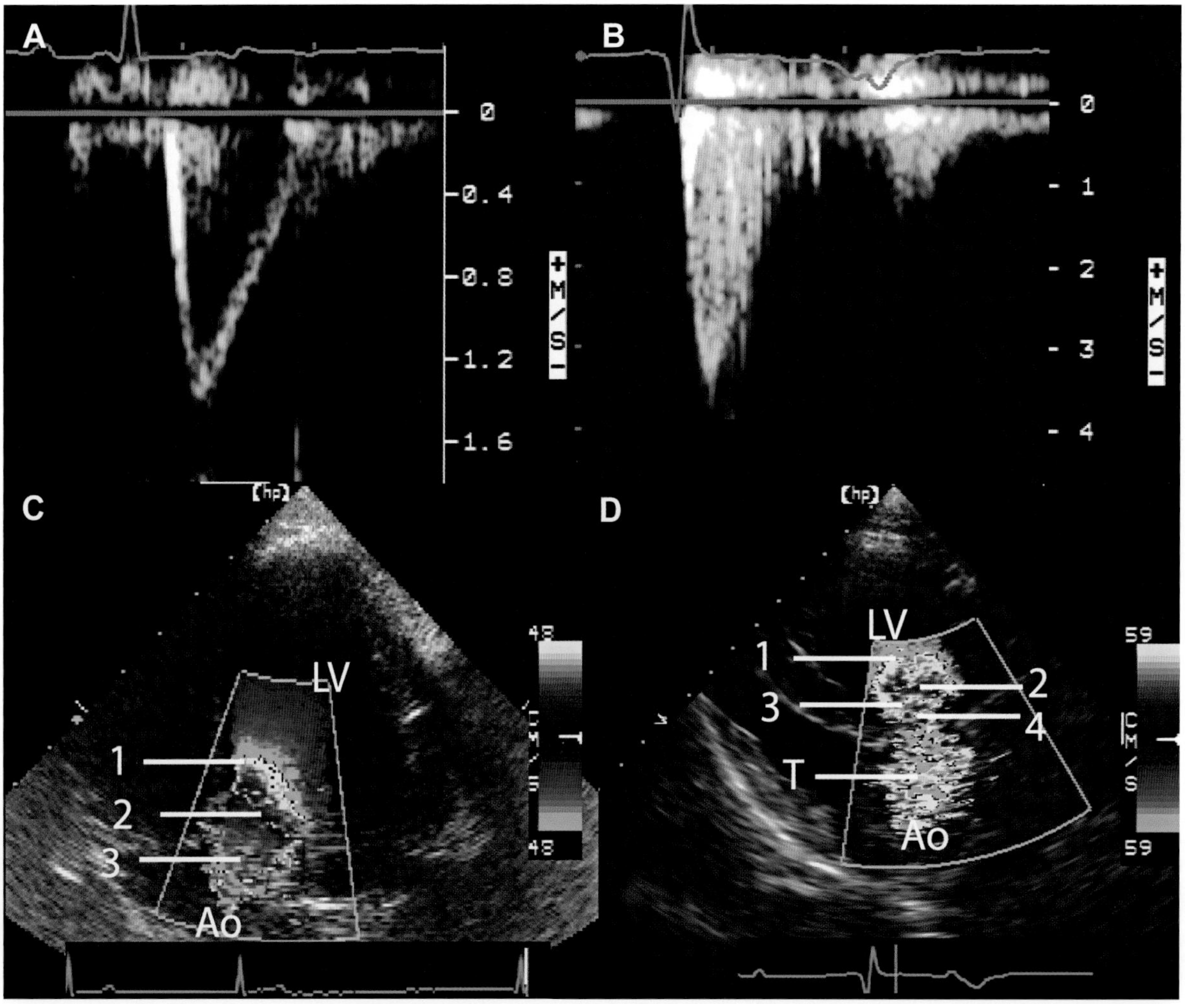

Figure 5.14.

dimension (LA/Ao_m). It is often preferable, however, to index cardiac linear dimensions in terms of the body weight (BW, in kilograms) raised to the one-third power. The weight-based aortic dimension, $Ao_w = 0.795\ BW^{1/3}$, is an estimate of a dog's aortic diameter, and expectations for LA/Ao_w are similar to the index derived using the measured aortic dimension (Figure 5.20). Similarly, the aortic area can be approximated as $AoA_w = \Pi Ao_w^2/4$, the area of a circle with radius $Ao_w/2$, and incorporated into various area ratio indices. In dogs, for example, LA area in the RPS short-axis orientation (SAx) image is normally 2–4 aortic areas in size, regardless of body size (LA area/AoA_w = 2–4).

The majority of published cardiac dimensional data for dogs and cats are from M-mode recordings. Many of these may be recast into the form of a ratio index that enables interpretation independent of body weight. Normal values for raw echocardiographic measurements and ratio indices are tabulated in the Appendix at the end of this chapter.

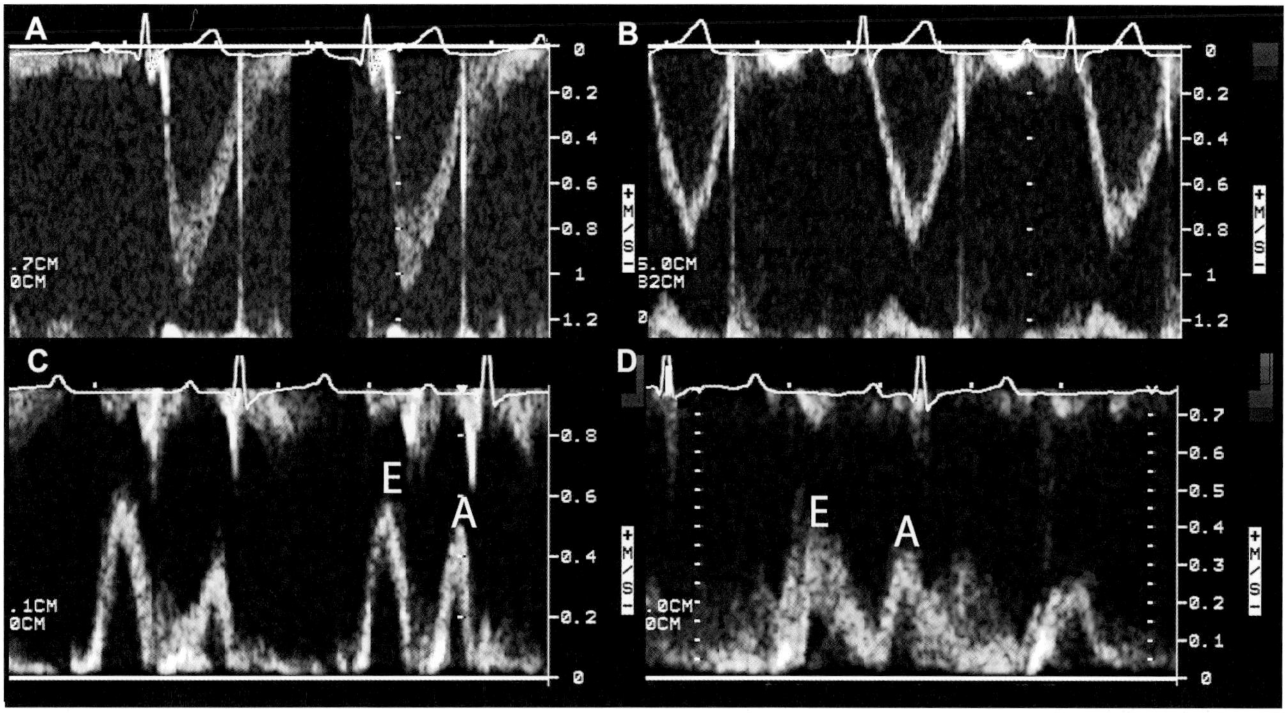

Figure 5.15. Normal PWD recordings. PWD recordings from a normal dog are shown for the Ao (**A**, LAp transducer position), pulmonic (**B**, RPS position), mitral (**C**, LAp position), and tricuspid (**D**, LAp position) valves. Characteristically, Ao ejection flow velocity peaks early in systole and may generate a dagger-shaped velocity envelope like the one shown. Inclusion of the valve itself in the velocity sampling volume generates a vertical artifact that marks the end of the ejection for both cardiac cycles shown. Normal mitral and tricuspid inflow occurs in two distinct phases (E and A waves as labeled) corresponding to M-mode designations.

Figure 5.14. Laminar versus turbulent flow. **A:** The PWD Ao ejection signal, recorded from the subcostal transducer position of a normal dog, demonstrates a laminar flow signal. **B:** In contrast, a CWD recording of a turbulent pattern from a dog with third-degree atrioventricular block and bradycardia causing a marked increase in stroke volume. This results in a wide range of Doppler frequencies (i.e., velocities) at each moment during the ejection and spectral broadening of the signal; the velocity envelope is filled in (white) throughout ejection. **C:** A CFD image from the normal dog (LAp transducer position) early in the Ao ejection phase. The color pattern is laminar but depicts color aliasing that occurs at position 1. Velocity continues to increase in the direction of the outflow and has aliased to black, at position 2, wrapping around to blue again at position 3. **D:** The CFD image of AO ejection for the bradycardic dog. Color aliasing occurs so that velocity can be seen to wrap around the color scale at least twice with a blue-yellow interface (Nyquist frequency) at positions 1 and 3, and indicated zero velocity at positions 2 and 4. A turbulent color flow pattern appears in the Ao (T), as represented by small juxtaposed islands of blue and yellow, also known as a mosaic pattern.

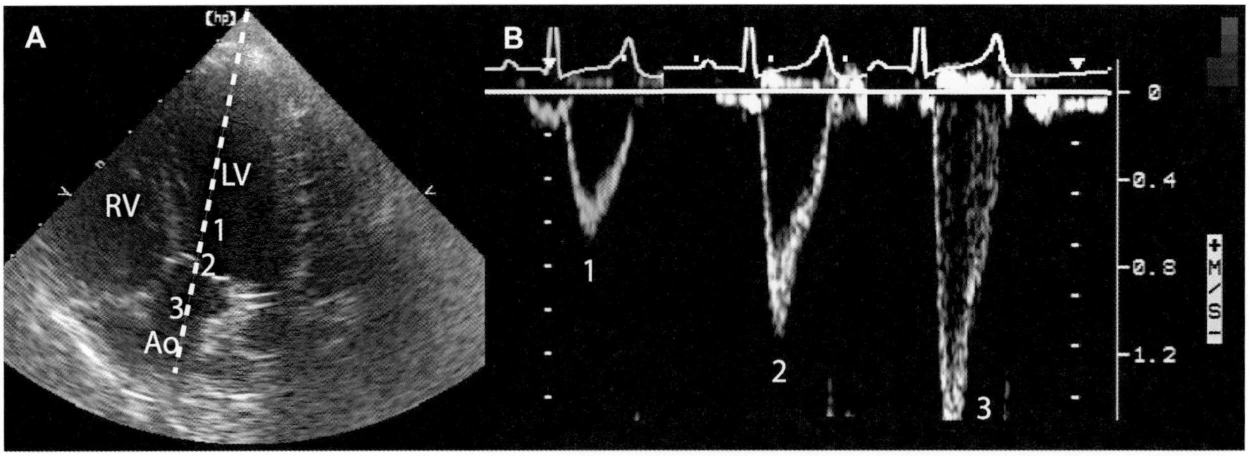

Figure 5.16. Variation of Ao ejection velocity with location. PWD recordings of Ao ejection with the LAp five-chamber image **(A)** showing sample volume locations. There is a marked progression of peak velocity from the subvalvular position (1) to the valvular (2) and supravalvular (3) positions. CWD recordings from the same transducer position (not shown) samples all velocities included along the chosen scan line (dotted). In **B**, the envelope of the CWD recording indicates the maximum velocity along the scan line throughout ejection, and there may be considerable spectral broadening because a wide range of velocities is present along the line at each moment in time.

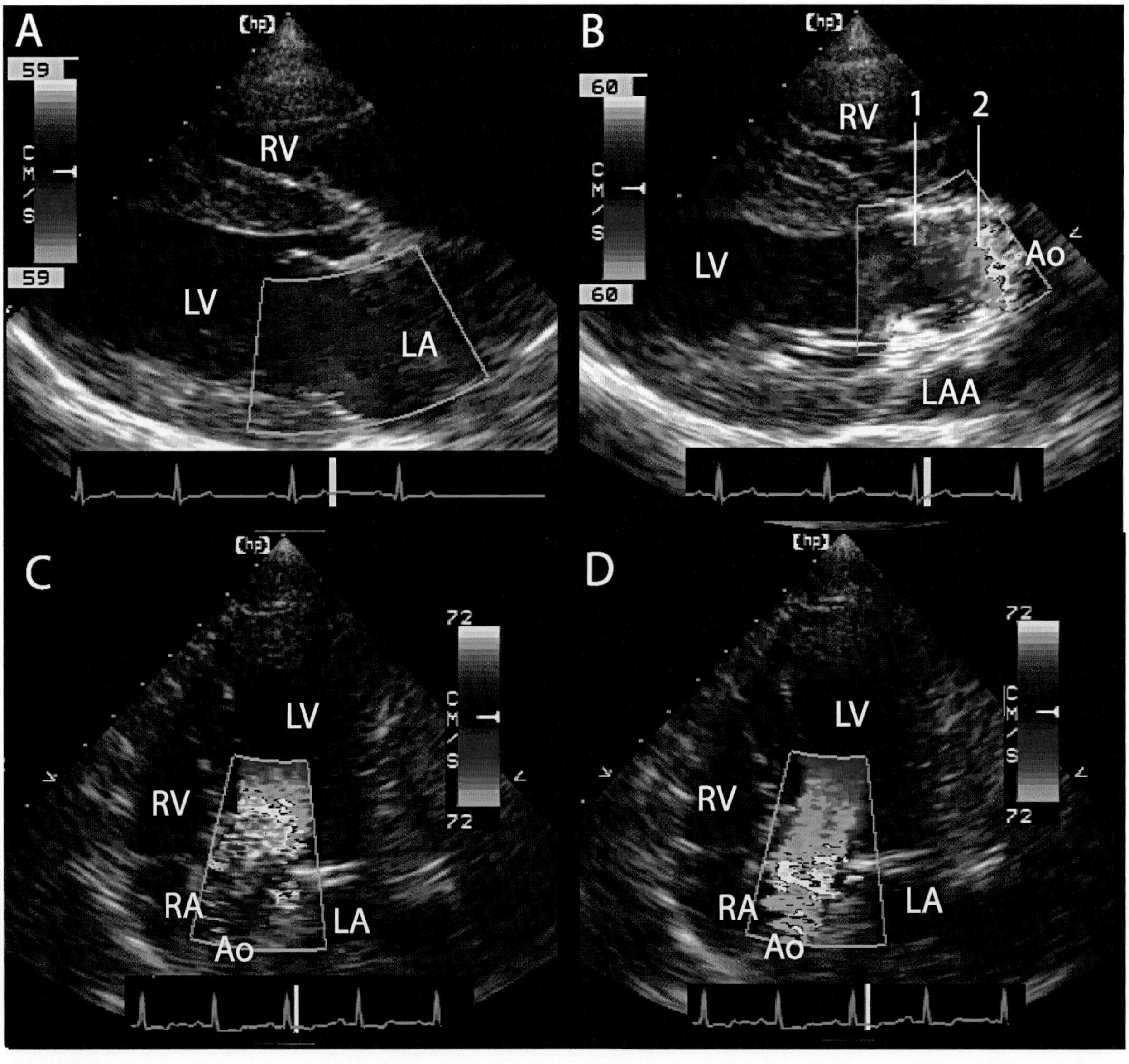

Figure 5.17.

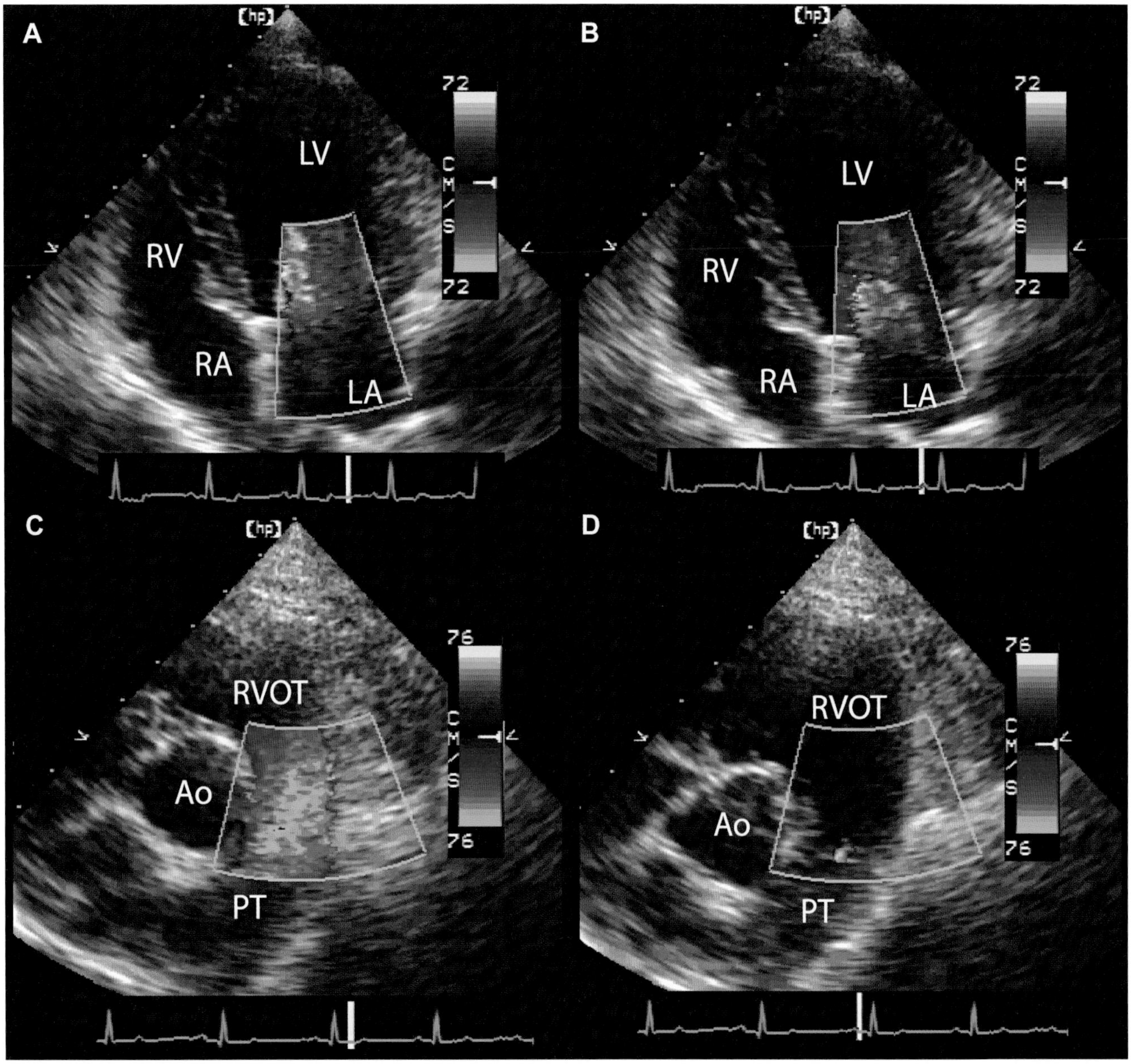

Figure 5.18. Normal CFD images of mitral and pulmonic flow. LV inflow, recorded from the LAp 4 chamber view, is shown for early diastole **(A)** and for atrial kick **(B)**, corresponding to the E and A waves of mitral inflow, respectively (Figure 5.32). RPS SAx images of pulmonic flow correspond to laminar systolic ejection **(C)** and mild PI **(D)**. The latter is a normal finding.

Figure 5.17. Normal CFD images of Ao flow. **A and B:** CFD images from the RPS position of a normal dog. Inflow **(A)** and outflow **(B)** velocities of the LV are not aligned with the direction of ultrasound propagation from the RPS position, and accurate quantification of these velocities is not achieved. **A:** Normal mitral inflow in early diastole is directed relatively toward the transducer and depicted in red in accordance with the color velocity map shown. **B:** LV ejection follows a bend in the Ao so that part of the flow is directed toward the transducer (red), part is directed away (blue), and velocity is completely perpendicular to the ultrasound beam at location 1, where velocity appears to be zero (black). Color aliasing occurs at location 2, where flow away from the transducer exceeds the Nyquist limit. Improved LV inflow and outflow alignment are achieved from the LAp position. **C:** Early peak Ao ejection, with color aliasing. **D:** Subsequent ejection at decreased velocity.

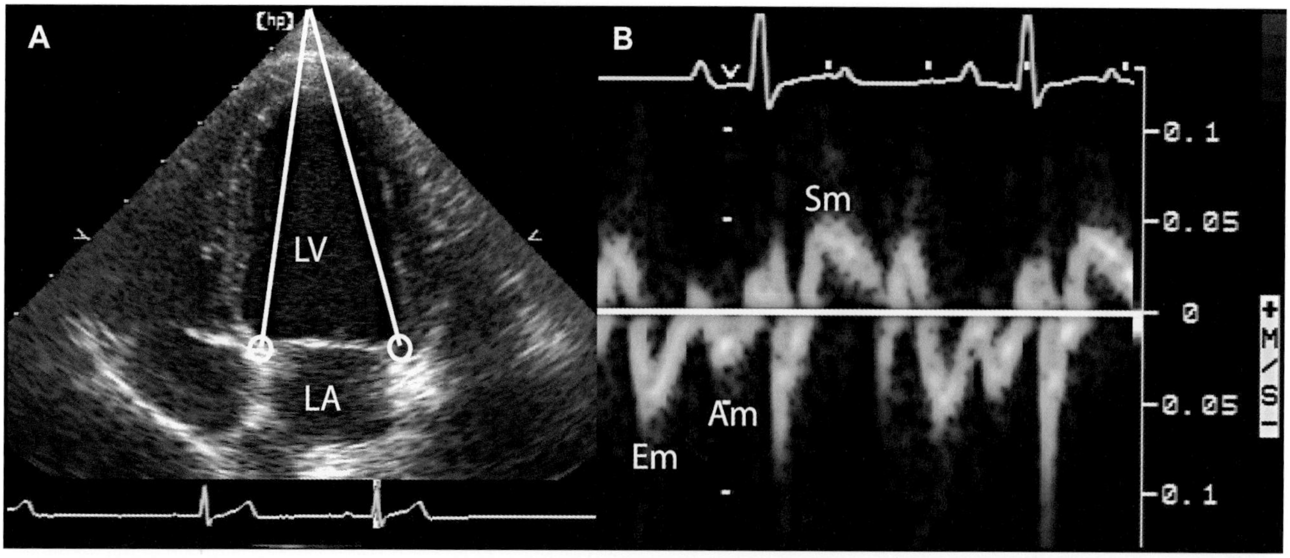

Figure 5.19. TD recording of mitral annular velocity. Velocity sampling locations are depicted in the LAp four-chamber image **(A)** to record either septal or lateral mitral annulus velocity **(B)**. Diastolic annular velocity measurements recapitulate the mitral inflow pattern with two distinct phases of filling. The LV expands longitudinally in both early and late diastole, resulting in annular velocity away from the transducer and generation of the E_m and A_m waves, respectively. LV contraction entails a longitudinal component that is directed toward the transducer and generation of the systolic TD wave (S_m).

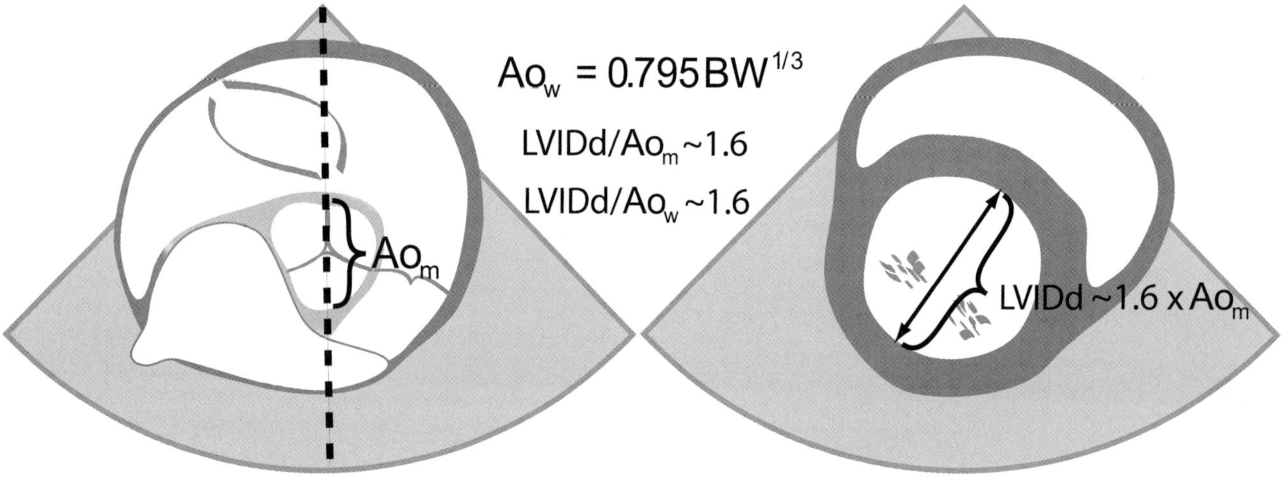

Figure 5.20. Ratio index normalization for body size. Size normalization of measured linear dimensions, area, volume, or mass can often be accomplished by using a ratio index. The measured Ao diameter (Ao_m), obtained from M-mode or 2DE recordings, has been used as a suitable reference length in echocardiography. The diastolic LV internal dimension (LVIDd), for example, ranges between 1.2 and 2.0 Ao diameters across in normal dogs, regardless of body size. However, the Ao dimension also may be estimated from body weight (kilograms), as shown, and often is superior statistically to Ao_m as a length standard.

Linear Dimensions

M-mode recordings suitable for accurate and reproducible linear measurements require 2DE guidance, both for transducer placement and cursor alignment. For LV measurements, the M-mode scan line should transect the LV central axis perpendicularly near the tips of the open mitral leaflets (Sahn et al. 1978; O'Rourke et al. 1984). M-mode linear measurements are made vertically along the *y*-axis of the strip chart, i.e., at a specific instant in time (Figure 5.21). A simultaneous electrocardiogram facilitates timing of the cardiac cycle where the QRS complex signals the end of diastole. It is typical for the maximum LV internal

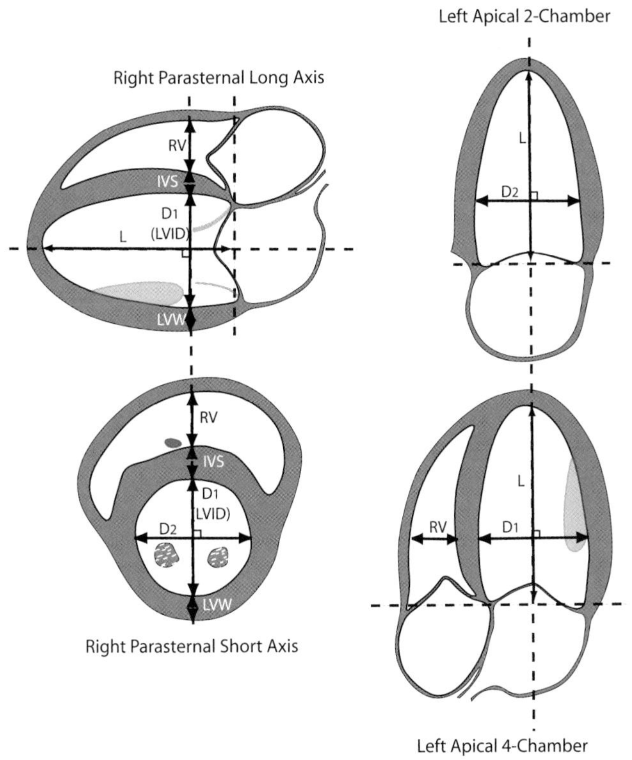

Figure 5.21. Linear ventricular measurements from 2DE. The D_1 short-axis dimension corresponds to the LV internal dimension (LVID) from M-mode, whereas D_2 must be determined from 2DE, from either the RPS SAx or LAp two-chamber image, as shown. LV length (L) is measured from the plane of the mitral annulus to the LV apex along the central LV axis (Schiller et al. 1989).

dimension to occur during the QRS complex, and it is often possible to observe a slight presystolic distension induced by atrial contraction. End systole occurs near the end of the electrocardiographic T wave, but the timing of the systolic measurement is determined from the echocardiogram itself at the occurrence of the minimum LV internal dimension. Normally, the interventricular septum moves away from the transducer during systole while the LV wall moves toward it, but motion may be slightly dyssynchronous in normal animals. There may be a brief interval near end systole where the septum and LV wall both move toward the transducer. Consequently, the minimal internal dimension need not coincide with maximal wall excursions with respect to the transducer. Linear measurement can be accomplished alternatively from single frame images of the 2DE, and this is preferable whenever M-mode cursor alignment is not attainable (O'Grady et al. 1986; Schiller et al. 1989) (Figure 5.22).

LA size embodies relevant diagnostic and prognostic information, but quantification is problematic because of the irregular three-dimensional shape (Rishniw and Erb 2000; Hansson et al. 2002). The measurement derived from M-mode recordings exemplifies this issue because it includes only a small portion of the structure—the atrial appendage—plus a variable thickness of adipose tissue that lies between the aorta and appendage. Body-size normalization of the M-mode measurement in dogs has been accomplished through

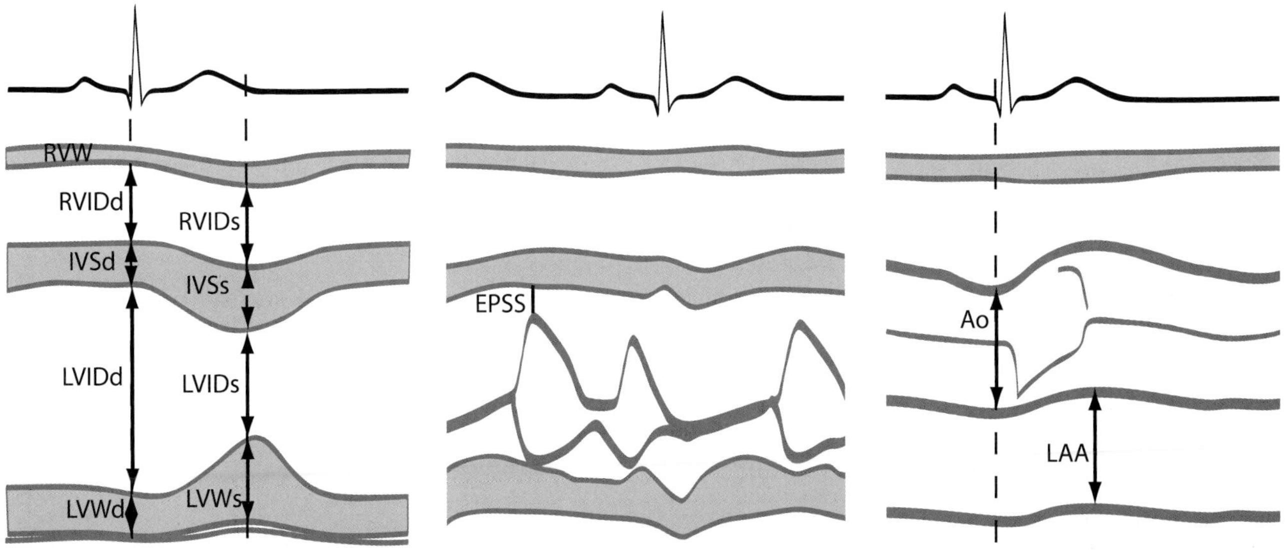

Figure 5.22. Linear ventricular measurements from M-mode echocardiography. 2DE guidance for transducer placement and M-mode scan-line selection is paramount for accurate and reproducible results. Subscripts d and s refer to diastolic and systolic determinations, respectively, where end diastole coincides with the greatest LV internal dimension (LVID), typically shortly after the onset of the QRS complex, and systole coincides with the smallest LVID. The Ao measurement is made at end diastole, coincident with maximal distance of the Ao from the transducer, and the LAA measurement is made at its maximal dimension in time, coinciding with end systole. Linear measurements are made vertically across the strip chart. EPSS, end point to septal separation distance; and RVID, RV internal dimension.

division by the measured aortic dimension (Ao_m). Mean values of this ratio are near 1.0 across the entire body-size spectrum but with normal maximum values up to 1.4, depending on breed (Appendix). The upper limit for the raw measurement in cats ranges from 1.2 to 1.7 cm, depending on the study (Appendix). Linear 2DE LA measurements from SAx and LAx images afford advantages in sensitivity over M-mode determinations (Figure 5.23). Like their M-mode counterparts, maximal 2DE LA size determinations are made at end systole, just prior to the mitral valve opening.

Measurements of aortic and pulmonary trunk diameter may be used to evaluate these outflow tracts for narrowing, stenosis, or dilation, and also are used for estimations of ventricular stroke volume and cardiac output in conjunction with Doppler velocity measurements (Figure 5.24).

Cardiac Volume and Mass

Numerous mathematical formulas have been proposed for the estimation of ventricular volume, which pertains importantly to cardiovascular diagnosis and prognosis.

Ejection fraction is a ratio index calculated from ventricular volume as (EDV – ESV)/EDV, where EDV and ESV are the end-diastolic volume and the end-systolic volume, respectively (Schiller et al. 1989). Many

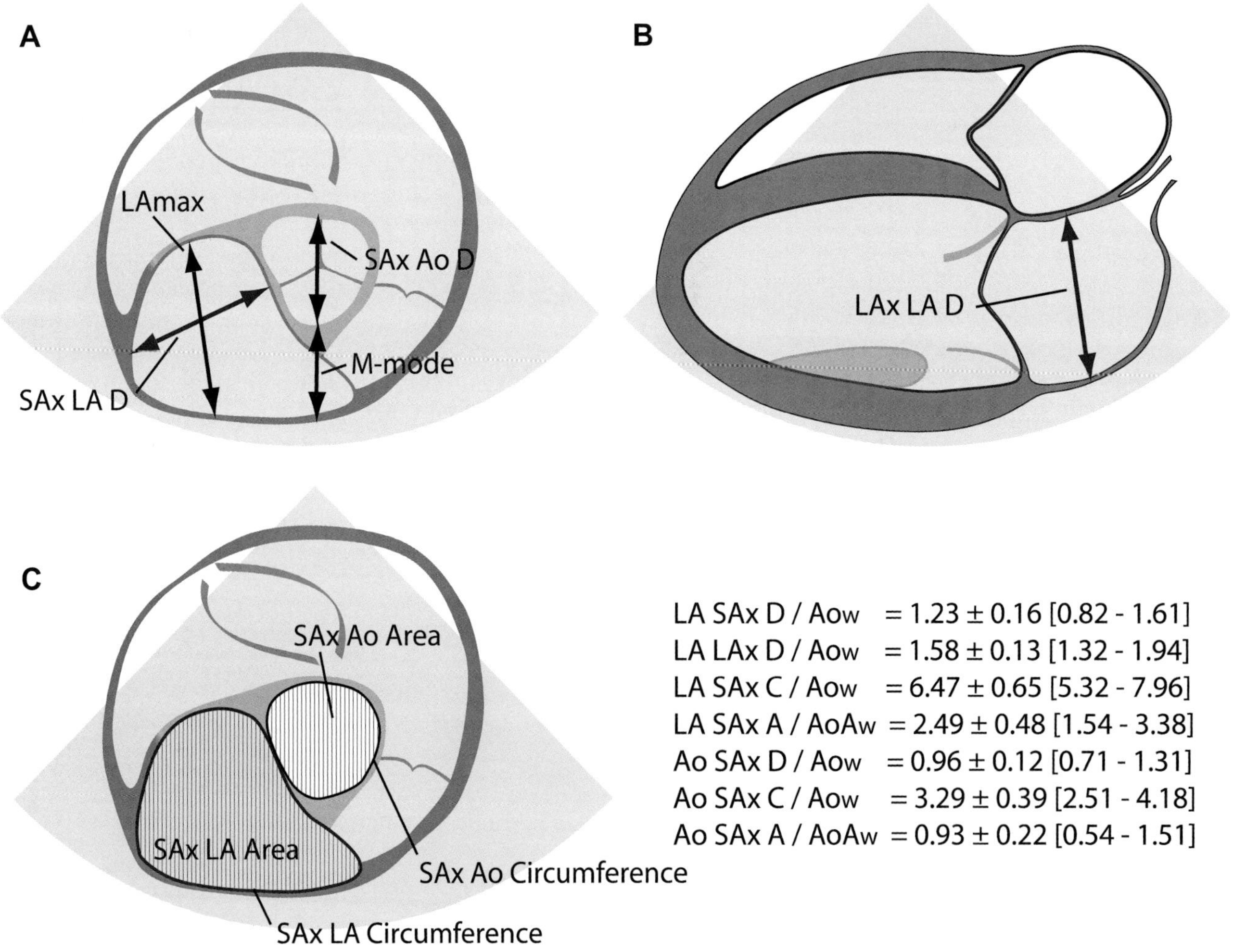

Figure 5.23. LA size determination. LA size determination is problematic because of the irregular three-dimensional shape. In dogs, the standard M-mode measurement includes only a small portion of the LA, i.e., the LAA **(A)**. Linear measurements made from the 2DE RPS SAx **(A)** and LAx **(B)** are more representative of atrial size but still suffer from angular dependence. The planimetered SAx LA area and circumference are less dependent on angle **(C)**. LA measurements studied by Rishniw and Erb may be conveniently expressed as a ratio index, dividing linear dimensions by the weight-based Ao diameter ($Ao_w = 0.795\ BW^{1/3}$) and area measurements by the weight-based Ao area ($AoA_w = \Pi\ Ao_w^2/4$). Each index exhibits minimal dependence on body size. Mean ± standard deviation and, in brackets, range for each index are shown. Original data supplied by Rishniw and Erb (2000). A, area; BW, body weight; C, circumference; D, diameter, and max, maximum.

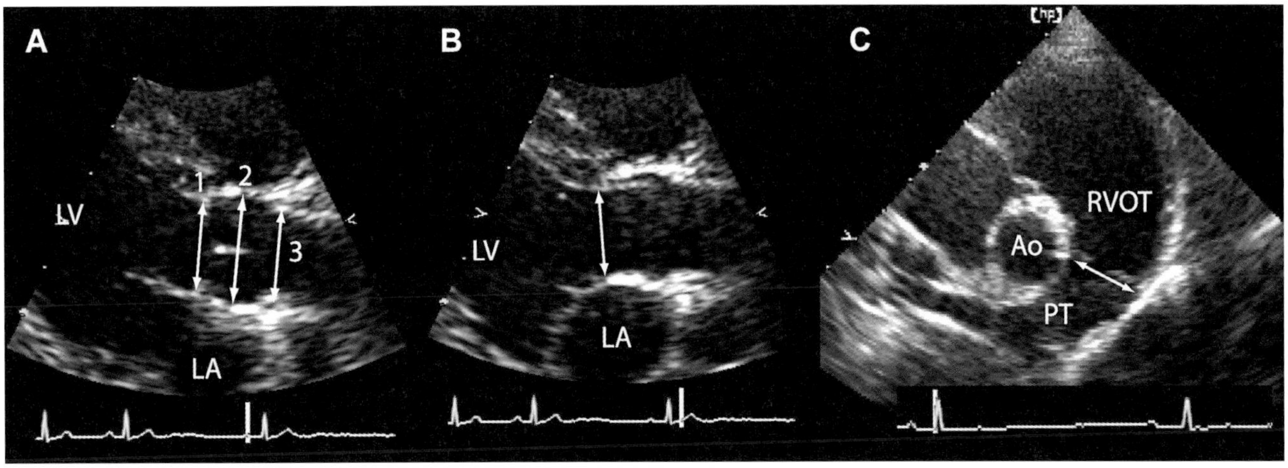

Figure 5.24. LVOT and RVOT diameters. RPS LAx (**A and B**) and SAx (**C**) images are shown. Measurements are made perpendicular to the vessel axes, and longitudinal vessel images show how dimensions vary in diameter with axial location. **A:** Position 1 depicts the Ao root diameter in diastole. **B:** The systolic dimension, where the measurement can be made between the right coronary cusp and Ao root wall to quantify the flow diameter. Position 2 in **A** corresponds to the dilation that occurs at the sinus of Valsalva, and position 3 is the sinotubular junction, a local minimum for the Ao diameter. **C:** The diameter of the PV orifice. Accurate determination of RVOT diameter is problematic because the ultrasound beam is nearly parallel to the reflecting surfaces.

cardiologists use the terms ejection fraction and systolic function synonymously. The one-dimensional analogue of ejection fraction is the fractional shortening, FS = (LVIDd – LVIDs)/LVIDd, determined usually from M-mode short-axis measurements of diastolic (LVIDd) and systolic (LVIDs) LV internal dimension. LV stroke volume (SV) may be estimated from the difference between diastolic and systolic volumes. A body-size normalized ratio index, wΔA (Table 5.3), is the estimated LV SAx stroke area divided by the weight-based aortic area. Values derived from M-mode measurements range from 0.8 to 2.8 in dogs and may be somewhat breed and body size dependent (Appendix). The M-mode index is simplistic but valuable for clinical quantification of LV volume overload or underload in the authors' experience. Relative echocardiographic ratio indices of the left ventricle and interventricular septum are defined in Table 5.4.

LV mass may be estimated by calculating the external volume of the left ventricle and subtracting the internal volume (Schiller et al. 1989) (Figure 5.25). Myocardial mass is normally proportional to body weight and thus requires normalization. Ratio indices wWΛd and wWAs correspond to normalized LV short-axis wall area in diastole and systole, respectively, where myocardial wall area is divided by the weight-based aortic area (Table 5.3). Normal values of wWAd in dogs range roughly from 1.8 to 5.5 but with

$$r_1 = \sqrt{\frac{A_1}{\pi}}, \ r_2 = \sqrt{\frac{A_2}{\pi}}, \ t = r_1 - r_2$$

$$1.05 \left\{ \left[\frac{5}{6} A_1 (a + d + t) \right] - \left[\frac{5}{6} A_2 (a + d) \right] \right\}$$

LV Mass - Area-Length

$$1.05\pi \left\{ r_1^2 \left[\frac{2}{3}(a+t) + d - \frac{d^3}{3(a+t)^2} \right] - r_2^2 \left[\frac{2}{3}a + d - \frac{d^3}{3a^2} \right] \right\}$$

LV Mass - Truncated Ellipsoid

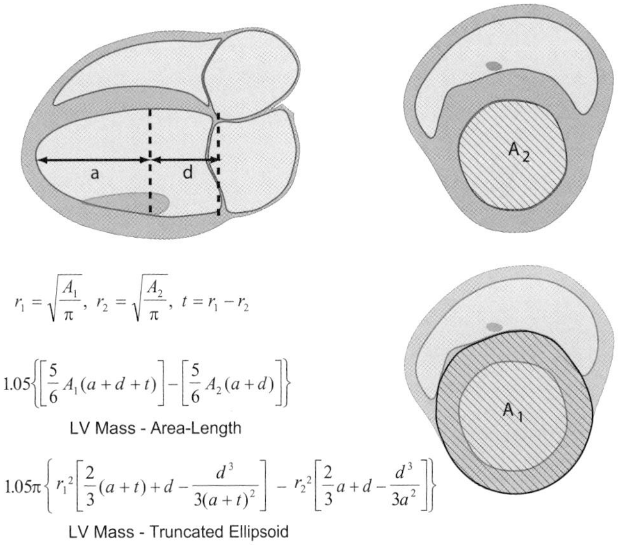

Figure 5.25. LV mass estimation by 2DE methods. Short-axis external (A_1) and internal (A_2) areas are determined by planimetry at the level of the mitral CT and used to determine geometric mean radii, both outer (r_1) and inner (r_2); constant wall thickness (t) is assumed. The major axis of the ellipsoid (a) is measured along the LV axis from the apex to the point of maximal radius, as shown; the distance (d) comprises the remainder of the LV length from the apex to the mitral annulus. The constant (1.05 g/cm³) is the density of normal soft tissue. LV mass values obtained by either equation require normalization for body size (Schiller et al. 1989).

Table 5.3.
Weight-based echocardiographic ratio indices

Index	Calculation	Description
wAo	Ao_m/Ao_w	Indexed aortic root dimension
wIVSd	$IVSd/Ao_w$	Indexed interventricular septal thickness, diastole
wLVIDd	$LVIDd/Ao_w$	Indexed left ventricular internal dimension, diastole
wLVWd	$LVWd/Ao_w$	Indexed left ventricular wall thickness, diastole
wIVSs	$IVSs/Ao_w$	Indexed interventricular septal thickness, systole
wLVIDs	$LVIDs/Ao_w$	Indexed left ventricular internal dimension, systole
wLVWs	$LVWs/Ao_w$	Indexed left ventricular wall thickness, systole
wLA	LA/Ao_w	Indexed left atrial dimension
wLVODd	$(IVSd + LVIDd + LVWd)/Ao_w$	Index of left ventricular outer dimension, diastole
wWTd	$(IVSd + LVWd)/Ao_w$	Index of combined septal and left ventricular wall thickness, diastole
wLVODs	$(IVSs + LVIDs + LVWs)/Ao_w$	Index of left ventricular outer dimension, systole
wWTs	$(IVSs + LVWs)/Ao_w$	Index of combined septal and left ventricular wall thickness, systole
wΔA	$(LVIDd^2 - LVIDs^2)/Ao_w^2$	Index of change in left ventricular internal area, i.e., short-axis stroke area
wWAd	$(LVODd^2 - LVIDd^2)/Ao_w^2$	Index of left ventricular short-axis myocardial wall area, diastole, i.e., hypertrophy
wWAs	$(LVODs^2 - LVIDs^2)/Ao_w^2$	Index of left ventricular short-axis myocardial wall area, systole, i.e. hypertrophy

A ratio index normalizes raw echocardiographic measurements for body size. Ao_w is the weight-based aortic dimension calculated as $Ao_w = kBW^{1/3}$ where k is a species-dependent constant equal to 0.795 in dogs and 0.567 in cats.

Table 5.4.
Relative echocardiographic ratio indices

Index	Calculation	Description
FS	(LVIDd – LVIDs)/LVIDd	Fractional shortening. Relative left ventricular internal wall motion or LV short axis deformation.
FWTd	(IVSd + LVWd)/LVODd	Fractional left ventricular myocardial wall thickness, diastole. Relative left ventricular wall thickness in diastole.
FWTs	(IVSs + LVWs)/LVODs	Fractional left ventricular myocardial wall thickness, systole. Relative left ventricular wall thickness in systole.
FΔA	$(LVIDd^2 - LVIDs^2)/LVIDd^2$	Fractional change in left ventricular internal area. Relative left ventricular internal wall motion or left ventricular short-axis deformation.
FWAd	$(LVODd^2 - LVIDd^2)/(LVODd^2)$	Fractional left ventricular myocardial wall area (short axis), diastole. Relative left ventricular wall area in diastole.
FWAs	$(LVODs^2 - LVIDs^2)/(LVODs^2)$	Fractional left ventricular myocardial wall area (short axis). Relative left ventricular wall area in systole.
IVSFT	(IVSs – IVSd)/IVSd	Intraventricular septum fractional thickening. Relative thickening of interventricular septum.
LVWFT	(LVWs – LVWd)/LVWd	Left ventricular wall fractional thickening. Relative thickening of left ventricular wall.
RWTd	2 LVWd/LVIDd	Relative left ventricular wall thickness, diastole. Relative left ventricular wall thickness to chamber dimension, diastole.
RWTs	2 LVWs/LVIDs	Relative left ventricular wall thickness, systole. Relative left ventricular wall thickness to chamber dimension, systole.

Fractional shortening is a better-known ratio index derived by dividing the change in left ventricular internal dimension by the diastolic value; it is common practice to multiply the result by 100 and express the value as a percentage (%ΔD). Relative ratio indices are normalized for some aspect of heart size, not for the size of the individual.

significant breed dependency; upper values in Italian greyhounds, whippets, and greyhounds range from 5.0 to 6.0 (Appendix). These are clinical indices derived from M-mode or planar 2DE measurements that do not estimate true myocardial mass. However, they may be superior indicators of hypertrophy compared with simple measurements of wall thickness, which can depend strongly on hemodynamic conditions.

Doppler Measurements and Systolic Time Intervals

Much of the quantitative value of Doppler studies stems from the application of fluid dynamic principles to the interpretation of measured velocities through the modified Bernoulli equation (Hatle and Angelsen 1985). The modified Bernoulli equation is expressed as $\Delta P = 4\ V^2$ for many clinical applications, where velocity (V) is in meters per second (m/s) and the calculated pressure is in millimeters of mercury (mm Hg). Velocity recordings are optimized accomplished at the time of the recording by diligent positioning of the transducer at the appropriate body-wall location, aided by cues from the CFD image and both visual and auditory feedback from the spectral Doppler display (Darke et al. 1993). Transducer position varies with the specific lesion to be evaluated, e.g., aortic stenosis versus mitral regurgitation (MR), as well as nuances specific to the individual.

Besides pressure gradients, valuable functional information is derived from spectral Doppler signals that enable the timing of cardiac cycle events and estimation of blood flow rate (Figure 5.26). Systolic time intervals have been employed for many years to evaluate cardiac function, predating the ultrasonic era, but Doppler signals are ideal for obtaining the required measurements. Systolic time intervals are determined from time measurements of the cardiac cycle and consequently are indices of global function; determinations are most commonly used to evaluate LV function. A ratio index of preejection period (PEP)–LV ejection time (PEP/LVET), is often used to help normalize raw time measurements for body size and heart rate. An additional index, the velocity of circumferential shortening, is equivalent to the fractional shortening divided by LV ejection time (FS/LVET) and so relates to the rate of cardiac deformation. Additional determinations made from either aortic or pulmonary flow-velocity signals include the acceleration time and the velocity time integral (VTI). Acceleration time is related to both myocardial function and afterload (Figure 5.26).

The aortic or pulmonary VTI is the planimetered area under the flow-velocity envelope. It has physical units of length (e.g., centimeters), corresponding to the integration of velocity with respect to time, and also has been termed the *stroke length* (Figure 5.30). Multiplication of the VTI by the effective orifice area (A_E) gives the volume of blood passing through the orifice during the ejection, i.e., the forward stroke volume ($SV = VTI \times A_E$). Multiplication of the stroke

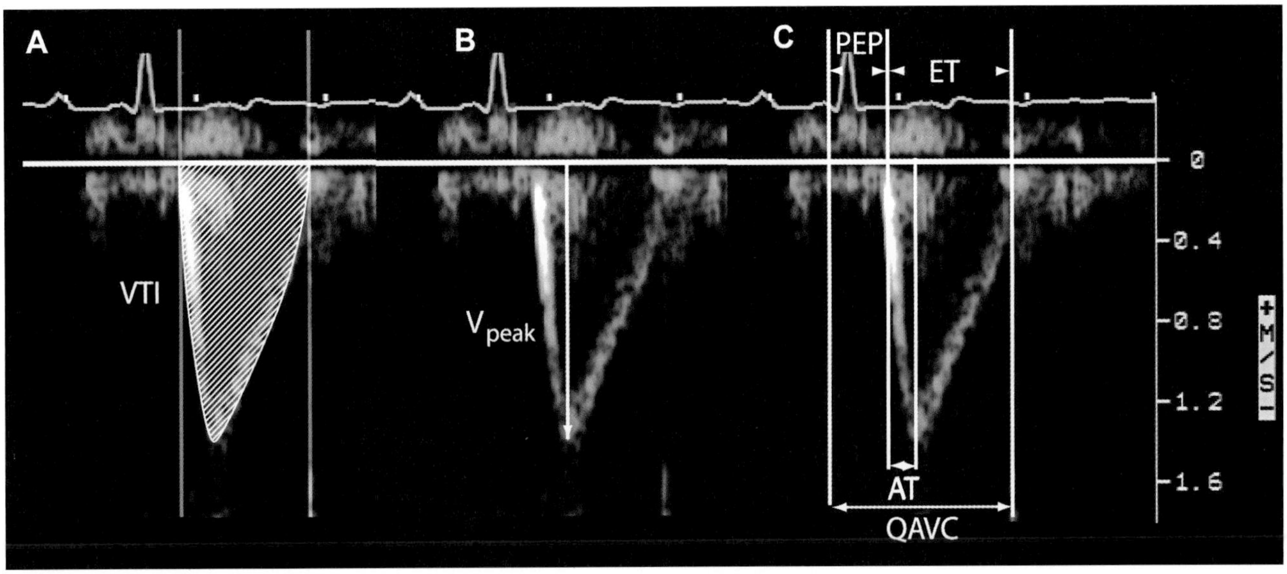

Figure 5.26. Measurements from Ao spectral Doppler signals. **A:** Planimetry of the area under the flow-velocity envelope yields the velocity-time integral (VTI), which has units of length (e.g., centimeters). **B:** Measurement of the temporal peak velocity (V_{peak}). **C:** Determination of timing intervals. The preejection period (PEP) is from the onset of the electrocardiographic QRS complex to the onset of ejection. Measurement of the ejection time (ET) is facilitated by inclusion of the Ao valve in the velocity sampling volume so that valve motion artifacts delineate the interval. Total electrical-mechanical systole is from the onset of the QRS to Ao valve closure (QAVC) and is the sum of PEP and ET. The acceleration time (AT) is the interval from the beginning of the ejection to the peak flow velocity. Average flow velocity (e.g., centimeters per second) can be determined by dividing the VTI by ET. Terminology applies to RV outflow signals, as well.

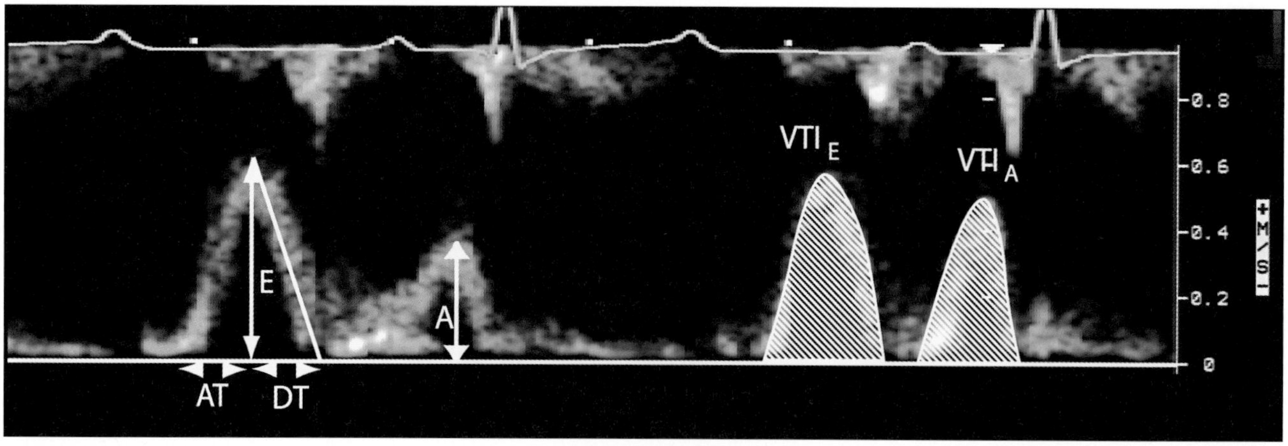

Figure 5.27. Measurements from mitral inflow signals. Measurements include peak velocities for the E and A waves and the velocity-time integrals (VTIs) of each. The E/A peak velocity ratio, normally greater than 1.0, or VTI_E/VTI_A may be used to quantify relative contributions of each to ventricular filling. Peak velocities are related to the peak atrial-ventricular pressure gradient through the Bernoulli equation and so may suggest valvular stenosis or increased LA pressure. The acceleration time (AT) is the interval from opening of the MV to peak velocity. The deceleration time (DT) is determined by extrapolating from peak E-wave velocity to baseline along the flow-velocity envelope, as shown; it is common for the A wave to intervene without the velocity envelope reaching zero. The slope of the deceleration may also be recorded.

volume by heart rate gives the cardiac output. The effective orifice area (A_E) may be estimated from 2DE images as just described for aortic and pulmonary outflow tracts by using the measured diameter (D) to compute the area of a corresponding circle ($A = \pi D^2/4$) (Figure 5.24).

Measurements from mitral and tricuspid inflow-velocity signals include the velocity magnitude of the E and A waves and the planimetered area (VTI) for each (Figure 5.27). Factors affecting the form of inflow velocities are complex and pertain to diastolic ventricular function.

Congenital Heart Disease

Valvular Diseases

Aortic Stenosis

Aortic stenosis (AS) signifies an obstruction to LV outflow. It may be valvular, subvalvular (subaortic stenosis [SAS]), or supravalvular. SAS is the most common congenital defect of large-breed dogs. Moderate to severe SAS causes characteristic, but variable, 2DE abnormalities, including discrete or diffuse narrowing of the LV outflow tract, poststenotic aortic dilation, and thickening of the aortic and anterior mitral valve leaflets (Figure 5.28). On the RPS LAx image, a subvalvular obstruction may appear as an echogenic ridge on the septum, mitral apparatus, or both, corresponding to a complete or incomplete hyperechoic ring of fibrocartilaginous tissue encircling the outflow tract (Bonagura and Herring 1985b). AS causes LV pressure overload and concentric hypertrophy of the left ventricle as quantified by septal and LV wall thickness and other indices of absolute or relative hypertrophy. The extent of hypertrophy is variably correlated with the severity of obstruction. Severe obstruction also may be accompanied by increased echogenicity of the papillary muscles and/or subendocardial myocardium, possibly secondary to ischemia of these regions and subsequent fibrosis or calcification. In severely affected cases, M-mode echocardiography of the aortic root may demonstrate premature systolic closure of the aortic valve.

CFD of the LV outflow tract in systole reveals a region of flow acceleration proximal to the obstructive lesion, and turbulent or disturbed flow with increased velocity distally (Moise 1989) (Figure 5.29). Arbitrary prognostic categories based on the pressure gradient are mild (<50 mm Hg), moderate (50–75 mm Hg), severe (75–100 mm Hg), and very severe (>100 mm Hg). The aortic flow-velocity envelope also becomes more rounded, and its acceleration time increases; that is, delayed peak velocity with increasing severity (Figure 5.30). The pressure gradient and peak velocity are flow-dependent indices of severity.

In the absence of shunts or significant semilunar valve insufficiency, the ratio of aortic (VTI_A) and pulmonary (VTI_P) VTIs approximates the ratio of effective

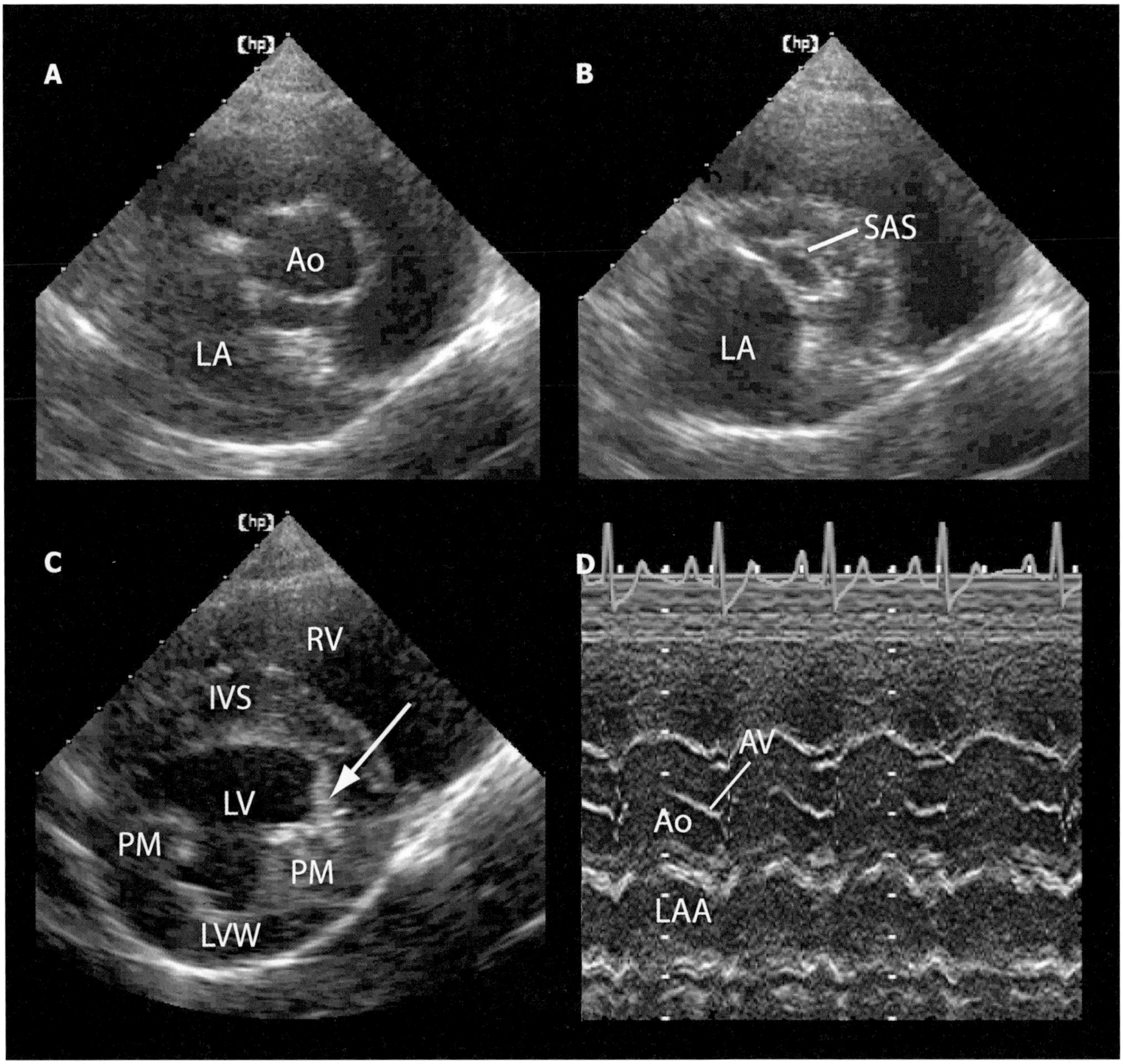

Figure 5.28. RPS SAx images from a dog with subaortic stenosis (SAS). The maximum Ao dimension occurs normally at the level of the Ao sinus of Valsalva **(A)**; valve leaflets are evident. The obstruction in SAS is most typically at the immediate subvalvular location, and the short-axis view may suggest the anatomical severity in terms of cross-sectional area relative to the Ao root **(B)**. **C:** Thickened LVW and LV septum, caused by concentric hypertrophy, are evident. There is an increase in subendocardial echogenicity (arrow) thought to represent fibrosis, secondary to ischemia. **D:** M-mode through the Ao root depicts Ao valve leaflets (AV) that separate partially in early systole, only to quickly return to the closed position. The leaflets may inscribe a diamond or double diamond within the confines of the Ao root.

orifice areas of the two tracts and is corrected for body size and flow rate. In the authors' experience, $VTI_A/VTI_P > 1.6$ (PWD at the valve level) is suggestive of mild SAS and is specific compared with velocity alone (Figure 5.30). Bicuspid aortic valve is a common congenital defect in human patients but a rare cause of stenosis in dogs and cats (Figure 5.31).

Pulmonic Stenosis

Pulmonic stenosis (PS) is the third most common congenital cardiac defect in dogs but is uncommon in cats. PS signifies an obstruction to RV outflow and may occur at subvalvular, supravalvular, or valvular locations, the latter being the most common site in

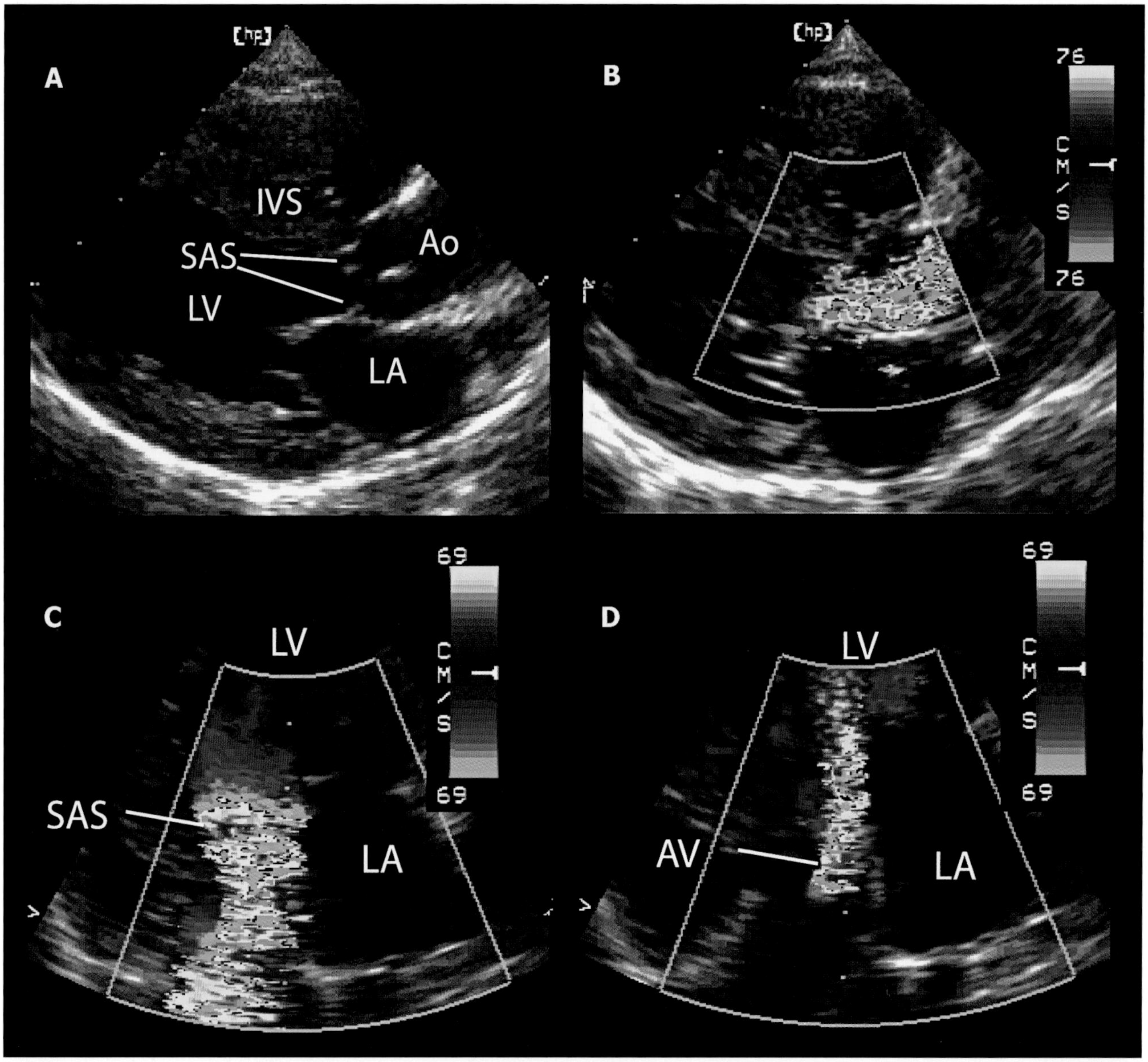

Figure 5.29. CFD images from a dog with subaortic stenosis (SAS). **A:** This RPS LAx 2DE image depicts the location of the obstruction immediately proximal to the AV and is confirmed by CFD in **B**. Although the example shown includes both septal and mitral aspects of the encircling obstruction, neither may be clearly evident, depending on the extent and location of the collar. **C and D:** CFD images obtained from the LAp five-chamber position. During systole **(C)**, the color halo of a *flow convergence zone* appears where flow acceleration and color aliasing occur proximal to the obstruction. A turbulent mosaic pattern is apparent distally in the Ao. **D:** Ao insufficiency present in the same patient during diastole. Here the flow convergence zone is in the Ao as blood accelerates toward the transducer at the location of the AV. CFD clearly demonstrates that the location of the obstruction is proximal to the valve in this instance. Mild to moderate Ao insufficiency commonly accompanies SAS.

dogs. Potential echocardiographic features in common with all forms of PS include RA enlargement, poststenotic dilation of the pulmonary trunk, and concentric hypertrophy of the right ventricle with increased thickness of the septum and RV wall. The RV papillary muscles may become prominent, as do trabeculae carnae, imparting an uneven appearance to the RV endocardial surface and contributing to obstruction. Increased echogenicity of the RV myocardium may be associated with severe obstruction and presumed ischemic myocardial damage. Severe RV pressure overload causes flattening of the interventricular septum and an ovoid LV cross section in the short-axis plane. LV volume underload in this circumstance may suggest

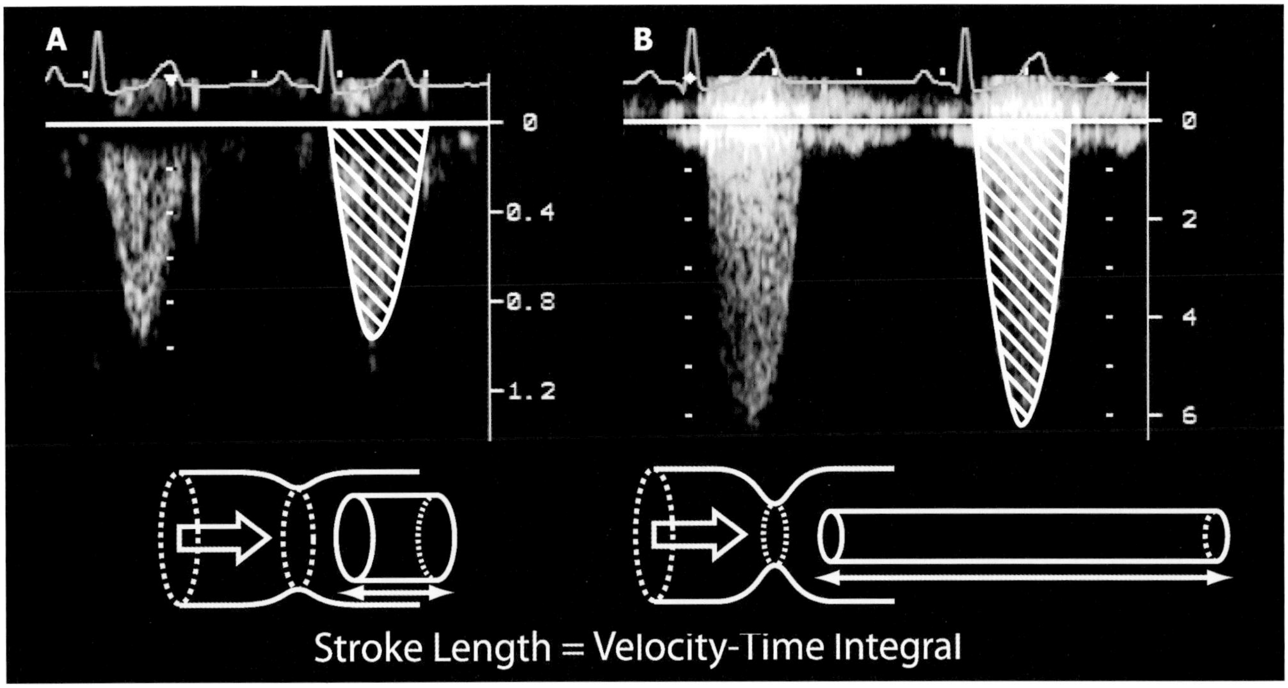

Figure 5.30. Spectral Doppler recordings in subaortic stenosis. Recordings from the pulmonary (**A**, RPS position) and Ao (**B**, subcostal position) outflow tracts of a dog. A temporal peak velocity of 6 m/s for the stenosis corresponds to a maximum pressure gradient of $4 \times 6^2 = 144$ mm Hg and a very severe stenosis. The area under each phasic velocity curve, indicated by hatching, is termed the *velocity-time integral* (VTI) and has physical units of length (e.g., centimeters). This quantity has also been termed the *stroke length*, corresponding to the length of a figure whose volume equals the cardiac stroke volume, and whose cross-sectional area is the effective orifice area the ventricle ejects through. If the stroke volumes of the two ventricles are the same, then the ratio of VTIs approximates the ratio of effective orifice areas and is an index of stenosis severity that is relatively flow independent.

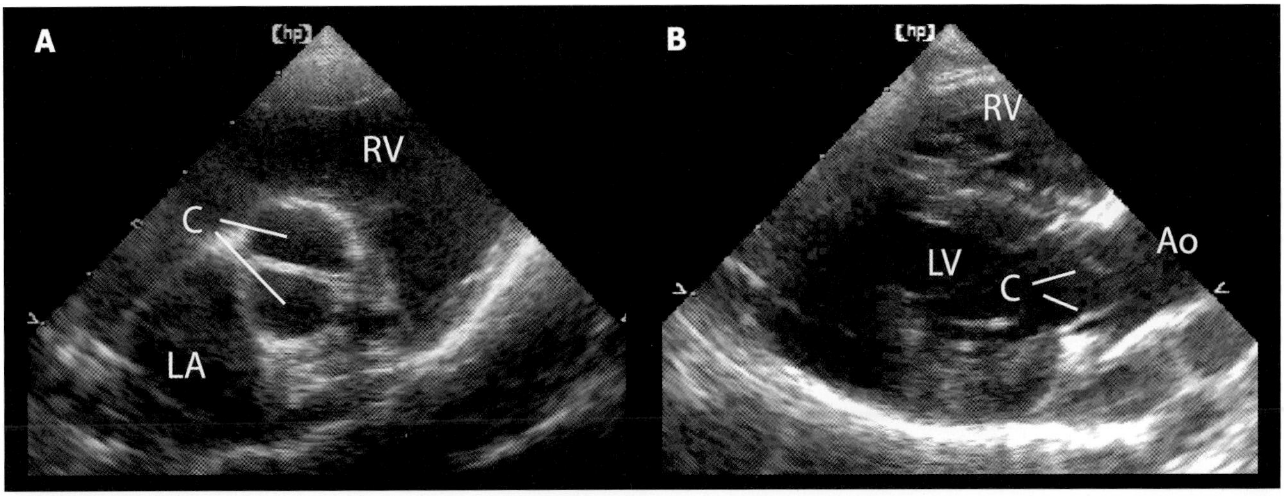

Figure 5.31. Valvular Ao stenosis. 2DE RPS SAx **(A)** and LAx **(B)** images from a dog with a bicuspid Ao valve. **A:** Only two cusps **(C)** are evident where there are normally three. **B:** A maximal opening excursion of the leaflets. Significant stenosis accompanied this unusual abnormality, as evidenced by the Doppler recordings (not shown).

concentric LV hypertrophy erroneously (pseudohypertrophy) with increased LV wall thickness and decreased LV and LA internal dimensions (Figure 5.32).

In valvular PS, leaflets may be thickened and/or fused at the commissures such that leaflet separation is impaired; the fused leaflets may form a valvular *dome* as they bulge into the pulmonary artery during systole. The outflow tract itself may be hypoplastic and echogenic in conjunction with valvular lesions. An unusual form of subvalvular PS is caused by a discrete fibromuscular partition separating the RV outflow tract from the RV; this condition has also been termed *double-chamber right ventricle* (Figure 5.33). Supravalvular obstructions also may be visualized.

Combined Doppler examination of the RV outflow tract enables peak gradient quantification (CWD) and confirms the location of the obstruction, indicated by the velocity step up (PWD) or flow convergence zone (CFD) just proximal to the lesion. Suggested prognostic categories based on the pressure gradient are mild (<50 mm Hg), moderate (50–100 mm Hg), and severe (>100 mm Hg). Specificity and sensitivity of these categories for specific outcomes have not been determined. Mild to moderate tricuspid regurgitation commonly coexists with significant pressure overload of the right heart. CWD evaluation of this jet velocity sometimes provides supplemental quantitative information, particularly when alignment with the PS jet is problematic.

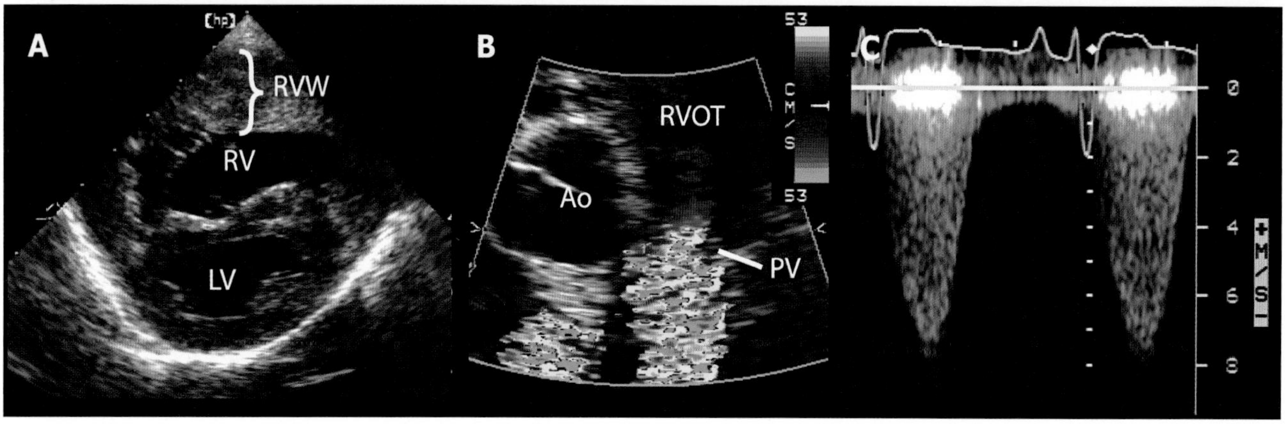

Figure 5.32. Valvular pulmonic stenosis in a dog. RPS SAx 2DE image **(A)**, RPS CFD at the PV **(B)**, and CWD of the pulmonic flow jet **(C)** from a dog with severe valvular pulmonic stenosis. The RVW is extremely thickened at more than twice that LVW thickness. The increased echogenicity of the myocardium is thought to be caused by ischemia and fibrosis. The septum is displaced toward the LV, thus causing an ovoid LV cross section because of the flattened septum. CFD confirms the location of the obstruction at the valve. A velocity of nearly 8.0 m/s corresponds to a peak pressure gradient of $4 \times 8^2 = 250$ mm Hg and severe obstruction.

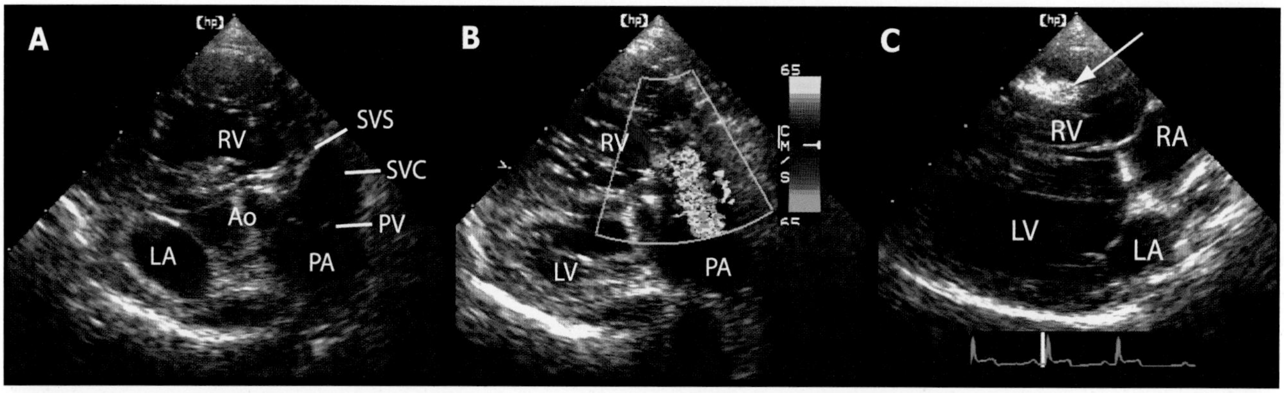

Figure 5.33. Subvalvular pulmonic stenosis in a dog. RPS SAx 2DE **(A)** and CFD **(B)** from the pulmonary outflow tract of a dog with *double-chamber RV*, a variant of subvalvular pulmonic stenosis. The PV is of normal thickness, but a discrete subvalvular stenosis (SVS) divides the RV proper from a subvalvular chamber (SVC). CFD confirms the location of the obstruction, proximal to the valve. **C:** This RPS LAx image illustrates marked thickening of the RVW and an area of increased echogenicity secondary to myocardial hypertrophy and fibrosis (arrow).

Tricuspid Dysplasia

Dysplasia of the tricuspid valve may entail a wide range of structural abnormalities. The condition is transmitted genetically in Labrador retrievers, the most frequently affected canine breed. Echocardiographic findings may include abnormal numbers or arrangement of papillary muscles; chordae tendinae may be foreshortened or papillary muscles may attach directly to a valve leaflet. Tricuspid leaflets may be elongated (Figure 5.34) or shortened and abnormally tethered to the septum or RV wall, thereby

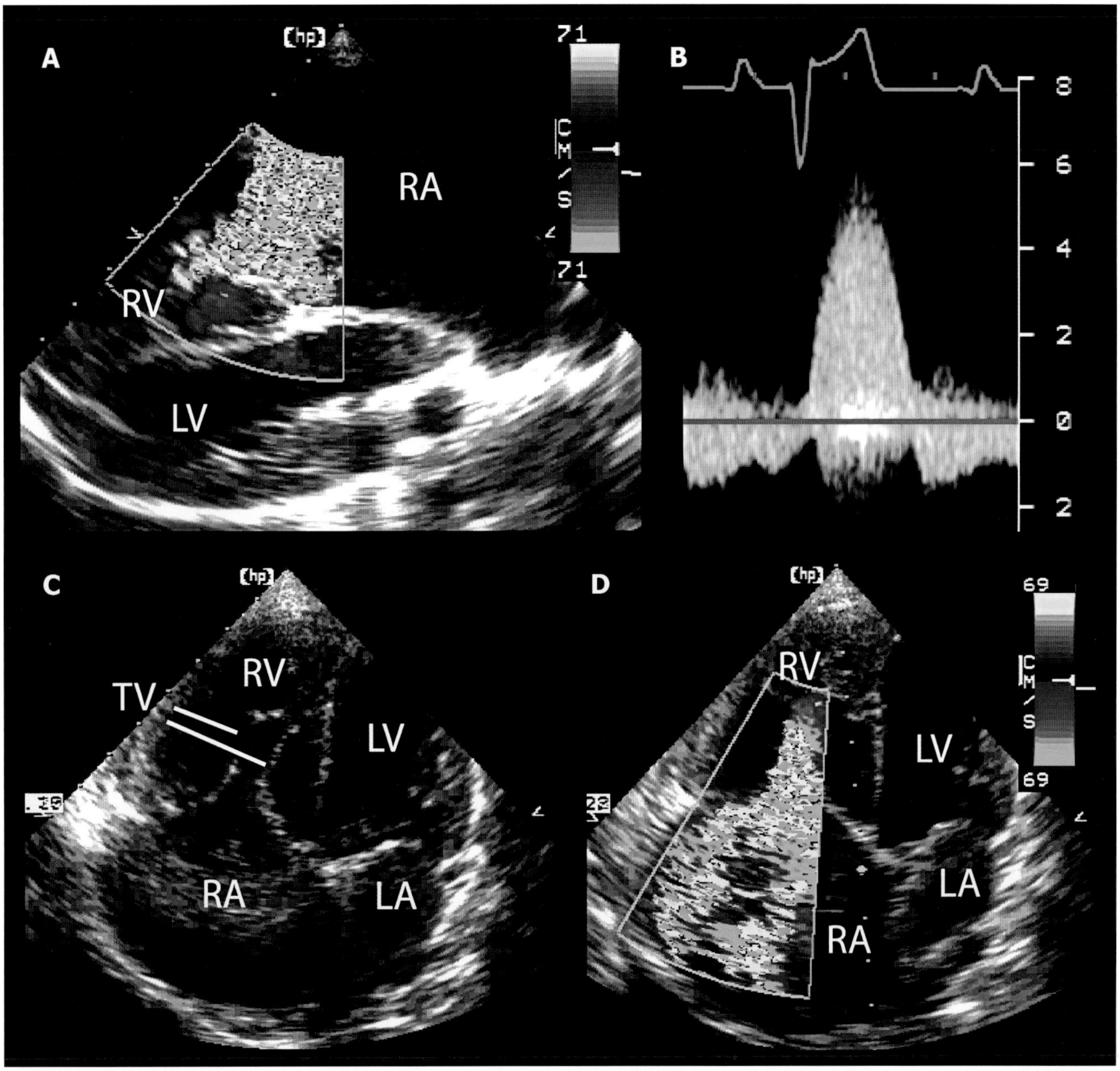

Figure 5.34. Tricuspid dysplasia and pulmonic stenosis in a Labrador retriever with RCHF. The RPS LAx CFD image **(A)** demonstrates marked TR. Unusually, the extreme RA dilation caused the RPS position to be suitable for TR velocity quantification with the jet directed toward the transducer **(B)**. A TR jet velocity of 5.0 m/s suggests a driving pressure of $4 \times 5^2 = 100$ mm Hg and is incompatible with normal RV pressure. In this case, RV pressure overload caused by pulmonic stenosis was responsible (not shown). The LAp four-chamber view **(C)** demonstrates extreme dilation of both the RA and RV. The TV leaflets are overlong and displaced toward the apex (compare with the position of the mitral leaflets). The CFD image from the same location **(D)** demonstrates marked TR and apical displacement of the flow convergence zone into the RV. Frame-by-frame visualization of the tricuspid apparatus revealed direct attachment of PMs to the tricuspid leaflets and a network of abnormal interconnecting CT, tethering the TV leaflets to the myocardial wall.

restricting motion and function; leaflet fusion may cause stenosis (Figure 5.35). The entire tricuspid apparatus may be displaced toward the cardiac apex, similar to Ebstein's malformation in human patients. Tricuspid dysplasia may cause valvular regurgitation and variable degrees of RV volume overload with dilation of the right ventricle and right atrium. Doppler examination reveals tricuspid regurgitation; the origin of this jet, determined from the flow convergence zone, may be displaced toward the RV apex.

Increased tricuspid regurgitation jet velocity (e.g., >3.0 m/s) should prompt consideration of concurrent pulmonary hypertension or PS, and atrial septal defect also may accompany the condition (Figure 5.34). Tricuspid stenosis also may be caused by dysplasia of this valve leading to a *diastolic* jet (e.g., >2.0 m/s) into the right ventricle.

Mitral Dysplasia

Mitral valve dysplasia (MD) may entail a wide range of structural and functional abnormalities, including abnormal numbers or origins of papillary muscles; excessively shortened, lengthened, or thickened chordae tendinae; and abnormal chordal attachments to nonvalvular structures (Figures 5.36 and 5.37).

Clinically relevant forms of MD cause hemodynamically significant MR (most commonly), mitral stenosis, or aortic outflow obstruction. The authors have encountered several cases of MD causing SAS directly where the anterior mitral leaflet was tethered to the septum. Subsequent rupture of the abnormal chordae caused spontaneous resolution of the stenosis.

Patent Ductus Arteriosus

Left to right patent ductus arteriosus (PDA) is the first or second most common congenital heart defect in dogs. Echocardiographic features of the condition include LV and LA dilation, LV hypertrophy, and increased stroke volume (*volume overload*) (Figure 5.38). Both the aorta and pulmonary trunk may be dilated in conjunction with increased blood flow. CFD examination of the pulmonary trunk reveals continuous turbulent flow and is useful in establishing the site of the ductus itself. Continuous-wave spectral Doppler velocity quantification reveals continuous flow into the pulmonary trunk and a peak velocity during systole of roughly 4.5–5.5 m/s, corresponding to the normal systolic aortic-pulmonic gradient of 80–120 mm Hg (Moise 1989). Velocities significantly lower than this

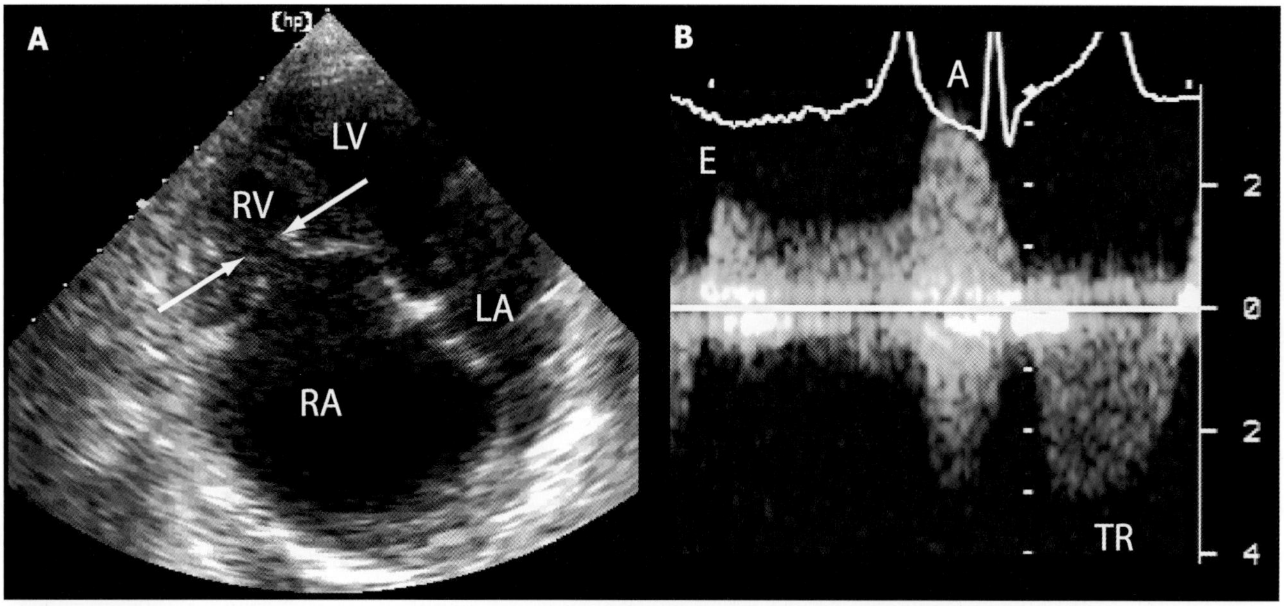

Figure 5.35. Tricuspid dysplasia with valvular stenosis and regurgitation. 2DE LAp four-chamber image **(A)** and CWD recording **(B)** from a Labrador retriever. Arrows indicate the position of tricuspid leaflets at maximal separation during diastole. A TR velocity of less than 3.0 m/s **(B)** is consistent with relatively normal TR driving pressure (RV pressure – RA pressure = ca. 36 mm Hg). However, actual peak RV pressure may be substantially greater in this case because the RA pressure is likely increased. The inflow recording demonstrates abnormal spectral broadening, and the velocity is elevated throughout diastole. A peak inflow gradient of 4×3.5^2 = ca. 50 mm Hg occurs at the Doppler A wave following a large P wave on the electrocardiogram. The E-F slope is flattened because of delayed pressure equalization between the atrium and ventricle.

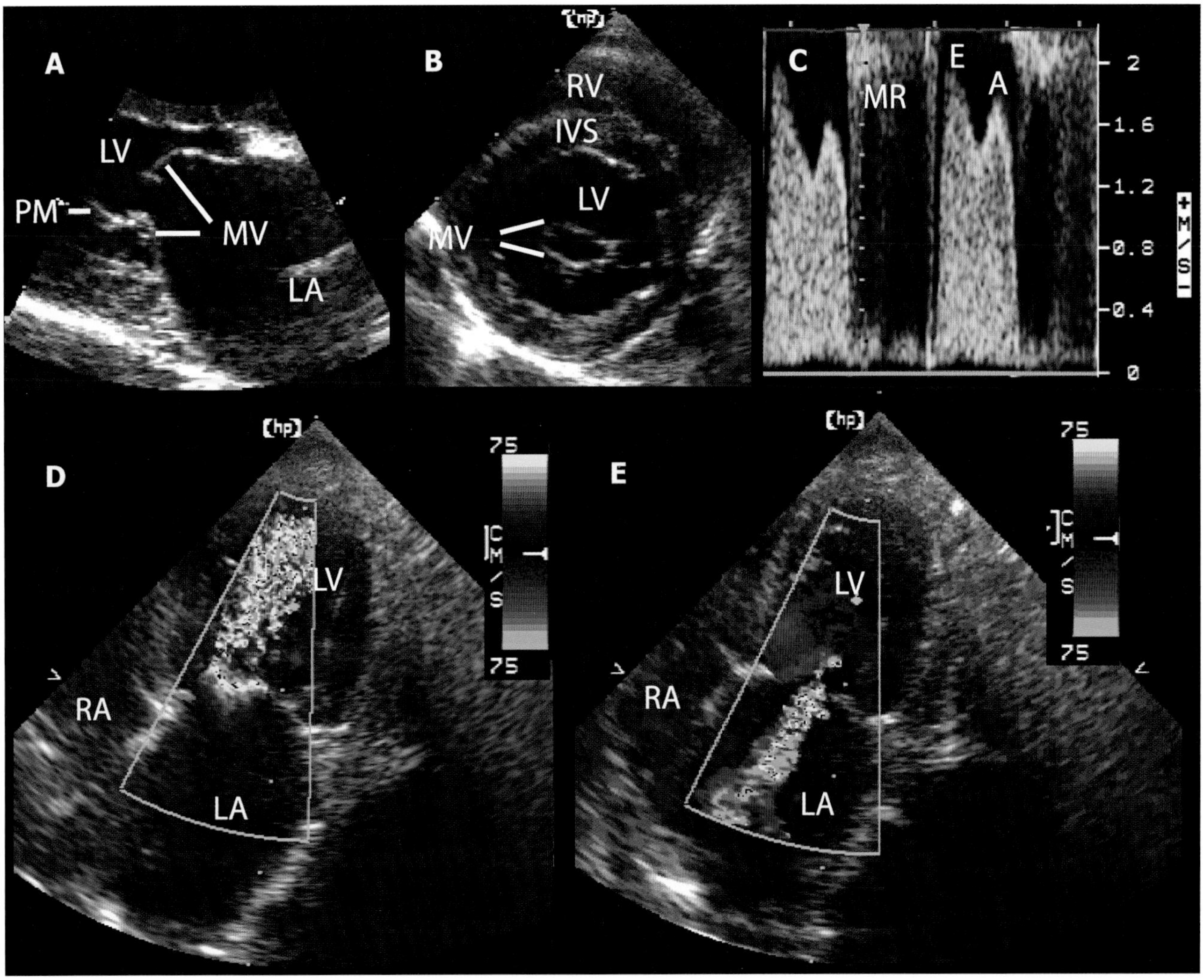

Figure 5.36. Mitral dysplasia with valvular stenosis and regurgitation in a cat. RPS LAx **(A)** and SAx **(B)** images obtained during maximal diastolic separation of the MV leaflets. **A:** The tip of the anterior leaflet is tethered, so that the valve cannot open normally, and bows toward the septum because of increased LA pressure. A PM attaches directly to the parietal (posterior) leaflet (i.e., extreme shortening of CT). **B:** The diminished maximal orifice area is suggested by the cross-sectional image at the level of the valve tips. **C:** The PWD recording (LAp transducer position) demonstrates a turbulent diastolic inflow signal, and the E wave approaches 2 m/s, corresponding to a 16-mm Hg gradient across the MV (modified Bernoulli equation). A turbulent MR signal with aliasing is also present. This example demonstrates a relatively mild case of stenosis, as suggested by the peak inflow velocity and also the rapid decline of velocity after the peak of the E wave (compare with E-F slope of the tricuspid dysplasia example in Figure 5.35). **D:** The LAp CFD image obtained during diastole demonstrates a flow convergence zone at the atrial side of the MV and a turbulent inflow jet within the LV. The systolic image **(E)** demonstrates the MR jet into the enlarged LA.

value may suggest pulmonary hypertension or a more complex lesion.

It is valuable to image the ductus directly and to determine carefully its suitability for interventional closure by coil embolization.

Right to left shunting patent ductus arteriosus (reverse PDA or RPDA) is uncommon but most typically occurs in dogs with a large ductus and persistent fetal circulation. Failure of the normal reduction of pulmonary vascular resistance at birth produces pulmonary pressures that approach or exceed aortic values and consequent reversal of the shunt flow direction and arterial desaturation, which may persist from birth. This scenario is consistent with echocardiographic findings of a thickened RV wall and septum typical of an RV pressure overload (Figure 5.39). The alternate RPDA scenario, i.e., left to right PDA producing progressive pulmonary hypertension and eventual

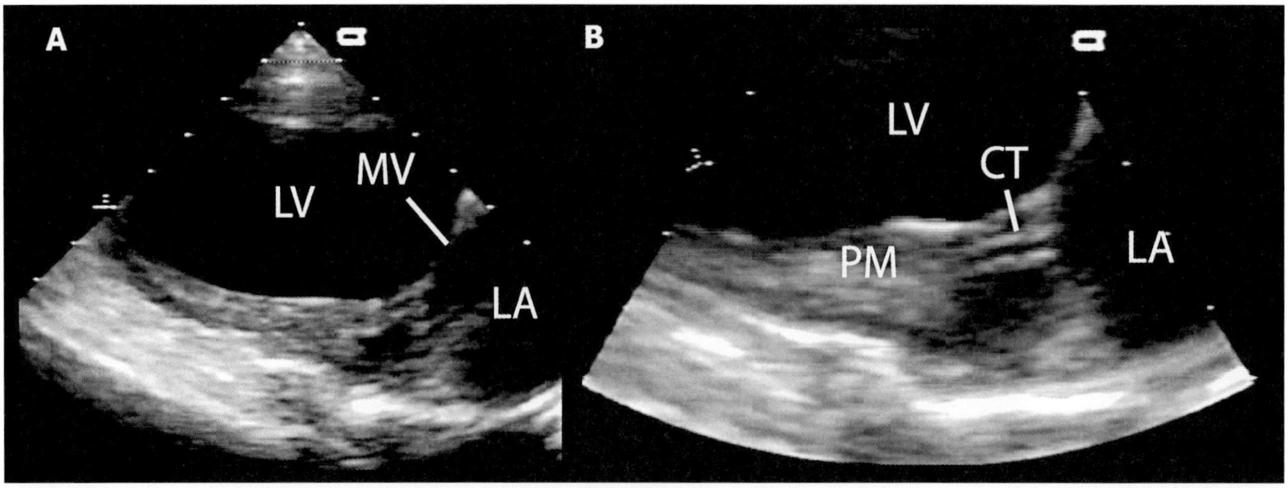

Figure 5.37. Mitral dysplasia in a Rottweiler puppy. **A and B:** The RPS LAx images depict marked LV and LA dilation. On the close-up **(B)**, a PM is visible giving rise to shortened CT that distract the MV abnormally toward the LVW. There was dramatic MR (not shown).

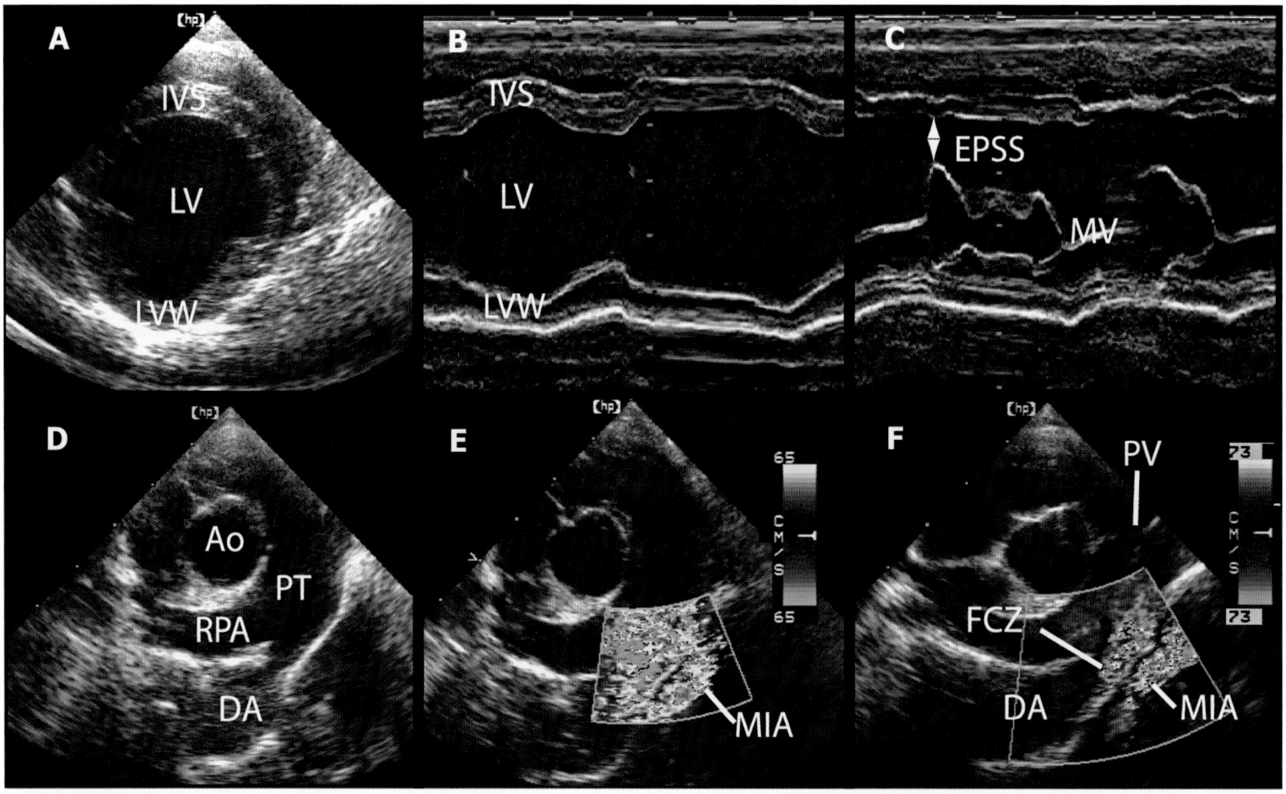

Figure 5.38. Left to right shunting patent ductus arteriosus (PDA). As suggested by the 2DE SAx LV image **(A)** and M-mode **(B)**, PDA causes LV dilation and stroke volume overload. Fractional shortening was depressed in this case, and the E-point to septal separation distance (EPSS) was increased **(C)**, suggestive of marked ventricular remodeling and deteriorating myocardial function. RPS SAx images **(D–F)** enable visualization of a large ductus (DA) that narrows at its entry into the pulmonary circulation. CFD images in systole **(E)** and diastole **(F)** facilitate the diagnosis by showing continuous flow from the PDA causing turbulence in the PT. A prominent CFD mirror-image artifact (MIA) is evident. Visualization and evaluation of the PDA is facilitated by the occurrence of a flow convergence zone (FCZ).

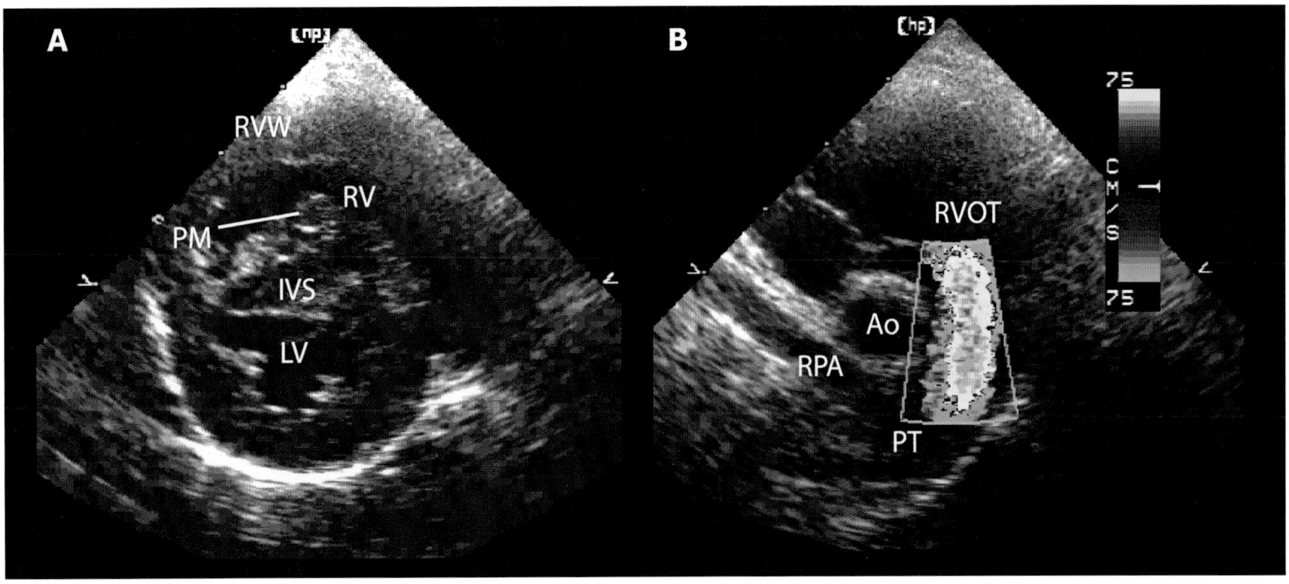

Figure 5.39. Reverse patent ductus arteriosus (RPDA or right to left PDA). The RPS SAx image **(A)** depicts marked RV hypertrophy, including dramatic thickening of the RVW and the trabecular and papillary muscles (PMs) of the interventricular septum. The LV appears somewhat small and thick walled because of volume underload and distortion by the RV. **B:** CFD imaging at the PV level depicts a laminar flow pattern with color aliasing in the central flow core. CFD interrogation of the RVOT, PT, and RPA yielded no evidence of stenosis, yet a dramatic increase in TR velocity confirmed increased RV pressure and pulmonary hypertension (not shown). 2DE echocontrast imaging of the abdominal Ao, following venous injection of micro-aerated saline, can be used to confirm the lesion if necessary.

shunt reversal, is less likely. The latter would be expected to include LV dilation secondary to LV stroke volume overload.

RPDA is suspected when there is clinical and echocardiographic evidence of RV pressure overload in the absence of an obstructive pulmonary lesion. The diagnosis may be confirmed by an echocontrast study (bubble study), if necessary. The method consists of injecting echogenic aerated saline into a peripheral vein (e.g., cephalic vein) while imaging the heart or great vessels. This technique enables determination of which vessels or cardiac chambers receive unoxygenated flow. In the case of RPDA, the abdominal aorta receives echocontrast within a few seconds of injection, having traversed the vena cava, right heart, pulmonary trunk, and ductus.

Abnormalities of Cardiac Septation

Failure of cardiac septation during embryogenesis results in a defect between the two hearts, including atrial septal defect (ASD), ventricular septal defect (VSD), or a combination of these two. Septation abnormalities may cause a wide spectrum of functional disease. Because of the normal distributions of intracardiac pressure and chamber compliance, both ASD and VSD most typically cause left to right shunting of blood and pulmonary overcirculation. Under these circumstances, ASD causes volume overload and consequent dilation of the right ventricle, whereas VSD necessitates increased stroke volume of the left ventricle. These abnormalities depend on the magnitude of the shunt.

Atrial Septal Defect

Deficiency of the septum secundum (septum secundum ASD) causes a defect near the normal position of the fossa ovalis in the midatrial wall (Figures 5.40 and 5.41). In distinction, a septum primum defect (septum primum ASD, endocardial cushion defect, or atrioventricular canal ASD) is located near the atrioventricular canal and may cause ASD, VSD, or both (Figure 5.42). *Sinus venosus* ASD, which is rare in small animals, occurs near the junction of the cranial vena cava. *Patent foramen ovale* is not an anatomical defect but results when functional closure of the foramen ovale at birth is not permanent. ASD flow typically is generated by a small pressure gradient with jet velocity less than 0.5 m/s.

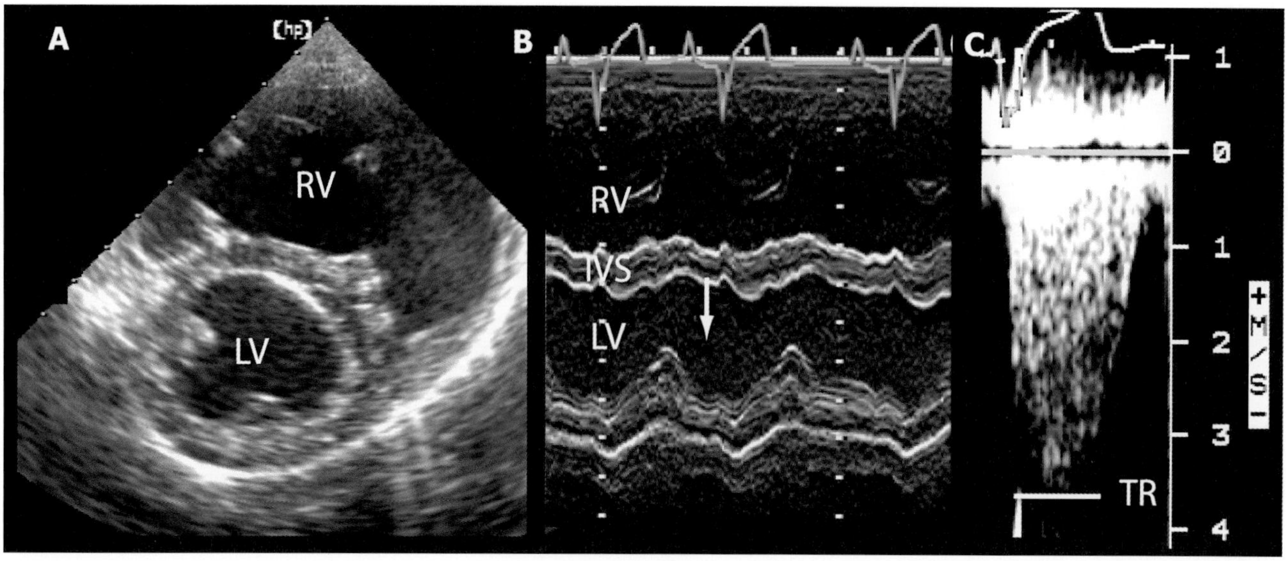

Figure 5.40. Secundum atrial septal defect (ASD). RPS SAx 2DE image **(A)** from a dog with a large-secundum-type ASD demonstrating RV dilation secondary volume overload. The RV dilation is also apparent on the M-mode recording **(B)** as is *paradoxical septal motion* (arrow) caused by displacement of the septum away from the transducer with diastolic filling of the enlarged RV. A CWD recording **(C)** of TR in this dog demonstrates a peak TV gradient of 4×3.5^2 m/s = ca. 50 mm Hg, consistent with either pulmonic stenosis or pulmonary hypertension. No pulmonic stenosis was evident, and pulmonary hypertension is a well-known sequela to chronic pulmonary overcirculation.

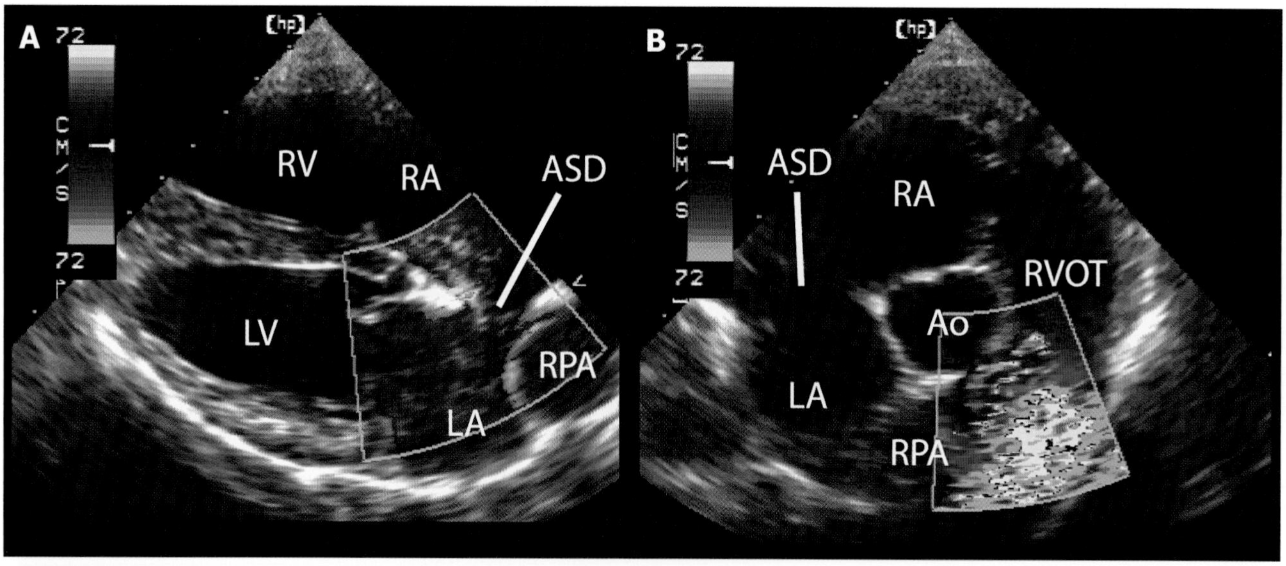

Figure 5.41. Secundum atrial septal defect (ASD). CFD RPS LAx **(A)** and SAx **(B)** images from the dog of the previous figure with secundum ASD (Figure 5.40). The RV and RA are dramatically dilated because of the volume overload generated by the defect, and there pulmonary overcirculation is suggested by marked enlargement of the RPA and increased velocity of blood flow in the main pulmonary artery. The LAx image demonstrates flow across the defect. Apparent ASD flow at this location must be differentiated from CaVC flow into the RA.

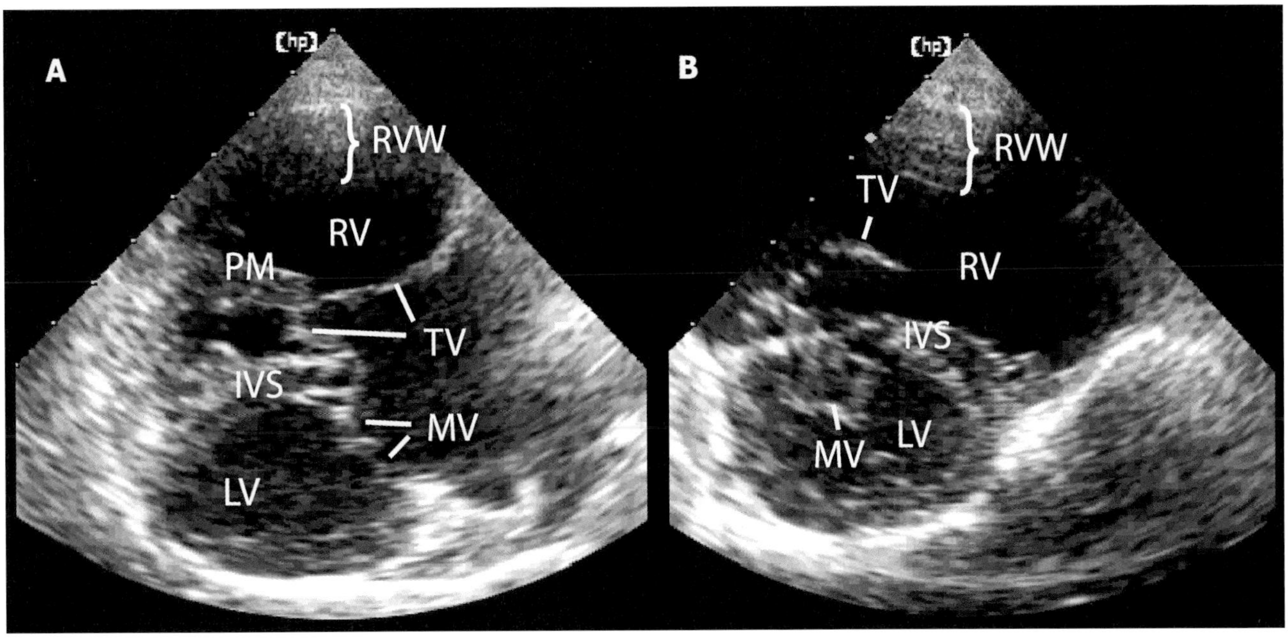

Figure 5.42. Primum atrial septal defect (ASD). LAx **(A)** and SAx **(B)** 2DE RPS images from a dog with a large-septum-primum ASD causing a so-called *common atrium*. The RV is dramatically enlarged because of volume overload, and a hypertrophied PM attaches directly to an elongated TV leaflet). RV hypertrophy is secondary to pulmonary overcirculation and hypertension in this case. The tricuspid and mitral apparatuses communicate through the defect, which involves the atrioventricular canal portion of the ventricular septum, as well (inlet VSD).

Ventricular Septal Defect

VSD also occurs with a range of anatomical and functional types. One aspect of classification relates to whether the VSD is small and *restrictive*, where the pressure gradient between the right and left ventricles is maintained and jet velocity is greater than 4 m/s, in contrast to *nonrestrictive*, where the large size of the defect approximates a single ventricle with pressure equilibration between the right and left sides (e.g., <3 m/s).

The most common form of VSD in dogs and cats is caused by a defect in the membranous (or conoventricular) septum located just proximal to the aortic root (Figure 5.43). Conversely, a defect in the conotruncal septum causes a VSD that is located distal to the crista supraventricularis (supracristal VSD, outlet VSD, or doubly committed VSD), including the specific type associated with tetralogy of Fallot (Figure 5.44). In the latter, the outlet septum is malaligned with the trabecular septum of the right ventricle, creating a septation defect (malalignment VSD) and disproportionate sizes of the two outflow tracts. The muscular outflow septum obstructs the RV outflow tract, causing a subvalvular PS, and the aorta is enlarged and straddles (overrides) the interventricular septum. Tetralogy of Fallot is the most common cyanotic congenital cardiac defect in small animals but is part of a spectrum of conditions ranging from mild outflow tract abnormalities to pseudotruncus arteriosus with pulmonary atresia, where conotruncal septal malalignment is so marked that the pulmonary outflow tract is functionally obliterated (Figure 5.45).

Miscellaneous and Complex Congenital Disease

A wide range of cardiac congenital defects and combination defects are possible, with varying severity and clinical importance of each. Echocardiographic principles are applied in each case to determine the presence of connections between vessels and chambers and pressure gradients between the connections.

Cor triatriatum is an unusual condition characterized by the presence of an accessory atrial chamber, separated from the atrium proper by a perforated membrane partition (Figure 5.46). Blood received by the accessory chamber must flow through the perforation, which may be restrictive. A significant pressure gradient across the membrane implies congestion of tissues and organs with venous drainage to the accessory chamber. Cor triatriatum may occur for the right atrium (cor triatriatum dexter) or the left (cor triatriatum sinister).

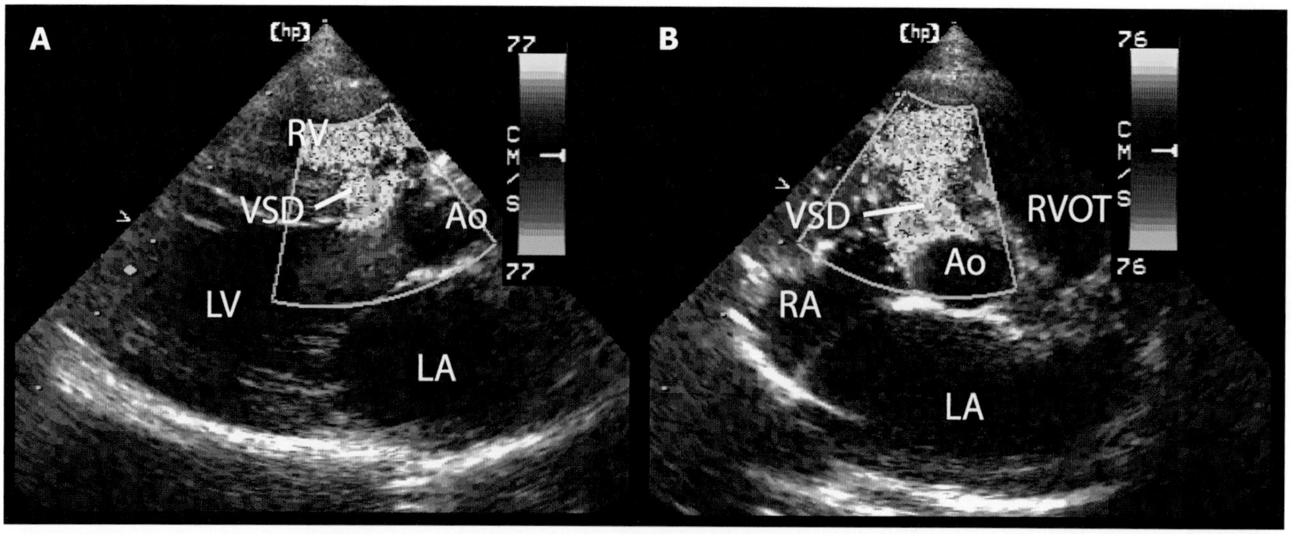

Figure 5.43. Membranous ventricular septal defect (VSD) in a cat. LAx **(A)** and SAx **(B)** CFD RPS images from a cat with membranous (or perimembranous) VSD. The location of the defect is identified by the color halo of the flow convergence zone, caused by color aliasing, where the blood accelerates through the defect; a turbulent mosaic color flow pattern is visible in the RV. The defect is immediately proximal to the Ao valve. This is the most common type of VSD in small animals.

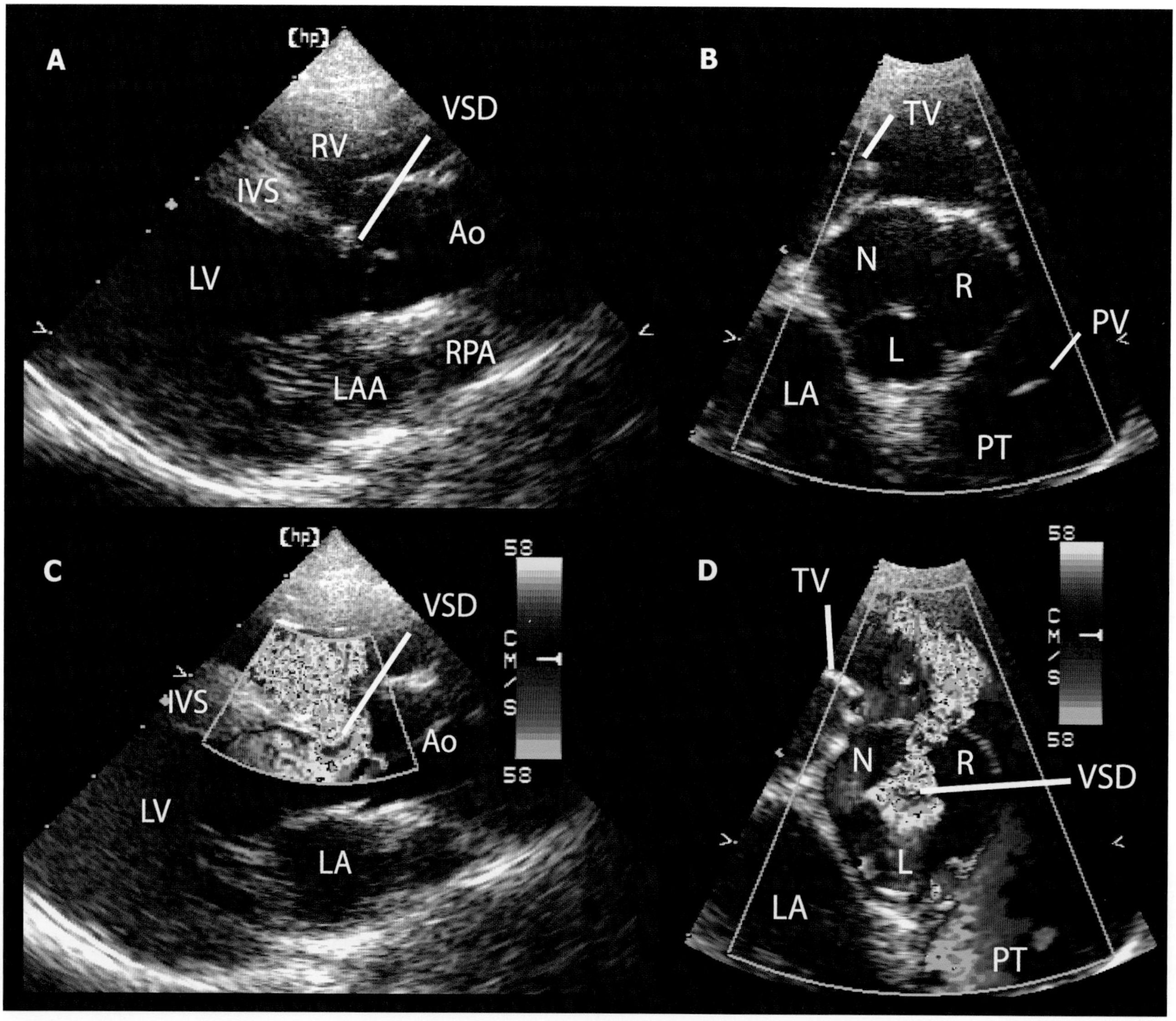

Figure 5.44.

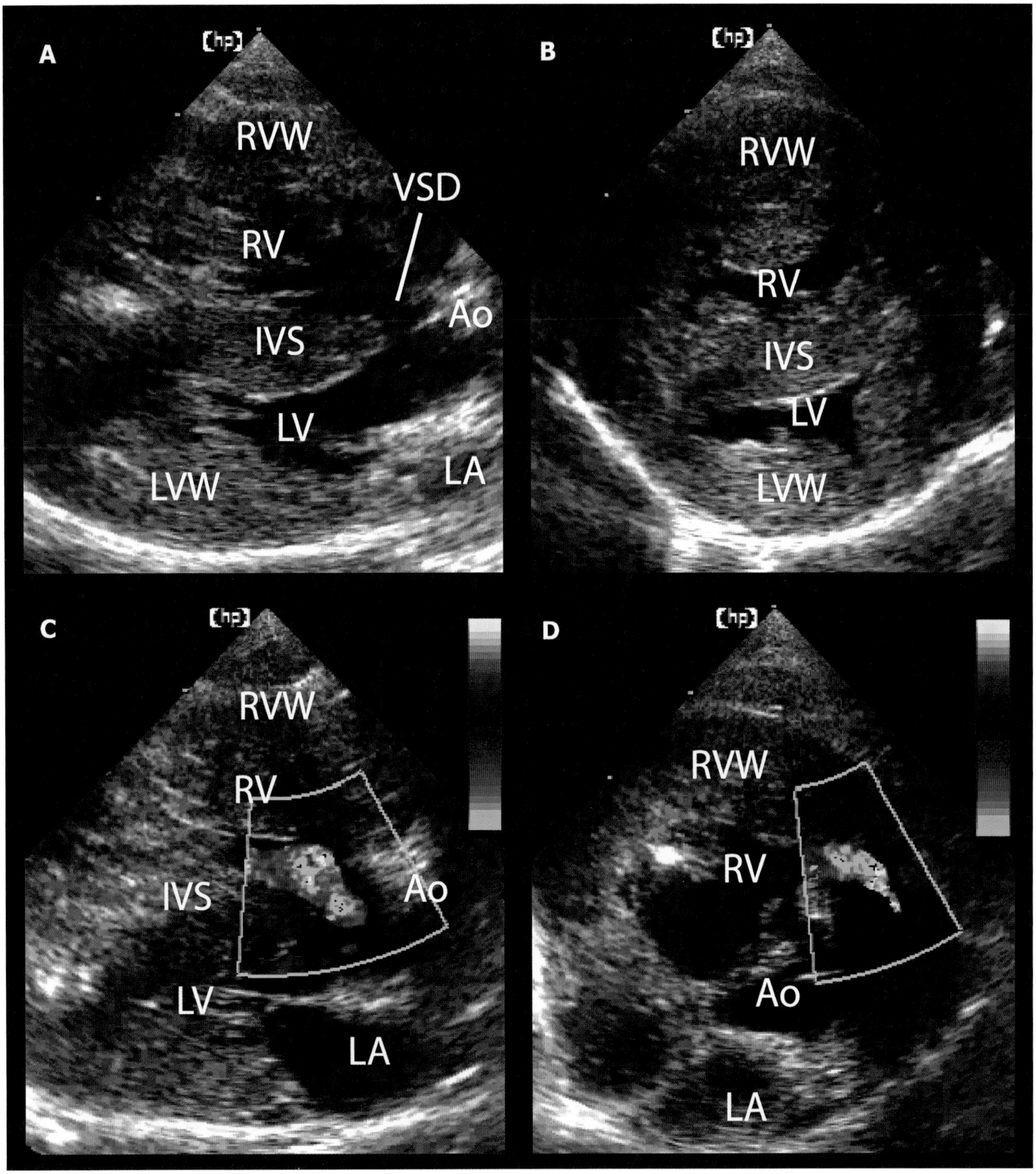

Figure 5.45. Tetralogy of Fallot (TF) in a cat. RPS 2DE LAx **(A)** and SAx **(B)** images depict extreme hypertrophy of the RVW. The LV appears diminutive and the LVW thickened as because of distortion and underloading caused by the extreme RV disease. The overriding Ao is demonstrated in image A where the Ao root appears to straddle the IVS immediately distal to the ventricular septal defect (VSD). **C and D:** Corresponding CFD images. The VSD was somewhat restrictive in this case, and image **C** demonstrates moderate velocity flow from the RV into the Ao caused by a significant pressure gradient. Hypertrophy was extreme to the extent that the RVOT could not be fully visualized. However, image **D** demonstrates flow convergence caused by infundibular stenosis.

Figure 5.44. Outlet ventricular septal defect (VSD). LAx **(A and C)** and SAx **(B and C)** 2DE **(A and C)** and CFD **(B and D)** RPS images from a dog with a left-to-right restrictive VSD in conjunction with an Ao that straddles the septum **(A)** (i.e., *overriding Ao*). The location of the defect is identified by the color halo of the flow convergence zone, caused by color aliasing, where the blood accelerates through the defect. Because the Ao straddles the septum, the defect lies directly beneath the Ao valve, particularly evident in **D**.

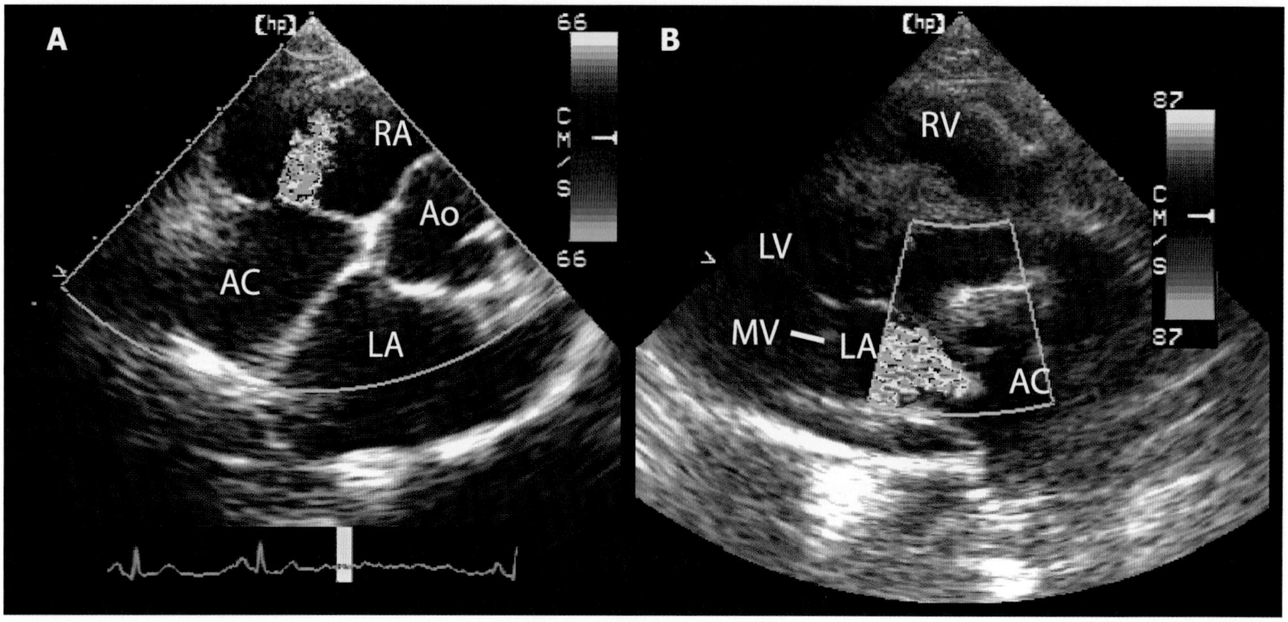

Figure 5.46. Cor triatriatum. RPS SAx CFD image of cor triatriatum dexter in a Labrador retriever **(A)** and LAx image of cor triatriatum sinister in a young cat **(B)**. In each case, an accessory chamber (AC) is separated from the atrium by a restrictive membrane. **A:** The dog also had tricuspid dysplasia, so the TV was displaced into the ventricle and is not visible. **B:** The MV is visible, and the flow convergence zone depicts the location of the restrictive membrane.

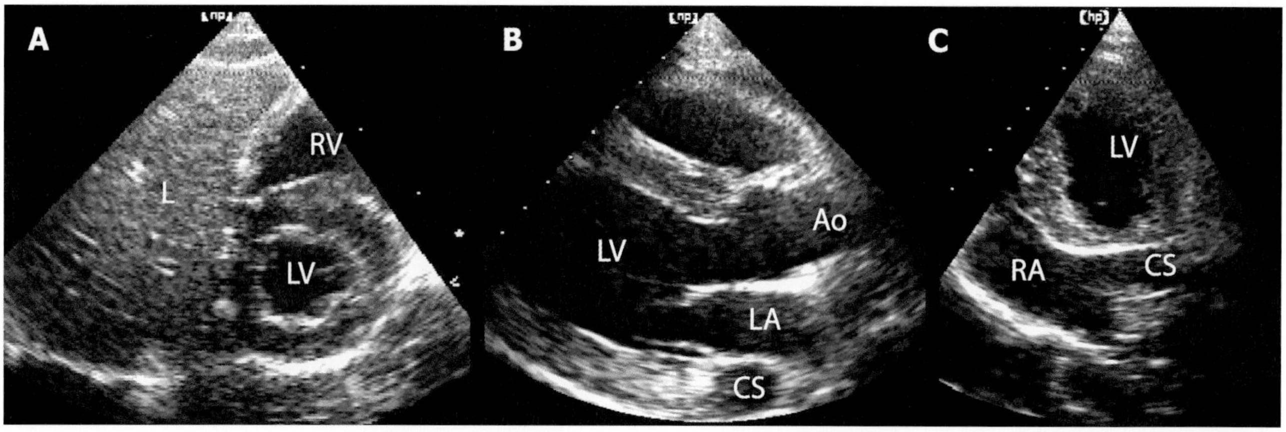

Figure 5.47. Miscellaneous and incidental abnormalities. **A:** The RPS SAx view from a cat with peritoneal-pericardial diaphragmatic hernia (PPDH). The liver (L) is juxtaposed to the heart, where normally there is intervening lung tissue and the diaphragm. The P does not appear to enclose the heart. The cat was presented for signs of respiratory distress, and a thoracic radiograph revealed a markedly enlarged cardiac silhouette, prompting cardiac evaluation. Respiratory signs were caused by bronchial disease and unrelated to the congenital pericardial abnormality. PPDH is often an incidental finding. Images **B** (RPS LAx) and **C** (LAp with caudal angulation) are from a dog with marked dilation of the coronary sinus (CS) likely caused by a persistent left CrVC. The view in image C shows the CS entering the RA at the caudal aspect of the heart.

Peritoneal-pericardial diaphragmatic hernia, which implies a communication between the pericardial space and the abdominal cavity, is likely related to abnormal fetal development of the septum transversum or pleuroperitoneal folds. The condition is most common in cats and may be diagnosed subsequent to the incidental discovery of an enlarged cardiac silhouette on thoracic radiography. Echocardiography reveals a range of abdominal organs within the pericardial space. Often, cardiac function is little affected, and determining whether clinical signs are related to the hernia may be difficult (Figure 5.47; see also Chapter 4 and Figures 4.54 and 4.55).

Eisenmenger physiology is caused by a shunt defect (ASD, VSD, or PDA) that results in right to left shunting subsequent to pulmonary vascular disease.

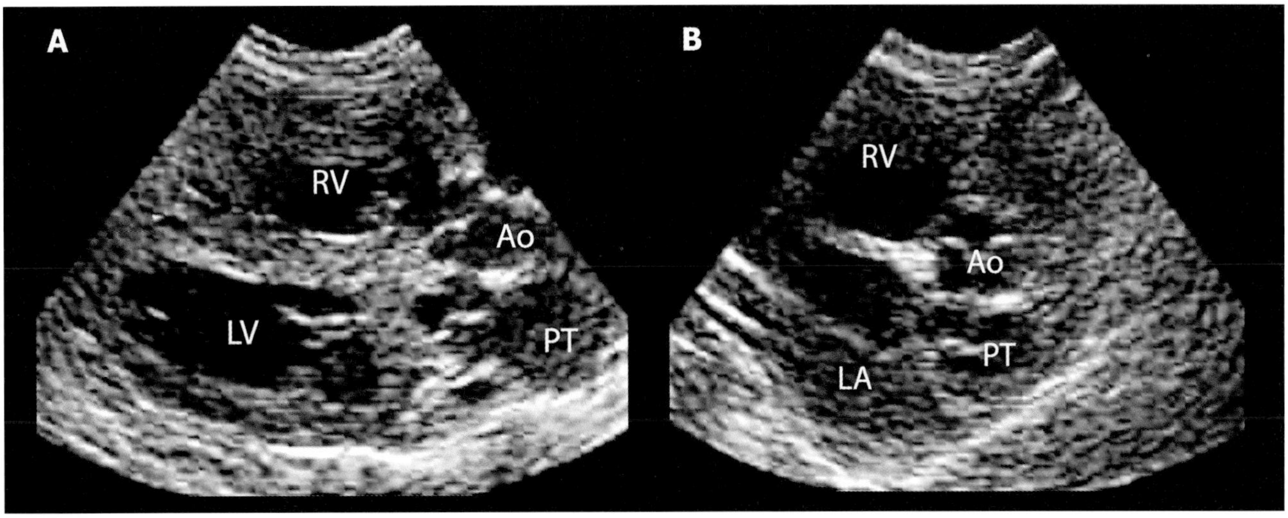

Figure 5.48. Uncorrected transposition of the great vessels (TGV). RPS LAx **(A)** and SAx **(B)** 2DE images from a rare case of uncorrected TGV in a cyanotic kitten (aorticopulmonary situs inversus). **A:** The Ao is evident leaving the RV while the PT joins the LV. Poststenotic dilation of the PT is visible because of a constriction at the junction of this vessel with the LV. **B:** This SAx image reveals simultaneous transverse views of both the Ao and PT. This does not occur in a normal heart because the two semilunar valves do not normally lie in the same plane. An atrial septal defect was the location of bidirectional shunting in this case. A shunt is necessary for survival beyond birth in uncorrected TGV because the pulmonary and systemic circulations are otherwise isolated from each other.

High-volume pulmonary overcirculation from a left to right shunt may initiate a well-described sequence of pulmonary vascular changes that ultimately causes elevation of right-sided pressures and shunt reversal. RV hypertrophy is present, and Doppler or echocontrast studies may assist in identifying the location and direction of the shunt.

Diagnosis of complex congenital heart disease is one of the most challenging applications of echocardiography and largely beyond the scope of this chapter. Potential abnormalities may include hypoplastic cardiac chambers, atretic great vessels, and situs inversus at the level of the abdomen, ventricles, or great vessels (Figure 5.48).

Acquired Heart Disease

Acquired Valvular Heart Disease

Endocardiosis

Endocardiosis, also known as chronic degenerative valve disease (CDVD), is the most common acquired heart disease of dogs and is particularly prevalent among smaller breeds. The mitral valve is the most commonly affected, but the tricuspid valve may be affected concurrently and/or preferentially in individuals. Exemplary 2DE echocardiographic findings of mitral CDVD include thickening, increased echogenicity, and prolapse of the valvular leaflets (Bonagura and Herring 1985a). Characteristic remodeling changes secondary to MR include progressively increasing LA and diastolic LV dimensions (Brown et al. 2005) (Figure 5.49). The end-systolic LV internal dimension (LVIDs) is characteristically preserved with the condition. This remodeling pattern coincides with a normal to increased fractional shortening, which is, consequently, a poor index for staging disease severity. In late-stage disease, LVIDs and E-point septal separation may begin to increase; these findings have been interpreted as evidence of myocardial dysfunction or failure (Kittleson et al. 1984).

Echocardiographic techniques for evaluation of MR range from qualitative measures to semiquantitative. One of the simplest methods is to evaluate the MR jet size by visual inspection on a CFD image. Alternatively, a ratio can be calculated (i.e., planimetered jet area divided by LA area) to provide a seemingly quantitative estimate of MR severity. Unfortunately, the extent of the MR jet is highly dependent on CFD control settings, jet and chamber geometry, and ambient hemodynamic conditions (Figure 5.50).

A semiquantitative Doppler method of MR evaluation involves estimation of the regurgitant fraction by using the proximal isovelocity surface area (PISA), which focuses on the flow convergence zone on the LV side of the regurgitant orifice (Kittleson and Brown 2003). Instantaneous blood flow rate across any

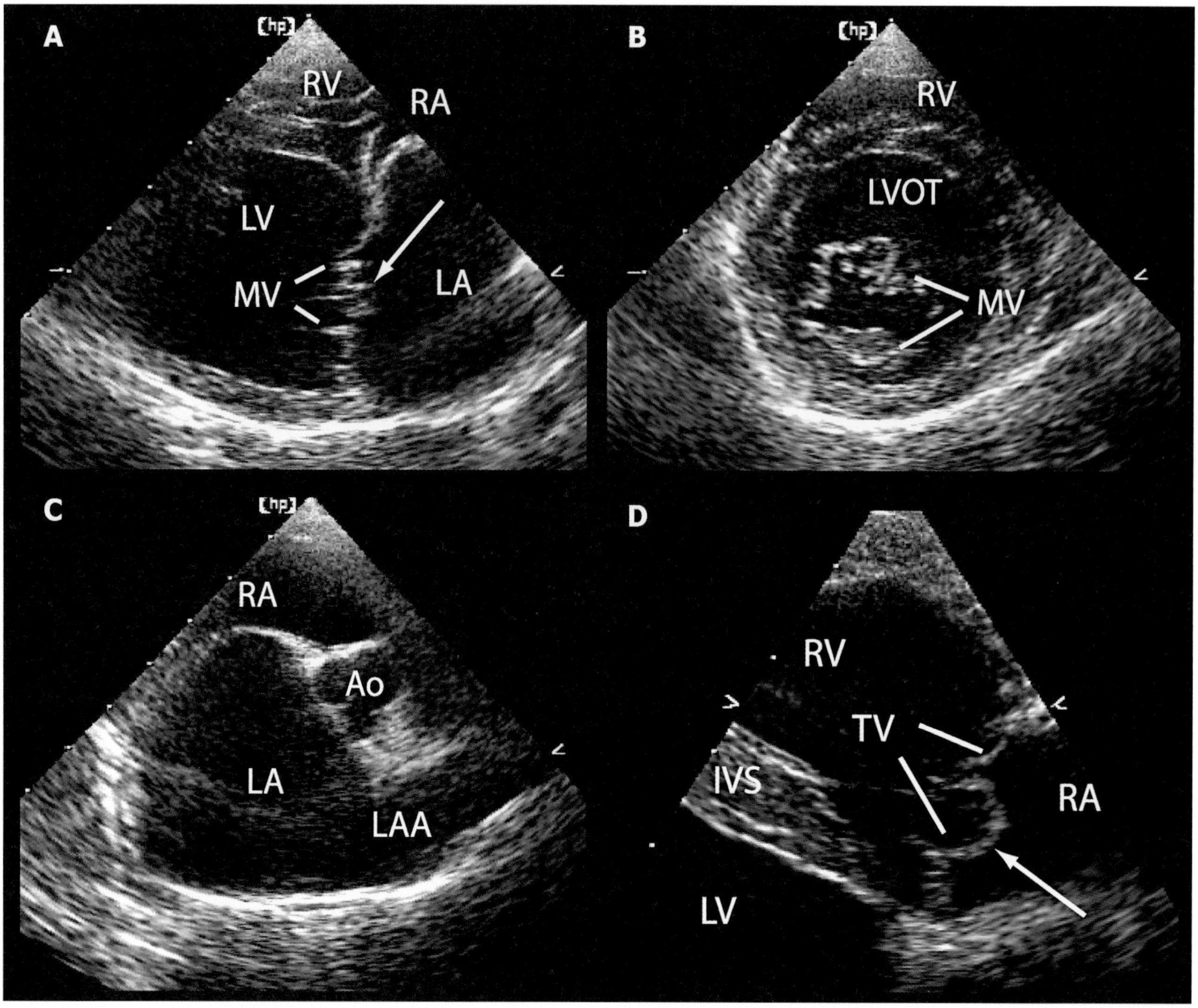

Figure 5.49. Chronic degenerative valve disease (CDVD [endocardiosis]). **A:** This RPS LAx view in early systole demonstrates dilation of the LV and LA along with prolapse of the AML, which appears as a displacement into the LA (arrow). **B:** This diastolic RPS SAx view portrays dramatic thickening of the leaflets. **C:** This SAx view at the level of the Ao root demonstrates dramatic LA dilation. **D:** This RPS LAx view of the TV demonstrates prolapse into the RA (arrow).

hemisphere is simply the product of blood velocity at that radius and the area of the hemisphere, $A = 2\pi r^2$. Radius and velocity are both determined from a CFD image, the radius being the distance from the orifice to the aliasing velocity (Figure 5.50). The PISA method is very sensitive to the radius measurement, and determining the location of the valvular orifice accurately can be difficult. Color M-mode can be helpful in increasing temporal resolution and enabling visual averaging of the radius during the regurgitant flow.

Using the maximal regurgitant flow rate (Q_r [PISA method]), the peak regurgitation velocity (V_p), and the VTI of the MR, the MR volume (V_r) can be calculated as follows: $V_r = (Q_r/V_p) \times VTI_r$. This value is used to calculate the regurgitant fraction after the LV forward stroke volume has been estimated ($V_{SV} = area_{Ao} \times VTI_{Ao}$). The regurgitant fraction is $V_r/(V_r + V_{SV})$.

Infective Endocarditis

Infective endocarditis is an unusual, but potentially devastating, consequence of bacteremia and/or sepsis most commonly affecting medium-sized and large dogs. Lesions most typically involve the aortic and/or mitral valves but can also extend to surrounding myocardial tissue, with possible periannular abscessation (Figure 5.51).

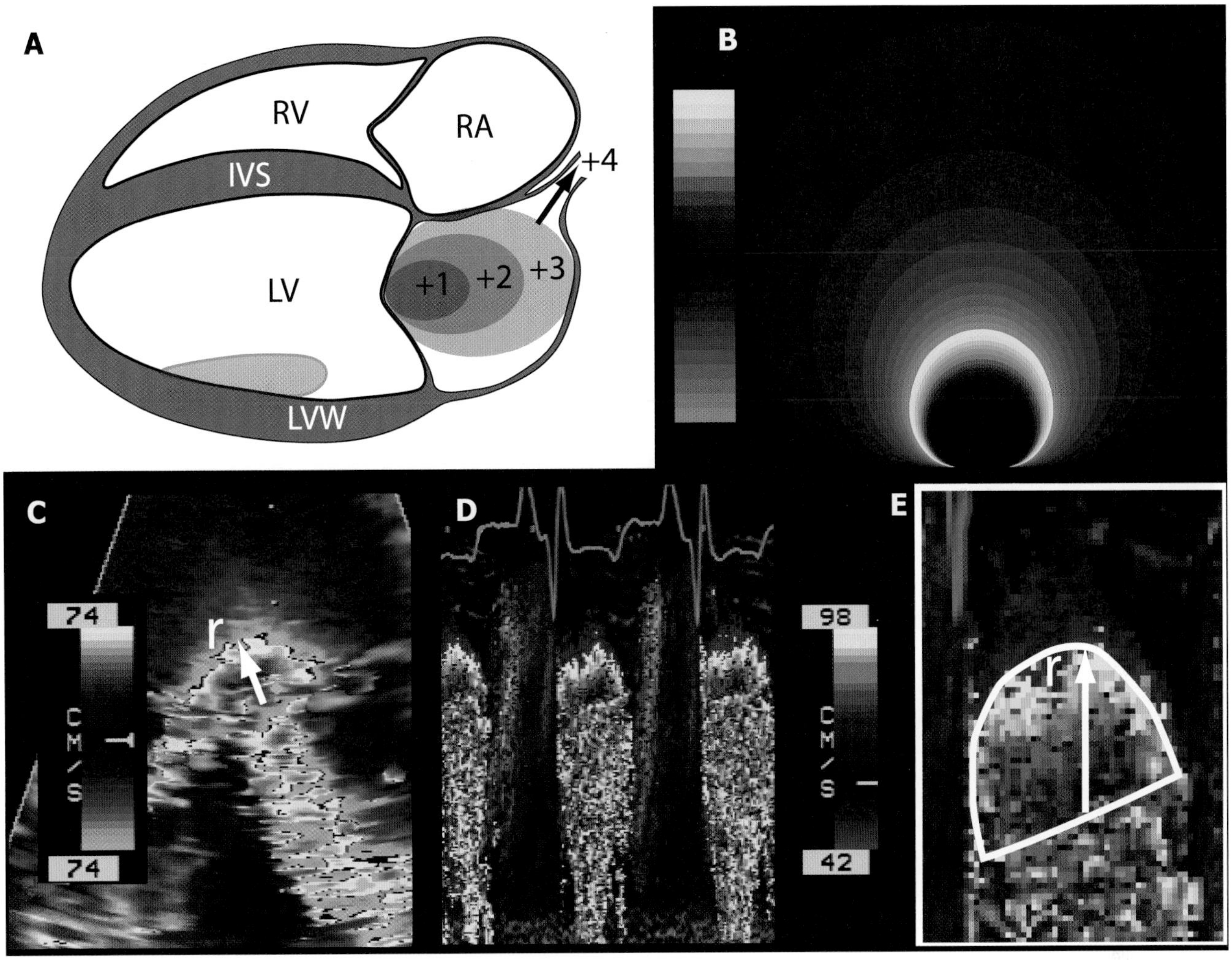

Figure 5.50. MR severity. Qualitative evaluation of MR can be made from CFD assessment of jet size **(A)**. +4 MR is associated with retrograde jet extension into the pulmonary veins. Semiquantitative methods assume that the regurgitant flow rate (cm^3/s) is approximated as the surface area of the hemispherical flow convergence zone ($A = 2\Pi r^2$) multiplied by the aliasing velocity (proximal isovelocity surface area method [PISA]). However, the computed mathematical solution of the assumed flow **(B)** results in infinite velocity at the infinitesimal orifice (inner black zone); PISA assumptions are not valid unless the hemisphere radius is large with respect to the orifice size. **C:** This LAp CFD image, which is from the regurgitant orifice of a dog with severe MR, was recorded at an aliasing velocity of 74 cm/s; the estimated radius of the hemisphere (r) is not large enough compared with the orifice. Requirements for the PISA determination are improved by adjusting the color baseline in the direction of flow, downward in this case, which decreases the aliasing velocity and increases the distance from the aliasing velocity contour to the orifice. This has been done for the color M-mode recording in image D, decreasing the aliasing velocity to 42 cm/s and increasing the hemisphere radius; the radius also can be estimated from the color M-mode recording **(E)**.

Nonspecific echocardiographic signs include thickened hyperechoic aortic and mitral valve leaflets, chordal rupture, and diastolic mitral valve fluttering or oscillation (Lombard and Buergelt 1983b). The diagnosis of endocarditis might be difficult if lesions are small or involve only the mitral valve of dogs predisposed to endocardiosis. Echocardiographic follow-up may be useful in these cases by revealing rapid valvular changes. Chronic vegetations may appear hyperechoic, with acoustic shadowing indicating calcification.

Large vegetative lesions may cause valvular stenosis, insufficiency, or both. The volume overload (insufficiency, either valve) or pressure overload (AS) is often acute. Hence, cardiac remodeling may not be apparent even though marked functional compromise is present. Doppler echocardiography enables confirmation and quantification of the valvular dysfunction.

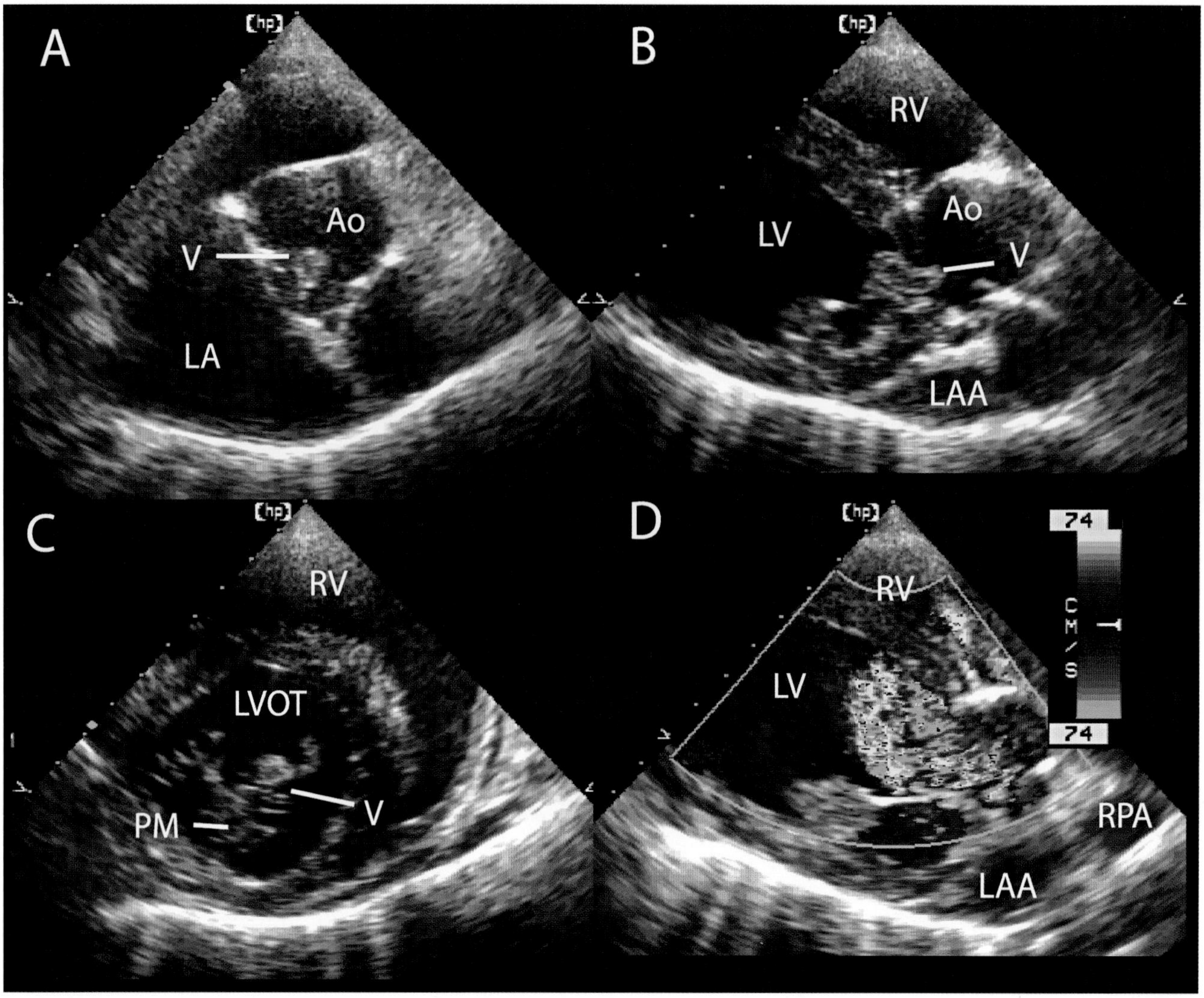

Figure 5.51. Endocarditis of the Ao and MVs. RPS SAx **(A and C)** and LAx **(B and D)** images from a dog with mitral and Ao endocarditis. The largest component of the vegetative lesion (V) is on the anterior leaflet of the MV and extends into the LVOT during systole. Nevertheless, the principal functional deficit in this case was Ao insufficiency, evident on the CFD image **(D)** as dramatic diastolic flow into the LV from the Ao.

Endocarditis is the most likely cause of substantial aortic insufficiency in dogs. Echocardiographic evidence of severe aortic insufficiency includes premature systolic mitral valve closure, an increasingly negative diastolic slope of the aortic regurgitation Doppler velocity envelope, and flow reversal in progressively distal segments of the aorta (Figure 5.52).

Myocardial Disease

Dilated Cardiomyopathy

Cardinal echocardiographic features of dilated cardiomyopathy (DCM) include chronically increased LV dimensions particularly in systole, and depressed fractional shortening and ejection fraction (Calvert et al. 1982) (Figure 5.53). Another fundamental diagnostic criterion is a decrease in the ratio of wall thickness to chamber dimension representing the inability of the myocardium to thicken appropriately. This decrease in relative wall thickness imparts the visual impression of dilation on 2DE images. Increased mitral E-point to septal separation distance is also noticed as a consequence of LV dilation, systolic dysfunction, and decreased peak mitral inflow.

LV echocardiographic changes are often most readily observed, but anatomical, pathological, and functional abnormalities are typically biventricular. As the name

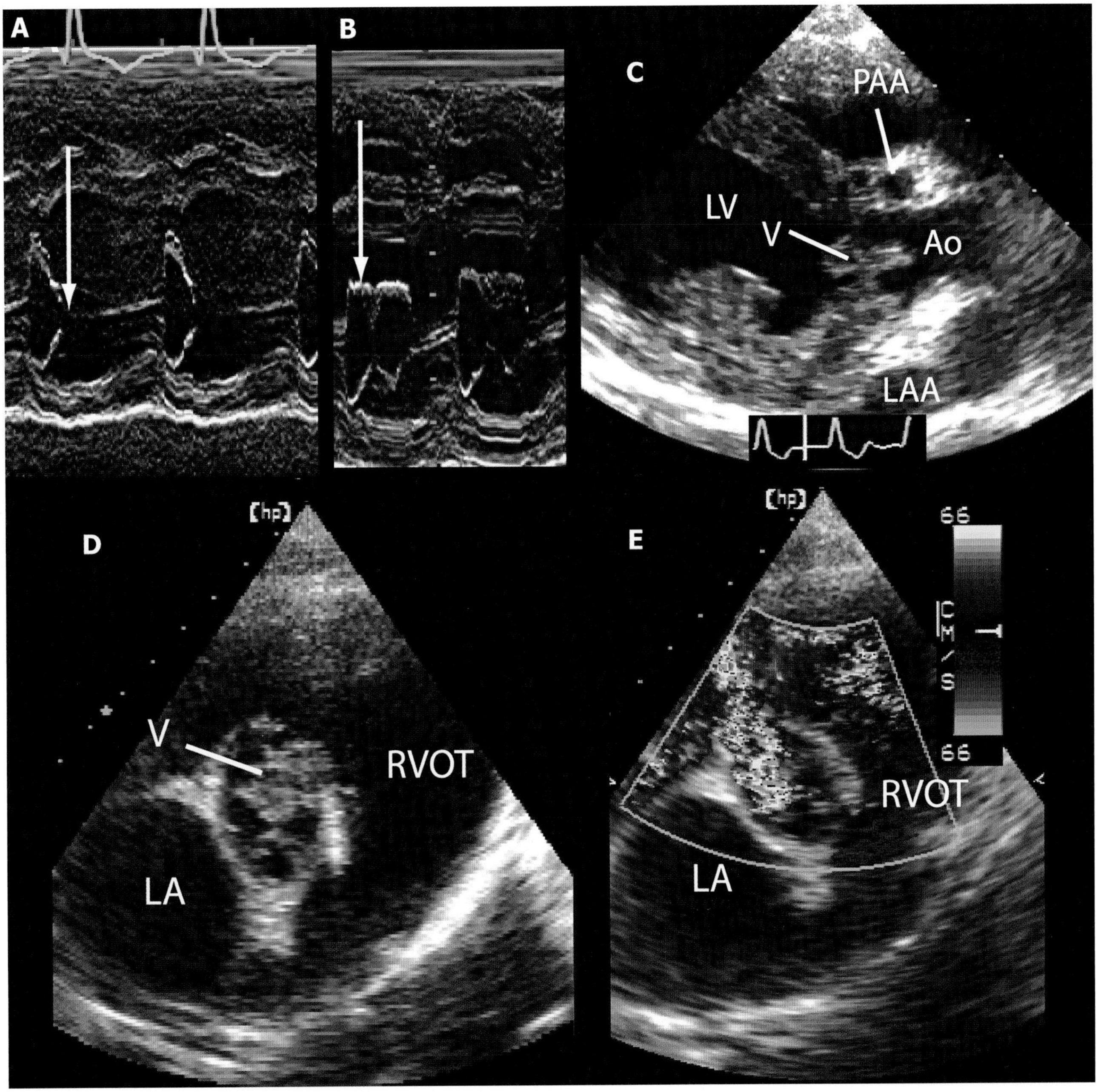

Figure 5.52. Miscellaneous findings with infective endocarditis. **A:** M-mode depicts early systolic closure of the MV (arrow) caused by severe Ao insufficiency leading to early diastolic equilibration of LV and LA pressures. **B:** Diastolic MV fluttering (arrow) is caused by the turbulent flow of Ao insufficiency past the valve. **C:** This RPS LAx image depicts a large vegetation (V) on the Ao valve and a para-annular abscess (PAA). **D and E:** These RPS SAx images (2DE and CFD, respectively) are from a dog with Ao valve endocarditis, vegetative lesions (V), and rupture of the sinus of Valsalva causing an acquired shunt. Continuous (systole and diastole) left to right flow occurred across this defect because of the persistent pressure gradient between the Ao and RV.

implies, the pathology of arrhythmogenic RV cardiomyopathy (ARVC) is initiated in the right heart but may cause global cardiac disease resembling the typical DCM. ARVC is common in boxers as a familial disease (also termed boxer cardiomyopathy) and has been reported in cats (Harvey et al. 2005).

Doppler studies most commonly demonstrate atrioventricular valve regurgitation in DCM relating to cardiac dilation and consequent dysfunction of the mitral and/or tricuspid apparatus (Figure 5.54). Typically, atrioventricular valvular regurgitation in DCM is not as voluminous as in CDVD, but both

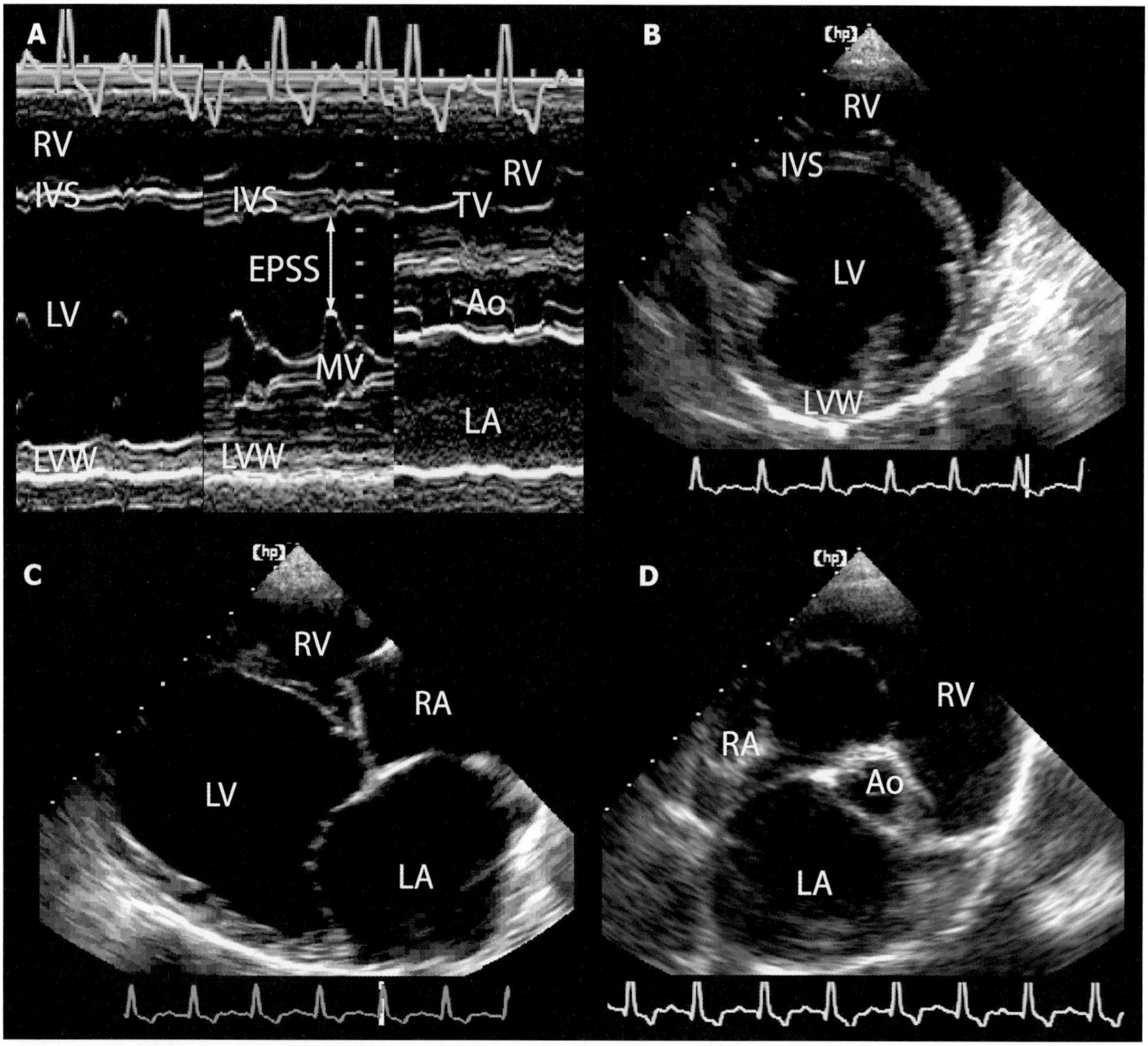

Figure 5.53. DCM in a boxer. **A:** RPS M-mode recordings demonstrate dramatic LV dilation and decreased fractional shortening. The E-point to septal separation distance (EPSS) is markedly increased, as is the LA/Ao. RPS SAx **(B and D)** and LAx **(C)** 2DE images depict marked dilation of all chambers.

diseases may occur in some individuals and produce a mixed echocardiographic pattern.

Hypertrophic Cardiomyopathy

Hypertrophic cardiomyopathy (HCM), defined as a primary myocardial abnormality, is the most common acquired heart disease in cats and is reported as a rare condition in dogs (Fox 1999). Echocardiographic abnormalities caused by feline HCM relate principally to myocardial hypertrophy including increased absolute (intraventricular septum [IVS] or LV wall [LVW]) or indexed wall thickness (wWT, wIVS, or wLVW), increased wall thickness relative to chamber dimension (RWT, FWT, or FWA [defined in Table 5.4]), and indices suggestive of an actual increase in muscle mass (wWA) (Moise et al. 1986) (Appendix). Increasing functional severity commonly is accompanied by progressive LA dilation (Figure 5.55).

M-mode echocardiography is useful in quantifying HCM changes but also suffers limitations. The LV wall thickness in diastole (LVWd) is less than 0.55 cm

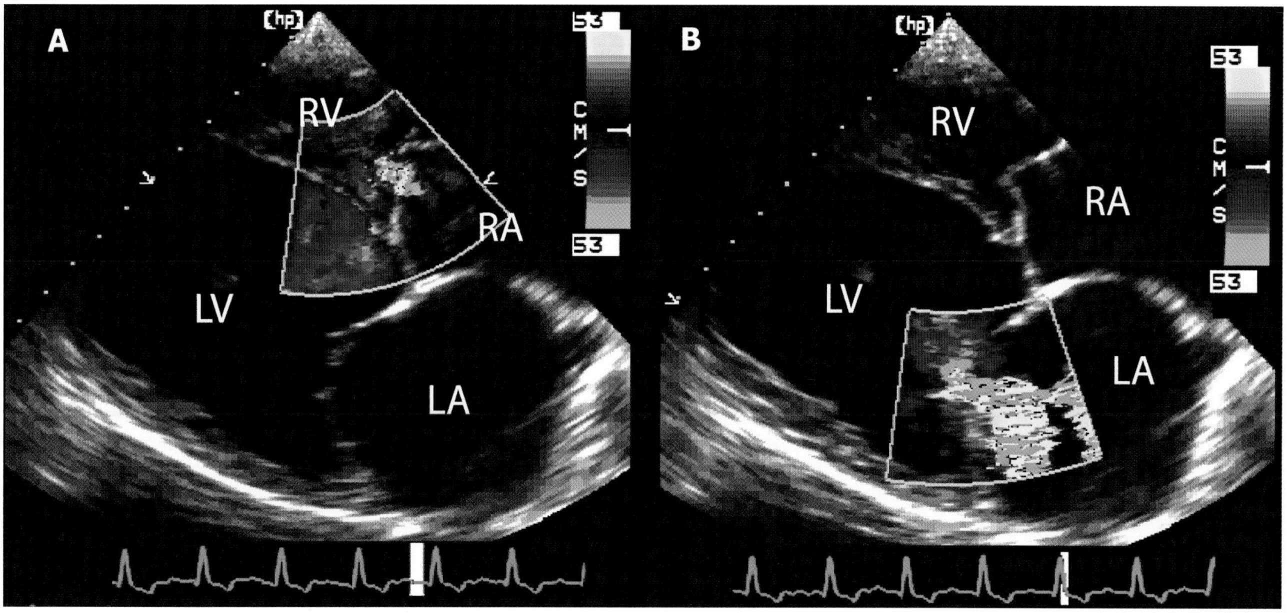

Figure 5.54. Valvular regurgitation with DCM. RPS LAx CFD images from the boxer in Figure 5.53. Marked cardiac dilation contributes to TR **(A)** and MR **(B)** commonly evident with the disease.

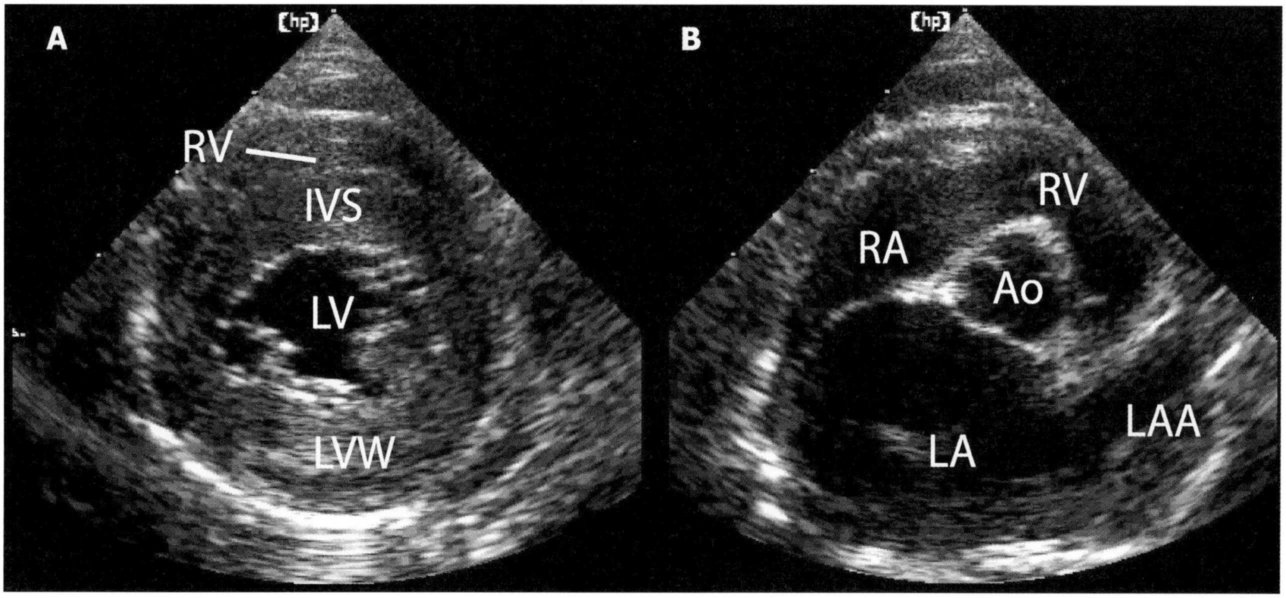

Figure 5.55. HCM. RPS SAx CFD images from a cat with HCM as suggested by thickening of the IVS and LVW, a decrease in LV internal dimension, and LA dilation.

normally, and values greater than 0.60 cm are suggestive of hypertrophy. However, subtle papillary muscle hypertrophy in mild cases or regional disparity in wall thickness may have no representation in an M-mode study. Systolic anterior motion (SAM) of the mitral valve is a functional abnormality, best identified on M-mode recordings, that typifies obstructive HCM. The result is dynamic outflow obstruction and subvalvular AS (Figure 5.56).

The obstructive aspect of HCM is best assessed with the addition of Doppler methods. While SAM is a common source of outflow obstruction, hypertrophy of papillary muscles or muscular trabeculae may cause intraventricular obstruction, observed as a turbulent

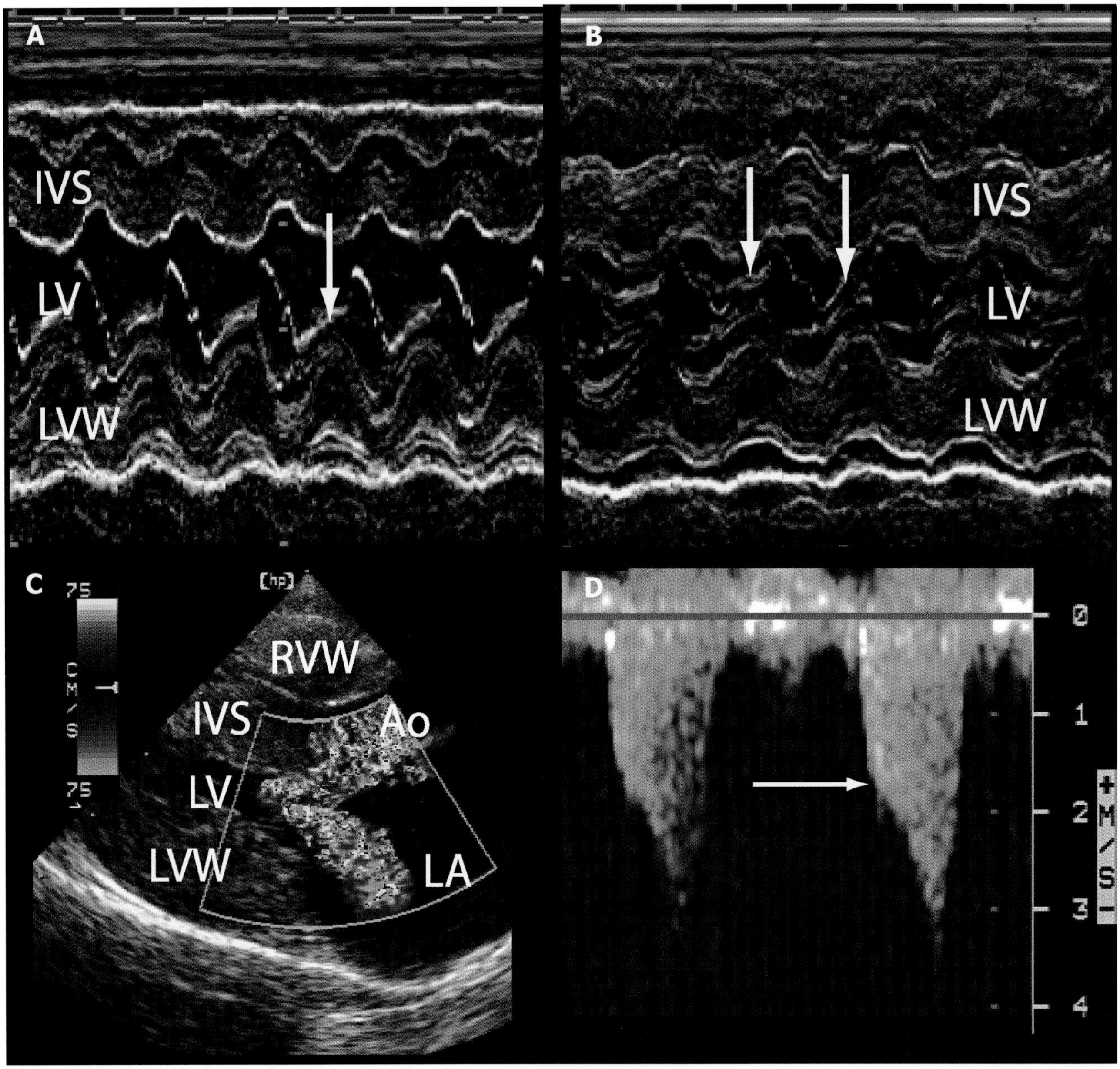

Figure 5.56. Dynamic LV outflow obstruction with HCM. M-mode recordings from cats with **(B)** and without **(A)** dynamic outflow obstruction secondary to HCM. There is pronounced thickening of the IVS and LVW in both cases. Arrows in both indicate the location of the MV during systole. **A:** Adequate separation between the IVS and MV coincides with an unobstructed LVOT. **B:** There is systolic anterior motion (SAM) of the MV; the MV is displaced into the LVOT and obstructs outflow. **C:** This RPS LAx CFD image displays the functional result of systolic obstruction, including both intra-Ao turbulence, caused by dynamic stenosis, and MR. **D:** This LAp CWD recording from the LVOT depicts spectral broadening caused by turbulence, increased peak velocity, and a dagger-shaped velocity envelope. Increasing proximity of the MV to the interventricular septum, beginning at the arrow, causes an abrupt change in the envelope as the degree of obstruction increases.

systolic jet emanating from within the ventricular chamber. Continuous-wave Doppler recording establishes the outflow tract blood flow velocity associated with an obstruction. Study of mitral inflow velocities may suggest impaired diastolic function and restrictive physiology (see the next section).

Development of intracardiac thrombi can sometimes be observed echocardiographically, particularly within the LA appendage (Figure 5.57). Stagnant blood flow can manifest echocardiographically as spontaneous echocontrast, so-called smoke within the left atrium, suggesting a high propensity for thrombus formation.

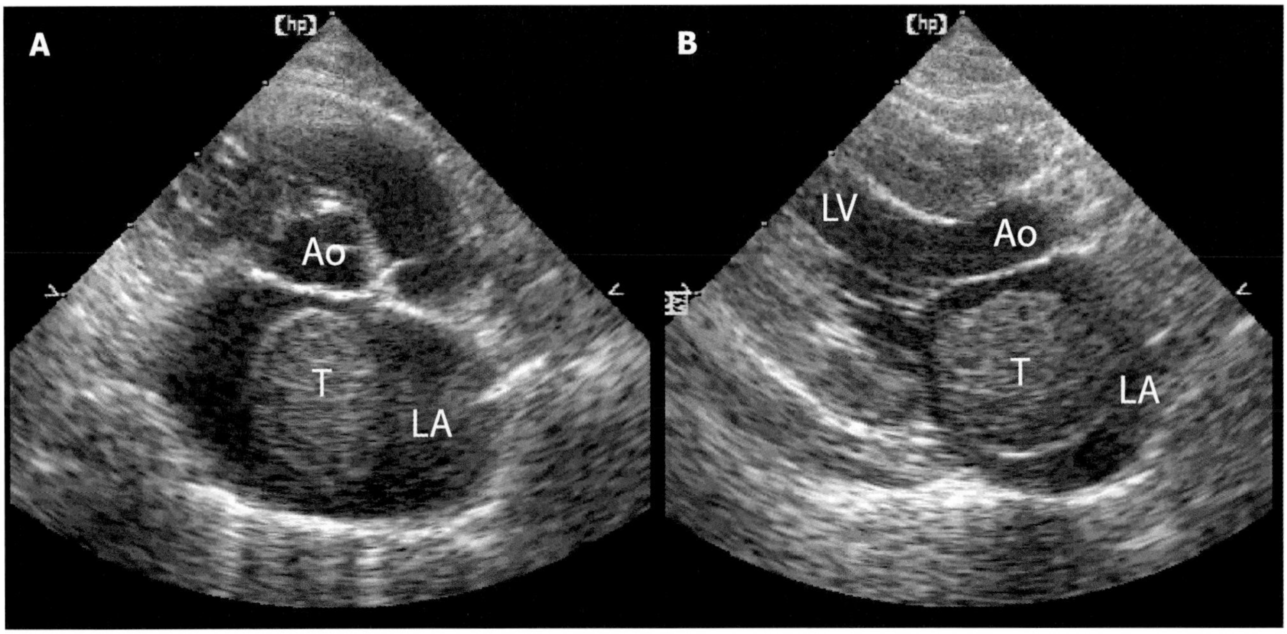

Figure 5.57. LA thrombus. RPS SAx **(A)** and LAx **(B)** images from a cat with restrictive cardiomyopathy demonstrating a free-floating echogenic thrombus (T) within the LA.

Restrictive Cardiomyopathy

Restrictive cardiomyopathy (RCM) includes a diverse array of disease that can cause loss of ventricular compliance, restrictive physiology and, ultimately, severe signs of congestive heart failure (Fox 1999). The source of restriction in RCM may reside within the myocardium (myocardial RCM) or be localized to the endocardium (endocardial RCM).

Feline myocardial RCM is associated with a restrictive flow pattern characterized in severe cases by increased velocity of the mitral E wave followed by an abrupt termination of inflow with a shortened deceleration time (Figure 5.58). This pattern may occur in the presence of normal fractional shortening and ejection fraction and normal wall thicknesses or only mild hypertrophy. Atrial dilation is often dramatic in RCM, particularly involving the left chamber, and predisposes patients to thromboembolic events (Figure 5.57). The LV endomyocardial form may include increased endocardial thickness and echogenicity, distortion and dysfunction of the mitral apparatus, or strands of echogenic tissue that bridge the ventricular chamber walls. RCM is often diagnosed by exclusion of typical DCM and HCM morphological characteristics in the presence of clearly significant heart disease. Hence, echocardiographic findings may entail a wide range of features, and a notable fraction of feline cardiomyopathies are not readily classified morphologically (unclassified cardiomyopathy).

Pulmonary Hypertension, Cor Pulmonale, and Heartworm Disease (Dirofilariasis)

Pulmonary hypertension (PHT) is excessive pulmonary arterial pressure and may be caused by elevated pulmonary venous pressure (left-sided congestive heart failure, pulmonary venous obstruction, mitral stenosis, or cor triatriatum sinister), pulmonary overcirculation (left to right shunts), or increased pulmonary vascular resistance (pulmonary thromboembolism, dirofilariasis, chronic respiratory disease and alveolar hypoxia, external vascular compression, vascular obliteration, persistent fetal circulation, or idiopathic PHT).

Cor pulmonale is RV hypertrophy and dysfunction caused by PHT not due to congenital heart disease or left heart failure causes. 2DE evidence of cor pulmonale may include thickening of the RV wall, papillary muscle, and trabeculae. RV and/or RA dilation may occur, particularly if significant tricuspid regurgitation results. The pulmonary trunk and main branches may be dilated, which is an assessment made by comparison with the aorta. The left ventricle may appear ovoid in cross section in the RPS short-axis image, with septal flattening because of compression and distortion imposed by the right heart; pseudohypertrophy of the left ventricle may occur from left-sided volume underload and septal hypertrophy. Paradoxical septal motion may be evident on M-mode recordings as

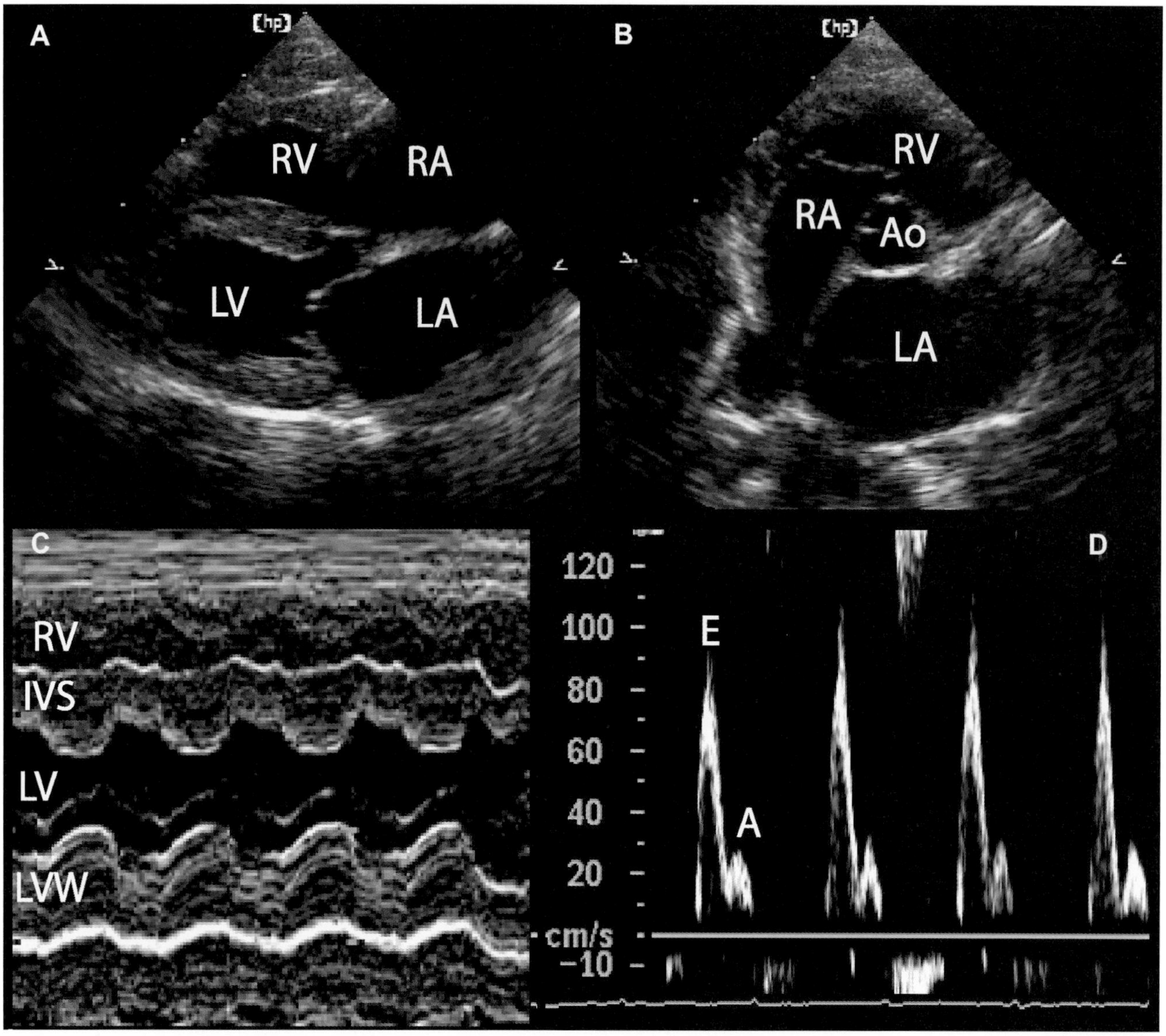

Figure 5.58. Restrictive cardiomyopathy (RCM). 2DE LAx **(A)** and SAx axis **(B)** images and M-mode **(C)** and PWD mitral inflow **(D)** recordings from a cat with RCM. There is dramatic atrial enlargement on the 2DE images, particularly of the left chamber; significant RV dilation is also present **(A)**. Nevertheless, wall thicknesses of all chambers are normal to mildly increased, the LV internal chamber dimensions and fractional shortening are within normal limits **(C)**. The PWD recording **(D)** demonstrates a restrictive flow pattern. In this example, the E wave of mitral inflow is prominent, with mildly increased velocity, and the A wave is nearly absent; atrial contraction causes little additional ventricular filling because of loss of compliance (i.e., restriction).

systolic LV pressure distends the septum toward the transducer (Figure 5.59). Doppler confirmation of PHT is made by CWD or at times by PWD quantification of tricuspid regurgitation or pulmonary insufficiency velocity; either or both may be caused by the excessive pressures and geometric distortion imposed by PHT.

Heartworm disease (HWD or dirofilarasis) is an important cause of PHT and cor pulmonale in dogs. In addition to the echocardiographic abnormalities already noted, adult parasites may be visualized directly within the pulmonary arteries, right ventricle or right atrium, or vena cavae (Lombard and Buergelt 1983a) (Figure 5.60). Echocardiography is an insensitive test for HWD in dogs because parasites may reside entirely within lobar and distal pulmonary arteries, which are inaccessible to 2DE examination. Nevertheless, when adults may be visualized in more proximal locations of the pulmonary circulation, 2DE facilitates qualitative evaluation of a parasite burden that becomes moderate to marked. *Vena cava syndrome*

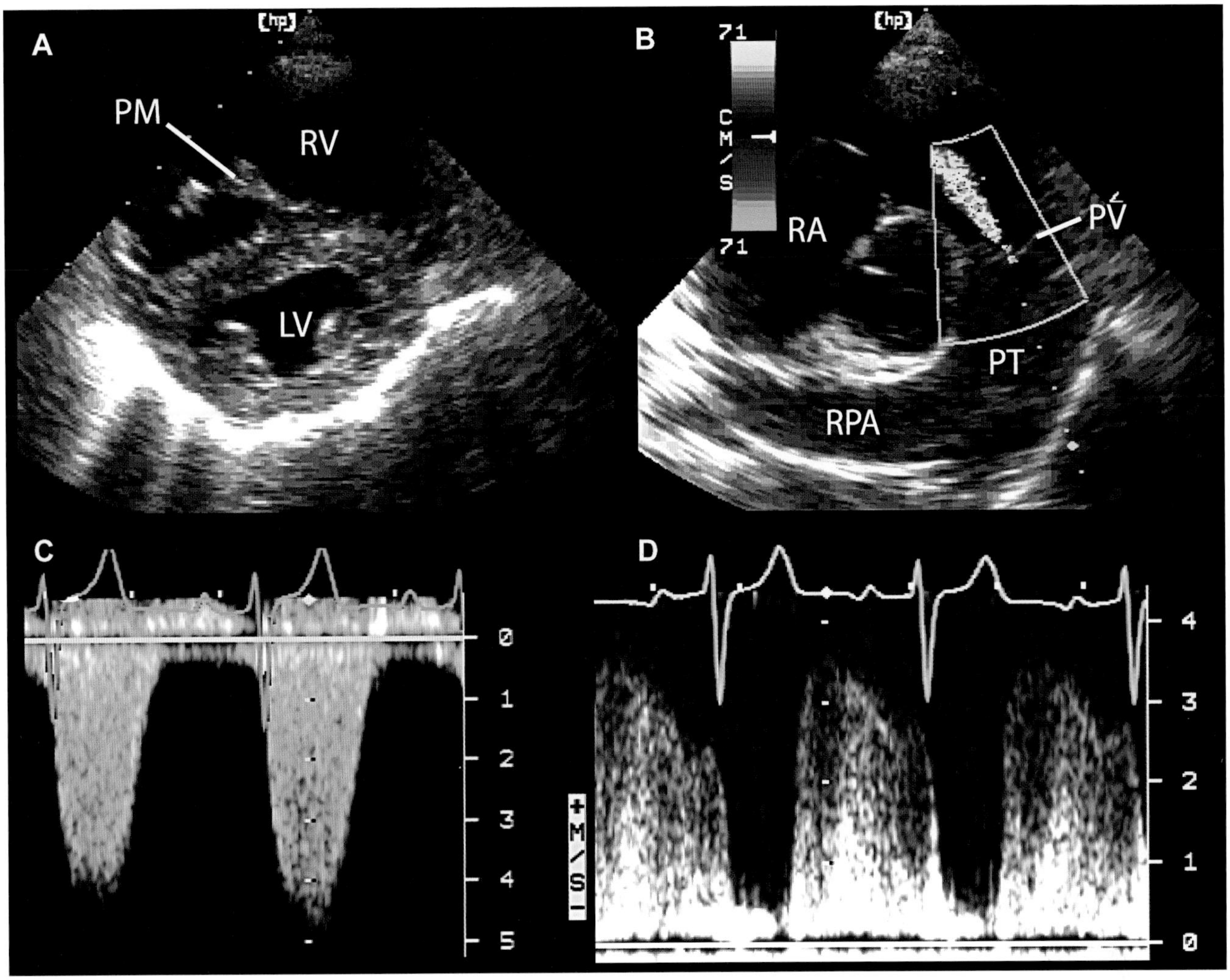

Figure 5.59. Cor pulmonale in a dog with chronic respiratory disease. **A:** This RPS SAx image depicts RV dilation, flattening of the IVS, and a small LV chamber. The RV PM is prominent because of hypertrophy, but RVW thickening is not dramatic. **B:** This CFD image demonstrates PV insufficiency, a normal finding except for the extent of the jet in this case, and dilation of the PT and RPA. CWD recordings of **(C)** TR and **(D)** pulmonary insufficiency confirm pulmonary hypertension. The peak TR velocity is greater than 4.5 m/s, which corresponds to a systolic driving pressure of greater than 80 mm Hg and peak pulmonary insufficiency velocity of 3.5 m/s, with a diastolic driving pressure of about 50 mm Hg.

is characterized by a dramatic parasite burden within the right ventricle, right atrium, and vena cavae.

Adult heartworms have a distinctive echocardiographic appearance because of the echogenicity of the parasite's cuticle relative to the gut (Figure 5.60). Although still an insensitive test, echocardiography is an important adjunct for the diagnosis of HWD in cats where visualization of a single adult parasite confirms the condition.

Pericardial Disease

Pericardial effusion (PE), which is the most common disorder involving the pericardium, is readily recognized echocardiographically. Effusions may be idiopathic (*benign idiopathic* PE), neoplastic, cardiogenic (congestive heart failure), inflammatory, infectious, or hemorrhagic in origin. PE typically appears as an anechoic or variably echogenic space between the epicardial surface of the heart and the echogenic parietal pericardium (Bonagura and Pipers 1981). Any significant fluid accumulation within the pericardium should prompt the ultrasonographer to search for a cause (advanced heart disease, neoplasia, or potential cardiac rupture) before completing the study. Cardiac tamponade results when PE accumulation is sufficient to elevate the intrapericardial pressure at the level of or above the right heart filling pressure. Tamponade is

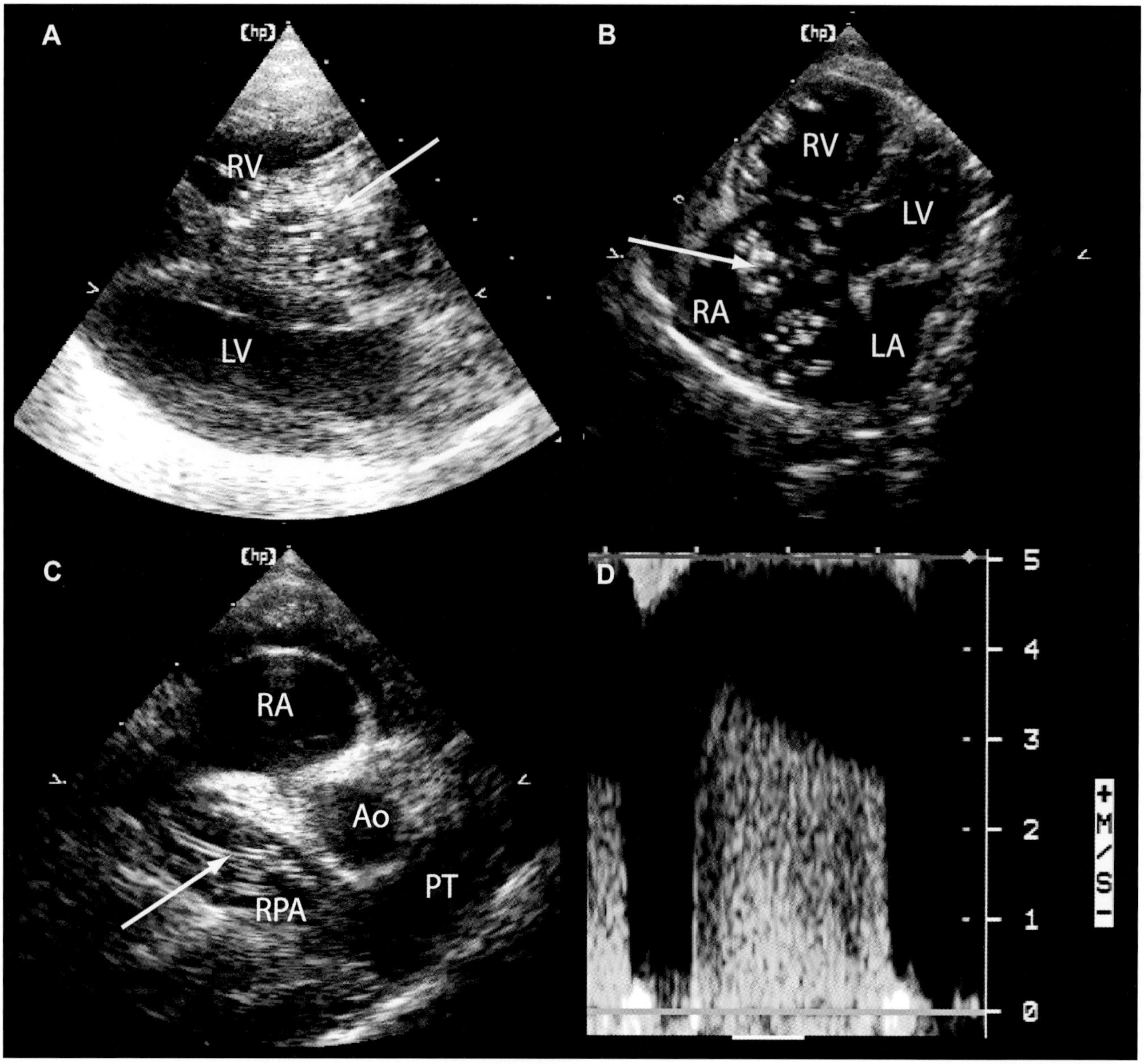

Figure 5.60. Heartworm disease (dirofilariasis). **A:** This RPS LAx image from a dog with vena cava syndrome depicts an extensive bolus of parasites flowing from the RA into the RV in early diastole (arrows indicate adult parasites in **A–C**). **B:** This LAp four-chamber image is from a rare case of vena cava syndrome from a cat with concurrent feline immunodeficiency virus infection. The RV and RA are dilated in both **A** and **B**. **C:** This RPS SAx image demonstrates parasites in a more typical location within the RPA. **D:** A continuous-wave Doppler recording of PI demonstrates a peak diastolic velocity of 3.5 m/s between the PT and RV, consistent with a driving pressure of 4×3.5^2 = ca. 50 mm Hg and pulmonary hypertension.

characterized echocardiographically by decreased ventricular size and early diastolic collapse of the right atrium, right ventricle, or both. With large effusions, the heart may exhibit a swinging motion within the pericardial space, typically on an every-other-beat basis. This motion coincides with the electrocardiographic occurrence of electrical alternans and is heart rate dependent (Figure 5.61).

Cardiac Neoplasia

Echocardiography is well suited for the diagnosis of cardiac neoplasia, which is common in dogs and a frequent cause of PE (Thomas et al. 1984). Hemangiosarcoma is the most common cardiac malignancy, with a strong site predilection for the RA appendage, right atrium, and RV wall. Small tumors

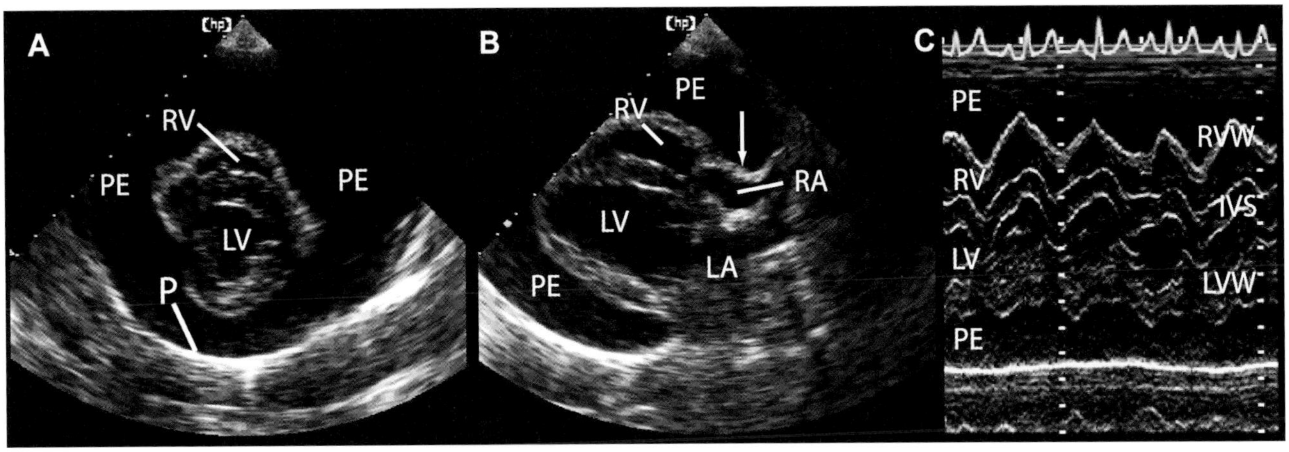

Figure 5.61. Pericardial effusion (PE) and tamponade. RPS SAx **(A)** and LAx **(B)** images from a dog with PE causing cardiac tamponade. There is a large anechoic space between the heart and the echogenic P. The LV and RV chambers are decreased in size. The RA exhibits early diastolic collapse in the LAx image (**B**, arrow). 2DE is superior for establishing the presence or absence of PE. However M-mode **(C)** is sometimes valuable for timing cardiac cycle events.

on the RA appendage often may be visualized from either the LPS or RPS transducer positions, and visualization may be improved by placing the transducer at the most cranial aspect of the imaging window. Neoplasia cannot be ruled out by echocardiography, however, and multiple transducer positions should be attempted if a tumor is suspected. PE may improve tumor visualization, providing an echo-free zone for contrast. Hemangiosarcoma may appear mottled or cavitated because of hypoechoic collections of blood within the tumor (Figure 5.62).

Chemodectoma (aortic body tumor), which is a common tumor of brachiocephalic breeds, arises from aortic chemoreceptor cells that are often situated near the base of the heart (heart base tumor) (Thomas et al. 1984). Chemodectomas range in appearance from a small nodule, seemingly adherent to the ascending aorta, to a large mass that partially or completely surrounds the great vessel. Tumors are most often biologically benign and cause clinical signs from PE or compression of the trachea or heart. Echocardiographic examination of a heart base tumor may necessitate imaging the ascending aorta far dorsal to the heart (Figure 5.63).

Thyroid carcinoma may arise from ectopic thyroid tissue, typically located at the heart base or within the RV outflow tract. Tumors may cause PE or obstruction of the RV ejection tract (Figure 5.63).

Mesothelioma involving the pericardium may be difficult to diagnose echocardiographically because it does not typically produce a discrete, echogenic mass. Pericardial and/or pleural effusion of unexplained origin must include this cell type as a differential.

Cardiac neoplasia in cats is uncommon. Lymphoma may occur within the heart, as one or more discrete masses, or as a diffuse, infiltrative lesion causing altered and irregular echogenicity.

Miscellaneous Acquired Disease

Echocardiography is an insensitive method for the detection of *pulmonary thromboembolism* but may provide evidence of chronicity (cor pulmonale) or hemodynamic severity (right-sided pressures, acute dilation, and RV stroke volume). Occasionally, thrombi may be visible in the pulmonary trunk or main branches (Figure 5.64). CFD or echocontrast may be valuable in delineating a thrombus and avoid overinterpretation.

Systemic hypertension (SHT), which is common in both dogs and cats, may cause nonspecific echocardiographic changes because of left-sided pressure overload. LV wall thickness and indices of LV hypertrophy may be increased with chronic SHT. Alterations can resemble mild to moderate HCM in cats and thus require blood-pressure determination for differentiation. Inconsistently, the aortic root and proximal aorta may be dilated with mild to moderate aortic insufficiency. In the absence of LV outflow obstruction, peak MR velocity greater than 6.3 m/s suggests SHT with peak systolic pressure greater than 160 mm Hg.

Hyperthyroidism is the most common endocrinopathy in cats, and concurrent, nonspecific echocardiographic abnormalities often are observed. LV wall thickening and hypertrophy may occur, and the

Figure 5.63. Cardiac neoplasia. **A and B:** RPS LAx and SAx views from a dog with a large mass (M) at the heart base. **C:** A thyroid carcinoma (M) is apparent on this RPS SAx view at a typical location in the RVOT. **D:** A SAx RPS image from a cat with echogenic cardiac metastases (M) from a carcinoma. A small amount of pericardial effusion (PE) is also evident.

condition may resemble HCM of mild to moderate severity echocardiographically (Moise et al. 1986). Tachycardia and increased indices of stroke volume (e.g., wΔA) may result with variable dilation of all cardiac chambers. Atrioventricular valvular regurgitation may accompany the condition if there is sufficient remodeling of the heart to impair valve function, and congestive heart failure with pulmonary edema and/or pleural effusion may occur in severe cases. Hyperthyroid cats are occasionally seen with cardiac changes resembling DCM, including marked chamber dilation and depressed fractional shortening.

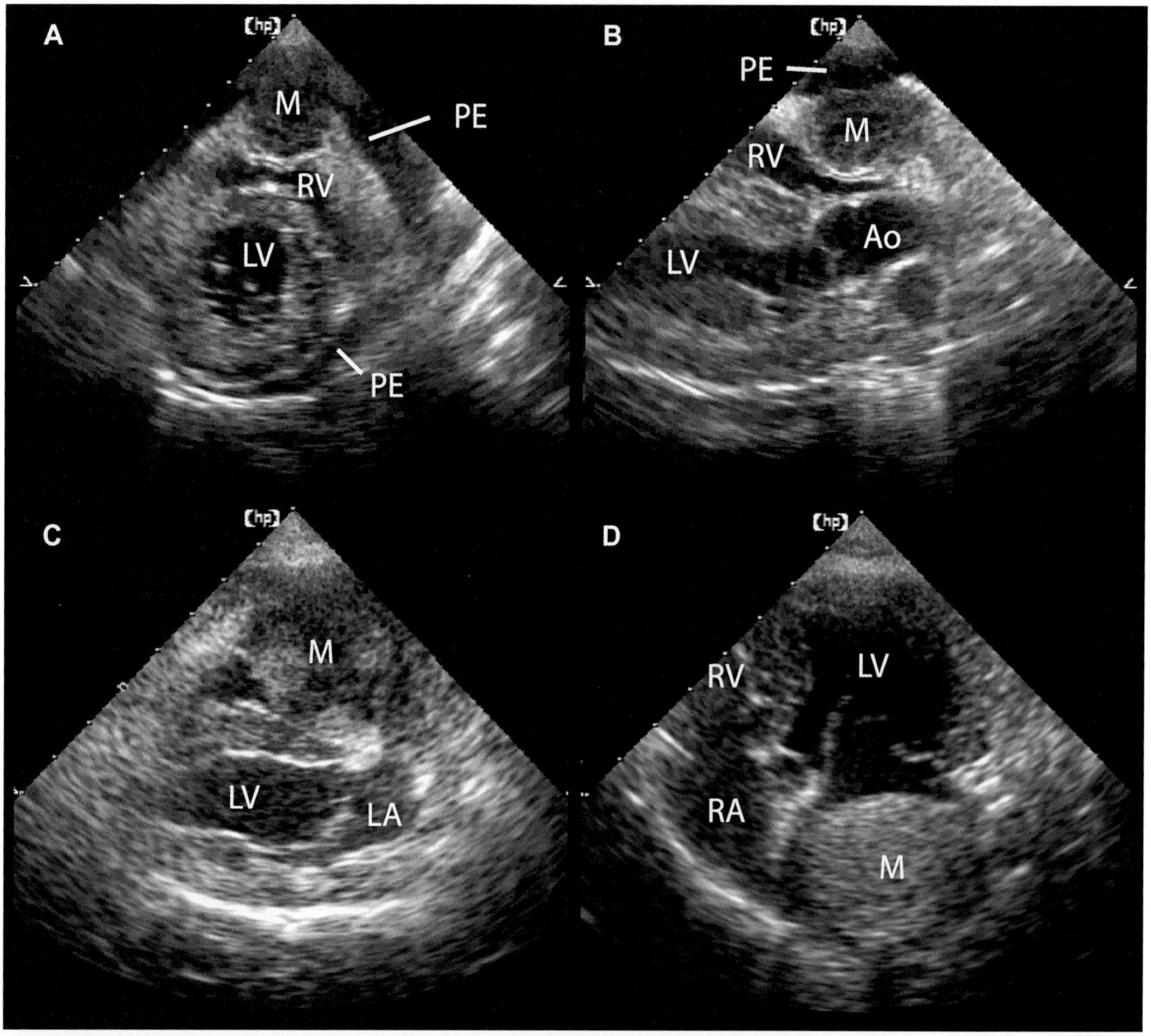

Figure 5.62. Hemangiosarcoma (HSA). RPS SAx **(A)** and LAx **(B)** 2DE images illustrate the typical location for HSA in a dog. A large mass (M) appears at the junction of the RVW and RA in this case. A small amount of pericardial effusion is evident (PE) because of extension of the tumor and bleeding into the pericardial space. **C and D:** Two variations of atypical cardiac HSA. In C, a large mass (M) fills the RV and RA in the RPS LAx image. In D, an LAp four-chamber view depicts a mass filling the LA.

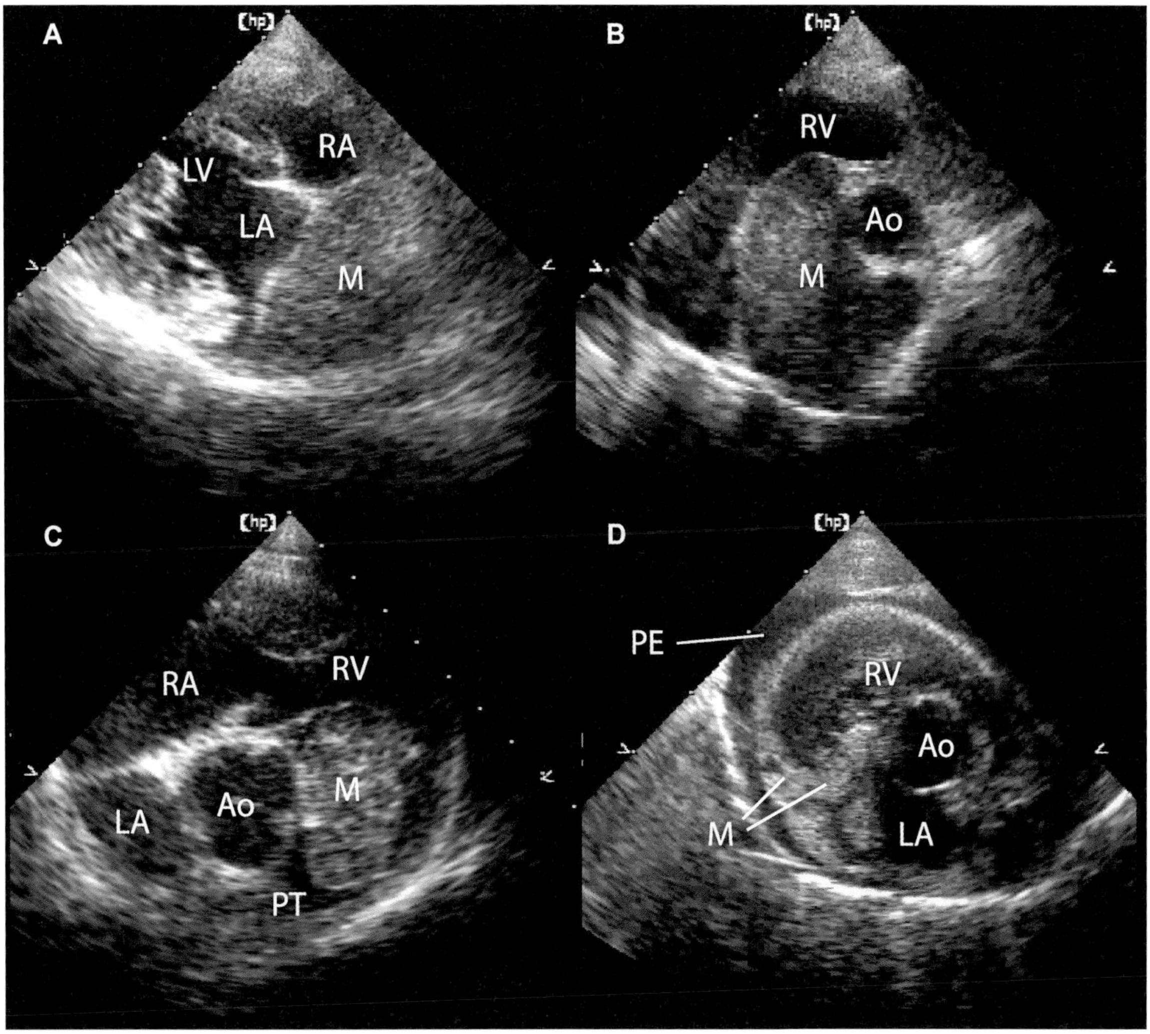

Figure 5.63.

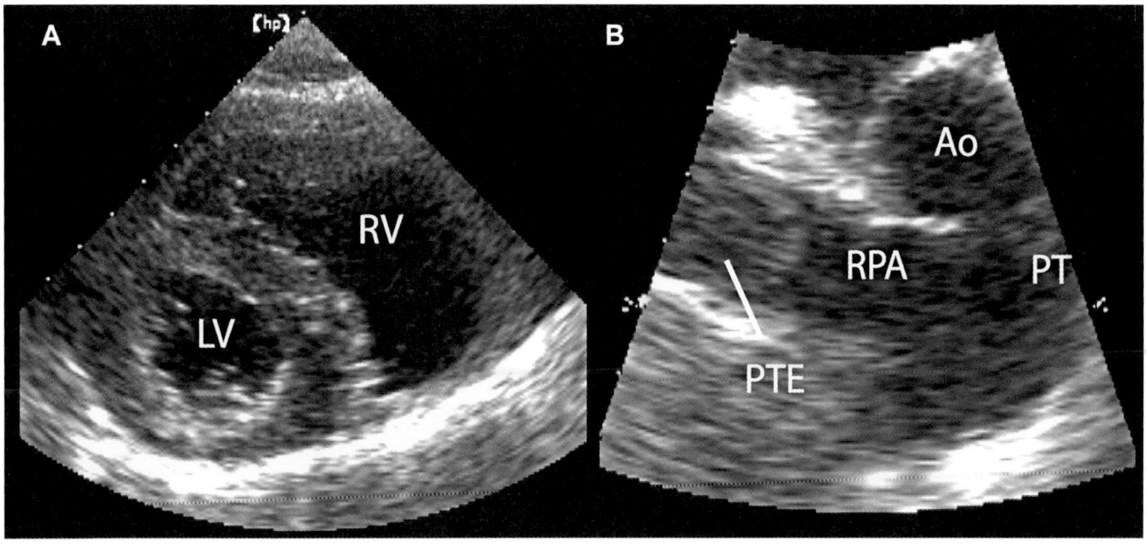

Figure 5.64. Pulmonary thromboembolism (PTE) in a dog. **A:** This RPS SAx image depicts RV dilation and hypertrophy, the latter suggesting chronicity. The LV appears small because of volume underloading. **B:** A thrombus (PTE) is evident in the dilated RPA.

Interventional Procedures

Pericardiocentesis (PC) is both a therapeutic and diagnostic procedure. Pericardial effusion (PE) associated with clinical signs due to cardiac compression (tamponade) is the major indication for PC. PC is also indicated in obtaining a sample of PE for diagnostic analysis.

Insufficient PE volume is the main contraindication for PC if the risk of the procedure outweighs potential benefits. Relative contraindications include hemorrhagic PE secondary to bleeding disorders or atrial tear, because reducing the pericardial pressure may perpetuate hemorrhage. Distension of the pericardium by solid tumors or abdominal contents as seen in peritoneal-pericardial diaphragmatic hernia is also a contraindication for PC.

The required equipment list includes a 14- to 18-gauge over-the-needle catheter (2–5 inches [5.08–12.7 cm], depending on patient size), syringes (3–50 mL), three-way stopcock, extension tubing, and collection tubes or apparatus for cytology (EDTA) and culture submission.

Sedation and local analgesia are useful and can be obtained with diazepam (0.2 mg/kg) intravenous (IV) in combination with either butorphanol (0.2 mg/kg) IV or oxymorphone (0.1 mg/kg) IV. Agents promoting hypotension must be avoided (e.g., acepromazine).

The patient is usually positioned in left lateral recumbency. Electrocardiographic monitoring for heart rate and rhythm during the procedure is essential. The catheter entry location is at the fifth to seventh intercostal space of the right ventral thorax, at the level of the costochondral junction (Figure 5.65). Ultrasound guidance is highly useful in directing the catheter, in confirming the distribution and amount of PE, in establishing the optimal catheter entry point and direction, and in confirming the catheter position. Needle entry should be near the center of the rib space to avoid puncture of the intercostal vessels and also catheter kinking and obstruction by a rib as the patient breathes.

Using aseptic technique, the operator attaches a sterile 3-mL syringe to the catheter, positions the point of the catheter at the predetermined location, and orients the direction of the catheter dorsocranially. The entire apparatus is advanced through the skin and thoracic wall while mild negative pressure (suction) is applied with the syringe. A burst of ventricular premature complexes on the electrocardiogram suggests that the catheter tip is in contact with the epicardium; this requires catheter retraction until the dysrhythmia resolves. The flexible catheter is advanced off the stylus into the pericardial space, and the metal catheter stylus is then fully withdrawn. Extension tubing is attached directly to the flexible catheter end, leading to a large syringe and interposed three-way stopcock operated by an assistant.

With tamponade, decompression of the pericardial space by even a small amount often causes an observable decrease in heart rate. A continual decrease in heart rate throughout the procedure is suggestive of

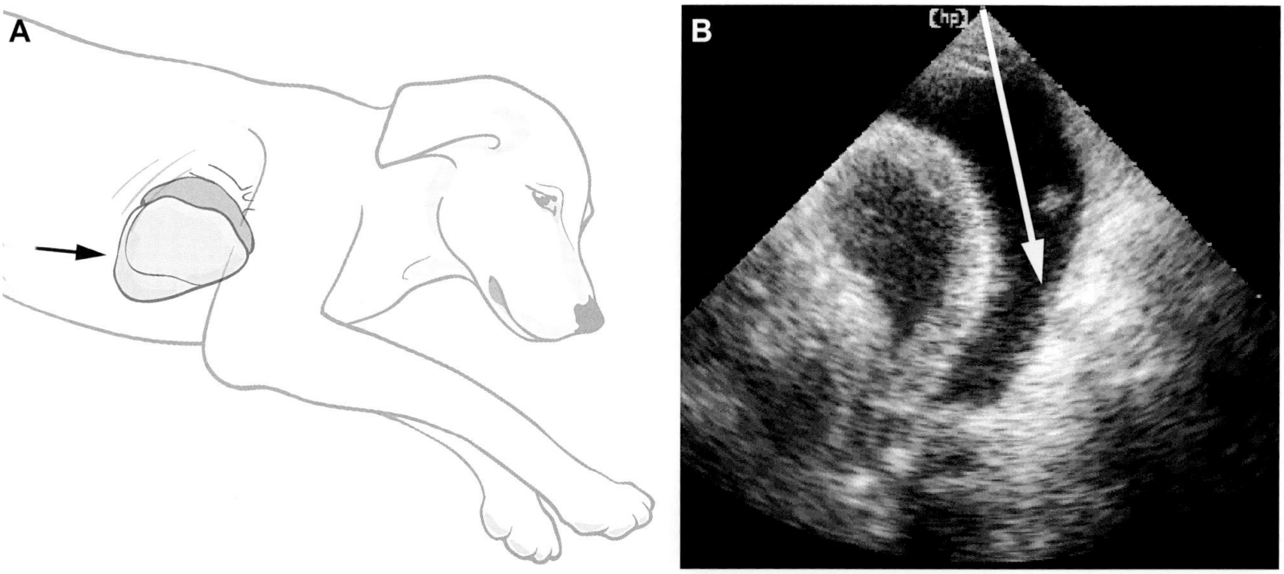

Figure 5.65. Pericardiocentesis in a dog. **A:** The catheter is placed at the fifth to seventh intercostal spaces of the right ventral thorax, at the level of the costochondral junction (arrow). **B:** The arrow indicates the orientation and position of an imaginary needle within the fluid-filled pericardial sac.

correct catheter placement, whereas any trend toward increased heart rate should prompt the operator to interrupt aspiration and reevaluate catheter position. Once the catheter-tip positioning within the pericardial space is assured, complete and rapid evacuation of PE may proceed (exceptions: atrial tear or bleeding disorder). Significant ventricular arrhythmias should prompt catheter repositioning and/or partial withdrawal. Intravenous administration of a 2% lidocaine bolus (2–4 mg/kg = 1–2 mL per 10 kg) should be considered if the dysrhythmia does not abate promptly.

Potential complications of PC include puncture of cardiac chambers or great vessels, cardiac dysrhythmia, coronary laceration, exsanguination, pulmonary laceration or hemorrhage, and pneumothorax. Complications are minimized by careful preparation and technique.

References

Abbott JA, MacLean HN (2003) Comparison of Doppler-derived peak aortic velocities obtained from subcostal and apical transducer sites in healthy dogs. Vet Radiol Ultrasound 44:695–698.

Bonagura JD (1983) M-mode echocardiography: Basic principles. Vet Clin North Am Small Anim Pract 13:299–319.

Bonagura JD, Herring DS (1985a) Echocardiography: Acquired heart disease. Vet Clin North Am Small Anim Pract 15:1209–1224.

Bonagura JD, Herring DS (1985b) Echocardiography: Congenital heart disease. Vet Clin North Am Small Anim Pract 15:1195–1208.

Bonagura JD, Miller MW (1998) Doppler echocardiography II: Color Doppler imaging. Vet Clin North Am Small Anim Pract 28:1361–1389.

Bonagura JD, Miller MW, Darke PGG (1998) Doppler echocardiography I. Pulsed-wave and continuous-wave examinations. Vet Clin North Am Small Anim Pract 28:1325–1359.

Bonagura JD, O'Grady MR, Herring DS (1985) Echocardiography: Principles of interpretation. Vet Clin North Am Small Anim Pract 15:1177–1194.

Bonagura JD, Pipers FS (1981) Echocardiographic features of pericardial effusion in dogs. J Am Vet Med Assoc 179:49–56.

Brown DJ, Rush JE, MacGregor J, Ross JN Jr, Brewer B, Rand WM (2005) Quantitative echocardiographic evaluation of mitral endocardiosis in dogs using ratio indices. J Vet Intern Med 19:542–552.

Calvert CA, Chapman WL Jr, Toal RL (1982) Congestive cardiomyopathy in Doberman pinscher dogs. J Am Vet Med Assoc 181:598–602.

Darke PGG (1992) Doppler echocardiography. J Small Anim Pract 33:104–112.

Darke PGG, Bonagura JD, Miller M (1993) Transducer orientation for Doppler echocardiography in dogs. J Small Anim Pract 34:2–8.

Fox PR (1999) Feline cardiomyopathies. In: Fox PR, Sisson D, Moise NS, eds. Textbook of Canine and Feline Cardiology: Principles and Clinical Practice, 2nd edition. Philadelphia: WB Saunders, pp 621–678.

Hansson K, Haggstrom J, Kvart C, Lord P (2002) Left atrial to aortic root indices using two-dimensional and M-mode echocardiography in cavalier King Charles spaniels with and without left atrial enlargement. Vet Radiol Ultrasound 43:568–575.

Harvey AM, Battersby IA, Faena M, Fews D, Darke PGG, Ferasin L (2005) Arrhythmogenic right ventricular cardiomyopathy in two cats. J Small Anim Pract 46:151–156.

Hatle LK, Angelsen B (1985) Physics of blood flow. In: Doppler Ultrasound in Cardiology: Physics, Principles, and Clinical Applications, 2nd edition. Philadelphia: Lea and Febiger, pp 8–31.

Henry WL, DeMaria A, Gramiak R, et al. (1980) Report of the American Society of Echocardiography Committee on Nomenclature and Standards in Two-dimensional Echocardiography. Circulation 62:212–217.

Kirberger RM, Bland-van den Berg P, Grimbeek RJ (1992) Doppler echocardiography in the normal dog. Part II: Factors influencing blood flow velocities and a comparison between left and right heart blood flow. Vet Radiol Ultrasound 33:380–386.

Kittleson MD, Brown WA (2003) Regurgitant fraction measured by using the proximal isovelocity surface area method in dogs with chronic myxomatous mitral valve disease. J Vet Intern Med 17:84–88.

Kittleson MD, Eyster GE, Knowlen GG, Olivier NB, Anderson LK (1984) Myocardial function in small dogs with chronic mitral regurgitation and severe congestive heart failure. J Am Vet Med Ass 184:455–459.

Lombard CW, Buergelt CD (1983a) Echocardiographic and clinical findings in dogs with heartworm-induced cor pulmonale. Compend Contin Educ Pract Vet 5:971–979.

Lombard CW, Buergelt CD (1983b) Vegetative bacterial endocarditis in dogs: Echocardiographic diagnosis and clinical signs. J Small Anim Pract 24:325–339.

Moise NS (1989) Doppler echocardiographic evaluation of congenital cardiac disease. J Vet Intern Med 3:195–207.

Moise NS, Dietze AE, Mezza LE, Strickland D, Erb HN, Edwards NJ (1986) Echocardiography, electrocardiography, and radiography of cats with dilatation cardiomyopathy, hypertrophic cardiomyopathy, and hyperthyroidism. Am J Vet Res 47:1476–1486.

O'Grady MR, Bonagura JD, Powers JD, Herring DS (1986) Quantitative cross-sectional echocardiography in the normal dog. Vet Radiol Ultrasound 27:34–49.

O'Rourke RA, Hanrath P, Henry WN, et al. (1984) Report of the Joint International Society and Federation of Cardiology/World Health Organization Task Force on recommendations for standardization of measurements from M-mode echocardiograms. Circulation 69:854A–857A.

Rishniw M, Erb HN (2000) Evaluation of four 2-dimensional echocardiographic methods of assessing left atrial size in dogs. J Vet Intern Med 14:429–435.

Sahn DJ, DeMaria A, Kisslo J, Weyman A (1978) Recommendations regarding quantitation in M-mode echocardiography: Results of a survey of echocardiographic measurements. Circulation 58:1072–1083.

Schiller NB, Shah PM, Crawford M, et al. (1989) Recommendations for quantitation of the left ventricle by two-dimensional echocardiography. American Society of Echocardiography Committee on Standards, Subcommittee on Quantitation of Two-dimensional Echocardiograms. J Am Soc Echocardiogr 2:358–367.

Thomas WP (1984) Two-dimensional, real-time echocardiography in the dog. Vet Radiol Ultrasound 25:50–64.

Thomas WP, Gaber CE, Jacobs GJ, et al. (1993) Recommendations for standards in transthoracic two-dimensional echocardiography in the dog and cat. J Vet Intern Med 7:247–252.

Thomas WP, Sisson D, Bauer TG, Reed JR (1984) Detection of cardiac masses in dogs by two-dimensional echocardiography. Vet Radiol Ultrasound 25:65–72.

Appendix

Canine breed-specific M-mode reference values: unindexed

Reference	Breed	N	BW (kg)	LVIDd (cm)	LVIDs (cm)	IVSd (cm)	IVSs (cm)	LVWd (cm)	LVWs (cm)	Ao (cm)	LA (cm)
Morrison et al. 1992	Miniature poodle	20	3.0[b] [1.4–9.0]	2.00[b] [1.60–2.80]	1.00[b] [0.80–1.60]	0.50[b] [0.40–0.60]	0.80[b] [0.60–1.00]	0.50[b] [0.40–0.60]	0.80[b] [0.60–1.00]	1.00[b] [0.80–1.30]	1.20[b] [0.80–1.80]
Della Torre et al. 2000[a]	Italian greyhound	20	5.4 ± 1.5 [3.2–8.4]	2.22 ± 0.27 [1.63–2.66]	1.28 ± 0.28 [0.84–1.76]	0.64 ± 0.11 [0.44–0.85]	0.91 ± 0.13 [0.69–1.15]	0.71 ± 0.09 [0.49–0.92]	1.02 ± 0.08 [0.86–1.19]		
Häggstrom[a] Cornell et al. 2004	Cavalier King Charles spaniel	57	8.9 ± 1.4 [5.5–11.9]	2.92 ± 0.31 [2.20–3.55]	1.96 ± 0.25 [1.50–2.70]			0.70 ± 0.09 [0.50–0.85]		1.60 ± 0.15 [1.20–2.00]	1.60 ± 0.19 [1.10–2.25]
Crippa et al. 1992	Beagle	20	8.9 ± 1.5 [5.9–11.9]	2.63 [1.95–3.31]	1.57 [0.89–2.25]	0.67 [0.45–0.89]	0.96 [0.66–1.26]	0.82 [0.44–1.20]	1.14 [0.76–1.52]		
Pedersen[a] Cornell et al. 2004	Dachshund	33	9.5 ± 1.9 [6.2–16.0]	2.84 ± 0.33 [2.20–3.60]	1.88 ± 0.29 [1.20–2.60]	0.70 ± 0.10 [0.50–0.80]	0.95 ± 0.11 [0.70–1.20]	0.68 ± 0.13 [0.40–0.90]	1.01 ± 0.14 [0.70–1.20]	1.82 ± 0.18 [1.50–2.30]	1.63 ± 0.23 [1.00–2.10]
Baade et al. 2002	West Highland white terrier	24	10.3 ± 0.9 [8.5–12.1]	2.88 [1.74–4.02]	2.00 [1.26–2.74]	0.69 [0.41–0.97]	1.02 [0.52–1.52]	0.64 [0.40–0.88]	0.98 [0.72–1.24]		
Gooding et al. 1986	English cocker spaniel	12	12.2 ± 2.4 [8.5–15.8]	3.38 ± 0.35 [2.90–4.00]	2.23 ± 0.29 [1.90–2.80]	0.82 ± 0.14 [0.50–0.90]		0.79 ± 0.12 [0.50–0.90]			
Morrison et al. 1992	Welsh corgi	20	15.0[b] [8.0–19.0]	3.20[b] [2.80–4.00]	1.90[b] [1.20–2.30]	0.80[b] [0.60–0.90]	1.20[b] [1.00–1.40]	0.80[b] [0.60–1.00]	1.20[b] [0.80–1.30]	1.80[b] [1.50–2.20]	2.10[b] [1.20–2.40]
Sisson and Schaeffer 1991	English pointer	16	19.2 ± 2.8 [13.6–24.9]	3.92 ± 0.24 [3.44–4.40]	2.53 ± 0.24 [2.05–3.01]	0.69 ± 0.11 [0.47–0.91]	1.06 ± 0.10 [0.86–1.26]	0.71 ± 0.07 [0.57–0.85]	1.15 ± 0.13 [0.89–1.41]	2.41 ± 0.17 [2.07–2.75]	2.26 ± 0.20 [1.86–2.66]
Morrison et al. 1992	Afghan hound	20	23.0[b] [17.0–36.0]	4.20[b] [3.30–5.20]	2.80[b] [2.00–3.70]	1.30[b] [0.80–1.80]	1.30[b] [0.80–1.80]	0.90[b] [0.70–1.10]	1.20[b] [0.90–1.80]	2.60[b] [2.00–3.40]	2.60[b] [1.80–3.50]
Page et al. 1993	Greyhound	16	26.6 ± 3.5 [20.7–32.5]	4.41 ± 0.30 [4.00–4.90]	3.25 ± 0.35 [2.90–3.80]	1.06 ± 0.17 [0.80–1.40]	1.34 ± 0.26 [1.00–1.70]	1.21 ± 0.17 [0.90–1.40]	1.53 ± 0.22 [1.20–1.80]		
Della Torre et al. 2000[a]	Greyhound	20	26.9 ± 3.3 [21.7–31.5]	4.27 ± 0.28 [3.88–4.92]	3.21 ± 0.25 [2.84–3.66]	1.19 ± 0.13 [0.9–1.51]	1.57 ± 0.13 [1.33–1.85]	1.29 ± 0.11 [1.13–1.49]	1.71 ± 0.13 [1.54–2.04]		
Snyder et al. 1995[a]	Greyhound	11	29.1 ± 3.7 [24.9–36.3]	4.69 ± 0.30 [3.98–4.98]	3.33 ± 0.26 [2.84–3.63]	1.34 ± 0.17 [1.04–1.61]		1.16 ± 0.17 [0.82–1.34]			
Vollmar[a] Cornell et al. 2004	Boxer	75	31.0 ± 4.8 [22.5–43.0]	4.13 ± 0.38 [3.27–5.08]	2.78± 0.31 [2.0–3.59]	0.97 ± 0.16 [0.65–1.27]	1.38 ± 0.22 [1.00–1.90]	0.98 ± 0.13 [0.66–1.26]	1.46 ± 0.18 [1.08–1.95]	2.28 ± 0.22 [1.82–3.00]	2.46 ± 0.31 [1.72–3.46]
Morrison et al. 1992	Golden retriever	20	32.0[b] [23.0–41.0]	4.50[b] [3.70–5.10]	2.70[b] [1.80–3.50]	1.00[b] [0.80–1.30]	1.40[b] [1.00–1.70]	1.00[b] [0.80–1.20]	1.50[b] [1.00–1.90]	2.40[b] [1.40–2.70]	2.70[b] [1.60–3.20]
Calvert and Brown 1986	Doberman pinscher	21	36.0 [31.0–42.0]	4.68 ± 0.42 [4.10–5.50]	3.08 ± 0.33 [2.50–3.60]	0.96 ± 0.06 [0.80–1.00]	1.43 ± 0.07 [1.30–1.50]	0.96 ± 0.06 [0.90–1.00]	1.41 ± 0.08 [1.30–1.50]	2.99 ± 0.23 [2.80–3.50]	2.66 ± 0.15 [2.20–2.80]
Bayon et al. 1994	Spanish mastiff	12	52.4 ± 3.3 [45.8–59.0]	4.77 ± 0.14 [4.50–5.04]	2.90 ± 0.11 [2.69–3.11]	0.98 ± 0.04 [0.89–1.06]	1.56 ± 0.05 [1.46–1.66]	0.97 ± 0.04 [0.90–1.04]	1.52 ± 0.04 [1.43–1.60]	2.76 ± 0.08 [2.61–2.91]	2.85 ± 0.09 [2.67–3.03]
Koch et al. 1996	Newfoundland	27	61.0 [47.0–69.5]	5.00 [4.40–6.00]	3.55 [2.90–4.40]	1.15 [0.70–1.50]	1.50 [1.10–2.00]	1.00 [0.80–1.30]	1.50 [1.10–1.60]	2.90 [2.60–3.30]	3.00 [2.40–3.30]
Koch et al. 1996	Great Dane	15	62.0 [52.0–75.0]	5.30 [4.40–5.90]	3.95 [3.40–4.50]	1.45 [1.20–1.60]	1.65 [1.40–1.90]	1.25 [1.00–1.60]	1.60 [1.10–1.90]	2.95 [2.80–3.40]	3.30 [2.80–4.60]
Vollmar[a] Cornell et al. 2004	Irish wolfhound	144	63.5 ± 8.3 [45.0–91.0]	5.07 ± 0.37 [4.30–5.97]	3.35 ± 0.33 [2.55–4.09]	1.11 ± 0.19 [0.56–1.67]	1.55 ± 0.22 [1.03–2.13]	1.06 ± 0.16 [0.66–1.44]	1.58 ± 0.19 [1.19–2.21]	3.29 ± 0.30 [2.71–4.13]	3.18 ± 0.31 [2.47–3.89]
Koch et al. 1996	Irish wolfhound	20	68.5 [50.0–80.0]	5.00 [4.60–5.90]	3.60 [3.30–4.50]	1.20 [0.90–1.45]	1.50 [1.10–1.70]	1.00 [0.90–1.30]	1.40 [1.10–1.70]	3.00 [2.90–3.10]	3.10 [2.20–3.50]

[a]Original data supplied by investigators. All others from referenced sources.

[b]Mean or median ± standard deviation [range].

Ao, aorta; BW, body weight; IVSd, interventricular septal thickness, diastole; IVSs, interventricular septal thickness, systole; LA, left atrium; LVIDd, left ventricular internal dimension, diastole; LVIDs, left ventricular internal dimension, systole; LVWd, left ventricular wall thickness, diastole; and LVWs, left ventricular wall thickness, systole.

Canine breed-specific M-mode reference values indexed for body size (weight-based ratio indices)

Reference	Breed	N	BW (kg)	wLVIDd	wLVIDs	wIVSd	wIVSs	wLVWd	wLVWs	wAo	wLA
Morrison et al. 1992	Miniature poodle	20	3.0[b] [1.4–9.0]	1.74[b] [1.40–2.44]	0.87[b] [0.70–1.40]	0.44[b] [0.35–0.52]	0.70[b] [0.52–0.87]	0.44[b] [0.35–0.52]	0.70[b] [0.52–0.87]	0.87[b] [0.70–1.13]	1.05[b] [0.70–1.57]
Della Torre et al. 2000[a]	Italian greyhound	20	5.4 ± 1.5 [3.2–8.4]	1.61 ± 0.18 [1.17–1.88]	0.93 ± 0.17 [0.62–1.22]	0.46 ± 0.06 [0.34–0.57]	0.66 ± 0.07 [0.52–0.80]	0.51 ± 0.05 [0.42–0.65]	0.74 ± 0.07 [0.61–0.86]		
Häggstrom[a] Cornell et al. 2004	Cavalier King Charles spaniel	57	8.9 ± 1.4 [5.5–11.9]	1.78 ± 0.16 [1.40–2.16]	1.19 ± 0.14 [0.91–1.60]			0.42 ± 0.05 [0.34–0.52]		0.98 ± 0.09 [0.78–1.19]	0.97 ± 0.10 [0.76–1.24]
Crippa et al. 1992	Beagle	20	8.9 ± 1.5 [5.9–11.9]	1.60 [1.18–2.01]	0.95 [0.54–1.37]	0.41 [0.27–0.54]	0.58 [0.40–0.76]	0.50 [0.27–0.73]	0.69 [0.46–0.92]		
Pedersen[a] Cornell et al. 2004	Dachshund	33	9.5 ± 1.9 [6.2–16.0]	1.70 ± 0.19 [1.32–2.37]	1.12 ± 0.16 [0.72–1.51]	0.42 ± 0.05 [0.29–0.53]	0.57 ± 0.06 [0.41–0.66]	0.41 ± 0.07 [0.24–0.53]	0.61 ± 0.08 [0.42–0.75]	1.08 ± 0.09 [0.90–1.25]	0.98 ± 0.14 [0.60–1.18]
Baade et al. 2002	West Highland white terrier	24	10.3 ± 0.9 [8.5–12.1]	1.66 [1.01–2.32]	1.16 [0.73–1.58]	0.40 [0.24–0.56]	0.59 [0.30–0.88]	0.37 [0.23–0.51]	0.57 [0.42–0.72]		
Gooding et al. 1986	English cocker spaniel	12	12.2 ± 2.4 [8.5–15.8]	1.85 ± 0.14 [1.62–2.04]	1.22 ± 0.14 [1.02–1.41]	0.45 ± 0.08 [0.25–0.55]		0.44 ± 0.08 [0.25–0.55]			
Della Torre et al. 2000[a]	Whippet	20	14.5 ± 2.1 [10.8–20.2]	1.86 ± 0.12 [1.56–2.03]	1.25 ± 0.14 [0.96–1.49]	0.44 ± 0.05 [0.32–0.52]	0.64 ± 0.06 [0.45–0.72]	0.46 ± 0.05 [0.40–0.60]	0.67 ± 0.10 [0.56–0.92]		
Morrison et al. 1992	Welsh corgi	20	15.0[b] [8.0–19.0]	1.63[b] [1.43–2.04]	0.97[b] [0.61–1.17]	0.41[b] [0.31–0.46]	0.61[b] [0.51–0.71]	0.41[b] [0.31–0.51]	0.61[b] [0.41–0.66]	0.92[b] [0.76–1.12]	1.07[b] [0.61–1.22]
Sisson and Schaeffer 1991	English pointer	16	19.2 ± 2.8 [13.6–24.9]	1.84 ± 0.11 [1.62–2.07]	1.19 ± 0.11 [0.96–1.41]	0.32 ± 0.05 [0.22–0.43]	0.50 ± 0.05 [0.40–0.59]	0.33 ± 0.03 [0.27–0.40]	0.54 ± 0.06 [0.42–0.66]	1.13 ± 0.08 [0.97–1.29]	1.06 ± 0.09 [0.87–1.25]
Wey[a] Cornell et al. 2004	Generic	47	20.8 ± 13.0 [2.2–47.4]	1.75 ± 0.16 [1.45–2.09]	1.16 ± 0.19 [0.62–1.42]	0.40 ± 0.06 [0.28–0.54]	0.56 ± 0.11 [0.38–0.92]	0.40 ± 0.05 [0.29–0.50]	0.57 ± 0.09 [0.39–0.78]		
Morrison et al. 1992	Afghan hound	20	23.0[b] [17.0–36.0]	1.86[b] [1.46–2.30]	1.24[b] [0.88–1.64]	0.57[b] [0.35–0.80]	0.57[b] [0.35–0.80]	0.40[b] [0.31–0.49]	0.53[b] [0.40–0.80]	1.15[b] [0.88–1.50]	1.15[b] [0.80–1.55]
de Madron 1983	Generic	27	24.4 ± 19.2 [2.7–95.0]	1.91 ± 0.16 [1.49–2.16]	1.29 ± 0.16 [0.99–1.68]	0.36 ± 0.08 [0.23–0.54]	0.52 ± 0.07 [0.36–0.65]	0.33 ± 0.07 [0.22–0.52]	0.51 ± 0.09 [0.32–0.72]	1.06 ± 0.15 [0.81–1.38]	1.05 ± 0.17 [0.39–1.26]

Brown et al. 2003	Generic	50	25.2 ± 17.4 [2.3–76.4]	1.59 ± 0.15 [1.30–1.85]	1.04 ± 0.16 [0.78–1.36]	0.44 ± 0.06 [0.28–0.57]	0.59 ± 0.09 [0.40–0.79]	0.41 ± 0.06 [0.29–0.57]	0.60 ± 0.08 [0.43–0.76]	1.00 ± 0.12 [0.81–1.43]	1.01 ± 0.11 [0.76–1.26]
Page et al. 1993	Greyhound	16	26.6 ± 3.5 [20.7–32.5]	1.86 ± 0.12 [1.69–2.06]	1.37 ± 0.15 [1.22–1.60]	0.45 ± 0.07 [0.34–0.59]	0.56 ± 0.11 [0.42–0.72]	0.51 ± 0.07 [0.38–0.59]	0.64 ± 0.09 [0.51–0.76]		
Della Torre et al. 2000[a]	Greyhound	20	26.9 ± 3.3 [21.7–31.5]	1.79 ± 0.13 [1.62–2.05]	1.35 ± 0.10 [1.22–1.58]	0.05 ± 0.04 [0.43–0.62]	0.66 ± 0.04 [0.54–0.74]	0.54 ± 0.04 [0.49–0.60]	0.72 ± 0.05 [0.65–0.90]		
Goncalves et al. 2002[a]	Generic	70	27.7 ± 19.5 [3.9–97.7]	1.52 ± 0.14 [1.21–1.79]	0.95 ± 0.13 [0.61–1.24]	0.52 ± 0.08 [0.38–0.70]	0.70 ± 0.09 [0.54–0.93]	0.42 ± 0.11 [0.29–1.15]	0.63 ± 0.10 [0.45–0.91]	0.93 ± 0.12 [0.71–1.48]	1.13 ± 0.14 [0.89–1.50]
Snyder et al. 1995[a]	Greyhound	11	29.1 ± 3.7 [24.9–36.3]	1.92 ± 0.12 [1.68–2.12]	1.37 ± 0.11 [1.20–1.54]	0.55 ± 0.07 [0.44–0.67]		0.48 ± 0.06 [0.34–0.55]			
Lombard[a] Cornell et al. 2004	Generic	23	30.1 ± 7.8 [21.0–44.0]	1.76 ± 0.17 [1.37–2.01]	1.10 ± 0.13 [0.82–1.34]			0.42 ± 0.04 [0.35–0.53]		1.01 ± 0.08 [0.80–1.17]	0.98 ± 0.13 [0.62–1.14]
Vollmar[a] Cornell et al. 2004	Boxer	75	31.0 ± 4.8 [22.5–43.0]	1.66 ± 0.14 [1.39–2.09]	1.12 ± 0.12 [0.84–1.43]	0.39 ± 0.06 [0.27–0.50]	0.55 ± 0.08 [0.41–0.77]	0.40 ± 0.05 [0.26–0.52]	0.59 ± 0.07 [0.42–0.81]	0.92 ± 0.08 [0.79–1.16]	0.99 ± 0.11 [0.73–1.30]
Morrison et al. 1992	Golden retriever	20	32.0[b] [23.0–41.0]	1.78[b] [1.47–2.02]	1.07[b] [0.71–1.39]	0.40[b] [0.32–0.51]	0.55[b] [0.40–0.67]	0.40[b] [0.32–0.48]	0.59[b] [0.40–0.75]	0.95[b] [0.55–1.07]	1.07[b] [0.63–1.27]
Calvert and Brown 1986	Doberman pinscher	21	36.0 [31.0–42.0]	1.78 ± 0.16 [1.56–2.09]	1.17 ± 0.13 [0.95–1.37]	0.37 ± 0.02 [0.30–0.38]	0.54 ± 0.02 [0.50–0.57]	0.37 ± 0.02 [0.34–0.38]	0.54 ± 0.03 [0.50–0.57]	1.14 ± 0.09 [1.07–1.33]	1.01 ± 0.06 [0.84–1.07]
Bayon et al. 1994	Spanish mastiff	12	52.4 ± 3.3 [45.8–59.0]	1.60 ± 0.05 [1.51–1.69]	0.97 ± 0.04 [0.90–1.05]	0.33 ± 0.01 [0.30–0.36]	0.53 ± 0.02 [0.49–0.56]	0.33 ± 0.01 [0.30–0.35]	0.51 ± 0.01 [0.48–0.54]	0.93 ± 0.03 [0.88–0.98]	0.96 ± 0.03 [0.90–1.02]
Koch et al. 1996	Newfoundland	27	61.0 [47.0–69.5]	1.60 [1.41–1.92]	1.13 [0.93–1.41]	0.37 [0.22–0.48]	0.48 [0.35–0.64]	0.32 [0.26–0.42]	0.48 [0.35–0.51]	0.93 [0.83–1.05]	0.96 [0.77–1.05]
Koch et al. 1996	Great Dane	15	62.0 [52.0–75.0]	1.68 [1.40–1.87]	1.26 [1.08–1.43]	0.46 [0.38–0.51]	0.52 [0.44–0.60]	0.40 [0.32–0.51]	0.51 [0.35–0.60]	0.94 [0.89–1.08]	1.05 [0.89–1.46]
Vollmar[a] Cornell et al. 2004	Irish wolfhound	144	63.5 ± 8.3 [45.0–91.0]	1.60 ± 0.12 [1.33–1.88]	1.06 ± 0.11 [0.83–1.29]	0.35 ± 0.06 [0.19–0.51]	0.49 ± 0.07 [0.32–0.67]	0.33 ± 0.05 [0.21–0.47]	0.50 ± 0.06 [0.37–0.65]	1.04 ± 0.09 [0.89–1.30]	1.01 ± 0.11 [0.73–1.26]
Koch et al. 1996	Irish wolfhound	20	68.5 [50.0–80.0]	1.54 [1.41–1.81]	1.11 [1.01–1.38]	0.37 [0.28–0.45]	0.46 [0.34–0.52]	0.31 [0.28–0.40]	0.43 [0.34–0.52]	0.92 [0.89–0.95]	0.95 [0.68–1.08]

[a]Original data supplied by investigators. All others estimated from referenced sources.
[b]Mean or median, ± standard deviation [range].
Index formulas from Table 5.3.

Canine breed-specific M-mode functional and relative indices

Reference	Breed	N	BW (kg)	FS	EF	wΔA	FWTd	FWAd	wWAd	wWAs
Della Torre et al. 2000[a]	Italian greyhound	20	5.4 [3.2–8.4]	0.43 [0.32–0.56]	0.80 [0.68–0.92]	1.75 [0.98–2.25]	0.38 [0.30–0.45]	0.61 [0.51–0.70]	4.11 [2.63–5.20]	4.58 [3.17–6.08]
Häggstrom[a] Cornell et al. 2004	Cavalier King Charles spaniel	57	8.9 [5.5–11.9]	0.33 [0.21–0.44]	0.69 [0.50–0.82]	1.74 [0.94–2.59]				
Crippa et al. 1992	Beagle	20	8.9 [5.9–11.9]	0.40 [0.22–0.58]						
Pedersen[a] Cornell et al. 2004	Dachshund	33	9.5 [6.2–16.0]	0.34 [0.19–0.53]	0.70 [0.46–0.89]	1.63 [0.86–4.35]	0.33 [0.25–0.39]	0.55 [0.44–0.62]	3.51 [1.71–4.36]	4.01 [1.90–5.13]
Baade et al. 2002	West Highland white terrier	24	10.3 [8.5–12.1]	0.35 [0.21–0.49]						
Gooding et al. 1986	English cocker spaniel	12	12.2 [8.5–15.8]	0.34 [0.29–0.43]	0.71 [0.64–0.82]	1.95 [1.52–2.53]	0.32 [0.20–0.38]	0.54 [0.36–0.62]	4.09 [2.26–5.33]	
Della Torre et al. 2000[a]	Whippet	20	14.5 [10.8–20.2]	0.33 [0.25–0.47]	0.69 [0.57–0.85]	1.88 [1.45–2.36]	0.33 [0.29–0.42]	0.55 [0.49–0.66]	4.20 [3.36–5.08]	4.96 [3.97–5.72]
Maschiro et al. 1976	Generic	16	17.6 [11.3–24.0]	0.31 [0.24–0.39]	0.67 [0.57–0.77]	1.72 [1.14–2.13]	0.25 [0.22–0.29]	0.44 [0.39–0.50]	2.59 [2.07–3.39]	
Sisson and Schaeffer 1991	English pointer	16	19.2 [13.6–24.9]	0.36 [0.28–0.44]						
Wey[a] Cornell et al. 2004	Generic	47	20.8 [2.2–47.4]	0.34 [0.23–0.59]	0.69 [0.54–0.93]	1.71 [0.91–2.71]	0.31 [0.25–0.37]	0.53 [0.43–0.61]	3.47 [2.50–4.90]	3.91 [2.46–6.37]
de Madron 1983	Generic	27	24.4 [2.7–95.0]	0.33 [0.22–0.46]	0.69 [0.53–0.84]	1.99 [1.20–2.60]	0.26 [0.19–0.32]	0.46 [0.35–0.54]	3.15 [1.95–5.12]	3.72 [2.21–5.25]
Brown et al. 2003	Generic	50	25.2 [2.3–76.4]	0.34 [0.25–0.50]	0.71 [0.58–0.87]	1.44 [0.78–2.01]	0.35 [0.28–0.44]	0.57 [0.48–0.68]	3.40 [2.21–5.05]	3.94 [2.63–5.13]
Della Torre et al. 2000[a]	Greyhound	20	26.9 [21.7–31.5]	0.25 [0.18–0.32]	0.57 [0.44–0.68]	1.40 [0.87–2.01]	0.37 [0.32–0.42]	0.60 [0.53–0.66]	4.83 [3.87–5.30]	5.62 [4.48–6.32]
Goncalves et al. 2002[a]	Generic	70	27.7 [3.9–97.7]	0.38 [0.30–0.57]	0.75 [0.66–0.92]	1.43 [0.80–2.21]	0.38 [0.30–0.54]	0.61 [0.52–0.79]	3.77 [2.44–7.31]	4.30 [2.81–5.88]
Snyder et al. 1995[a]	Greyhound	11	29.1 [24.9–36.3]	0.29 [0.24–0.37]	0.64 [0.56–0.75]	1.82 [1.39–2.30]	0.35 [0.32–0.40]	0.57 [0.54–0.64]	4.99 [4.04–5.98]	
Lombard[a] Cornell et al. 2004	Generic	23	30.1 [21.0–44.0]	0.38 [0.30–0.49]	0.75 [0.66–0.87]	1.93 [0.95–2.75]				
Vollmar[a] Cornell et al. 2004	Boxer	75	31.0 [22.5–43.0]	0.33 [0.26–0.41]	0.69 [0.59–0.79]	1.50 [0.94–2.35]	0.32 [0.24–0.39]	0.54 [0.42–0.63]	3.23 [1.93–4.47]	3.85 [2.58–5.72]
Bayon et al. 1994	Spanish mastiff	12	52.4 [45.8–59.0]							
Koch et al. 1996	Newfoundland	27	61.0 [47.0–69.5]	0.30 [0.22–0.37]						
Koch et al. 1996	Great Dane	15	62.0 [52.0–75.0]	0.25 [0.18–0.36]						
Vollmar[a] Cornell et al. 2004	Irish wolfhound	144	63.5 [45.0–91.0]	0.34 [0.25–0.45]	0.71 [0.58–0.84]	1.45 [0.95–2.36]	0.30 [0.20–0.36]	0.51 [0.36–0.59]	2.68 [1.56–4.30]	3.09 [1.94–4.19]
Koch et al. 1996	Irish wolfhound	20	68.5 [50.0–80.0]	0.28 [0.20–0.34]						

[a]Original data supplied by investigators. All others from referenced sources.
[b]Mean or median, ± standard deviation [range].
Index formulas from Table 5.3.

Feline M-mode echocardiographic reference values

	References						
	Jacobs et al. 1985	Pipers et al. 1979	Sisson et al. 1991	Moise et al. 1986	Allen and Downey 1983	Allen 1982	Fox et al. 1985
Conditions	Unanesthetized	Unanesthetized	Unanesthetized	Unanesthetized	Xylazine–sodium pentobarbital	Sodium pentobarbital	Ketamine hydrochloride
N	30	25	79	11	8	10	30
BW (kg)	[1.96–6.26]	[2.30–6.80]	[2.70–8.20]	4.30 ± 0.50	3.50 ± 0.41	3.64 ± 0.66	[2.05–6.80]
HR (/min)	[147–242]	[120–240]	[120–240]	182 ± 22	163 ± 13	175 ± 20	[160–300]
RVIDd (cm)	[0.00–0.70]						[0.12–0.75]
IVSd (cm)	[0.22–0.40]	[0.28–0.60]	[0.30–0.60]	0.50 ± 0.07		0.40 ± 0.03	[0.22–0.49]
LVIDd (cm)	[1.20–1.98]	[1.12–2.18]	[1.08–2.14]	1.51 ± 0.21	1.29 ± 0.09	1.30 ± 0.12	[1.07–1.73]
LVWd (cm)	[0.22–0.44]	[0.32–0.56]	[0.25–0.60]	0.46 ± 0.05		0.40 ± 0.40	[0.21–0.45]
RVWs (cm)	[0.23–0.43]						
RVIDs (cm)	[0.27–0.94]						
IVSs (cm)	[0.47–0.70]		[0.40–0.90]	0.76 ± 0.12			
LVIDs (cm)	[0.52–1.08]	[0.64–1.68]	[0.40–1.12]	0.69 ± 0.22	0.88 ± 0.08	0.86 ± 0.16	[0.49–1.16]
LVWs (cm)	[0.54–0.81]		[0.43–0.98]	0.78 ± 0.10			
Ao (cm)	[0.72–1.19]	[0.40–1.18]	[0.60–1.21]	0.95 ± 0.15		0.90 ± 0.07	[0.71–1.15]
LA (cm)	[0.93–1.51]	[0.45–1.12]	[0.70–1.70]	1.21 ± 0.18		1.00 ± 0.07	[0.72–1.33]
LA/Ao	[0.95–1.65]		[0.88–1.79]	1.29 ± 0.23			[0.73–1.64]
FS	[0.39–0.61]	[0.23–0.56]	[0.40–0.67]	0.55 ± 0.10	0.31 ± 0.47	0.35 ± 0.25	[0.30–0.60]
EPSS (cm)	[0.00–0.21]		[0.00–0.20]	0.04 ± 0.07			

Mean ± standard deviation [range].

Canine Doppler outflow reference values

	References						
	Kirberger et al. 1992	Kirberger et al. 1992	Brown et al. 1991	Darke et al. 1993	Gaber 1987	Yuill and O'Grady 1991	Bonagura and Miller 1989
Method	CWD	PWD	PWD		PWD	CWD	PWD
Aortic V_{peak} (m/s)	1.49 ± 0.27 [0.99–2.10]	1.57 ± 0.33 [1.06–2.29]	1.06 ± 0.21 [0.65–1.37]	1.19 ± 0.24	1.19 ± 0.18	1.18 ± 0.11 [1.04–1.38]	1.20 [–1.70]
Aortic VTI (m)			0.146 ± 0.029				
Aortic AT (s)		0.055 ± 0.015		0.050 ± 0.010			
Aortic ET (s)		0.182 ± 0.029	0.205 ± 0.015				
Aortic PEP (s)		0.058 ± 0.012					
Aortic PEP/ET				0.22 ± 0.06			
Aortic acceleration (cm/s)		32.00 ± 14.00		34.00 ± 16.00			
Pulmonic V_{peak} (m/s)	1.25 ± 0.26 [0.60–1.91]	1.20 ± 0.20 [0.88–1.20]	0.84 ± 0.17 [0.34–1.29]	0.99 ± 0.22	1.00 ± 0.15	0.98 ± 0.09 [0.76–1.22]	1.07 [–1.30]
Pulmonic VTI (m)			0.131 ± 0.028				
Pulmonic AT (s)		0.08 ± 0.02		0.07 ± 0.02			
Pulmonic ET (s)		0.184 ± 0.028	0.219 ± 0.018				
Pulmonic PEP (s)		0.051 ± 0.010					
Pulmonic PEP/ET				0.14 ± 0.03			

Mean ± standard deviation [range].

Canine Doppler inflow reference values

	References					
	Yuill and O'Grady 1991	Gaber 1987	Kirberger et al. 1992	Darke et al. 1993	Bonagura and Miller 1989	Yamamoto and Masuyama 1993
Mitral E_{peak} (m/s)	0.86 ± 0.10 [0.70–1.08]	0.75 ± 0.12	0.91 ± 0.15 [0.59–1.18]	0.65 ± 0.18	0.76 [–1.00]	0.56 ± 0.18
Mitral A_{peak} (m/s)			0.63 ± 0.13 [0.33–0.93]	0.43 ± 0.13	0.49 [–0.75]	0.44 ± 0.11
Mitral E_{peak}/A_{peak}			1.48 ± 0.31 [1.04–2.42]	1.55 ± 0.36		1.30 ± 0.30
Mitral VTI (m)						0.094 ± 0.032
Tricuspid E_{peak} (m/s)	0.69 ± 0.08 [0.52–0.92]	0.56 ± 0.16	0.86 ± 0.20 [0.49–1.31]	0.57 ± 0.15	0.60 [–0.80]	
Tricuspid A_{peak} (m/s)			0.58 ± 0.16 [0.33–0.94]	0.37 ± 0.15	0.48 [–0.60]	
Tricuspid E_{peak}/A_{peak}			1.60 ± 0.56 [0.69–3.08]	1.62 ± 0.36		

Systolic time interval reference values (canine and feline)

	References		
	Boon et al. 1983	Atkins and Snyder 1992	Atkins and Snyder 1992
Species	Canine	Canine	Feline
HR (/min)	98 ± 24	124 ± 23	226 ± 25
LVET (s)	0.178 ± 0.017	0.159 ± 0.015	0.116 ± 0.019
PEP (s)	0.057 ± 0.018	0.054 ± 0.007	0.046 ± 0.005
PEP/LVET	0.32 ± 0.11	0.24 ± 0.05	0.40 ± 0.05
Vcf (/s)	2.21 ± 0.40	2.48 ± 0.50	4.00 ± 0.90

References

Allen DG (1982) Echocardiographic study of the anesthetized cat. Can J Comp Med 46:115–122.

Allen DG, Downey RS (1983) Echocardiographic assessment of cats anesthetized with xylazine–sodium pentobarbital. Can J Comp Med 47:281–283.

Atkins CE, Snyder PS (1992) Systolic time intervals and their derivatives for evaluation of cardiac function. J Vet Intern Med 6:55–63.

Baade H, Schober K, Oechtering G (2002) Echocardiographic reference values in West Highland White Terriers with special regard to right heart function. Tierarztl Prax 30:172–179.

Bayon A, Fernandez del Palacio MJ, Montes AM, Gutierrez Panizo C (1994) M-mode echocardiography study in growing Spanish mastiffs. J Small Anim Pract 35:473–479.

Bonagura JD, Miller MW (1989) Veterinary echocardiography. Am J Cardiovasc Ultrasound Allied Tech 6:229–264.

Boon J, Wingfield WE, Miller CW (1983) Echocardiographic indices in the normal dog. Vet Radiol 24:214–221.

Brown DJ, Knight DH, King RR (1991) Use of pulsed-wave Doppler echocardiography to determine aortic and pulmonary velocity and flow variables in clinically normal dogs. Am J Vet Res 52:543–550.

Brown DJ, Rush JE, MacGregor J, Ross JN, Brewer B, Rand W (2003) M-mode echocardiographic ratio indices in normal dogs, cats, and horses: A novel quantitative method. J Vet Intern Med 17:653–662.

Calvert CA, Brown J (1986) Use of M-mode echocardiography in the diagnosis of congestive cardiomyopathy in Doberman pinschers. J Am Vet Med Assoc 189:293–297.

Cornell CC, Kittleson MD, Della Torre P, et al. (2004) Allometric scaling of M-mode variables in normal adult dogs. J Vet Intern Med 18:311–321.

Crippa L, Ferro E, Melloni E, Brambilla P, Cavalletti E (1992) Echocardiographic parameters and indices in the normal beagle dog. Lab Anim 26:190–195.

Darke PGG, Fuentes VL, Champion SR (1993) Doppler echocardiography in canine congestive cardiomyopathy. In: 11th ACVIM Forum, pp 531–534.

de Madron E (1983) M-mode echocardiography in the dog (L'echocardiographie en mode M chez le chien normal) 76: Ecole Nationale Veterinaire d'Alfort.

Della Torre PK, Kirby AC, Church DB, Malik R (2000) Echocardiographic measurements in greyhounds, whippets, and Italian greyhounds: Dogs with similar conformation but different size. Aust Vet J 78:49–55.

Fox PR, Bond BR, Peterson ME (1985) Echocardiographic reference values in healthy cats sedated with ketamine hydrochloride. Am J Vet Res 46:1479–1484.

Gaber C (1987) Normal pulsed Doppler flow velocities in adult dogs. In: 5th ACVIM Forum, p 923.

Goncalves AC, Orton EC, Boon JA, Salman MD (2002) Linear, logarithmic, and polynomial models of M-mode echocardiographic measurements in dogs. Am J Vet Res 63:994–999.

Gooding JP, Robinson WF, Mews GC (1986) Echocardiographic assessment of left ventricular dimensions in clinically normal English cocker spaniels. Am J Vet Res 47:296–300.

Jacobs G, Knight DH (1985) M-mode echocardiographic measurements in nonanesthetized healthy cats: Effects of body weight, heart rate, and other variables. Am J Vet Res 46:1705–1711.

Kirberger RM, Bland-van den Berg P, Grimbeek RJ (1992) Doppler echocardiography in the normal dog: Part II. Factors influencing blood flow velocities and a comparison betwen left and right heart blood flow. Vet Radiol Ultrasound 33:380–386.

Koch J, Pedersen HD, Jensen AL, Flagstad A (1996) M-mode echocardiographic diagnosis of dilated cardiomyopathy in giant breed dogs. J Vet Med 43:297–304.

Maschiro I, Nelson RR, Cohn JN, Franciosa JA (1976) Ventricular dimensions measured noninvasively by echocardiography in the awake dog. J App Physiol 41:953–959.

Moise NS, Dietze AE, Mezza LE, Strickland D, Erb HN, Edwards NJ (1986) Echocardiography, electrocardiography, and radiography of cats with dilatation cardiomyopathy, hypertrophic cardiomyopathy, and hyperthyroidism. Am J Vet Res 47:1476–1486.

Morrison SA, Moise NS, Scarlett J, Mohammed H, Yeager AE (1992) Effect of breed and body weight on echocardiographic values in four breeds of dogs of differing somatotype. J Vet Intern Med 6:220–224.

Page A, Edmunds G, Atwell RB (1993) Echocardiographic values in the greyhound. Aust Vet J 70:361–364.

Pipers FS, Reef V, Hamlin RL (1979) Echocardiography in the domestic cat. Am J Vet Res 40:882–886.

Sisson D, Schaeffer D (1991) Changes in linear dimensions of the heart, relative to body weight, as measured by M-mode echocardiography in growing dogs. Am J Vet Res 52:1591–1596.

Sisson DD, Knight DH, Helinski C, et al. (1991) Plasma taurine concentrations and M-mode echocardiographic measures in healthy cats and in cats with dilated cardiomyopathy. J Vet Intern Med 5:232–238.

Snyder PS, Sato T, Atkins CE (1995) A comparison of echocardiographic indices of the nonracing healthy greyhound to reference values from other breeds. Vet Radiol Ultrasound 36:387–392.

Yamamoto K, Masuyama TJT (1993) Effects of heart rate on the left ventricular filling dynamics: Assessment from simultaneous recordings of pulsed Doppler transmitral flow velocity pattern and haemodynamic variables. Cardiovasc Res 27:935–941.

Yuill CDM, O'Grady MR (1991) Doppler-derived velocity of blood flow across the cardiac valves in the normal dog. Can J Vet Res 55:185–192.

CHAPTER SIX

LIVER

Marc-André d'Anjou

PREPARATION AND SCANNING TECHNIQUE

Hair clipping of animals should cover the entire cranial abdomen and ideally the last one or two intercostal spaces, particularly in deep-chested dogs or if microhepatica is suspected. Animals can be scanned in dorsal, left, or right recumbency after acoustic gel application. The ability to visualize the liver in small animals is related to body conformation, liver size, and overlying gastrointestinal content. In small dogs and cats, the liver can usually be entirely scanned in transverse and longitudinal planes by means of a subcostal approach (Figure 6.1), as long as the stomach is not overly distended with ingesta or gas. The transverse colon can also limit hepatic visibility, particularly if filled with gas or feces, or if the liver is small. In these instances, an intercostal approach can provide a useful alternative. In large deep-chested dogs, the liver is completely hidden by the rib cage, routinely requiring the use of an intercostal approach to reach all parts of the liver. In these dogs, and especially if the liver is atrophied, several other structures, such as the spleen, can move under the costal arch and should not be confused for a portion of the liver. In obese animals, the presence of a large amount of falciform fat can also reduce hepatic visibility by increasing the distance between the sonographic probe and the organ and by degrading image quality because of beam scattering.

The appropriate probe must be chosen based on the size and depth of the liver. In small or medium-sized dogs and cats, a medium-frequency probe (5 MHz and higher) can be used unless the liver is markedly enlarged, whereas a probe with more penetration (5 MHz and lower) is required in larger dogs. Sectorial or convex probes are preferred over linear probes because of the triangular shaped scanned field of view that enables larger portions of the liver to be imaged. A smaller footprint also enables most parts of the liver to be reached through limited acoustic windows such as intercostal spaces. Gain settings and focal zones must be constantly adjusted during the exam in order to optimize ultrasonographic penetration and image quality (Figure 6.2).

ULTRASONOGRAPHIC ANATOMY OF THE NORMAL LIVER

Parenchyma and Size

In dogs and cats, the liver is composed of four lobes, four sublobes, and two processes: left lobe (lateral and medial), quadrate lobe, right lobe (lateral and medial), and caudate lobe (caudate and papillary processes) (Evans 1993a; Hudson and Hamilton 1993), which cannot be easily distinguished unless separated by peritoneal effusion (Figure 6.3).

The left lobe forms a third to nearly a half of the entire liver mass and contacts the left portion of the gallbladder (GB). The quadrate lobe is relatively central and partially encircles the GB. The right portion of the GB is in contact with the right medial lobe. The caudate process of the caudate lobe is the most caudal extension of the liver, on the right side, and extends to the level of the right kidney. The hepatic and portal veins (PVs) of each of these hepatic lobe divisions are relatively constant in dogs and can represent useful ultrasonographic landmarks (Carlisle et al. 1995).

A large part of the liver is beneath the costal arch, just cranial to the stomach, in dogs and cats. Its cranial margin lies against the diaphragm and lung interface. The diaphragm appears as a curved hyperechoic line, sometimes associated with a mirror-image artifact (Figure 6.4).

Caudally, the liver is often in contact with the spleen on the left side and with the right kidney on the right side at the level of the renal fossa of the caudate lobe. The hepatic volume is difficult to evaluate objectively in cats and dogs, mainly because of the variability in body conformation. As with radiography, the costal arch and location of the stomach can help in

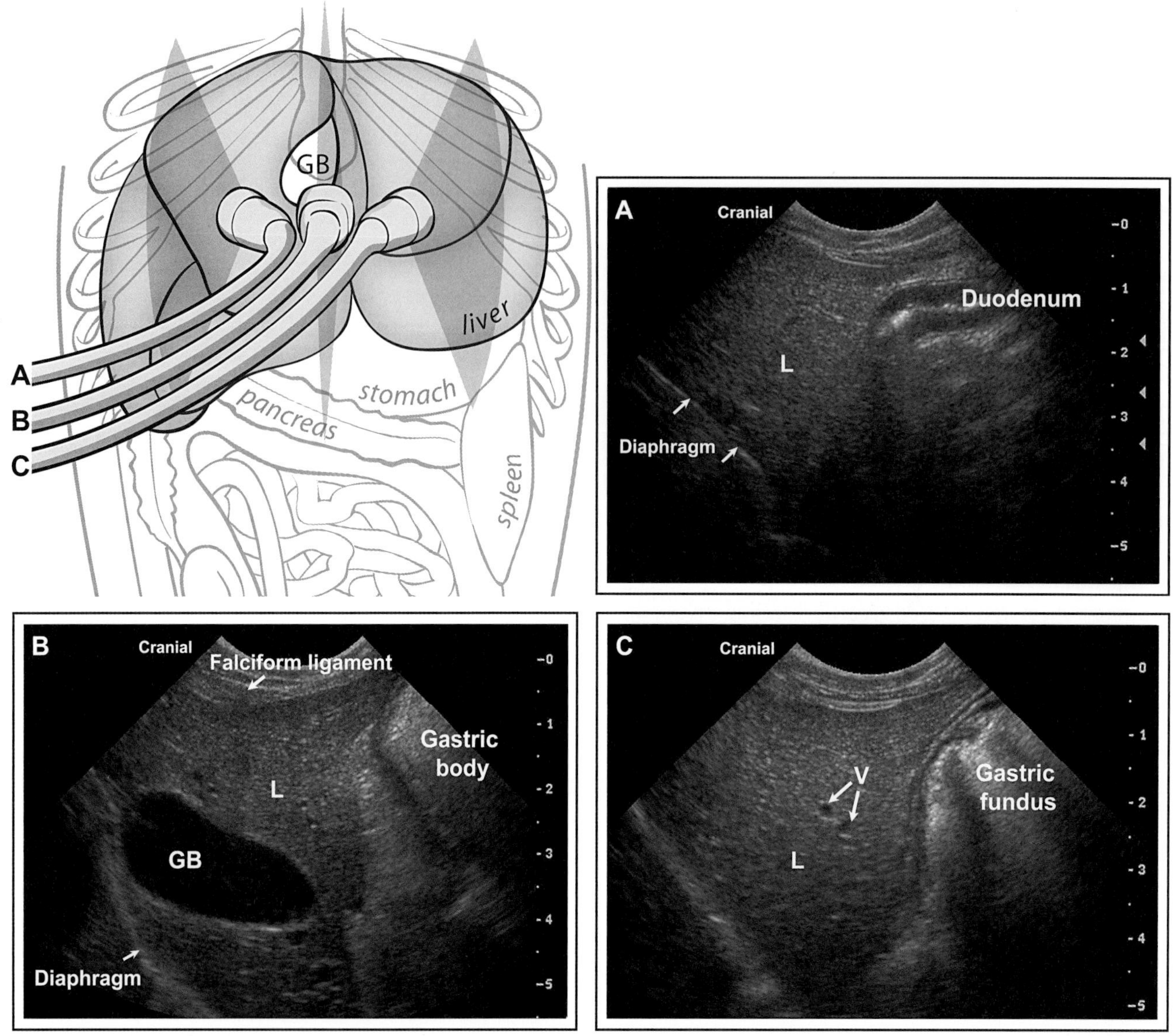

Figure 6.1. Ultrasonographic approach and anatomy of the normal liver. Illustration of the scanning technique using a subcostal approach with a dog or a cat in dorsal recumbency. The ultrasound probe must be moved in order to cover the entire liver, sequentially in sagittal **(A–C)** and transverse **(D–F)** planes. The additional use of oblique planes, as well as an intercostal approach, can be necessary in some patients. **A–C:** Using a longitudinal plane in a dog, the probe is sequentially moved from the right **(A)** to the left **(C)** of the liver (L). The intimate relation between the duodenum-stomach and the liver is visualized. The falciform ligament, which can vary in size because of fat deposition, is in the near field. Hepatic vessels (V) appear as round, anechoic structures on cross section. The gallbladder (GB), located to the right of the midline, is a useful landmark. **D–F:** By using a transverse plane, the liver is also entirely scanned, from its cranioventral portion **(D)** to its caudodorsal portion **(F)**. The gallbladder is seen on the right in the midportion of the liver **(E)**. Branching portal veins (PV) with hyperechoic boundaries are also recognized.

subjectively evaluating liver size, taking into account body conformation. The caudal extension of the hepatic lobes can be compared with the location of the last pair of ribs (Figure 6.5A). In deep-chested dogs, the liver does not usually reach the costal arch, and the stomach is often cranially located. Conversely, in small dog breeds and in cats, the liver normally extends to the costal arch. The caudal tips of the hepatic lobes normally are pointed. With severe hepatomegaly, these tips are rounded and can extend beyond the right kidney and/or reach the left kidney, depending on the symmetry of the enlargement (Figure 6.5B).

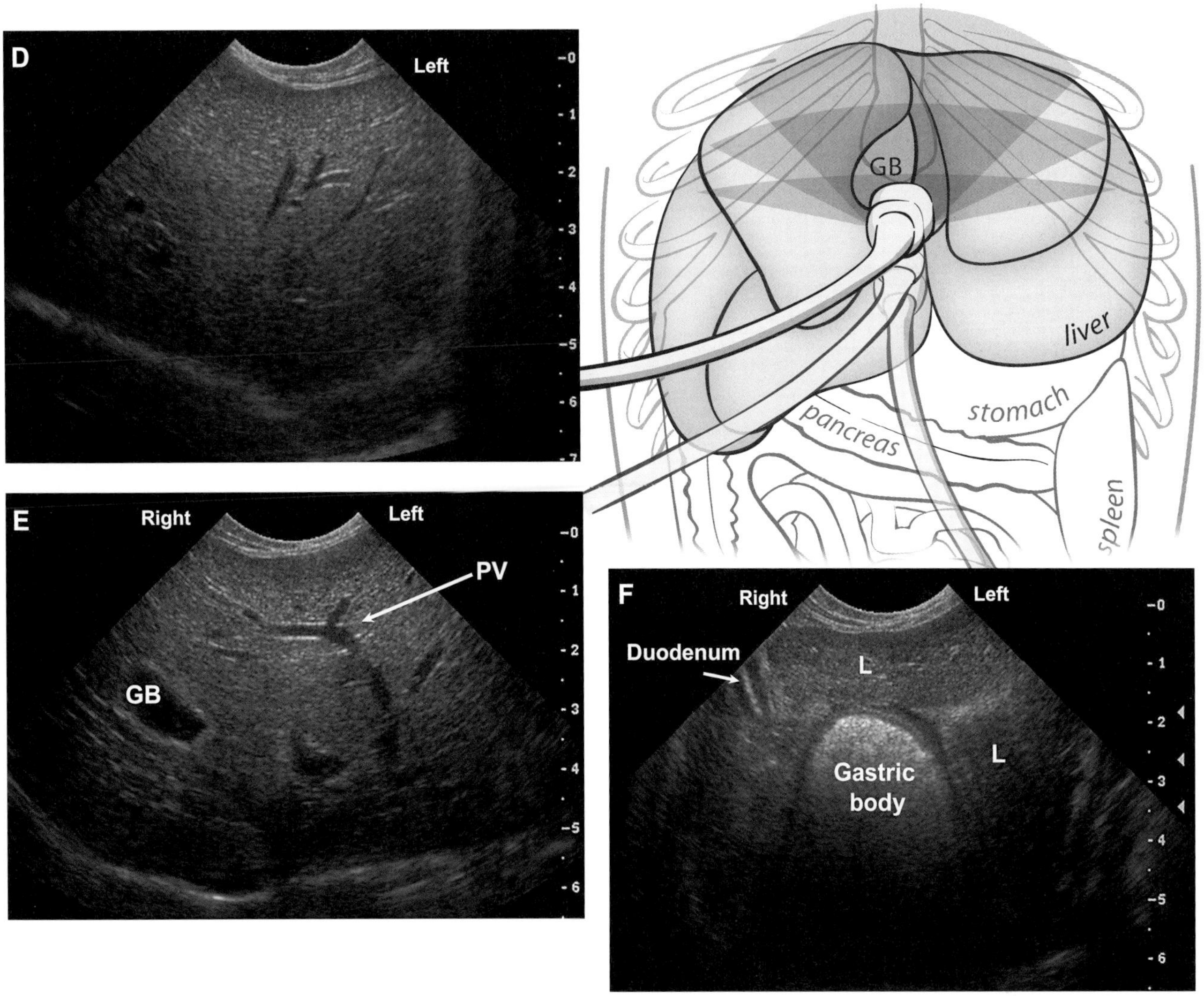

Figure 6.1. *Continued*

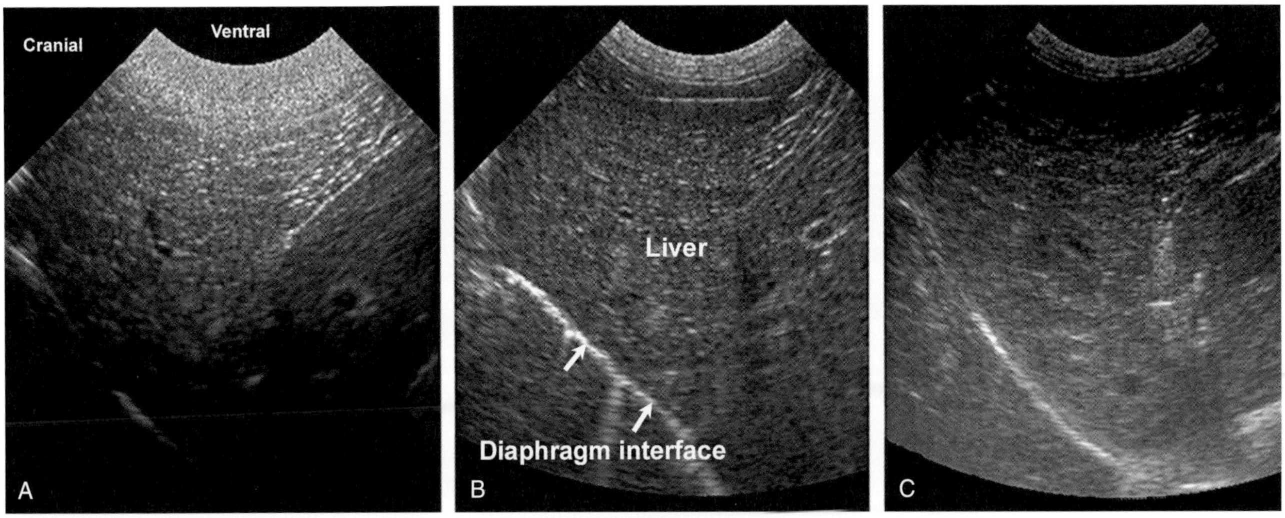

Figure 6.2. Gain setting. Because of the attenuation of the ultrasound beam as it travels through soft tissues, the amplification of echoes received must be adjusted according to tissue type and depth. This modulation can be made using time-gain compensation bars or far/near/general gain knobs. These three images show the variation in echogenicity of a normal liver with **(A)** excessive near gain and insufficient far gain, **(B)** well-adjusted near and far gains, and **(C)** insufficient near gain and excessive far gain.

The falciform ligament filled with a variable amount of fat is ventral to the liver and protrudes between the right and left portions, dorsal to the xiphoid process (Figure 6.6). This poorly defined structure is usually isoechoic or hyperechoic to the liver and presents a coarse echotexture relative to the liver. However, clinically obese cats may have a liver that is hyperechoic to the falciform fat (Nicoll et al. 1998). The normal hepatic parenchyma is uniformly hypoechoic, with a coarser echotexture, when compared with the spleen. Its echogenicity relative to the renal cortices is more variable, although usually hyperechoic (Figure 6.7).

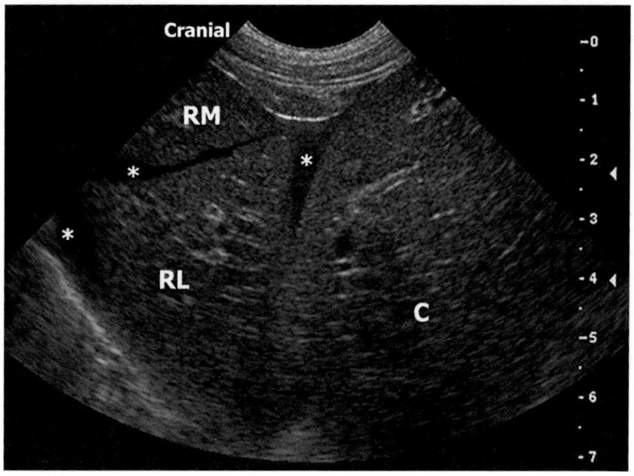

Figure 6.3. Effusion separating hepatic lobes. Longitudinal oblique image of the right portion of the liver with three distinct separate lobes well outlined by peritoneal effusion (*). C, caudate lobe; RL, right lateral; and RM, right medial.

Biliary System

The biliary system is relatively similar in dogs and cats. The GB, occasionally bilobed in cats (Figure 6.8), represents the bile reservoir and is an anechoic teardrop-shaped structure with a conical extension: the cystic duct. The GB can vary markedly in size among animals and becomes enlarged in anorexic animals. Therefore, its volume alone cannot be used as a reliable sign of biliary obstruction. The wall of the normal GB is thin and smooth, measuring less than 1 mm thick in cats (Hittmair et al. 2001) and less than 2–3 mm in dogs (Spaulding 2003). Biliary sludge can accumulate in normal GB and is usually considered nonsignificant, particularly in dogs (Bromel et al. 1998)

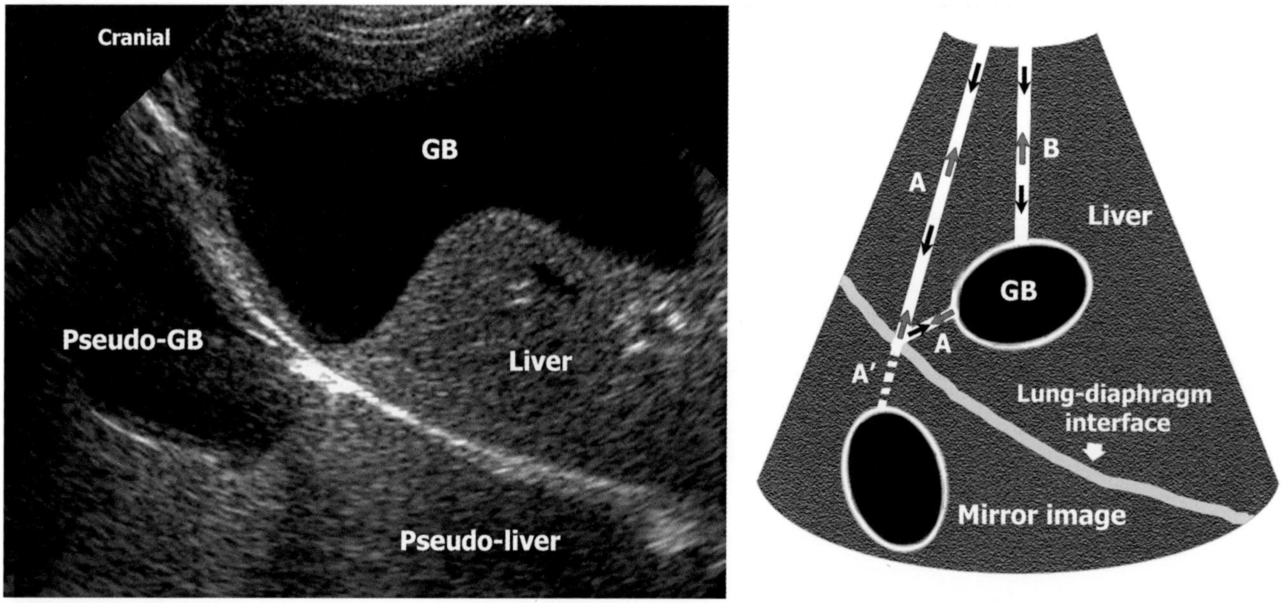

Figure 6.4. Mirror image of liver and gallbladder. Sagittal ultrasonographic and schematic images of a mirror artifact commonly visualized at the lung-diaphragm interface. Hepatic structures including the gallbladder (GB) are artifactually reflected beyond the lung surface. The smooth, curved, lung-diaphragm interface acts as a mirror intensely reflecting the ultrasound waves (black arrows along path A) back to the liver and the gallbladder. This relatively intense beam interacts again with the hepatic structures and is partially reflected back to the diaphragm and eventually to the ultrasound probe along the same path (gray arrows). Because of the increased travel time, the spatial localization of these multireflected echoes appears deeper beyond the diaphragm in the animal. In fact, the computer assumes that the reflected path A is actually located at A′. This mirror image is added to the accurately localized structures (path B). Care must be taken not to confuse a mirror image with a thoracic pathology.

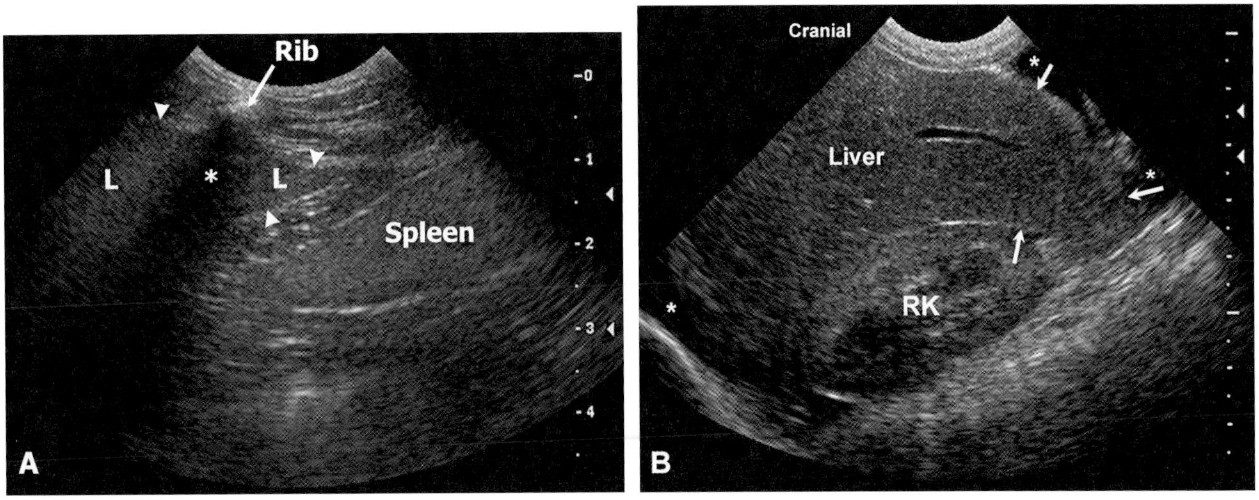

Figure 6.5. Evaluation of liver size. **A: Normal liver.** Left parasagittal image of the cranial abdomen in a normal small-breed dog with the caudal tip of the liver (L and arrowheads) extending slightly beyond the last rib. Acoustic shadowing (*) is noted deep to this hyperattenuating structure. The tip of the liver appears smooth and pointy. **B: Hepatomegaly.** On this sagittal image of the liver obtained in the right cranial abdomen of a dog, a liver lobe (arrows) extends caudal to the right kidney (RK) and has a rounded tip consistent with enlargement. Passive hepatic congestion was diagnosed, and peritoneal effusion (*) was also detected.

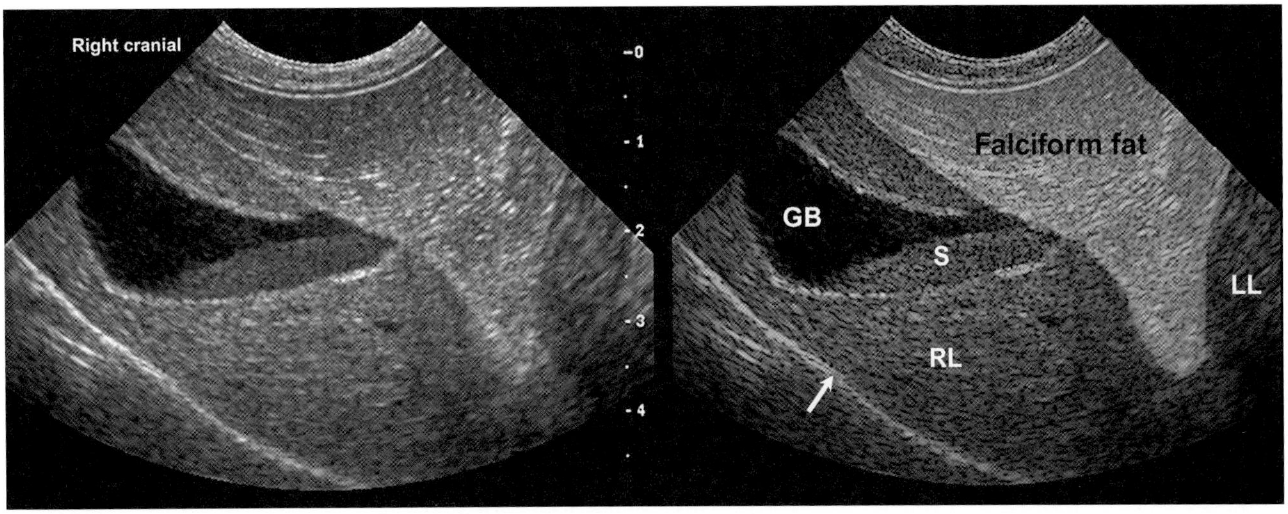

Figure 6.6. Falciform ligament. On these sagittal oblique ultrasonographic and corresponding schematic images of the liver, the falciform fat appears as a triangular hyperechoic structure with a coarse echotexture protruding between the right and left portions of the liver. The gallbladder (GB) contains a small amount of biliary sludge (S) in its dependent portion (dorsal recumbency). The arrow points to the lung-diaphragm interface. LL, left liver; and RL, right liver.

(Figure 6.9). The sludge is then mobile, sometimes giving the impression of an aggregate mimicking a soft-tissue mass. However, the movement of the echogenic substance should respond to gravity after the animal is repositioned. Additionally, because of the relatively low attenuation of the ultrasound beam through the bile, acoustic enhancement is commonly observed beyond the GB (Figure 6.9). This artifact must be differentiated from a focal hyperechoic hepatic lesion.

The intrahepatic biliary tree, composed of biliary canaliculi and larger biliary ducts, is not seen in normal patients. The common bile duct (CBD), which represents the continuation of the connecting GB cystic duct and biliary ducts, can be seen more easily in normal cats than in normal dogs. The CBD can be visualized

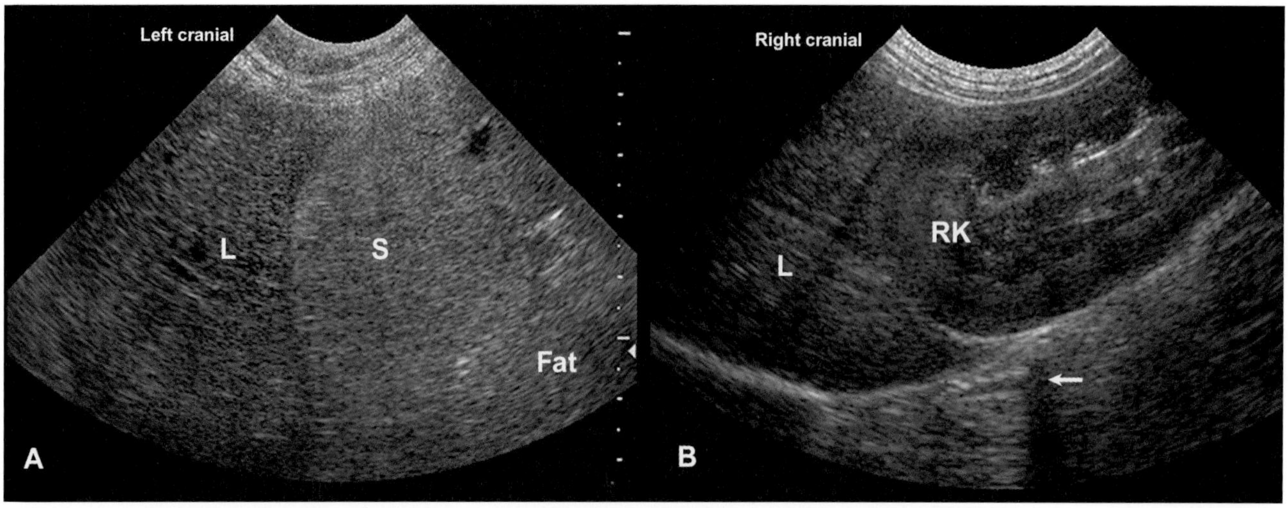

Figure 6.7. Liver, spleen, and kidney relative echogenicities and echotextures. **A:** Sagittal image obtained in the left cranial abdomen of a normal dog. The liver (L) is in contact with the spleen (S), and is relatively hypoechoic and more granular in echotexture. **B:** Sagittal image obtained in the right cranial abdomen of a normal dog. The liver (L) appears relatively isoechoic to the cortex of the right kidney (RK). Acoustic shadowing (arrow) is caused by one of the last ribs.

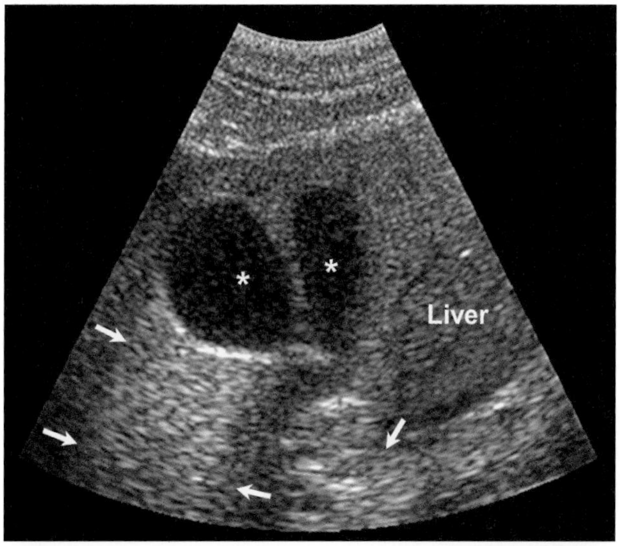

Figure 6.8. Bilobed gallbladder in a cat. On this transverse image obtained in the right-central portion of the liver of a normal cat, the gallbladder is partially divided into two compartments (*). This represents an incidental finding in cats. Far acoustic enhancement is noted in the liver dorsal to these fluid-filled cavities (arrows).

between the proximal duodenum (ventrally) and the PV (dorsally) (Figure 6.10). It can be up to 3 mm wide in normal dogs (Zeman et al. 1981) and 4 mm wide in normal cats (Léveillé et al. 1996). It parallels the PV over a few centimeters before entering into the duodenum through the major duodenal papilla.

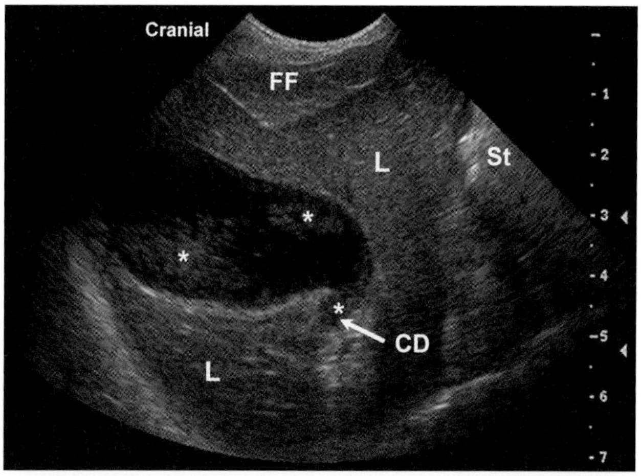

Figure 6.9. Biliary sludge. Longitudinal image of the right-central portion of the liver of a normal dog with the GB and cystic duct (CD) containing poorly defined echogenic material consistent with biliary sludge. The mobility of this sludge was confirmed by repositioning the animal during the exam. FF, falciform fat; L, liver; and St, stomach.

Hepatic Vasculature

The afferent vascular flow to the liver is dual, with a larger proportion coming from the PV (80%) and the rest coming from the hepatic arteries (Evans 1993a) (Figure 6.11). The efferent flow follows the hepatic veins into the caudal vena cava (CVC). This particular vascular pattern is divided into all hepatic lobes and can aid in distinguishing these lobes. When using

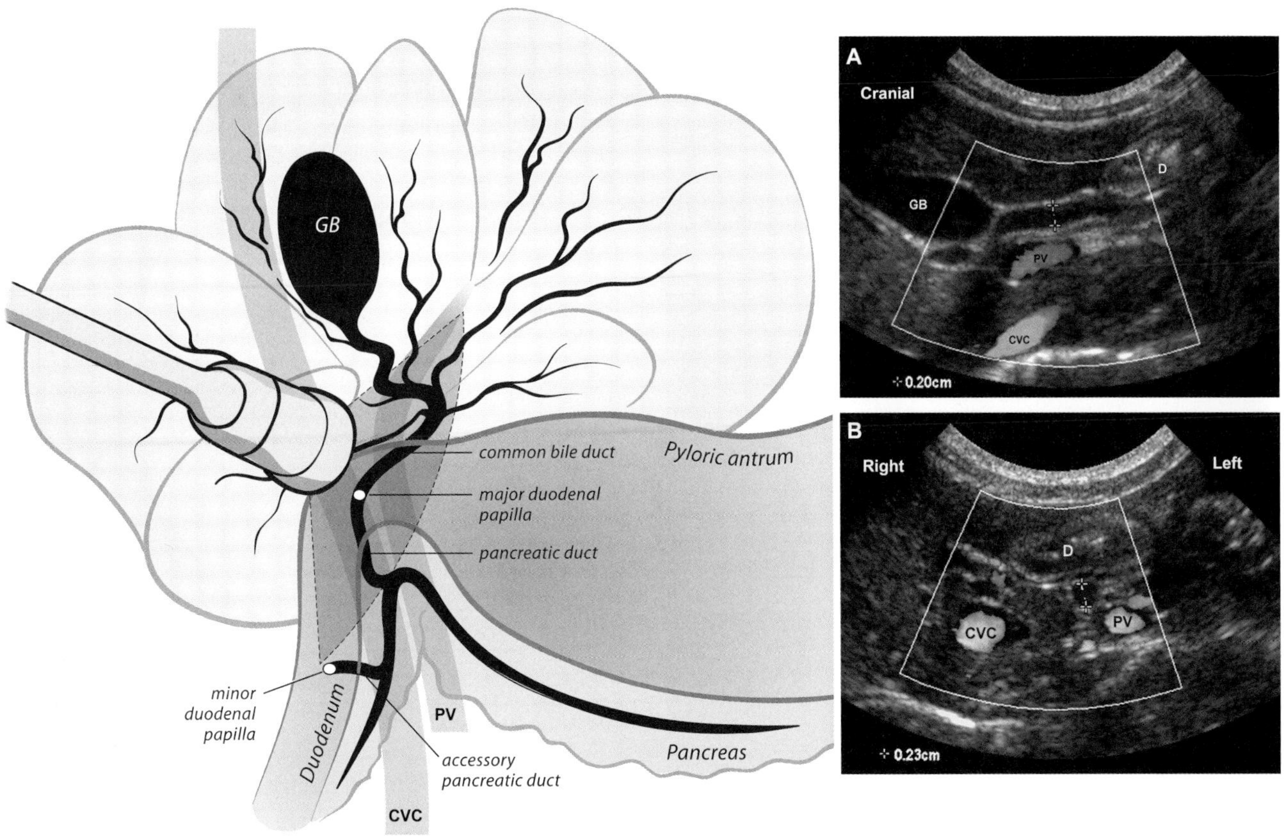

Figure 6.10. Scanning technique for the common bile duct in a cat. Schematic representation of the regional anatomy and landmarks of the biliary tract in the cat, with the ultrasound probe placed to obtain a longitudinal view **(A)** of the common bile duct. The probe is then rotated to obtain a transverse plane **(B)**. The common bile duct (2 mm wide) is found just ventral to the portal vein (PV) and dorsal to the proximal duodenum (D). This duct can sometimes be followed to the level of the major duodenal papilla, at the same level as the pancreatic duct termination. CVC, caudal vena cava; and GB, gallbladder.

B-mode imaging, only the hepatic and PVs (larger than the arteries) can be seen as anechoic, branching, smoothly tapering tubular structures. The walls of the PVs appear hyperechoic, regardless of the orientation of the ultrasonographic beam, facilitating their identification (Figure 6.12). However, the walls of the hepatic veins can also appear hyperechoic when the ultrasonographic beam is directed perpendicularly (see Figure 6.71).

The visibility of the larger and smaller branches of these veins is influenced by patient size, vascular luminal diameter, portal flow, pressure in the CVC, hepatic parenchymal echogenicity, and image quality and resolution. When measured at the same depth, the hepatic and portal branches should be relatively symmetrical in diameter (Figure 6.12B).

The use of color Doppler facilitates the identification and distinction of hepatic vessels. When using standard color-map settings, portal flow directed from the center to the periphery appears as a red signal, whereas hepatic venous flow appears as a blue signal (Figure 6.12B). Arterial flow, also directed from the center to the periphery, can also demonstrate a red signal, depending on the size of the arteries and the Doppler settings, such as gain and filtration threshold.

Extrahepatic Portal Vasculature

The extrahepatic portion of the PV is relatively central in the abdomen, ventral to the CVC, and ventral and to the right of the aorta (Figure 6.13). The main PV is more tortuous than the CVC and aorta, and curves slightly to the right side before entering the liver. When measured at the level of the porta hepatis, its luminal diameter varies between 3.4 and 5.0 mm in normal cats and between 3.3 and 10.5 mm in normal dogs. When comparing the maximal luminal diameter of the PV and the aorta, PV-aorta ratios of 0.71–1.25 are normally expected in these two species (d'Anjou et al. 2004).

The main PV is formed by the confluence of the cranial and caudal mesenteric veins and splenic vein,

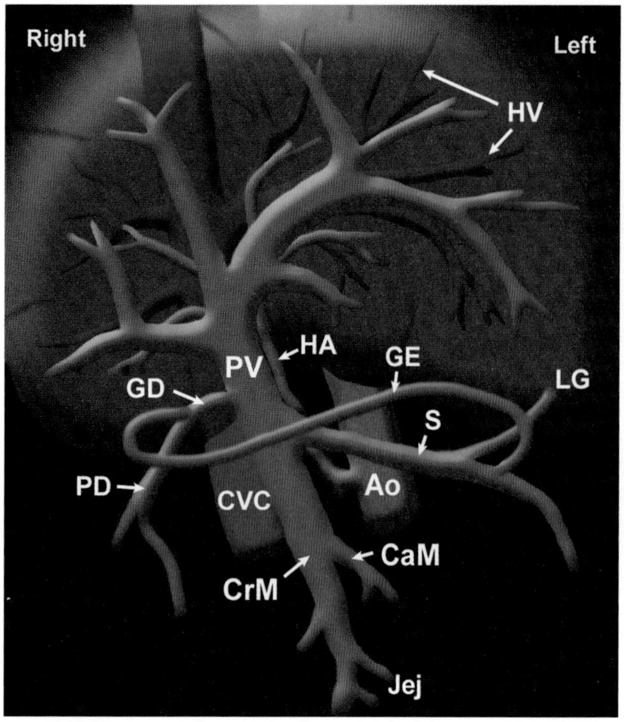

Figure 6.11. Portal vascular system. Schematic illustration of the hepatic vasculature and extrahepatic portal system of dogs and cats, as seen from a ventral approach. The liver receives its vascular supply through the portal vein (PV) and hepatic arteries (HA). The portal vein receives several smaller veins draining most abdominal viscera. The relationship with the caudal vena cava (CVC) and aorta (Ao) is also illustrated. HV, hepatic veins. Veins of the portal system: CaM, caudal mesenteric; CrM, cranial mesenteric; GD, gastroduodenal; GE, gastroepiploic; Jej, jejunal; LG, left gastric, PD, pancreaticoduodenal; and S, splenic.

and therefore drains most abdominal organs (Evans 1993b) (Figure 6.11). It also receives a smaller tributary, the gastroduodenal vein, only a few centimeters caudal to the hepatic entrance. The gastroduodenal vein connects to the right-ventral aspect of the PV after receiving the pancreaticoduodenal and gastroepiploic veins. A few centimeters more caudally, the main PV receives the splenic vein on the left side, which follows the left limb of the pancreas after receiving the left gastric vein. The cranial mesenteric vein receiving all jejunal branches represents the caudal extension of the main PV after the entry of the smaller caudal mesenteric vein another few centimeters caudal to the splenic vein. These portal tributaries enlarge as they approach the main PV, and the flow of all is directed toward the liver (*hepatopetal flow*). The portal flow contained in these tributaries, as well as in the main PV, is normally parabolic and relatively constant, giving a characteristic spectral Doppler pattern (Figure 6.14). Portal flow mean velocity can be measured with spectral Doppler, after the use of an insonation angle correction of less than 60°. Portal flow mean velocity can be calculated by the ultrasound system by using the uniform insonation technique, which requires the application of a sample gate volume that fills the entire width of the main PV. Alternatively, a sample gate volume that fills approximately half of the vessel lumen placed in its center can be used to obtain maximal flow velocity. Because of the parabolic behavior of the portal flow, mean portal flow velocity can then be estimated by multiplying this result by 0.57. Mean portal flow velocities have been reported to vary between 15 ± 3

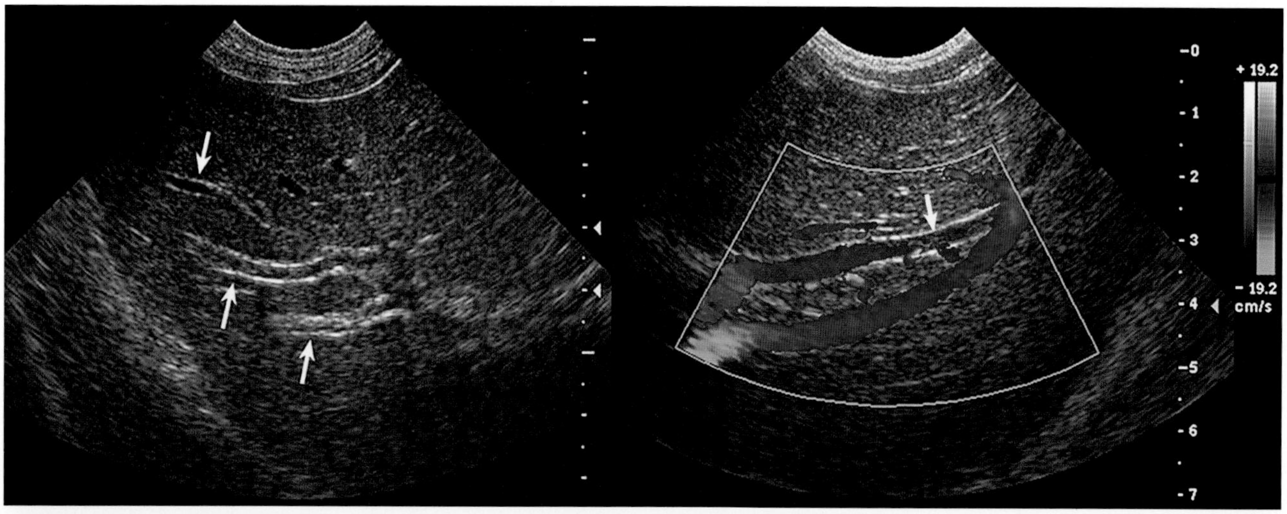

Figure 6.12. Hepatic vasculature. Portal veins can be differentiated from hepatic veins because of the consistent hyperechogenicity of their walls (arrows), regardless of the ultrasound-beam orientation. With conventional color Doppler, portal venous flow appears as a red signal directed toward the transducer, compared with a blue signal for the hepatic veins that drain in the caudal vena cava (i.e., away from the transducer). Smaller hepatic arteries are not normally seen.

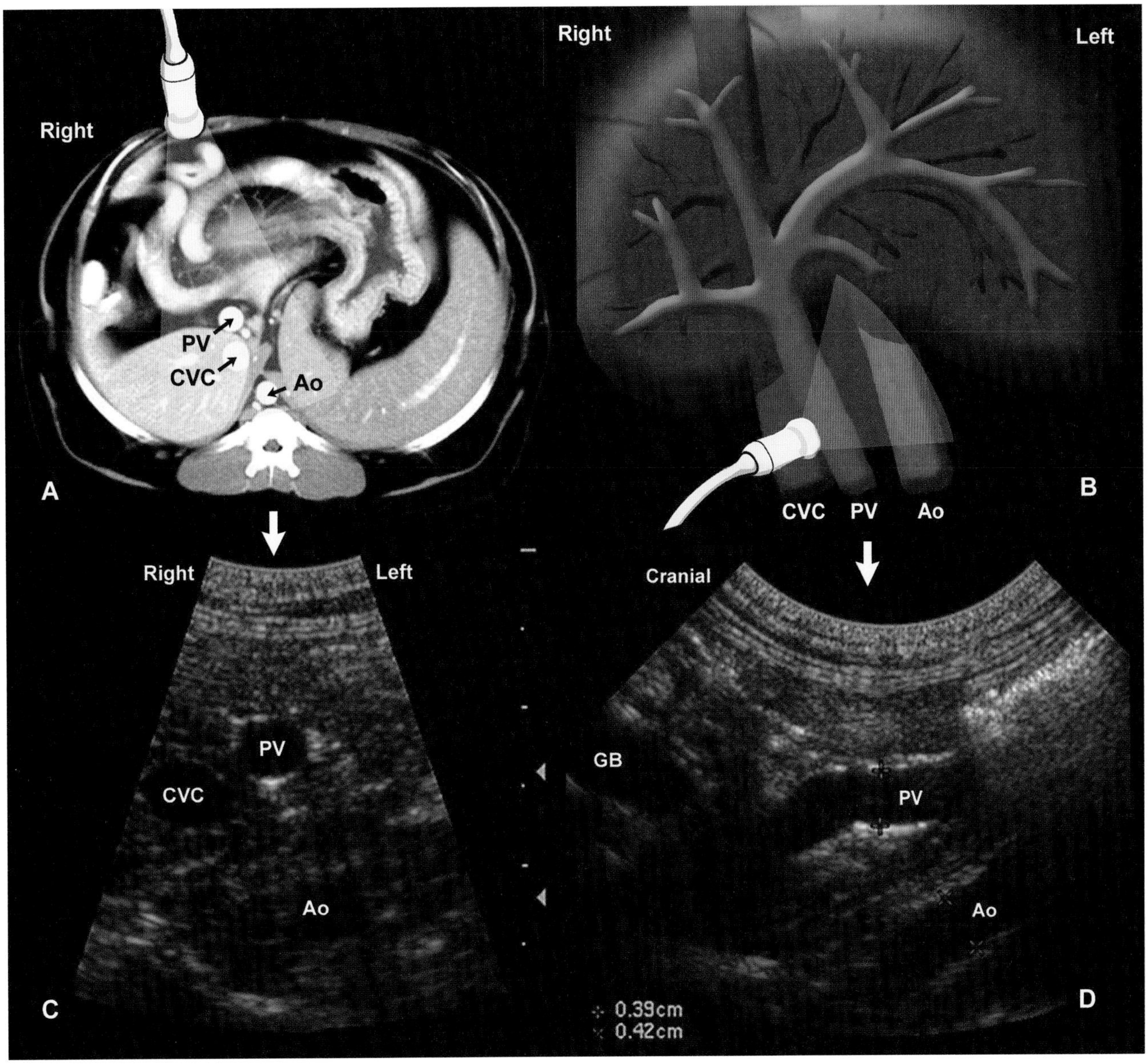

Figure 6.13. Ultrasonographic approach to the hepatic vasculature. Transverse computed tomographic image **(A)** and ventral schematic image **(B)** of the hepatic vasculature showing the relationship between the portal vein (PV), caudal vena cava (CVC), and aorta (Ao). On transverse **(C)** and longitudinal **(D)** ultrasonographic images obtained at the porta hepatis, these three vessels can usually be well visualized in normal dogs and cats, and should be similar in size. When measured at the caudal margin of the liver, the portal vein should not be less than 65% of the diameter of the aorta. GB, gallbladder. Computed tomographic image courtesy of Matthew Winter, University of Florida.

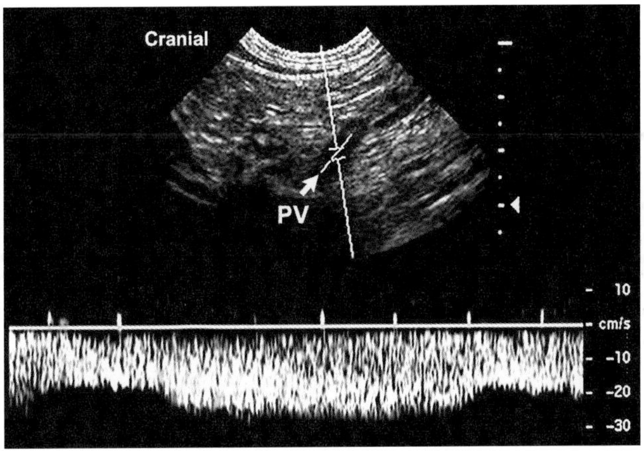

Figure 6.14. Spectral Doppler pattern of the portal flow. With spectral Doppler, the flow within the portal vein (PV) can be assessed after placing the sample-volume gate in the center of the vascular lumen and correcting for the angle of flow direction. The flow spectrum observed in this normal dog is broad and relatively linear, with some variations occurring because of movement of the sample volume during respiration in regard to the center of the vessel, where maximal velocity is reached. Mean flow velocity is calculated by multiplying the maximal velocity (25 cm/s) by a factor of 0.57, which equals 14.3 cm/s. The angle of sample volume correction was 50°.

and 18 ± 8 cm/s in normal dogs and 10–18 cm/s in normal cats (Nyland and Fisher 1990; Lamb and Mahoney 1994; Lamb 1998; d'Anjou et al. 2004). However, these measurements are susceptible to inaccurate estimations, especially with higher correction angles (more than 60°), and must therefore be used cautiously.

Ultrasonographic Features of Hepatic Disorders

Several hepatic disorders are found in dogs and cats and cause focal, multifocal, or diffuse parenchymal alterations. The evaluation of the liver must include several parameters: liver size and contour, parenchymal echogenicity, and ultrasound-beam attenuation, as well as the distribution of abnormalities. Although some of these disorders have characteristic ultrasonographic features, most changes are not pathognomonic of one particular process. A more definite diagnosis is usually based on the combination of clinical presentation, blood-test results, ultrasonographic findings, and cytological or histopathologic results.

Diffuse Hepatic Parenchymal Disorders

Diffuse hepatic disorders can be difficult to differentiate from poorly defined multifocal diseases. Typically, these disorders affect all lobes, although not always symmetrically. The parenchymal echogenicity can be increased, reduced, or unaffected. These disorders can also affect the parenchymal uniformity and distort the hepatic margin. The evaluation of the liver contour is facilitated by the presence of peritoneal effusion (Figure 6.3). With the exception of congenital portal vascular anomalies such as portosystemic shunting, chronic hepatitis, and cirrhosis, most disorders tend to be associated with symmetrical or asymmetrical hepatomegaly. Two or more hepatic disorders, such as hepatitis, vacuolar hepatopathy, or nodular hyperplasia, can be found in the same patient, complicating the ultrasonographic diagnosis and justifying fine-needle aspiration or biopsy in most cases. Table 6.1 lists the typical diagnostic differential for diffuse changes in hepatic parenchymal echogenicity, and Table 6.2 lists the causes of diffuse or focal/asymmetrical hepatomegaly.

Vacuolar Hepatopathies and Nodular Hyperplasia

Hepatic lipidosis and steroid hepatopathies are common. Miscellaneous vacuolar hepatopathies are

Table 6.1.
Diagnostic differentials for diffuse alterations in hepatic parenchymal echogenicity

Diffuse Hyperechogenicity	Diffuse Hypoechogenicity	Mixed Echogenicity
Steroid hepatopathy	Passive congestion	Steroid hepatopathy associated with benign hyperplasia, or other combinations of processes
Lipidosis	Acute hepatitis or cholangiohepatitis	Hepatitis
Other vacuolar hepatopathies	Lymphoma	Lymphoma
Chronic hepatitis	Leukemia	Hepatocellular carcinoma
Fibrosis	Histiocytic neoplasms	Metastasis
Cirrhosis	Amyloidosis	Necrosis
Lymphoma		Amyloidosis
Mast cell tumor		

Table 6.2.
Diagnostic differentials for alterations in hepatic volume

Diffuse Hepatomegaly	Focal or Asymmetrical Hepatomegaly	Small Liver
Steroid hepatopathy	Primary or metastatic neoplasia	Congenital portosystemic shunting
Lipidosis	Abscess	Microvascular dysplasia or primary portal vein hypoplasia
Hepatitis or cholangiohepatitis	Cyst(s)	Cirrhosis
Passive congestion	Granuloma	Fibrosis
Round-cell neoplasia: lymphoma, malignant histiocytosis, and mast cells	Thrombosis	Severe hypovolemia
Massive hepatocellular carcinoma or metastases	Lobar torsion	
Amyloidosis	Hematoma	

often present with other primary disorders in dogs (Wang et al. 2004). These hepatopathies are usually associated with a diffuse increase in parenchymal echogenicity and hepatomegaly (Nyland and Park 1983; Biller 1992) (Figures 6.15–6.17). The parenchyma can also appear hyperattenuating, i.e., result in excessive sound-beam attenuation (Figures 6.16 and 6.17). Consequently, the far gain must be increased in many of these patients to be able to evaluate the deepest portions of the liver. Additionally, the parenchyma can appear heterogeneous or contain hypoechoic or hyperechoic nodular foci, possibly because of concurrent nodular hyperplasia (Figure 6.17).

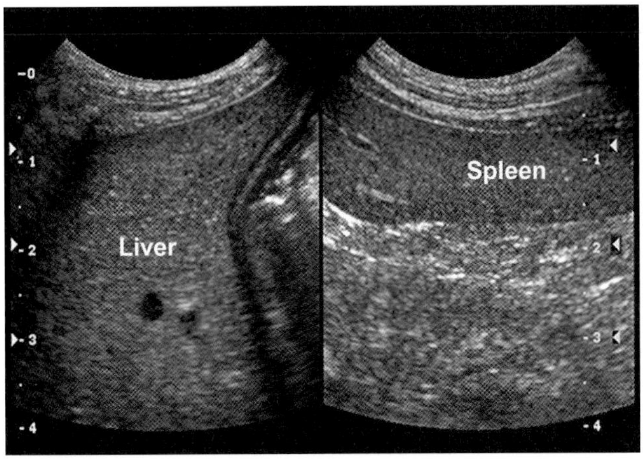

Figure 6.15. Hyperechoic liver. Dual images of the liver and spleen of a dog that were obtained with identical settings (depth, gain, and focus), allowing hepatic and splenic parenchymal echogenicities to be compared. Hepatic lipidosis that caused a diffusely hyperechoic liver, isoechoic to the spleen, was diagnosed.

Hepatitis, Cholangiohepatitis, and Cirrhosis

Diffuse hepatic inflammatory processes can show variable ultrasonographic features. In cats, cholangiohepatitis is most commonly associated with a decrease in parenchymal echogenicity and an increased visibility of the portal vasculature (Newell et al. 1998) (Figure 6.18). Additionally, this process is often associated with biliary anomalies, such as biliary sludge, cholelithiasis, or wall thickening. In dogs, acute hepatitis also tends to cause diffuse liver hypoechogenicity (Biller 1992), as seen with leptospirosis (Figure 6.19).

Chronic hepatitis, on the other hand, tends to be associated with fibrosis, which is typically associated with an increased echogenicity (Biller 1992). The presence of chronic active inflammation, consisting of a mixture of inflammatory cells, edema, fibrosis, necrosis, as well as regenerative nodules (hyperplasia) can cause a markedly heterogeneous liver with variable echogenicity (Figure 6.20). Although cirrhosis classically causes the liver to appear small, hyperechoic, and irregular in contour (Biller 1992) (Figure 6.21), its appearance can vary and sometimes mimic neoplasia. However, chronic hepatitis and its ultimate outcome, cirrhosis, usually do not cause hepatic enlargement, as opposed to the effect of massive neoplastic infiltration.

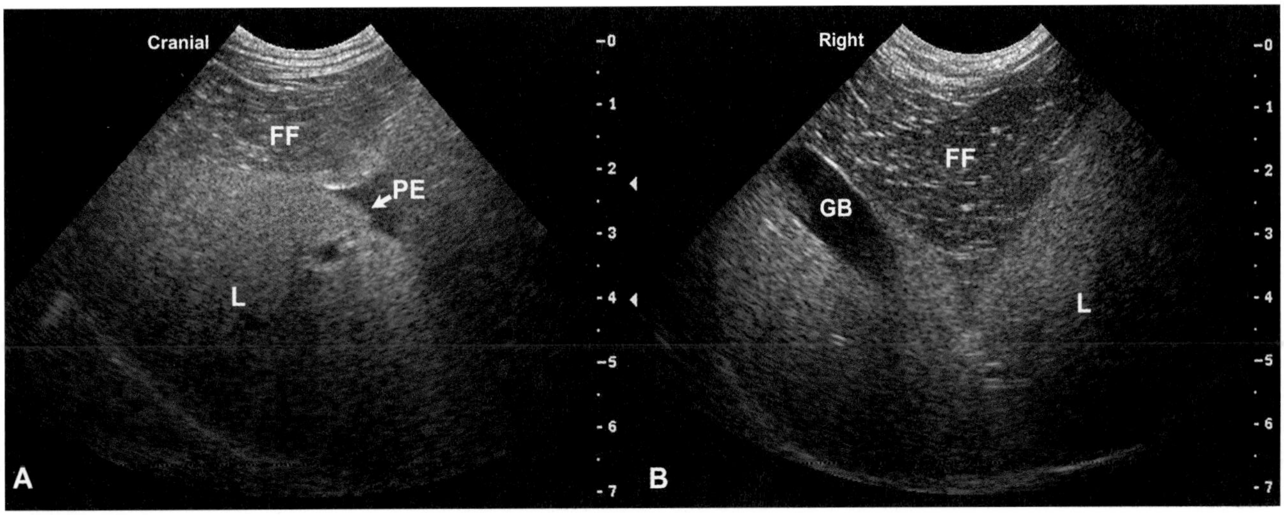

Figure 6.16. Feline hepatic lipidosis. Sagittal **(A)** and transverse **(B)** images of the liver in a cat with diffuse hyperechogenicity and ultrasonographic beam hyperattenuation. The liver (L) is markedly hyperechoic to the falciform fat (FF), at least superficially. The echoes coming from the deepest portions of the liver were reduced and could only be partially compensated for by increasing far gain. A small volume of peritoneal effusion (PE) is noted between liver lobes. GB, gallbladder.

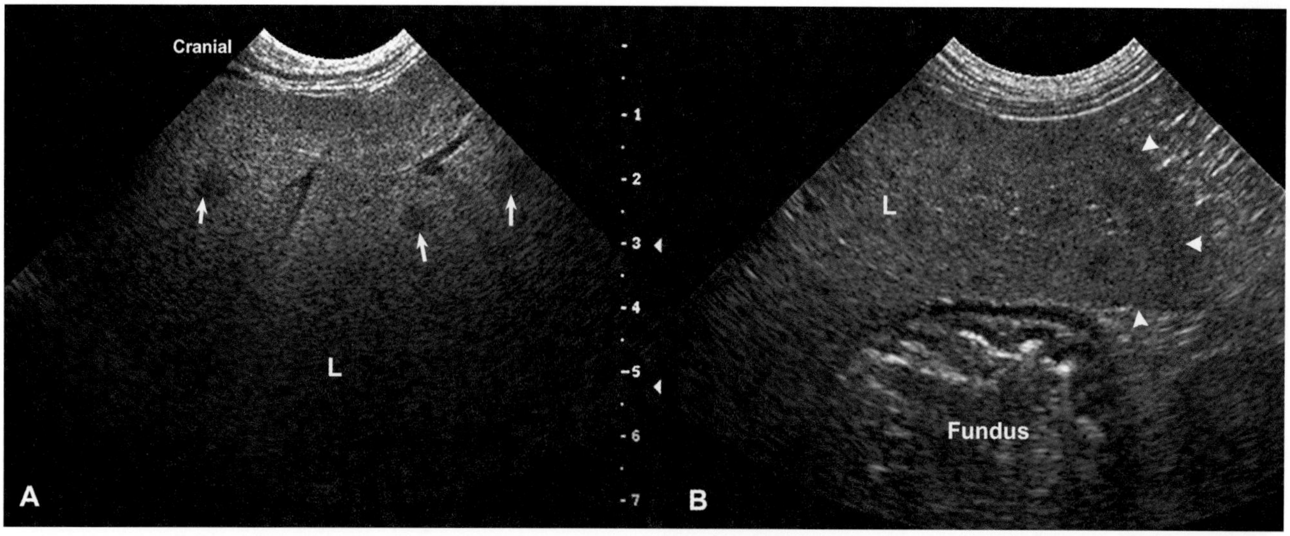

Figure 6.17. Steroid hepatopathy. Longitudinal images of the left portion of the liver in a dog with pituitary-dependent hyperadrenocorticism. The liver (L) is enlarged, diffusely hyperechoic, and heterogeneous. Multiple hypoechoic nodular foci, less than 1 cm wide, are noted in the liver in **A** (arrows). **B**. The liver contour is rounded (arrowheads) and extends beyond the gastric fundus. In **A**, the deep portion of the liver is difficult to assess because of increased ultrasound-beam attenuation. Ultrasound-guided biopsy indicated vacuolar hepathopathy and benign nodular hyperplasia.

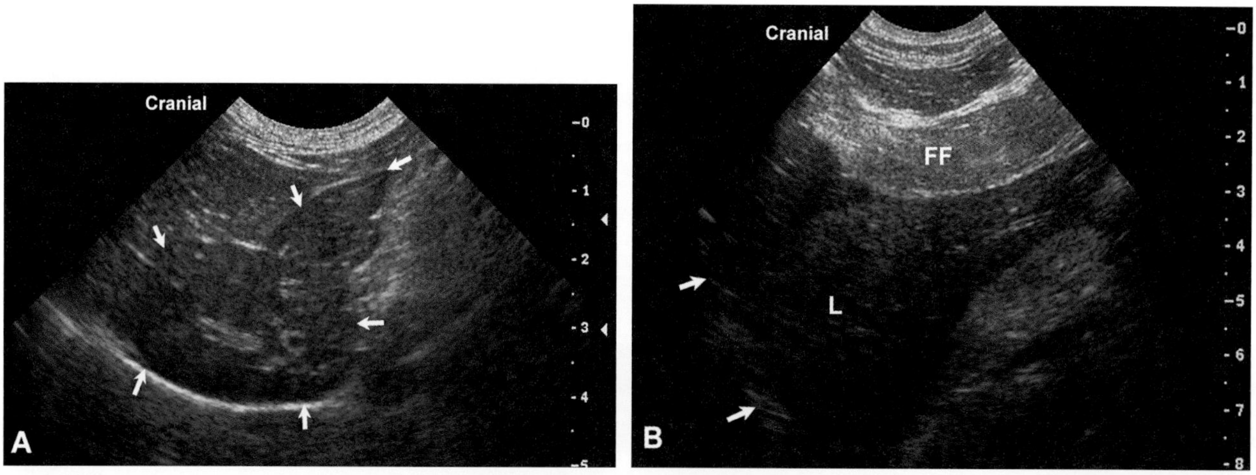

Figure 6.18. Feline cholangiohepatitis. **A:** Longitudinal image of the left portion of the liver (arrows) of a cat with fever and icterus. The liver parenchyma is diffusely hypoechoic, and the portal vein margins appear prominent. These features are suggestive of cholangiohepatitis in cats. **B:** Longitudinal image of the central portion of the liver in another cat with cholangiohepatitis. Similar features are observed. The liver (L) is significantly hypoechoic when compared with the falciform fat (FF) located ventrally. Arrows delineate the cranial hepatic border.

Hepatic Neoplasia

Although several primary and secondary neoplastic processes can affect the liver in dogs and cats, diffuse hepatic involvement is less common and is usually caused by diffuse round-cell infiltration. Hepatomegaly is expected in most types of diffuse neoplasia, although its magnitude can vary with the level of infiltration.

Lymphoma can involve the liver without detectable ultrasonographic changes or cause diffuse parenchymal hypoechogenicity, hyperechogenicity, or mixed echogenicity, with or without hypoechoic nodules (Whiteley et al. 1989; Lamb et al. 1991) (Figure 6.22). Histiocytic neoplasms are more commonly associated with hypoechoic nodules and masses, although diffuse hepatic hypoechogenicity has been reported (Cruz-

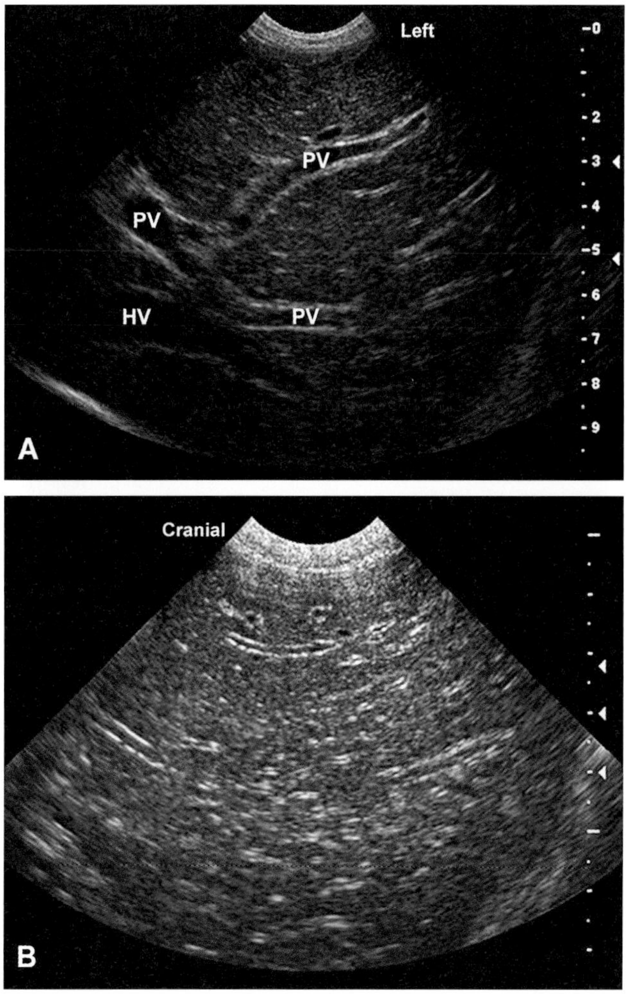

Figure 6.19. Canine acute hepatitis. **A:** Transverse oblique image of the left side of the liver in a dog with acute hepatitis with prominent portal veins (PV) because of diffuse parenchymal hypoechogenicity. The main left hepatic vein (HV) is also observed, but its wall is less apparent. The prominence of the PV boundaries may have also been related to the inflammatory process. **B: Leptospirosis.** Ultrasonographic image of a portion of the liver in a dog with acute leptospirosis. The liver is diffusely hypoechoic, and its portal walls are prominent, appearing as double lines and "donuts" throughout the parenchyma. These findings are common in dogs with leptospirosis.

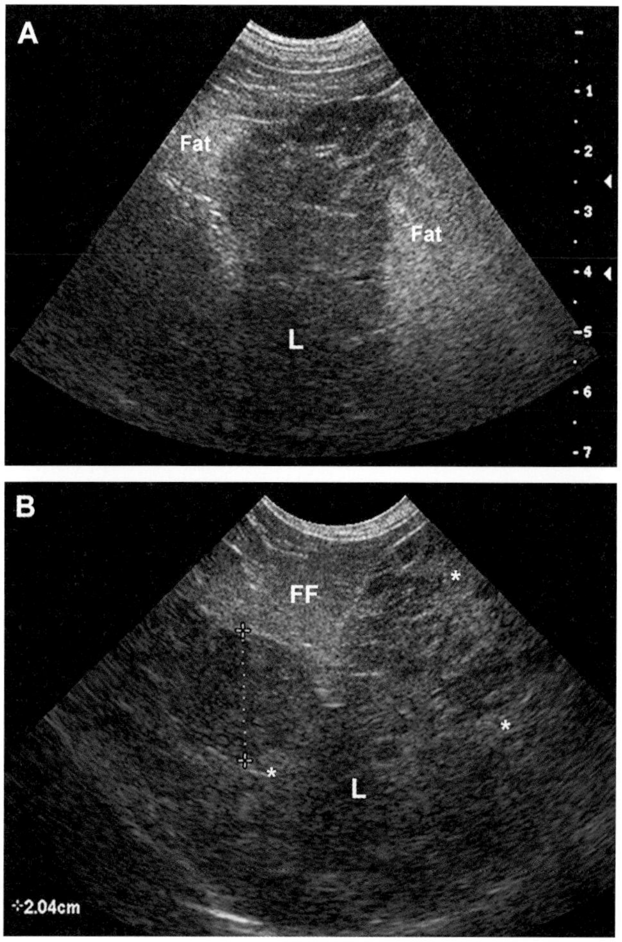

Figure 6.20. Chronic active hepatitis and nodular hyperplasia. **A:** Longitudinal image of the left portion of the liver (L), which appears diffusely hypoechoic, and with irregular and ill-defined contours. The adjacent fat is hyperechoic. Chronic active hepatitis was diagnosed on fine-needle aspiration and ultrasound-guided biopsy. **B:** Transverse oblique image of the left portion of the liver (L) in another dog with diffuse parenchymal heterogeneity. Several hypoechoic coalescing nodules are found that reach up to 2 cm deep, as well as hyperechoic patches (*). Ultrasound-guided biopsy confirmed chronic hepatitis with fibrosis and nodular hyperplasia. FF, falciform fat.

Arambulo et al. 2004) (see Figure 6.33). Conversely, mast cell infiltration of the liver tends to cause diffuse hyperechogenicity (Sato and Solano 2004). Hepatic carcinomas can also be diffuse, or involve multiple lobes, with a variable ultrasonographic appearance that depends on the presence of necrosis, inflammation, hemorrhage, or cavitation. A mixed pattern of echogenicity is common with these malignant tumors (Figure 6.23).

Miscellaneous Diffuse Hepatic Disorders

Other types of hepatopathies can be encountered in small animals, although less commonly. Amyloidosis, primarily affecting shar-peis and Abyssinian and Siamese cats, can cause hepatic enlargement and parenchymal ultrasonographic changes. In cats, the liver tends to become diffusely heterogeneous with mixed hyperechoic and hypoechoic foci (Beatty et al. 2002). Spontaneous hepatic rupture and hemoabdomen can also be caused by massive hepatic

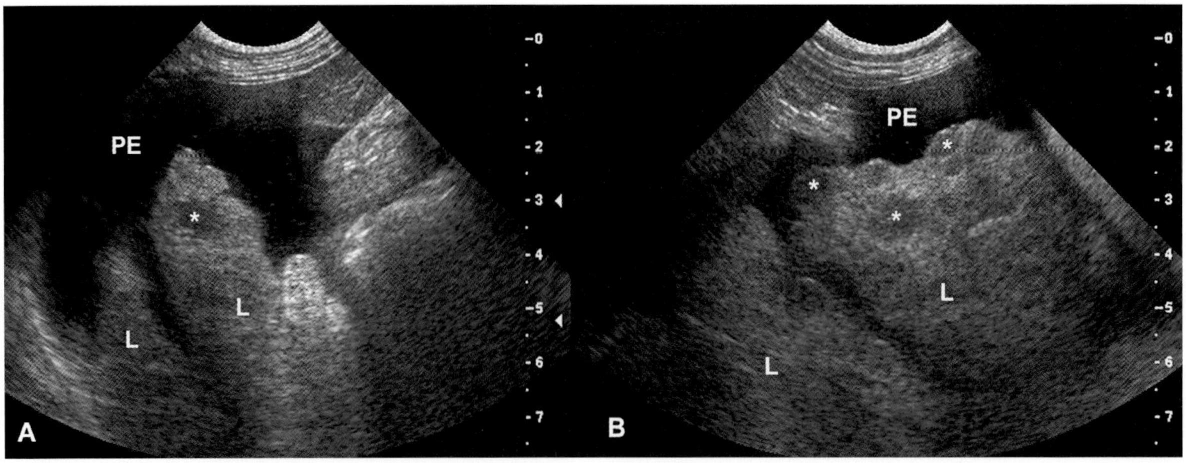

Figure 6.21. Hepatic cirrhosis. Transverse oblique images of the right **(A)** and left **(B)** portions of the liver (L) in a dog with chronic hepatic insufficiency. All lobes are small and hyperechoic. Hypoechoic nodules (*) are found throughout the parenchyma, irregularly deforming its contours. These contours are visualized because of the presence of a large volume of anechoic peritoneal effusion (PE). These findings are common in end-stage cirrhosis in dogs.

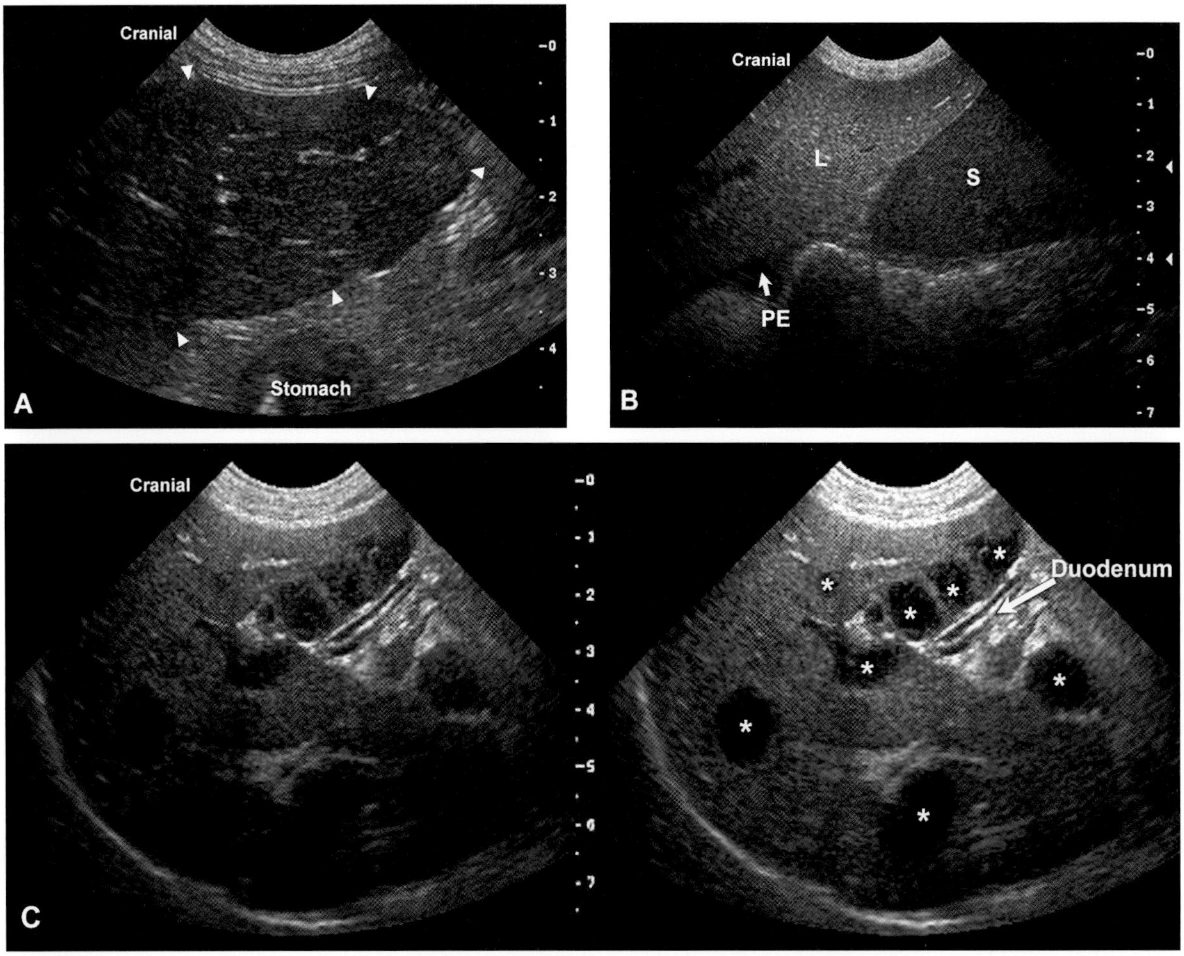

Figure 6.22. Canine lymphoma. **A:** Transverse oblique image of the left portion of the liver in a dog with multicentric lymphoma. The portal vein walls are prominent because of diffuse parenchymal hypoechogenicity. The left lateral hepatic lobe is enlarged (arrowheads), extending several centimeters caudal to the stomach, and its caudal tip is rounded. **B:** Lymphoma can also cause diffuse hepatic hyperechogenicity (L), as seen in this other dog. The spleen (S) is relatively hypoechoic. Both organs are enlarged, and their borders are rounded. Peritoneal effusion is also present (PE). **C:** Sonographic and schematic images. In this other dog with lymphoma, multiple, well-defined, hypoechoic nodules (*) are noted throughout the liver. Image C courtesy of D. Penninck.

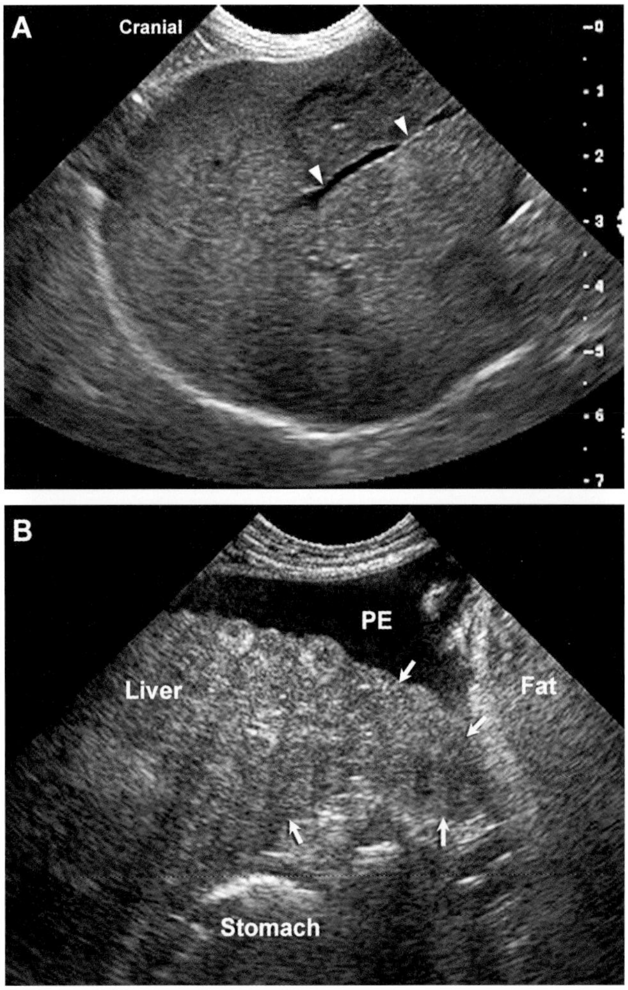

Figure 6.23. Diffuse hepatic carcinomas. **A: Hepatic adenocarcinoma in a cat.** The liver is moderately enlarged and mildly inhomogeneous, with several ill-defined hypoechoic areas. The neoplastic infiltration deforms the vasculature (arrowheads). Image courtesy of D. Penninck. **B: Hepatocellular carcinoma in a dog.** Longitudinal image of the left lateral hepatic lobe in a dog with diffuse hepatocellular carcinoma. This lobe extending caudal to the stomach (arrows) is hyperechoic and presents a nodular border. Marked peritoneal effusion is also evident ventrally (PE).

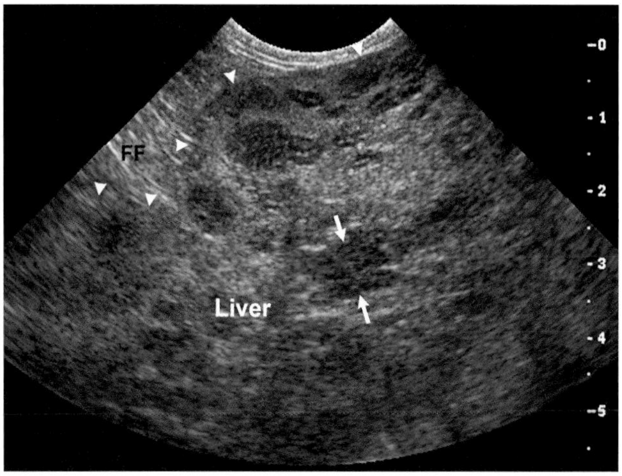

Figure 6.24. Hepatocutaneous syndrome. Transverse image of the left central portion of the liver of a dog with superficial necrolytic dermatitis. Diffusely distributed hypoechoic irregular foci (arrows) are surrounded by hyperechoic parenchyma, giving a honeycomb pattern. Histological evaluation revealed tissue necrosis and mild inflammation. The arrowheads delineate the rounded margins of the liver.

amyloidosis. In dogs with hepatocutaneous syndrome (superficial necrolytic dermatitis), the liver can become highly hyperechoic with diffusely distributed 0.5- to 1.5-cm-wide hypoechoic regions, producing a honeycomb pattern (Nyland et al. 1996) (Figure 6.24).

Focal Hepatic Parenchymal Disorders

The improvement in ultrasound equipment technology has increased the sensitivity of ultrasonography in detecting focal hepatic lesions. It has been suggested that hepatomas exceeding 5 mm can be detected in ideal imaging conditions in people (Nyman et al. 2004). The conspicuity of a focal lesion is also greatly influenced by its imaging characteristics. Hence, for a given size, an anechoic cyst is more likely to be detected than a soft-tissue nodule of echogenicity similar to one of adjacent normal parenchyma. Although many different types of focal lesions can be detected with ultrasonography, the appearance of several of these processes is quite variable, resulting in limited diagnostic specificity. The advances in contrast harmonic ultrasonography have helped to increase the overall diagnostic accuracy and may prove to be useful in clinical settings (Nyman et al. 2004; O'Brien et al. 2004). This topic, though, is beyond the scope of this chapter.

Table 6.3 lists the diagnostic differential for focal hepatic lesions, based on their typical appearance. Although some trends in ultrasonographic appearance have been reported for some of these processes, a definitive diagnosis usually requires fine-needle aspiration or biopsy.

Benign Hyperplasia and Neoplasia

Benign nodular hyperplasia is common, particularly in dogs, and accounts for many focal hepatic lesions identified with ultrasonography. Although these regenerative nodules can vary in echogenicity and size, they tend to appear as hypoechoic nodules measuring less than 5–15 mm wide (Stonewater et al. 1990;

Table 6.3.
Diagnostic differentials for focal hepatic lesions with ultrasonography

Anechoic	Hypoechoic	Hyperechoic	Mixed Echogenicity
Cyst	Nodular hyperplasia	Nodular hyperplasia	Nodular hyperplasia
Cystic tumor	Metastasis	Primary neoplasia	Primary neoplasia
Necrosis	Lymphoma	Metastasis	Metastasis
Abscess	Primary hepatic neoplasia	Mineralization or cholelithiasis	Abscess
Hematoma	Abscess	Abscess	Hematoma
	Necrosis	Fat or myelolipoma	
	Hematoma	Granuloma	
	Complex cyst	Gas	
		Metallic clip	

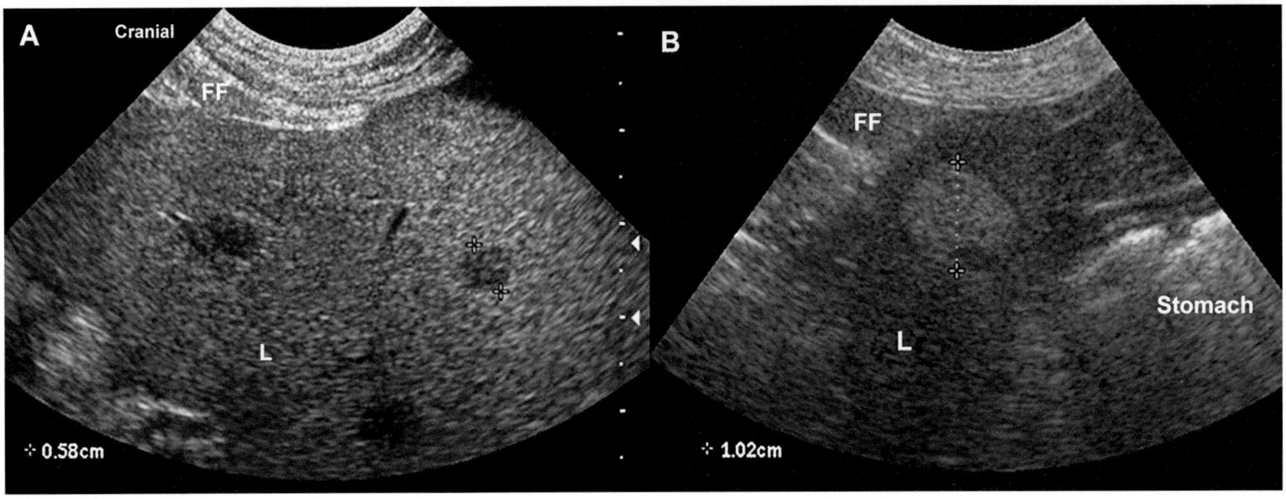

Figure 6.25. Nodular hyperplasia. Longitudinal images of the left portion of the liver (L) in two dogs with a variable appearance of regenerative nodules. **A:** Several poorly defined hypoechoic foci, less than 1 cm wide are noted. **B:** Conversely, the regenerative nodule is hyperechoic and well defined. FF, falciform fat.

O'Brien et al. 2004) (Figure 6.25). As for most other types of focal lesions, their margin can be well circumscribed or poorly defined. Benign hepatic adenomas or hepatomas can appear as a focal mass of variable size and usually hyperechoic (O'Brien et al. 2004) (Figure 6.26).

Malignant Neoplasia

The liver is a common target for metastasis, mainly through the portal system, which drains most abdominal structures. Primary hepatic neoplasms such as hepatocellular carcinomas can also be seen as focal or multifocal masses, although less frequently than metastasis. The variable tissue characteristics of primary and metastatic neoplastic processes, including tissue density, vascular pattern, necrosis, liquefaction, and calcification, cause variable ultrasonographic appearances (Nyland and Park 1983; Whiteley et al. 1989; O'Brien et al. 2004) (Figures 6.27–6.31 and 6.36–6.38). Focal hypoechoic lesions with a hyperechoic center, also termed *target lesions*, are more commonly associated with metastasis (Figure 6.29 and 6.32), although benign processes, such as nodular hyperplasia, can cause a similar pattern (Cuccovillo and Lamb 2002; O'Brien et al. 2004). It has been reported that the finding of at least one target lesion in the liver or spleen had a positive predictive value of 74% for malignancy in small animals (Cuccovillo and Lamb 2002).

Histiocytic neoplasms and lymphoma can demonstrate similar imaging characteristics. Although findings can vary, particularly with lymphoma, multifocal nodules or masses, hypoechoic or mixed in echogenicity, are commonly found with these processes (Cruz-Arambulo et al. 2002; Ramirez et al. 2002) (Figures 6.33 and 6.34). Significant hepatic lymphade-

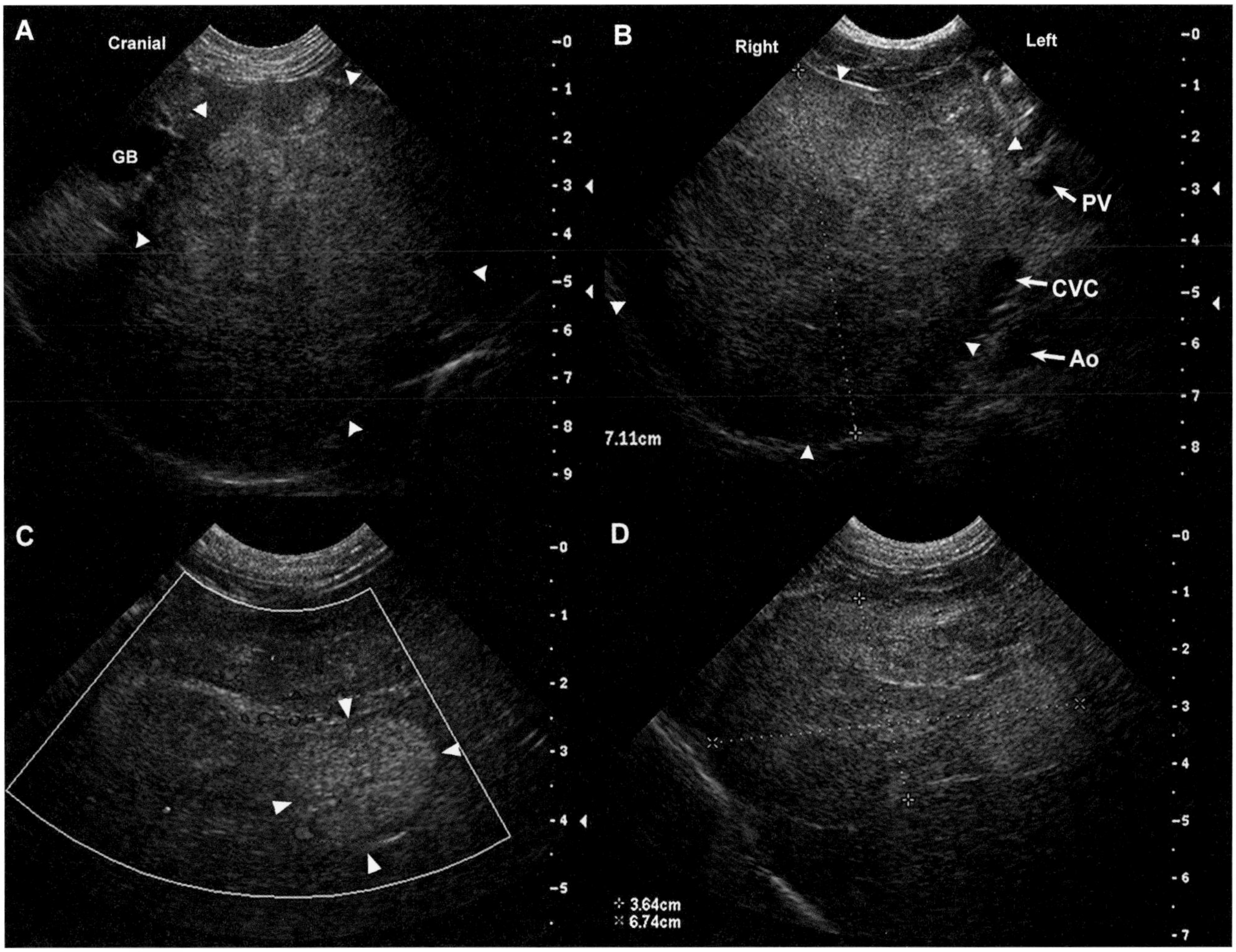

Figure 6.26. Benign liver tumors. **A and B: Hepatoma.** Longitudinal **(A)** and transverse **(B)** images of the right portion of the liver of a dog with increased liver enzymes. In these images, a large, mildly hyperechoic and mildly heterogeneous mass (arrowheads), measuring at least 7 cm wide, is in the right portion of the liver and in contact with the gallbladder (GB), portal vein (PV), and caudal vena cava (CVC), and close to the aorta (Ao). The extent of this mass and the lack of vascular invasion could not be confirmed with the ultrasonographic exam and required computed tomography. **C and D: Adenoma or hepatoma.** Longitudinal images of two separate hyperechoic masses found in the liver of a clinically normal dog. The smaller mass **(C, arrowheads)** presents a thin hypoechoic halo, and the larger mass **(D, cursors)** is mildly inhomogeneous. The findings on fine-needle aspiration were consistent with benign liver tumors (adenoma or hepatoma).

nopathy is also common with these neoplasms of round-cell origin and their presence often helps in diagnosing these processes.

Cavitary Lesions

Hepatic and biliary cysts are sometimes identified in dogs and cats and appear as well circumscribed, regular or irregular, anechoic foci, typically associated with far-enhancement artifact (Nyland and Park 1983) (Figure 6.35). In these benign cysts, the adjacent parenchyma is usually normal. These cavitary lesions must be differentiated from cystic tumors, such as biliary cystadenomas and cystadenocarcinomas, commonly demonstrating a multilocular pattern and a change in tissue appearance around the anechoic cavitations (Nyland and Park 1999) (Figures 6.36 and 6.37). Although more common in cats, cystic or cavitary tumors can also be seen in dogs (Figure 6.38).

Hepatic abscesses, which are uncommon in dogs and cats, tend to appear as round to oval, regular or irregular, hypoechoic lesions that are often cavitated (Schwarz et al. 1998). Enhancement artifact, abdominal effusion, regional lymphadenopathy, and hyperechoic perihepatic fat are commonly seen in affected animals (Figure 6.39A). Abscesses can also show pus

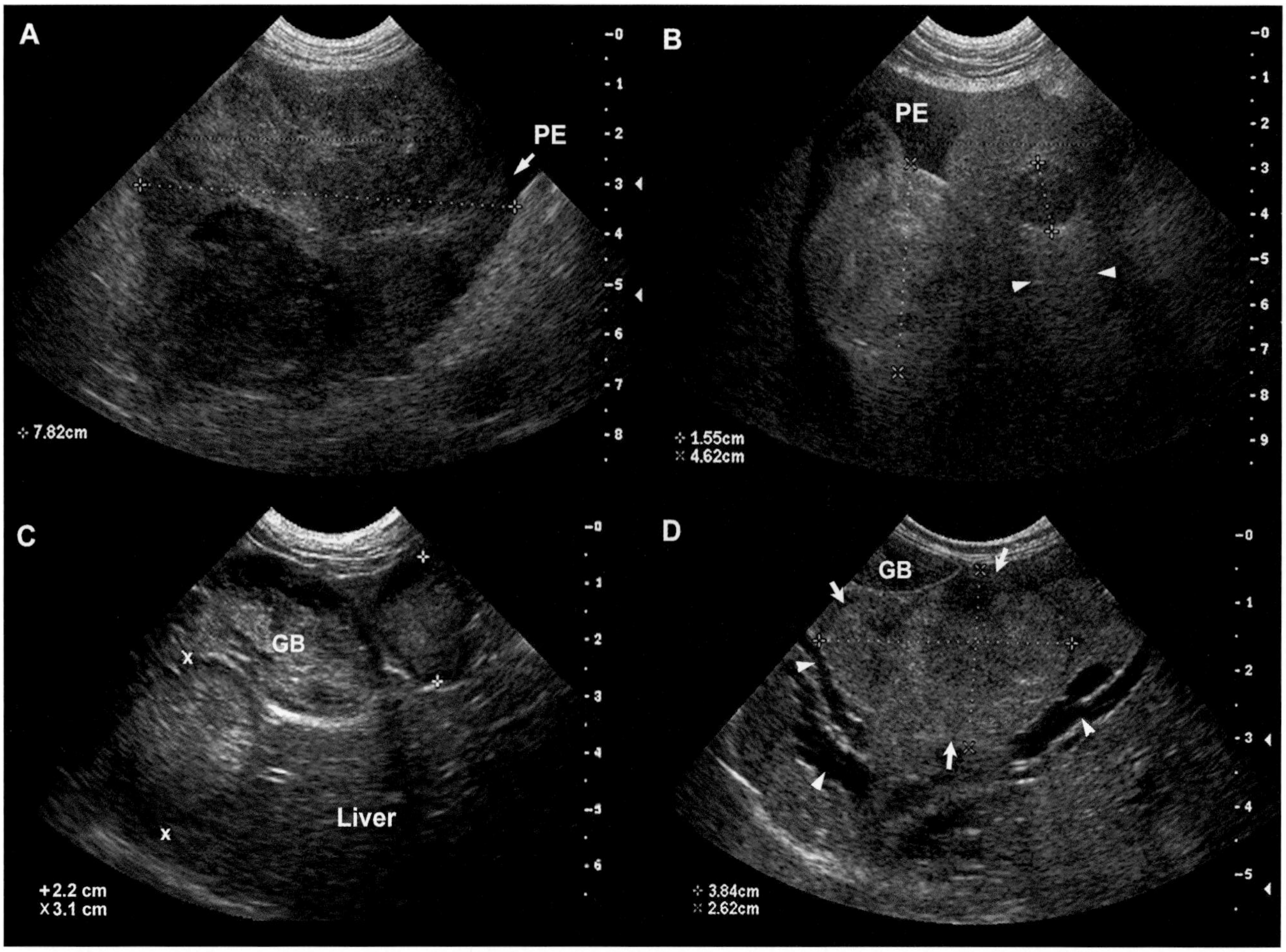

Figure 6.27. Primary liver carcinomas. **A: Hepatocellular carcinoma in a dog.** Transverse image obtained in the right cranial abdomen of a dog with a hemoabdomen. An irregular, inhomogeneous and poorly defined mass (7.8 cm wide) is deforming the architecture of a liver lobe. A small amount of fluid is noted around the mass. PE, peritoneal effusion. **B: Hepatic adenocarcinoma and metastasis in a dog.** A spherical, hyperechoic mass (4.6 cm) is deforming the contour of a liver lobe and surrounded by mildly echogenic peritoneal effusion (PE). Another small, hypoechoic nodule (1.6 cm) in the same lobe is associated with acoustic enhancement in the far field (arrowheads). **C: Neuroendocrine carcinoma in a dog.** Multiple mildly hyperechoic masses (2.2–3.1 cm) demonstrating a hypoechoic halo were found in the liver of this dog, with a histological diagnosis of neuroendocrine carcinoma. GB, gallbladder. Image courtesy of D. Penninck. **D: Biliary carcinoma in a cat.** Transverse image of the liver in a cat with icteria. A lobulated, mildly hyperechoic, inhomogeneous mass (arrows and cursors) is displacing the gallbladder (Ga) ventrally. Irregular, anechoic, tubular structures (arrowheads) are also noted throughout the liver, consistent with dilated intrahepatic biliary ducts.

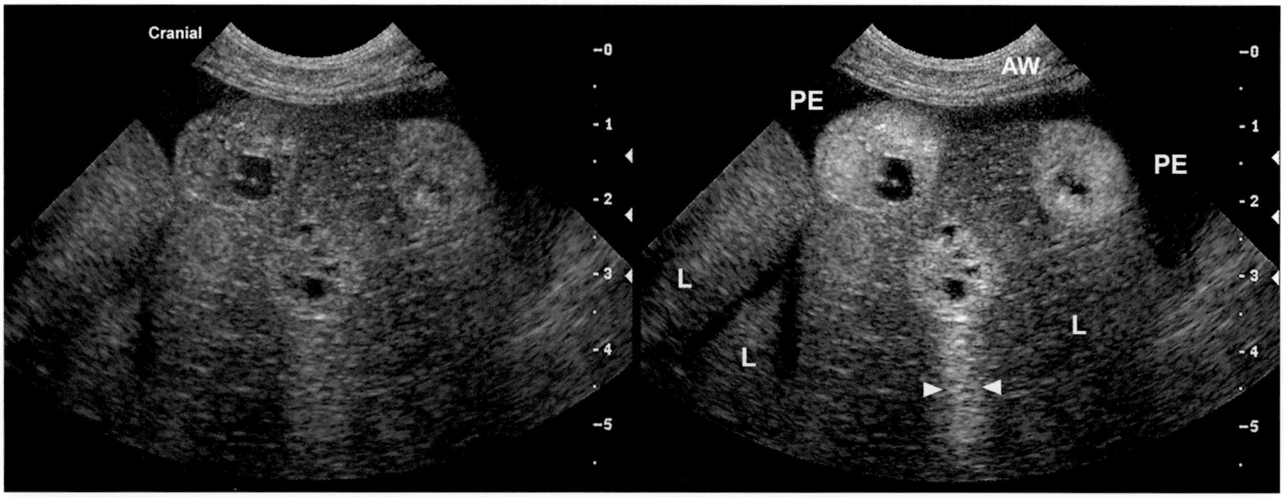

Figure 6.28.

sedimentation in the central cavitations or appear as complex or more echogenic masses (Figure 6.39B). Hyperechoic foci with reverberation consistent with gas can also be observed (Figure 3.69C). Cellular debris or hemorrhage accumulating in benign hepatic cysts can mimic abscesses, although these lesions typically show a thinner, more well-defined rim. Parasitic cysts occurring with liver flukes or hydatid disease can look similar to abscesses with the addition of mineralization (Nyland et al. 1999). Fine-needle aspiration can be

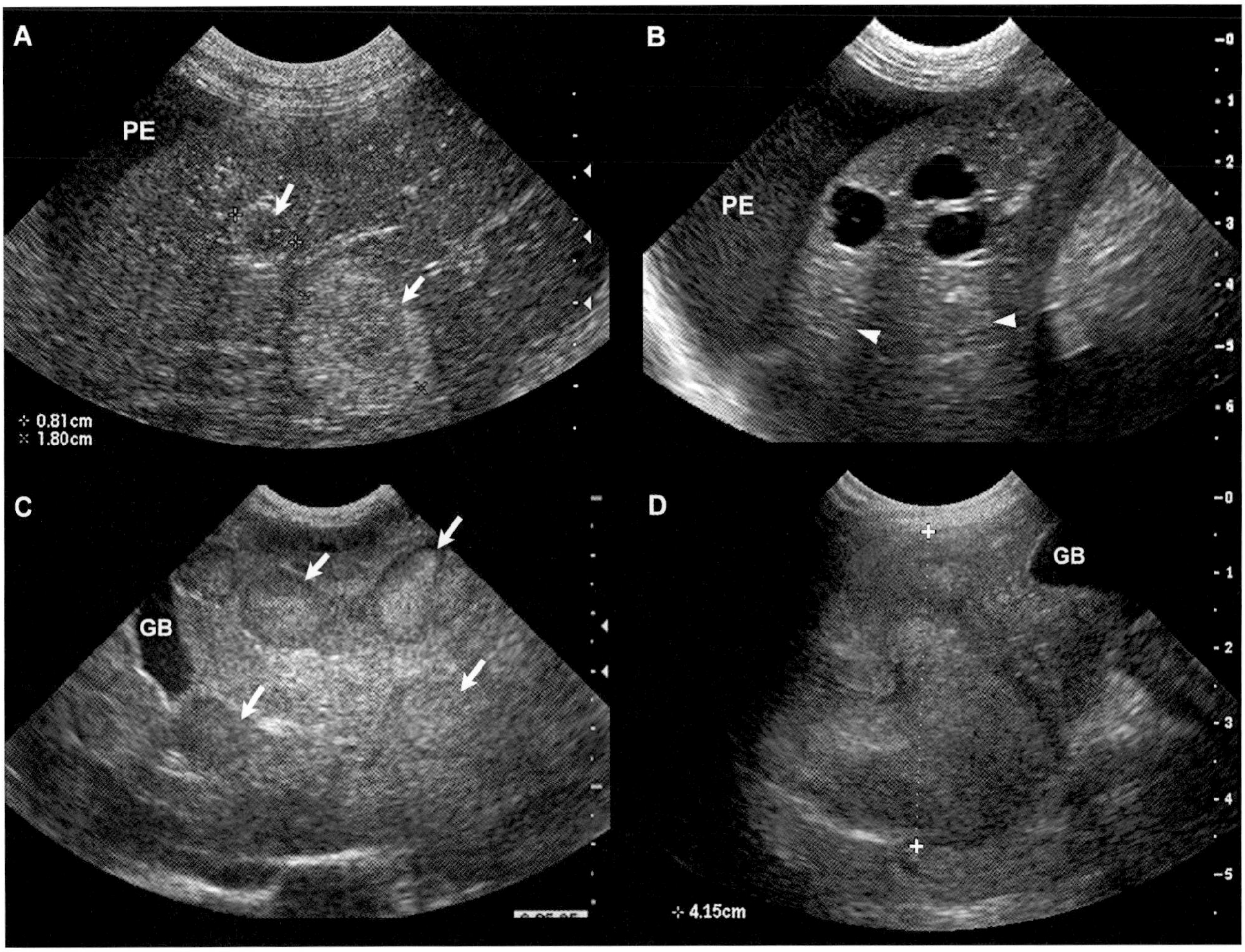

Figure 6.29. Hepatic metastases. **A: Pancreatic adenocarcinoma.** Oblique image of the left hepatic lobe with two distinct metastatic nodules (arrows). A smaller hypoechoic nodule with a thin hyperechoic rim and a larger hyperechoic nodule are present, measuring 0.8 cm and 1.8 cm wide, respectively. Hypoechoic peritoneal effusion (PE) is present. **B: Splenic hemangiosarcoma.** Well-defined, anechoic cavitary metastases are seen in the liver of this other dog with splenic hemangiosarcoma and severe, echogenic peritoneal effusion (PE) consistent with hemorrhage. Acoustic enhancement (arrowheads) is noted distal to these fluid-filled lesions. **C: Thyroid carcinoma.** Multiple "target" lesions (arrows) are seen throughout the liver of this dog with thyroid carcinoma. The hypoechoic halo seen at the periphery of these rather hyperechoic nodules is a feature that is most commonly observed with metastases. GB, gallbladder. **D: Pancreatic adenocarcinoma.** A 4-cm inhomogeneous mass is in the liver of this other dog with malignant pancreatic neoplasia. The findings on fine-needle aspiration supported a diagnosis of pancreatic metastasis. GB, gallbladder. Images B and C courtesy of D. Penninck.

Figure 6.28. Hepatic metastases. On these ultrasonographic and corresponding schematic images, three irregular hyperechoic nodules, 1.0–1.5 cm wide, are found in the liver of a dog with splenic hemangiosarcoma. Hypoechoic to anechoic cavitary foci are found in some of these nodules and are associated with far enhancement (arrowheads) Peritoneal effusion (PE) delineates the liver lobes (L). Hepatic metastases were confirmed at surgery. AW, abdominal wall.

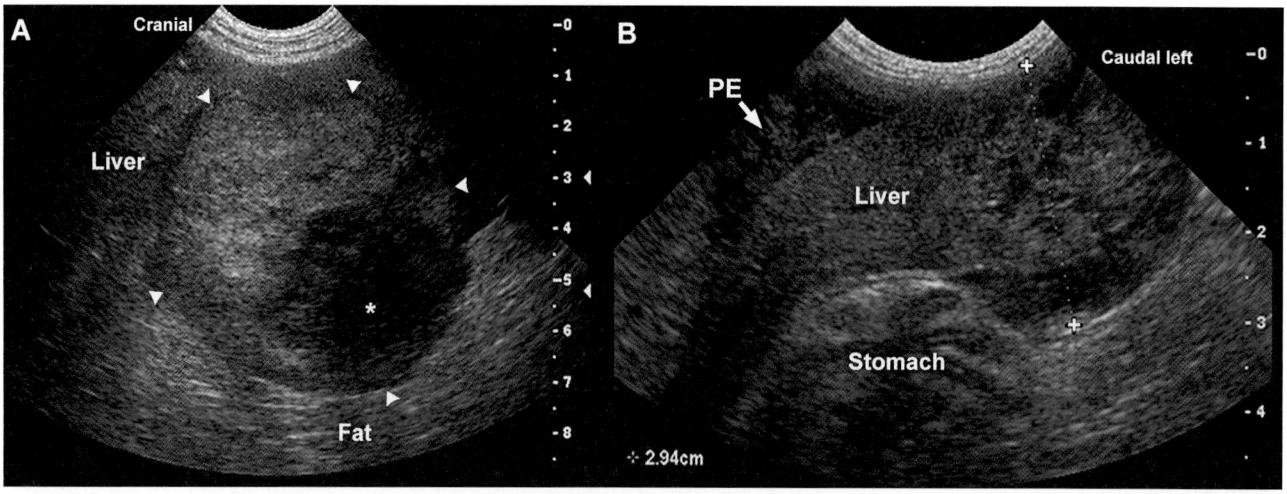

Figure 6.30. Hepatic hemangiosarcoma. **A:** Longitudinal image obtained of the left portion of the liver in a dog with acute hemoabdomen. A large hyperechoic mass (arrowheads) with a hypoechoic necrotic area (*) involves the margin of a hepatic lobe. These features are common with malignant tumors. **B:** Oblique image of the left portion of the liver in a cat with hemoabdomen. A 3-cm-wide inhomogeneous mass with small anechoic cavitary portions is at the caudal tip of the left lateral liver lobe. Peritoneal effusion (PE) with echogenic floating structures is identified in the cranioventral abdomen, consistent with hemorrhage.

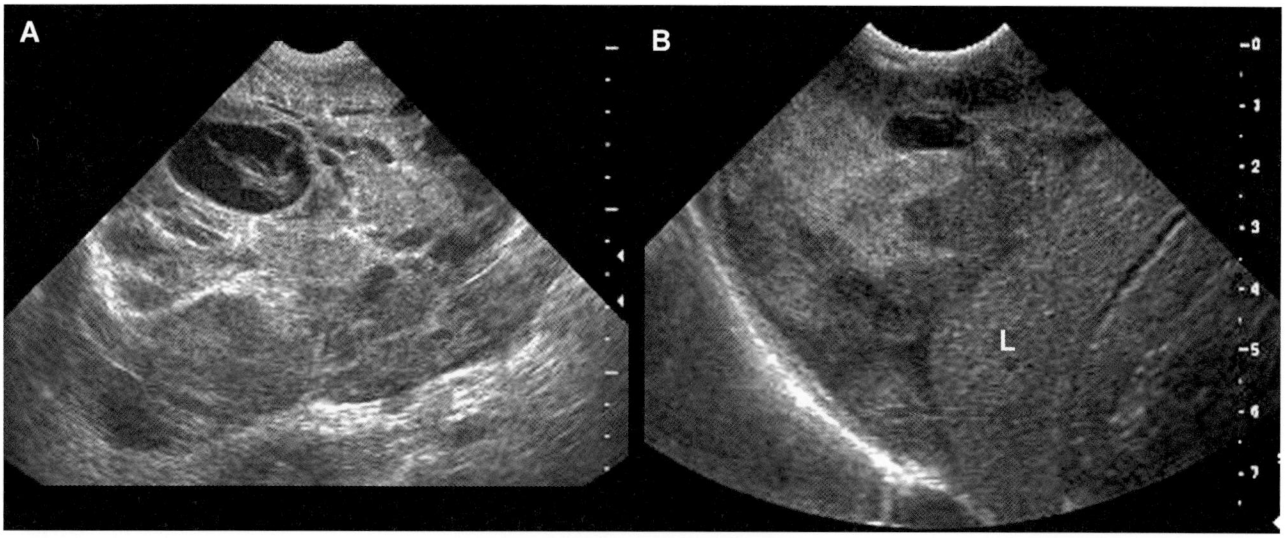

Figure 6.31. Myxosarcoma in a dog. **A:** A large, markedly heterogeneous, cavitated mass in the liver of this dog is disturbing most of the hepatic architecture. **B:** Longitudinal image of the same tumor obtained 3 months later. In this image, a clear distinction is made between the heterogeneous mass and the normal liver (L). Image courtesy of D. Penninck.

useful in confirming the nature of the fluid contained in cavitary lesions and enable drainage of abscesses.

Granulomas, Hematomas, and Mineralization

Hepatic granulomas or pyogranulomas can sometimes occur in dogs and cats, particularly with fungal diseases or with feline infectious peritonitis (Figure 6.40). In people, granulomatous lesions tend to appear as hyperechoic nodules (Mills et al. 1990). Hepatic hemorrhage is rare in dogs and is usually related to hemangiosarcoma or trauma (Whiteley et al. 1989). Hepatic hematomas can also develop following ultrasound-guided procedures such as biopsies and demonstrate variable ultrasonographic changes related to clot organization and resorption (Nyland and Park 1983)

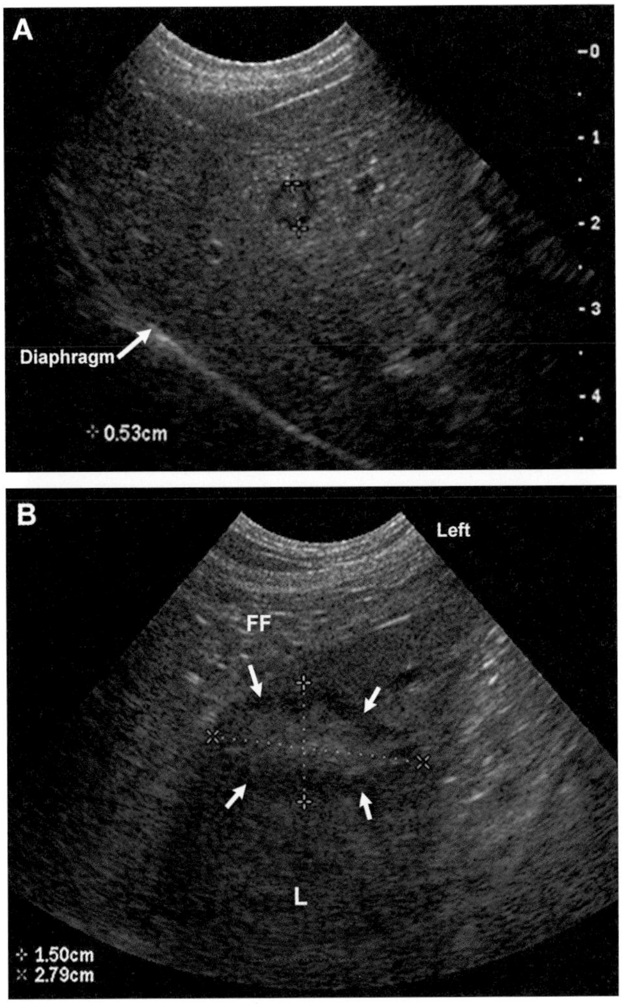

Figure 6.32. Target lesions. **A:** Longitudinal image of the midportion of the liver in a dog with intestinal carcinoma, on which a small nodule outlined by a peripheral hypoechoic halo is seen. The central portion of this lesion is more echogenic, giving the impression of a target. **B:** Longitudinal oblique image of the left portion of the liver of a dog with a primary hepatocellular carcinoma identified in the right lateral lobe. An ovoid nodule with a peripheral hypoechoic halo and a more echogenic center (arrows), consistent with a metastasis, is in the liver (L). Smaller but similar target lesions were found in the rest of the liver. FF, falciform fat.

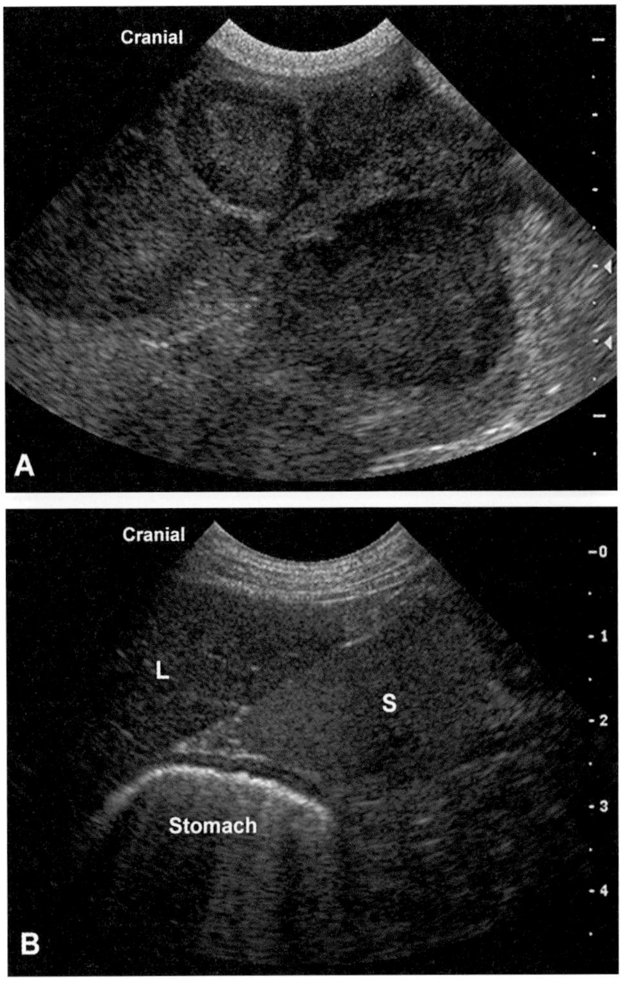

Figure 6.33. Disseminated histiocytic sarcoma (malignant histiocytosis). **A:** Multiple hypoechoic nodules and masses (more than 3 cm wide) are in the liver of this Bernese mountain dog. These lesions are relatively well circumscribed and have a mildly echogenic center. The liver was also enlarged. **B:** In this other dog with disseminated histiocytic sarcoma, the liver (L) is uniformly hypoechoic and enlarged. The difference between the hepatic and splenic (S) echogenicities was considered excessive.

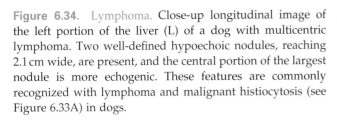

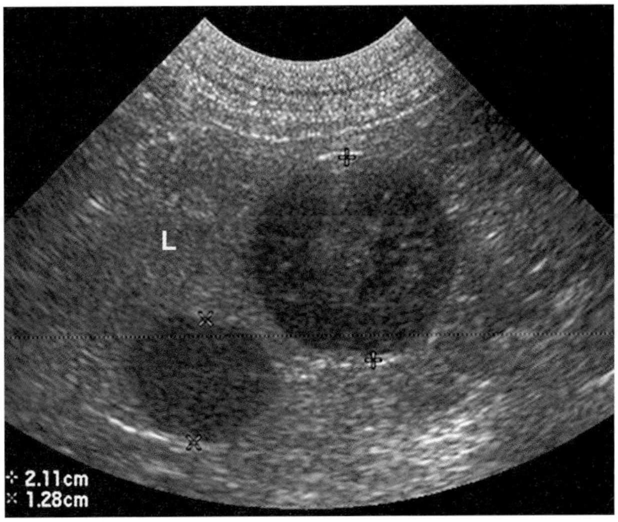

Figure 6.34. Lymphoma. Close-up longitudinal image of the left portion of the liver (L) of a dog with multicentric lymphoma. Two well-defined hypoechoic nodules, reaching 2.1 cm wide, are present, and the central portion of the largest nodule is more echogenic. These features are commonly recognized with lymphoma and malignant histiocytosis (see Figure 6.33A) in dogs.

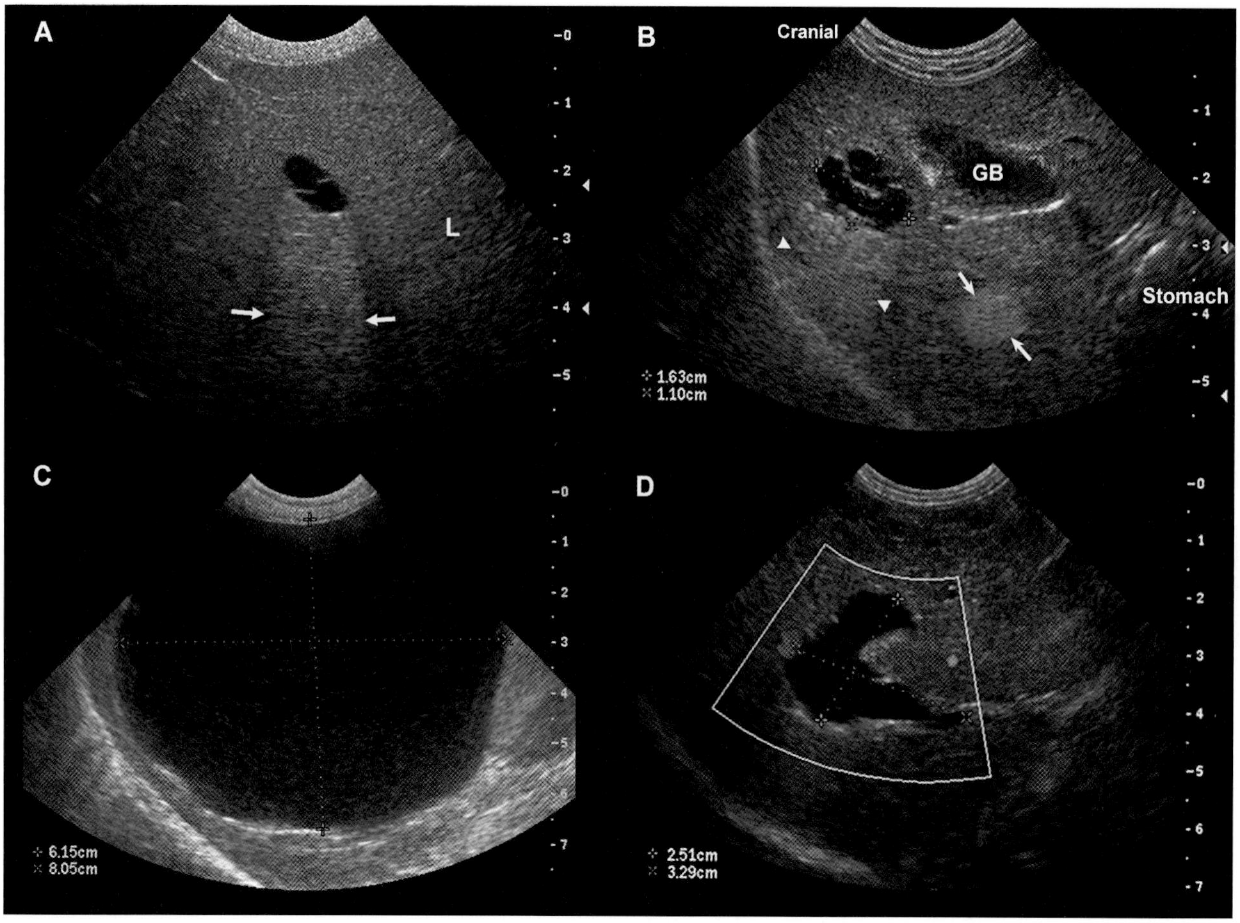

Figure 6.35. Benign hepatic cyst-like lesions. **A:** Transverse image of the liver (L) of a dog with a discrete anechoic structure (approximately 1 cm wide) that is septated and associated with far acoustic enhancement (arrows), consistent with hypoattenuating content. A clear fluid was aspirated with ultrasound guidance. The peripheral hepatic parenchyma is homogeneous. **B:** Longitudinal image of the liver of a dog with a well-circumscribed, loculated, anechoic structure. Irregular contours and far enhancement (arrowheads) are present. Bile was aspirated. The clinical significance of this finding was not determined in this patient. A hyperechoic regenerative nodule (arrows) is also present. The gallbladder wall is thickened and irregular (GB), presumably because of cholecystitis. **C and D:** Ultrasound images of a large liver cyst in a dog with abdominal pain that were obtained before **(C)** and after **(D)** ultrasound-guided drainage. The peripheral liver parenchyma is normal.

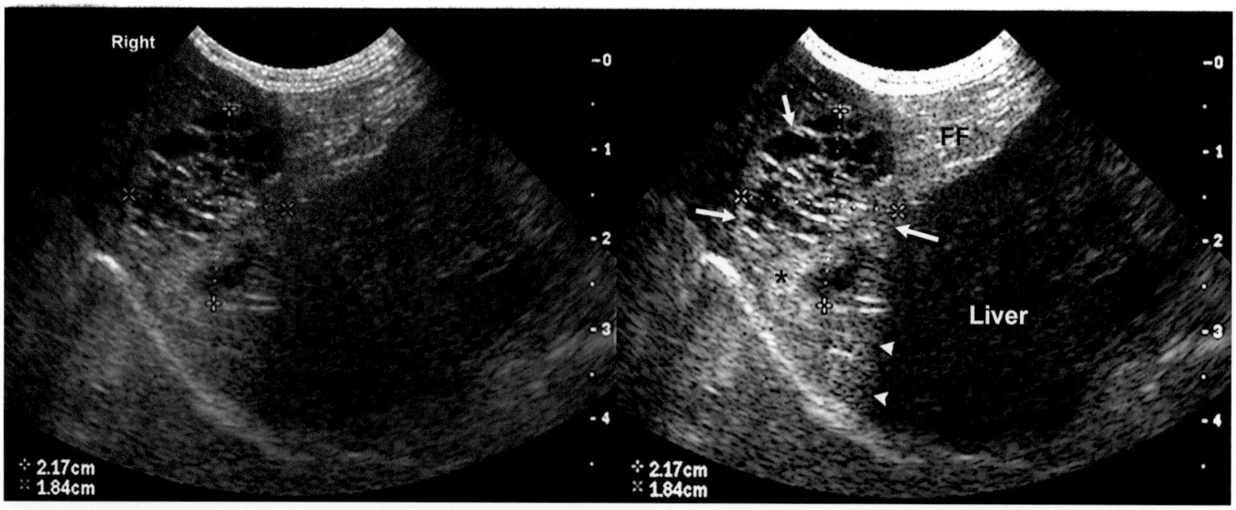

Figure 6.36. Biliary cystadenocarcinoma in a cat. Transverse ultrasonographic and corresponding schematic images of the liver of a cat with increased hepatic enzymes. A multiloculated mass (arrows and cursors) with a more solid dorsal component (*) is identified in the right portion of the liver. Far acoustic enhancement is noted (arrowheads) because of the presence of hypoattenuating fluid-filled cavities. A malignant tumor was confirmed through ultrasound-guided biopsy. FF, falciform fat.

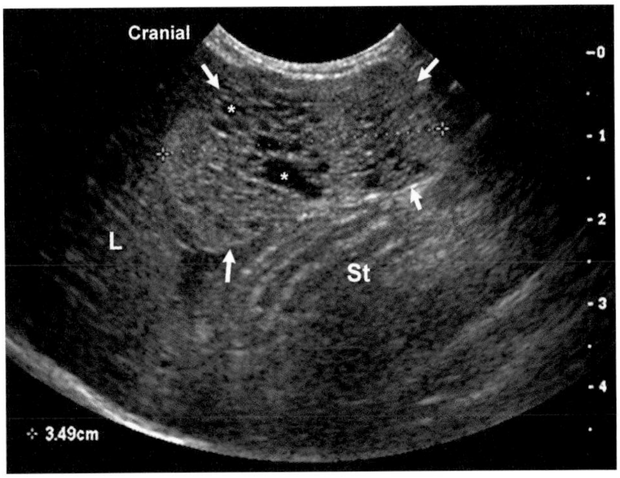

Figure 6.37. Biliary cystadenoma in a cat. Longitudinal oblique image of the left portion of the liver of a cat with a palpable mass in the cranioventral abdomen. A multiloculated hyperechoic mass (arrows) is ventral to the stomach (St) and connected to the liver (L). Within this mass are multiple anechoic cavities (*), consistent with biliary cystadenoma.

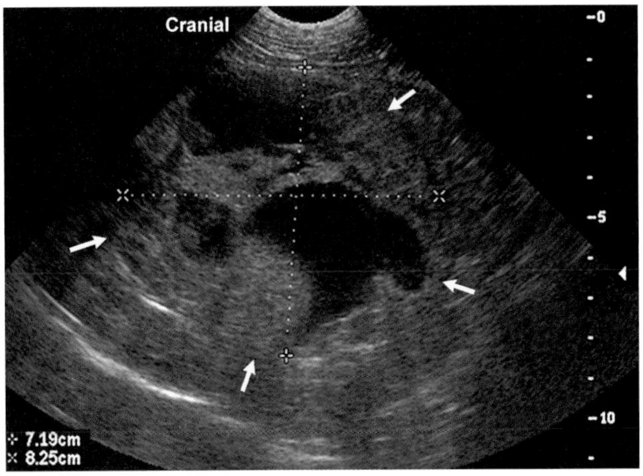

Figure 6.38. Biliary carcinoma in a dog. Longitudinal image of the right portion of the liver in an icteric dog with a large cavitated mass. This poorly defined mass (arrows) contains irregular hypoechoic and anechoic cavitations. The findings on ultrasound-guided fine-needle aspiration of the more solid portions of the mass were suggestive of biliary carcinoma.

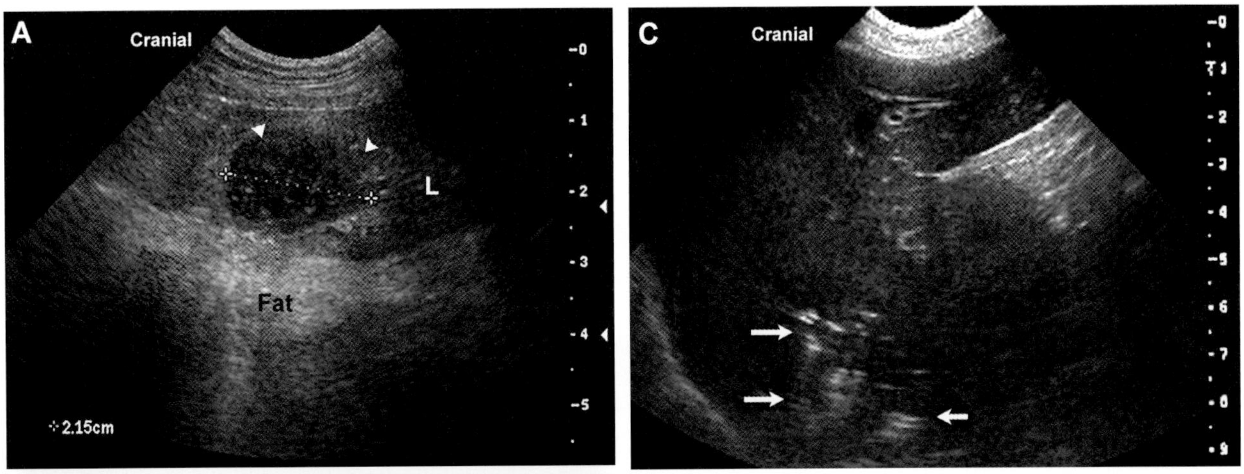

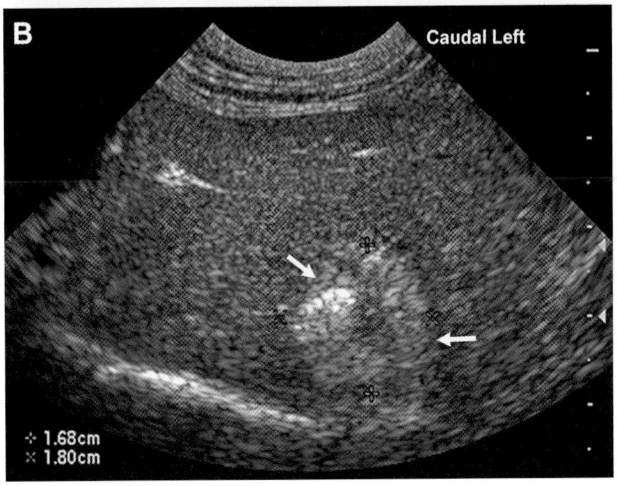

Figure 6.39. Hepatic abscesses. **A:** Longitudinal image of the left portion of the liver in a febrile dog with abdominal pain. An irregular hypoechoic lesion (arrowheads) can be seen. The abdominal fat adjacent to the liver (L) border is hyperechoic and hyperattenuating, suggesting steatitis. Ultrasound-guided fine-needle aspiration confirmed the presence of an abscess. **B:** Longitudinal oblique image of the left portion of the liver in a febrile dog. A poorly defined hyperechoic nodule (arrows) with a hypoechoic center is found at the dorsal margin of this lobe, which was indicative of a septic abscess. **C:** Longitudinal image of the liver of a Airedale terrier in which a hepatic abscess was identified. The abscessed region (arrows), deep in the liver, is poorly marginated and contains several reverberating, hyperechoic foci consistent with gas. Image C courtesy of D. Penninck.

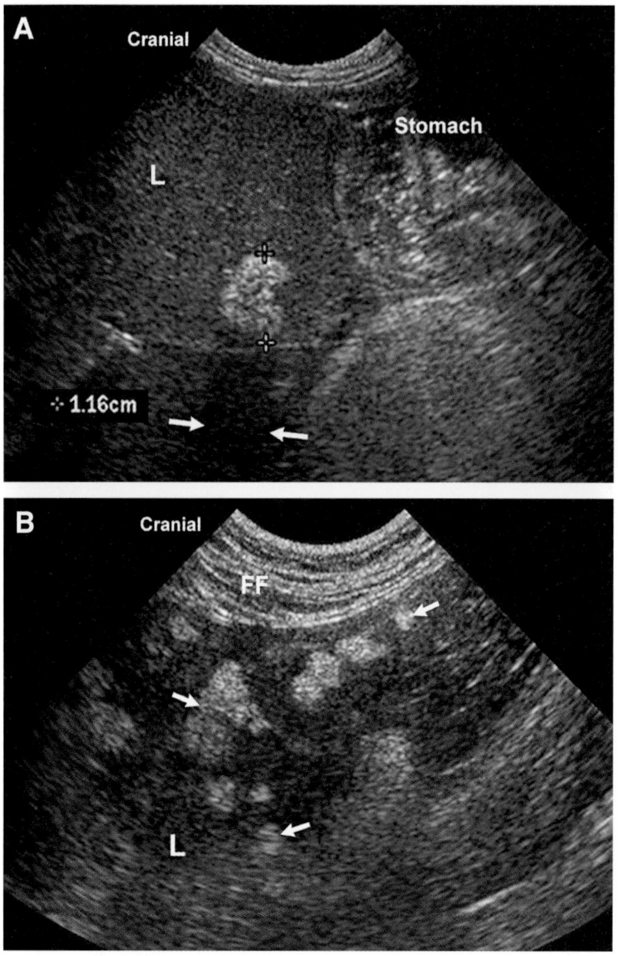

Figure 6.40. Hepatic granulomas. **A:** Longitudinal image of the left portion of the liver (L) in a dog with a relatively well-defined hyperechoic focus associated with acoustic shadowing (arrows). A granuloma was diagnosed, although no underlying etiology could be identified. This granuloma was thought to be an incidental finding. **B:** Longitudinal image of the right portion of the liver in an icteric cat with irregular hyperechoic nodules (arrows) dispersed within a hypoechoic liver (L). The diagnosis was pyogranulomatous cholangiohepatitis in relation to feline infectious peritonitis. FF, falciform fat.

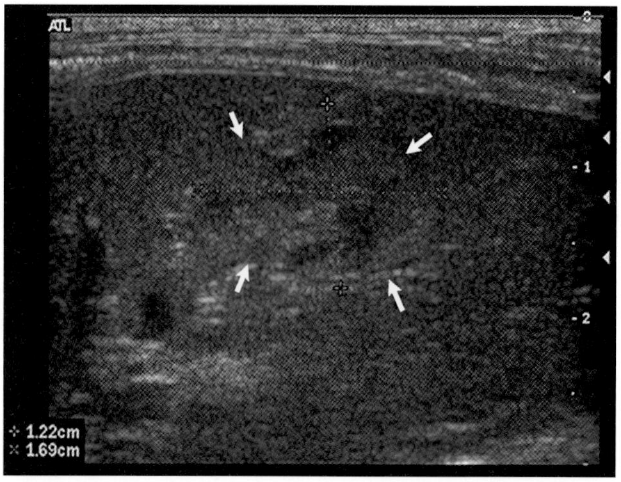

Figure 6.41. Hepatic hematoma. Longitudinal image of the left portion of the liver in small-breed dog that was bitten by a larger dog 3 days earlier. An ill-defined, irregular area of mixed echogenicity (arrows and cursors), consistent with a traumatic hematoma, is found in the superficial portion of the liver.

(Figure 6.41). With time, hematomas tend to develop a cystic component following clot lysis. This feature, as well as the progressive reduction in size on follow-up exams, should help in differentiating spontaneous hematomas from neoplastic processes. Hepatic mineralization other than cholelithiasis can accompany benign processes (such as hematoma or granuloma) or malignant processes. Mineralization typically appears as strongly hyperechoic foci associated with acoustic shadowing (Figure 6.42). However, the visibility or magnitude of the shadowing is influenced by several factors, such as the size of the mineral foci relative to the size of the ultrasound beam, image contrast, and equipment settings (probe frequency, gain, and focal zone). Furthermore, other types of hyperattenuating material, such as fibrous tissue or a migrating foreign body, can also be associated with acoustic shadowing.

Hepatic Lobe Torsion, Infarction, and Gas

Liver-lobe torsion, which leads to lobar congestion, hemorrhage, and necrosis, can show variable signs that can mimic neoplasia or abscess formation. In a recent report, the affected lobe was hypoechoic (more commonly) or mixed in echogenicity, and Doppler assessment of the lobe revealed reduced vascularity in many dogs (Hinkle Schwartz et al. 2006) (Figure 6.43). Spontaneous infarction is less common in the liver when compared with the spleen, but can show a similar pattern of an irregular and poorly echogenic area with reduced flow on color Doppler or power Doppler (Figure 6.44). Hyperechoic foci associated with reverberating artifact, consistent with gas, can be seen in the liver, most often in the biliary tract, following surgery. Gas can also form because of bacterial infection (Figure 6.45). Metallic clips used with surgical biopsies appear as short, strongly hyperechoic lines with reverberation, mimicking gas. A radiograph can be used, if needed, to differentiate gas from metal.

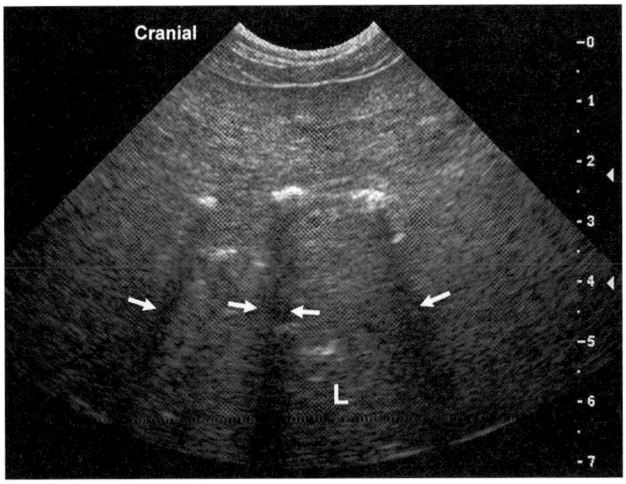

Figure 6.42. Parenchymal mineralization. Longitudinal image of the left portion of the liver (L) in a dog with chronic hepatitis. The liver parenchyma is diffusely hyperechoic, with several small, hyperechoic, irregular foci associated with acoustic shadowing (arrows).

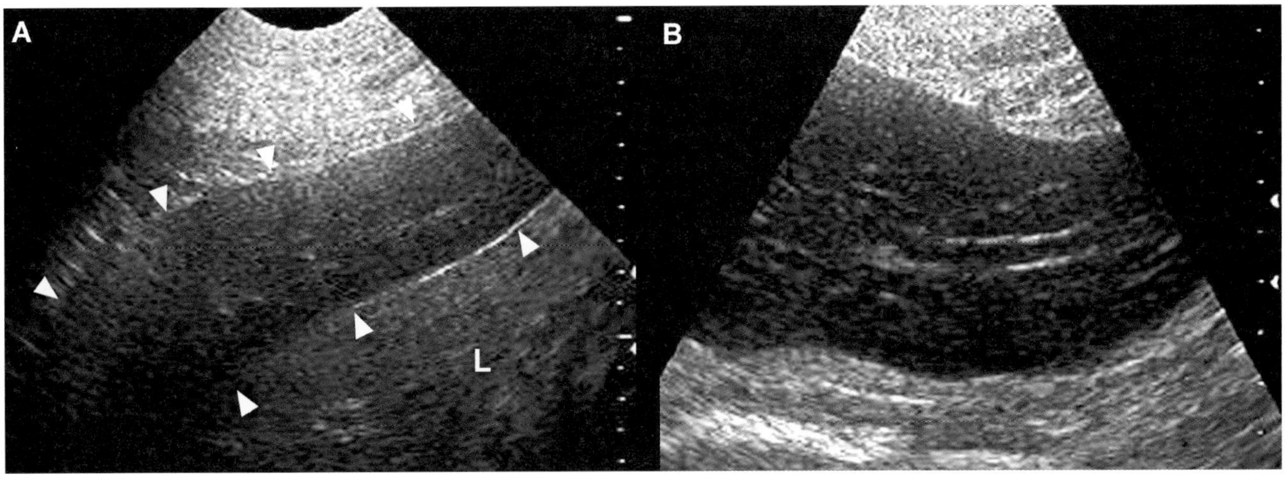

Figure 6.43. Hepatic lobe torsion. **A:** The twisted left lateral liver lobe is diffusely hypoechoic (arrowheads), contrasting with the underlying left medial lobe (L). **B:** A close-up view of the affected lobe. There was no evidence of flow through the visible vessels. The lobe margins are rounded. The surrounding fat is hyperechoic. Images courtesy of D. Penninck.

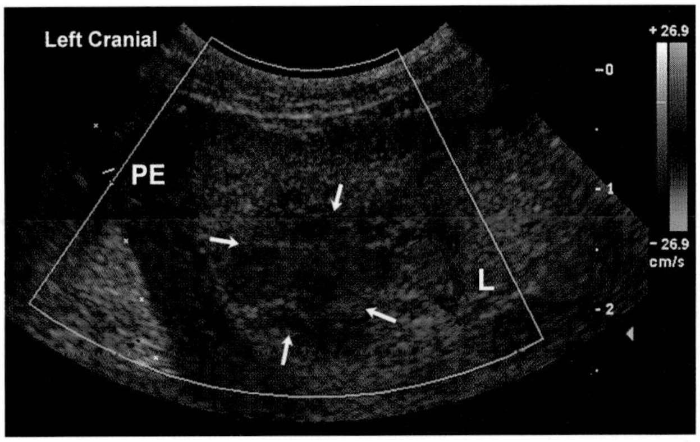

Figure 6.44. Hepatic infarction. Longitudinal oblique image of the left portion of the liver (L) of dog with increased liver enzymes. Within the liver is an irregular hypoechoic region (arrows) with peripheral vascular signal. Ultrasound-guided biopsy revealed infarction of uncertain origin. Peritoneal effusion (PE) is also noted.

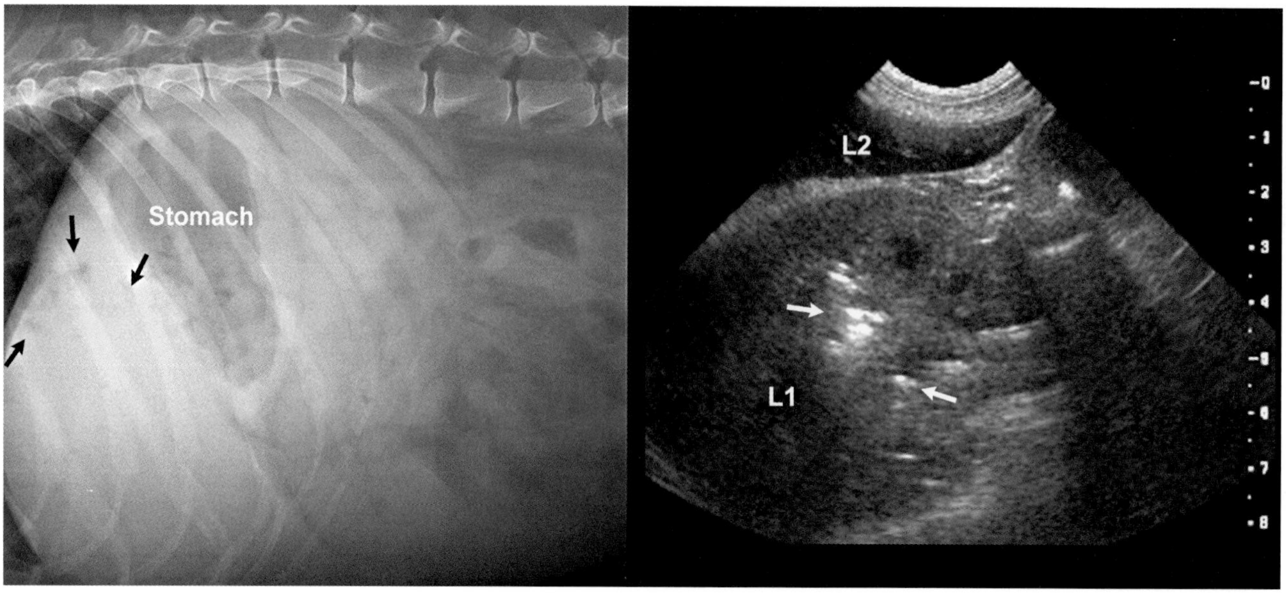

Figure 6.45. Emphysematous hepatitis. Corresponding lateral abdominal radiograph and sonogram of a dog with emphysematous hepatitis. Gas foci (arrows) are radiotransparent on the radiograph and hyperechoic with reverberation artifacts on the ultrasound image. The affected lobe (L1) is enlarged, hyperechoic, and heterogeneous when compared with an adjacent lobe (L2). Images courtesy of D. Penninck.

Disorders of the Biliary System

Biliary Obstruction

Ultrasonography has become an important investigative tool in assessing icteric dogs and cats with biliary obstruction. After complete obstruction of the CBD, retrograde dilatation is expected that initially affects the CBD and GB, followed by the extrahepatic ducts and intrahepatic ducts (Nyland and Gillett 1982). With extrahepatic biliary obstruction, the cystic duct and CBD dilate and often become tortuous proximal to the site of obstruction (Figures 6.46–6.51). A CBD more than 4mm wide is usually predictive of obstruction in cats (Léveillé et al. 1996). This is probably also true in dogs, although it has not been described. Within 5–7 days, irregular and tortuous anechoic tubes with hyperechoic walls can be found in the liver, following the more linear PVs and unassociated with color flow, indicating dilated hepatic ducts. This sign, also referred to as the "too many tubes" sign, is usually indicative of complete obstruction (Figures 6.47C and 6.48). Additionally, these anechoic tubes can be associated with acoustic far enhancement, which is not expected with vessels than contain a more attenuating fluid (Nyland and Gillett 1982). Although the GB can be dilated with biliary obstruction, wall contraction or inflammation possibly associated with fibrosis can limit its capacity to distend. Furthermore, reduced compliance of the peripheral liver parenchyma may limit GB dilatation. Thus, the absence of GB distension should not be used to rule out biliary obstruction.

Extrahepatic biliary obstruction more commonly involves the CBD, mainly in its distal segment, in proximity to the major duodenal papilla. Pancreatitis is often responsible for CBD obstruction, particularly in dogs, because of edema, inflammation, and fibrosis involving the duodenal wall and major papilla and/or the CBD (Fahie and Martin 1995; Léveillé et al. 1996; Mayhew et al. 2002) (Figure 6.49). Chronic duodenitis or cholecystitis can also be associated with fibrous tissue proliferation and subsequent stenosis. Inflammatory processes involving the biliary tract can be associated with cholelithiasis (Mayhew et al. 2002). The CBD must be evaluated thoroughly for the presence of hyperechoic and hyperattenuating choleliths, possibly lodged in the distal CBD (Figure 6.50). Choleliths can also form secondary to partial or complete biliary obstruction (Mayhew et al. 2002), thus complicating the ultrasound identification of the source of the obstruction.

Several types of neoplasia (predominantly carcinomas) involving the biliary tract, the duodenum, or the pancreas can cause biliary obstruction (Fahie and Martin 1995). Nodules or masses of variable echo-

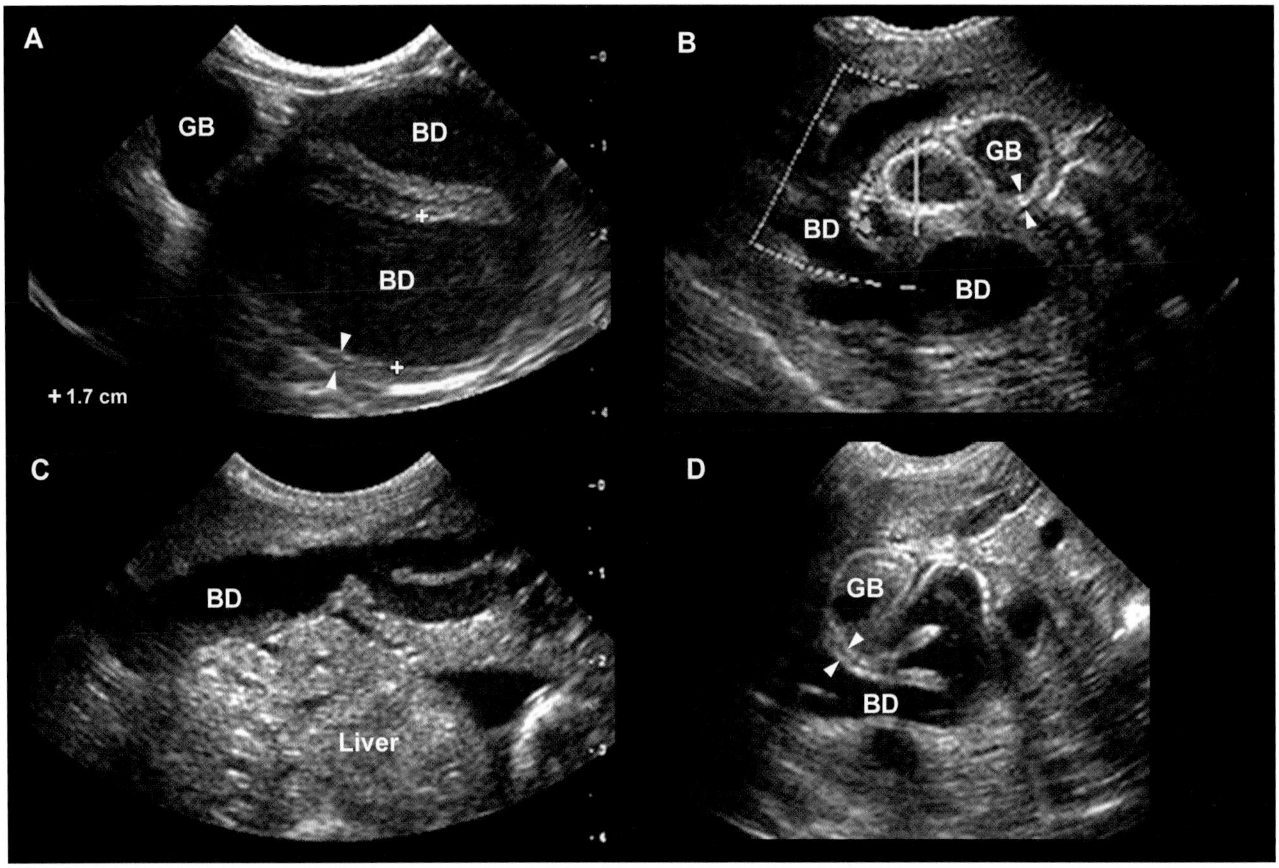

Figure 6.46. Congenital malformation with biliary ectasia in two cats. **A:** Sagittal image at the porta hepatis in a 2-year-old cat with biliary obstruction. Numerous bile ducts (BD), including the common bile duct, are markedly dilated (lumen between the cursors) and show a thickened wall (arrowheads). The bile content is also more echogenic than normal. Extensive biliary tree fibrosis and stenosis were identified, and an underlying congenital defect was suspected. GB, gallbladder. **B–D:** Similar changes observed in a 8-month-old cat. The bile ducts are distended and irregular. The gallbladder (GB) contains echogenic sludge and shows a thickened, hyperechoic wall (arrowheads). Color Doppler **(B)** was used to confirm the absence of flow in these bile ducts (BD), distinguishing those from hepatic vessels. A congenital defect such as hypoplasia or atresia of the common bile duct was suspected at necropsy. Images courtesy of D. Penninck.

genicity, sometimes with a cystic component, can be observed (Figure 6.51). Evaluation of the rest of the abdomen, especially the liver parenchyma and lymph nodes, can help in differentiating benign from malignant processes. Fine-needle aspiration or biopsy is recommended if the abnormal tissue can be safely reached.

Gallbladder and Common Bile Duct Wall Anomalies

GB wall thickening (greater than 1 mm in cats and greater than 2–3 mm in dogs) can be caused by inflammation (cholecystitis), edema (portal hypertension, hypoalbuminemia, biliary obstruction, or inflammation), cystic mucosal hyperplasia, or rarely neoplasia (Nyland and Park 1983; Spaulding 1993; Hittmair et al. 2001). With cholecystitis, the chronicity and severity of the inflammatory process influence the appearance of the wall. Although it can appear normal, thickening is often seen, along with a double-rim pattern (particularly in more acute cases) or diffuse wall hyperechogenicity, sometimes associated with dystrophic mineralization, particularly in chronic cholecystitis (Figure 6.52). The double-rim pattern is often seen in wall edema (Figure 6.53). Changes in the GB wall may be more evident with concurrent parenchymal hypoechogenicity, such as in many cases of feline cholangiohepatitis.

Thickening of the CBD wall, along with luminal dilatation, is also common with cholecystitis (Figure 6.54). In fact, it can be difficult to differentiate obstructive dilation of the CBD from dilatation associated with stasis secondary to chronic inflammation of the

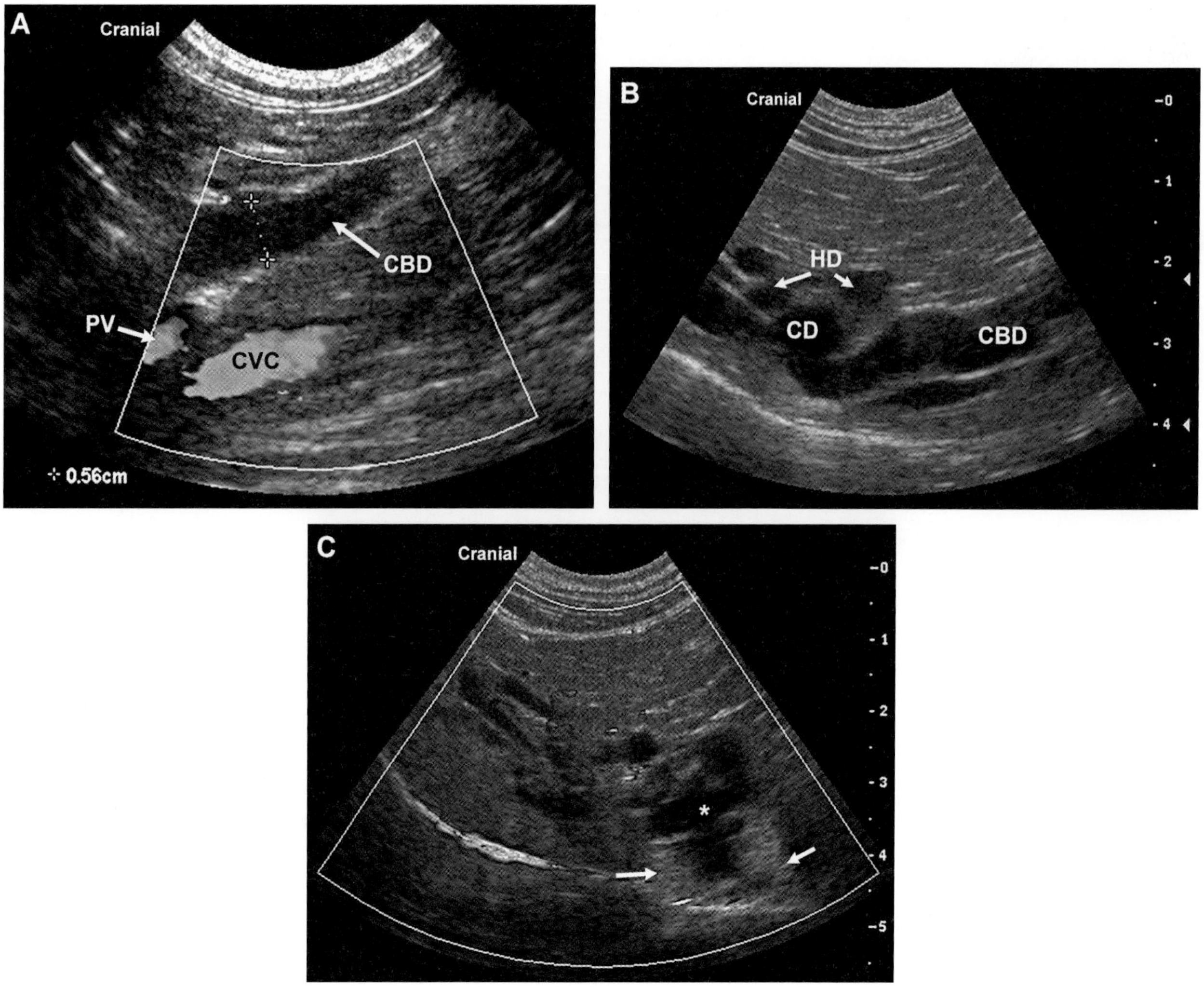

Figure 6.47. Extrahepatic biliary obstruction. **A:** Longitudinal image obtained just caudal to the porta hepatis of a dog with a dilated common bile duct (CBD) ventral to the portal vein (PV) and caudal vena cava (CVC). The lumen of the CBD reaches 5.6mm wide, indicating an obstruction located more distally. **B:** Longitudinal image obtained in the central perihilar region of the liver of an icteric cat. Tortuous hypoechoic to anechoic tubular structures representing dilated hepatic duct (HD), cystic duct (CD), and common bile duct (CBD) indicate extrahepatic biliary obstruction. **C:** Longitudinal image (with power Doppler) of the right portion of the liver in a cat with an obstructive mass involving the common bile duct. Multiple anechoic, tortuous, tubular structures without evidence of flow that are indicative of intrahepatic bile ducts are found in the liver. A lobulated anechoic structure at the porta hepatis is associated with far acoustic enhancement (arrows) consistent with a dilatation of the junction of the extrahepatic biliary ducts, the cystic duct, and the common bile duct.

Figure 6.50. Obstructive cholelith. Longitudinal ultrasonographic and schematic images obtained in a cat with icterus. A small hyperechoic structure, consistent with a cholelith (arrow), is found in the distal portion of the common bile duct (CBD). The common bile duct and cystic duct (CD) are dilated and thickened (1.7mm) because of cholecystitis and biliary obstruction. The stone is casting an acoustic shadow (*).

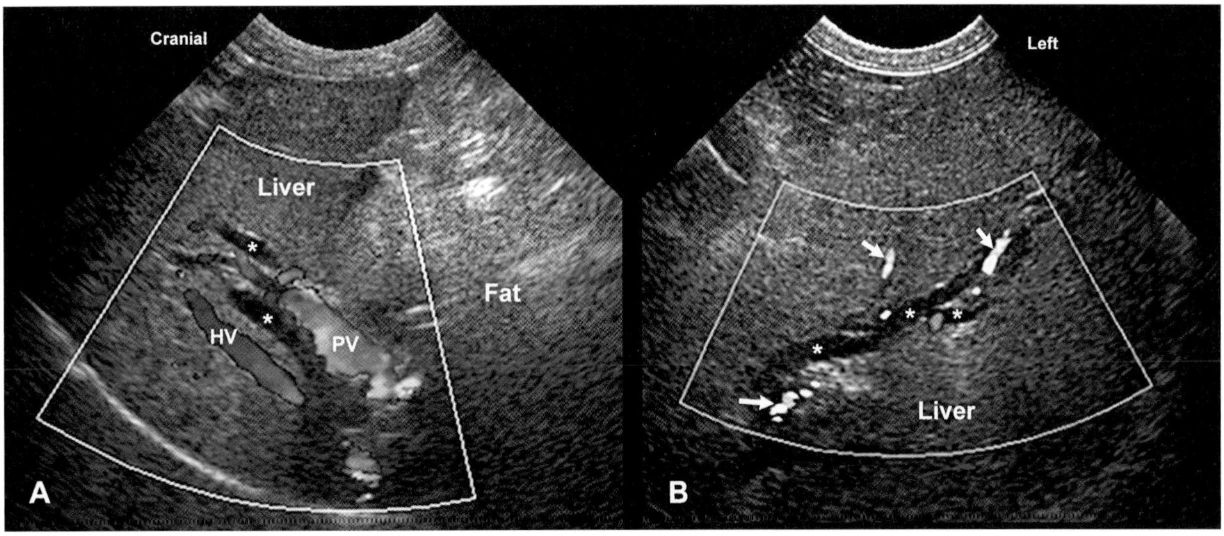

Figure 6.48. Chronic extrahepatic biliary obstruction. Longitudinal **(A)** and transverse **(B)** images of the liver of a dog with tortuous, anechoic, tubular structures (*) near the portal veins (PV and arrows). Power Doppler was used to confirm the absence of flow in these tubes, indicating intrahepatic biliary duct distension. The hyperechoic and hyperattenuating fat caudal to the liver seen in longitudinal image **A** was consistent with steatitis. Chronic pancreatitis was diagnosed.

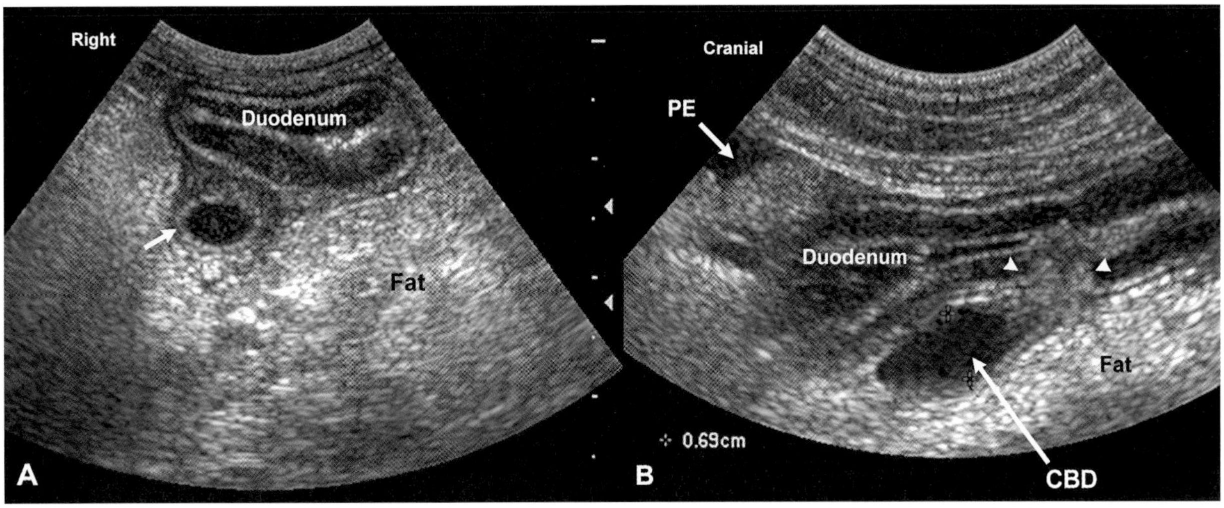

Figure 6.49. Pancreatitis and biliary obstruction. Transverse **(A)** and longitudinal **(B)** images of the proximal duodenum of a dog with pancreatitis. The distal portion of the common bile duct (CBD) is dilated. The peripheral fat is markedly hyperechoic, and a small amount of peritoneal effusion is noted (PE). The duodenal papilla (arrowheads) is hyperechoic and subjectively enlarged, and the wall of the common bile duct appears thickened. These changes suggest an extension of the inflammatory process to these structures that causes biliary obstruction. In **A,** the arrow points to the thickened common bile duct wall.

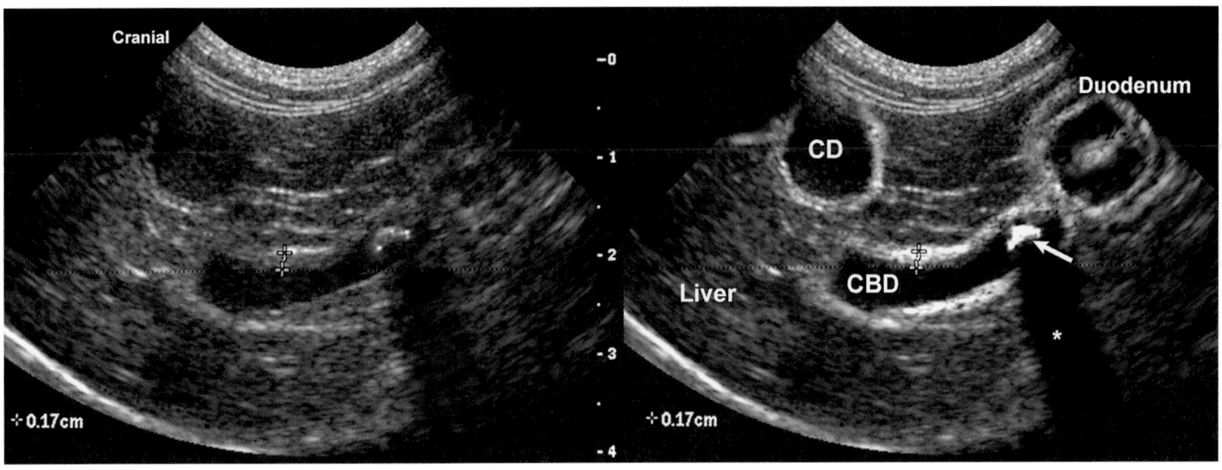

Figure 6.50.

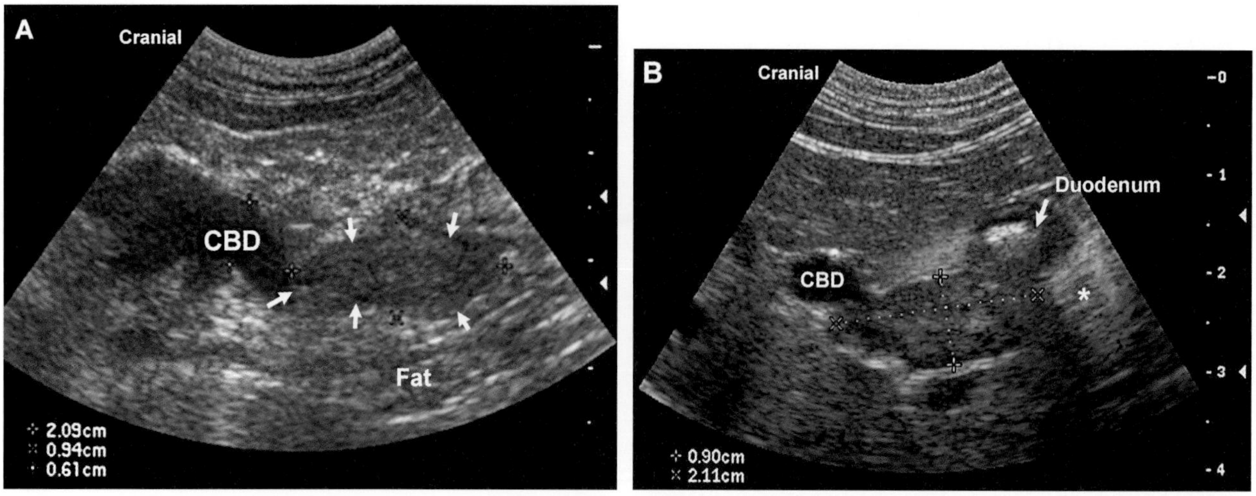

Figure 6.51. Biliary obstruction by a mass. **A: Biliary carcinoma in a cat.** Longitudinal image of a cat's common bile duct (CBD) with a uniform, mildly echogenic mass (arrows and cursors) obliterating the lumen of the CBD. These features can indicate chronic cholecystitis with fibrosis, or a neoplastic process. Biliary carcinoma was identified at surgery. **B: Chronic cholecystitis and common bile duct obstruction.** Longitudinal image of the common bile duct in a cat with chronic suppurative cholangiohepatitis and cholecystitis. Within the distal common bile duct (CBD) is a mass (cursors) that suggests a neoplastic process. However, this mass was confirmed to represent pyogranulomatous inflammation associated with fibrous tissue. Adjacent hyperechoic fat (*) is consistent with steatitis.

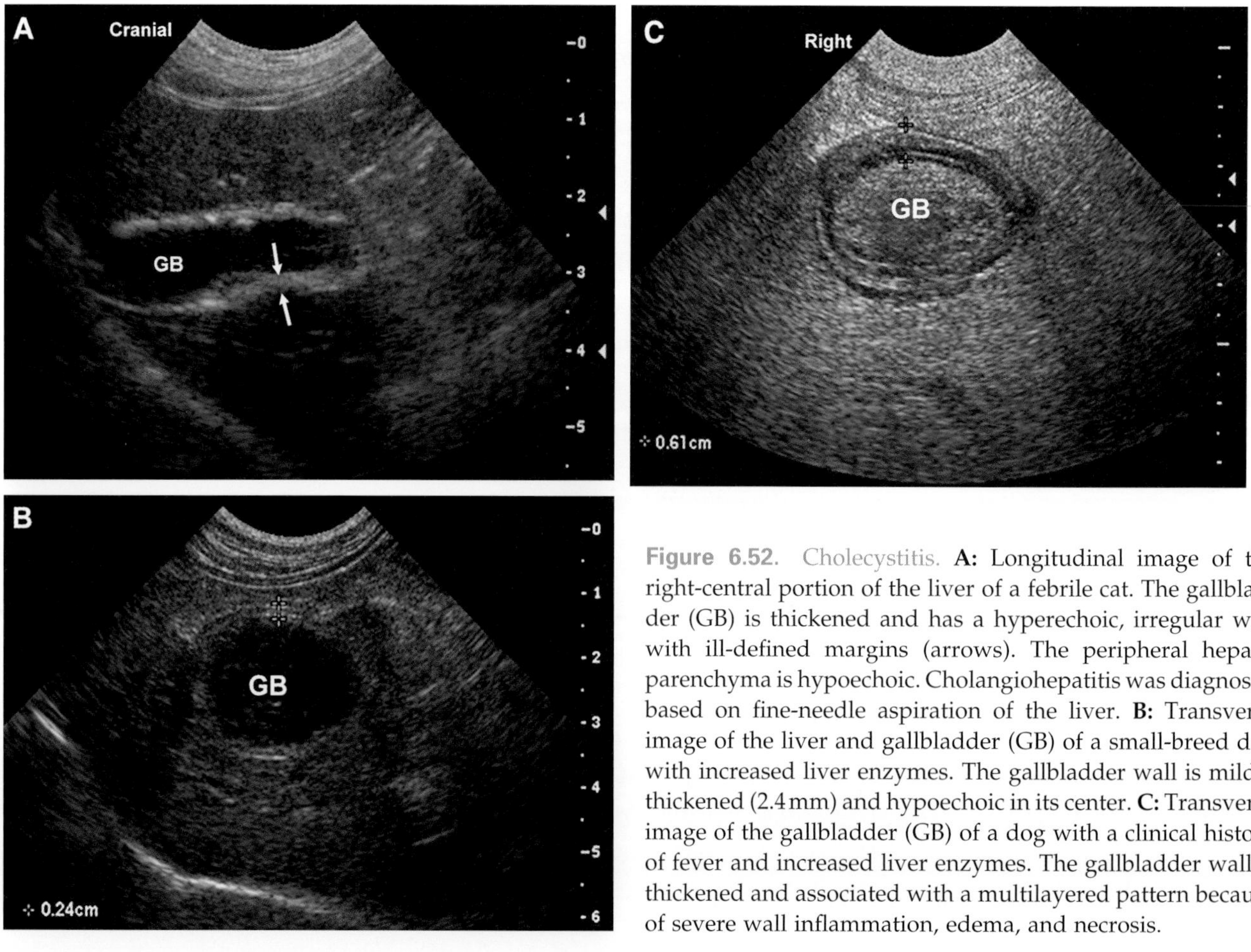

Figure 6.52. Cholecystitis. **A:** Longitudinal image of the right-central portion of the liver of a febrile cat. The gallbladder (GB) is thickened and has a hyperechoic, irregular wall with ill-defined margins (arrows). The peripheral hepatic parenchyma is hypoechoic. Cholangiohepatitis was diagnosed based on fine-needle aspiration of the liver. **B:** Transverse image of the liver and gallbladder (GB) of a small-breed dog with increased liver enzymes. The gallbladder wall is mildly thickened (2.4 mm) and hypoechoic in its center. **C:** Transverse image of the gallbladder (GB) of a dog with a clinical history of fever and increased liver enzymes. The gallbladder wall is thickened and associated with a multilayered pattern because of severe wall inflammation, edema, and necrosis.

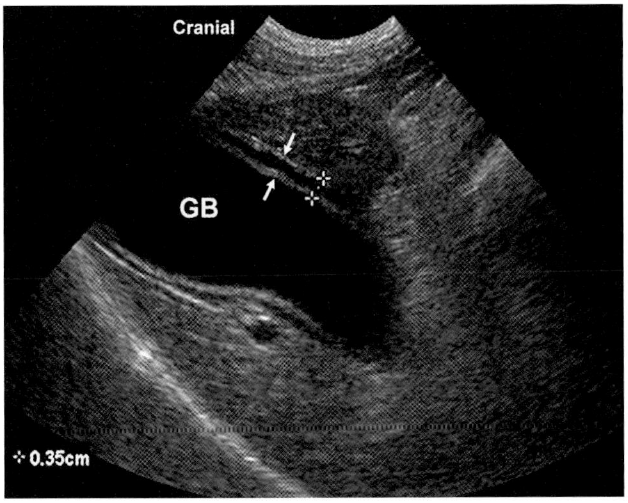

Figure 6.53. Gallbladder wall edema. Longitudinal image of the gallbladder (GB) in a dog with hypoalbuminemia. The gallbladder wall is thickened, with a double rim (arrows) consistent with edema. Cholecystitis could be not excluded based on the image (see Figure 6.52B).

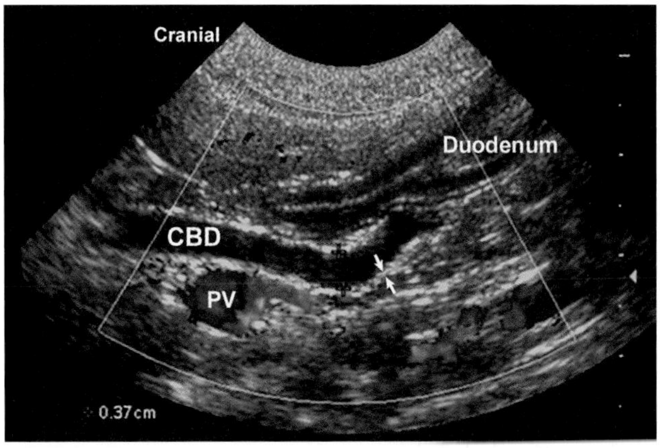

Figure 6.54. Common bile duct thickening. Longitudinal image of the common bile duct (CBD) of a cat with elevated liver enzymes and vomiting. The lumen of the common bile duct is well visualized, while less than 4 mm wide. The duct wall (arrows) is thickened and hyperechoic, suggesting an inflammatory process. The cat responded to medical treatments for cholecystitis. PV, portal vein.

biliary system (Léveillé et al. 1996). Furthermore, in chronic outflow obstruction, the CBD can remain dilated even after the cause of obstruction has been alleviated.

GB wall polyps and malignant neoplastic processes, although rarely seen in dogs and cats, can be associated with biliary obstruction. Although it can be difficult to differentiate these processes, pedunculated echogenic masses protruding into the GB lumen are more typical of polyps.

GB mucoceles are being increasingly recognized in dogs, particularly in older dogs of small and medium-sized breeds, now representing an important cause of biliary obstruction (Besso et al. 2000). This complex pathology is characterized by an excessive accumulation of mucus within the GB lumen, progressively leading to overdistension and wall necrosis and rupture. Intraluminal mucinous plugs can extend or migrate into the CBD and cause obstruction. In affected GB, a characteristic accumulation of hypoechoic mucus is seen boarding the inner margin of the wall, centrally displacing the echogenic biliary sludge, which becomes independent of gravity. As the mucocele is progressively formed in the GB, a *stellate pattern* is seen initially, followed by the appearance of immobile hyperechoic radiating striations that lead to the appearance of a *kiwifruit-like pattern* (Figures 6.55–6.57) (Besso et al. 2000). The GB wall may also appear thickened, hyperechoic, and irregular because of edema, inflammation, and/or necrosis. A discontinuity in the GB wall is an important sign of rupture, along with the presence of hyperechoic fat at the periphery of the GB and the presence of peritoneal effusion (Figure 6.57). These signs generally indicate a surgical emergency. Fragments of mucoceles may also migrate within the peritoneal cavity (Figure 6.57B). Although most affected dogs have concurrent clinical evidence of hepatobiliary disease, GB mucocele can be found incidentally on ultrasound.

Cholelithiasis

Choleliths are often incidental within any portion of the biliary tract in dogs and cats. An underlying or consecutive inflammatory process (cholecystitis or cholangiohepatitis) is more commonly recognized in cats (Eich and Ludwig 2002). These calculi typically appear as well-defined, hyperechoic, shadowing foci with a tendency to form linear tracts when located in the hepatic ducts or a sediment in the GB lumen and cystic duct (Figure 6.58). Consecutive intrahepatic or extrahepatic biliary obstruction can be observed, although choleliths may also form because of an obstruction (Mayhew et al. 2002).

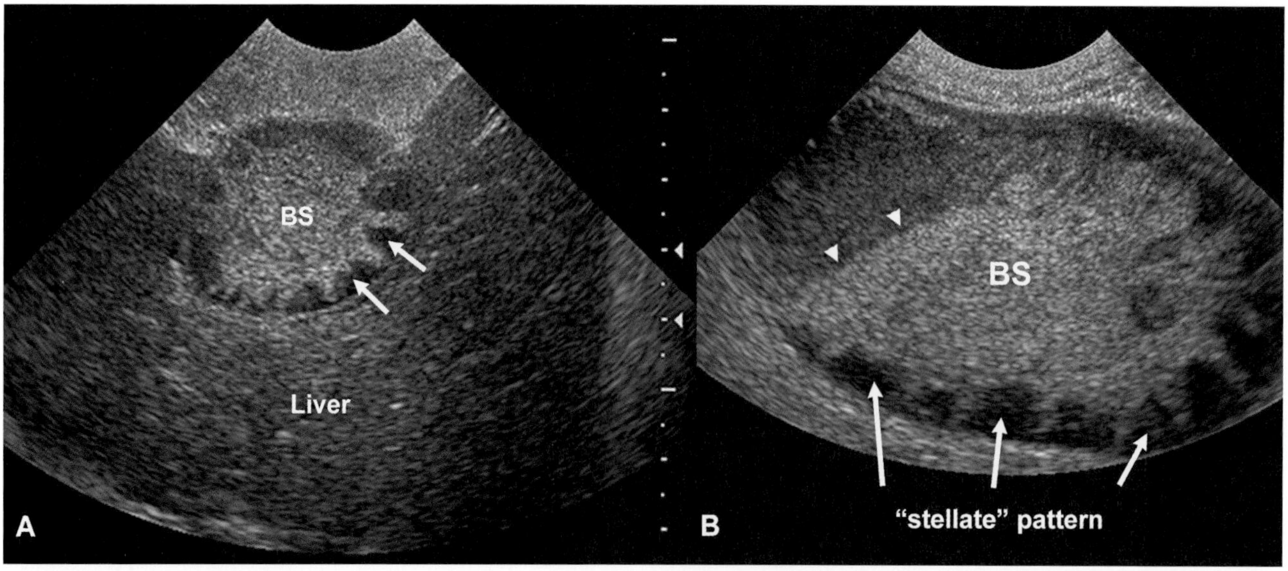

Figure 6.55. Partial gallbladder mucocele. Transverse **(A)** and longitudinal **(B)** images of the gallbladder of a dog with increased liver enzymes. The gallbladder is distended with echogenic biliary sludge (BS) in the dependent portion of the lumen (arrowheads at horizontal level). An interrupted and irregular, hypoechoic to anechoic rim is visible at the inner periphery of the gallbladder, consistent with mucus. The triangular shape of these hypoechoic foci (arrows) has been referred as the *stellate pattern*.

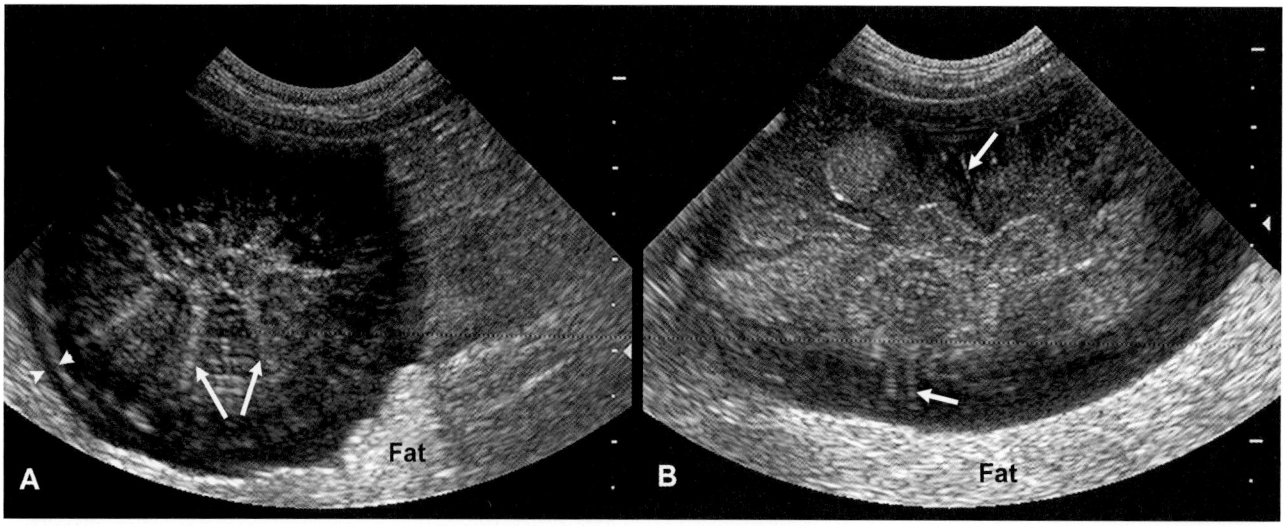

Figure 6.56. Complete gallbladder mucocele. Transverse **(A)** and longitudinal **(B)** images of the gallbladder of a dog with icterus and acute abdominal pain. The gallbladder is distended and shows a pattern of hyperechoic striations (arrows) radiating toward its center. The central hyperechoic area is heterogeneous and completely immobile. These features are described as a *kiwifruit-like pattern*, which is a pathognomonic sign for gallbladder mucocele. The gallbladder wall is also thickened (arrowheads) and the adjacent fat is hyperechoic, suggesting imminent or recent wall rupture.

Figure 6.58. Cholelithiasis. **A:** Longitudinal image of the central portion of the liver (L) in a small dog with acute pancreatitis. Several rounded hyperechoic structures (*) associated with acoustic shadowing (arrowheads), consistent with choleliths, are in the gallbladder (GB) neck. Small hyperechoic foci, associated with some reverberation (arrow), are in the nondependent ventral region of the gallbladder. These foci could indicate small choleliths adhered to the wall or indicate gas. There was no increase in liver enzymes in this dog. The gallstones were not considered clinically significant. **B:** A larger volume of cholelithiasis (*) is in the dependent portion of the gallbladder (GB) of this other larger dog with Cushing's disease. Similar ultrasound features are observed. **C:** Transverse oblique image of the left portion of the liver of a cat with increased liver enzymes. Several linear hyperechoic tracts (short arrows), causing acoustic shadowing (arrowheads), are parallel to the portal veins (PV). These features suggest cholelithiasis within the intrahepatic biliary ducts. Cholangiohepatitis was diagnosed with ultrasound-guided aspiration and biopsy.

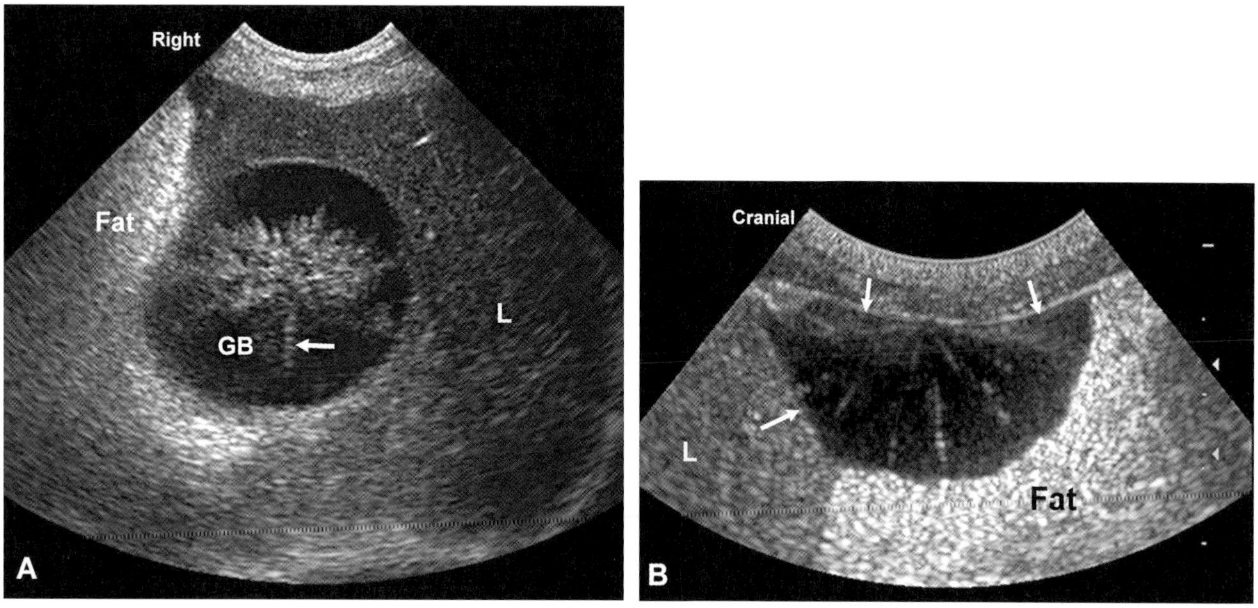

Figure 6.57. Gallbladder rupture. **A: Transverse image of the gallbladder in a dog** with signs of acute abdominal pain. A *kiwifruit-like pattern* of striations, consistent with mucocele, is noted (arrow) in the gallbladder (GB). The fat at the right and ventral aspects of the gallbladder is markedly hyperechoic and hyperattenuating, highly suggestive of wall perforation and was confirmed with surgical exploration. L, liver. **B: Migrating mucocele.** Longitudinal image of the region just caudoventral to the liver (L) in a dog with gallbladder mucocele. A crescent-shaped anechoic structure with fine radiating striations (arrows) is found at the caudal margin of the liver. This structure represents a fragment of mucocele that migrated after gallbladder rupture. Consecutive bile peritonitis was present, associated with hyperechoic fat.

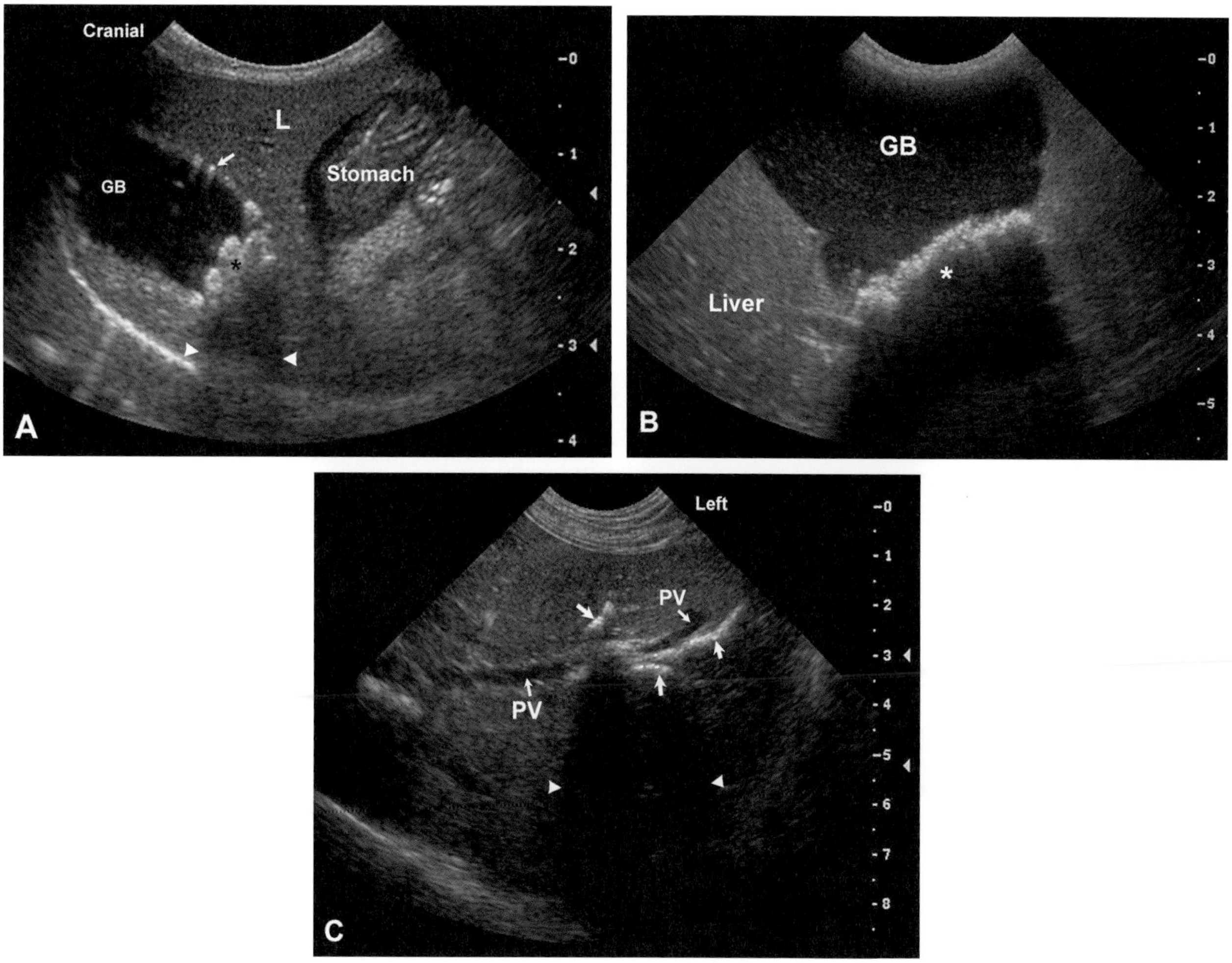

Figure 6.58.

Disorders of the Hepatic and Portal Vasculature

Congenital Portosystemic Shunts

Portosystemic shunts (PSS), which represent one of the most common vascular anomalies in dogs and cats, connect the portal system to the systemic circulation through the CVC or azygos vein. The use of ultrasonography in the detection and characterization of these anomalies has been well described (Lamb 1996 and 1998; Lamb et al. 1996a; d'Anjou et al. 2004; Szatmari et al. 2004). Most PSS are congenital in dogs and cats, and more commonly detected in juvenile animals; however, a certain number of these shunts can remain undetected for several years in dogs and particularly in cats.

Because of the common reduction in hepatic volume in affected animals, a complete evaluation of the intrahepatic and extrahepatic portal vasculature can be challenging to achieve (Figure 6.59). A right-lateral approach through the 11th or 12th intercostal spaces may be required in order to visualize the liver and porta hepatitis, as well as the region of the CVC, without overlying gastrointestinal content.

Congenital PSS are most often single. Double-shunting loops anastomosing before entering the systemic circulation were reported to be more common with shunts originating from the right gastric vein in dogs (Szatmari et al. 2004). Schematic morphological differences among congenital PSS are depicted in Figure 6.60.

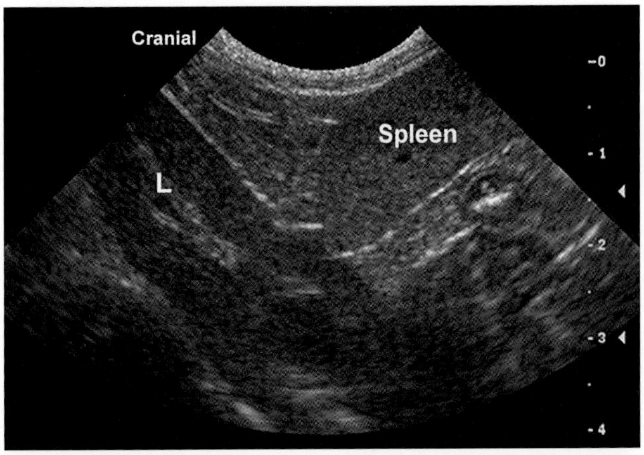

Figure 6.59. Microhepatica. Longitudinal image of the central portion of the liver (L) of a dog with a congenital extrahepatic portosystemic shunt. Because of the significant reduction in hepatic volume, the spleen is displaced cranially and the portal vein cannot be easily followed to the liver.

Extrahepatic portosystemic shunts, arising from the main PV or a tributary (for example, the splenic, right gastric, left gastric, or gastroepiploic vein), represent the most common type of PSS and are most prevalent in small breeds of dogs and in cats (Lamb 1996 and 1998; Lamb et al. 1996a; d'Anjou et al. 2004; Szatmari et al. 2004). An anomalous tortuous vessel, containing hepatofugal flow and with a maximal diameter similar to the one of the aorta, is typically seen originating from a branch of the portal system (Figure 6.61). A termination into the CVC is often visualized in association with focal flow turbulence that appears as a mosaic pattern on color Doppler (Lamb 1996; d'Anjou et al. 2004) (Figure 6.61D).

Portocaval shunts typically terminate in the CVC cranial to the right renal vein (Figure 6.61C). The shunt termination can be more difficult to visualize when a shunt connects to the azygos vein. Portoazygos shunts typically dive craniodorsally, in the direction of the aortic hiatus, after originating from one of the portal branches (Figure 6.62). The anomalous vessel can be followed dorsally and cranially to the transverse colon and stomach, unless this window is blocked by acoustic shadowing and/or reverberation caused by the presence of gas, ingesta, or feces. In some cases, a dilated vessel adjacent and parallel to the aorta can be seen that contains venous flow directed cranially. The visualization of such a vessel, which can indicate either the shunt or a dilated azygos vein, is considered specific for portoazygos shunting (Figure 6.62C).

Intrahepatic portosystemic shunts are more prevalent in large-breed dogs and are defined as left-divisional, central divisional, or right-divisional. Left-divisional shunts, caused by a patent ductus venosus, represent the most common form of intrahepatic shunt (Szatmari et al. 2004) (Figure 6.60). With this type of PSS, a large tortuous vessel is seen originating from the intrahepatic PV and curving into the left portion of the liver before entering the CVC (Figure 6.63A). Morphologically, these shunts typically connect to the left hepatic vein, which drains into the CVC. Right-divisional shunts often appear as a mirror image of patent ductus venosus PSS, but instead curve into the right liver before connecting to a right hepatic vein or to the CVC (Figure 6.63B and C). Central divisional shunts often present as a window-type shunt between a closely aligned intrahepatic PV and CVC. The PV is commonly dilated at the site of the foramen, and flow turbulence can be observed in the CVC (Figure 6.63D).

The PV size has a significant predictive value in shunt investigation. In fact, because of flow diversion, the size of the PV cranial to the shunt origin is

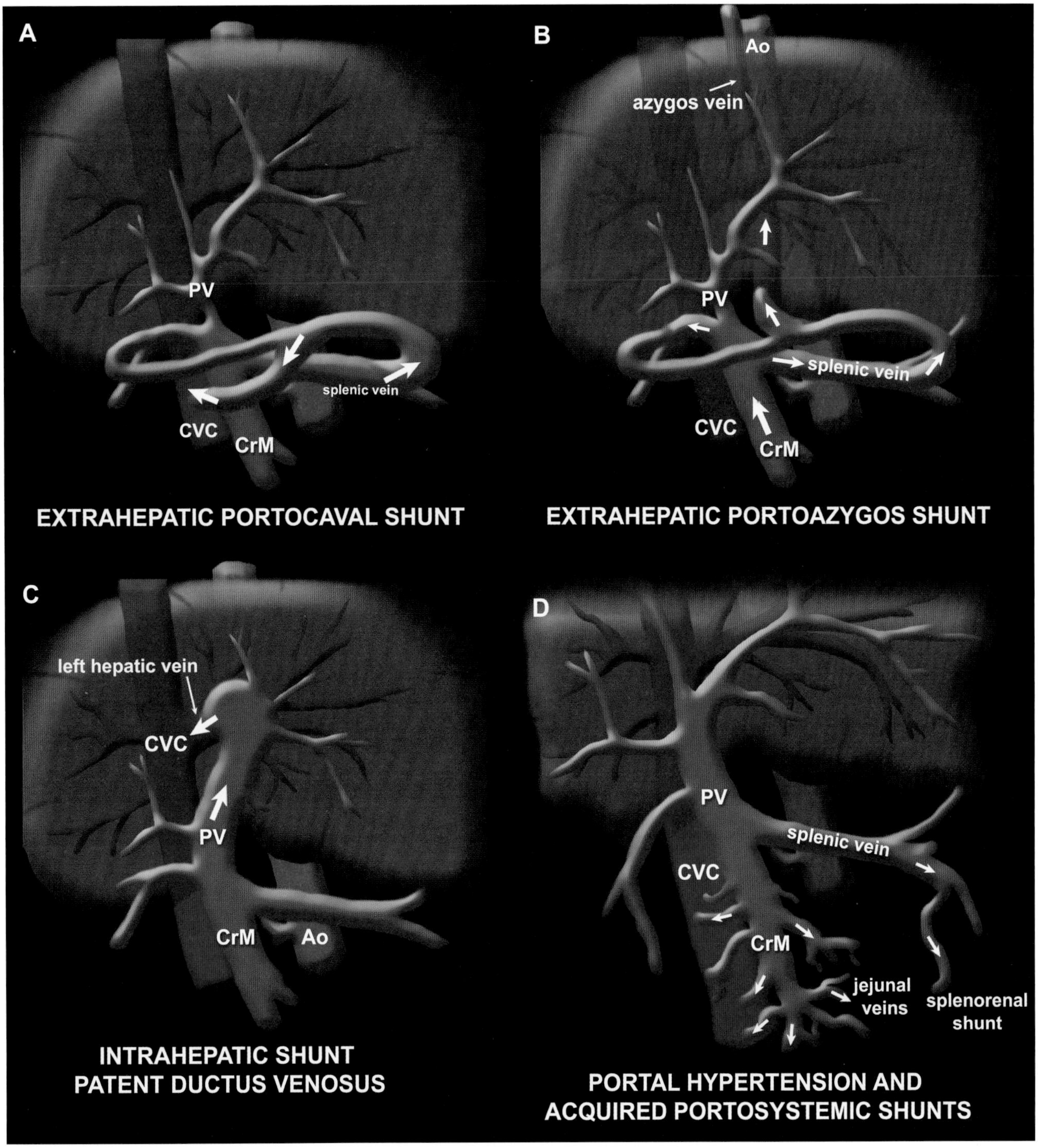

Figure 6.60. Categories of portosystemic shunts. Schematic illustrations of typical categories of portosystemic shunts showing the direction of shunting flow (arrows) in dogs and cats. **A and B:** Congenital extrahepatic shunts can terminate into the caudal vena cava or azygos vein. In either case, the diameter of the portal vein (PV) cranial to the origin of the shunt is significantly reduced because of flow diversion. A portoazygos shunt can be followed in the direction of the aortic hiatus, along the aorta (Ao), but its termination can be difficult to visualize. On the other hand, most portocaval shunt terminations can be seen with ultrasonography. **C:** Left-sided intrahepatic shunts (patent ductus venosus) represent the most common type of intrahepatic shunts. This shunt typically terminates into an "ampula" formed by the confluence of this shunt and a left hepatic vein, just before the caudal vena cava (CVC). PV, portal vein. **D:** Multiple acquired shunts most commonly are caused by chronic liver disease and secondary portal hypertension. Small tortuous vessels can usually be identified in the central abdomen around the caudal vena cava (CVC), as well as between the spleen and the left kidney (splenorenal anastomosis). Intrahepatic veins can also be distorted and reduced in diameter. With chronic hepatitis or cirrhosis, the liver is typically irregular in contour and heterogeneous. CrM, cranial mesenteric vein; and PV, portal vein. Illustrations by M.A. d'Anjou.

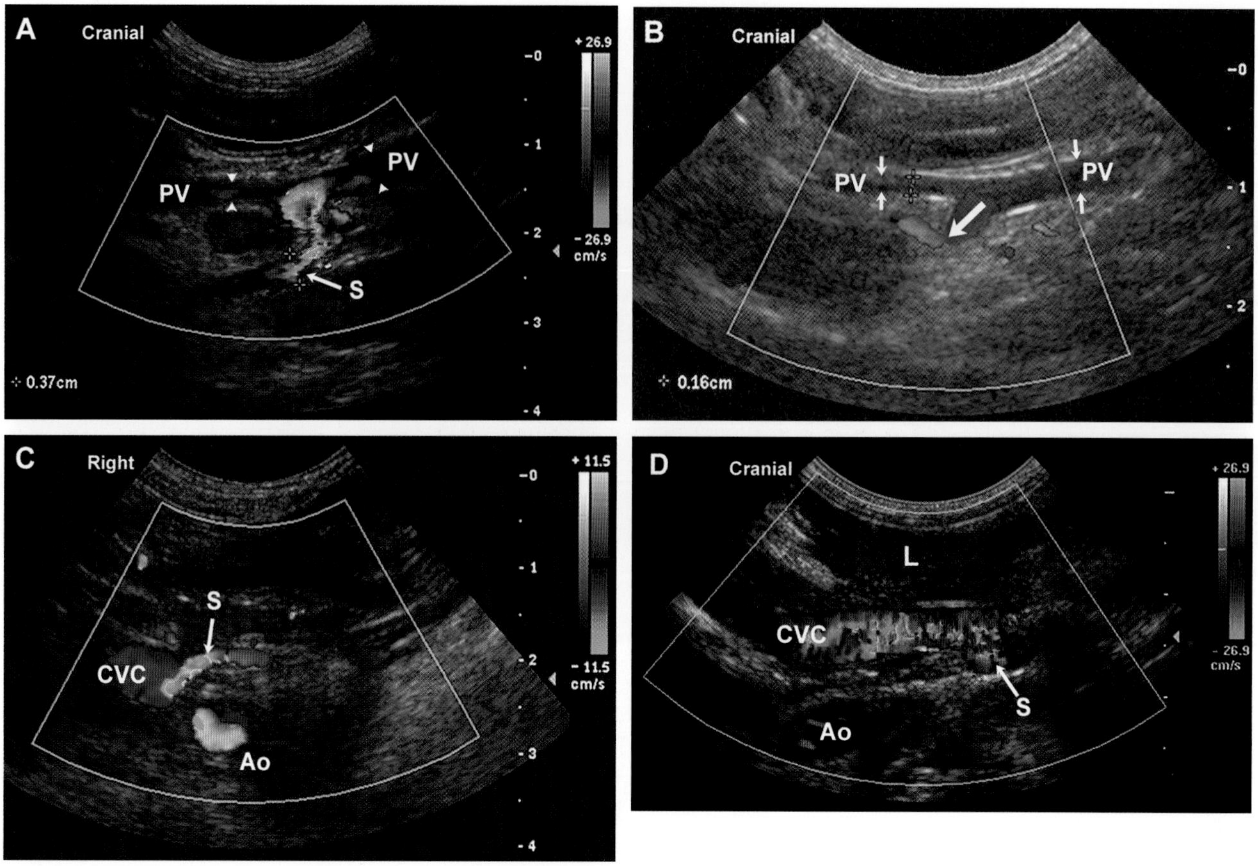

Figure 6.61. Extrahepatic portocaval shunts. **A:** Longitudinal color Doppler image of the abdomen of a Yorkshire terrier. An anomalous shunting vein (S) just caudal to the stomach is seen originating from the main portal vein. This vessel contains hepatofugal flow and is directed craniodorsally. The portal vein diameter (PV) is significantly reduced cranial to the shunt origin (arrowheads). **B:** Longitudinal sonogram of the abdomen of a Maltese terrier with an anomalous vein, just caudal to the stomach, that originates from the main portal vein (PV). The portal vein diameter (small arrows) is significantly reduced cranial to the shunt origin (large arrow) when compared with caudal to the shunt. **C:** Transverse color Doppler image obtained in the craniodorsal abdomen of a 8-year-old small dog with a small aberrant vessel (S) connecting to the caudal vena cava (CVC), just cranial to the site of the right renal vein. This shunting vessel was followed to the splenic vein compatible with an extrahepatic splenocaval shunt. Ao, aorta. **D:** Longitudinal color Doppler ultrasound image obtained in the craniodorsal abdomen of a dog with extrahepatic portocaval shunting. A mosaic pattern observed in the caudal vena cava (CVC) is consistent with flow turbulence at the site of shunt termination (S). Ao, aorta; and L, liver.

significantly reduced (d'Anjou et al. 2004; Szatmari et al. 2004) (Figures 6.61A and B and 6.64). A congenital extrahepatic shunt is suspected if the main PV is smaller in diameter when compared with its tributaries. The search for the origin of the PSS is focused on the region where the PV, or a tributary, abruptly diminishes in size. A ratio comparing the luminal diameter of the PV, just before entering the liver, with the maximal luminal diameter of the aorta, obtained in the cranial abdomen, was investigated to predict the likelihood of an extrahepatic PSS in dogs and cats (d'Anjou et al. 2004). Based on these results, a PV-aorta ratio of ≤0.65 predicts the presence of an extrahepatic shunt (Figure 6.65), whereas a ratio ≥0.8 excludes this type of PSS (Figure 6.15). However, a low PV-aorta ratio could also be found in dogs with primary PV hypoplasia (idiopathic noncirrhotic portal hypertension), leading to multiple acquired PSS because of portal hypertension. PV-aorta ratios of ≥0.8 are seen only in animals with a normal portal system, microvascular dysplasia, intrahepatic PSS, or portal hypertension caused by chronic liver disease.

Several other findings can be observed in dogs and cats affected with congenital PSS. Besides the reduction in liver volume observed in most patients (particularly in dogs), the visibility of intrahepatic portal

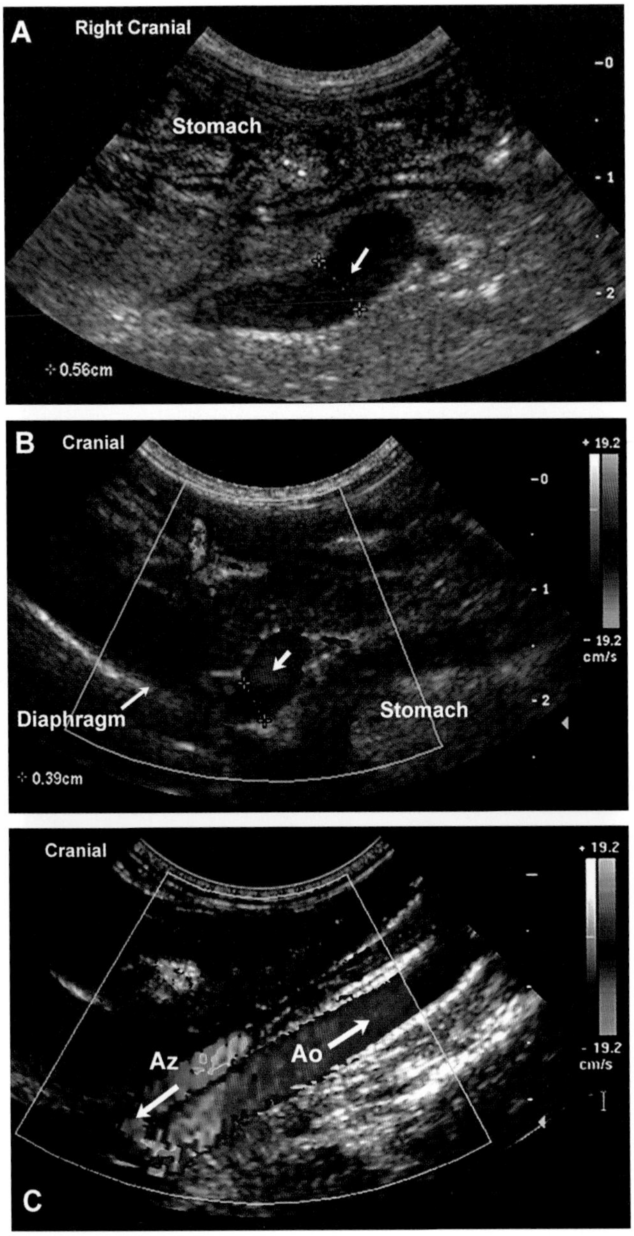

Figure 6.62. Portoazygos shunts. **A:** Transverse image obtained in the craniodorsal abdomen of a small-breed dog with a large vessel dorsal to the stomach in the direction of the aortic hiatus. This vein contained hepatofugal flow (arrow) and could be followed to the diaphragm. A portoazygos shunt was confirmed at surgery. **B:** Longitudinal oblique color Doppler image obtained in the craniodorsal abdomen of a young Yorkshire terrier. An aberrant vein with hepatofugal flow (short arrow) is next to the gastric cardia and diaphragm. A portoazygos shunt was surgically confirmed. **C:** Longitudinal color Doppler image obtained in the craniodorsal abdomen of a young cat with a right azygos vein (Az) abnormally apparent. A shunt was detected connecting to this vein in the midabdomen. Ao, aorta.

branches is often reduced because of hypoperfusion. When evaluated with spectral Doppler, the portal flow is commonly irregular because of cardiac cycle influence on the normally relatively constant portal flow (Lamb 1996 and 1998; d'Anjou et al. 2004) (Figure 6.65). The kidneys are commonly enlarged, especially in dogs, and uroliths are often recognized. The combination of microhepatica, renomegaly, and urolithiasis is highly predictive of PSS in young dogs with clinically suspected shunting (d'Anjou et al. 2004).

A systematic approach is recommended in the detection of congenital and acquired PSS in animals (Figure 6.66).

Portal Hypertension and Acquired Portosystemic Shunts

Chronic liver disease, particularly involving fibrosis and diffuse nodular regeneration (cirrhosis) or infiltrative neoplasia, can cause reduced PV compliance and increased pressure. Portal hypertension can also be caused by congenital or developmental PV hypoplasia (also termed noncirrhotic portal hypertension), arterioportal fistula, portal thrombosis, or PV compression from an extraluminal mass. Ultrasonographically, portal hypertension can be manifested by the presence of ascites and signs of edema involving several structures, such as the GB wall and pancreas. Portal hypertension is suspected when the portal flow is significantly reduced in velocity (mean <10 cm/s) or reversed (*hepatofugal*), especially if the vein is normal in size or dilated (Nyland and Fisher 1990; d'Anjou et al. 2004) (Figures 6.65B and 6.67). However, flow reduction or reversal may not be observed at the time of the exam.

Sustained portal hypertension leads to the opening of preexisting collateral vessels that connect the portal system to the systemic circulation (Figure 6.60D). Of these collaterals in dogs, a splenorenal anastomosis is commonly observed that originates from the splenic vein and has a flow directed caudally and coursing caudally along the dorsal splenic border (Figure 6.68A) (d'Anjou et al. 2004). The caudal termination of this collateral can be difficult to visualize. However, in the same region, multiple small tortuous vessels are often seen that connect to the left renal vein or directly to the CVC (Figure 6.68B). The visualization of a vein connecting to the left renal vein, consistent with a dilated gonadal vein, has been described as a specific sign of acquired PSS (Szatmari et al. 2004) and indicates the termination of the splenorenal anastomosis (Figure 6.68D). Small, tortuous, aberrant vessels can

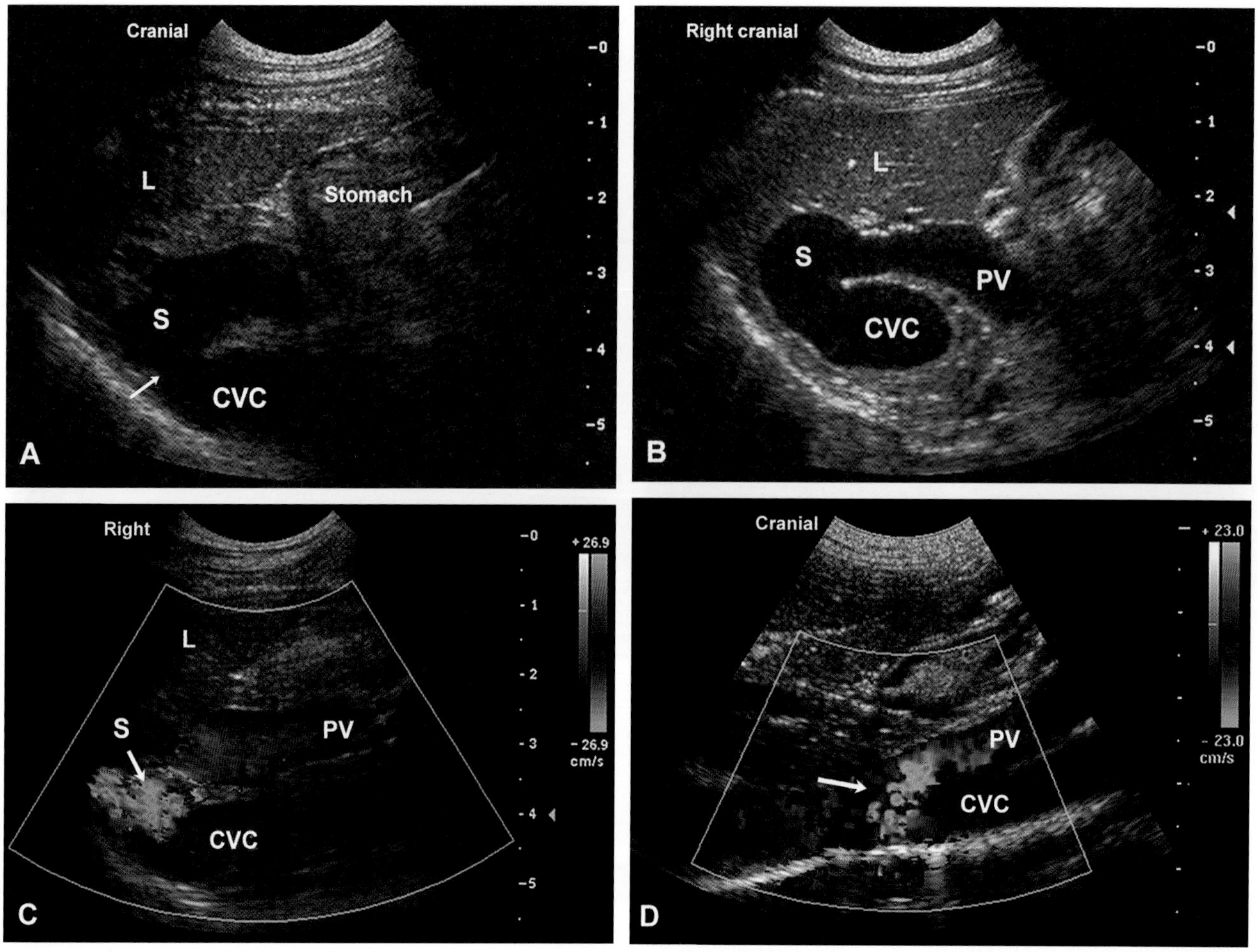

Figure 6.63. Intrahepatic shunts. **A: Patent ductus venosus.** Longitudinal oblique ultrasound image obtained in the left cranial abdomen of a young golden retriever. A large tortuous vein apparent in the liver connects to the caudal vena cava (CVC and arrow). Hepatofugal flow observed on color Doppler was consistent with a left-divisional intrahepatic shunt (S). The liver (L) is also reduced in volume. **B: Right-divisional shunt.** Transverse ultrasound image of the liver (L) obtained through the right 12th intercostal space (S) in a young Bernese mountain dog with suspected portosystemic shunting. A large, intrahepatic, tortuous vein connects the portal vein (PV) to the caudal vena cava (CVC). **C: Right-divisional shunt.** Longitudinal oblique ultrasound image obtained through the right 12th intercostal space in a young Akita with suspected portosystemic shunting. A large tortuous vein (S) is between the portal vein (PV) and the caudal vena cava (CVC) in the liver (L). Turbulent flow is obvious, as manifested by a mosaic pattern on color mode at the site of communication of the shunt (arrow) with the caudal vena cava. **D: Central divisional intrahepatic shunt.** Longitudinal color Doppler image obtained in the craniodorsal abdomen of a young large-breed dog with suspected portosystemic shunting. The intrahepatic portal vein (PV) dives dorsally and a "window" (arrow) containing turbulent flow (mosaic pattern) is seen connecting to the caudal vena cava (CVC).

also be observed in the mesentery and surrounding the CVC, particularly when color or power Doppler is used (Figure 6.68C). Flow turbulence is typically seen in the CVC at the site of shunt entry.

Arterioportal Fistulas

Congenital or acquired connections between PVs and hepatic arteries, termed arterioportal fistulas, can dramatically increase the pressure within the portal system and lead to rapidly progressive hypertension and the eventual opening of portosystemic collaterals (acquired PSS). Ultrasonographically, the PV can become markedly enlarged, and flow reversal can be observed with Doppler (Szatmari et al. 2004) (Figure 6.69). Intrahepatic portal branches typically become dilated and tortuous in the affected lobe, which can be more difficult to identify.

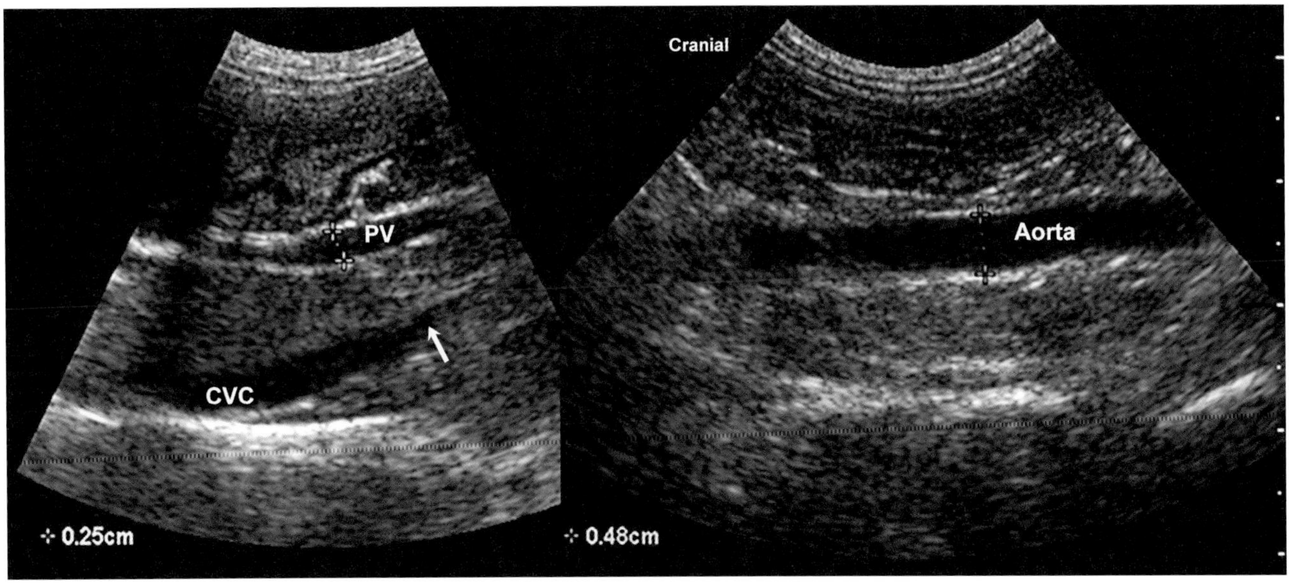

Figure 6.64. Reduced portal vein–aorta ratio. In these longitudinal images of the portal vein (PV) and aorta, obtained at the level of the porta hepatis, the portal vein appears significantly smaller. The portal vein–aorta ratio was calculated as 0.52. A congenital extrahepatic shunt was detected caudal to the site of measurement of the portal vein. The caudal vena cava (CVC) can be collapsed easily during the exam (arrow).

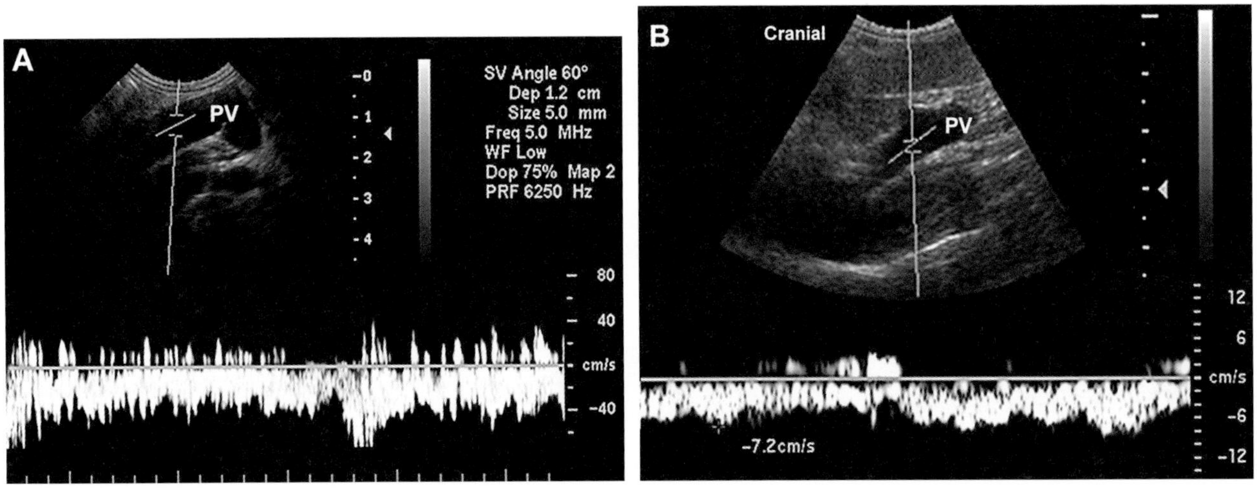

Figure 6.65. Portal flow alterations. **A: Intrahepatic shunt.** Spectral Doppler evaluation of the portal flow characteristics in a dog with intrahepatic shunting. The flow velocity is markedly irregular in the main extrahepatic portal vein (PV) because of the retrograde influence of pressure variations in the caudal vena cava. **B: Portal hypertension.** Spectral Doppler evaluation of the portal flow in a dog with chronic liver disease. The flow velocity is reduced (maximal 7.2 cm/s) in the extrahepatic portal vein (PV) because of intrahepatic hypertension. Multiple acquired shunts were detected.

Portal Venous Thrombosis

Thrombosis can form because of a hypercoagulable state, vascular stasis, or damage to the vascular endothelium (Lamb et al. 1996b). Local neoplasia or inflammation can lead to PV thrombosis. Significant portal thrombosis causes portal hypertension and consequently the formation of multiple acquired PSS, particularly if the thrombosis is long-standing. Portal thrombosis can also extend caudally into the cranial mesenteric vein or splenic vein and cause congestion that can lead to life-threatening infarction.

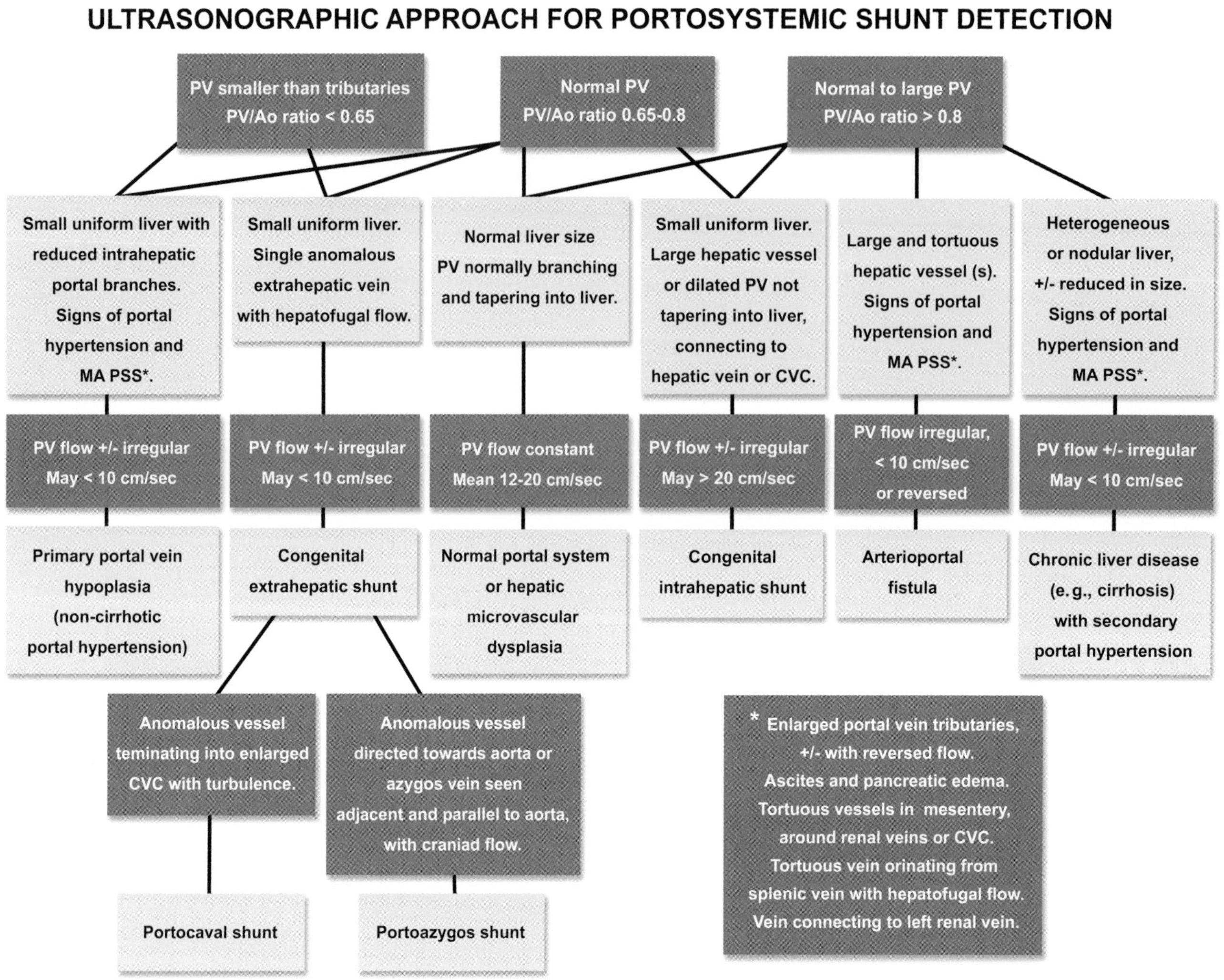
ULTRASONOGRAPHIC APPROACH FOR PORTOSYSTEMIC SHUNT DETECTION
PV smaller than tributaries PV/Ao ratio < 0.65
Normal PV PV/Ao ratio 0.65-0.8
Normal to large PV PV/Ao ratio > 0.8
Small uniform liver with reduced intrahepatic portal branches. Signs of portal hypertension and MA PSS*.
Small uniform liver. Single anomalous extrahepatic vein with hepatofugal flow.
Normal liver size PV normally branching and tapering into liver.
Small uniform liver. Large hepatic vessel or dilated PV not tapering into liver, connecting to hepatic vein or CVC.
Large and tortuous hepatic vessel (s). Signs of portal hypertension and MA PSS*.
Heterogeneous or nodular liver, +/- reduced in size. Signs of portal hypertension and MA PSS*.
PV flow +/- irregular May < 10 cm/sec
PV flow +/- irregular May < 10 cm/sec
PV flow constant Mean 12-20 cm/sec
PV flow +/- irregular May > 20 cm/sec
PV flow irregular, < 10 cm/sec or reversed
PV flow +/- irregular May < 10 cm/sec
Primary portal vein hypoplasia (non-cirrhotic portal hypertension)
Congenital extrahepatic shunt
Normal portal system or hepatic microvascular dysplasia
Congenital intrahepatic shunt
Arterioportal fistula
Chronic liver disease (e.g., cirrhosis) with secondary portal hypertension
Anomalous vessel teminating into enlarged CVC with turbulence.
Anomalous vessel directed towards aorta or azygos vein seen adjacent and parallel to aorta, with craniad flow.
Portocaval shunt
Portoazygos shunt
* Enlarged portal vein tributaries, +/- with reversed flow. Ascites and pancreatic edema. Tortuous vessels in mesentery, around renal veins or CVC. Tortuous vein orinating from splenic vein with hepatofugal flow. Vein connecting to left renal vein.

Figure 6.66. Portosystemic shunt search algorithm. Typical findings observed with different categories of portosystemic shunts (PSS) are shown. The main portal vein (PV) is evaluated and measured just caudal to its insertion into the liver. In that process, care most be taken not to confuse a portal tributary or an aberrant vein for the main portal vein. CVC, caudal vena cava; MA PSS, multiple acquired portosystemic shunts; and PV/Ao (aorta) ratio, ratio between the luminal diameter of the main portal vein and aorta.

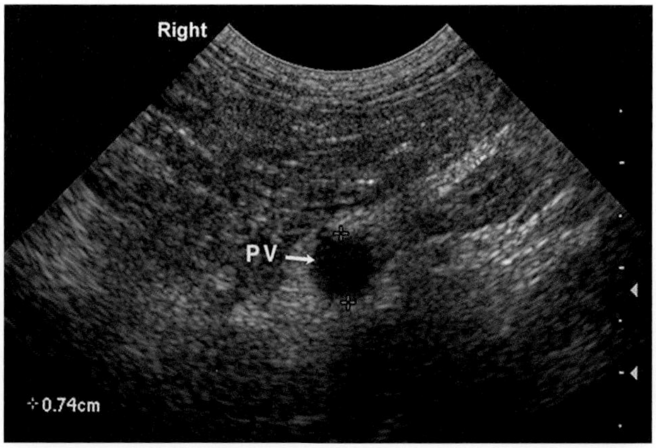
Right
PV
0.74cm

Figure 6.67. Portal hypertension. Transverse image obtained in the midcranial abdomen, caudal to the liver, of a small-breed dog. The portal vein (PV) is enlarged. The flow velocity is reduced because of portal hypertension. Hepatic cirrhosis was diagnosed.

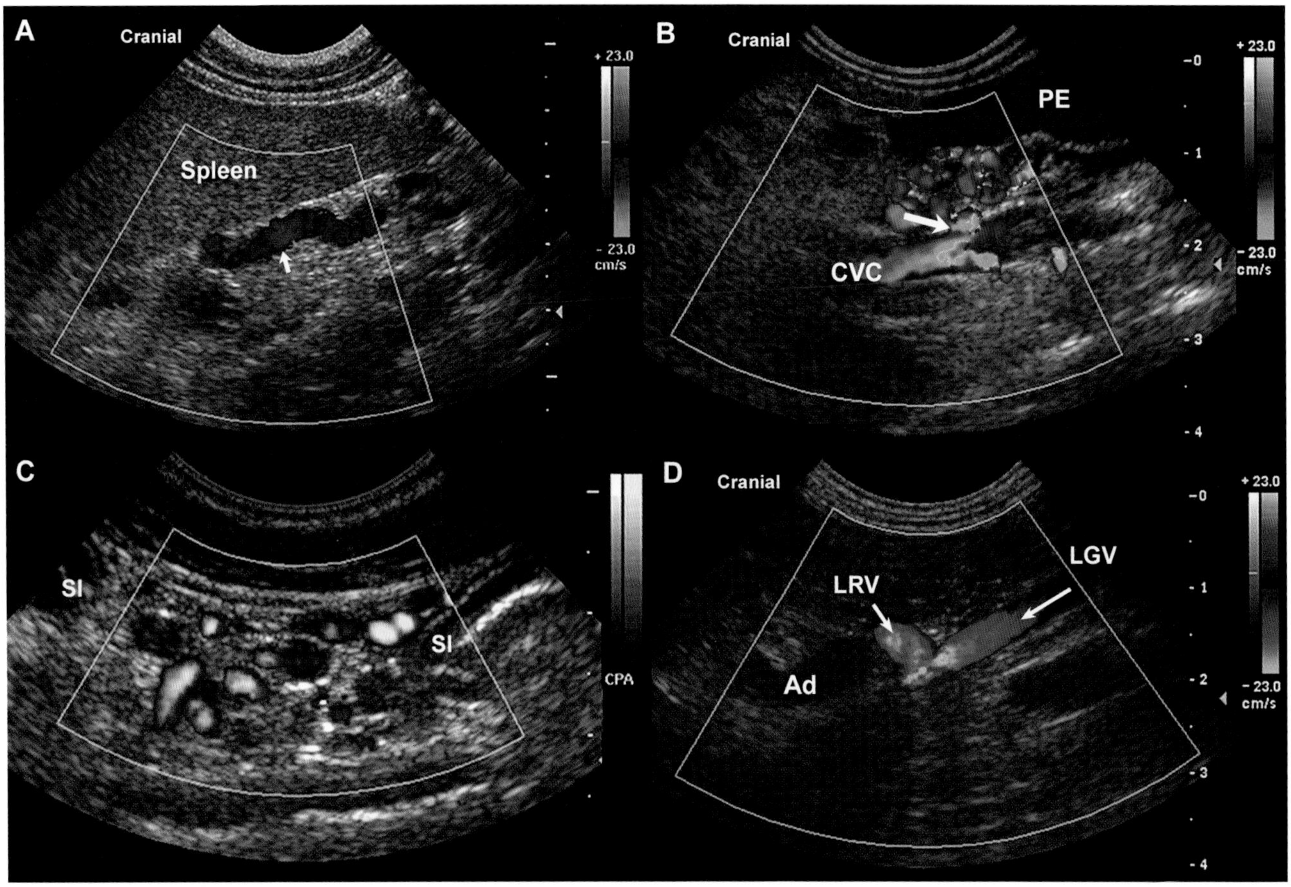

Figure 6.68. Multiple acquired portosystemic shunts. **A:** Longitudinal image obtained at the level of the spleen. A tortuous vein (arrow) containing flow directed caudally was connected to the splenic vein cranially and could be followed to the level of the right renal vein, caudally, consistent with an acquired splenorenal anastomosis. This dog had primary portal vein hypoplasia. **B:** Longitudinal image of a dog with portal hypertension obtained in the midabdomen, at the level of the caudal vena cava (CVC). Multiple small tortuous vessels are seen in the mesentery, in proximity to the CVC, with a direct connection observed (arrow). Anechoic peritoneal effusion (PE) is also detected. **C:** Longitudinal image obtained in the midabdomen, at the level of the omentum and small intestine (SI), of a dog with portal hypertension. Multiple small tortuous vessels are seen in the mesentery. **D:** Longitudinal image obtained at the level of the left adrenal gland (Ad) in a dog with portal hypertension caused by portal venous thrombosis. An aberrant vein is seen connecting with the left renal vein (LRV), consistent with an enlarged left gonadal vein (LGV). This feature is specific of acquired portosystemic shunt in dogs. Images courtesy of D. Penninck.

Ultrasonographically, thrombi are characterized by a lack of flow in the affected region of the vein, as well as by the presence of an immobile, mildly echogenic structure within the vessel lumen (Lamb et al. 1996b) (Figure 6.70). The vein can be dilated, particularly caudal to the stenosis and involving the peripheral portal tributaries. Vascular congestion can be better assessed with spectral Doppler. Color Doppler and power Doppler are also useful in confirming the magnitude of the thrombosis, particularly when thrombi are initially formed and hypoechogenic. Power Doppler, which is more sensitive and not direction dependent, helps to better assess the presence of flow around or within the thrombus, particularly when the vessel is aligned perpendicularly to the probe or if the flow is significantly reduced.

Hepatic Congestion

Hepatic venous congestion is more commonly caused by right-sided heart insufficiency, such as cardiac tamponade, leading to increased pressure within the CVC and consequently within hepatic veins. The CVC and hepatic veins appear dilated, and the liver is typically enlarged and diffusely hypoechoic (Biller 1992) (Figure 6.71).

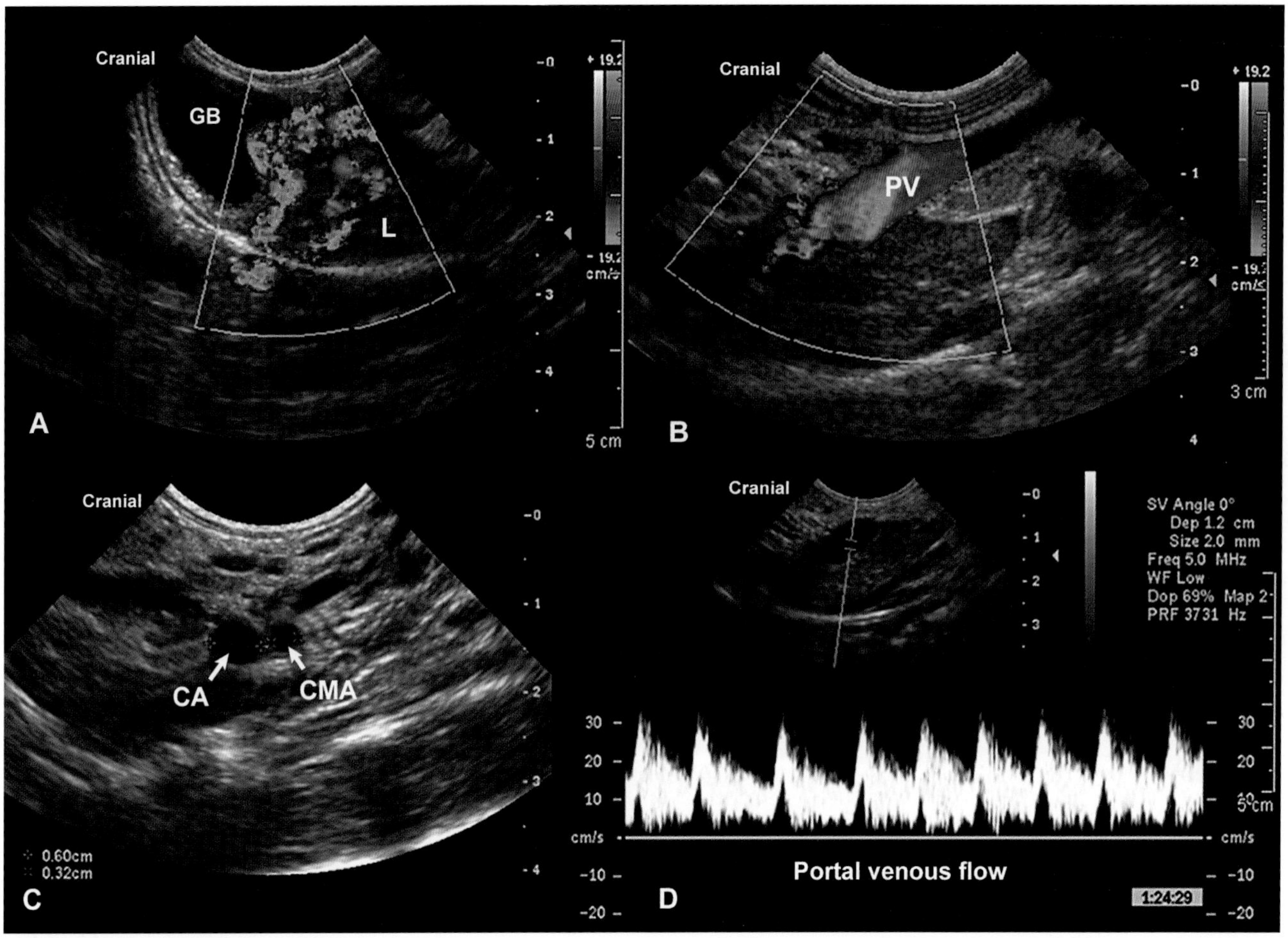

Figure 6.69. Arterioportal fistula. **A:** On this longitudinal color Doppler image obtained in a young dog with suspected portosystemic shunting, a markedly tortuous vascular structure with turbulent flow is observed within the liver (L), just caudal to the gallbladder (GB). The portal vein (PV) is distended and associated with reversed flow (hepatofugal; red signal) on color Doppler **(B)** and abnormal pulsatility on spectral Doppler **(D)**. These signs indicate the presence of an arterioportal fistula in the liver. **C:** Additionally, the celiac artery (CA) is noted to be much larger than the cranial mesenteric artery (CMA). Multiple acquired shunts were detected during the exam (not shown). Images courtesy of D. Penninck

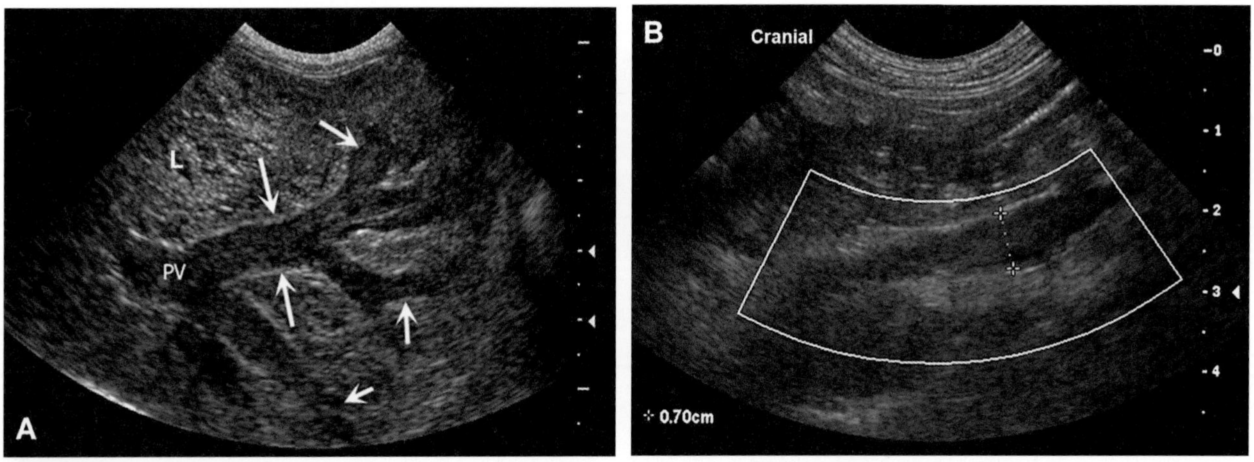

Figure 6.70. Portal venous thrombosis. **A:** Transverse image of the left portion of the liver (L) in a dog with severe chronic hepatitis. The intrahepatic portal venous lumens (arrows) appear hyperechoic. Color Doppler confirmed the absence of flow and the presence of massive thrombosis. Secondary portal hypertension was also identified. PV, portal vein. **B:** Longitudinal image of the portal vein in a small dog with protein-losing nephropathy and signs of portal hypertension. The portal vein is enlarged (cursors) and presents a mildly hyperechoic luminal content without evidence of flow on color Doppler, indicating thrombosis. The surrounding fat is mildly hyperechoic. Multiple acquired shunting vessels were also identified.

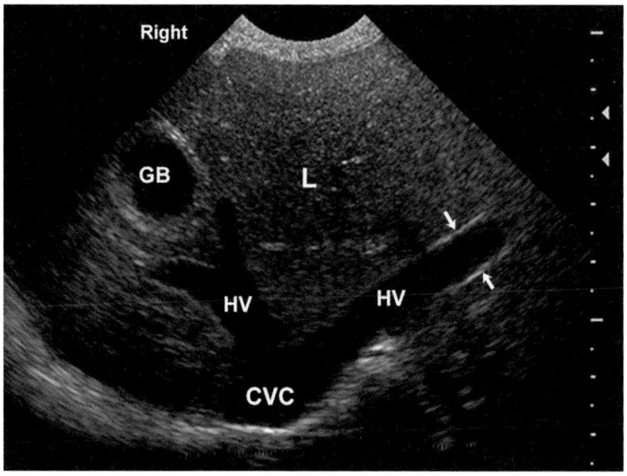

Figure 6.71. Passive hepatic venous congestive. Transverse image of the central portion of the liver (L) of a dog with cardiac tamponade. The caudal vena cava (CVC) and hepatic veins (HV) are dilated, and the hepatic parenchyma is diffusely mildly hypoechoic. The gallbladder (GB) wall has a double rim because of edema. The left hepatic vein has hyperechoic walls (arrows) because of their perpendicular position relative to the ultrasound beam.

Interventional Procedures

Ultrasound-guided fine-needle aspiration and biopsy have become routine procedures complementing hepatic ultrasonography (Penninck and Finn-Bodner 1998). The choice of needle size (gauge) and length depends on the size, the vascularity, and the depth of the targeted tissue. Typically, 20- to 22-gauge needles are used for fine-needle aspiration, and 14- to 18-gauge needles are used for automated core biopsy. Fine-needle aspiration can usually be performed with patients under minimal sedation, whereas biopsy usually requires general anesthesia. Aspiration can be performed with a customized biopsy-needle guide placed on the probe or by using a freehand technique. The latter, which is more commonly used especially on superficial lesions, can usually be performed more quickly and limits possible lacerations (Figure 6.72). Although freehand aspiration is relatively safe and easy to perform in cases of diffuse hepatic disorders, it can be more challenging if small, deep lesions are targeted. With the assisted technique, the needle is placed through the biopsy guide tunnel and introduced along a precise path, which, however, cannot be modified (Figure 6.73).

Vacuolar hepatopathies, such as lipidosis and hyperadrenocorticism, are reliably diagnosed through cytological specimens obtained with fine-needle aspiration (Wang et al. 2004). Some neoplastic processes, such as lymphoma, and inflammatory processes can also be diagnosed through cytological examination, although a more confident diagnosis may require biopsy. Fine-needle drainage of cavitary lesions, such as cysts or abscesses, can also be performed as a diagnostic and/or therapeutic procedure (Figure 6.35C and D).

Hemorrhage represents the most common complication observed with ultrasound-guided aspiration

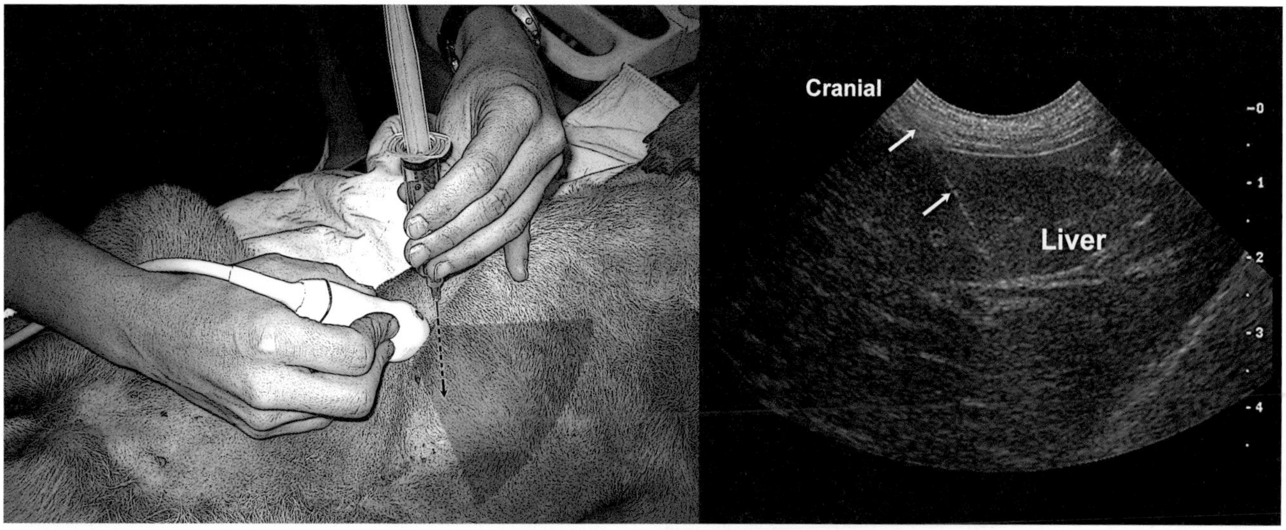

Figure 6.72. Ultrasound-guided fine-needle aspiration. On this photograph, a freehand, ultrasound-guided, fine-needle aspiration is performed. The needle is inserted through the skin just caudal to the xiphoid process and costal arch, and through the left portion of the liver. This technique is preferred when diffuse processes are suspected, because it prevents inadvertent gallbladder puncture. The corresponding ultrasound image is also shown. The hyperechoic fine needle can be seen obliquely into the parenchyma (arrows).

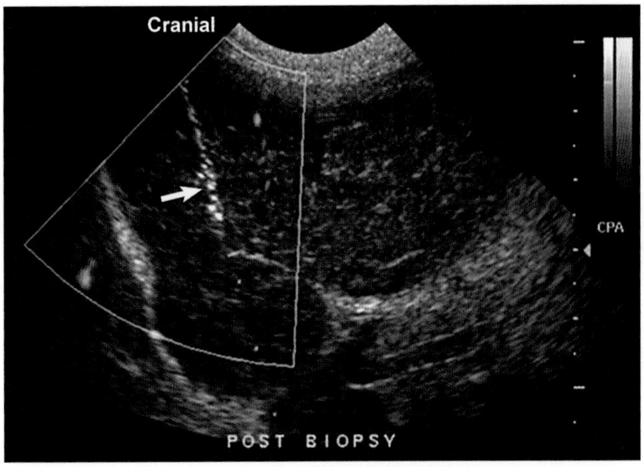

Figure 6.73. Ultrasound-guided percutaneous biopsy. Longitudinal image obtained using power Doppler after biopsy of the left portion of the liver of a dog with suspected hepatitis. A hyperechoic needle tract can be seen along the biopsy guide path (small aligned dots at the arrow) without evidence of hemorrhage. The left portion of the liver was chosen to avoid the gallbladder.

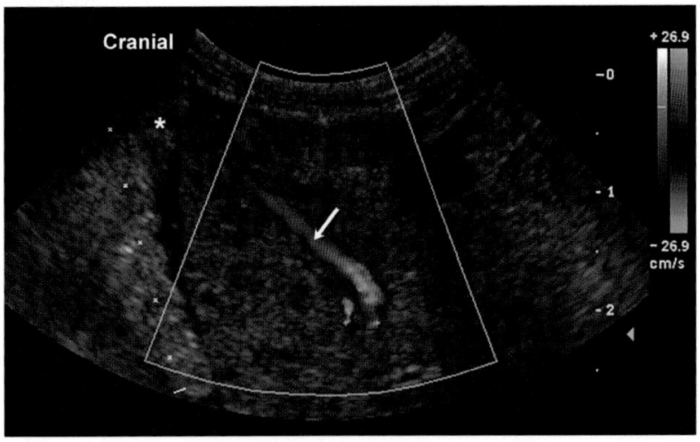

Figure 6.74. Postbiopsy hemorrhage. Longitudinal image obtained after ultrasound-guided biopsy of the left portion of the liver of a dog with chronic active hepatitis. A red-signal linear tract (arrow), consistent with retrograde hemorrhage, is observed along the biopsy tract. Echogenic peritoneal effusion is at the cranial aspect of the biopsy site (*), consistent with peritoneal hemorrhage.

and biopsy, particularly if the liver is friable and/or if a coagulopathy is present. Preinterventional coagulation profiles are recommended in most cases. Additionally, postinterventional ultrasonographic examination should be performed to monitor the presence of hemorrhage (Figure 6.74).

Needle-tract implantation of neoplastic or infectious processes, although not well investigated in small animals, can represent a limiting factor, particularly if surgical excision is planned.

Ultrasound-guided cholecystocentesis can be used to obtain a sample of bile for culture or for GB decompression in animals with extrahepatic biliary obstruction secondary to an inflammatory process, such as pancreatitis (Center 1996; Herman et al. 2005). Although infrequent, bile leakage and subsequent peritonitis, as well as peritoneal hemorrhage, represent potential complications. Risks of complications are increased if the GB is distended or if its wall is diseased. The transhepatic approach is considered to be the safest percutaneous method of bile aspiration, enabling the liver parenchyma to seal the area of GB Puncture (Center 1996).

Intraoperative ultrasonography can also help in the localization of an intrahepatic shunt and assist surgical ligation or placement of embolization coils.

References

Beatty JA, Barrs VR, Martin PA, et al. (2002) Spontaneous hepatic rupture in six cats with systemic amyloidosis. J Small Anim Pract 43:355–363.

Besso JG, Wrigley RH, Gliatto JM, Webster CRL (2000) Ultrasonographic appearance and clinical findings in 14 dogs with gallbladder mucocele. Vet Radiol Ultrasound 41:261–271.

Biller DS (1992) Ultrasonography of diffuse liver disease: A review. J Vet Intern Med 6:71–76.

Bromel C, Barthez PY, Léveillé R, Scrivani PV (1998) Prevalence of gallbladder sludge in dogs as assessed by ultrasonography. Vet Radiol Ultrasound 9:206–210.

Carlisle CH, Wu JX, Heath TJ (1995) Anatomy of the portal and hepatic veins of the dog: A basis for systematic evaluation of the liver by ultrasonography. Vet Radiol Ultrasound 36:227–233.

Center SA (1996) Diseases of the gallbladder and biliary tree. In: Guilford WG, Center SA, Strombeck DR, Williams DA, Meyer DJ, eds. Strombeck's Small Animal Gastroenterology, 3rd edition. Philadelphia: WB Saunders, pp 860–882.

Cruz-Arambulo R, Wrigley R, Powers B (2004) Sonographic features of histiocytic neoplasms in the canine abdomen. Vet Radiol Ultrasound 45:554–558.

Cuccovillo A, Lamb CR (2002) Cellular features of sonographic target lesions of the liver and spleen in 21 dogs. Vet Radiol Ultrasound 43:275–278.

d'Anjou MA, Penninck D, Cornejo L, Pibarot P (2004) Ultrasonographic diagnosis of portosystemic shunting in dogs and cat. Vet Radiol Ultrasound 45:424–437.

Eich CS, Ludwig LL (2002) The surgical treatment of cholelithiasis in cats: A study of nine cases. J Am Anim Hosp Assoc 38:290–296.

Evans HE (1993a) Chapter 7: The Digestive Apparatus and Abdomen. In: Evans HE, Christensen GC, eds. Miller's Anatomy of the Dog, 3rd edition. Philadelphia: WB Saunders, pp 385–462.

Evans HE (1993b) Veins. In: Evans HE, Christensen GC, eds. Miller's Anatomy of the Dog, 3rd edition. Philadelphia: WB Saunders, pp 682–716.

Fahie MA, Martin RA (1995) Extrahepatic biliary tract obstruction: A retrospective study of 45 cases (1983–1993). J Am Anim Hosp Assoc 31:478–482.

Herman BA, Brawer RS, Murtaugh RJ, Hackner SG (2005) Therapeutic percutaneous ultrasound-guided cholecystocentesis in three dogs with extrahepatic biliary obstruction and pancreatitis. J Am Vet Med Assoc 227:1782–1786.

Hinkle Schwartz SG, Mitchell SL, Keating JH, Chan DL (2006) Liver lobe torsion in dogs: 13 cases (1995–2004). J Am Vet Med Assoc 228:242–247.

Hittmair KM, Vielgrader HD, Loupal G (2001) Ultrasonographic evaluation of gallbladder wall thickness in cats. Vet Radiol Ultrasound 42:149–155.

Hudson LC, Hamilton WP, eds. (1993) Atlas of Feline Anatomy for Veterinarians, 1st edition. Philadelphia: WB Saunders, 287 pp.

Lamb CR (1996) Ultrasonographic diagnosis of congenital portosystemic shunts in dogs: Results of a prospective study. Vet Radiol Ultrasound 37:281–288.

Lamb CR (1998) Ultrasonography of portosystemic shunts in dogs and cats. Vet Clin North Am Small Anim Pract 28:725–753.

Lamb CR, Forster-van Hijfte MA, White RN, McEvoy FJ, Rutgers HC (1996a) Ultrasonographic diagnosis of congenital portosystemic shunt in 14 cats. J Small Anim Pract 35:205–209.

Lamb CR, Hartzband LE, Tidwell AT, Pearson SH (1991) Ultrasonographic findings in hepatic and splenic lymphosarcoma in dogs and cats. Vet Radiol Ultrasound 32:117–120.

Lamb CR, Mahoney PN (1994) Comparison of three methods for calculating portal blood flow velocity in dogs using duplex-Doppler ultrasonography. Vet Radiol Ultrasound 35:190–194.

Lamb CR, Wrigley RH, Simpson KW, et al. (1996b) Ultrasonographic diagnosis of portal vein thrombosis in four dogs. Vet Radiol Ultrasound 37:121–129.

Léveillé R, Biller DS, Shiroma JT (1996) Sonographic evaluation of the common bile ducts in cats. J Vet Intern Med 10:296–299.

Mayhew PD, Holt DE, McLear RC, Washabau RJ (2002) Pathogenesis and outcome of extrahepatic biliary obstruction in cat. J Small Anim Pract 43:247–253.

Mills P, Saverymuttu S, Fallowfield M, Nussey S, Joseph AE (1990) Ultrasound in the diagnosis of granulomatous liver disease. Clin Radiol 41:113–115.

Newell SM, Selcer BA, Girard E, Roberts GD, Thompson JP, Harrison JM (1998) Correlations between ultrasonographic findings and specific hepatic diseases in cats: 72 cases (1985–1997). J Am Vet Med Assoc 213:94–98.

Nicoll RG, O'Brien R, Jackson MW (1998) Quantitative ultrasonography of the liver in obese cats. Vet Radiol Ultrasound 39:47–50.

Nyland TG, Barthez PY, Ortega TM, Davis CR (1996) Hepatic ultrasonographic and pathologic findings in dogs with canine superficial necrolytic dermatitis. Vet Radiol Ultrasound 37:200–205.

Nyland TG, Fisher PE (1990) Evaluation of experimentally induced canine hepatic cirrhosis using duplex Doppler ultrasound. Vet Radiol Ultrasound 31:189–194.

Nyland TG, Gillett NA (1982) Sonographic evaluation of experimental bile duct ligation in the dog. Vet Radiol Ultrasound 23:252–260.

Nyland TG, Koblik PD, Tellyer SE (1999) Ultrasonographic evaluation of biliary cystadenomas in cats. Vet Radiol Ultrasound 40:300–306.

Nyland TG, Park RD (1983) Hepatic ultrasonography in the dog. Vet Radiol Ultrasound 24:74–84.

Nyman HT, Kristensen AT, Flagstad A, McEvoy FJ (2004) A review of the sonographic assessment of tumor metastases in liver and superficial lymph nodes. Vet Radiol Ultrasound 45:438–448.

O'Brien RT, Iani M, Delaney F, Young K (2004) Contrast harmonic ultrasound of spontaneous liver nodules in 32 dogs. Vet Radiol Ultrasound 45:547–553.

Penninck D, Finn-Bodner ST (1998) Updates in interventional ultrasonography. Vet Clin North Am Small Anim Pract 28:1017–1040.

Ramirez S, Douglass JP, Robertson ID (2002) Ultrasonographic features of canine abdominal malignant histiocytosis. Vet Radiol Ultrasound 43:167–170.

Sato A, Solano M (2004) Ultrasonographic findings in abdominal mast cell disease: A retrospective study of 19 patients. Vet Radiol Ultrasound 45:51–57.

Schwarz LA, Penninck DG, Leveille-Webster C (1998) Hepatic abscesses in 13 dogs: A review of the ultrasonographic findings, clinical data and therapeutic options. Vet Radiol Ultrasound 39:357–365.

Spaulding KA (1993) Ultrasound corner: Gallbladder wall thickness. Vet Radiol Ultrasound 34:270–272.

Stonewater JL, Lamb C, Shelling SH (1990) Ultrasonographic features of canine hepatic nodular hyperplasia. Vet Radiol Ultrasound 31:268–272.

Szatmari V, Rothuizen J, van den Ingh GA, van Sluijs FJ, Voorhout G (2004) Ultrasonographic findings in dogs with hyperammonemia: 90 cases (2000–2002). J Am Vet Med Assoc 224:717–727.

Wang KW, Panceria DL, Al-Rukibat RK, Radi AZ (2004) Accuracy of ultrasound-guided fine-needle aspiration of the liver and cytologic findings in dogs and cats: 97 cases (1990–2000). J Am Vet Med Assoc 224:75–78.

Whiteley MB, Feeney DA, Whiteley LO, Hardy RM (1989) Ultrasonographic appearance of primary and metastatic canine hepatic tumors: A review of 48 cases. Ultrasound Med 8:621–630.

Zeman RK, Taylor KJ, Rosenfield AT, Schwartz A, Gold JA (1981) Acute experimental biliary obstruction in the dog: Sonographic findings and clinical implications. Am J Roentgenol 136:965–967.

CHAPTER SEVEN

Spleen

Silke Hecht

Preparation and Scanning Technique

Ultrasonographic examination of the spleen is usually performed with the animal in dorsal recumbency. For evaluation of the craniodorsal extremity (head) of the spleen in large and deep-chested dogs it, may be beneficial to position the dog in right lateral recumbency and use a left intercostal approach. The abdomen and, if necessary, the left caudal thoracic wall are clipped, and acoustic coupling gel is applied. Depending on the size of the animal, a 5- to 10-MHz curvilinear or sector transducer is routinely used. Alternatively, because of the superficial location of the spleen, use of a linear transducer may be feasible, particularly in small dogs or in cats.

The cranial extremity of the spleen is located in the left craniodorsal abdomen immediately caudal to the stomach and adjacent to the body wall. Its position varies with gastric filling. The position of splenic extremities and splenic size are highly variable in dogs, necessitating modification of the ultrasonographic approach in individual patients (Figure 7.1). After examination of the cranial extremity of the spleen through a ventral abdominal or left intercostal approach, the spleen is traced to the hilus and caudal extremity, which can be done by positioning the transducer in a plane transverse to the long axis of the spleen. However, since the spleen extends beyond the transducer's field of view in most dogs, a thorough examination of the abdomen with meandering probe movement is usually necessary to facilitate examination of the entire organ. In cats, the spleen is smaller and more consistent in size and location.

Sonographic Anatomy of the Normal Spleen

The spleen is elongated and tongue-shaped in the long-axis view and triangular on cross section. Whereas the position of the spleen is variable in dogs, the cranial extremity (head) is in a very dorsal location and commonly seen to form a "hook" between gastric fundus and left kidney (Figure 7.2). The splenic parenchyma is homogeneous and of a fine echotexture and is covered by a thin, very hyperechoic capsule (Figure 7.3). In comparison with liver and renal cortices, the spleen is usually hyperechoic (Nyland et al. 1995) (Figure 7.4). Branches of the splenic vein are seen as tubular anechoic structures within the splenic parenchyma and exit the spleen at the hilus (Figure 7.5). Splenic arteries are usually not seen.

Sonographic Findings in Splenic Disorders

Splenomegaly (Normal Echogenicity)

Ultrasonographic assessment of splenic size is subjective. In dogs, the margins of the spleen appear rounded, and the organ extends further caudally and to the right side of the abdomen. In cats, folding of the spleen upon itself indicates splenic enlargement (Hanson et al. 2001). Splenomegaly with normal echogenicity is a frequent finding in dogs sedated with acepromazine (O'Brien et al. 2004) (Figure 7.6). However, it may also be encountered secondary to extramedullary hematopoiesis, infectious diseases, splenic torsion, or malignant infiltration such as occurs in lymphoma and mast cell tumors (Nyland et al. 1995; Saunders et al. 1998; Hanson et al. 2001; Sato and Solano 2004) (Figure 7.7).

Diffuse Echogenic Changes of the Splenic Parenchyma

Generalized splenomegaly with parenchymal heterogeneity or hypoechogenicity can be observed in a variety of splenic disorders, including extramedullary hematopoiesis, nodular hyperplasia, neoplastic infiltration (e.g., mast cell or lymphoma) (Figures 7.8 and 7.9), infection (Figure 7.10), and vascular compromise (Figures 7.11–7.13). A diffuse, lacy, hypoechoic

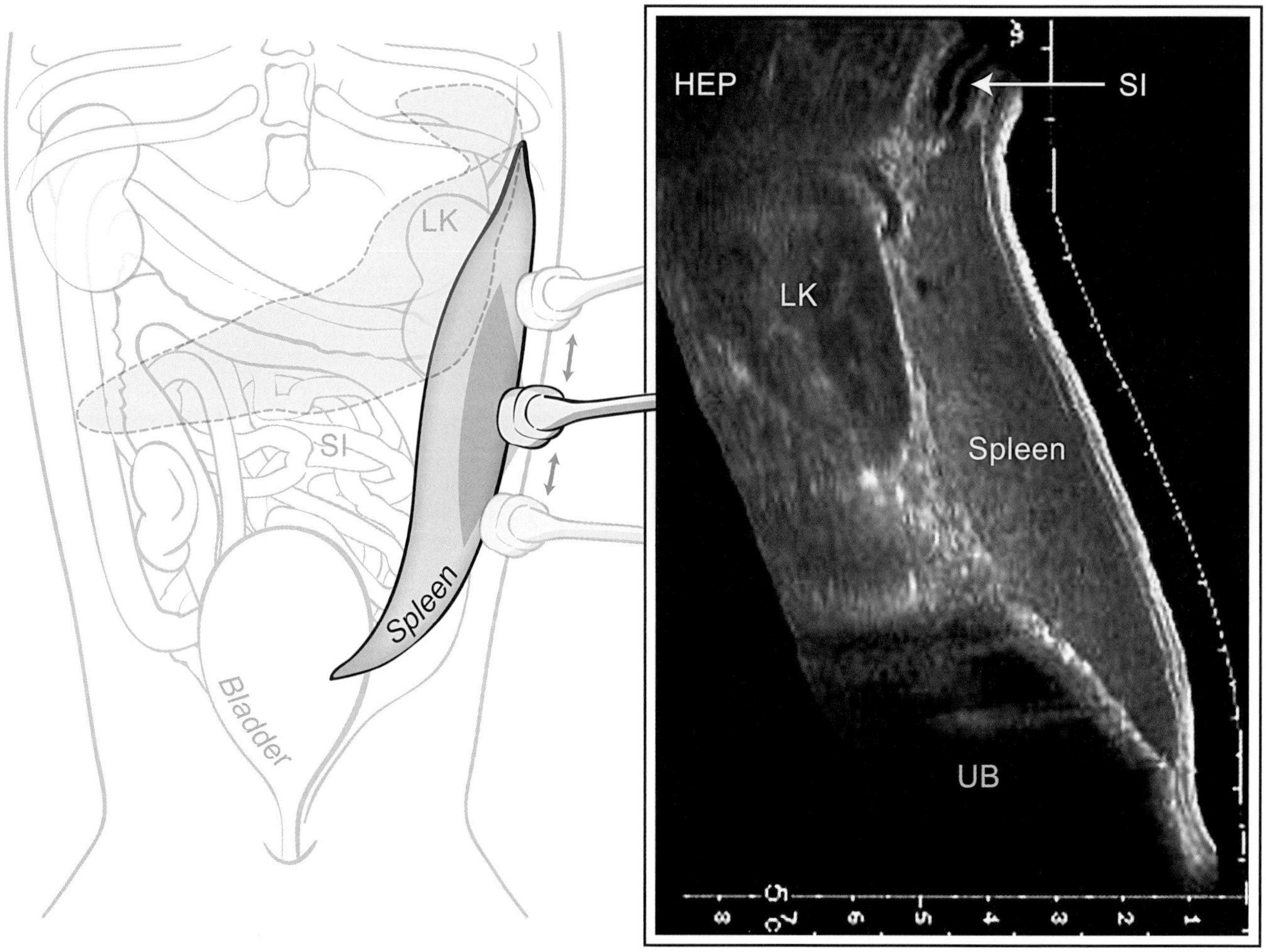

Figure 7.1. Normal anatomy and scanning technique in a dog. **Left:** A schematic representation of the spleen and its variable position in the abdomen. Ultrasound-probe positioning has to be adapted to accommodate the situation in the individual patient. LK, left kidney; and SI, small intestine. **Right:** A panoramic ultrasonographic view of the spleen, displaying its relationship to the liver (HEP), small intestine (SI), left kidney (LK), and urinary bladder (UB).

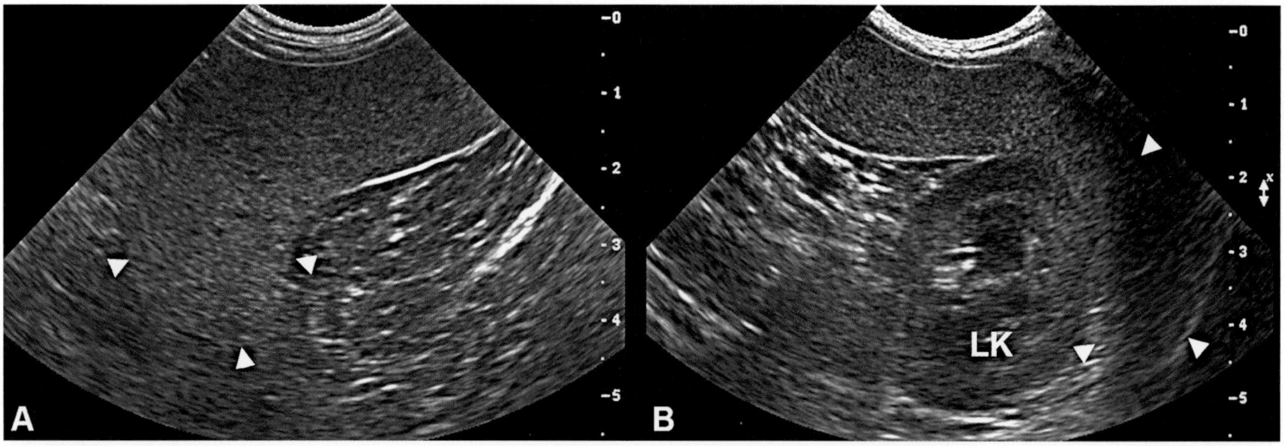

Figure 7.2. Normal ultrasonographic appearance of the craniodorsal extremity of the spleen in a dog. **A:** Image obtained with sagittal transducer orientation. The cranial portion of the spleen courses dorsally (arrowheads). Part of the central portion of the spleen is in the near field. **B:** Image obtained with transverse transducer orientation. The cranial extremity of the spleen (arrowheads) courses along the left abdominal wall laterally to the left kidney (LK), which is visible on cross section. The central portion of the spleen is seen in the near field.

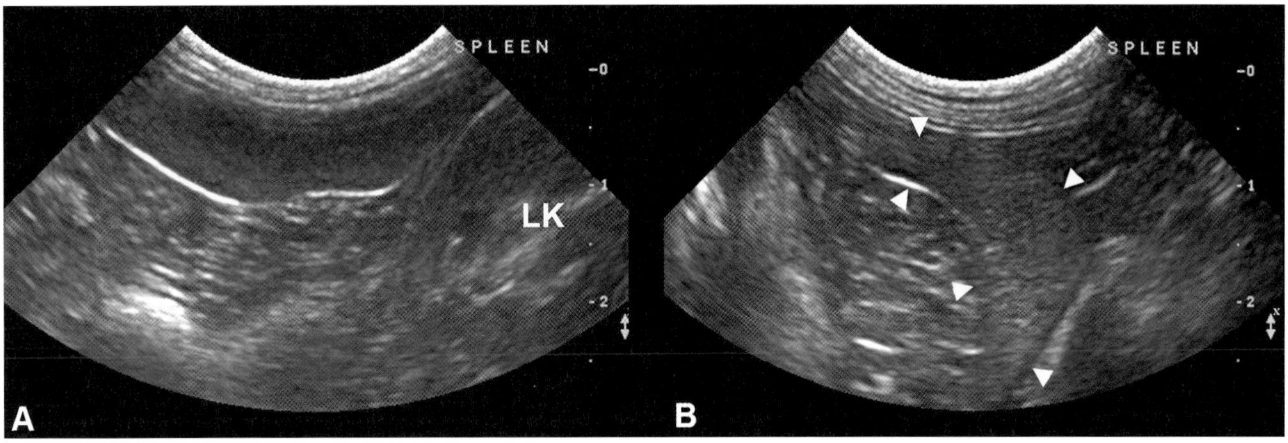

Figure 7.3. Normal feline spleen. **A:** Sagittal sonogram of a normal spleen. The spleen is visible in the near field as a homogeneous tongue-shaped organ with a very hyperechoic capsule. The caudal extremity of the spleen is to the right of the image, close to the left kidney (LK). **B:** Transverse sonogram of a normal spleen. The spleen (arrowheads) appears as a sharply marginated triangular structure of homogeneous echotexture in the left cranial abdomen.

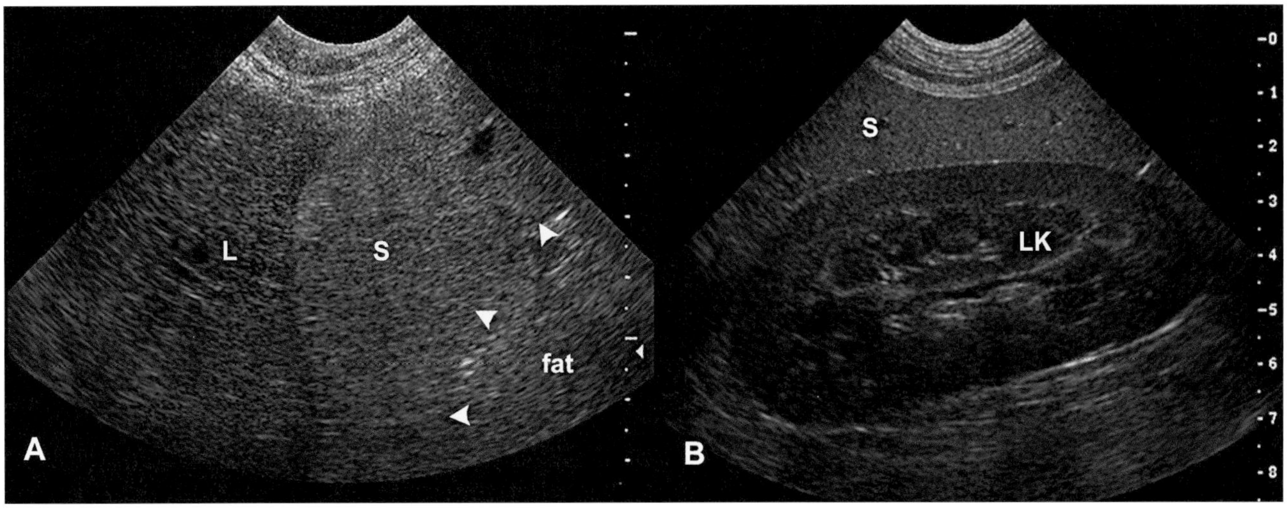

Figure 7.4. Normal splenic echogenicity in a 3-year-old large breed dog. **A:** Comparison between normal splenic and hepatic parenchyma. The cranial extremity of the spleen (S and arrowheads) curves dorsally along the liver (L) and is relatively hyperechoic to this organ. Its echotexture is also finer than the one of the liver. **B:** Comparison between normal splenic and renal echogenicity. The spleen (S) in the near field is hyperechoic to the left kidney (LK). Images courtesy of M.A. d'Anjou.

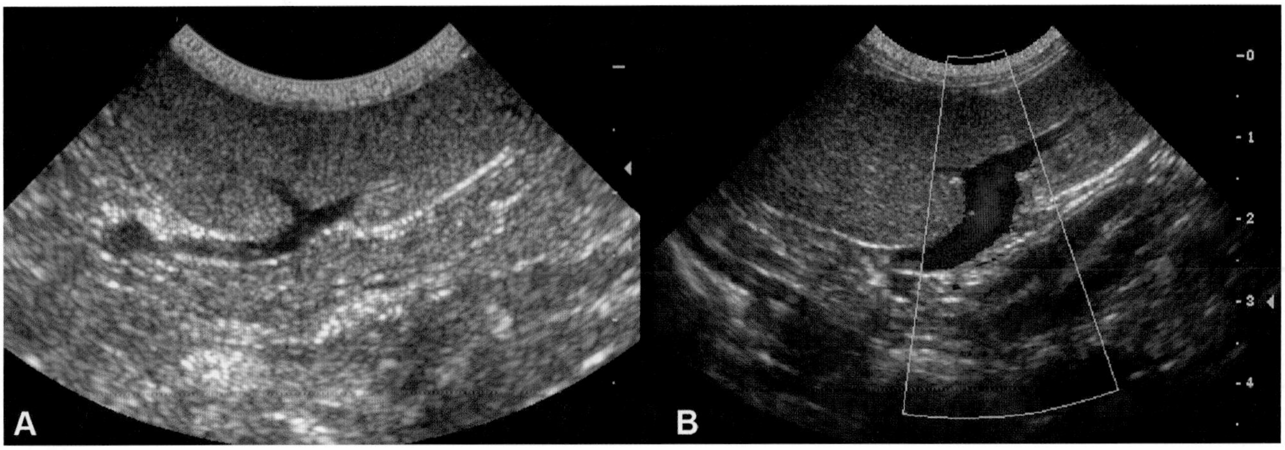

Figure 7.5. Normal splenic veins in two dogs. **A:** Normal spleen in a 13-year-old shi tzu. A branch of the splenic vein is leaving the spleen at the splenic hilus. **B:** Color Doppler image of a branch of the splenic vein leaving the hilus in a 12-year-old springer spaniel. There is normal low-velocity flow without evidence of turbulence or thrombosis. As it moves away from the transducer, this flow appears blue on the color map.

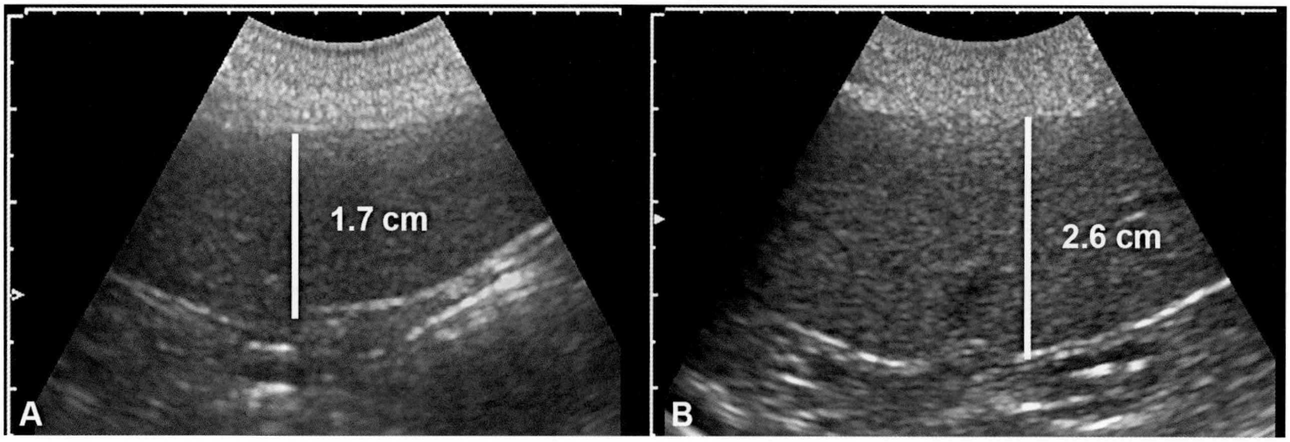

Figure 7.6. Splenomegaly following sedation in a 7-year-old mixed-breed dog. **A:** Image of the spleen prior to sedation. Maximum thickness of the spleen is 1.7 cm. **B:** Splenic enlargement is seen approximately 15 min after administration of acepromazine. Maximum thickness of the spleen is 2.6 cm.

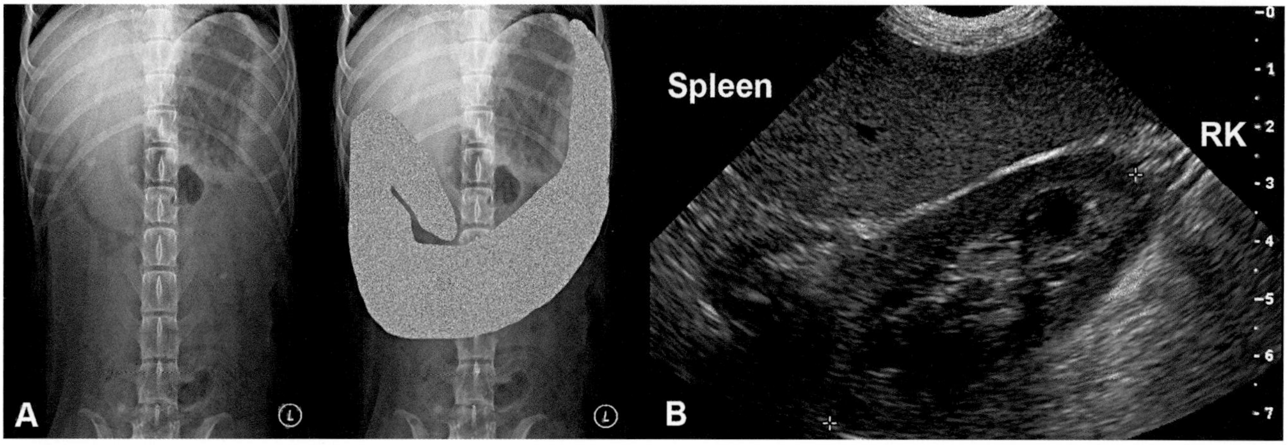

Figure 7.7. Splenomegaly in a 7-year-old mixed-breed dog with lymphoma. **A:** On the ventrodorsal radiograph of the abdomen, the spleen extends across midline into the right abdomen and folds on itself at the level of the right kidney. **B:** Ultrasonographic image of the spleen at the level of the right kidney (RK). The spleen is enlarged, within normal limits for echogenicity, and smoothly marginated.

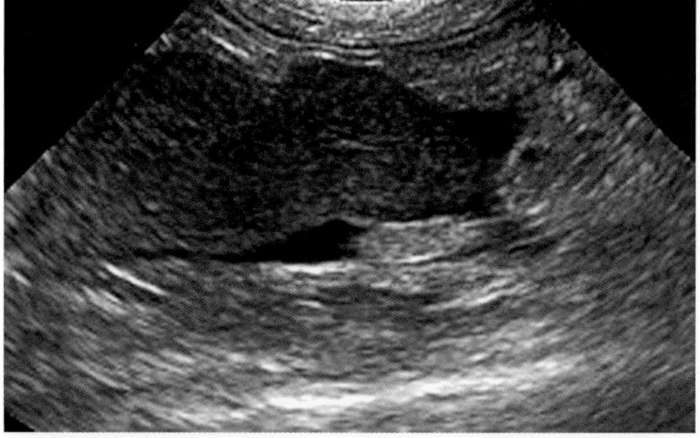

Figure 7.8. Splenic mast cell tumor in a 9-year-old domestic shorthair cat. The spleen is enlarged and has irregular contours. A small amount of anechoic peritoneal effusion outlines the margins of the spleen. Image courtesy of D. Penninck.

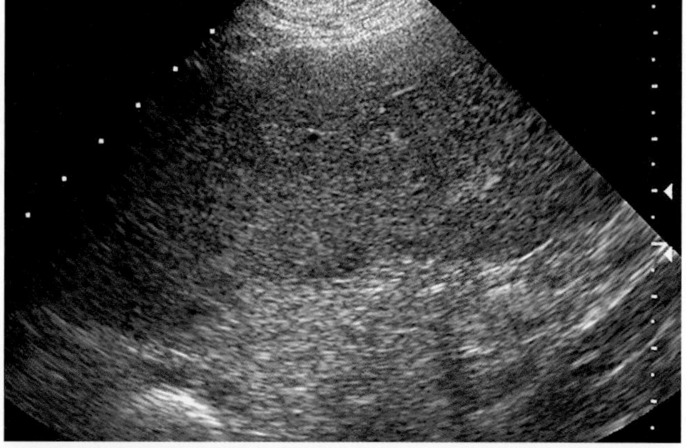

Figure 7.9. Splenic lymphoma in a 10-year-old mixed-breed dog. The spleen is enlarged, slightly inhomogeneous, irregular, and hypoechoic.

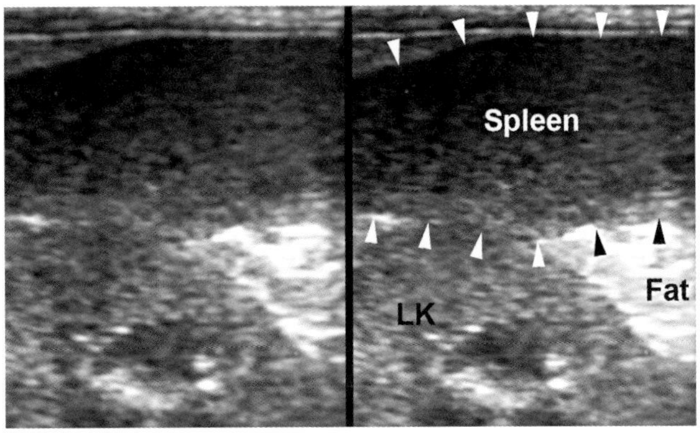

Figure 7.10 Splenic histoplasmosis in an 11-year-old miniature schnauzer. The spleen (arrowheads) is hypoechoic to the adjacent left kidney (LK) and inhomogeneous.

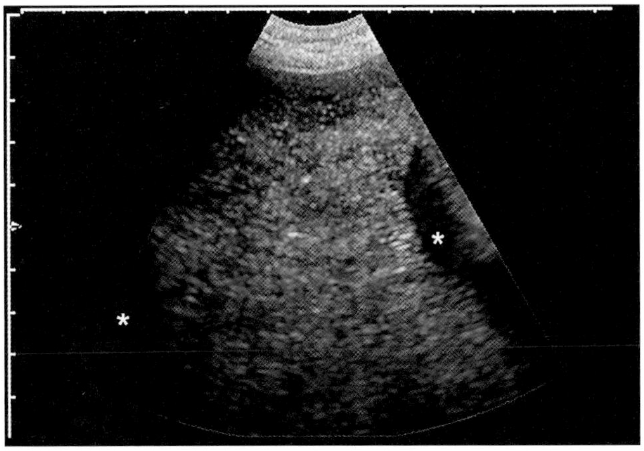

Figure 7.11. Splenic infarction and necrosis in a 6-year-old German shepherd. Enlarged and inhomogeneous spleen outlined by anechoic abdominal effusion (*) caused by massive infarction of undetermined etiology.

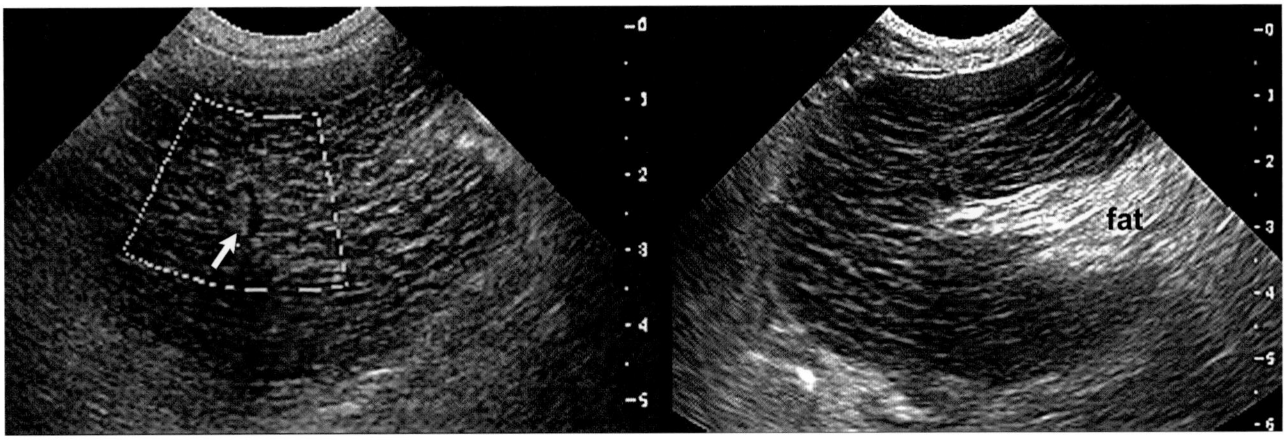

Figure 7.12. Splenic torsion in a 9-year-old standard poodle. Common features of splenic torsion. **Left:** Sonographic image of the spleen at the hilus, showing an echogenic thrombus obliterating the vessel lumen. Upon Doppler examination, no flow was detected in the splenic veins. **Right:** Sonographic image of the splenic parenchyma. The spleen is enlarged and has a diffuse lacy hypoechoic echotexture. The adjacent abdominal fat is hyperechoic. Images courtesy of D. Penninck.

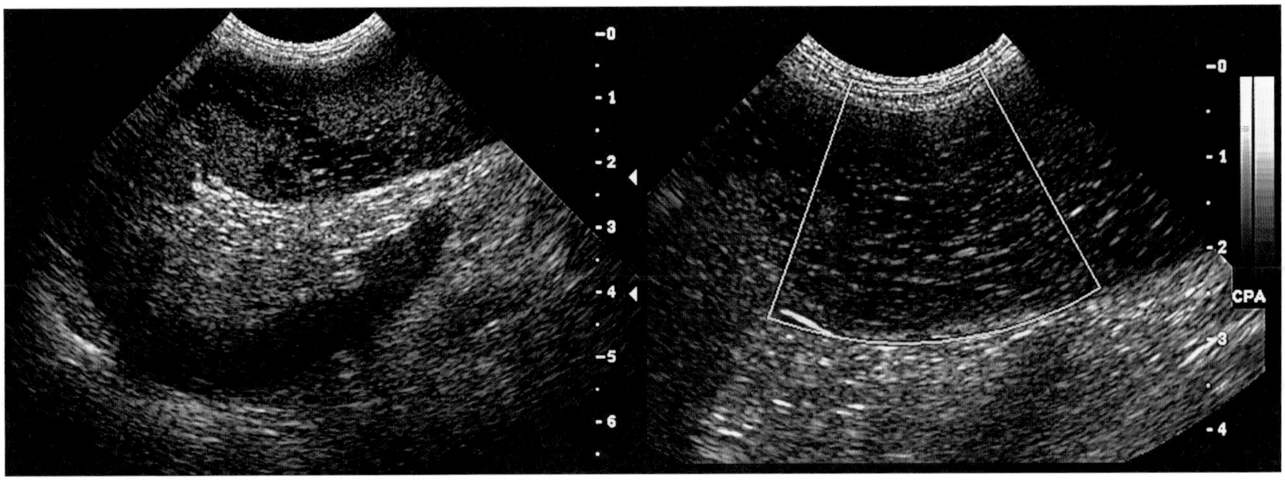

Figure 7.13. Splenic torsion in a 10-year-old Labrador retriever with acute abdominal pain. B-mode and power Doppler images of the torsed spleen. Several regions show a characteristic anechoic, lacey echotexture consistent with infarction and necrosis. Power Doppler revealed reduced blood flow. Images courtesy of M.A. d'Anjou.

echotexture of the spleen is commonly encountered in dogs with splenic torsion (Saunders et al. 1998) and can be seen with extensive venous thrombosis. However, the appearance of the spleen may vary with the degree of torsion and change over time.

Focal and Multifocal Abnormalities of the Splenic Parenchyma

Splenic nodules of variable echogenicity and size are a common and nonspecific finding. Differential diagnoses include nodular hyperplasia, extramedullary hematopoiesis (Figures 7.14–7.16), hematoma (Figure 7.17), infection (Figure 7.18), infiltrative neoplasia such as lymphoma, mast cell disease or disseminated histiocytic or poorly differentiated sarcoma (Figures 7.19 and 7.20), and metastatic disease (Figures 7.21–7.23) (Wrigley et al. 1988; Lamb et al. 1991; Crevier et al. 2000; Hanson et al. 2001; Ramirez et al. 2002; Sato and Solano 2004).

A spotted echotexture of the spleen with multiple small hypoechoic nodules is highly suggestive of

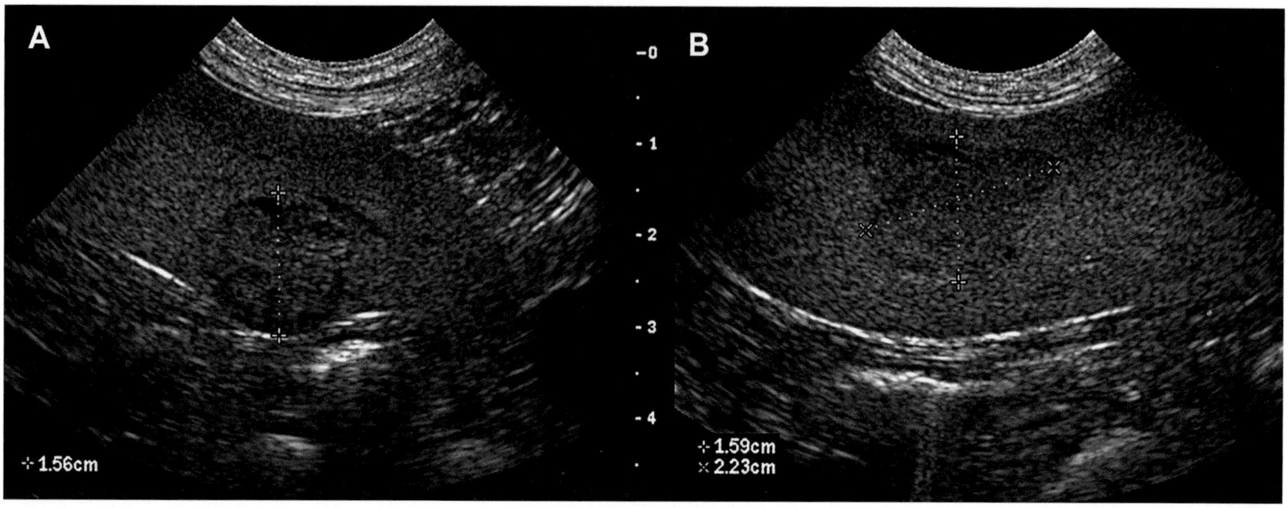

Figure 7.14. Nodular hyperplasia and extramedullary hematopoiesis in a dog. Ultrasonographic images of the spleen obtained during abdominal staging for hind-leg mast cell tumor. Two nodular lesions were observed. **A:** One of these nodules (between the cursors) has a smooth, well-defined, mildly hypoechoic border displacing the splenic capsule. **B:** The second nodule (between the cursors) is more irregular and only slightly hypoechoic to the normal splenic parenchyma. Fine-needle aspiration revealed the presence of nodular hyperplasia and extramedullary hematopoiesis involving these two separate lesions. Images courtesy of M.A. d'Anjou.

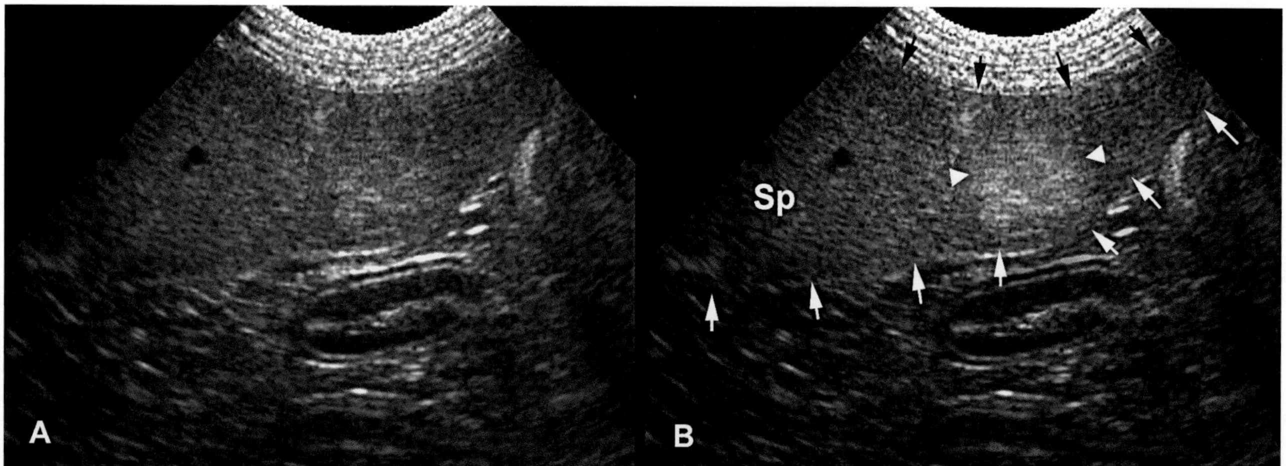

Figure 7.15. Nodular hyperplasia in a 12-year-old golden retriever. On these longitudinal sonographic **(A)** and schematic **(B)** images is a poorly defined, isoechoic to hyperechoic nodule (approximately 1-cm diameter) associated with the splenic parenchyma (arrowheads) and deforming the contour (arrows) of the spleen (Sp).

lymphoma (Figure 7.24), although it can also be seen in benign and other malignant conditions (Figure 7.23).

Strongly hyperechoic nodules along the mesenteric border of the spleen, with or without distal acoustic shadowing, are a common incidental finding especially in older dogs. These lesions represent myelolipomas (Schwarz et al. 2001) (Figures 7.25–7.27). These benign lesions can also appear deeper in the splenic parenchyma, commonly along vessels. Their size and number vary greatly. In rare instances, these lesions can grow significantly (Figure 7.27).

Splenic masses cause deformation of the splenic border. They are of variable shape, margination, and echogenicity and may be cavitated (Saunders 1998). As

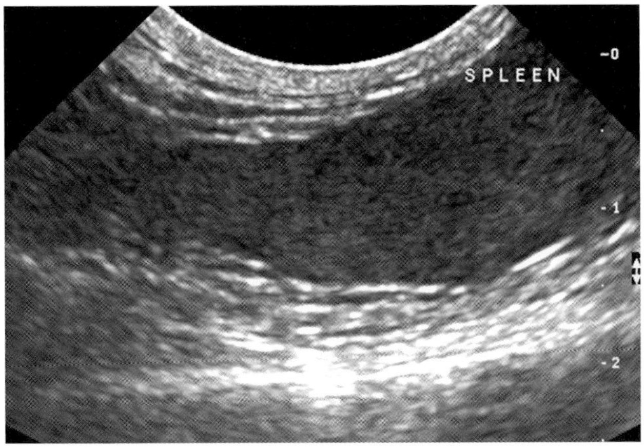

Figure 7.16. Extramedullary hematopoiesis in a 4-year-old cat. The spleen is enlarged, and multiple ill-defined hypoechoic nodules and foci are associated with the splenic parenchyma.

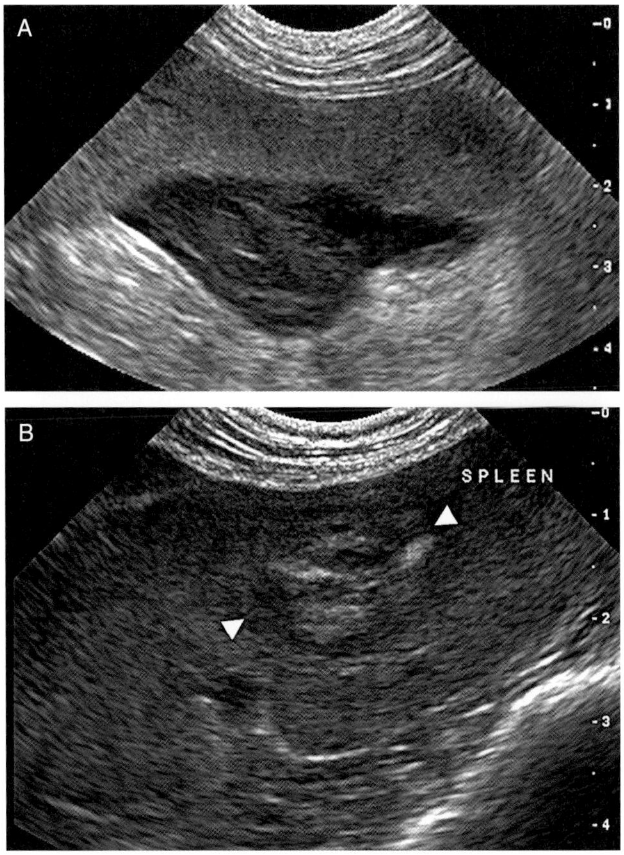

Figure 7.17. Splenic hematomas in two dogs. **A:** Longitudinal sonogram of the distal tip of the spleen, outlined on its visceral surface by an irregularly hypoechoic region. This lesion represents a subcapsular hematoma in this dog recently hit by a car. Image courtesy of D. Penninck. **B:** Splenic hematoma in a 13-year-old Labrador retriever. An approximately 1.5-cm, mixed echogenic nodule (arrowheads) is associated with the splenic parenchyma.

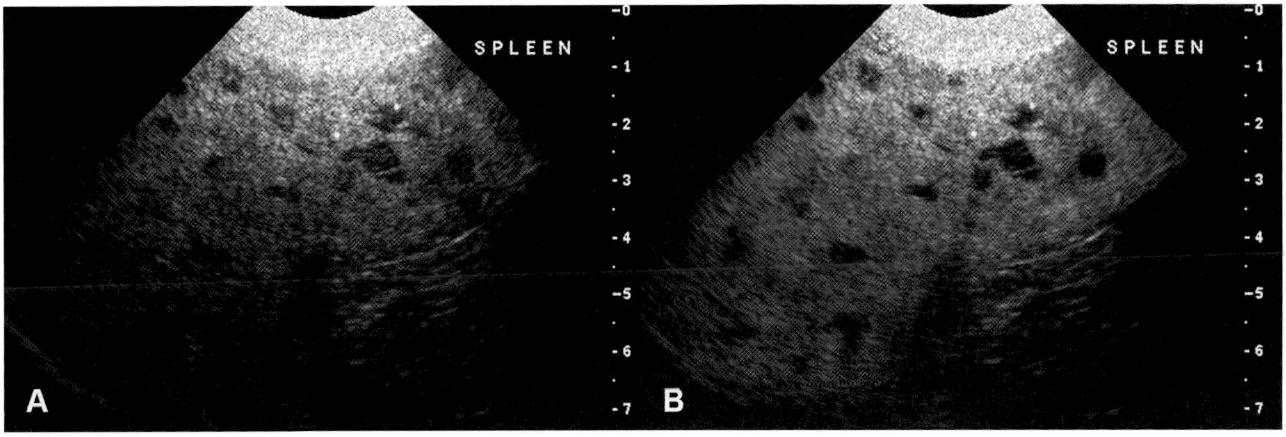

Figure 7.18. Pyogranulomatous splenitis of undetermined etiology in a 5-year-old Rottweiler. Ultrasound **(A)** and schematic **(B)** images of the spleen, in which it appears enlarged and diffusely hyperechoic with dispersed hypoechoic nodules and ill-defined foci. On the ultrasound image, the affected parenchyma is also hyperattenuating, resulting in hypoechogenicity in the far field.

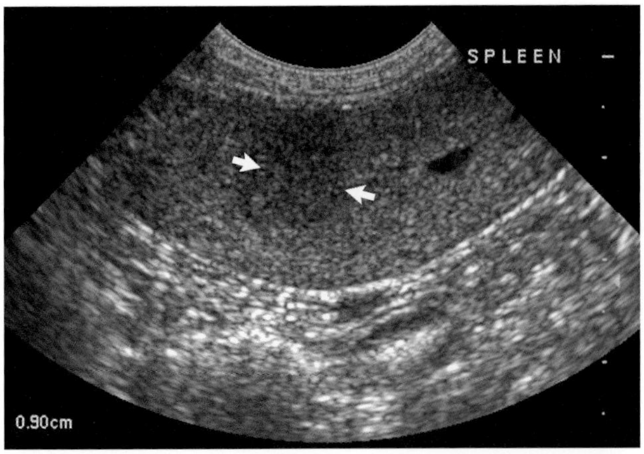

Figure 7.19. Lymphoma in a shi tzu. There is a 0.9 cm hypoechoic nodule (arrows) associated with the spleen.

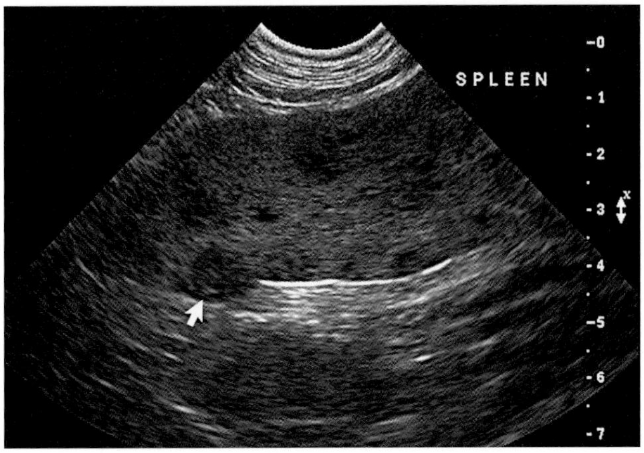

Figure 7.20. Disseminated histiocytic sarcoma in a 7-year-old Bernese mountain dog. There are multiple hypoechoic nodules throughout the spleen, some of which deform the splenic border (arrow).

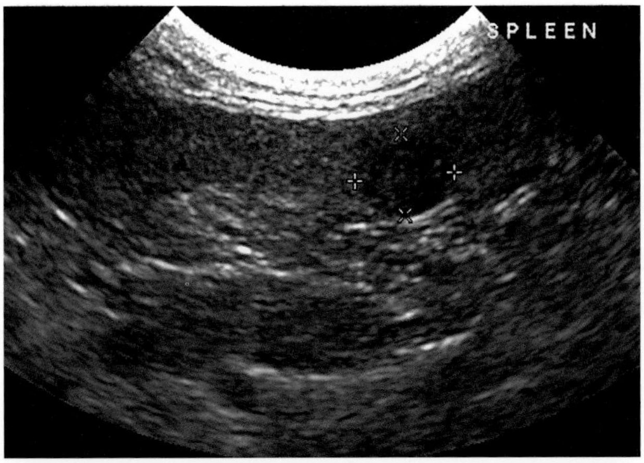

Figure 7.21. Malignant splenic epithelial neoplasm (presumably metastatic) in a cat. Several hypoechoic nodules are in the spleen. The one displayed on this image measures 0.8 × 0.6 cm (between the cursors).

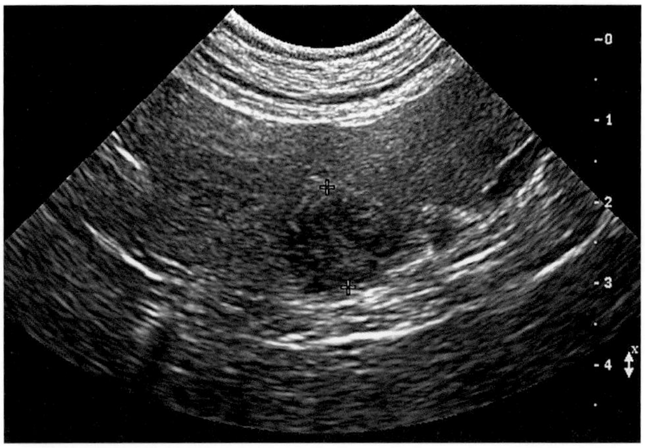

Figure 7.22. Malignant splenic epithelial neoplasm (presumably metastatic) in a 10-year-old golden retriever. There were several hypoechoic nodules associated with the spleen, one of which is shown and measures 1.3 cm in diameter (between the cursors).

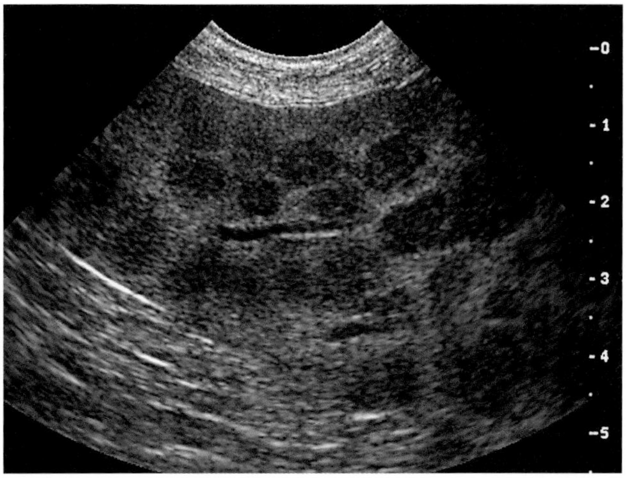

Figure 7.23. Metastatic anal sac adenocarcinoma in a dog. The spleen is enlarged and has extensively distributed hypoechoic nodules. Fine-needle aspiration revealed epithelial metastatic disease throughout the spleen, liver, and abdominal lymph nodes, although lymphoma was initially expected based on the ultrasonographic features. Image courtesy of M.A. d'Anjou.

in the case of splenic nodules, splenic masses may be benign or malignant and cannot be differentiated based on their ultrasonographic appearance. Differential diagnoses include benign lesions such as nodular hyperplasia and hematomas (Figures 7.28–7.31), and malignancies such as hemangiosarcoma, other sarcomas, round-cell neoplasms, and metastases (Figures 7.32–7.41). According to recent publications, benign splenic mass lesions are more common than malignant mass lesions in dogs (Fife et al. 2004). Although rupture of a splenic mass with subsequent

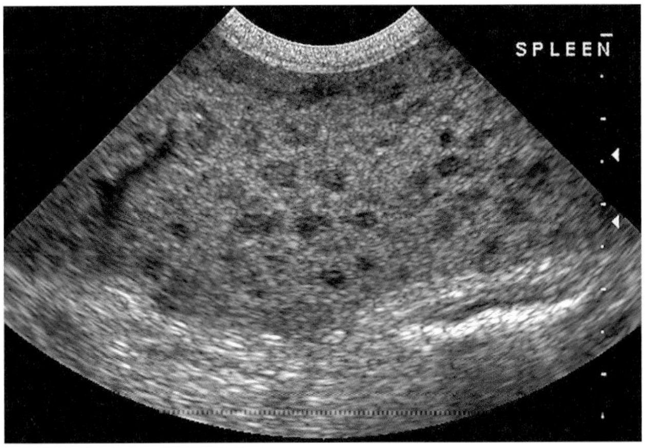

Figure 7.24. Lymphoma in a 6-year-old pit bull. There are numerous small hypoechoic nodules throughout the spleen, causing a spotted echotexture. This pattern is most commonly seen with lymphoma.

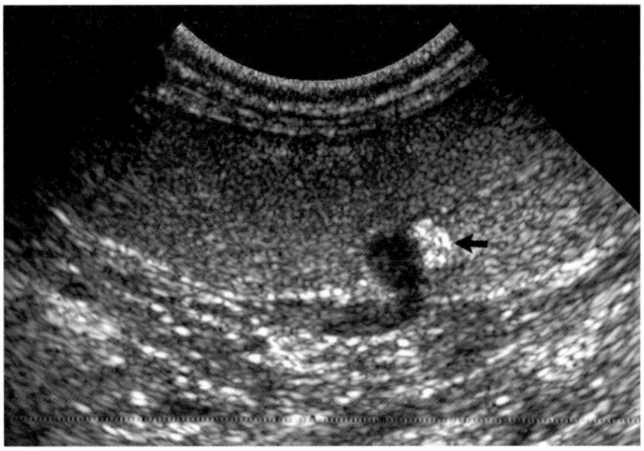

Figure 7.25. Splenic myelolipoma in an 11-year-old collie. Close to a branch of the splenic vein is a focal, strongly hyperechoic nodule associated with the visceral border of the spleen (arrow).

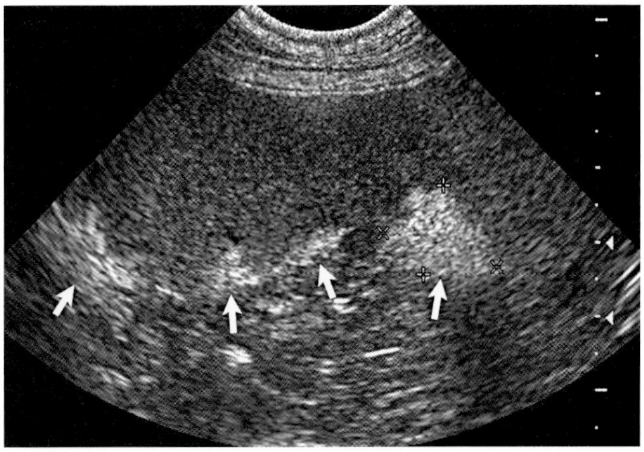

Figure 7.26. Splenic myelolipomas in a 12-year-old mixed-breed dog. Multiple strongly hyperechoic nodules are associated with the visceral border of the spleen (arrows). The largest nodule (between the cursors) measures 1.2 × 1.7 cm.

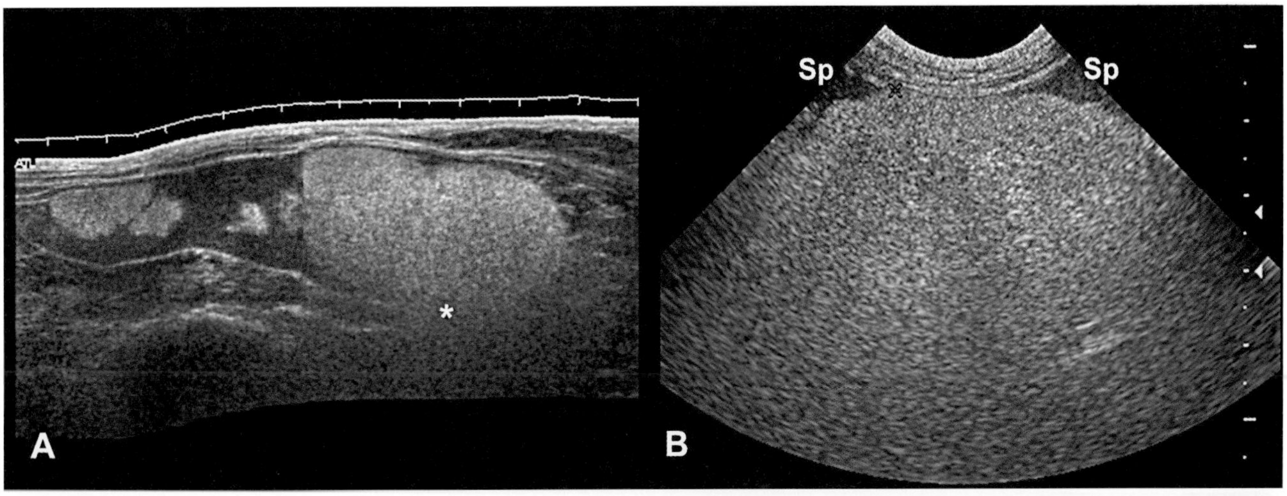

Figure 7.27. Large splenic myelolipomas in a cat and a dog. **A:** Panoramic view of the spleen of a 8-year-old domestic shorthair cat. Multiple strongly hyperechoic nodules and mass lesions are associated with the splenic parenchyma, deforming the capsule. The largest of these masses is associated with acoustic scattering in the far field (*), blurring the dorsal border of the spleen and mass. **B:** A similar but larger hyperechoic mass, originating from the spleen (Sp), is seen in this dog referred for a possible splenic hemangiosarcoma. A benign myelolipoma reaching 13 cm wide was confirmed histologically after splenectomy. Image B courtesy of M.A. d'Anjou. Image A courtesy of D. Penninck.

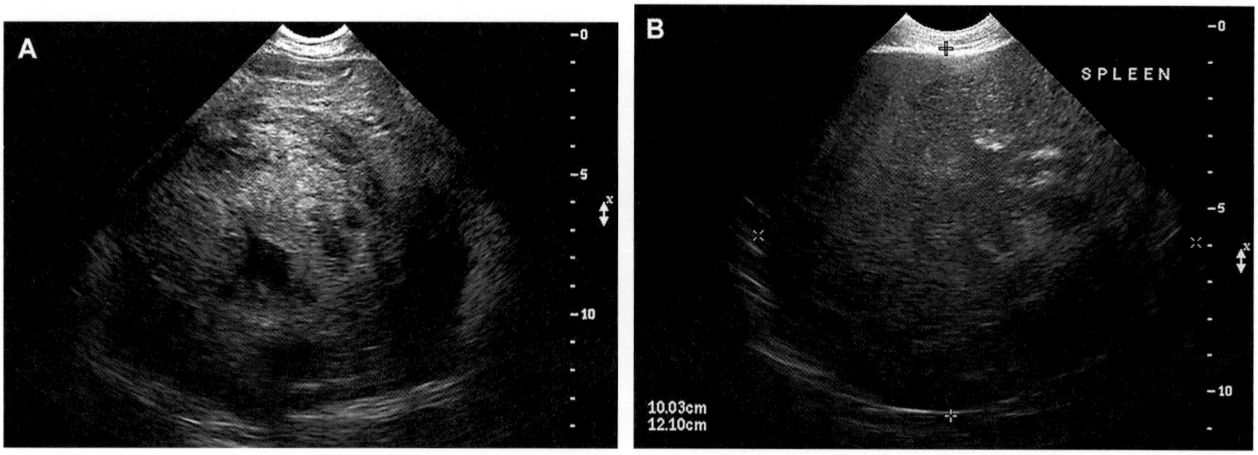

Figure 7.28. Large benign splenic masses in two dogs. **A:** Splenic nodular hyperplasia in an 11-year-old Labrador retriever. An approximately 15 cm mixed echogenic mass is associated with the cranial extremity of the spleen. Histopathologic examination indicated no evidence of malignancy. **B:** Nodular hyperplasia and hematoma in a 14-year-old mixed-breed dog. A relatively homogeneous mass of 10 × 12 cm (between the cursors) is associated with the spleen.

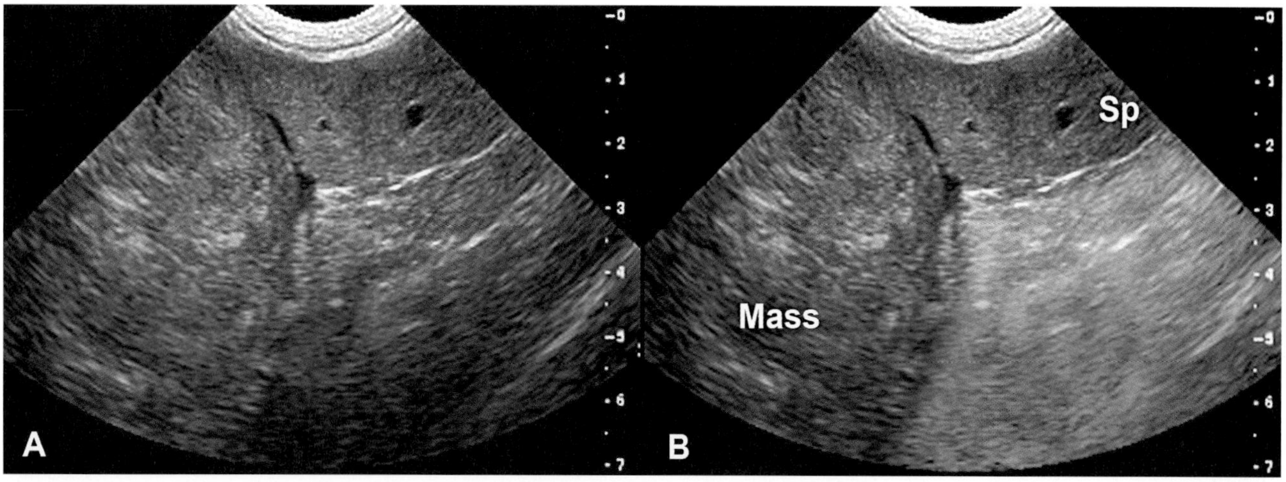

Figure 7.29. Large benign splenic mass in a dog. Longitudinal sonographic **(A)** and schematic **(B)** images of a large splenic mass (Sp). The histopathologic diagnosis was nodular hyperplasia and extramedullary hematopoiesis.

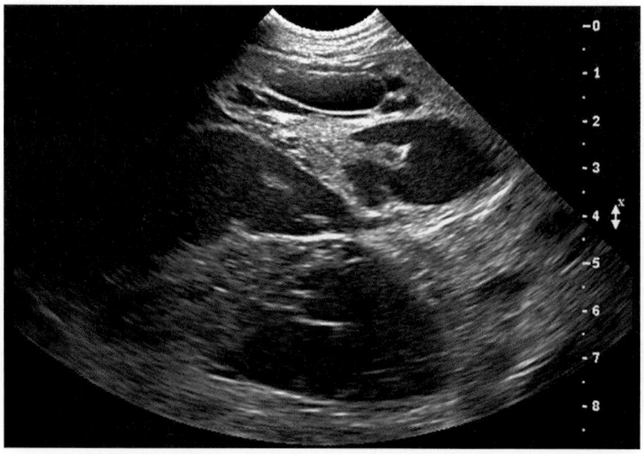

Figure 7.30. Splenic nodular hyperplasia, hemorrhage, and infarction in a 9-year-old Labrador retriever. An ill-defined, more than 10-cm, mixed echogenic and cavitated mass is associated with the spleen. There was no evidence of malignancy on histopathologic examination.

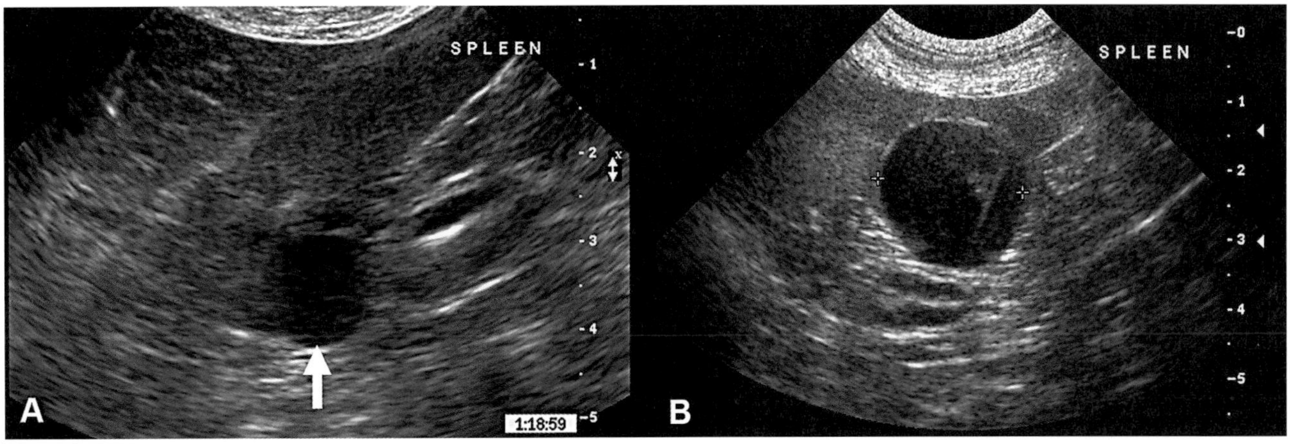

Figure 7.31. Splenic nodular hyperplasia and hemorrhage in a 13-year-old Labrador retriever. Follow up images of the spleen in this dog previously diagnosed with hemangiosarcoma of the thoracic wall. **A:** The initial examination shows a well-circumscribed hypoechoic nodule of approximately 1-cm diameter associated with the spleen (arrow). **B:** Examination 3 weeks later shows that the nodule (between the cursors) has doubled in size (2.2-cm diameter) and is almost anechoic, indicating cavitation. There was no evidence of malignancy on histopathologic examination.

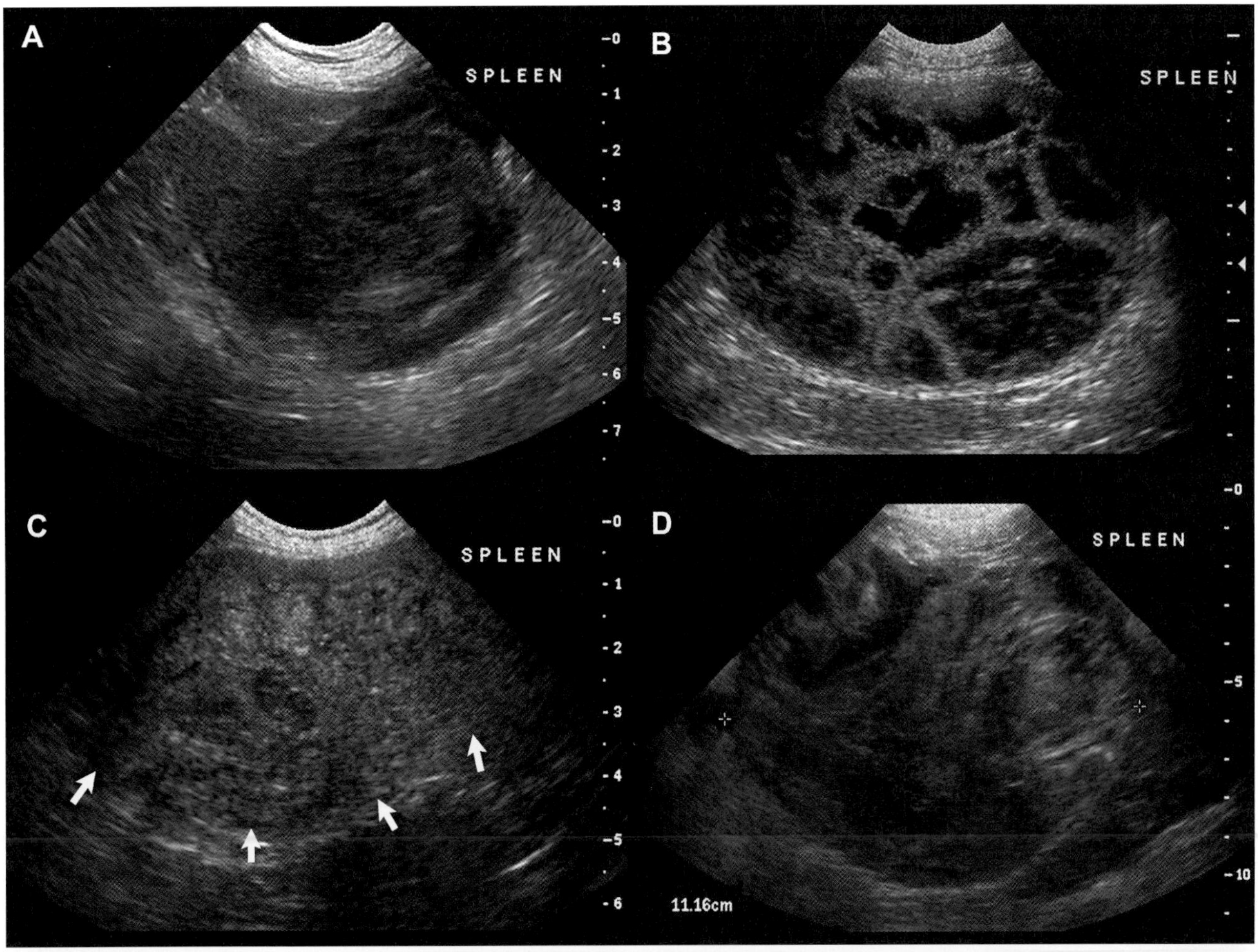

Figure 7.32. Variable appearances of splenic hemangiosarcoma in dogs. **A:** An approximately 6-cm-wide, mixed echogenic and mainly hypoechoic mass was identified in this 12-year-old Border collie. **B:** A round, well-circumscribed, mixed echogenic and cavitated mass of 8-cm diameter was identified in this 4-year-old golden retriever. **C:** Ill-defined, mixed echogenic mass (arrows) associated with the spleen of this 9-year-old golden retriever, replacing most of the normal parenchyma. **D:** Mixed echogenic mass of more than 11-cm diameter associated with the spleen (between the cursors) in this 8-year-old German shepherd.

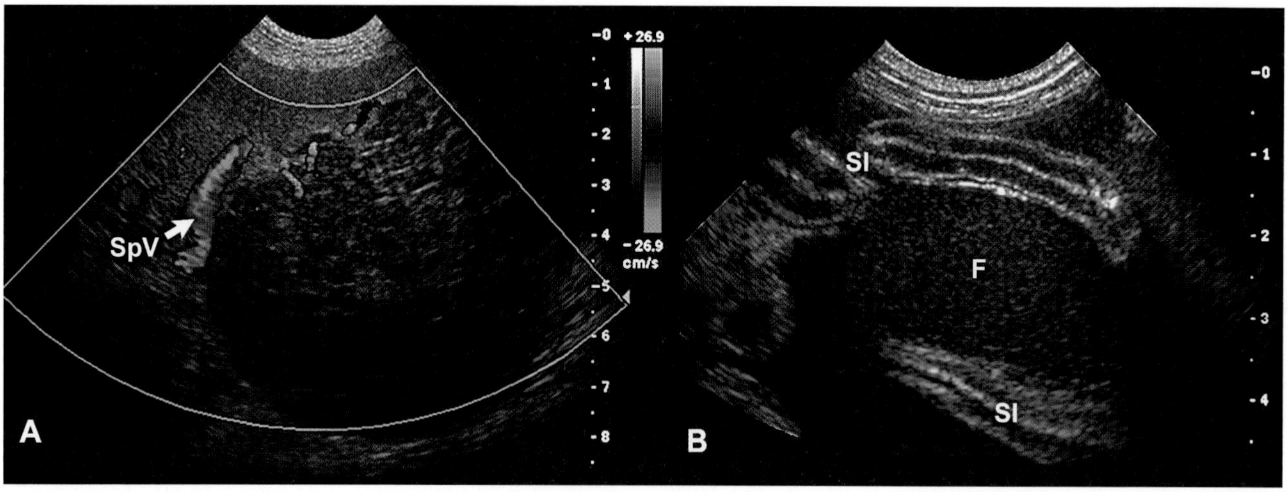

Figure 7.33. Splenic hemangiosarcoma and hemoabdomen in a large-breed dog. **A:** Ultrasound image of the spleen in which an abdominal mass was palpated. An irregular, well-defined, hypoechoic mass measuring approximately 7 cm wide is attached to spleen. Using color Doppler, numerous short vessels connecting the mass with the spleen are seen in the near field, which confirms the origin of this mass. The main splenic vein (SpV) is displaced by the mass. **B:** Severe, echogenic, peritoneal effusion (F) is also present, consistent with hemorrhage. SI, small intestine. Images courtesy of M.A. d'Anjou.

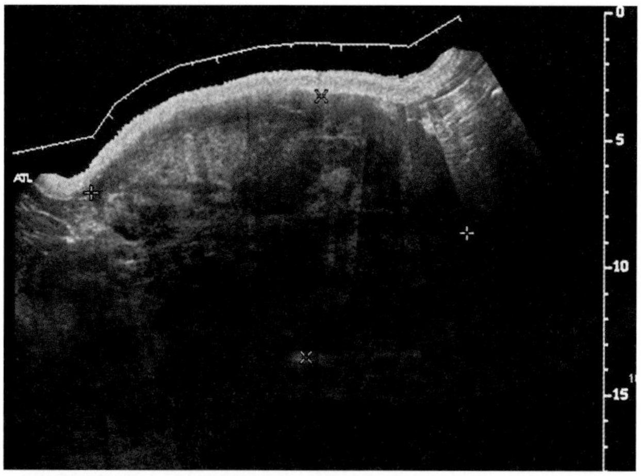

Figure 7.34. Malignant fibrous histiocytoma in a dog. On this panoramic ultrasound view, a solid, mixed echogenic mass (between the cursors) over 8 cm long is associated with the cranial aspect of the spleen.

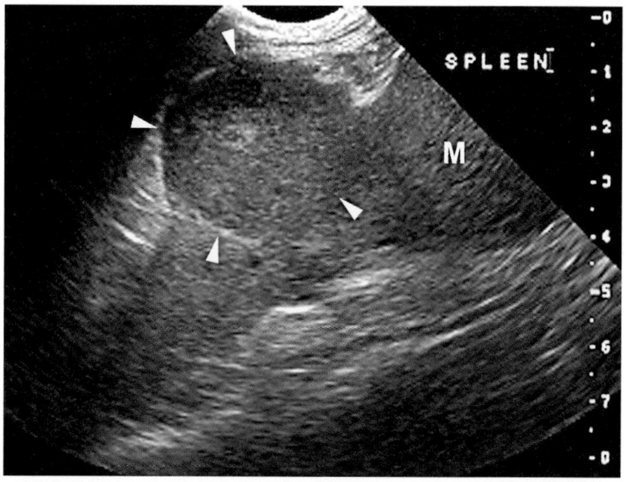

Figure 7.35. Histiocytic sarcoma in a 9-year-old golden retriever. A large, nearly isoechoic splenic mass (M) and a similar echogenic nodule (arrowheads) deforming the splenic contour are present. The histopathologic diagnosis was histiocytic sarcoma. Image courtesy of D. Penninck.

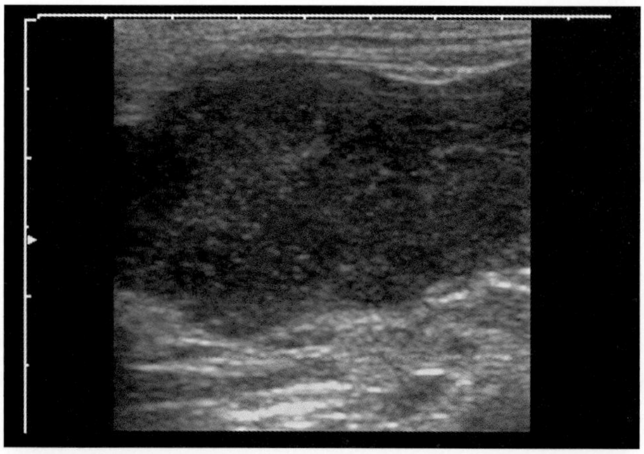

Figure 7.36. Presumptive malignant fibrous histiocytoma in a 12-year-old cat. There are multiple hypoechoic nodules in the spleen, each measuring up to 2 cm in maximum diameter.

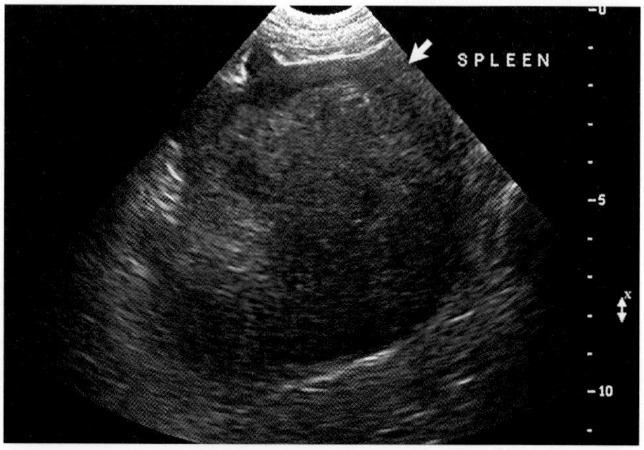

Figure 7.37. Poorly differentiated splenic sarcoma in an 8-year-old boxer. There is an approximately 10 cm mainly hypoechoic and inhomogeneous mass associated with the spleen. Normal spleen is present in the near field (arrow).

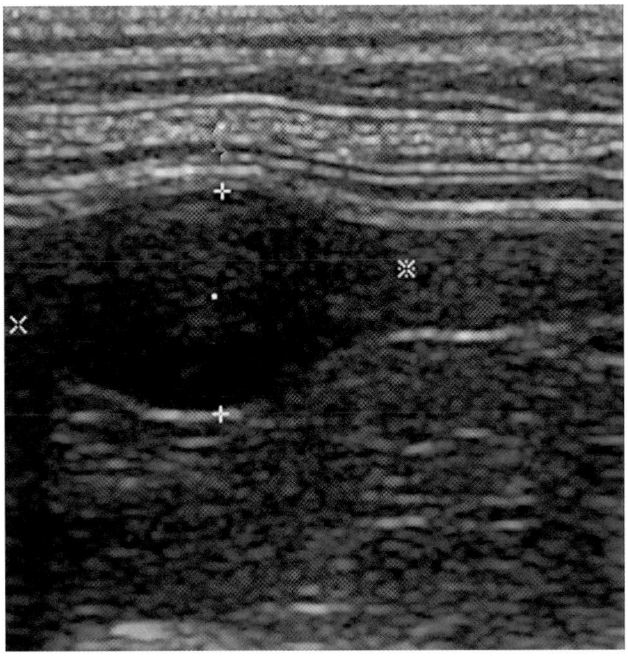

Figure 7.38. Splenic sarcoma in a 10-year-old cat. A homogeneous hypoechoic nodule (between the cursors) associated with the spleen is deforming the splenic border.

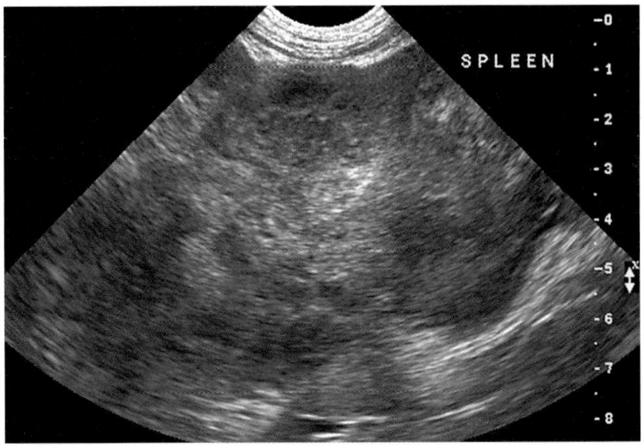

Figure 7.39. Round-cell tumor of the spleen in a 10-year-old coonhound. There is severe generalized splenomegaly, and the normal parenchyma is replaced by numerous ill-defined mass lesions of variable echogenicity.

hemoabdomen is more frequently encountered in cases of splenic malignancies (Figures 7.33, 7.37, 7.40, and 7.41), it also occurs in benign lesions. Splenic cysts and abscesses are rare and manifest as fluid-filled cavities of variable echogenicity within the splenic parenchyma, similar to hepatic cysts and abscesses. These cannot be differentiated from hematomas or cavitated masses based on their ultrasonographic appearance.

Nodules or masses with a hypoechoic rim and a hyperechoic to isoechoic center, which have been

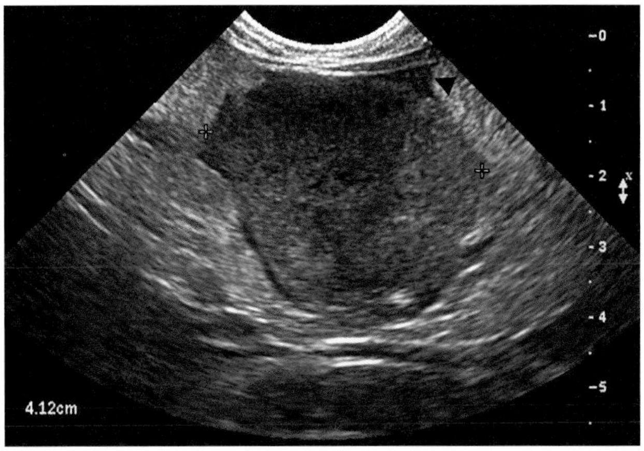

Figure 7.40. Splenic mast cell tumor in a cat. A homogeneous mass of medium echogenicity is associated with the spleen, which measures more than 4 cm in diameter (between the cursors). A small volume of abdominal effusion is at the periphery of this mass, particularly in the near field (arrowhead).

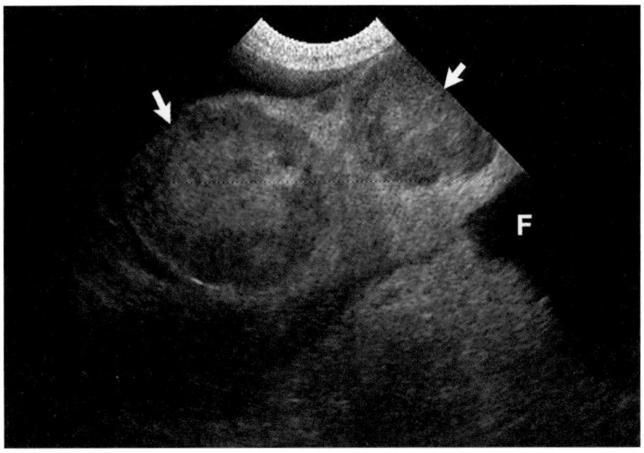

Figure 7.41. Splenic hemangiosarcoma and hemoabdomen in an 8-year-old Labrador retriever. There are two masses (arrows), which are characterized by a hypoechoic rim and a hyperechoic center (target lesions). A large volume of echogenic abdominal effusion (F) is noted.

described as target lesions, are more commonly associated with malignant processes such as metastasis (Cuccovillo and Lamb 2002) (Figure 7.41). However, these may also be seen with benign processes such as nodular hyperplasia. Malignant neoplasms may occasionally disrupt the splenic capsule and invade the adjacent mesentery (Figure 7.42).

Vascular Disorders

Thrombosis of splenic vein branches is occasionally encountered as the result of altered blood flow or

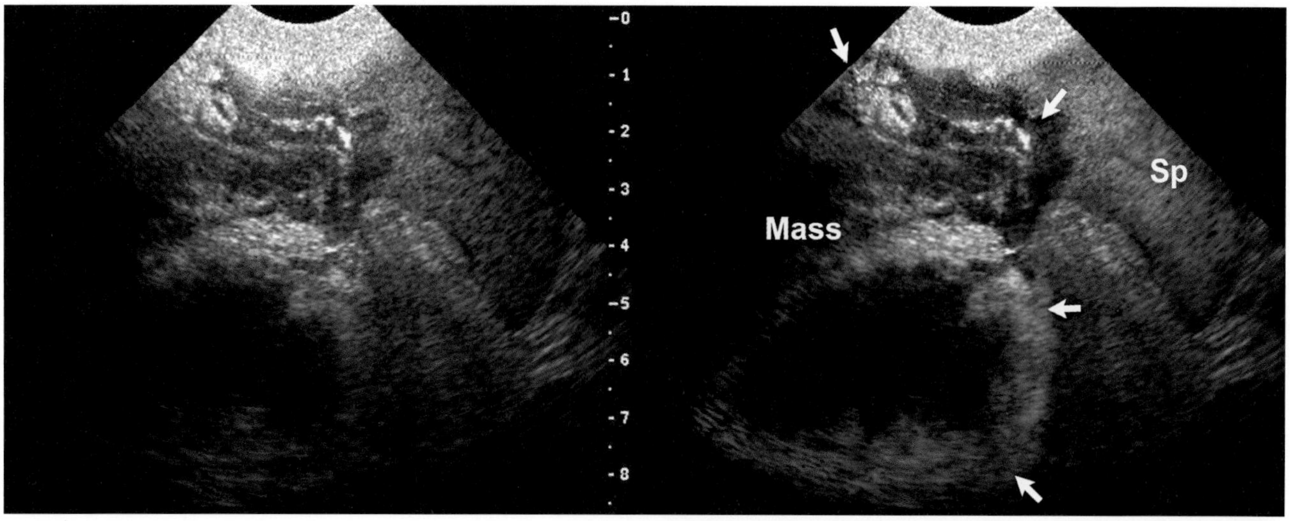

Figure 7.42. Poorly differentiated carcinoma in a 7-year-old Labrador retriever. **Left:** An ill-defined mixed echogenic mass suspected to be infiltrating the adjacent hyperechoic mesentery (arrows). **Right:** The corresponding modified labeled sonogram. Sp, spleen.

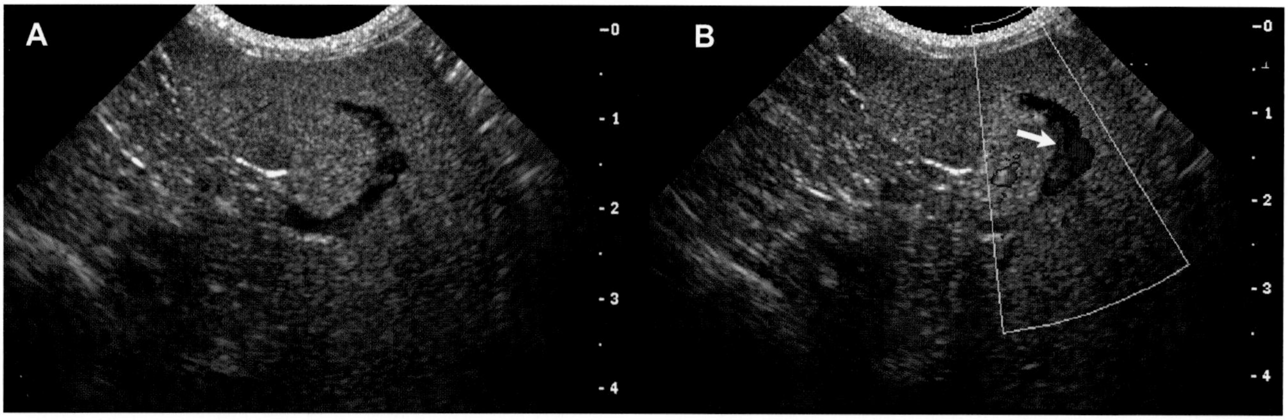

Figure 7.43. Splenic vein thrombus without evidence of splenic infarction in a 12-year-old springer spaniel. **A:** Echogenic material is associated with one of the branches of the splenic vein. The splenic parenchyma is within normal limits. **B:** On color Doppler examination, blood flow is noted around the thrombus (arrow), indicating incomplete vascular occlusion.

coagulation (Hardie et al. 1995). It manifests as echogenic material within the otherwise anechoic lumen of the vessel. Thrombi may remain inconsequential if occlusion of the vessel is incomplete or collateral vessels provide venous drainage of the affected areas (Figures 7.43 and 7.44). Occasionally, malignant splenic tumors invade splenic vessels and cause splenic vein thrombosis and splenic infarction (Figure 7.45).

When splenic infarction occurs, the affected areas appear hypoechoic, sharply demarcated from the adjacent parenchyma, and show decreased or absent blood flow on color Doppler or power Doppler examination. In contrast to splenic masses, infarcts do not tend to distort the normal organ contour, although this can be seen (Figures 7.46–7.48).

Splenic torsion is a rare disorder in dogs. Usually, there is progressive enlargement of the spleen, with decreased to absent blood flow. The parenchymal echogenicity and echotexture can vary as the congestion, hemorrhage, or infarction progresses. The parenchyma is typically mottled, and lacy anechoic to hypoechoic areas are observed, focally or diffusely, throughout the spleen (Saunders et al. 1998; Mai 2006) (Figures 7.12, 7.13, and 7.49). Static, echogenic thrombi can sometimes be seen in vascular lumens (Figure 7.49). Additionally, the bordering fat can become hyperechoic, and a hilar, perivenous, hyperechoic triangle has been described as a relatively specific sign of acute splenic torsion in dogs (Mai 2006) (Figure 7.50). However, these changes can also be found with

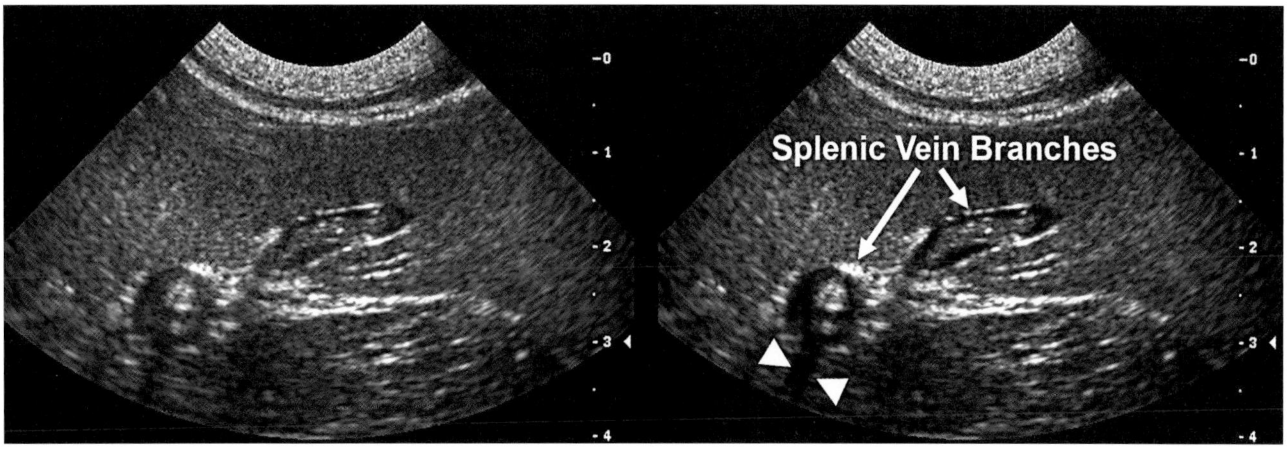

Figure 7.44. Chronic splenic vein thrombosis in an 11-year-old Labrador retriever. Strongly echogenic material is within the lumen of the splenic vein branches (arrows). Ultrasound-beam attenuation is distal to one of the thrombi (arrowheads), indicating fibrosis and/or mineralization of the clot. There is no evidence of parenchymal changes suggesting infarction.

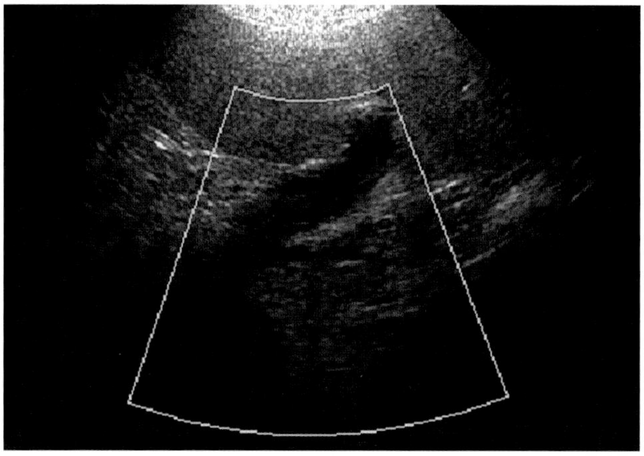

Figure 7.45. Poorly differentiated carcinoma with vascular invasion in a 7-year-old Labrador retriever (the same dog as in Figure 7.44). On power Doppler examination, no blood flow is detected within the affected splenic vein branch, even though the lumen appears hypoechoic.

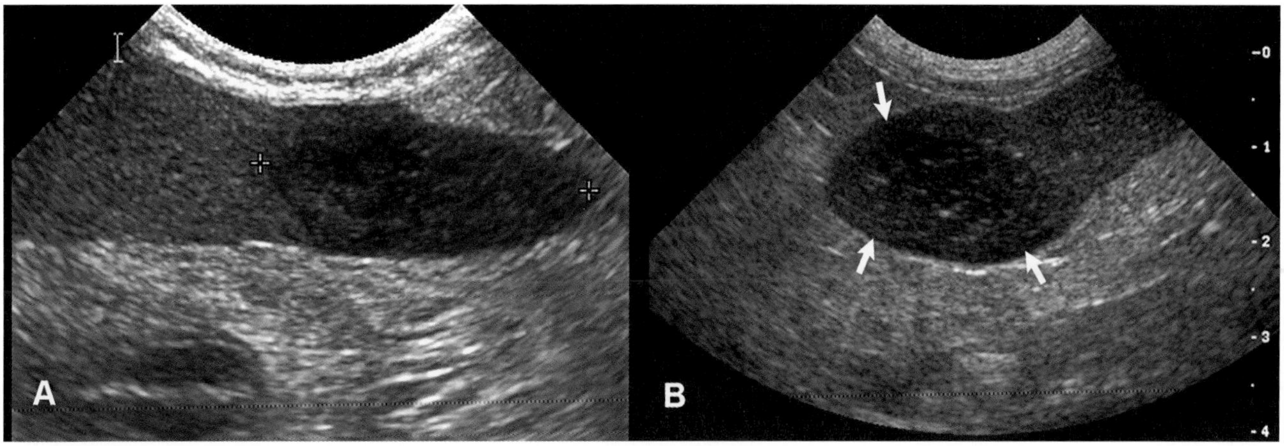

Figure 7.46. Splenic infarcts in two dogs. **A:** In a 10-year-old Australian shepherd, a sharply demarcated, lacy hypoechoic area is observed at the caudal extremity of the spleen (between the cursors), which is confined to the normal splenic border without evidence of a mass effect. **B:** In another dog, the infarcted area presents a mass effect at the tip of the spleen (arrows). Image B courtesy of M.A. d'Anjou.

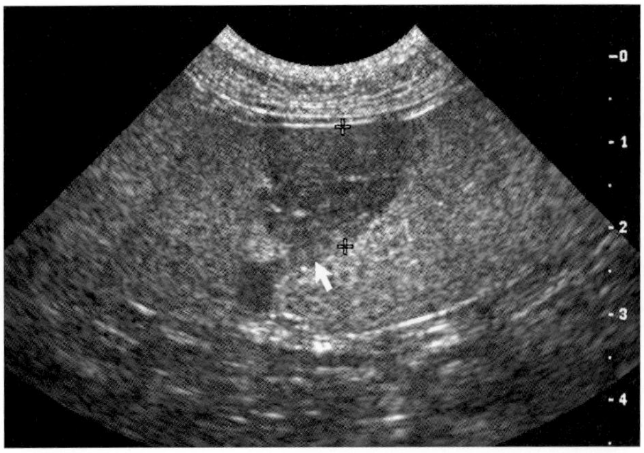

Figure 7.47. Splenic infarct in a 4-year-old Australian shepherd. A sharply demarcated hypoechoic area is associated with the body of the spleen (between the cursors). Echogenic material, consistent with a thrombus, is within the lumen of the contributing splenic vein (arrow).

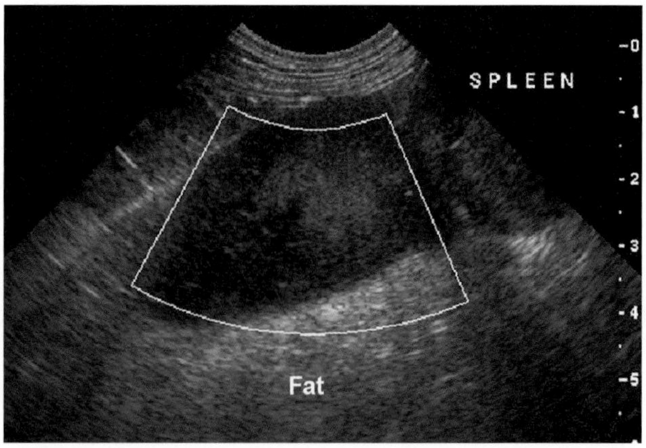

Figure 7.48. Splenic infarct in a 15-year-old golden retriever. An inhomogeneous lacy hypoechoic area within the spleen does not show blood flow on color Doppler examination. The fat at the dorsal margin of the spleen is hyperechoic.

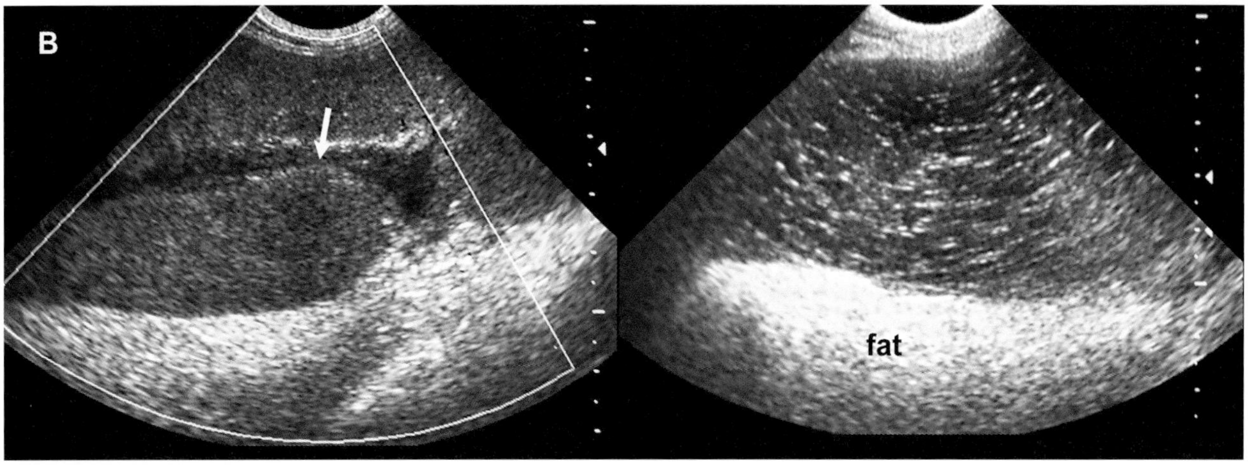

Figure 7.49. Splenic torsion in a 6-year-old standard poodle. **Left:** Sonographic image of the spleen at the time of presentation. The spleen is homogeneously hypoechoic and within normal limits for size. Upon Doppler examination, no flow was detected in the splenic veins, and a hyperechoic thrombus is seen (arrow). **Right:** Sonographic image of the splenic parenchyma 2 days later. The spleen is enlarged and has a diffuse, lacy hypoechoic echotexture. The adjacent fat is hyperechoic.

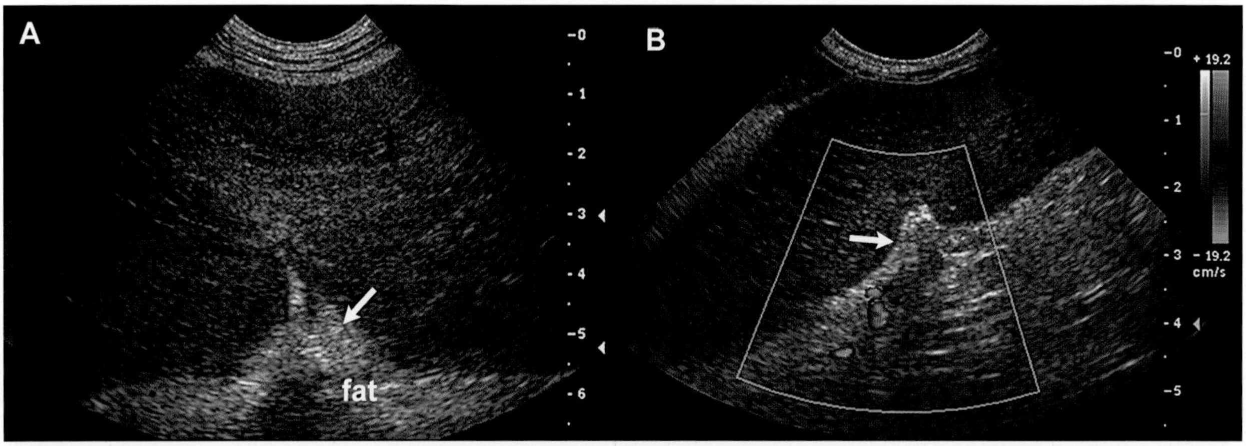

Figure 7.50. Perivenous hyperechoic triangle at the level of the splenic hilus in two dogs. A hyperechoic triangle (arrows) is a common feature observed with splenic torsion, as seen in **A**. This feature can also be observed with massive splenic infarction, as seen in **B**. This second dog was suffering from severe necrotic pancreatitis and progressively developed splenic infarction. At surgery, the spleen was not twisted, but was removed because of the complete venous thrombosis. In each case, the adjacent fat was hyperechoic. Images courtesy of M.A. d'Anjou.

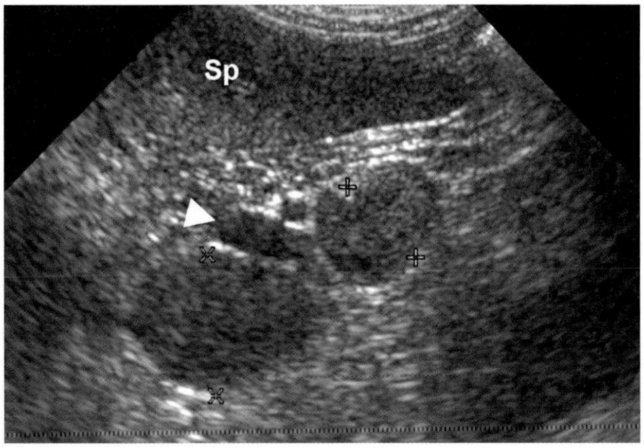

Figure 7.51. Lymphoma in a shi tzu. In the far field to the spleen (Sp) are two enlarged lymph nodes (0.9 and 1.3 cm in diameter, respectively; between the cursors) adjacent to a branch of the splenic vein (arrowhead).

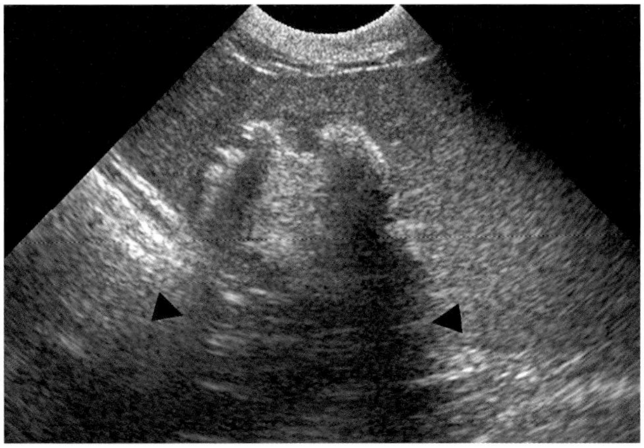

Figure 7.52. Extraskeletal osteosarcoma in a 10-year-old German shepherd. An irregularly marginated hyperechoic mass lesion associated with the splenic parenchyma shows strong distal ultrasound-beam attenuation (arrowheads).

extensive venous thrombosis and/or diffuse neoplastic infiltration (e.g., lymphoma).

Other Abnormalities

Normal splenic lymph nodes are usually not seen ultrasonographically. Enlarged lymph nodes may be visualized in cases of metastatic neoplasia as isoechoic to hypoechoic, rounded, soft-tissue nodules along the splenic vessels close to the hilus (Figure 7.51).

Strongly hyperechoic areas with strong distal acoustic shadowing are indicative of dystrophic mineralization or a mineralized neoplasm such as extraskeletal osteosarcoma (Figure 7.52).

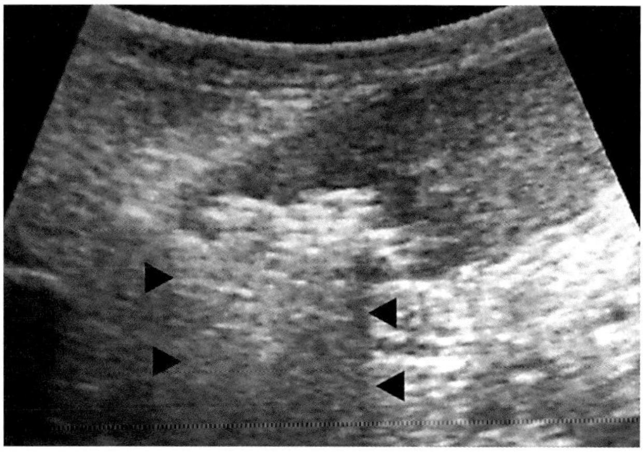

Figure 7.53. Clostridial splenitis in a 10-year-old greyhound. Multiple small confluent hyperechoic foci are associated with the cranial portion of the spleen. The inhomogeneous hypoechoic area distal to this lesion (dirty shadowing, arrowheads) is consistent with gas inclusions within the splenic parenchyma.

Gas inclusions in the spleen, though rarely seen, are indicative of infection with gas-producing bacteria (Gaschen et al. 2003) (Figure 7.53). Gas typically appears as hyperechoic foci with reverberation artifacts.

Interventional Procedures

Fine-needle aspiration of the spleen is routinely performed and is particularly useful in the diagnosis of diffuse infiltrative disorders. In most cases, freehand aspiration is possible because of the spleen's superficial location. A guide may be useful in cases of deep focal lesions. Tissue-core biopsy of a splenic lesion is not routinely performed. However, in cases of inconclusive fine-needle aspiration, biopsy of poorly vascularized mass lesions may be considered. Aspiration of fluid-filled splenic mass lesions such as hemangiosarcomas or hematomas frequently remains inconclusive because of blood dilution.

References

Crevier FR, Wrigley RH (2000) The sonographic features of splenic lymphoid hyperplasia in 31 dogs: A retrospective study (1980–2000) [Abstract]. Vet Radiol Ultrasound 41:566.

Cuccovillo A, Lamb CR (2002) Cellular features of sonographic target lesions of the liver and spleen in 21 dogs and a cat. Vet Radiol Ultrasound 43:275–278.

Fife WD, Samii VF, Drost WT, Mattoon JS, Hoshaw-Woodard S (2004) Comparison between malignant and nonmalignant splenic masses in dogs using contrast-enhanced computed tomography. Vet Radiol Ultrasound 45:289–297.

Gaschen L, Kircher P, Venzin C, Hurter K, Lang J (2003) Imaging diagnosis: The abdominal air-vasculogram in a dog with splenic torsion and clostridial infection. Vet Radiol Ultrasound 44:553–555.

Hanson JA, Papageorges M, Girard E, Menard M, Hebert P (2001) Ultrasonographic appearance of splenic disease in 101 cats. Vet Radiol Ultrasound 42:441–445.

Hardie EM, Vaden SL, Spaulding K, Malarkey DE (1995) Splenic infarction in 16 dogs: A retrospective study. J Vet Intern Med 9:141–148.

Lamb CR, Hartzband LE, Tidwell AS, Pearson SH (1991) Ultrasonographic findings in hepatic and splenic lymphosarcoma in dogs and cats. Vet Radiol Ultrasound 32:117–120.

Mai W (2006) The hilar perivenous hyperechoic triangle as a sign of acute splenic torsion in dogs. Vet Radiol Ultrasound 47:487–491.

Nyland TG, Mattoon JS, Herrgesell ER, Wisner ER (1995) Spleen. In: Nyland TG, Mattoon JS, eds. Small Animal Diagnostic Ultrasound. Philadelphia: WB Saunders, pp 128–143.

O'Brien RT, Waller KR, Osgood TL (2004) Sonographic features of drug-induced splenic congestion. Vet Radiol Ultrasound 45:225–227.

Ramirez S, Douglass JP, Robertson ID (2002) Ultrasonographic features of canine abdominal malignant histiocytosis. Vet Radiol Ultrasound 43:167–170.

Sato AF, Solano M (2004) Ultrasonographic findings in abdominal mast cell disease: A retrospective study of 19 patients. Vet Radiol Ultrasound 45:51–57.

Saunders HM (1998) Ultrasonography of abdominal cavitary parenchymal lesions. Vet Clin North Am Small Anim Pract 28:755–775.

Saunders HM, Neath PJ, Brockman DJ (1998) B-mode and Doppler ultrasound imaging of the spleen with canine splenic torsion: A retrospective evaluation. Vet Radiol Ultrasound 39:349–353.

Schwarz LA, Penninck DG, Gliatto J (2001) Canine splenic myelolipomas. Vet Radiol Ultrasound 42:347–348.

Wrigley RH, Konde LJ, Park RD, Lebel JL (1988) Ultrasonographic features of splenic lymphosarcoma in dogs: 12 cases (1980–1986). J Am Vet Med Assoc 193: 1565–1568.

CHAPTER EIGHT

Gastrointestinal Tract

Dominique Penninck

Preparation and Scanning Procedure

Animals can be scanned while they are in dorsal recumbency, right or left recumbency, or standing position, if needed, to optimize an acoustic window by displacing the intraluminal fluid to the region of interest. Left lateral recumbency helps with the evaluation of the fundus, whereas right lateral recumbency improves the evaluation of the pylorus and duodenum. The standing position can be helpful for evaluating the ventral aspect of the pylorus and body of the stomach. However, the results of these positional studies also depend on a dog's conformation, the degree of stomach dilation, the nature of gastric contents, and patient cooperation.

A real-time scanner with a high-frequency (7.5 MHz and higher) sectorial, curvilinear, or linear transducer is recommended. High-frequency probes optimize the evaluation of the gastrointestinal (GI) wall layering. Curvilinear probes with a small footprint are useful because they can more easily be placed below the rib cage or between ribs for the assessment of the stomach and proximal duodenum. Transverse and longitudinal views of the GI segments are required to fully assess the thickness and the extent of a suspected lesion (Figure 8.1).

Little preparation is needed; a fast of 12 h can reduce interference with gastric contents and the associated gas, but the results are inconsistent. Gas in the GI tract is the most common cause of imaging artifacts such as reverberation, comet tail, and acoustic shadowing (Figure 8.2).

Ultrasonographic Anatomy of the Normal Gastrointestinal Tract

The wall thickness and layering, and relative motility of different segments of the GI tract, can be evaluated. The thickness of the GI tract can be measured by placing calipers on the outer aspect of the serosa and on the mucosal inner border.

Table 8.1 lists the range of normal thickness of the GI wall in dogs and cats (Penninck et al. 1989; Newell et al. 1999; Goggin et al. 2000; Delaney et al. 2003).

The gastric wall is challenging to measure mainly when the stomach is collapsed. There is significant difference between the thicknesses of the rugal folds and interrugal folds. The thickness varies depending on the degree of distension and the size of the dog. The mean of the observed rate of peristalsis is 4–5 contractions per minute in dogs. The descending duodenum in dogs is thicker than is the remainder of the small bowel. The ileum in cats can easily be identified by its prominent and bright submucosal layer.

The colon, often gas or feces filled, has a thinner wall than the small bowel in dogs and cats. Composite images of the main segments of the GI tract in dogs and cats illustrate their main features (Figures 8.3 and 8.4).

Five ultrasonographic layers can be identified throughout the GI tract. From the lumen to the serosal surface, one can identify the hyperechoic

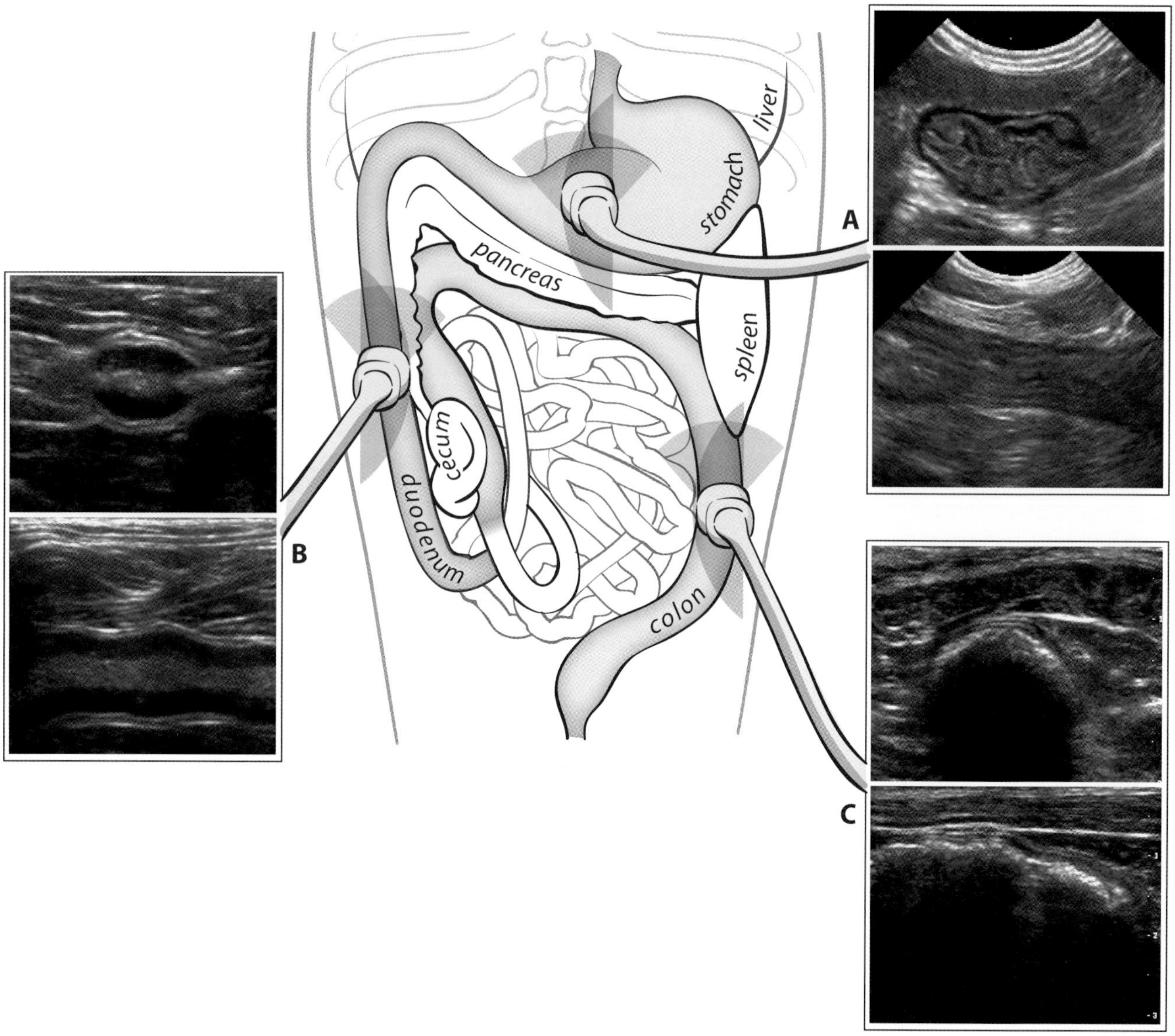

Figure 8.1. Ultrasonographic anatomy of the normal canine gastrointestinal tract in dorsal recumbency. Illustration of the location of the main gastrointestinal segments, with placements of the probe to fully evaluate some of these segments. **Plan A** shows the position of the probe on the stomach. Both transverse (top sonographic image) and longitudinal images (bottom sonographic image) are obtained by sliding the probe along the long axis of the stomach. **Plan B** shows the position of the probe on the descending duodenum. Both transverse (top sonographic image) and longitudinal images (bottom sonographic image) of this bowel segment are displayed. **Plan C** shows the position of the probe on the descending colon. Both transverse (top sonographic image) and longitudinal images (bottom sonographic image) of the colon are displayed.

Figure 8.3. Sonograms of normal gastrointestinal segments in dogs. **A:** On transabdominal approach, the esophagus is rarely seen. In this 10 year-old corgi, the most distal portion of the esophagus (E) is visible. In the same image is a transverse view of the aorta (Ao) and the fundus of the stomach. **B:** The stomach is easily recognized by its location, the presence of rugal folds, and its peristaltic activity. When the stomach is collapsed like in this dog, it is difficult to assess the wall thickness accurately. Note the adjacent transverse colon (C) located caudal to the stomach body. **C:** The proximal duodenum (D) is a superficial and rectilinear segment coursing along the right lateral abdominal wall. The duodenum has a thicker wall than the remaining small bowel. Another fluid-filled intestinal segment is in the near field, consistent with a segment of jejunum (J) **D:** In the proximal portion of the descending duodenum, the duodenal papilla, seen on transverse plane on this picture (between the cursors) can easily be identified. Occasionally, as in this dog, a small anechoic (fluid filled) lumen can be seen. **E:** Jejunal segments are freely looping in the midabdomen. The wall layering is visible. **F:** The ileocecocolic junction is difficult to identify because gas is often collected at that location. In this dog, a small amount of fluid at the junction facilitated its identification on a transverse plane. Note the smaller-diameter segment of the ileum (I) joining the ascending colon (C). **G:** The colon, often gas or feces filled, has a thinner wall than the small bowel. In this dog, the finely layered colonic wall is 1.5 mm thick.

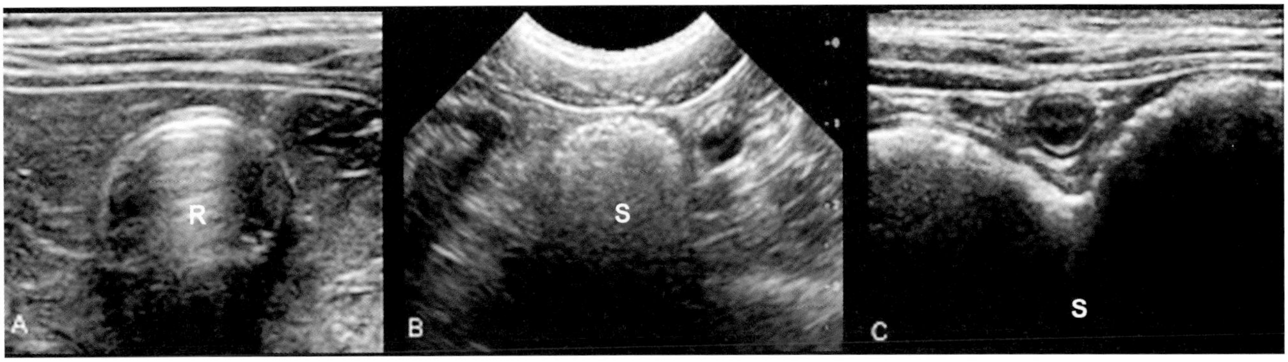

Figure 8.2. Artifacts commonly seen associated with the gastrointestinal tract. **A:** Gas in the colon of this dog creates a reverberation artifact (R) masking most of the far wall. The sound is entirely reflected back from the gas and then bounces back and forth between the probe and the gas, creating multiple echoes from one ultrasound pulse. **B and C:** The mixture of gas and fecal material in the gastrointestinal tract often creates acoustic shadowing (S) appearing as an area of low-amplitude echoes created by highly attenuating structures. The shadowing can be dirty **(B)** or clean **(C)**, depending on its homogeneity.

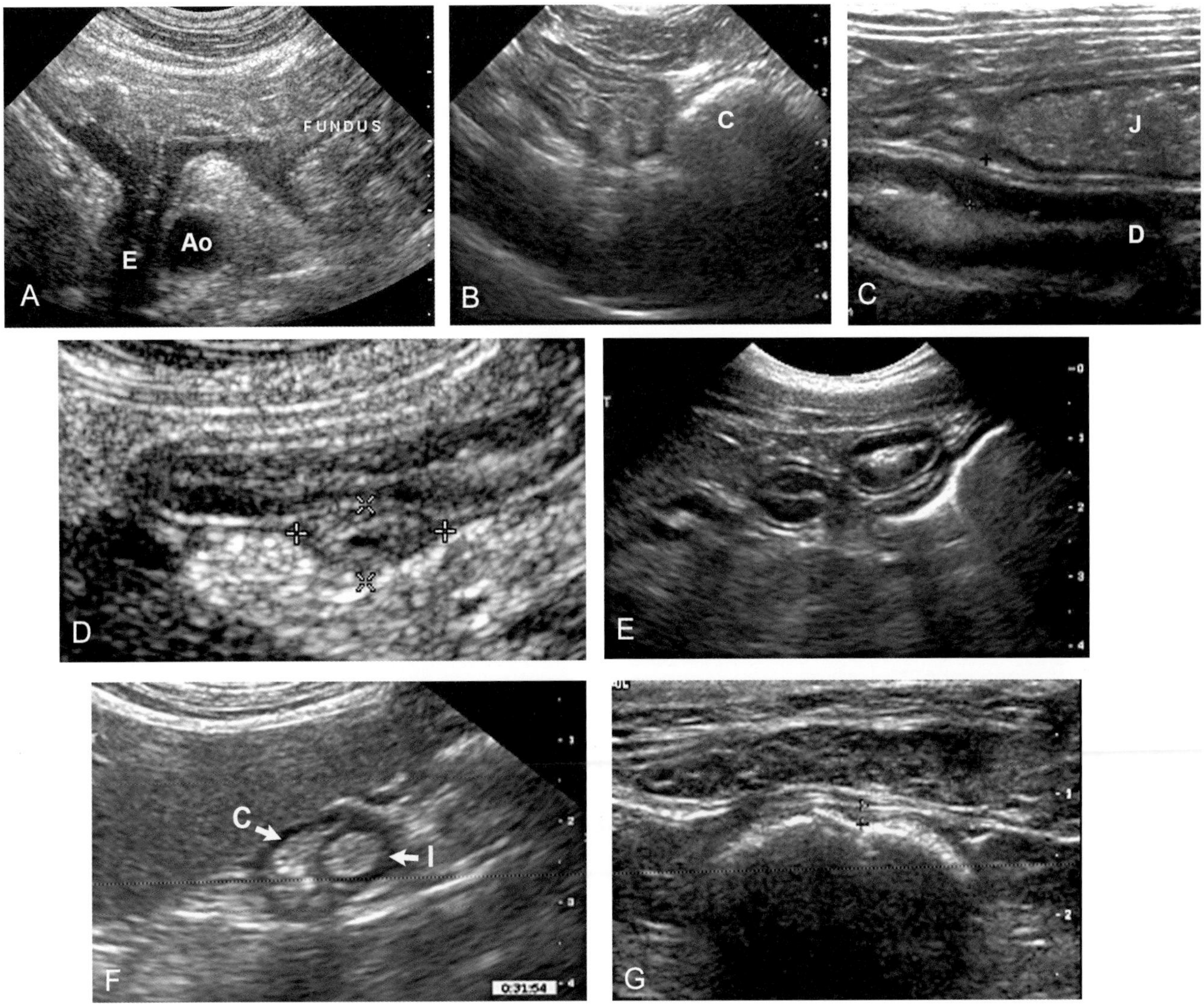

Figure 8.3.

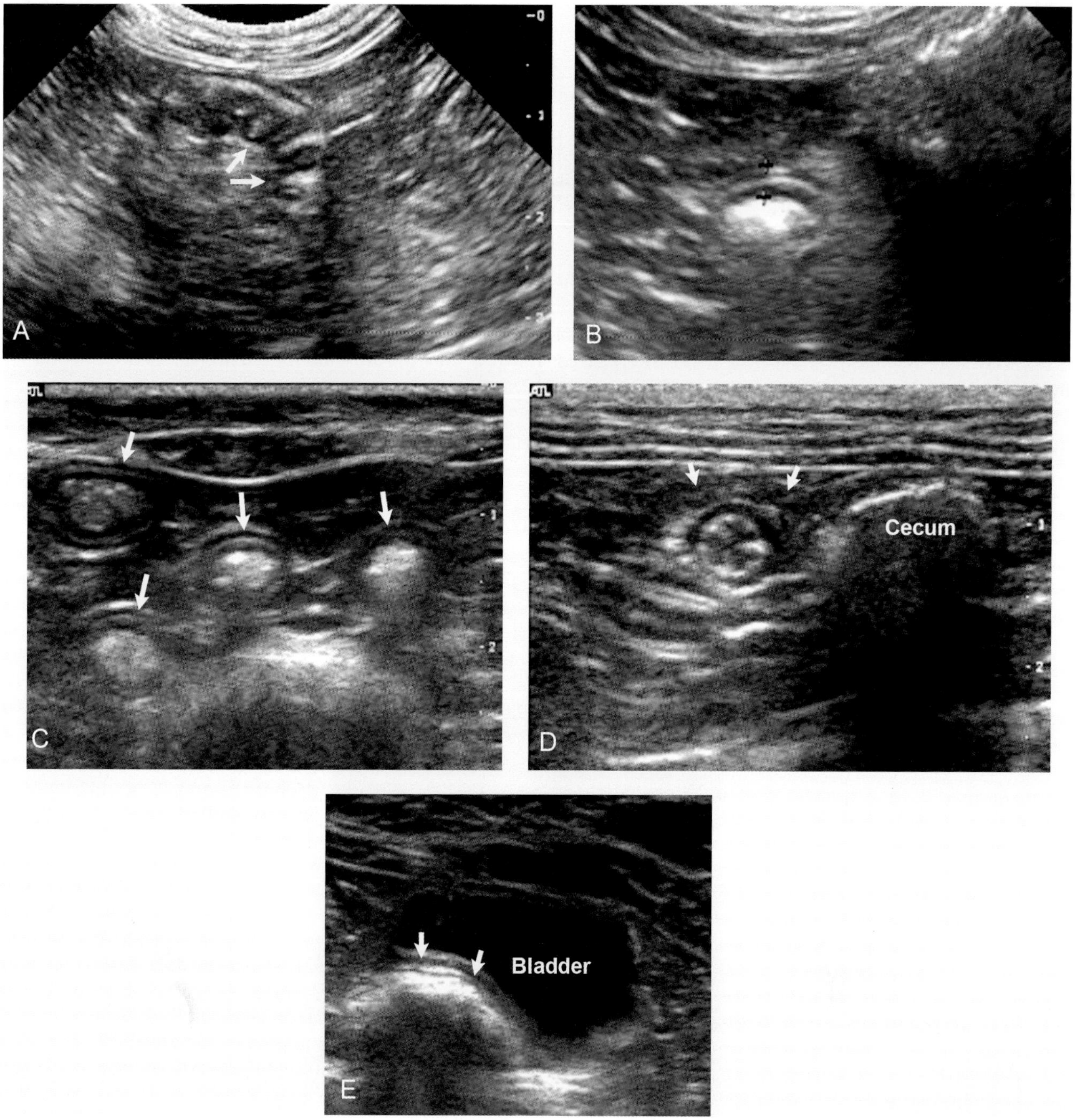

Figure 8.4. Sonograms of normal gastrointestinal segments in cats. **A:** Transverse sonogram of the collapsed gastric fundus in an adult cat. A small amount of gas in the lumen prevents complete assessment of the far wall. Rugal folds protrude into the lumen (arrows). **B:** Transverse sonogram of the descending duodenum (between the cursors). The wall layering is visible. The gas-filled colon associated with shadowing is on the right side of the duodenum. **C:** Several loops of jejunum, containing fluid and gas, are present in this sonogram (arrows). There is no significant difference between the thickness of duodenum and jejunum in cats. **D:** Transverse sonogram of the ileum. The gas-filled cecum is on the right of the ileum, and the ileum is entering the echogenic fluid-filled ascending colon (arrows). This short segment of bowel has more prominent submucosa and muscularis than the remaining bowel segments in cats. These characteristic features have been referred as the "wagon-wheel" sign in cats. **E:** Transverse sonogram of the feces-filled descending colon in a normal cat. The thin wall and its layering are barely visible (arrows), just ventral to the hyperechoic interface created by the presence of feces and its associated shadow in the far field.

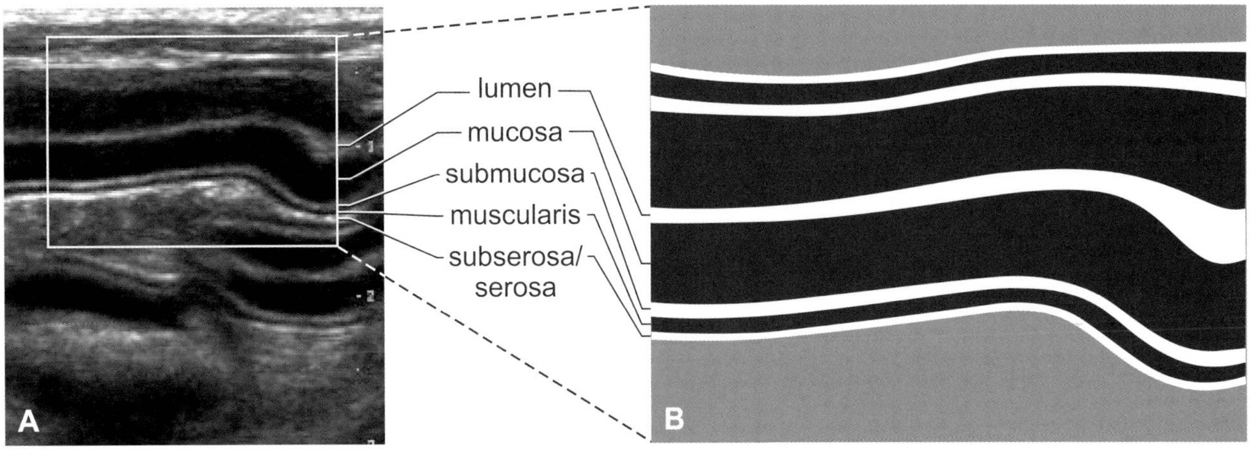

Figure 8.5. Normal intestinal layers. **A:** Longitudinal sonogram of a normal jejunal segment. Five ultrasonographic layers can easily be identified. **B:** Schematic representation of the bowel wall layers. The lumen is a bright interface in the center of the bowel, surrounded by the relatively thick mucosa (hypoechoic), thin submucosa (hyperechoic), thin muscularis (hypoechoic), and thin subserosa/serosa (hyperechoic).

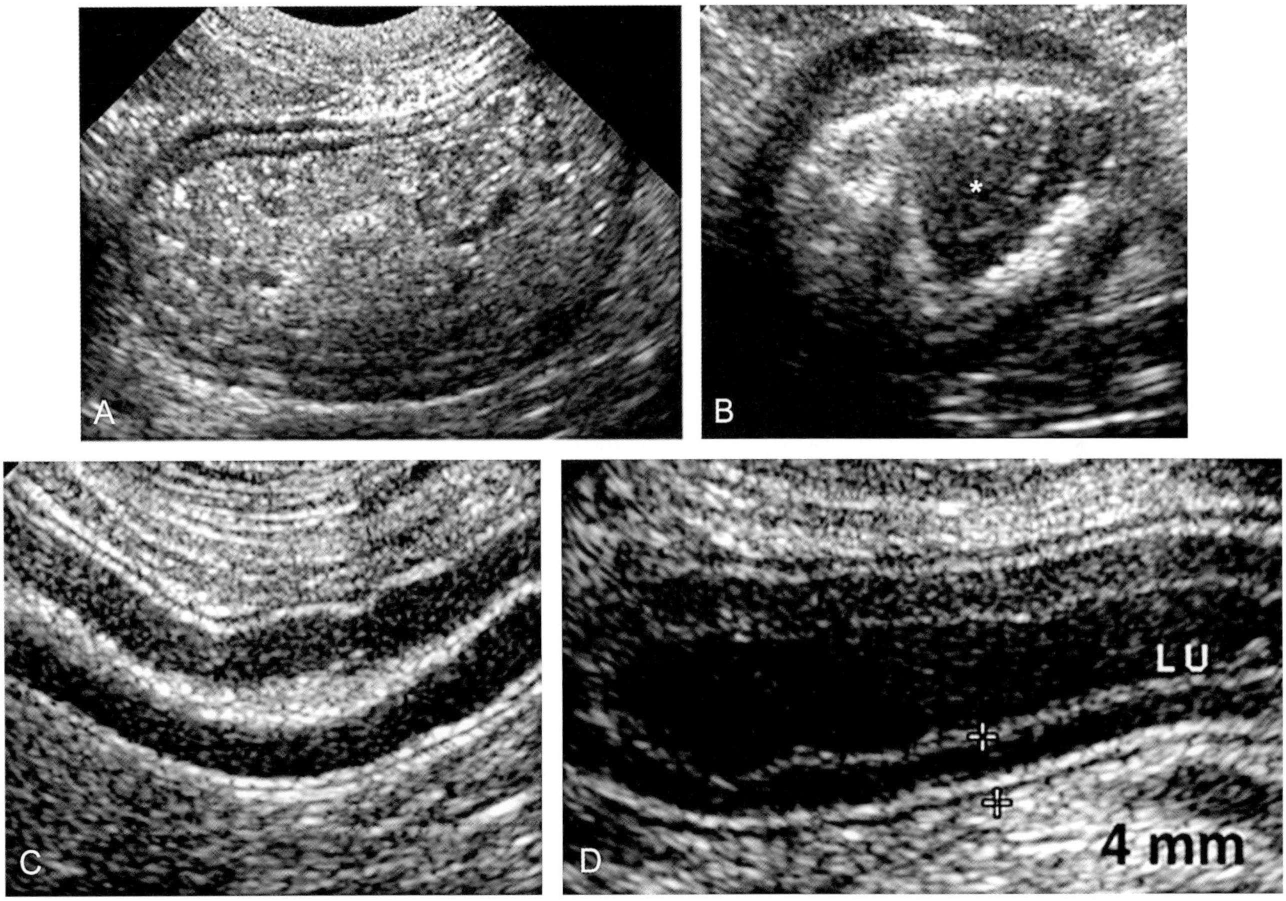

Figure 8.6. Normal luminal contents. **A:** The alimentary pattern consists of food particles of variable size and shape in the gastric lumen. It may or may not be associated with imaging artifacts. In this dog, small, rounded, echogenic balls of food can be identified in the gastric lumen. **B:** A large amount of food or large pieces of food can occasionally mimic a mass in the stomach. A large poorly echogenic "mass" was seen in this dog presented because of vomiting (*). The "mass" was surrounded by a small amount of gas and mucus. During the real-time examination, the content was moving within the gastric lumen. A mural mass was considered less likely, but a gastric foreign body could not be ruled out. A repeat examination, after fast, showed an empty normal stomach. **C:** The mucous pattern appears as a bright interface in the lumen of this jejunal segment. Note the absence of artifact with this pattern. The gastrointestinal wall can be fully evaluated. **D:** The fluid pattern is characterized by anechoic to uniformly echogenic luminal contents. This pattern optimizes the visualization of the wall layers on each side of the lumen. LU, lumen of the bowel. **E:** The gas pattern appears as an intraluminal, hyperechoic, reflective surface with acoustic shadowing and prevents evaluation of deeper structures. At the ileocolic junction in this cat, a small amount of gas is seen in the ascending colon. The gas is associated with a reverberation artifact.

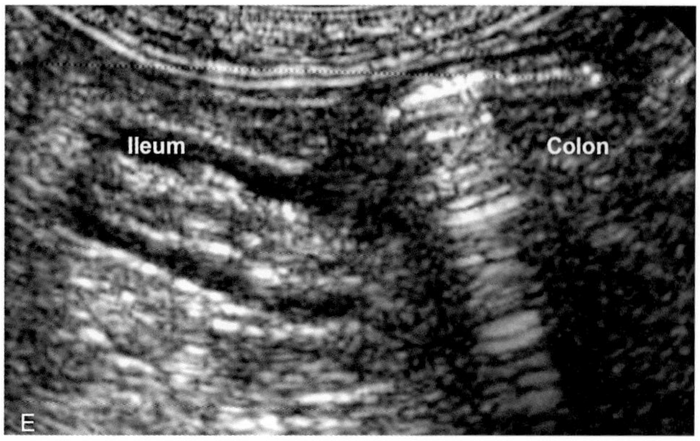

Figure 8.6. *Continued*

Table 8.1.
Reference table for normal range of wall thickness for the different segments of the gastrointestinal tract in dogs and cats

Wall Thickness	Dog	Cat
Stomach	2–5 mm[a]	1.7–3.6 mm
Duodenum	3–6 mm[b]	2.0–2.5 mm
Jejunum	2–5 mm[b]	2.0–2.5 mm
Ileum	2–4 mm	2.5–3.2 mm
Colon	2–3 mm	1.4–2.5 mm

[a]Varies with distension of the stomach and measurements taken at the rugal or the interrugal level.
[b]Body weight correlation exists (Delaney et al. 2003).

mucosal interface in contact with the lumen, the hypoechoic mucosa, the hyperechoic submucosa, the hypoechoic muscular layer, and the hyperechoic subserosa and serosa (Figure 8.5). The mucosal layer often is thicker than the muscularis layer, but mucosa and muscularis can be of equal thickness during peristaltism.

There is a good morphological correlation between the ultrasonographic appearance and the histological layers.

The normal luminal contents can vary and consist of food, mucus, fluid, or gas (Figure 8.6).

The distal esophagus, which can be occasionally seen on ultrasound in small dogs (Figure 8.3A), is difficult to access because its position is cranial to the diaphragm and because of the interposition of gas in the surrounding lungs.

The stomach, which is the largest portion of the GI tract, can be identified easily by its rugal folds (Figures 8.1A, 8.3B, and 8.4A).

The descending duodenum (Figures 8.1B and 8.3C), which is the thickest segment of small bowel in dogs, has a superficial and rectilinear course along the right lateral abdominal wall.

The duodenal papilla (Figure 8.3D) is identified easily in the proximal portion of the descending duodenum.

The ileum in cats (Figure 8.4D) is a short bowel segment that has prominent submucosa and muscularis. The ileocecocolic junction can be challenging to identify in dogs because the cecum is most commonly gas filled (Figure 8.3F). In cats, the ileocecocolic junction (Figure 8.4D) can be more easily recognized. The colon (Figures 8.1C, 8.2, 8.3G, 8.4E, and 8.6E) has a thin, layered wall and often contains gas and feces.

Sonographic Features of Gastrointestinal Disorders

Intussusception

The main ultrasonographic feature of an intussusception is the multilayered appearance of the wall (called also *concentric rings* or *ring sign*) representing the superimposed wall layers of the intussusceptum and intussuscipiens (Figure 8.7).

In dogs and cats (Lamb and Mantis 1998; Patsikas et al. 2003), the appearance of intussusception varies somewhat with the location and length of the GI segment involved, the duration of the process, and the orientation of the scan plane relative to the axis of the intussusception. The intussuscipiens (outer bowel segment) is often thickened, edematous, and hypoechoic, whereas the thickness and layering of the intussusceptum may appear normal. The invaginated portion can involve different segments of the GI tract, such as the stomach (Figure 8.8), small bowel (Figures 8.9 and 8.10), or colon (Figures 8.11 and 8.12).

Gastric intussusception is rare, but when encountered can be challenging to diagnose ultrasonographically (Hoffman et al. 2003; Lee et al. 2005). Frequently, invaginated mesenteric fat is associated with the intus-

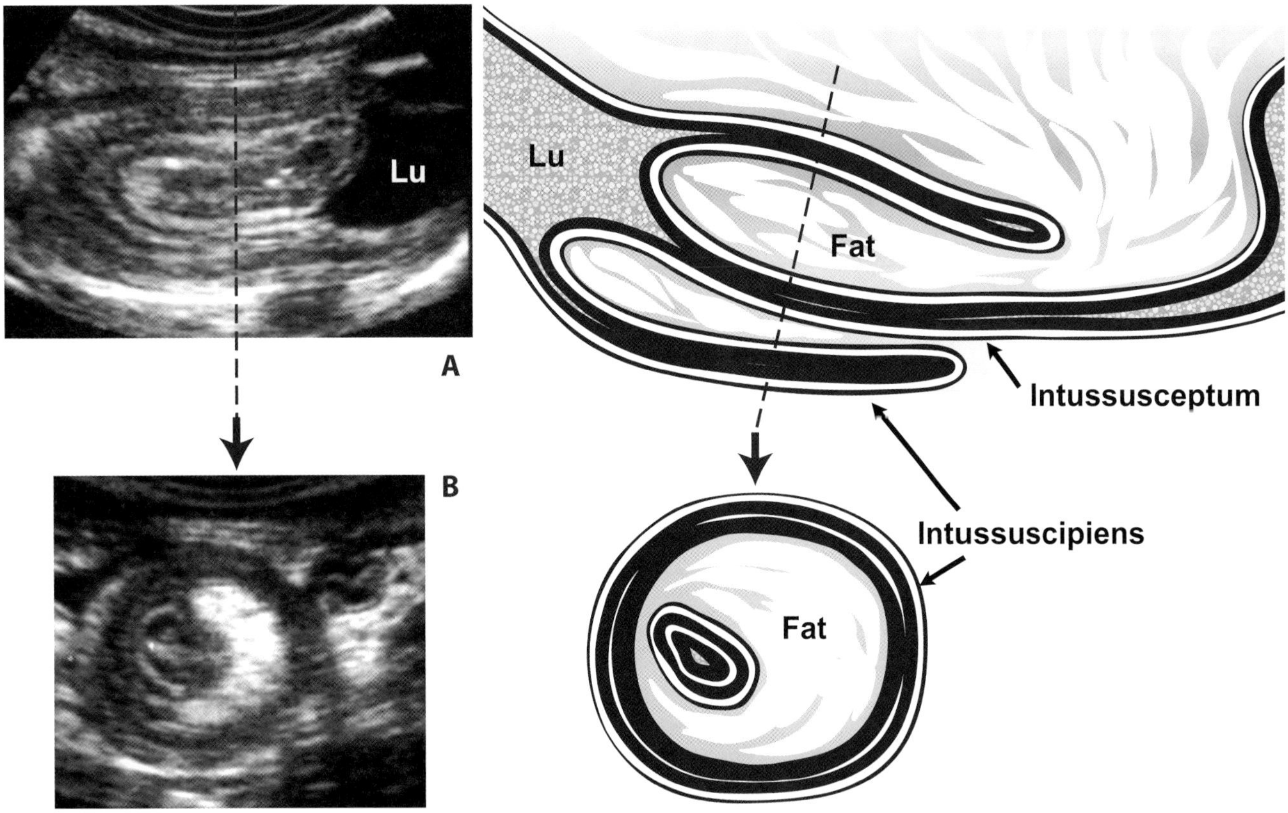

Figure 8.7. Intussusception in a cat. Illustrations of the relationship of the intussuscipiens, intussusceptum, and surrounding structures. On the top **(A)** is the longitudinal sonogram of a jejunoileal intussusception and its corresponding schematic illustration. On the bottom **(B)** is the transverse sonogram of a jejunoileal intussusception and its corresponding schematic illustration. The intestinal lumen (Lu) is dilated with fluid because of mechanical obstruction, and hyperechoic fat is invaginated with the intussusceptum within the intussuscipiens.

suscipiens. On occasions, inflammatory pseudocysts, enlarged lymph nodes (Figure 8.12B), foreign bodies (Figure 8.9), or tumoral mass (Figure 8.13) in older patients can be seen within or near the intussusception site.

At times, complex lesions affecting the GI tract, such as redundant or hyperplastic mucosa protruding into the its lumen, can simulate the pattern of intussusception (Figure 8.14). By evaluating the lesion in several planes, one can avoid such pitfalls.

Foreign Bodies

GI foreign bodies greatly vary in size, shape, and echogenicity. Segmental fluid or gas accumulation within the stomach or part of the intestinal tract is an indicator of mechanical ileus (obstruction). When present, abnormal fluid distension facilitates the detection of foreign material (Figure 8.15).

Balls are easily identified because of their characteristic curvilinear interface. They may vary in echogenicity, depending on the makeup of their material (Figure 8.16).

Independently from the type of foreign body, the presence of bright interface associated with strong shadowing is highly suggestive of a foreign material (Tidwell and Penninck 1992). Feces in the colon can simulate foreign material, and compact fecal material is similarly associated with shadowing. It is thus critical to identify accurately the segment of the intestinal tract, especially differentiating small bowel from colon (Figure 8.2). Occasionally, the contour of the interface can enable the identification of the type of foreign body (Figure 8.17).

Linear foreign bodies present as bright linear interfaces, commonly associated with shadowing, and the affected bowel segment often appears plicated (Figure 8.18). The degree of plication varies with duration and severity. Intestinal distension often is less pronounced than with larger obstructive foreign bodies. Linear foreign bodies vary in diameter, contour, and length and can be associated with larger

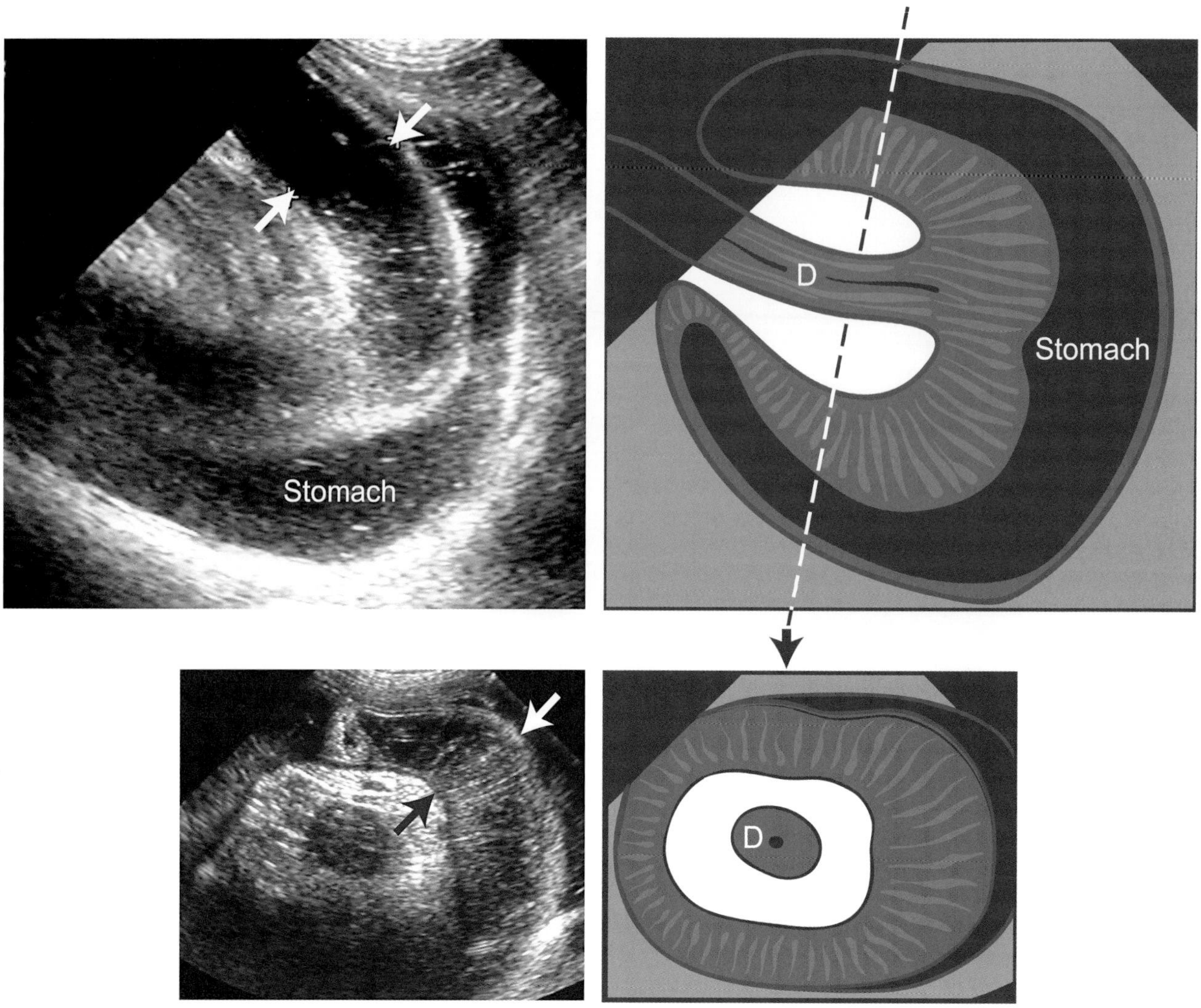

Figure 8.8. Duodenogastric intussusception. Illustration of a duodenogastric intussusception in a 6-year-old male Labrador retriever with glomerulonephritis and presented because of severe, acute vomiting. The most proximal portion of the duodenum is invaginated within the pylorus, which protrudes within the fluid-filled gastric body (Stomach). The gastric wall was severely thickened and hypoechoic because of severe edema (arrows). This change was misinterpreted as a mass. D, duodenum.

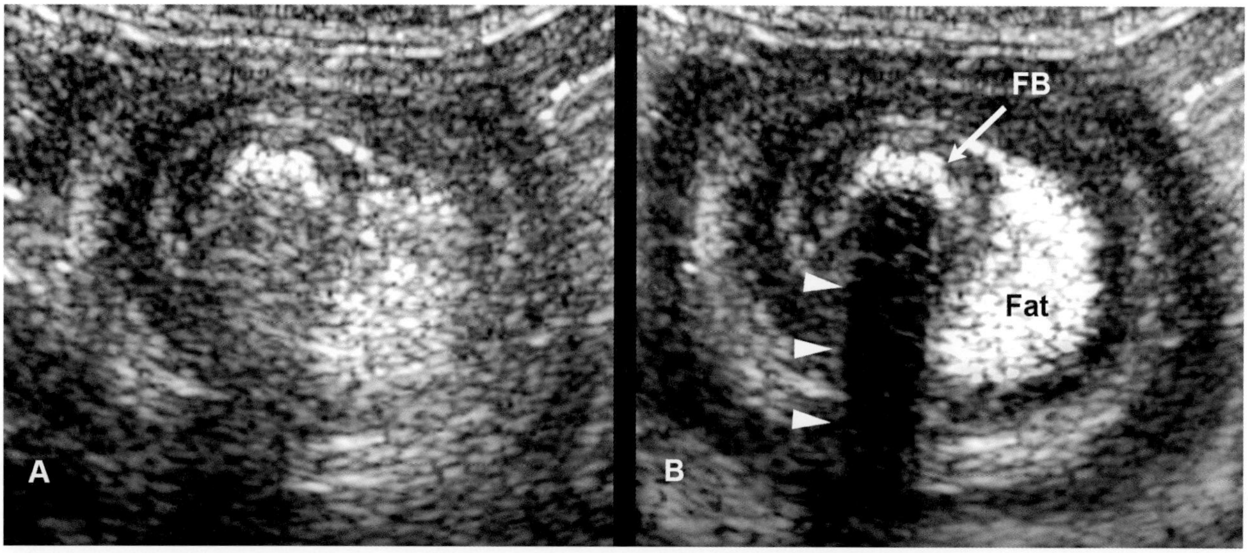

Figure 8.9. Jejunal intussusception and linear foreign body. Transverse sonographic **(A)** and schematic **(B)** images of a jejunojejunal intussusception identified in a 3-year-old standard poodle. The intussuscepted segment contains a linear foreign body (FB) associated with acoustic shadowing (arrowheads). The invaginated hyperechoic fat is crescent shaped at the center of the intussusception. Note the concentric hypoechoic rings consistent with an intussusception.

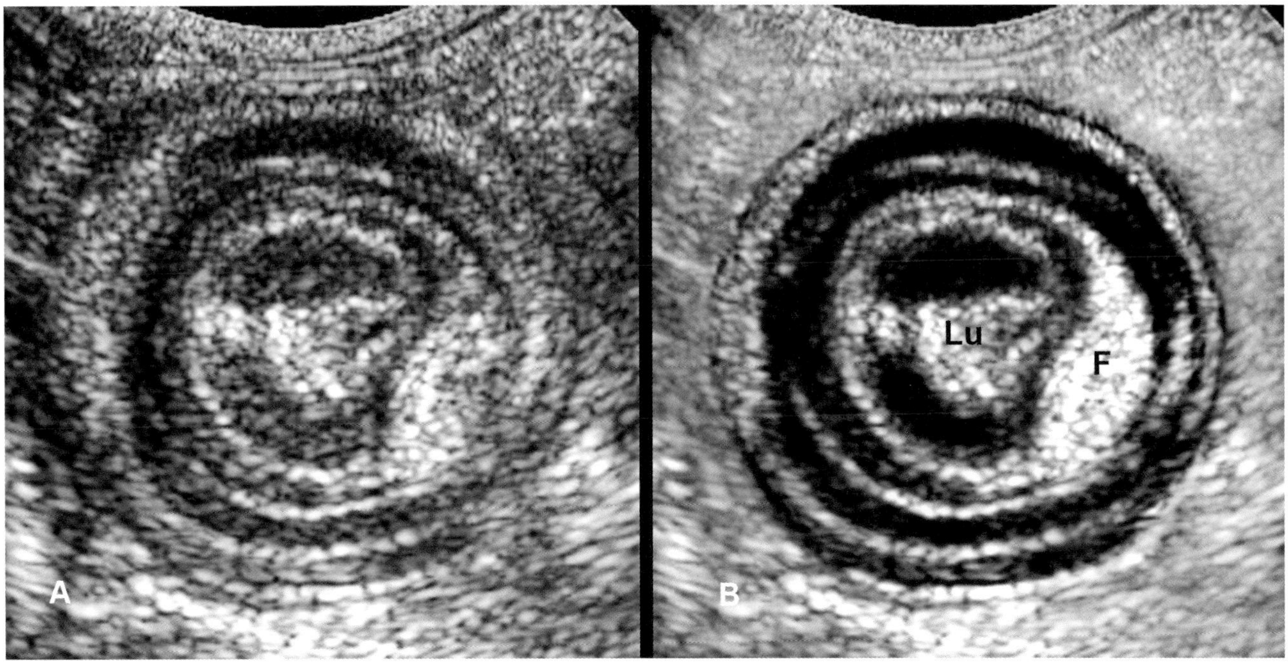

Figure 8.10. Jejunal intussusception. Transverse sonographic **(A)** and schematic **(B)** images of a jejunoduodenal intussusception diagnosed in this 6-year-old Maltese terrier, which had progressive weight loss and inappetence over the previous 2 months. A foreign body was identified in the stomach and proximal duodenum (not seen in this image). The layers of both segments of bowel are mostly intact. Only a small amount of fat (F) is invaginated. Lu, lumen of the intussuscepted segment.

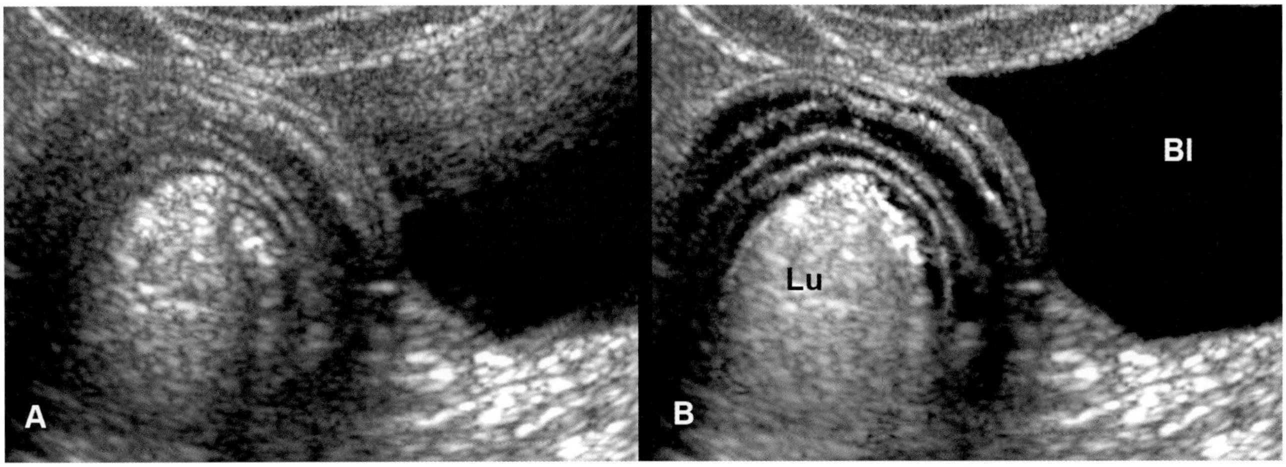

Figure 8.11. Colonic intussusception. Transverse sonographic **(A)** and schematic **(B)** images of a distal colocolonic intussusception detected in this 13-year-old cat, which had a history of 3 months straining to defecate and bloody stool. A multilayered appearance of the colon is noted. Bl, bladder; and Lu, lumen of intussuscepted colonic segment.

portions that can remain anchored in the pyloric antrum.

The presence of GI parasites can mimic the appearance of linear foreign bodies. Roundworms (*Ascaris*) appear as smooth, tubular hyperechoic structures (Figure 8.19). Shadowing is usually not observed with these adult parasites.

Gastric trichobezoars, commonly referred to as *hairballs*, are commonly seen in cats. These compact foreign bodies appear as irregular bright interfaces with a strong, uniform, clean acoustic shadow (Figure 8.20A). In dogs and cats, Several foreign bodies can be encountered that have variable size, shape, echogenicity, and acoustic shadowing. The ultrasound

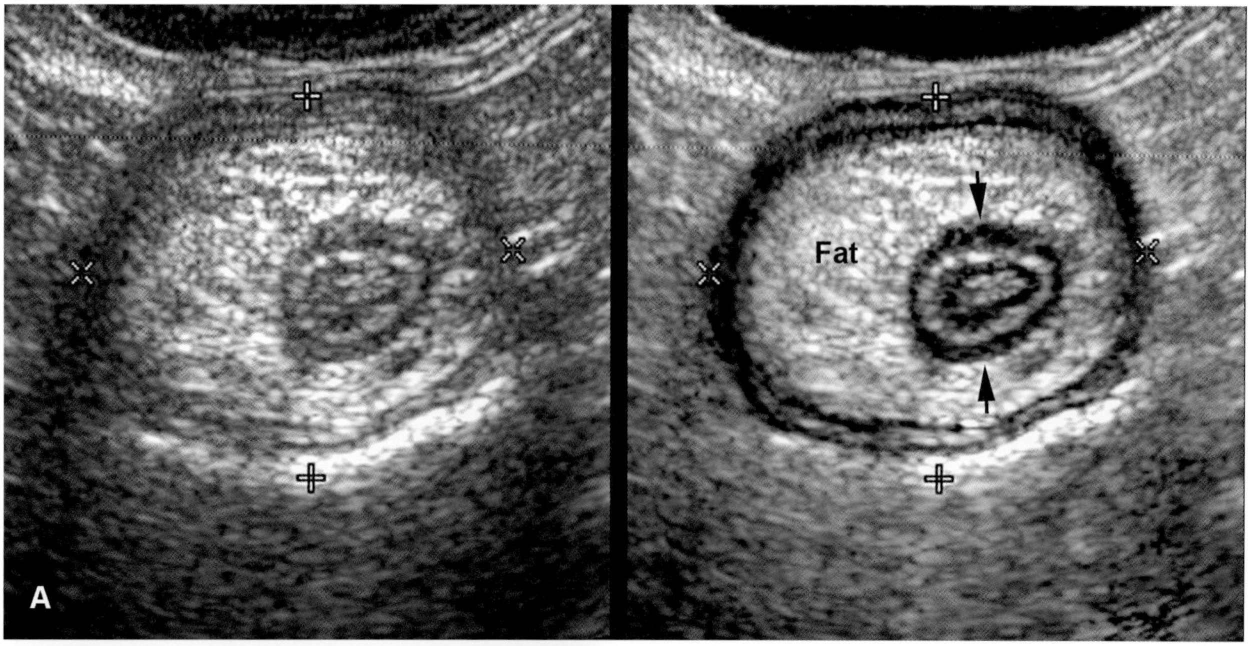

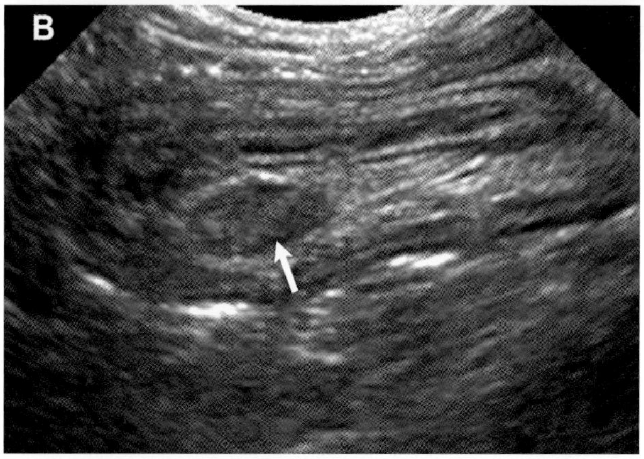

Figure 8.12. Intussusceptions. **A:** Corresponding transverse ultrasonographic **(left)** and schematic **(right)** images of an ileocolic intussusception (cursors) in a cat. The ileum (arrows) is identified as the intussuscepted segment within the colon. Note the hyperechoic intussuscepted fat asymmetrically distributed around the intussuscepted ileum. **B:** Longitudinal ultrasonographic image of a jejunojejunal intussusception in a Siamese cat. A mesenteric lymph node (arrow) is identified in the intussusception.

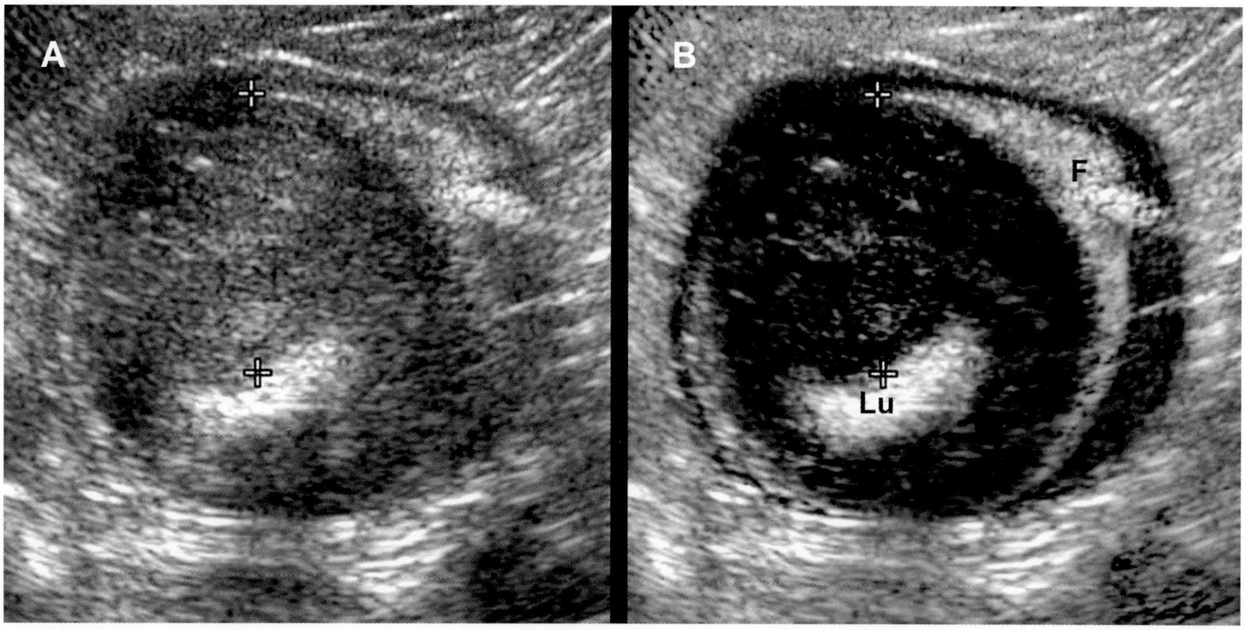

Figure 8.13. Intussusception and intestinal mass. Transverse sonographic **(A)** and schematic **(B)** images of a large poorly echogenic mass associated with an intussusception in a 13-year-old golden retriever. The mass was diagnosed as a colonic adenocarcinoma (cursors). F, invaginated fat; and Lu, lumen of intussusceptum.

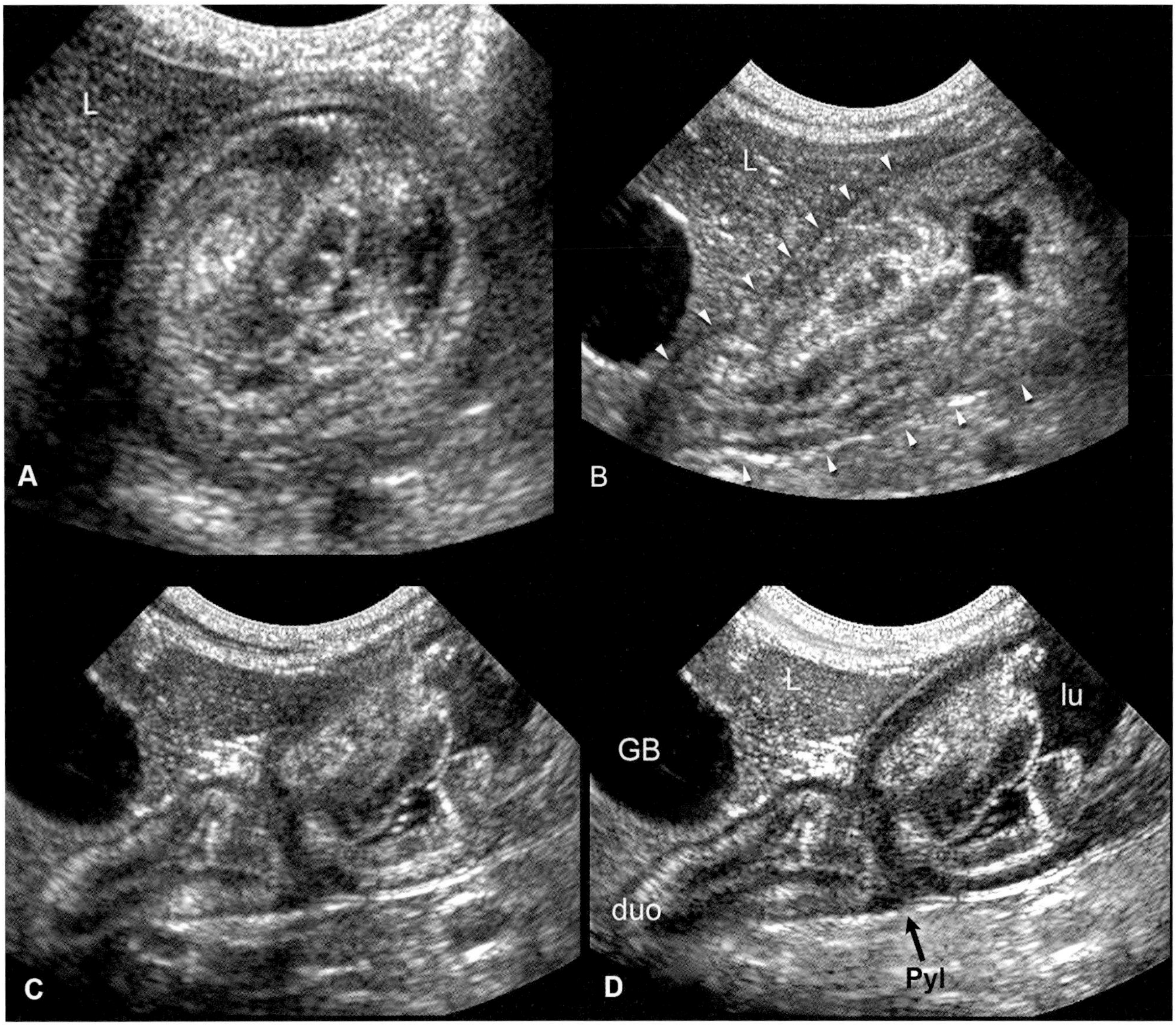

Figure 8.14. Chronic mucosal hyperplasia in a young French bulldog. Transverse **(A)** and sagittal **(B)** sonograms of an exuberant nodular lesion at the pylorus of this 4-month-old French bulldog with a history of lethargy and regurgitation. In these images is a multilayered pattern suggestive of intussusception. The arrowheads outline the serosal margins of the stomach. However, on one of the parasagittal planes (**C**, and corresponding schematic image **D**), the asymmetrical but circumferential lesion protruding into the gastric lumen is more clearly defined as originating from the pyloric wall. The final diagnosis after surgical resection was chronic mucosal hyperplasia. Duo, duodenum; GB, gallbladder; L, liver; lu, lumen of pyloric antrum; and Pyl, pylorus.

features depend on the physical properties of the material.

Perforating foreign bodies, such as ingested teriyaki sticks, are usually anchored within the stomach and may affect the surrounding soft tissue within and outside the cranial abdominal cavity (Penninck and Mitchell 2003) (Figure 8.21). The perforated wall is locally thickened, and focal loss of layering is common.

At times, foreign material accumulates at a pathologically narrowed intestinal site. The narrowing can be caused by intussusception (Figure 8.10), posttraumatic or surgical stricture, or focal neoplastic infiltrate (Figure 8.22).

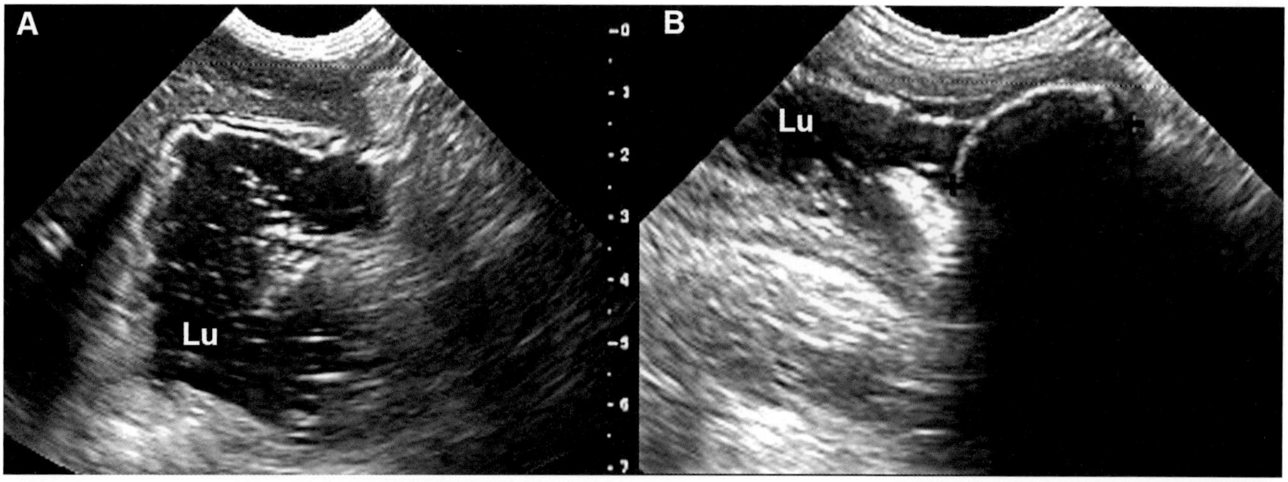

Figure 8.15. Duodenal obstructive foreign body. **A:** Transverse sonogram of the fluid distended stomach of an 8-year-old Lhapsa apso that had suffered 3 days of vomiting and a painful abdomen. Decreased gastric motility is noted during the examination. Lu, lumen of stomach. **B:** The descending duodenum is also fluid distended up to the level of the foreign material (about 2 cm wide [cursors]). Note the strong, uniform acoustic shadowing beyond the bright interface of the foreign body. Lu, lumen of descending duodenum.

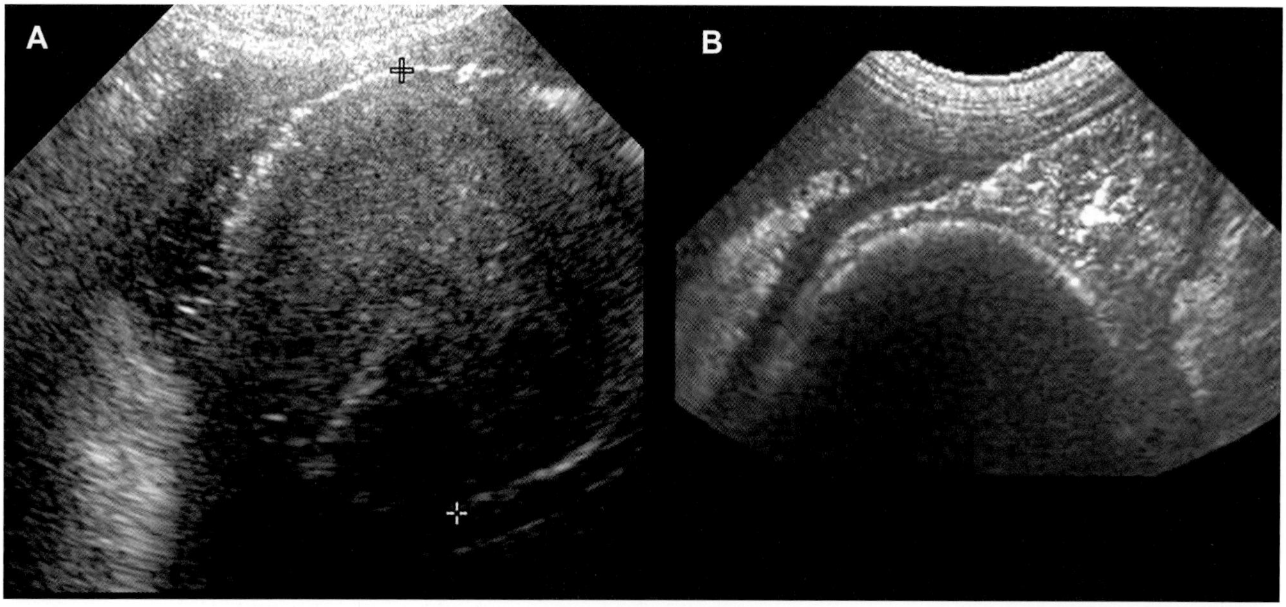

Figure 8.16. Gastric foreign bodies: play balls. **A:** Longitudinal sonogram of the pyloric region of a dog presented because of vomiting. A large (4.6-cm diameter), rounded, poorly echogenic structure, associated with moderate acoustic shadowing, is between the cursors. A spongy ball was retrieved endoscopically. **B:** In this other dog, the ball appears as a bright curvilinear interface associated with strong acoustic shadowing.

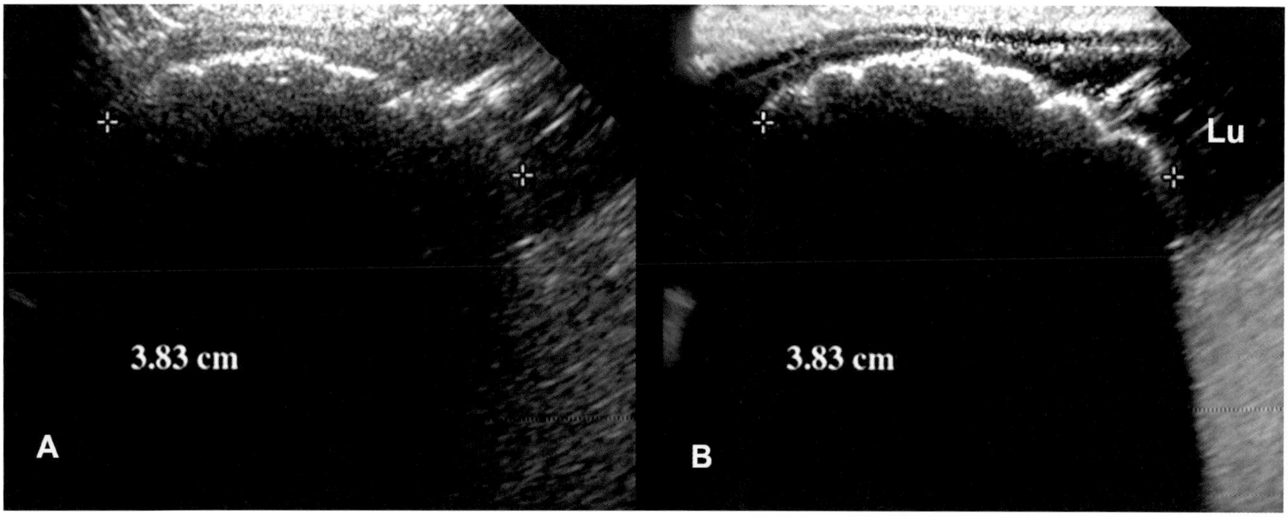

Figure 8.17. Intestinal foreign body: peach pit. Longitudinal sonographic **(A)** and schematic **(B)** images of a bowel segment of a 5-year-old cocker spaniel that had acute vomiting. A peach pit is in the lumen (Lu) of a mildly fluid-distended bowel segment and has a characteristic curved interface with evenly spaced small protuberances in the near field. Note the uniform strong acoustic shadow associated with the foreign body.

Inflammatory Diseases

Wall thickening is the most common finding in inflammatory diseases, but this finding is not specific. The severity of the thickening is not a reliable feature for distinguishing different inflammatory from neoplastic diseases. Symmetry, extent of the wall thickening, and layer identification are useful parameters in distinguishing inflammation from neoplasia (Penninck et al. 2003). Inflammation is usually characterized by extensive and symmetrical wall thickening with preserved layering. However, depending on the severity of the inflammation and the presence of wall edema or hemorrhage, layering can be altered as seen by change in echogenicity or relative thickness of one or more layers.

In gastritis, diffuse or localized wall thickening with decreased motility can be identified. Commonly the stomach is collapsed during the ultrasound evaluation, limiting accurate assessment of the wall thickness. In severe gastritis, the wall thickening can be associated with increased echogenicity or decreased visualization of the wall layers (Figure 8.23).

Gastric ulcers may be identified as discrete, mucosal defects outlined by hyperechoic microbubbles accumulated at the crater site (Figure 8.24A–C). Hyperechoic speckles consistent with dissecting gas can also be observed in the affected wall in some animals (Figure 8.24C and D). Fluid accumulation and decreased gastric motility are common findings in ulcerative disease (Penninck et al. 1997). Ulcers can be seen in both inflammatory and neoplastic diseases. As there is often marked focal thickening with loss of layering, the underlying disorder cannot be characterized reliably.

Gastric wall edema, which is commonly associated with underlying inflammation and ulceration, appears as extensive and moderate thickening with altered layering. A thin inner hypoechoic layer borders the remaining finely striated wall (Figure 8.25). Because of the degree of thickening and the disrupted layering, this condition could easily be mistaken for a tumor.

Uremic gastritis or gastropathy is commonly encountered in patients with chronic uremia. The ultrasonographic features are a moderately thickened gastric wall with prominent rugal folds and a hyperechoic line at the mucosal-luminal interface secondary to mineralization of the mucosa (Grooters et al. 1994) (Figure 8.26).

Common intestinal inflammatory diseases such as lymphocytic-plasmacytic enteritis are associated with mild to moderate wall thickening that most commonly affects several or all intestinal segments with a variable degree of severity. Different ultrasonographic features are encountered: mild to moderate wall thickening affecting primarily the mucosa, the submucosa, and/or the muscular layer; diffuse increased echogenicity of the mucosa; or presence of bright mucosal speckles (Baez et al. 1999; Penninck et al. 2003) (Figure 8.27A and B). Loss of wall layer integrity can also be encountered with ulcerative enteritis (Figure 8.27C). Smooth muscle thickening can be present in chronic

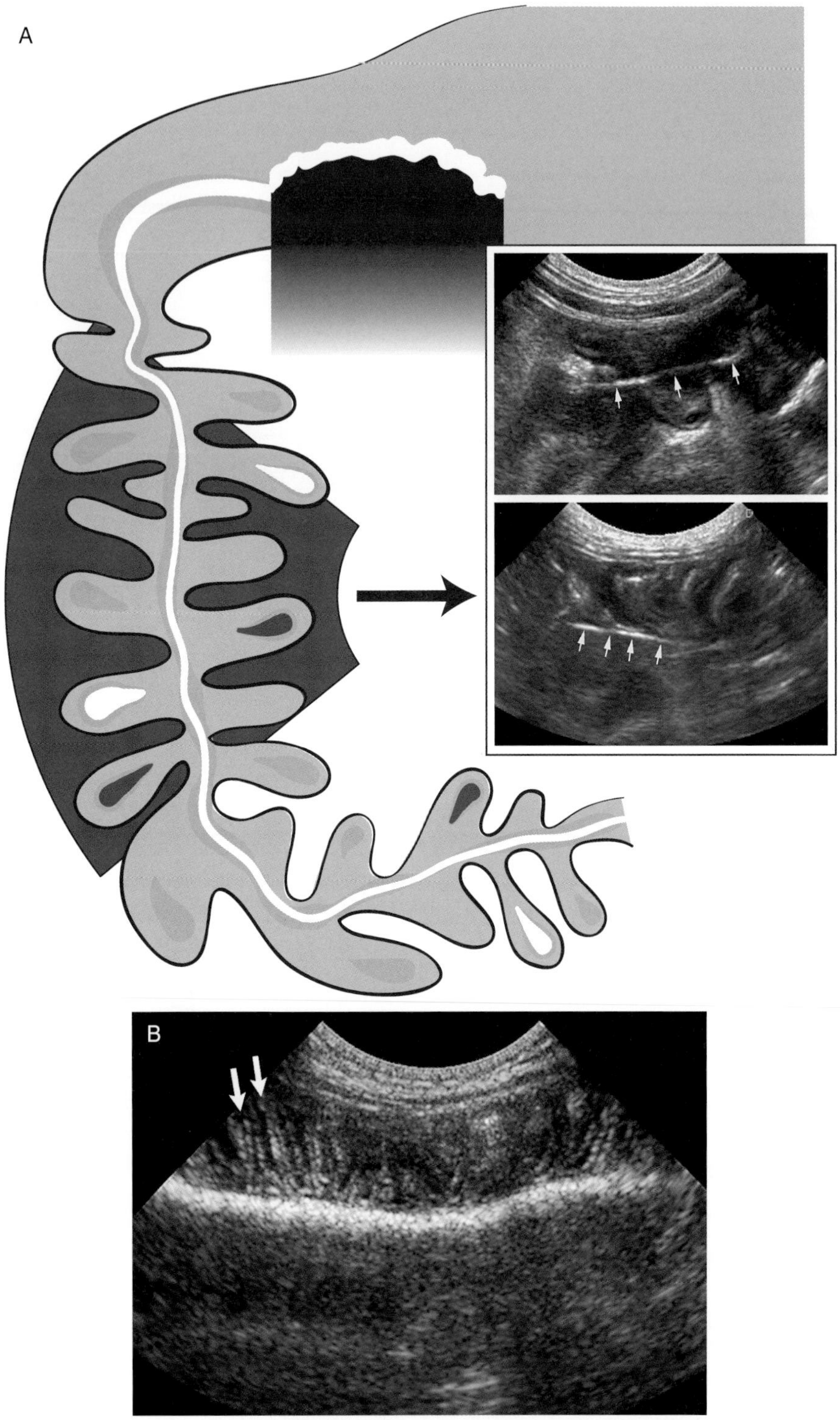

Figure 8.18. Linear foreign bodies in dogs. **A:** Illustration of linear foreign material in the stomach and extending into the descending duodenum, and the corresponding longitudinal sonograms. The linear foreign body itself often appears as a bright linear interface (arrows) intermittently associated with shadowing. **B:** Linear foreign body associated with marked intestinal plication (near field). The linear foreign body is the bright, nearly rectilinear interface seen in the lumen of this severely corrugated jejunal segment. Note the perpendicular hyperechoic striations (arrows) associated with the redundant submucosal layer.

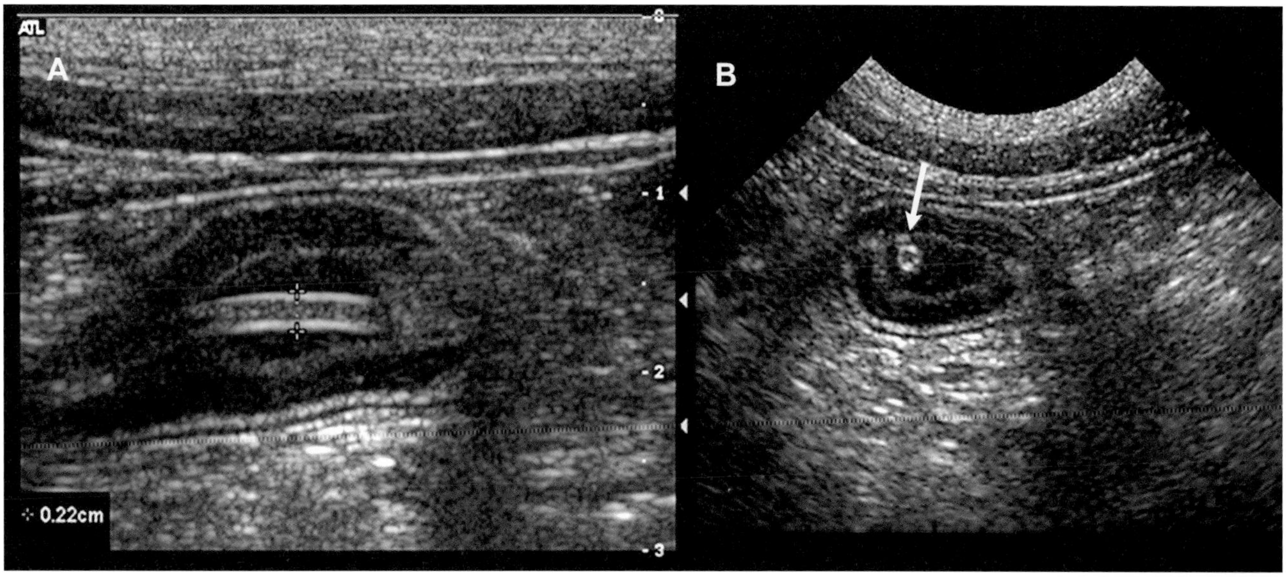

Figure 8.19. Roundworms. Longitudinal **(A)** and transverse **(B)** sonograms of a roundworm in a jejunal segment of a young dog with chronic diarrhea. Several other worms were identified throughout the intestinal tract, in association with fluid accumulation. These worms appear as tubular, double-interfaced, hyperechoic structures (between the cursors and at the arrow) in the lumen of the gastrointestinal tract. During real-time evaluation, the worms can be seen moving if they are alive. Images courtesy of M.A. d'Anjou.

enteritis, particularly in cats, but this finding is not specific and also can be present in other disorders, such as mechanical obstruction secondary to foreign material or tumoral infiltration (Penninck 2002; Diana et al. 2003) (Figure 8.27D).

Linear hyperechoic lines within the mucosa and aligned perpendicular to the lumen axis most likely represent dilated lacteols (Figure 8.28). This finding is commonly associated with protein-losing enteropathy and lymphangiectasia, and occasionally this pattern can be associated with diffusely infiltrative tumors (Sutherland-Smith et al. 2007).

Corrugation of the small bowel appears as regular waves of undulated bowel segments (Figure 8.29). This nonspecific finding can be seen in association with regional inflammation such as enteritis, pancreatitis, peritonitis, or abdominal neoplasia, or bowel ischemia (Moon et al. 2003).

In cases of severe inflammatory changes encountered with lymphoplasmacytic, eosinophilic, or granulomatous enteritis, edema, hemorrhage, and fibrosis can severely disrupt the wall layering and be associated with mass lesions suggestive of a tumoral process (Figure 8.30).

Inflammation, such as pancreatitis and duodenitis, can also be caused by regional extension of affected adjacent tissue (Figure 8.31).

Colonic inflammatory changes are challenging to detect ultrasonographically. Redundancy of the folds tends to cause one to overestimate the degree of wall thickening. Wall layering is often less distinct because of a thin wall (Figure 8.32A and B). In ulcerative colitis, the luminal mucosal border is irregular because of the numerous small superficial ulcers affecting the mucosa (Figure 8.32C).

Parasitic infestations such as peritoneal cestodiasis are rare. Cystic subserosal lesions have been found on the GI tract of affected dogs or cats (Venco et al. 2005) (Figure 8.33).

Perforation and Dehiscence

In perforation secondary to foreign-body migration, deep ulceration, or postoperative dehiscence, the affected wall is thickened and hypoechoic, and there is local loss of layering (Boysen et al. 2003). At times, a hyperechoic tract can be seen crossing the wall, and the adjacent mesenteric is significantly increased in echogenicity because of focal steatitis or peritonitis (Figures 8.34–8.37). Fluid accumulation can often be seen near the perforation or dehiscence site, and free peritoneal gas can sometimes be detected as short, bright, linear interfaces in the most upper portion of

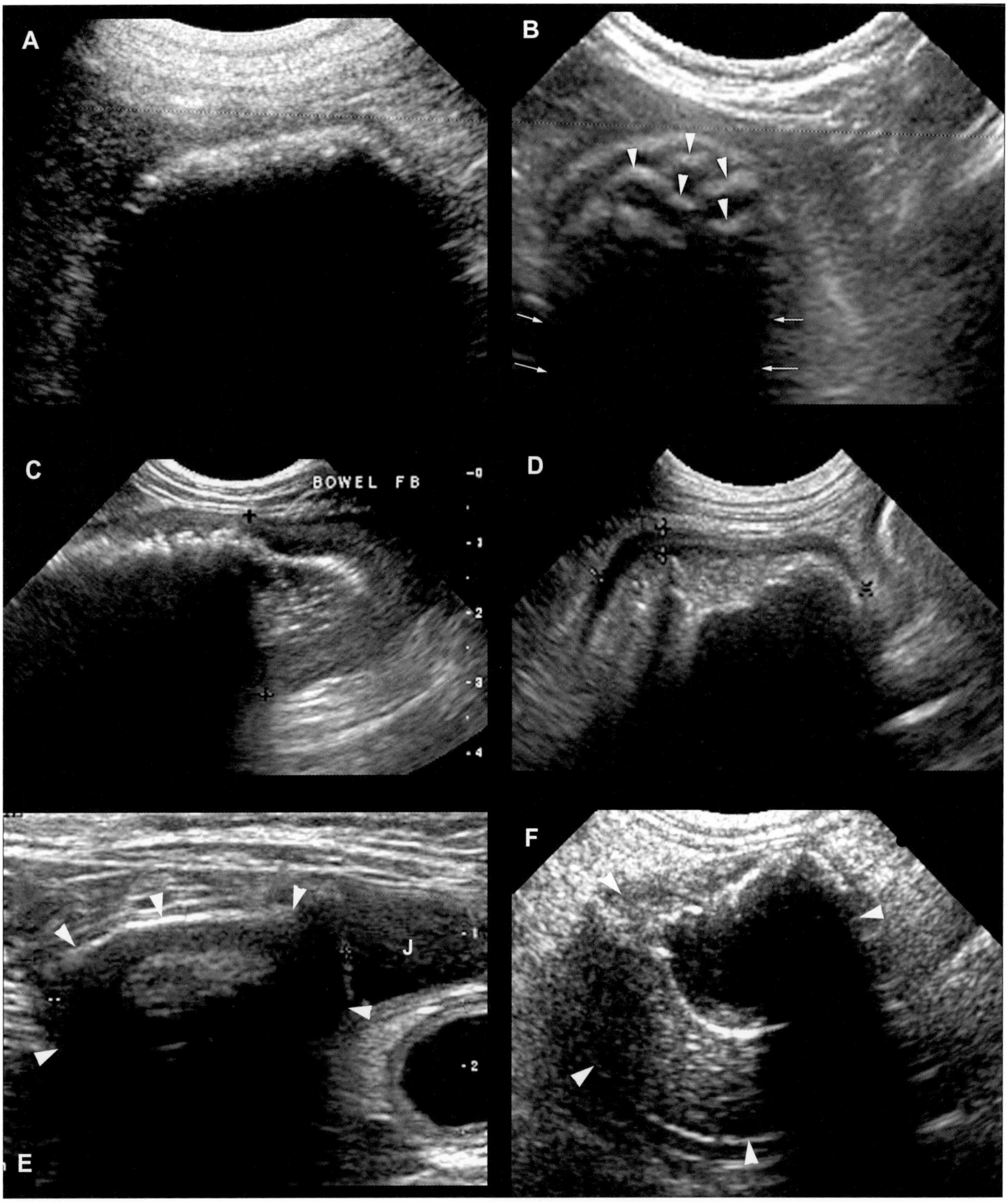

Figure 8.20. Intestinal foreign bodies. A wide range of foreign material can be found in the gastrointestinal tract. Most of them are associated with strong acoustic shadowing. **A:** Trichobezoars are compact foreign bodies with a bright interface and a uniform and clean acoustic shadow, as seen in this 6-year-old long-hair domestic cat with a large hairball in its stomach. **B:** Elastic bands in the stomach of a young cat mimic prominent rugal folds (arrowheads). The spacing and the uniform shadowing (arrows) supported the presence of foreign material. **C:** A large piece of corncob is in this dilated and thickened jejunal segment. **D:** Several irregular interfaces with uniform shadowing are in this moderately distended jejunum. **E:** A poorly echogenic object with echogenic center (arrowheads) is noted in the fluid dilated jejunum (J) of a cat. A piece of a plastic toy was removed surgically. **F:** A rounded and nearly layered structure (arrowheads) is in a dilated segment of small intestine. At first, this appearance was confused for a thickened bowel segment. At surgery, a large fragment of a "Kong" toy was removed.

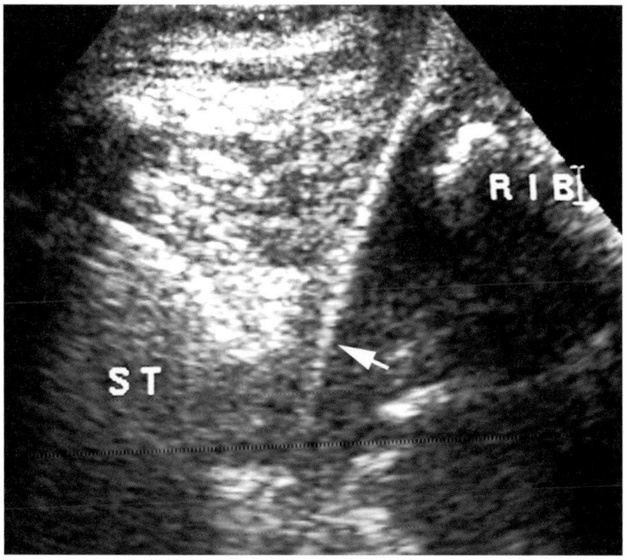

Figure 8.21. Perforating teriyaki stick. Teriyaki sticks appear as long, linear, bright interfaces, commonly associated with shadowing, within the gastrointestinal tract. In this young dog with a history of left cranial flank swelling, partially responsive to antibiotherapy, a long teriyaki stick (arrow) was identified in the fundus of the stomach. The stick was perforating the gastric wall and aiming toward the caudal chest wall (cranial the left 12th rib). The lumen of the stomach (ST) is at the left of the image.

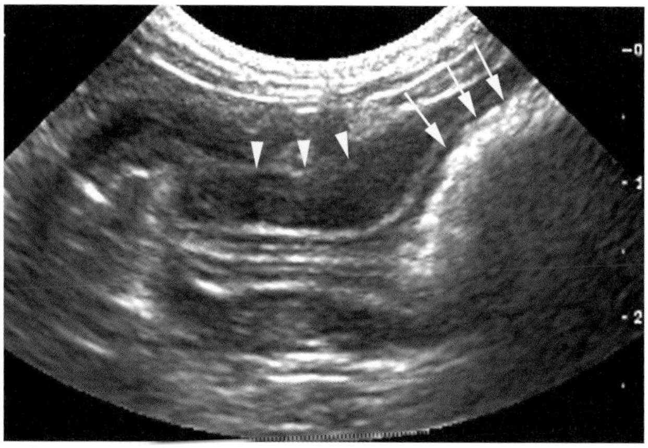

Figure 8.22. Partially obstructive intestinal adenocarcinoma. Foreign material (arrows) accumulated proximal to the focally thickened (arrowheads) jejunal segment. Surgical resection was performed and the histopathological diagnosis was adenocarcinoma.

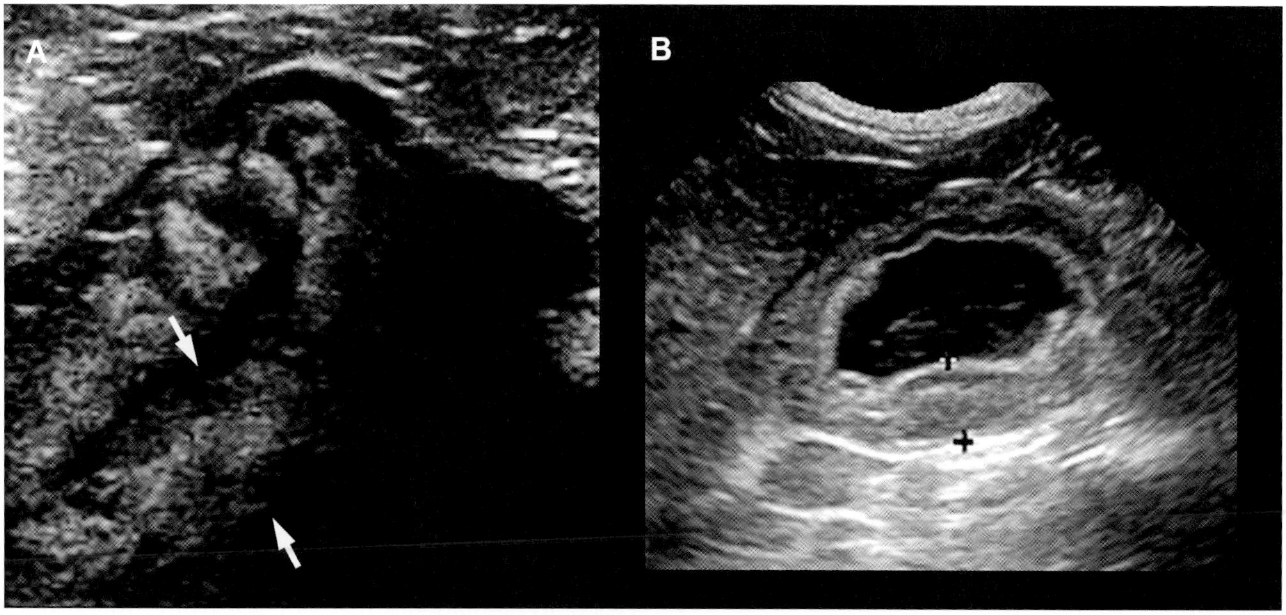

Figure 8.23. Severe gastritis. **A:** Despite a collapsed stomach, there is marked thickening (10mm [arrows]) of the wall in this 11-year-old Maltese terrier that was diagnosed as having eosinophilic gastritis. The mucosa is diffusely increased in echogenicity. **B:** A moderately thickened (8mm [cursors]) wall is noted in this 1-year-old cat that had severe chronic ulcerative mucosal and mural gastritis. The wall is also hyperechoic.

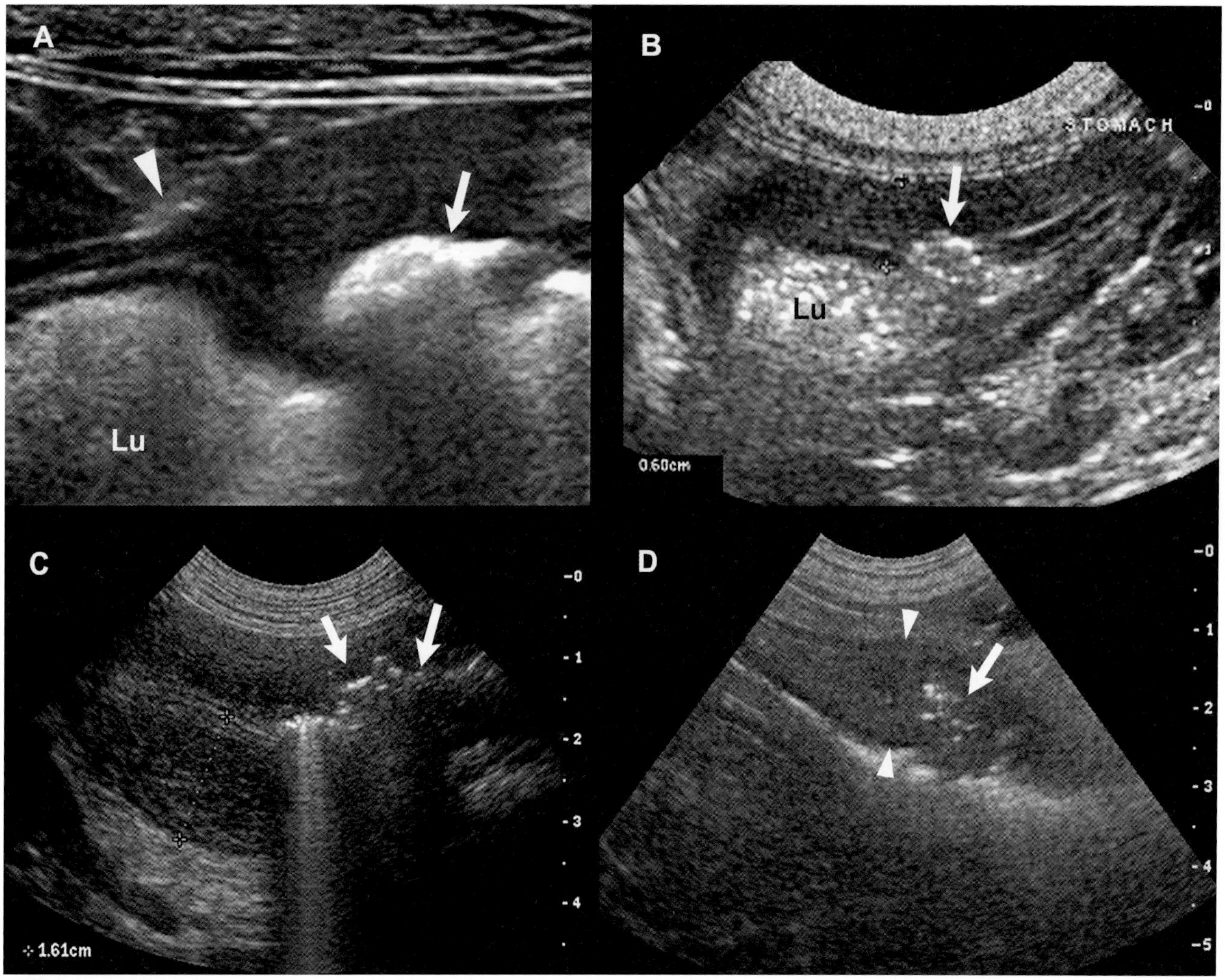

Figure 8.24. Gastric ulcers. **A:** Marked focal gastric wall thickening with loss of layering is noted in this 6-year-old springer spaniel. Within the thickest portion of the wall is a central crater (arrow). There is clear demarcation between the layered and affected wall segments (arrowhead). These features can be seen in both severe inflammatory and neoplastic processes. Lu, lumen. **B:** A small amount of echogenic fluid is seen in the gastric lumen (lu) of this young cat with chemically induced gastritis. The wall is thickened (between the cursors), and its layers are focally indistinct. A discrete mucosal crater (arrow) is noted. **C:** Hyperechoic speckles (arrows), consistent with gas, are found in the thickened wall of this dog with uremic gastritis and ulcerations. The layers are ill-defined. The wall opposite to the ulceration reaches 1.6 cm in thickness (between the cursors). **D:** Malignant ulcer in a 10-year-old Labrador retriever with gastric adenocarcinoma. Hyperechoic speckles (arrows) are in the thickened portion of the wall (arrowheads), infiltrated with the epithelial neoplasm. The layers are indistinct. Images C and D courtesy of M.A. d'Anjou.

the abdomen and be associated with comet-tail artifacts (Figure 8.34B).

In postoperative enterotomy or enterectomy, the surgical site can be identified by the regular alignment of sutures, which appear as small bright interfaces along or around the bowel, depending on the choice of surgical procedure (Figure 8.38A). Focal thickening of the bowel with loss of layering is commonly seen, but is expected to resolve partially over time (Figure 8.38).

At times, a stricture can be seen at a previous enterotomy or enterectomy site. Abnormal fluid, gas, or food accumulation is then noted proximal to the stricture site (Figure 8.39).

A fluid pocket representing a sterile seroma may accumulate near or at a recent surgical or ultrasound-guided biopsy site (Figure 8.40). This is a rare and transient complication of surgical intestinal biopsies.

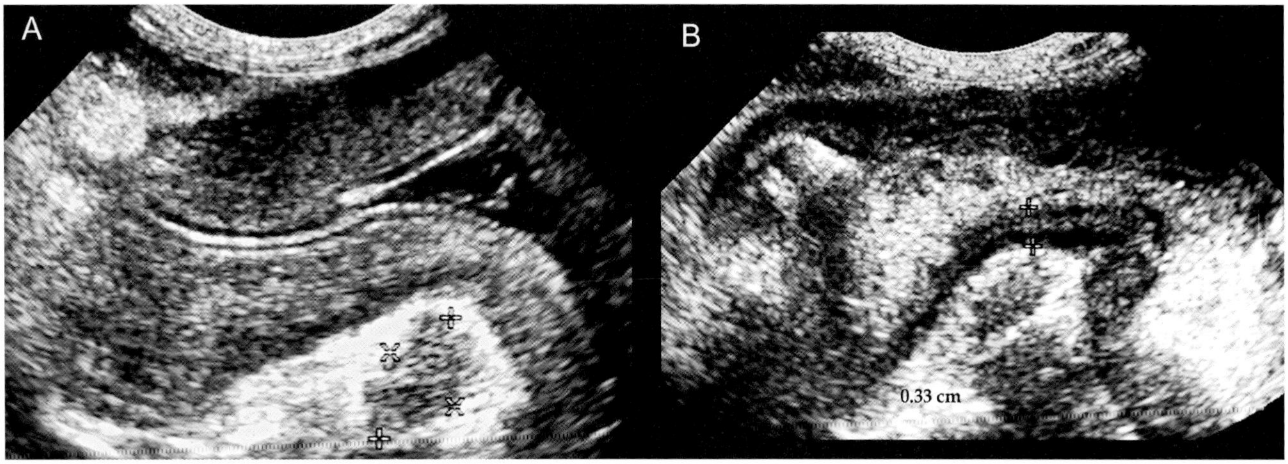

Figure 8.25. Pyogranulomatous gastritis. **A:** Longitudinal sonogram of the pyloric antrum of a 2-year-old Chihuahua with moderate to severe pyogranulomatous gastritis. Wall edema obliterates the normal wall layering, and only a thin and discrete anechoic band is on the inner mucosa. A small amount of fluid is in the gastric lumen. Mild regional lymphadenopathy is noted (cursors). **B:** Recheck sonogram 3 days later showing near complete resolution of the edema, but the wall layering remains affected.

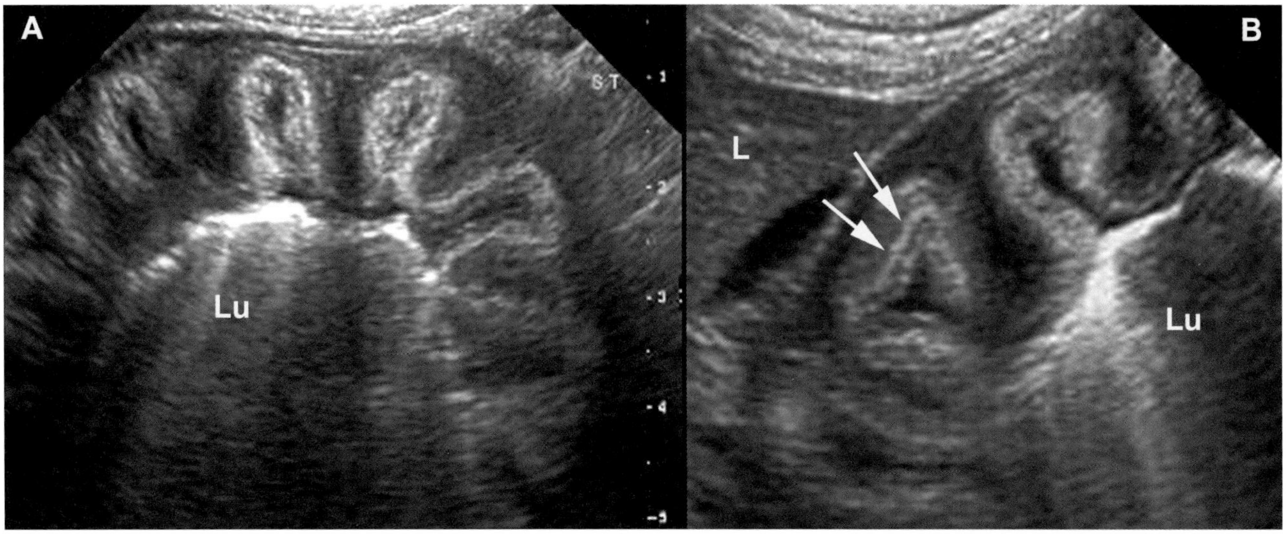

Figure 8.26. Uremic gastropathy. **A:** Uremic gastropathy is seen in dogs or cats suffering from chronic uremia. Thickening of the wall with a hyperechoic line (arrows) along the gastric mucosa and mineralization at the mucosal-luminal interface are common findings. **B:** Enlarged view with labels of the gastric wall changes. L, liver; Lu, lumen.

Gastrointestinal Tumors

GI neoplasia is often associated with motility disturbances that produce luminal fluid accumulation, which optimizes visualization of the lesion (Penninck 1998).

In dogs and cats, the most common ultrasonographic findings in GI lymphoma are transmural thickening associated with the diffuse loss of normal wall layering, reduced wall echogenicity, decreased localized motility and regional lymphadenopathy (Penninck et al. 1994). These features are similar in the stomach and along the intestinal tract (Figure 8.41). Gastric masses may be masked by the presence of air in the lumen, particularly when located on the lesser curvature (Figure 8.42). The thickening of the GI wall can range widely, from 5 mm to over 25 mm (Figures 8.43 and 8.44). Mesenteric lymphadenopathy is a common finding in intestinal lymphoma and in some instances

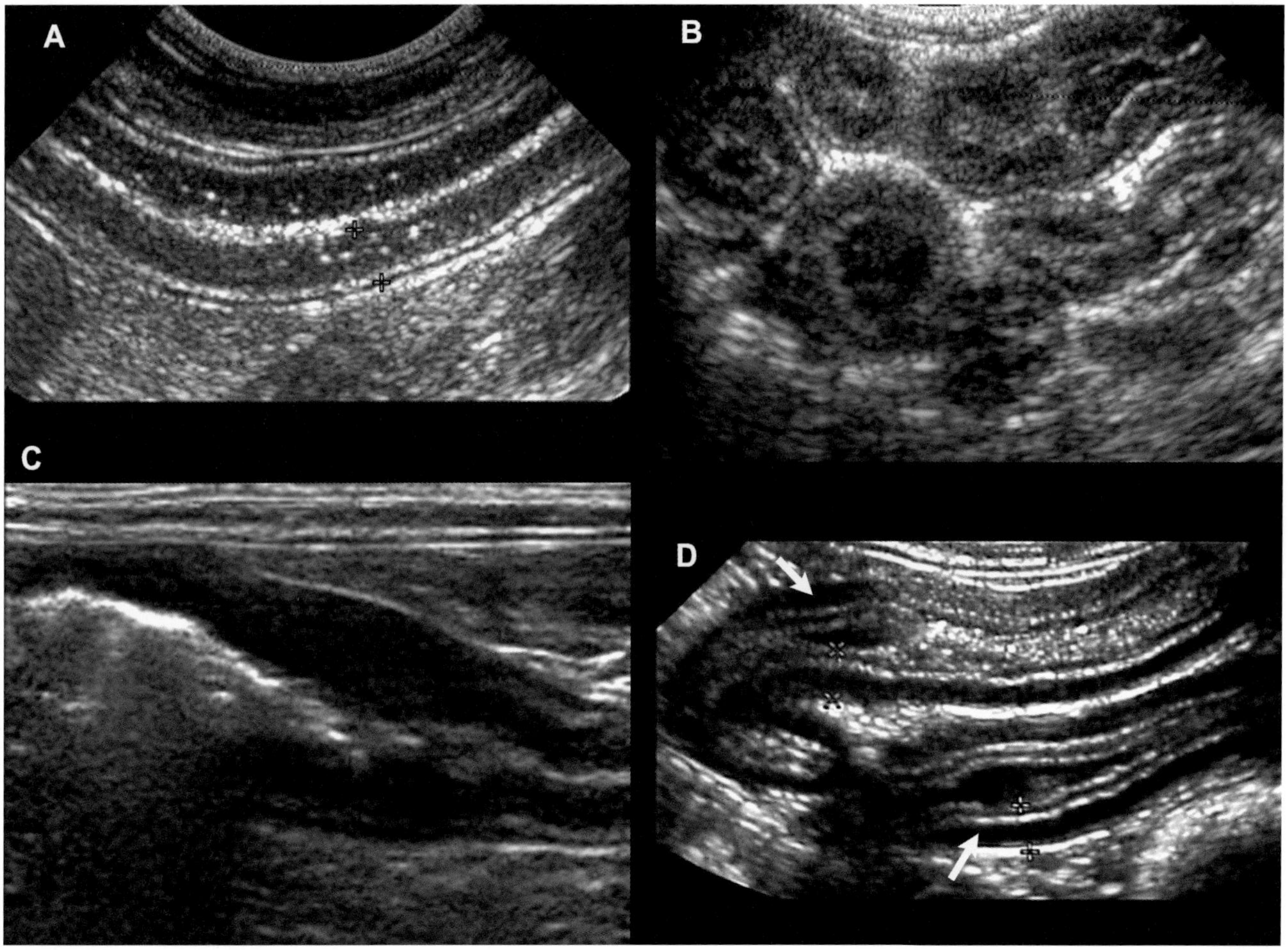

Figure 8.27. Inflammatory bowel disease. **A:** Longitudinal sonogram of a mildly thickened jejunal segment of a dog with lymphocytic-plasmacytic enteritis. Several bright speckles are unevenly distributed within the prominent mucosal layer, but the wall layers can still be identified. **B:** In this dog with eosinophilic enteritis, several intestinal segments were thickened, hypermotile, and partially fluid filled. The wall layers were visible, but the mucosa appeared hyperechoic and ill-defined. **C:** Longitudinal sonogram of a focally thickened jejunum in a corgi with severe ulcerative eosinophilic enteritis. The submucosa appears subjectively more prominent than normal. **D:** Several thickened (6 mm) intestinal loops with altered layering were seen in this cat with severe lymphocytic-plasmacytic enteritis. In this patient, the muscular layer is thicker (arrows) than the corresponding mucosa. A small amount of fluid is noted in the bowel, and the intestinal motility was reduced during the live exam.

can be responsible for most of the midabdominal mass effect (Figure 8.44). Ulcerated lymphoma can be encountered as an irregular mucosal surface or as a large defect centered on the affected portion of the GI tract (Figure 8.45). In cats, alimentary lymphoma can affect the intestinal tract without fully disrupting the wall layering (Figure 8.46).

The most common ultrasonographic finding in gastric carcinoma is wall transmural thickening that is associated with altered wall layering (Penninck et al. 1998). This altered layering appears as a moderately echogenic zone surrounded by outer and inner, poorly echogenic lines and is present in many dogs (Figure 8.47). However, other associated mural changes, such as edema, inflammation, fibrosis, or hemorrhage, can mask this hallmark feature. Because of the particular appearance and to avoid confusion with the term *layered wall*, which is usually reserved to describe the normal appearance of the GI wall, we call this feature *pseudolayering*. This pseudolayering most likely correlates with the unevenly layered tumor distribution noted histopathologically. This particular ultrasonographic feature is strongly suggestive of gastric carcinoma (Figure 8.47).

Intestinal carcinomas have been documented in dogs and cats, although it is encountered less frequently in cats. The most common ultrasonographic findings are transmural thickening with a complete

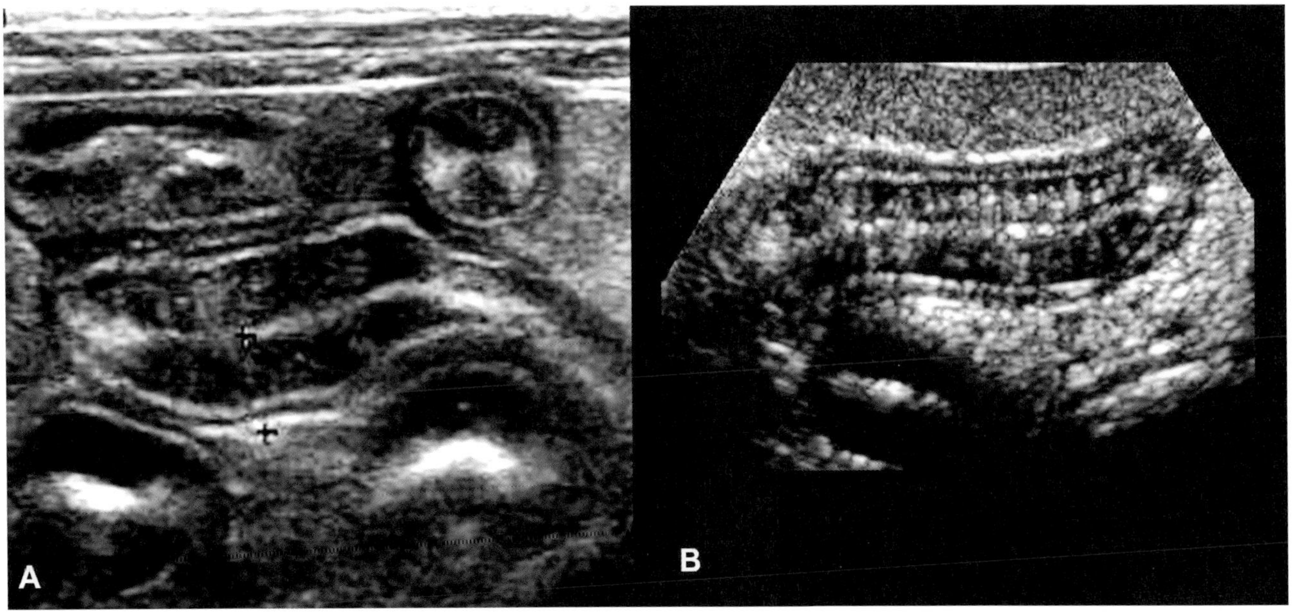

Figure 8.28. Mucosal hyperechoic striations. **A:** Longitudinal sonogram of mildly thickened jejunal segments (between the cursors) with hyperechoic linear striations within the mucosal layer. The bright mucosal striations in this 13-year-old Pomeranian with a confirmed diagnosis of moderate eosinophilic enteritis with multifocal lymphangiectasis and focal mural lipogranuloma represent dilated lacteals. **B:** Similar findings are present in this dog with severe lymphoplasmacytic enteritis.

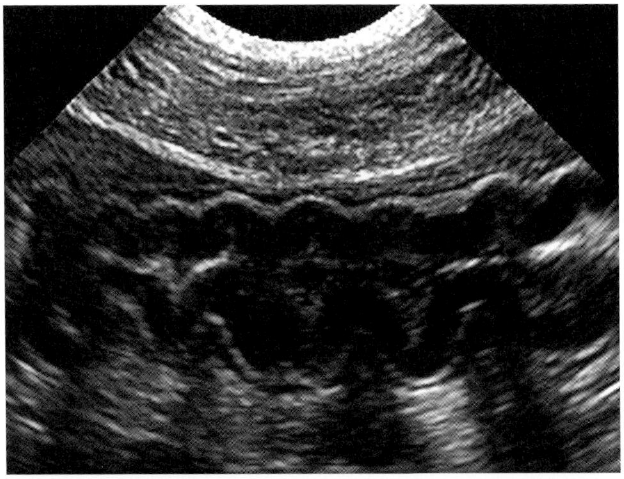

Figure 8.29. Bowel corrugation caused by peritonitis. Several corrugated bowel segments are present in this 5-year-old Weimaraner. Chronic peritonitis secondary to multifocal perforation of the jejunum was present at surgery.

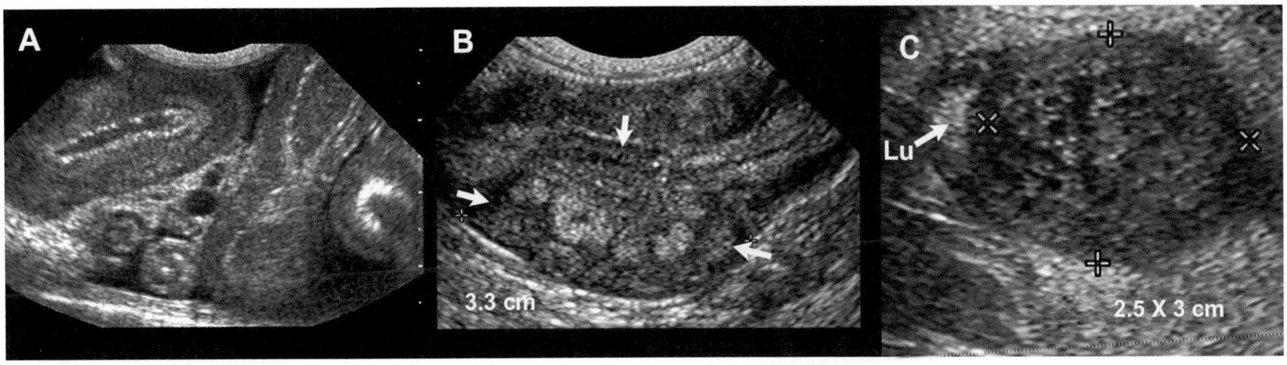

Figure 8.30. Granulomatous enteritis. **A:** In this cat, there is diffuse loss of layering of most jejunal segments. Moderate peritoneal effusion is present around the intestine. The surgical biopsies were diagnostic for toxoplasmosis. **B:** Longitudinal sonogram of severe recurrent granulomatous enteritis in a cat. Marked thickening and inhomogeneity of the intestinal wall is present, with the formation of mass lesions (arrows). **C:** Transverse sonogram of a granuloma secondary to a previously migrating foreign body in a dog. The lesion created this eccentric mass (cursors), deforming the intestinal lumen (Lu).

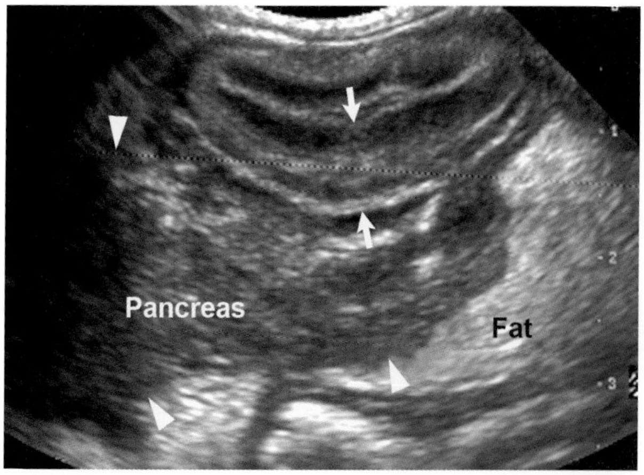

Figure 8.31. Duodenitis and pancreatitis in a dog. The duodenum is thickened, and the wall layering appeared affected but still visible (arrows). The adjacent right limb of the pancreas is enlarged and hypoechoic (arrowheads). Hyperechoic mesenteric fat outlines the margins of the inflamed pancreas.

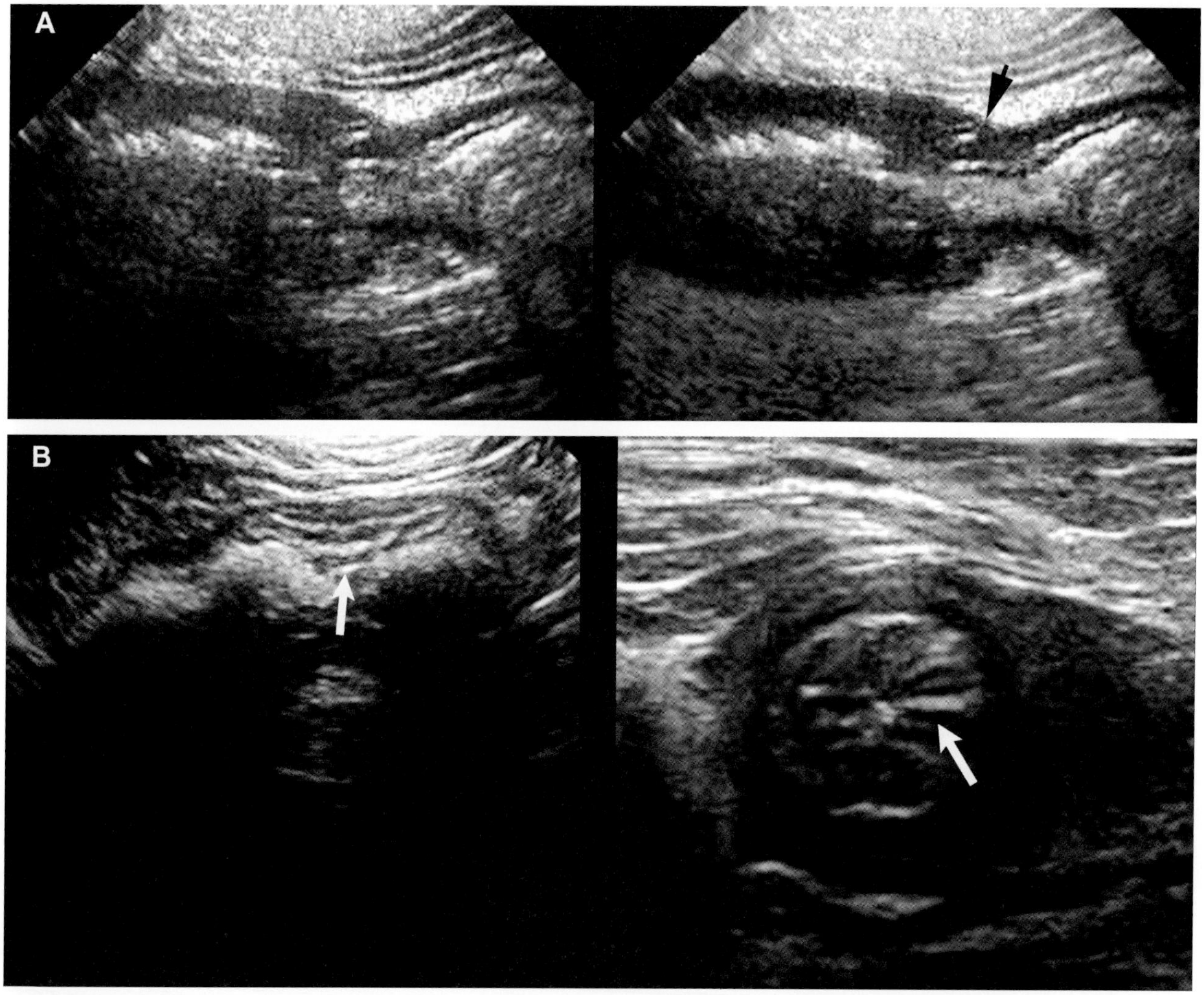

Figure 8.32. Colonic wall thickening and ulcers. **A:** Longitudinal sonographic **(left)** and schematic **(right)** images of the ileocecocolic junction of a dog with parasitic (hookworm) colitis. The wall is circumferentially thickened, and the wall layering is lost at the junction between the ileum and cecum and/or colon (arrow). **B:** True thickening should not be confused with colonic wall redundancy as seen in this cat presented for obstipation. Numerous folds can be identified (arrows) on the longitudinal **(left)** and transverse **(right)** planes. **C:** Longitudinal **(left)** and transverse **(right)** sonograms of a segment of the descending colon in a cat with severe ulcerative colitis. The wall is diffusely, severely thickened, which particularly involves the mucosa. This mucosa is hyperechoic (arrowheads) and presents irregular, hyperechoic, craterlike lesions consistent with ulceration (arrows). The mucosal surface is irregular in the rest of the segment, also consistent with erosions. Image C courtesy of M.A. d'Anjou.

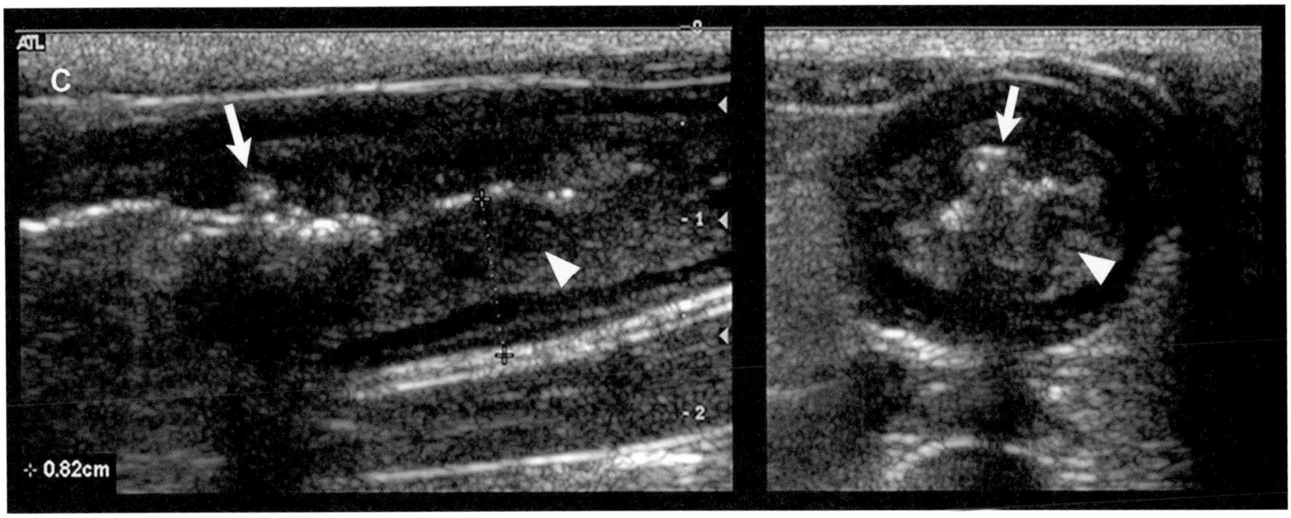

Figure 8.32. *Continued*

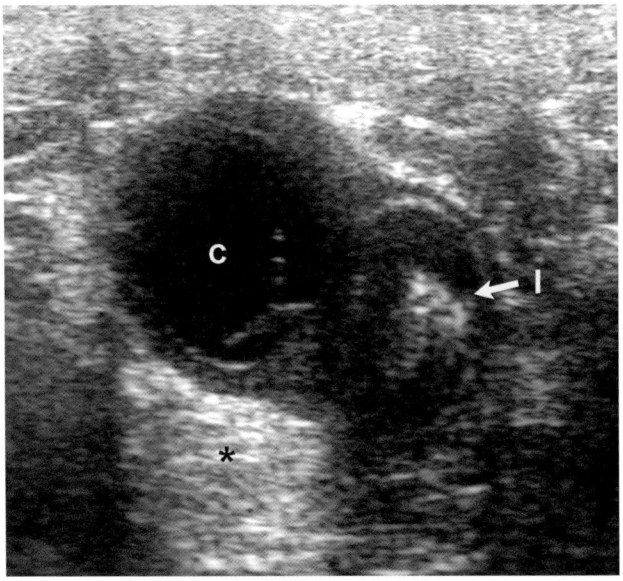

Figure 8.33. Peritoneal cestodiasis. Peritoneal cestodiasis in this 6-year-old mixed-breed dog is associated with a round, anechoic cystic lesion (C) associated with the serosal surface of an intestinal segment (I). Far enhancement is noted beyond the hypoattenuating fluid as a hyperechoic band (*). This sonographic image was obtained with a transverse plane. Image reprinted with permission (Venco et al. 2005).

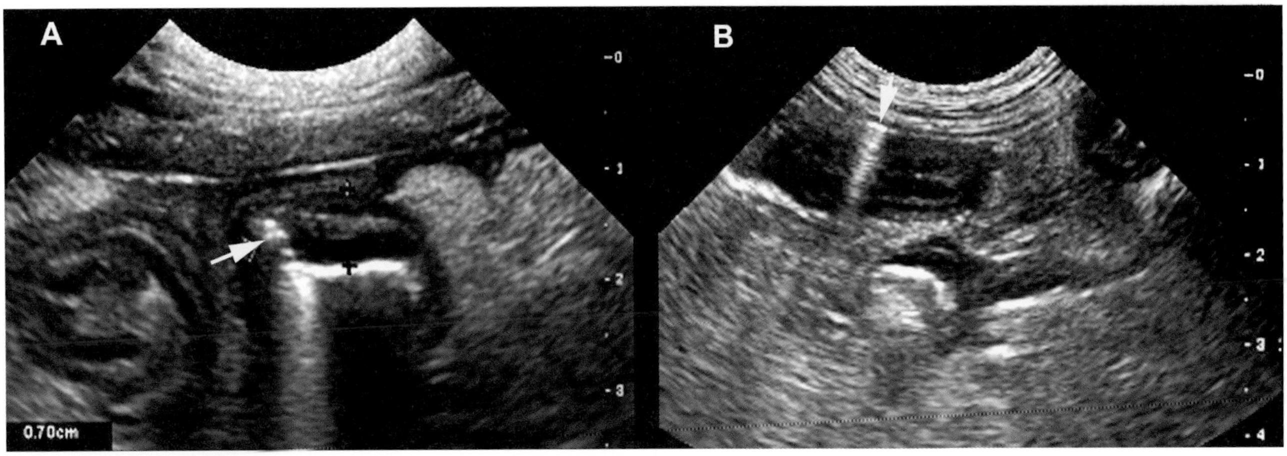

Figure 8.34. Intestinal perforation. **A:** A jejunal perforation secondary to foreign bodies (hairpins) was surgically confirmed in this 5-year-old Weimaraner. A hyperechoic gas tract (arrow) dissects the focally thickened jejunal segment (between the cursors). **B:** Free gas (arrow) and a moderate amount of echogenic fluid (not seen on this image) in the abdomen indicate perforation.

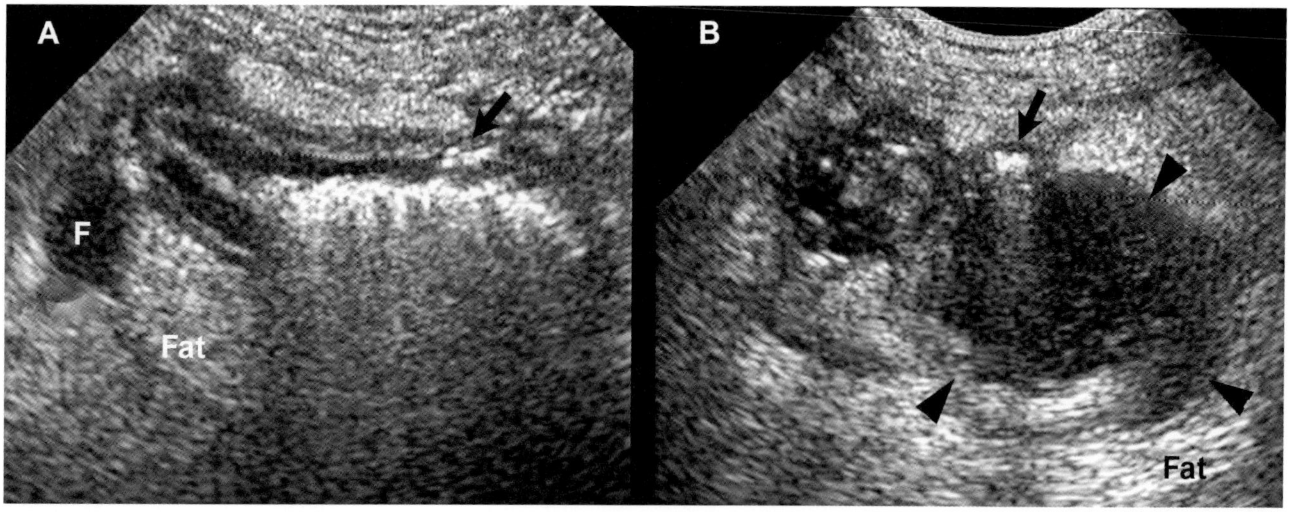

Figure 8.35. Intestinal perforation and peritoneal abscess. This 11-year-old English setter had a septic abdomen. **A:** A bright tract dissects the bowel wall (arrow). Peritoneal fluid (F) is noted and the mesenteric fat is bright. Free gas was also identified (not shown). **B:** A localized fluid pocket representing an abscess cavity (arrowheads) is near the perforation site (arrow). At surgery, the perforation, local abscessation, and peritonitis were confirmed.

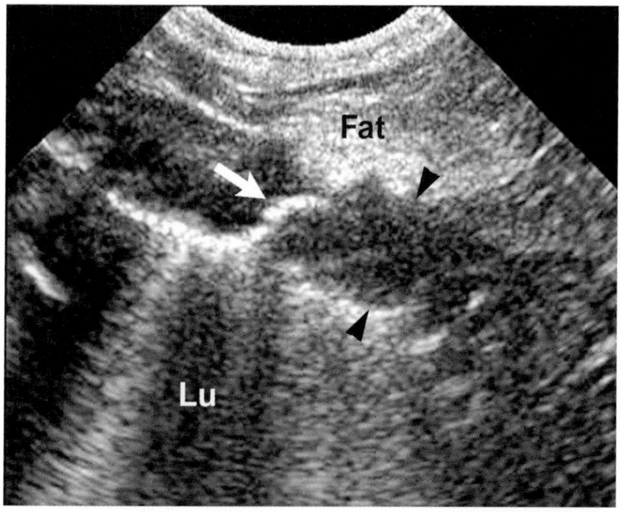

Figure 8.36. Perforating ulcer. Gastric ulceration and perforation were confirmed surgically in this 15-year-old mixed-breed dog that had experienced vomiting. On ultrasound, a discrete hyperechoic tract (white arrow) is seen crossing the thickened and hypoechoic gastric wall (arrowheads). The fat adjacent to the perforation site is hyperechoic, indicative of focal steatitis or peritonitis. Lu, gastric lumen.

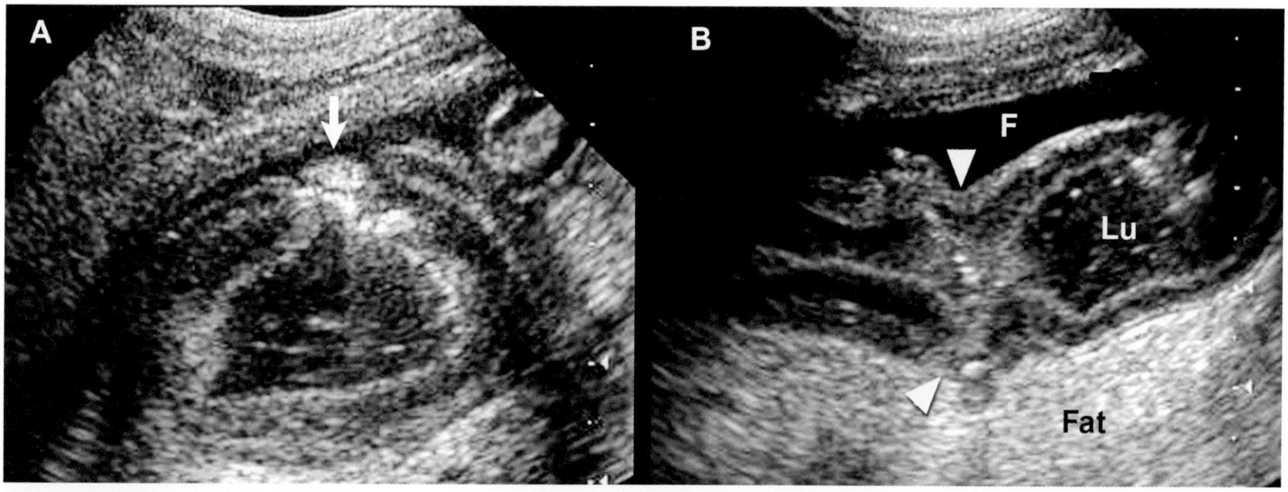

Figure 8.37. Intestinal dehiscence. **A:** There is dehiscence at the duodenal suture site in this 4-year-old Jack Russell terrier. Fluid accumulation (F) and bright fat are centered at the dehiscence site. Discontinuity of the duodenal wall is identified (arrow). **B:** The duodenum is hypomotile and fluid filled. Deformity of the duodenum axis is noted at the level of the suture line (arrowheads). Lu, lumen.

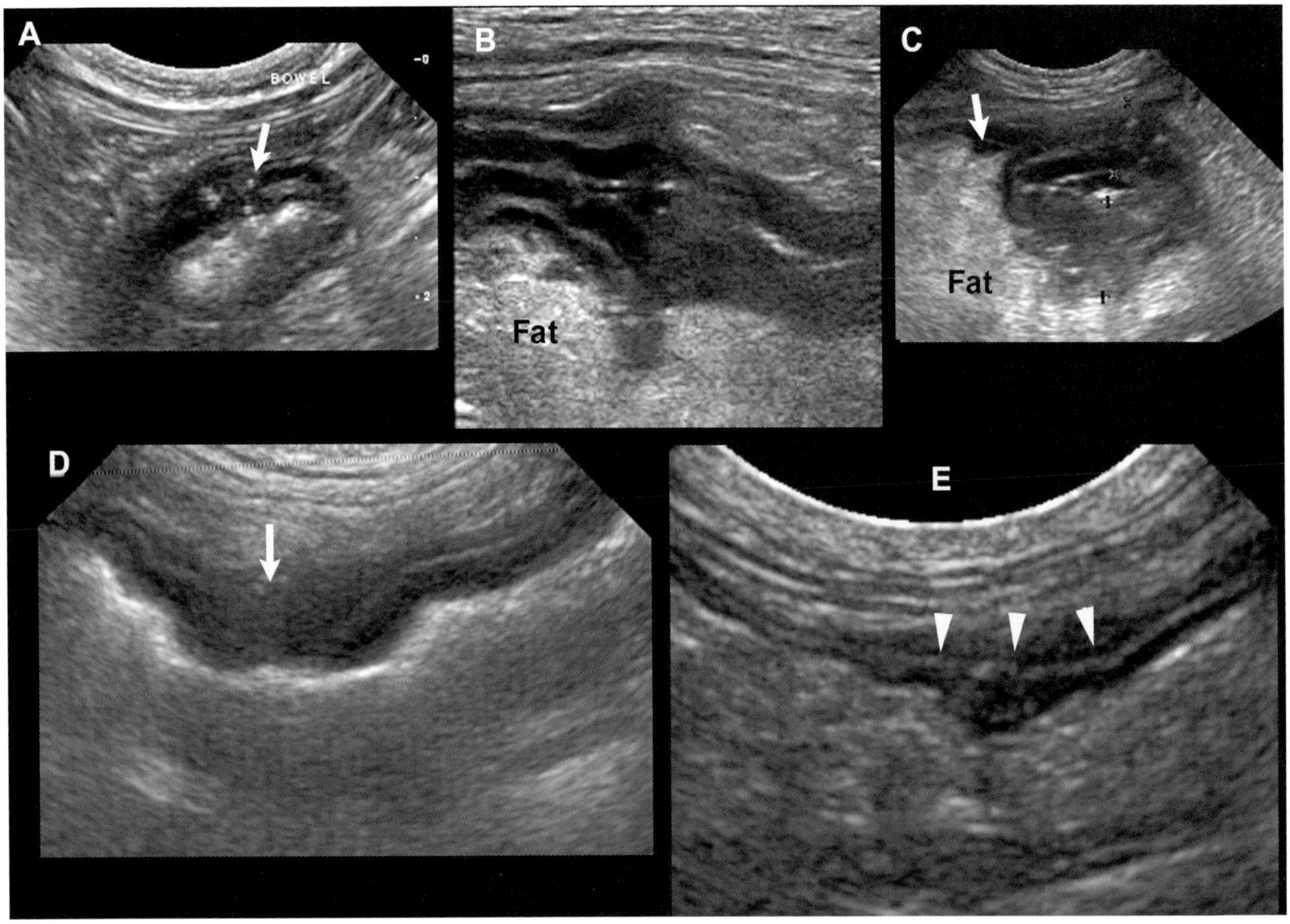

Figure 8.38. Postoperative enterotomy. **A:** Normal immediate postoperative sonogram of an enterotomy site in a dog. The sutures appear as discrete, small, bright interfaces (arrow). **B and C:** Longitudinal **(B)** and transverse **(C)** planes obtained at the site of anastomosis. The wall layering is disrupted, and the wall margins are deformed (between the cursors). Free gas and free fluid (arrow) are commonly encountered. The surrounding fat is bright. **D:** Several days later, the wall layering remains disrupted (arrow) in this longitudinal sonogram. **E:** Several weeks after surgery, despite a persistent focal thickening, the submucosa layer can be seen crossing the previous surgical site (arrowheads) in this dog with no gastrointestinal signs.

Figure 8.39. Intestinal stricture. Severe fluid distension (F) is noted proximal to the stricture site (arrows) in this dog with previous enterectomies for intestinal foreign bodies. Suboptimal peristaltic activity was noted throughout the intestinal tract. Stricture at the surgical site was diagnosed surgically.

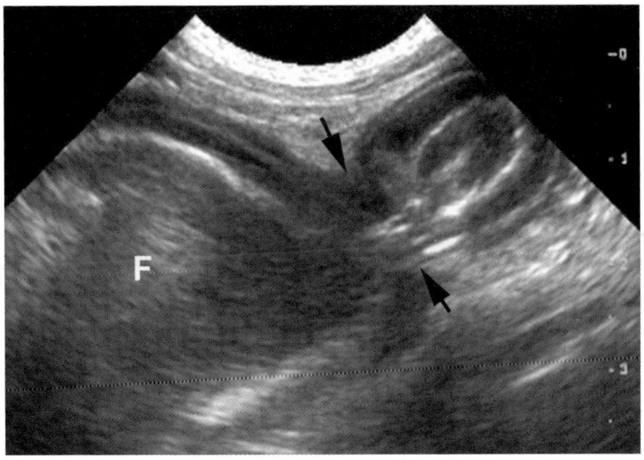

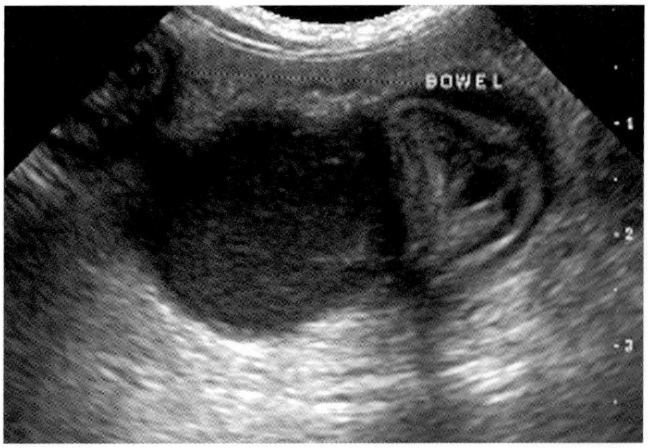

Figure 8.40. Subserosal seroma following biopsy. A discrete, rounded and hypoechoic fluid cavity associated with acoustic enhancement is deforming the adjacent intestinal wall and lumen. This represents a cystic seroma secondary to a recent surgical intestinal biopsy. The dog had no clinical signs related to this finding.

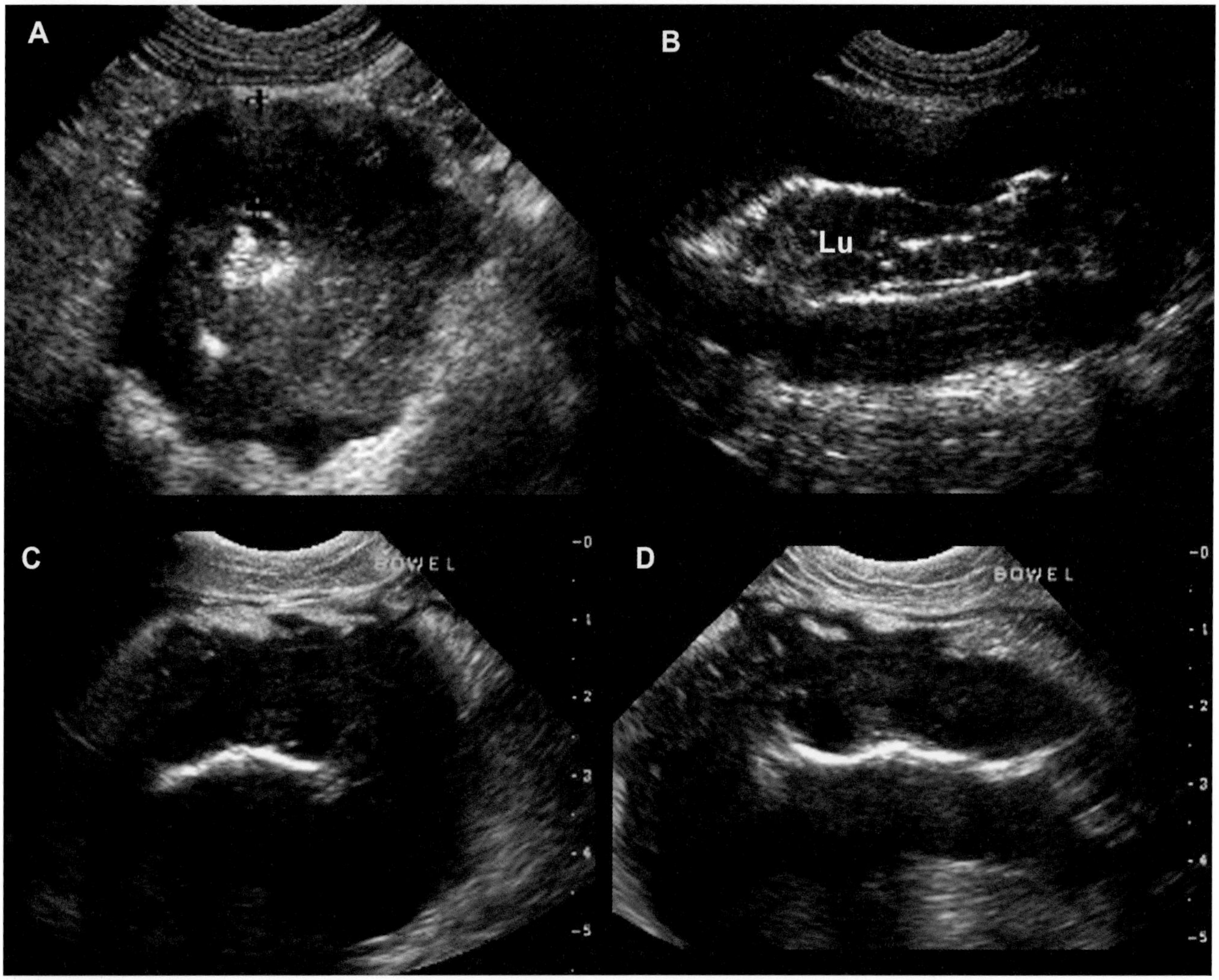

Figure 8.41. Intestinal lymphoma. **A and B:** Transverse **(A)** and longitudinal **(B)** sonograms of the thickened duodenum of a 10-year-old golden retriever with lymphoma. There is circumferential, irregular thickening (between the cursors: 1.3 cm) of a segment of small intestine, with extensive loss of wall layering. Fluid is noted in the lumen (Lu). **C and D:** Transverse **(C)** and longitudinal **(D)** sonograms of a long jejunal segment in an anorectic 15-year-old cat with lymphoma. Marked thickening of the wall and loss of layering are noted, as well as poorly marginated serosal margins surrounded by bright fat. This latter finding may represent neoplastic infiltrate within the mesentery. The bright, linear interface in the center of the mass indicates the presence of the gas-filled lumen and helps in confirming the intestinal origin.

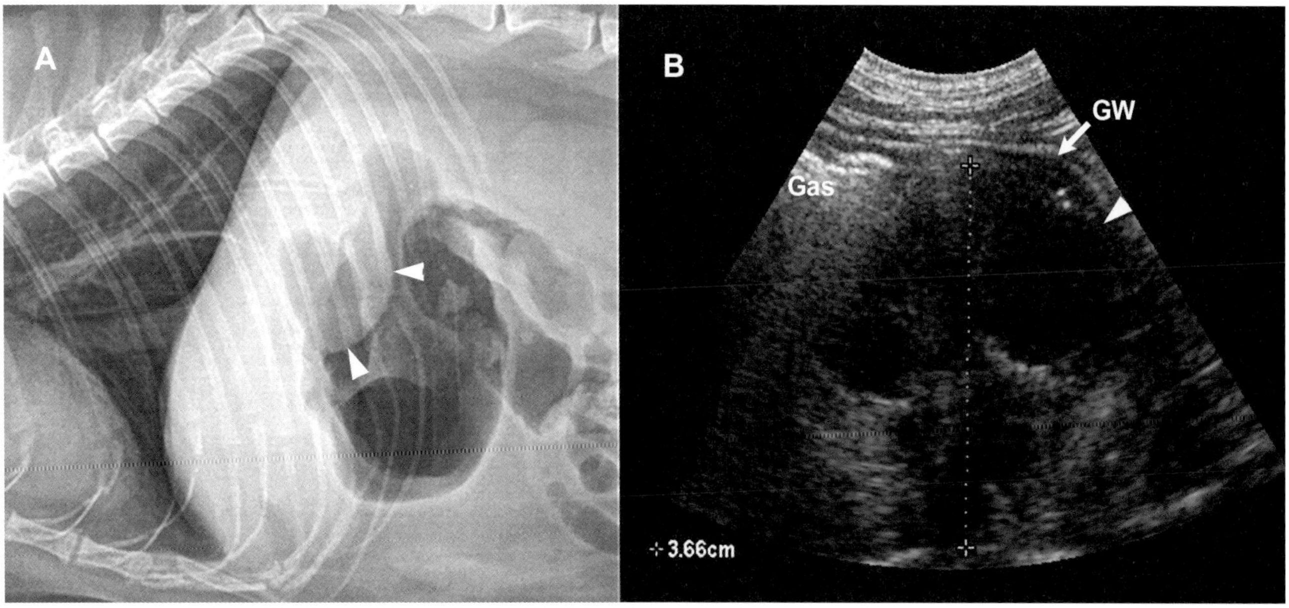

Figure 8.42. Gastric lymphoma. **A:** Lateral radiograph of a cat with chronic weight loss and vomiting. A smooth soft-tissue mass (arrowheads) protrudes into the gas-filled gastric lumen. **B:** Longitudinal sonogram obtained at the level of the gastric fundus. A 3.7-cm, hypoechoic, mildly inhomogeneous mass (cursors) that protrudes into the gastric lumen is partially masked by the presence of gas and its related reverberation artifacts. The arrowhead points to the level of transition between the normal gastric wall (GW), with intact layering, and the level of mass infiltration, with altered layers. Images courtesy of M.A. d'Anjou.

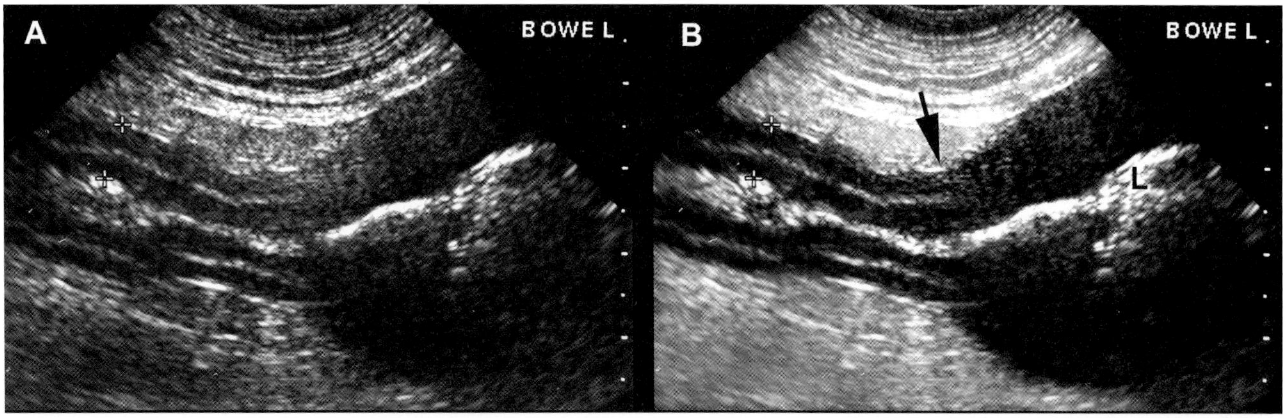

Figure 8.43. Intestinal lymphoma. Longitudinal sonographic **(A)** and schematic **(B)** sonograms of an intestinal segment of a cat with lymphoma. The wall was circumferentially thickened (1 cm thick) (cursors). The layers of the left portion of the bowel are still visible but irregular. The muscular layer is significantly thicker than normal, suggesting idiopathic hypertrophy or hyperplasia. On the right portion of the image, the wall is significantly thicker, with complete loss of layering at the place of tumoral infiltration. On the schematic image, the arrow points to the transition between layered wall and complete loss of layering. L, lumen.

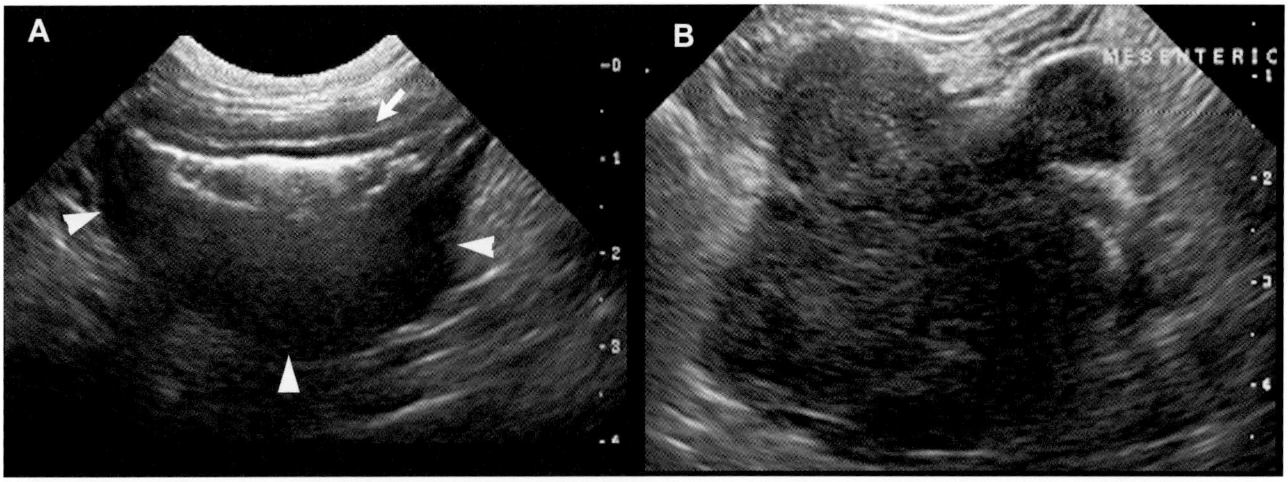

Figure 8.44. Intestinal lymphoma. **A:** Longitudinal sonogram of an asymmetrically thickened (1.5 cm) bowel segment in an 11-year-old cat diagnosed with alimentary lymphoma. The loss of layering involved mostly one side of the wall (arrowheads). The muscular layer appears particularly thickened in the opposite wall (arrow) **B:** The mesenteric lymph nodes were markedly enlarged (4.5 cm thick), lobulated, and hypoechoic.

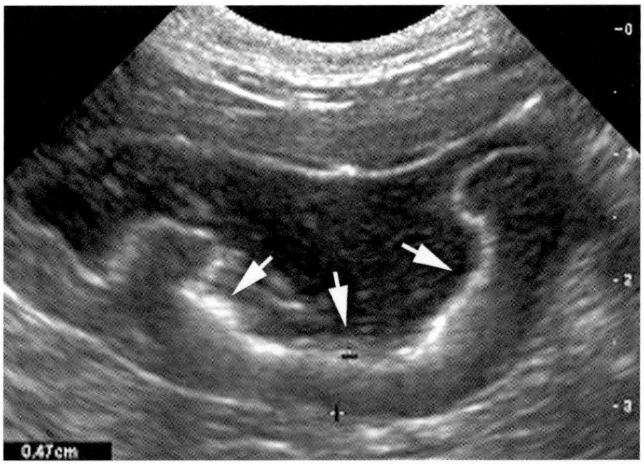

Figure 8.45. Ulcerated lymphoma. Longitudinal sonogram of an ulcerated lymphoma in a 15-year-old cat with vomiting and depression. Part of the gastric wall was moderately thickened, with complete loss of layering. The mucosal surface appears irregular, and a layer of hyperechoic microbubbles has accumulated at the site of the extensive ulceration (arrows). The stomach is filled with fluid and was hypomotile during the exam.

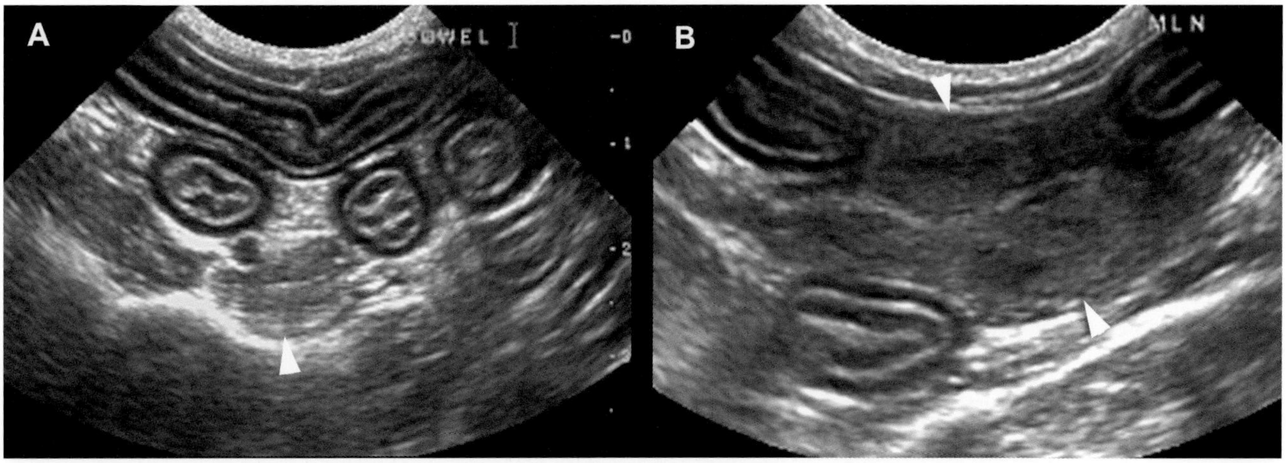

Figure 8.46. Feline lymphoma without loss of layering. **A:** Feline lymphoma occasionally is not associated with complete loss of wall layering, as in this 10-year-old cat with diffusely, mildly thickened bowel loops (4 mm). The muscular layer is particularly prominent. **B:** The mesenteric lymph nodes are moderately enlarged (up to 2.2 cm wide) (arrowheads).

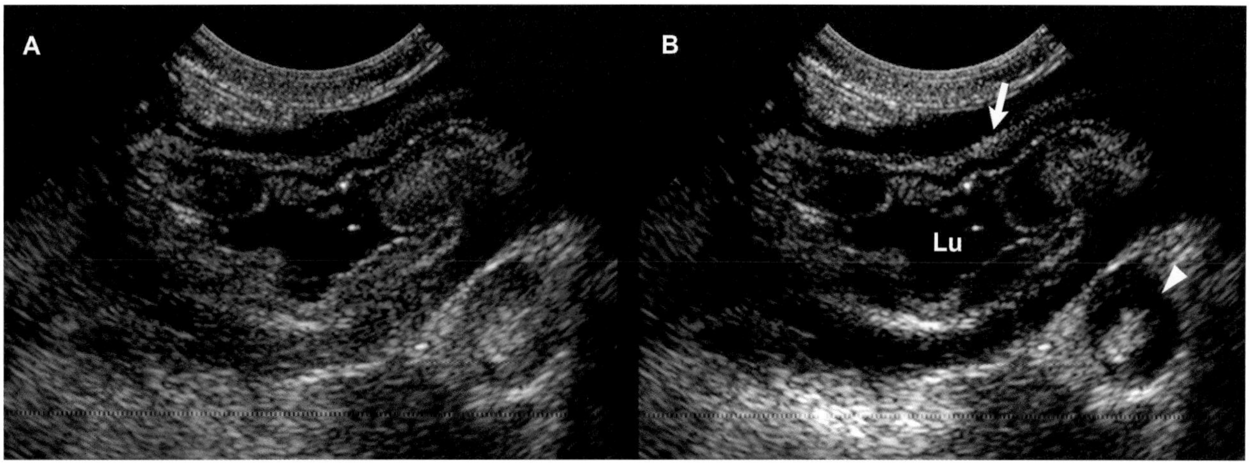

Figure 8.47. Gastric pseudolayering sign with adenocarcinoma. Longitudinal sonographic **(A)** and schematic **(B)** images of the pyloric antrum of a dog with carcinoma. The markedly thickened wall (up to 1.3 cm) displayed a pseudolayering pattern (arrow) suggestive of carcinoma. A mild amount of fluid is noted in the lumen (Lu). The gastric lymph node is enlarged (0.8 × 1.3 cm) (arrowhead) and has a target appearance (a hypoechoic rim around a bright center).

loss of layering, which is often associated with lymphadenopathy (Paoloni et al. 2002) (Figure 8.48). In the majority of these cases, evidence of fluid accumulation is proximal to the intestinal thickening or mass associated with a localized ileus. Intestinal carcinoma shares some of the ultrasonographic features seen in intestinal lymphoma, but the length of the lesion tends to be shorter in carcinoma than lymphoma, and mechanical ileus is more common in carcinoma than in lymphoma (Figures 8.48–8.50).

Several ultrasonographic features of GI smooth muscle tumors are helpful in differentiating them from other types of GI neoplasia. Leiomyosarcomas are often large (over 3 cm) intramural lesions growing out of the serosa as large eccentric or extraluminal masses (Myers and Penninck 1994) (Figures 8.51–8.54). Uncommonly they invade or project into the GI lumen. Because of their common exophytic distribution and their large size, it is difficult to assess the anatomical origin of the mass and even more so to determine the precise layer of tumor origin. During real-time evaluation, it is important to identify within the mass any gas and/or the small amount of fluid located in the distorted lumen.

Commonly the presence of a reverberation artifact indicates the presence of gas, and attempts to connect this artifact to an adjacent bowel segment should be made to confirm the GI origin. Large GI leiomyosarcomas tend to be heterogeneous with a mixed echogenic pattern. The presence of anechoic and hypoechoic foci within the mass may correlate with the areas of central degeneration and necrosis frequently found in these large lesions.

Other tumors have been reported, such as carcinoid, neurilemoma, nerve-sheath tumor, histiocytic sarcoma, mast cell tumor, hemangiosarcoma, and extraskeletal osteosarcoma (Stimson et al. 2000). The lesions tend to appear as poorly echogenic masses or as focal thickening with loss of layering. No specific ultrasonographic feature helps in differentiating the different tumors (Figure 8.55).

Miscellaneous Gastrointestinal Disorders

Congenital GI disorders are rare in small animals. Enteric duplication is rare, but has been reported in the literature (Spaulding et al. 1990).

In small-breed dogs, chronic hypertrophic pyloric stenosis can be encountered (Figure 8.56). The hypertrophic and/or hyperplastic changes primarily affect the smooth muscle layer of the pylorus (Biller et al. 1994). Because of this chronic condition, the stomach tends to be flaccid, and a moderate amount of fluid or food accumulates in it.

At times, the hypertrophic mucosal or hyperplastic glandular changes of the gastric wall may appear as a discrete nodule or mass. Exuberant hyperplastic or hypertrophic mucosal or muscular changes cannot be differentiated from benign polyps based on their imaging or gross appearance. Gastric polyps can appear as large, moderately echogenic nodules or masses projecting into the gastric lumen (Figure 8.57). They often are asymptomatic unless located in the pylorus and thus creating a gastric outflow disturbance.

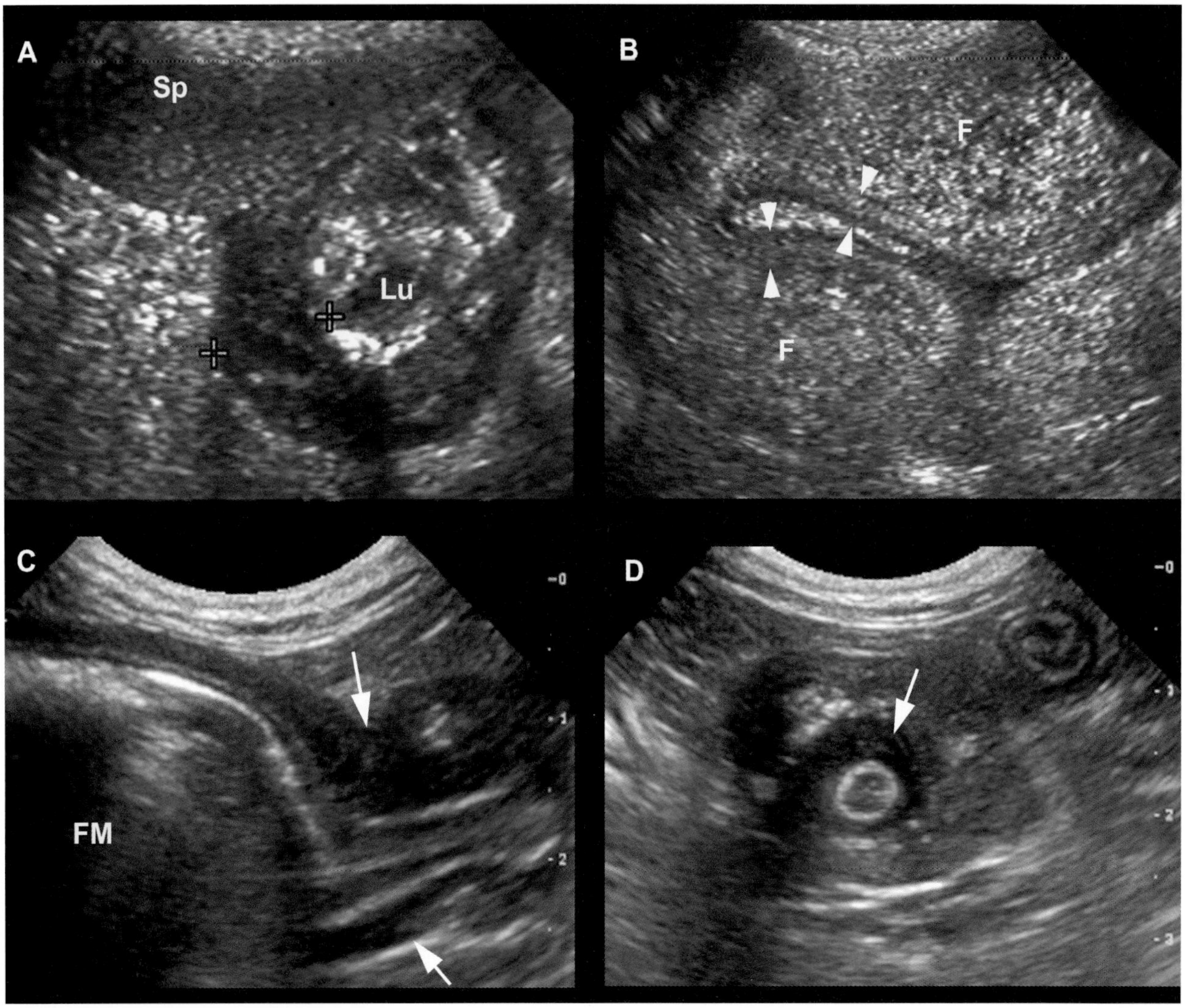

Figure 8.48. Jejunal adenocarcinomas causing partial obstruction. **A:** Sonogram of a circumferentially thickened bowel segment in a dog with jejunal adenocarcinoma. At the tumor site, the wall is hypoechoic, with absent layering. The length of the lesion was estimated to be less than 5 cm. Lu, lumen; and Sp, spleen. **B:** Moderate echogenic fluid accumulation (F) is present proximal to the lesion. This fluid is almost confluent with the distended walls (arrowheads) **C:** longitudinal sonogram of an intestinal adenocarcinoma in a cat that had experienced weight loss and anorexia. Proximal to the obstruction site is intestinal distension and foreign-material accumulation (FM). The arrows point to the narrowed and affected bowel segment. **D:** Transverse sonogram of the same lesion. The arrow points to the thickened ileum.

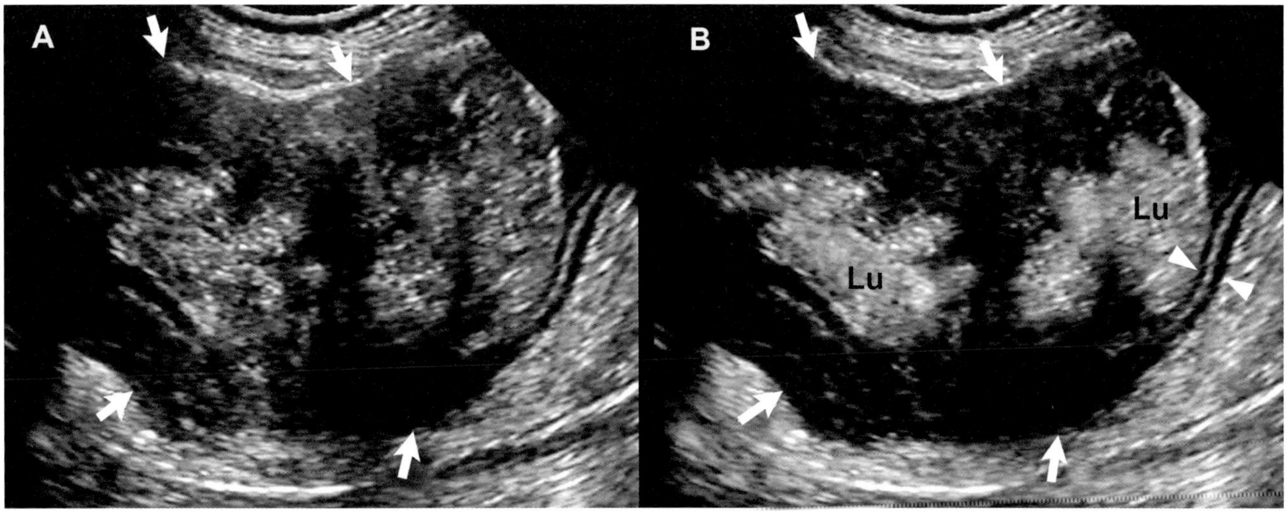

Figure 8.49. Jejunal adenocarcinoma. Longitudinal sonographic **(A)** and schematic **(B)** images of a focally invasive and unevenly circumferential adenocarcinoma invading the jejunum in this dog (arrows). Note the intact wall at the margin of the mass (arrowheads). Lu, lumen.

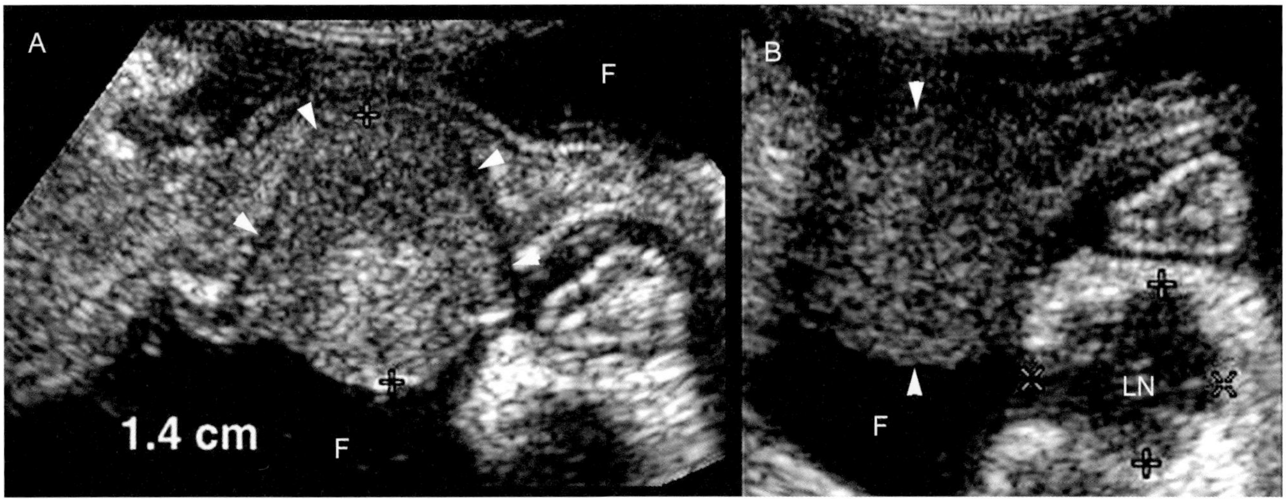

Figure 8.50. Colonic carcinoma. **A:** Longitudinal sonogram of the colon of a 20-year-old cat. A 1.4-cm, asymmetrical, moderately echogenic mass is noted involving the colonic wall and protruding into the lumen (arrowheads). A large amount of peritoneal fluid (F) is present. **B:** An enlarged regional lymph node (LN) is also present. The final diagnosis was colonic carcinoma with metastases to local lymph nodes. F, peritoneal fluid. The arrowheads point to the mass.

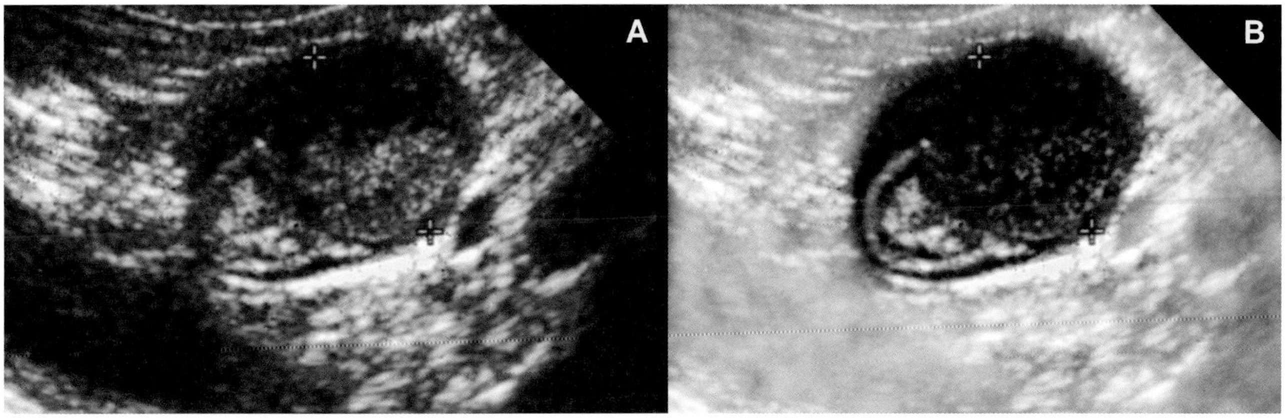

Figure 8.51. Leiomyoma. Transverse sonographic **(A)** and schematic **(B)** images of a small mass located at the pyloroduodenal angle in a dog. The mass is hypoechoic and homogeneous, deforming the outer contour of the duodenum, and protrudes into its lumen. The layers are focally indistinct. Mucosal polyp, hyperplastic nodule, and smooth-muscle tumor can look alike.

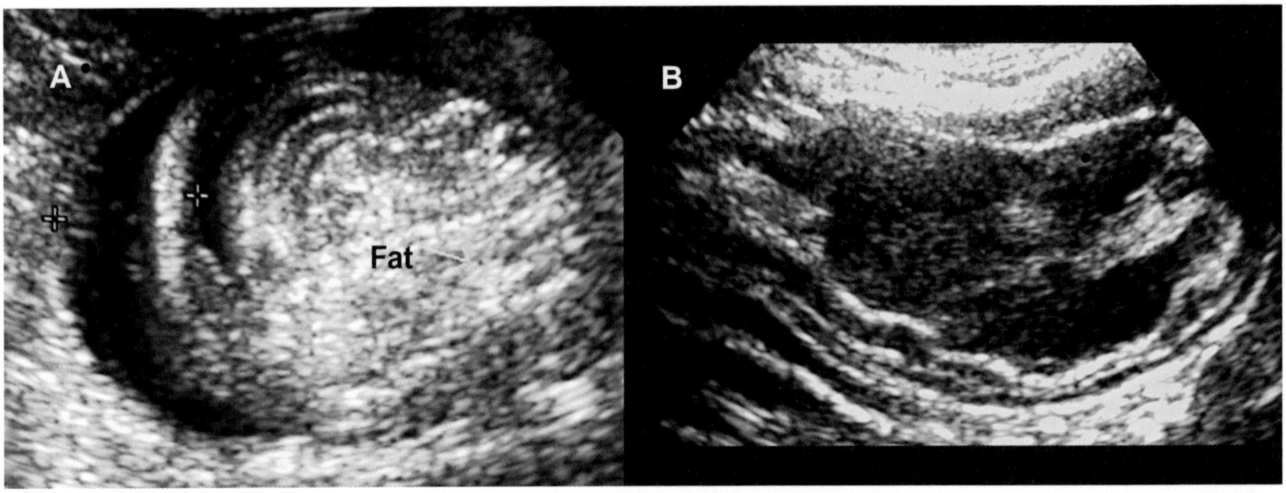

Figure 8.52. Smooth-muscle tumor and intussusception. Occasionally, smooth-muscle tumors are seen associated with an intussusception, as seen in this dog. **A:** The intussusceptum has a focally thickened wall (between the cursors). The outer hypoechoic layer representing the muscular layer seems to be the most affected. Differential diagnoses for this focal change seen at the intussusceptum may be smooth-muscle tumor, focal inflammation, edema, or hemorrhage of the wall. The fat is invaginated. **B:** The longitudinal sonogram centered on the thickening reveals a large hypoechoic mass imbedded in the intussusception.

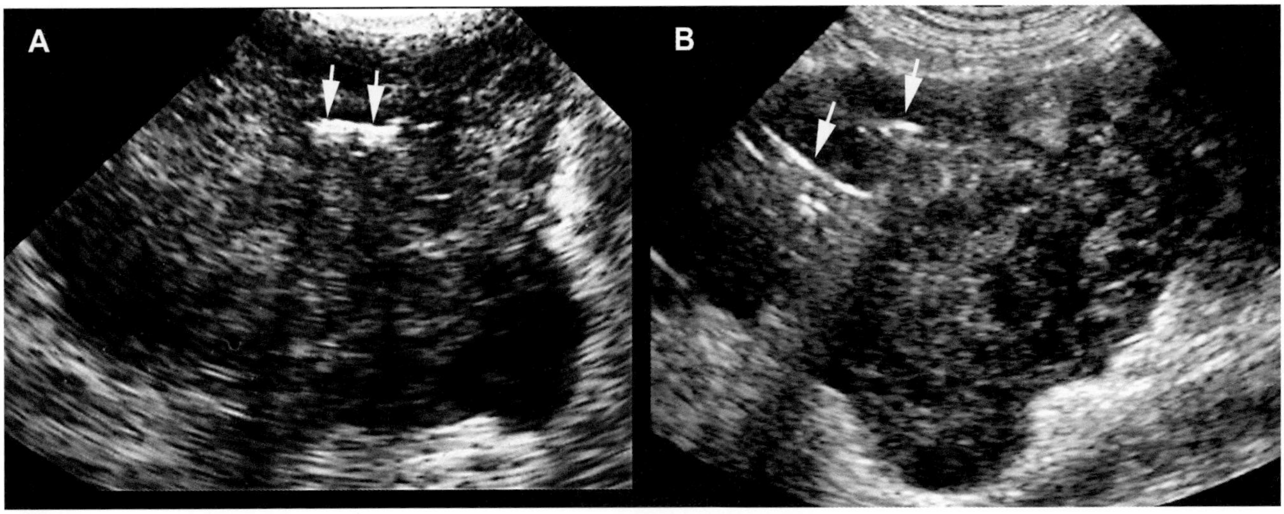

Figure 8.53. Intestinal leiomyosarcoma in two dogs. **A:** Sonogram of a jejunal leiomyosarcoma. The mass is large (approximately 8cm long by 5cm high). The irregular bright echoes seen in the near field (arrows) represent gas in the distorted intestinal lumen. The mass is inhomogeneous; a few hypoechoic areas seen within the mass most likely are areas of central degeneration and necrosis. **B:** Similar features of a large, eccentric, inhomogeneous mass noted in this other dog diagnosed with intestinal leiomyosarcoma. The arrows point to the lumen of the affected segments.

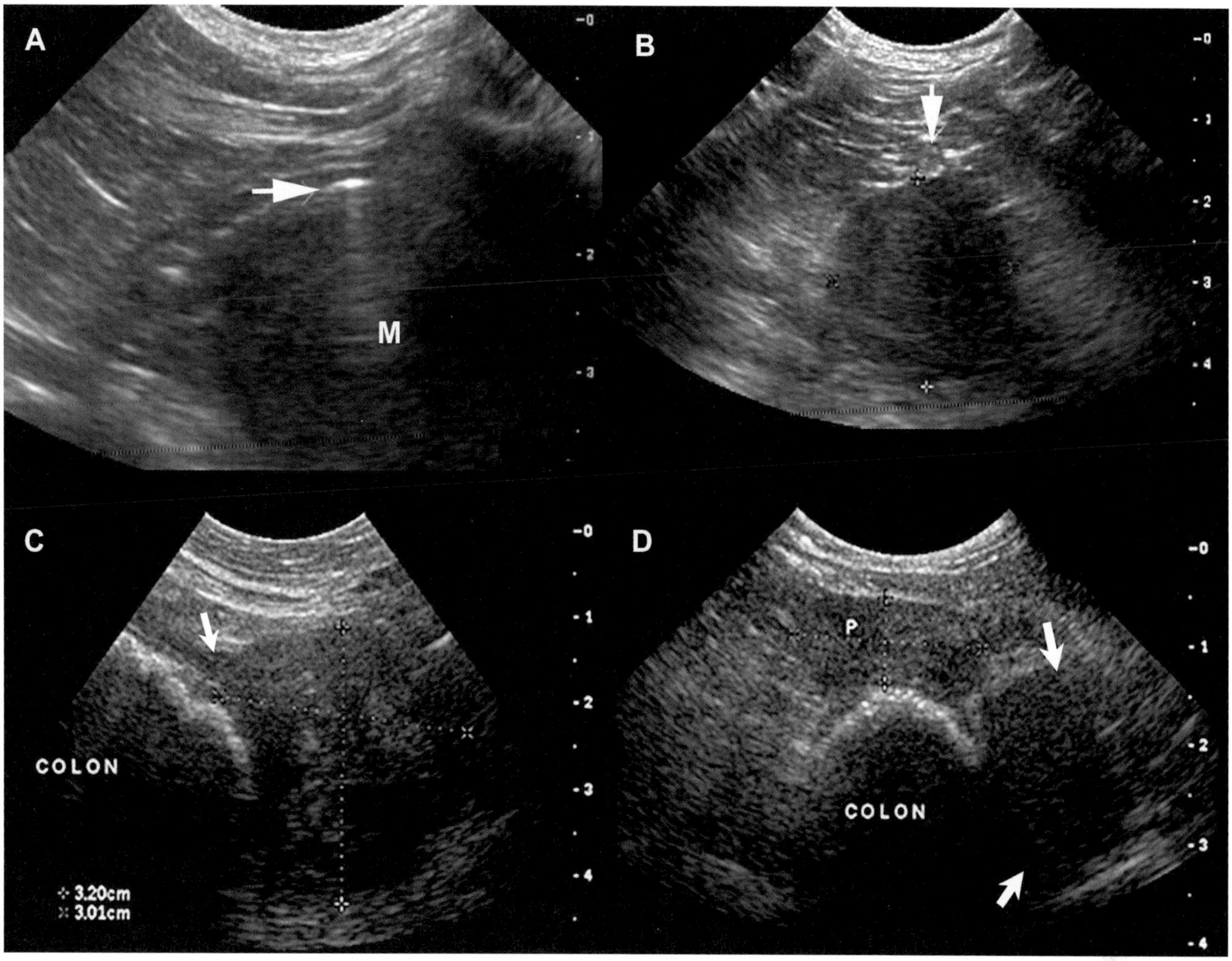

Figure 8.54. Colonic smooth-muscle tumors. Longitudinal **(A)** and transverse **(B)** images of a large, hypoechoic mass extending into the pelvic canal. The pubis prevents a complete ultrasonographic assessment of the contour and margins of the lesion. The lumen (arrow) of the colon is collapsed, and a small amount of trapped gas is associated with reverberation. In **B**, in the near field, the arrow points to the intact urethra, located ventral to the round mass (between the cursors). Longitudinal **(C)** and transverse **(D)** images of another smooth-muscle tumor in a dog with obstipation. The mass is eccentric, inhomogeneous, and appears to communicate with the muscularis of the adjacent colonic wall (arrow in **C**). Large shadowing feces are noted within the colonic lumen, partially compressed by mural mass (arrows). The prostate is located ventrally (P). Images C and D courtesy of M.A. d'Anjou.

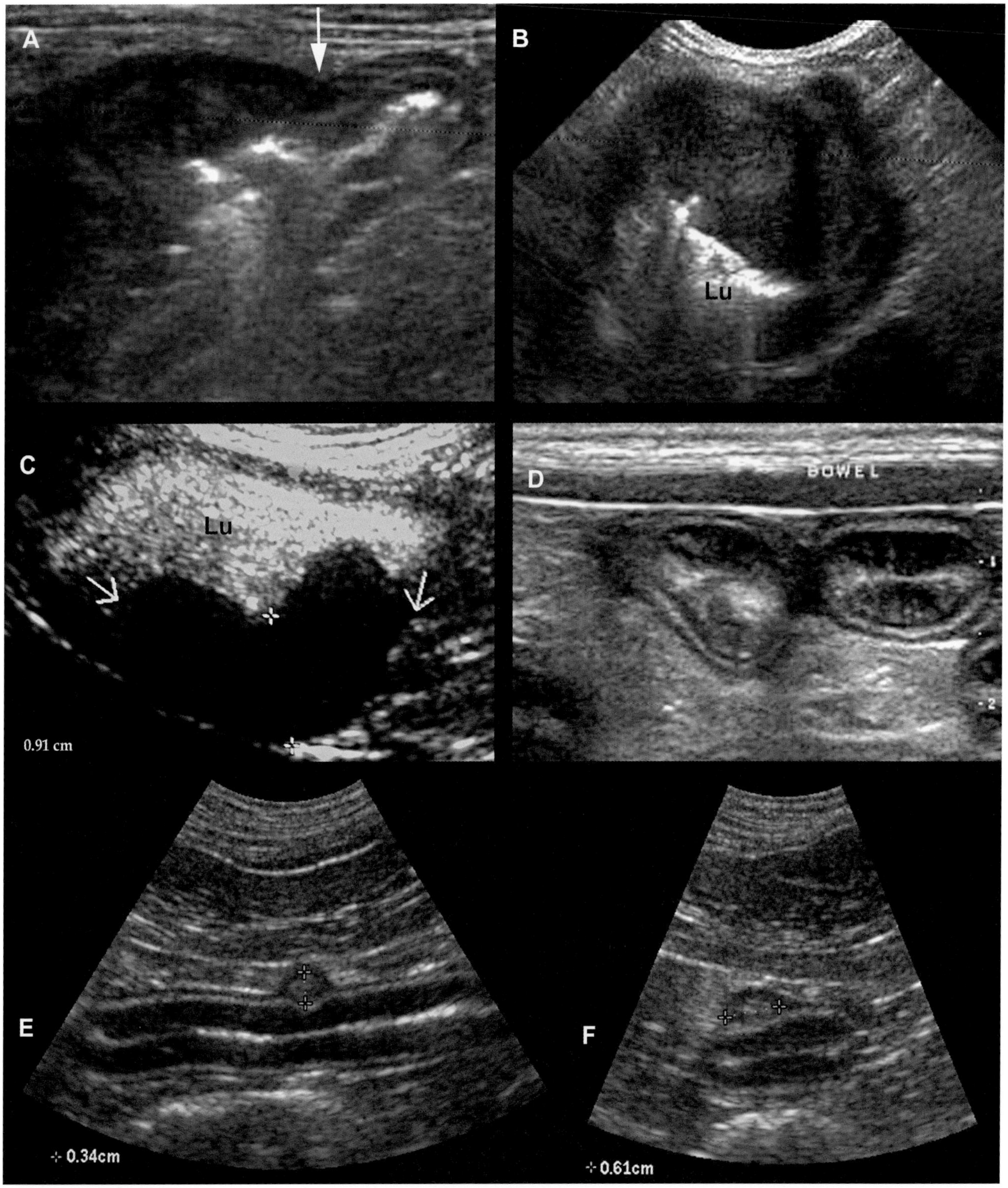

Figure 8.55. Unusual intestinal tumors. **A:** Longitudinal sonogram of a large, hypoechoic mass invading this midjejunal segment. The arrow points to the level of transition between the abnormally thickened wall with loss of layering and the normal wall. A poorly differentiated sarcoma was diagnosed. **B:** Transverse sonogram of the same lesion. The lumen (Lu) is eccentrically located. **C:** A hypoechoic mass (arrows) projecting within the lumen of this bowel segment was noted in this 11-year-old German shepherd. The mass is boomerang shaped, and there is loss of wall layering. The surgical biopsy sample was diagnosed as jejunal mast cell tumor. **D:** Diffusely thickened intestinal tract in a 10-year-old cocker spaniel–poodle mix with a poorly differentiated round-cell neoplasm (suspected of histiocytic origin). Note that the wall layering is maintained, and there are multiple, hyperechoic, linear mucosal striations consistent with lacteal dilation. **E and F:** Longitudinal and transverse images of a segment of jejunum in a Bernese mountain dog with disseminated histiocytic sarcoma. A small, well-defined, hyperechoic nodule is present within the muscularis, deforming the contour of the submucosa. Similar lesions were observed in other intestinal segments. All nodules, including those in the liver were hyperechoic. Images E and F courtesy of M.A. d'Anjou.

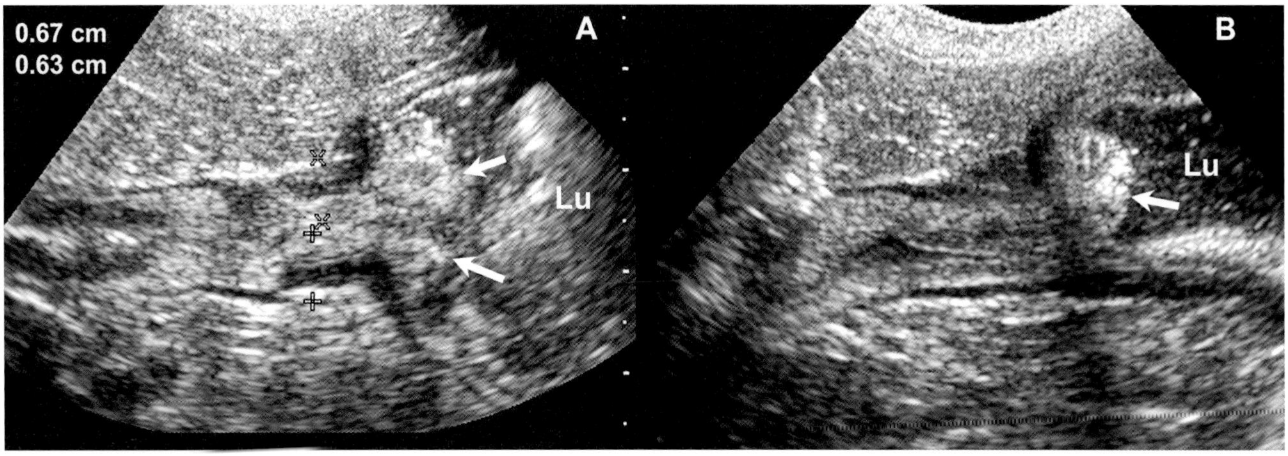

Figure 8.56. Pyloric hypertrophy. **A and B:** There is moderate thickening of the pyloric sphincter in this 9-year-old shih tzu. The hypertrophied walls (between the cursors) protrude as two rounded projections (arrows) into the fluid-filled pyloric antrum (Lu). The wall layers are still visible.

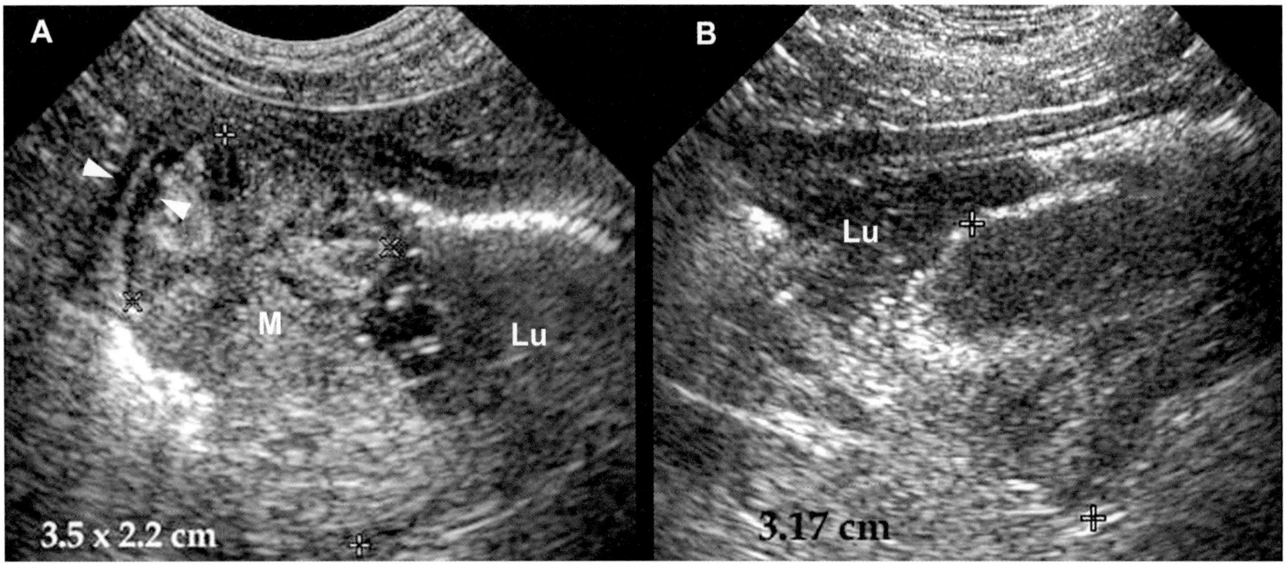

Figure 8.57. Gastric polyps. **A:** The stomach of a 9-year-old Lhasa apso with intermittent vomiting is distended with echogenic and amorphous food material compromising full evaluation of the stomach. However, near the pyloroduodenal angle, a moderately echogenic mass (M) protrudes into the gastric lumen (Lu), along an intact wall (arrowheads). Other hyperechoic masses were seen projecting into the gastric lumen (not shown here). They all were diagnosed as gastric polyps. **B:** There is an outflow obstruction secondary to a large (over 3 cm thick) gastric mass in this 7-year-old giant schnauzer that had experienced vomiting. A lobulated mass is seen protruding into the lumen (Lu), opposite to the intact wall of the greater curvature. The histopathologic diagnosis was inflamed, benign, mucosal polyp.

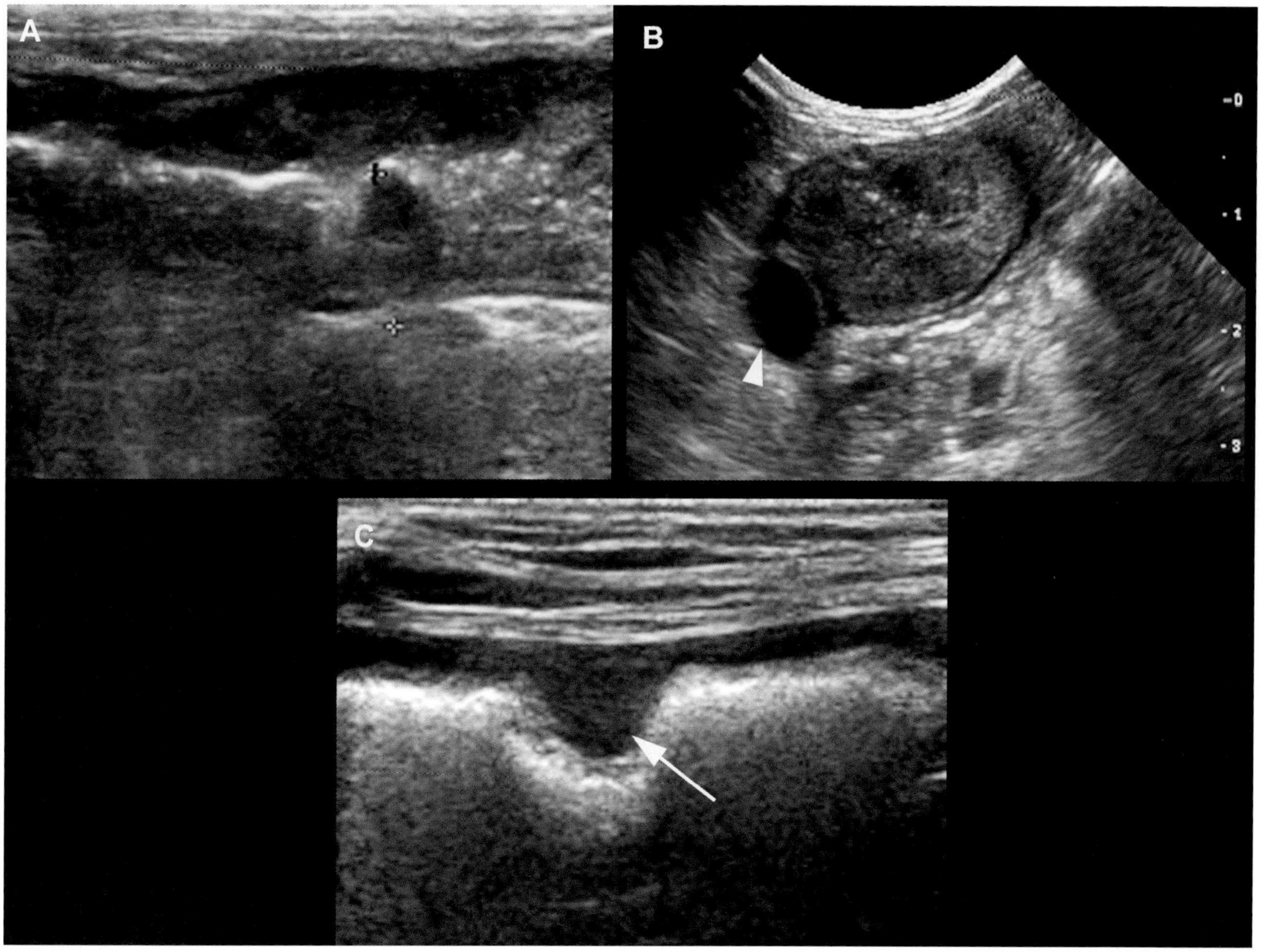

Figure 8.58. Duodenal mucosal hyperplasia evolving into adenocarcinoma. **A and B:** Longitudinal **(A)** and transverse **(B)** images of marked diffuse duodenal thickening (between the cursors) in a 13-year-old cat. The papilla is fluid dilated (arrowhead). Initial surgical biopsies were diagnostic of extensive tubulovillous, adenomatous, mucosal hyperplasia. Drastic surgical resection was performed 7 months later, and the final histopathologic diagnosis was duodenal adenocarcinoma. The sonographic features had not progressed during this long period. **C:** There is diffuse thickening with loss of layering along several jejunal segments in this corgi diagnosed with moderate eosinophilic erosive and polypoid enteritis. The arrow points to one polyp. Notice the loss of wall layering.

Extensive hyperplastic changes can be found at other locations along the GI tract. If located within the proximal portion of the descending duodenum, these changes may induce outflow obstruction or compromise the bile flow (Figure 8.58A). Focal lesions along the intestinal tract mimic tumoral nodules (Figure 8.58B).

GI vascular disorders such as infarction or ischemia or angiodysplasia are uncommon and very challenging to diagnose (Fan et al. 1999; Wallack et al. 2003). Bowel infarction can initially display normal layering of a focally dilated small bowel segment. Subsequent (72h after presentation) thickening and loss of wall layering and adjacent hyperechoic fat suggestive of peritonitis can then be observed.

Interventional Procedures

Percutaneous ultrasound-guided fine-needle aspiration and automated microcore biopsy of GI lesions are safe alternative procedures to use instead of endoscopic or surgical biopsy. The guided techniques of fine-needle aspiration using either a 22- or 20-gauge spinal needle, and/or microcore automated biopsy using an 18-gauge Tru-Cut needle, assisted by an automated biopsy gun, are efficient and safe methods of

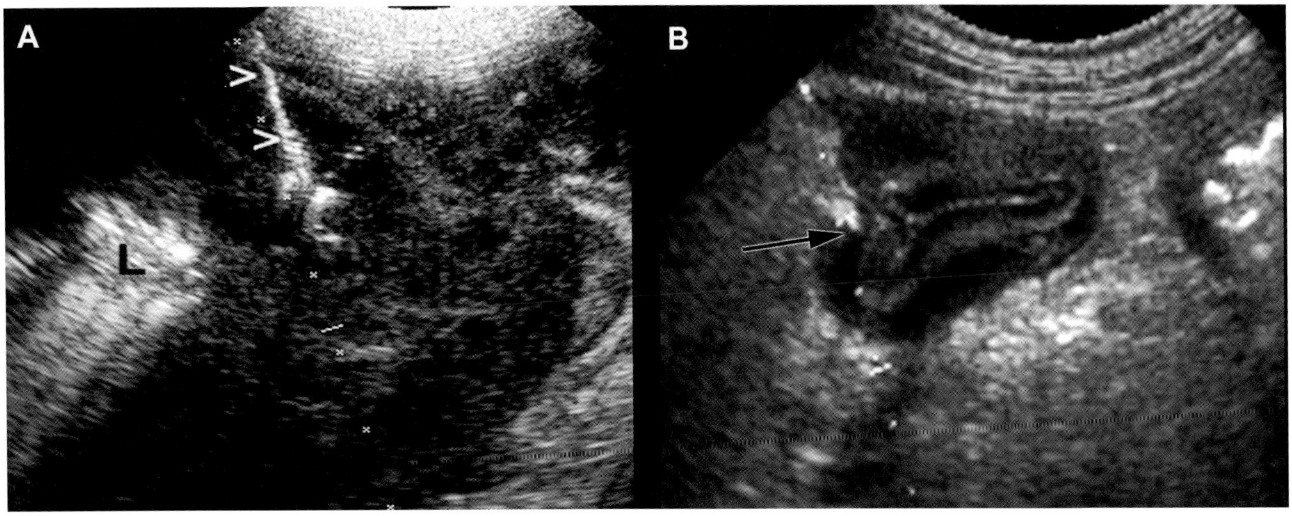

Figure 8.59. Ultrasound-guided biopsy and fine-needle aspiration. **A:** An ultrasound-guided core biopsy was performed on this markedly thickened and distorted intestinal wall of a dog diagnosed with lymphoma. The visible needle path enables careful placement of the needle (>), far away from the intestinal lumen (L). **B:** Fine-needle aspiration can also be performed safely. Notice the needle tip (black arrow) engaged in this mildly thickened bowel segment.

obtaining a diagnostic sample (Penninck et al. 1993) (Figure 8.59).

They are especially useful when lesions are not accessible endoscopically and when surgical resection is not a safe option for a compromised patient. One paramount safety rule is to carefully locate and avoid the lumen.

In presence of a GI lesion associated with regional lymphadenopathy, it is recommended to target both structures to increase the chance of obtaining one or more diagnostic sample.

Complications such as local hemorrhage or seroma collection are rare. Intestinal content leakage, which can be a serious complication, can be avoided by careful selection of the biopsy site.

References

Baez JB, Hendrick MJ, Walker LM, Washabau RJ (1999) Radiographic, ultrasonographic, and endoscopic findings in cats with inflammatory bowel disease of the stomach and small intestine: 33 cases (1990–1997). J Am Vet Med Assoc 215:349–354.

Biller DS, Partington BP, Miyabayashi T, Leveille R (1994) Ultrasonographic appearance of chronic hypertrophic pyloric gastropathy in the dog. Vet Radiol Ultrasound 35:30–33.

Boysen SR, Tidwell AS, Penninck DG (2003) Sonographic findings in dogs and cats with intestinal perforation: A retrospective study (1995–2001). Vet Radiol Ultrasound 44:556–564.

Delaney F, O'Brien RT, Waller K (2003) Ultrasound evaluation of small bowel thickness compared to weight in normal dogs. Vet Radiol Ultrasound 44: 577–580.

Diana A, Pietra M, Guglielmini C, Boari A, Bettini G, Cipone M (2003) Ultrasonographic and pathologic features of intestinal smooth muscle hypertrophy in four cats. Vet Radiol Ultrasound 44:566–569.

Fan TM, Simpson KW, Polack E, Dykes N, Harvey J (1999) Intestinal haemorrhage associated with colonic vascular ectasia (angiodysplasia) in a dog. J Small Anim Pract 40:25–30.

Goggin JM, Biller DS, Debey BM, Pickar JG, Mason D (2000) Ultrasonographic measurement of gastrointestinal wall thickness and the ultrasonographic appearance of the ileocolic region in healthy cats. J Am Anim Hosp Assoc 36:224–228.

Grooters AM, Miyabayashi T, Biller DS, Merryman J (1994) Sonographic appearance of uremic gastropathy in four dogs. Vet Radiol Ultrasound 35:35–40.

Hoffman KL (2003) Sonographic signs of gastroduodenal linear foreign body in 3 dogs. Vet Radiol Ultrasound 44:466–469.

Lamb CR, Mantis P (1998) Ultrasonographic features of intestinal intussusception in 10 dogs. J Small Anim Pract 39:437–441.

Lee H, Yeon S, Lee H, et al. (2005) Ultrasonographic diagnosis: Pylorogastric intussusception in a dog. Vet Radiol Ultrasound 46:317–318.

Moon ML, Biller DS, Armbrust LJ (2003) Ultrasonographic appearance and etiology of corrugated small intestine. Vet Radiol Ultrasound 44:199–203.

Myers NC, Penninck DG (1994) Ultrasonographic diagnosis of gastrointestinal smooth muscle tumors in the dog. Vet Radiol Ultrasound 35:391–397.

Newell SM, Graham JP, Roberts GD, Ginn PE, Harrison JM (1999) Sonography of the normal feline gastrointestinal tract. Vet Radiol Ultrasound 40:40–43.

Paoloni MC, Penninck DG, Moore AS (2002) Ultrasonographic and clinicopathologic findings in 21 cases of canine intestinal adenocarcinoma. Vet Radiol Ultrasound 43:562–567.

Patsikas MN, Papazoglou LG, Papaioannou NG, Savvas I, Kazakos GM, Dessiris AK (2003) Ultrasonographic findings of intestinal intussusception in seven cats. J Feline Med Surg 5:335–343.

Penninck DG (1998) Ultrasonographic characterization of gastrointestinal tumors. Vet Clin North Am 28:777–797.

Penninck DG (2002) Gastrointestinal tract. In: Nyland T, Mattoon J, eds. Small Animal Diagnostic Ultrasound, 2nd edition. Philadelphia: WB Saunders, pp 207–230.

Penninck DG, Crystal MA, Matz ME, Pearson SH (1993) The technique of percutaneous ultrasound guided fine-needle aspiration biopsy and automated microcore biopsy in small animal gastrointestinal diseases. Vet Radiol Ultrasound 34:433–436.

Penninck DG, Matz M, Tidwell AS (1997) Ultrasonographic detection of gastric ulceration. Vet Radiol Ultrasound 38:308–312.

Penninck D, Mitchell SL (2003) Ultrasonographic detection of ingested and perforating wooden foreign bodies in four dogs. J Am Vet Med Assoc 223:206–209.

Penninck DG, Moore AS, Gliatto J (1998) Ultrasonography of canine gastric epithelial neoplasia. Vet Radiol Ultrasound 39:342–348.

Penninck DG, Moore AS, Tidwell AS, Matz ME, Freden GO (1994) Ultrasonography of alimentary lymphosarcoma in the cat. Vet Radiol Ultrasound 35:299–304.

Penninck DG, Nyland TG, Fisher PE, Kerr LY (1989) Normal ultrasonography of the canine gastrointestinal tract. Vet Radiol Ultrasound 30:272–276.

Penninck DG, Smyers B, Webster CRL, Rand W, Moore AS (2003) Diagnostic value of ultrasonography in differentiating canine enteritis from intestinal neoplasia. Vet Radiol Ultrasound 44:570–575.

Spaulding KA, Cohn LA, Miller RT, Hardie EM (1990) Enteric duplication in two dogs. Vet Radiol Ultrasound 31:83–88.

Stimson EL, Cook WT, Smith MM, Forrester SD, Moon ML, Saunders GK (2000) Extraskeletal osteosarcoma in the duodenum of a cat. J Am Anim Hosp Assoc 36:332–336.

Sutherland-Smith J, Penninck DJ, Keating JH, Webster CRL (2007) The morphological significance of ultrasonographic intestinal hyperechoic striations in dogs. Vet Radiol Ultrasound 48:51–57.

Tidwell AS, Penninck DG (1992) Ultrasonography of gastrointestinal foreign bodies. Vet Radiol Ultrasound 33: 160–169.

Venco L, Kramer L, Pagliaro L, Genchi C (2005) Ultrasonographic features of peritoneal cestodiasis caused by *Mesocestoides* sp. in a dog and in a cat. Vet Radiol Ultrasound 46:417–422.

Wallack ST, Hornof WJ, Herrgesell EJ (2003) Ultrasonographic diagnosis: Small bowel infarction in a cat. Vet Radiol Ultrasound 44:81–85.

CHAPTER NINE

Pancreas

Dominique Penninck

Preparation and Scanning Procedure

The pancreas is a thin, elongated organ located along the greater curvature of the stomach and the mesenteric border of the descending duodenum. Gas in the gastrointestinal tract often hampers complete evaluation. A 12-h fast may reduce gas interference.

The anatomical landmarks used to locate the right pancreatic lobe are the right kidney; the descending duodenum, with its straight course along the right abdominal wall; and the pancreaticoduodenal vein paralleling the descending duodenum (Figure 9.1). The right pancreatic lobe can be imaged from a ventral or lateral approach, with a longitudinal scan-plane orientation used to find the descending duodenum and right kidney (Saunders 1991). Using the ventral approach, the transducer is placed under the last rib of the animal and angled dorsally to image the right kidney. The scan plane is then moved medially until the descending duodenum is imaged medial to the right kidney. Alternatively, the ventral approach can start caudal to the xiphoid process. In a longitudinal scan plane, the stomach is identified, and the scan plane is moved laterally toward the right following the pyloric antrum into the descending duodenum.

The lateral approach is preferred to locate the descending duodenum in deep-chested dogs. Once the descending duodenum is located by using the ventral or lateral approach, the right pancreatic lobe and the pancreaticoduodenal vein can be identified. In large and deep-chested dogs, it is often necessary to use an intercostal window to access the most cranial portion of the descending duodenum and the corresponding portion of the pancreas. On occasion, the right pancreatic lobe is best scanned from the right side, with the animal in a right lateral recumbency as gastric fluid moves in the dependent pyloric antrum.

The pancreatic body can be imaged from ventrally or from the right side, with the animal in a dorsal, left, or right lateral recumbent position, by moving the scan plane craniomedially to the proximal descending duodenum and caudally to the pyloric antrum. The portal vein represents a useful landmark because it is located just dorsal and to the left of the body of the pancreas (Figure 9.1). A transverse scan just caudal to the porta hepatis and pylorus may be used to locate this vein and the body of the pancreas. The left pancreatic lobe is more difficult to image in dogs because of gas interference in the adjacent stomach and transverse colon. However, in cats, the left limb is larger and can be more easily identified than the right limb.

High-frequency transducers (greater than 7.5 MHz) are recommended to evaluate the pancreas, especially in cats and small to medium-sized dogs. The small contact area of sectorial, narrow curvilinear or microconvex transducers facilitates access to the right cranial abdominal quadrant for imaging under or between the right ribs.

Ultrasonography of the Normal Pancreas

In Dogs

The pancreas is thin, amorphous, and poorly distinct from the adjacent mesenteric fat. The pancreas is divided into three portions: right lobe, left lobe, and body (Figure 9.1). The right lobe lies in the mesoduodenum dorsomedial to the descending duodenum, ventral to the right kidney, and ventrolateral to the portal vein. Only the veins draining the right lobe are seen ultrasonographically (Saunders 1991). The body lies caudal to the pyloric region, craniomedial to the right kidney, and ventral to the portal vein. The pylorus is in the right cranial abdomen. The left lobe originates at the pancreatic body, lies dorsocaudal to the gastric antrum, and continues across the midline between the stomach and the transverse colon. The normal left lobe occasionally is seen in the triangular region defined by the spleen, stomach, and left kidney. The normal pancreas is homogeneous and is isoechoic or slightly hyperechoic to the caudate liver lobe. On rare occasions, a normal pancreas can be diffusely hyperechoic

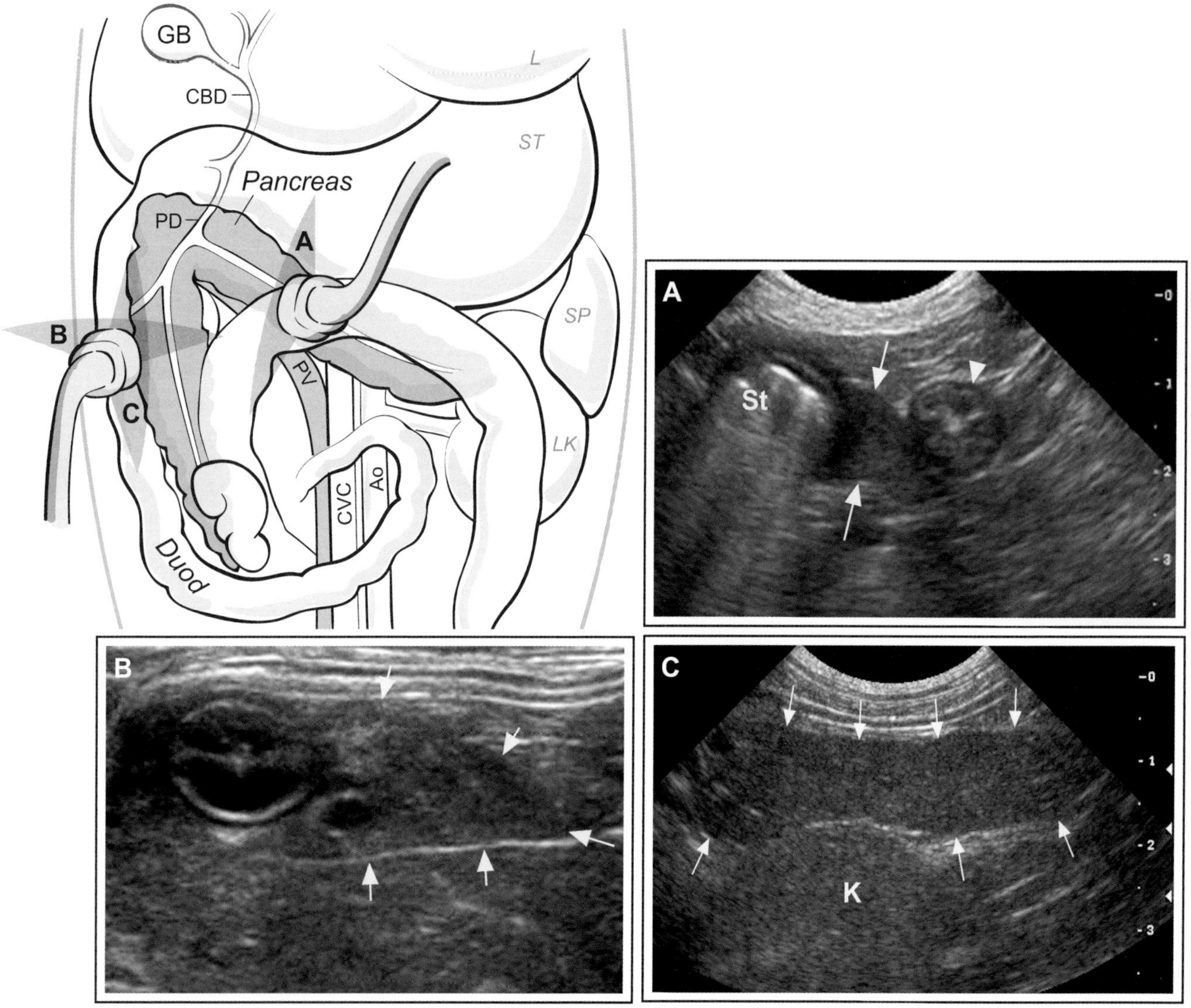

Figure 9.1. Approach to the normal canine pancreas. Illustration of the pancreas within the abdominal cavity, with the probe positioned along the left and right lobes of this organ at locations A, B, and C. Ao, aorta; CBD, common bile duct; CVC, caudal vena cava; Duod, duodenum; GB, gallbladder; L, liver; LK, left kidney; PD, pancreatic duct; PV, portal vein; SP, spleen; and ST, stomach. **A:** Transverse sonogram of the left lobe (arrows) seen between the stomach (St) and the collapsed transverse colon (arrowhead). **B:** Transverse sonogram of the right lobe of the pancreas (arrows). The layered descending duodenum is lateral to the pancreas. The pancreaticoduodenal vein appears as an anechoic rounded structure within the lobe. **C:** Longitudinal sonogram of the right pancreatic lobe (arrows) near the right kidney (K). Image C courtesy of M.A. d'Anjou.

but within normal range for size (Figure 9.2). The pancreaticoduodenal vein is seen clearly in the right lobe and can be followed into the gastroduodenal vein and portal vein.

In Cats

In contrast to dogs, the distal third of the feline right limb curves cranially, giving it a hooklike appearance (Etue et al. 2001). The pyloroduodenal angle and the pancreatic body are more centrally located, and the angle formed by the left and right lobes with the pancreatic body is smaller. The normal sonographic appearance of the feline pancreas is isoechoic to slightly hyperechoic to the adjacent liver lobes and nearly isoechoic to the surrounding mesenteric fat (Figure 9.3).

The mean thickness measurements for each part of the pancreas and the pancreatic duct in cats are summarized in Table 9.1.

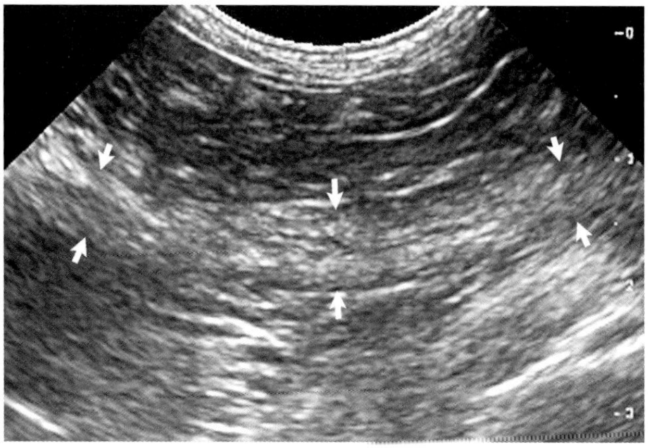

Figure 9.2. Normal pancreas in an old dog. Longitudinal sonogram of the left lobe of the pancreas in this 12-year-old Yorkie. The pancreas (arrows) is diffusely increased in echogenicity but maintains a normal size. The histopathology of the pancreas was unremarkable.

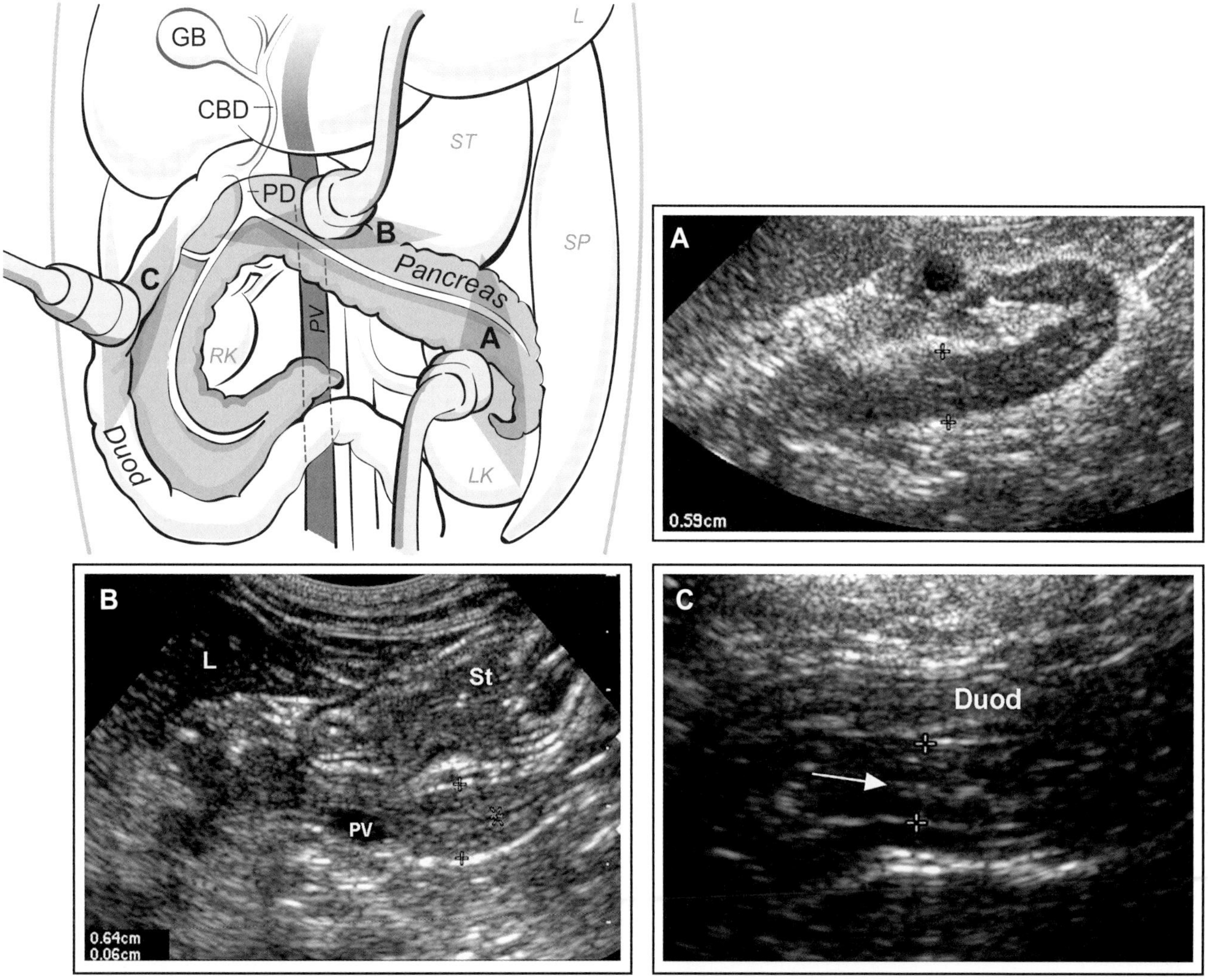

Figure 9.3. Approach to the normal feline pancreas. Illustration of the pancreas within the abdominal cavity with the probe positioned along the left (A) and right lobes (C) and body (B) of this organ. CBD, common bile duct; Duod, duodenum; GB, gallbladder; L, liver; LK, left kidney; PD, pancreatic duct; PV, portal vein; RK, right kidney; SP, spleen; and ST, stomach. **A:** Longitudinal sonogram showing the hook-shaped distal extremity of the left lobe. **B:** Longitudinal sonogram of the body. Notice the portal vein (PV) dorsal to the body (cursors). L, liver; and St, stomach. **C:** Longitudinal sonogram of the right lobe of the pancreas (cursors). Duod, duodenum. The arrow points to the pancreatic duct.

Table 9.1.
Pancreatic measurements in normal cats

Normal Cats	Left Lobe Mean (Range)	Body Mean (Range)	Right Lobe Mean (Range)	PD Mean (Range)
20[a] 1–9 years	5.4 mm (3.4–9.0)	6.6 mm (4.7–9.5)	4.5 mm (2.8–5.9)	0.8 mm (0.5–1.3)
84[b] 3 months to 16 years	5.4 mm (2.9–9.5*)	5.6 mm (3.3–9.4*)	NR	1.1 mm (0.65–2.5)
15[c] >10 years	6.5 mm (4.6–10.3)	6.4 mm (4.6–9.0)	4.3 mm (3.0–5.7)	1.13 mm (0.6–2.4)

PD, pancreatic duct; and NR, not reported.
[a]Etue et al. 2001.
[b]Moon et al. 2005.
[c]Hecht et al. 2006.
*Values represent the lower and upper limits of the 95% reference interval.

Ultrasonographic Features of Pancreatic Disorders

Pancreatitis

Pancreatitis has various ultrasonographic appearances, depending on the severity, duration, and extent of pancreatic and peripancreatic tissue inflammation.

In acute pancreatitis, the pancreas appears enlarged and diffusely hypoechoic while the surrounding fat appears moderately hyperechoic as the result of fat saponification (Figure 9.4). In dogs, the right limb of the pancreas tends to be most commonly affected (Nyland et al. 1983), whereas, in cats, the changes tend to be more severe in the body and left limb.

In cats, similar changes can be seen (Figure 9.5A and D), but pancreatic enlargement and diffuse changes in pancreatic and surrounding fat echogenicity are often less obvious (Figure 9.5B and C).

Pancreatitis in cats has been reported associated with hepatic lipidosis, inflammatory bowel disease, and cholangiohepatitis (Akol et al. 1993). Thickened gastric and/or duodenal wall and regional peritoneal effusion can be seen in association with pancreatitis (Saunders et al. 2002) (Figures 9.4–9.6). The thickening of the gastric and duodenal wall is usually not associated with complete loss of layering, although the wall layers can be altered (Figure 9.6B).

In severe hemorrhagic, necrotizing pancreatitis, irregular hypoechoic area(s) represent necrosis and hemorrhage of part of the pancreas and peripancreatic tissue (Figure 9.7). The pancreatic margins can be ill-defined, and the pancreas appears amorphous. The adjacent mesentery is hyperechoic because of inflammation and edema.

Pancreatic edema appears as numerous hypoechoic stripes demarcating pancreatic lobulation and dissecting the enlarged pancreas (Figure 9.8). Pancreatic edema may be associated with pancreatitis (Figure 9.8A and B), although it can also be caused by hypoalbuminemia or portal hypertension (Figure 9.8C) (Lamb 1999).

Focal pancreatic lesions caused by acute pancreatitis contain combined areas of pancreatic necrosis, hemorrhage, and surrounding inflamed mesentery (Edwards et al. 1990). The hypoechoic and anechoic areas corresponding to collections of hemorrhage and necrotic tissue may, with chronicity, become more organized and develop into pseudocyst or abscess. Pseudocysts are fluid-filled lesions caused by pancreatitis that are surrounded by a capsule of fibrous tissue. The fluid is composed of pancreatic secretions originating from a ruptured duct. Pancreatic pseudocysts are anechoic to poorly echogenic rounded lesions, occasionally associated with acoustic enhancement in the far field. They are reported in both dogs and cats (Rutgers et al. 1985; Hines et al. 1996; VanEnkevort et al. 1999) (Figure 9.9).

Retention cysts are caused by pancreatic duct blockage and cannot be differentiated from congenital cysts or pseudocysts (Figure 9.10).

Pancreatic abscesses are a circumscribed collection of pus, usually located within the pancreas or close to it, containing little or no pancreatic necrosis (Salisbury et al. 1988). They are more common in dogs (Figure 9.11) than in cats (Figure 9.12). Ultrasonographic differentiation among these different fluid-filled pancreatic lesions is impossible. Abscesses with echogenic fluid may also mimic masses.

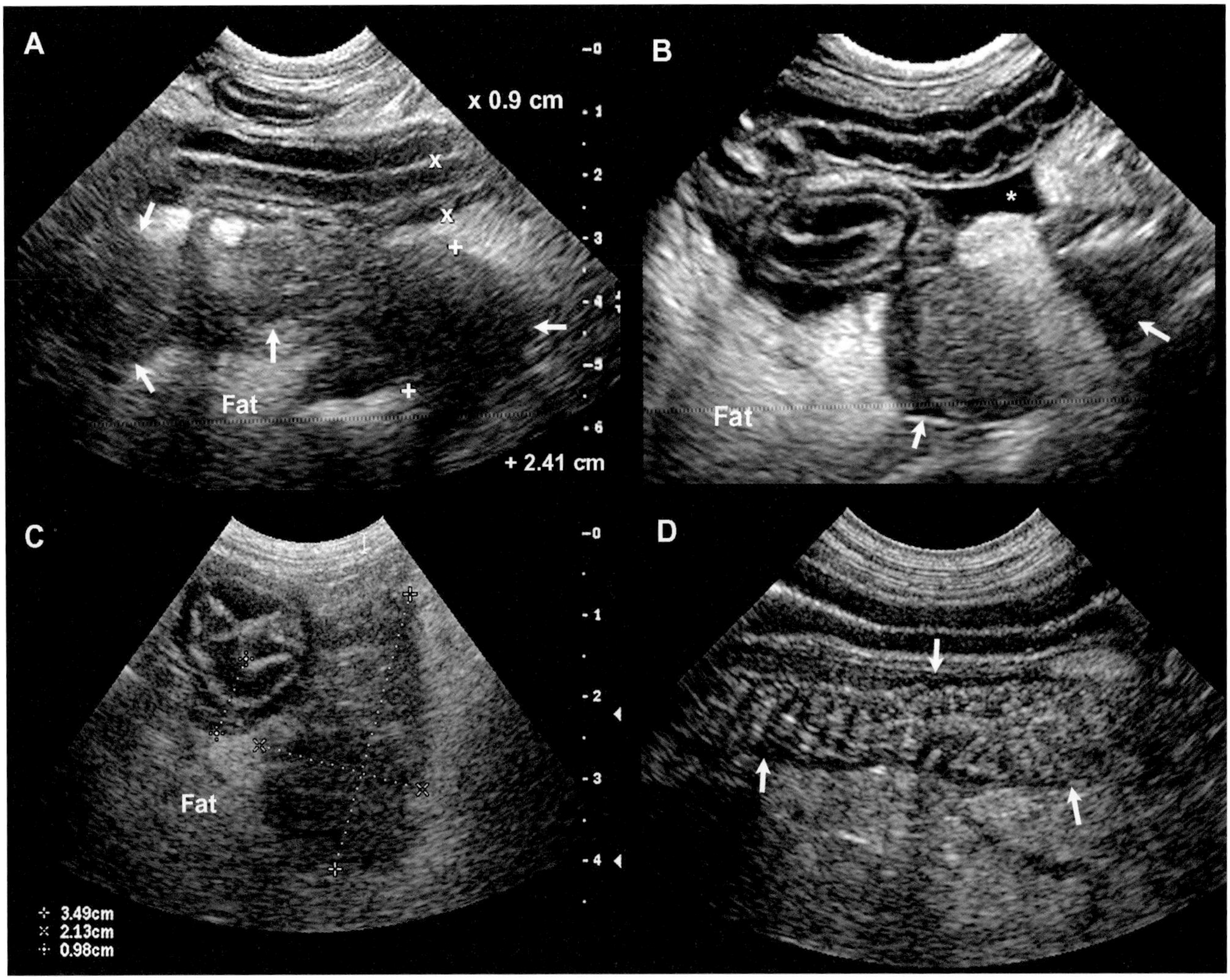

Figure 9.4. Acute pancreatitis in dogs. **A:** Longitudinal sonogram of the thickened (2.4 cm, cursors +), irregular, hypoechoic right lobe of the pancreas (arrows) surrounded by hyperechoic mesenteric fat. The descending duodenum is also thickened (9 mm, cursors ×), but its layers are still visible. **B:** Transverse sonogram of the same lobe (arrows). Notice the extension of the bright fat and the small amount of anechoic effusion (*) between the bowel loops. The bowel segment in the near field is corrugated. **C:** Transverse sonogram of the right limb of the pancreas of a dog with acute abdominal pain and vomiting. The pancreas (cursors) is enlarged, hypoechoic, irregular, and ill-defined. The surrounding fat is hyperechoic and hyperattenuating, hampering the visualization of deeper structures (not shown). The descending duodenum is also significantly thickened (1 cm), but layers remain distinct. **D:** In the same dog, the colon (arrows) was markedly corrugated. A normal bowel loop is in the near field. Images C and D courtesy of M.A. d'Anjou.

Ultrasound-guided fine-needle aspiration is recommended to determine the nature of the collection. Peritoneal effusion secondary to pancreatitis is more common with the severe, hemorrhagic, necrotizing form of pancreatitis. The effusion is more commonly a small volume of fluid that accumulates in small pockets between the pancreas and adjacent mesentery.

Bile duct obstruction secondary to pancreatic inflammation and subsequent fibrosis can cause gallbladder and bile duct distension. In these cases, the common bile duct (CBD) is dilated and tortuous (Figure 9.13). In dogs, the normal CBD is not seen, whereas, in cats, the CBD often is visible and considered within normal limits when up to 4 mm in diameter (Léveillé et al. 1996). Serial ultrasonographic examinations of the biliary tract can be necessary to document progressive mechanical obstruction. Progressive dilation of the biliary tract from the common bile duct to the peripheral intrahepatic ducts occurred 1 week after experimental bile duct ligation (Nyland and Gillette 1982).

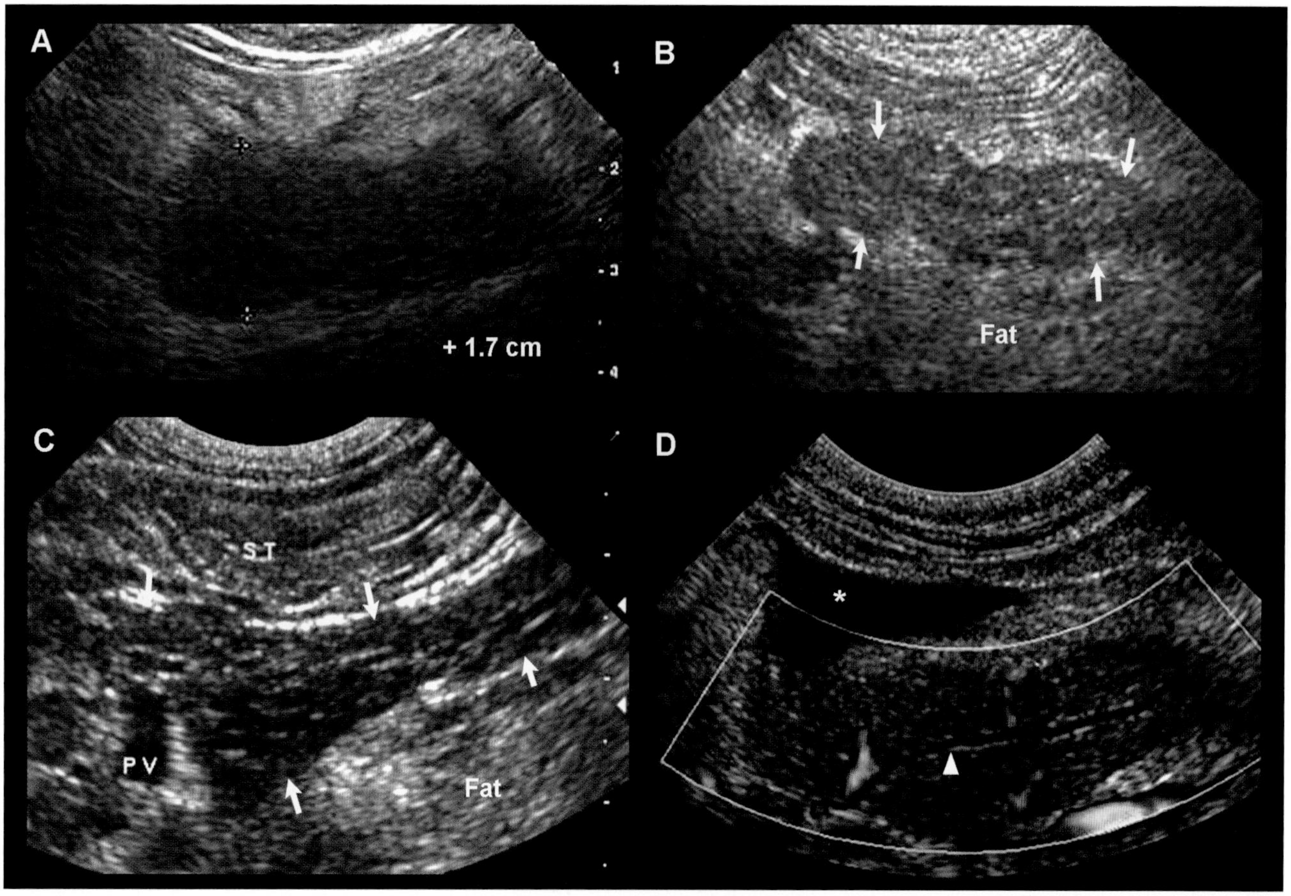

Figure 9.5. Acute pancreatitis in cats. **A:** Longitudinal sonogram of the left lobe of the pancreas. The lobe is markedly thickened, hypoechoic, and surrounded by hyperechoic local fat. **B:** In this other cat, the pancreas is only mildly thickened, but the surrounding fat is bright, outlining the pancreatic contours (arrows). **C:** The body and left lobe of the pancreas are within the upper limits of normal for size but appear hypoechoic. PV, portal vein; and ST, stomach. **D:** Power Doppler longitudinal image of the right limb of the pancreas in another cat. The pancreas is enlarged, hypoechoic, and surrounded by hyperechoic fat and focal anechoic peritoneal effusion (*). The pancreatic duct is clearly delineated (arrowhead) and not associated with flow, in comparison with nearby vessels.

Dilation of the extrahepatic bile ducts and gallbladder can remain despite reestablishment of normal bile flow after obstruction.

The mass effect created by an inflamed hypoechoic pancreas and hyperechoic peripancreatic tissue can displace the descending duodenum. Because the right pancreatic lobe is located dorsomedial to the descending duodenum, this loop of bowel is often displaced ventrolaterally (Murtaugh et al. 1985). In subacute to chronic active pancreatitis, the pancreas remains a distinct, well-defined hypoechoic structure that contrasts with the slightly hyperechoic peripancreatic mesentery (Figure 9.14A). At times, irregular margins of the pancreas and foci of mineralization can be seen (Figure 9.14B). Chronic pancreatitis characterized by interstitial fibrosis with acinar atrophy and lymphocytic infiltrates is rarely suspected clinically. Most cases encountered have vague clinical signs and nonspecific laboratory values. In these cases, the pancreas can be within normal range for size, and the parenchyma often is inhomogeneous (Figure 9.15). In cats, chronic pancreatitis is twice more frequent than acute pancreatitis. As this condition is often subclinical, it is very difficult to confirm the pancreatic changes histopathologically. On ultrasound, the changes can be similar to those described in dogs or subtle to inexistent (Figure 9.16). Acute necrotizing pancreatitis from chronic nonsuppurative pancreatitis cannot reliably be differenti-

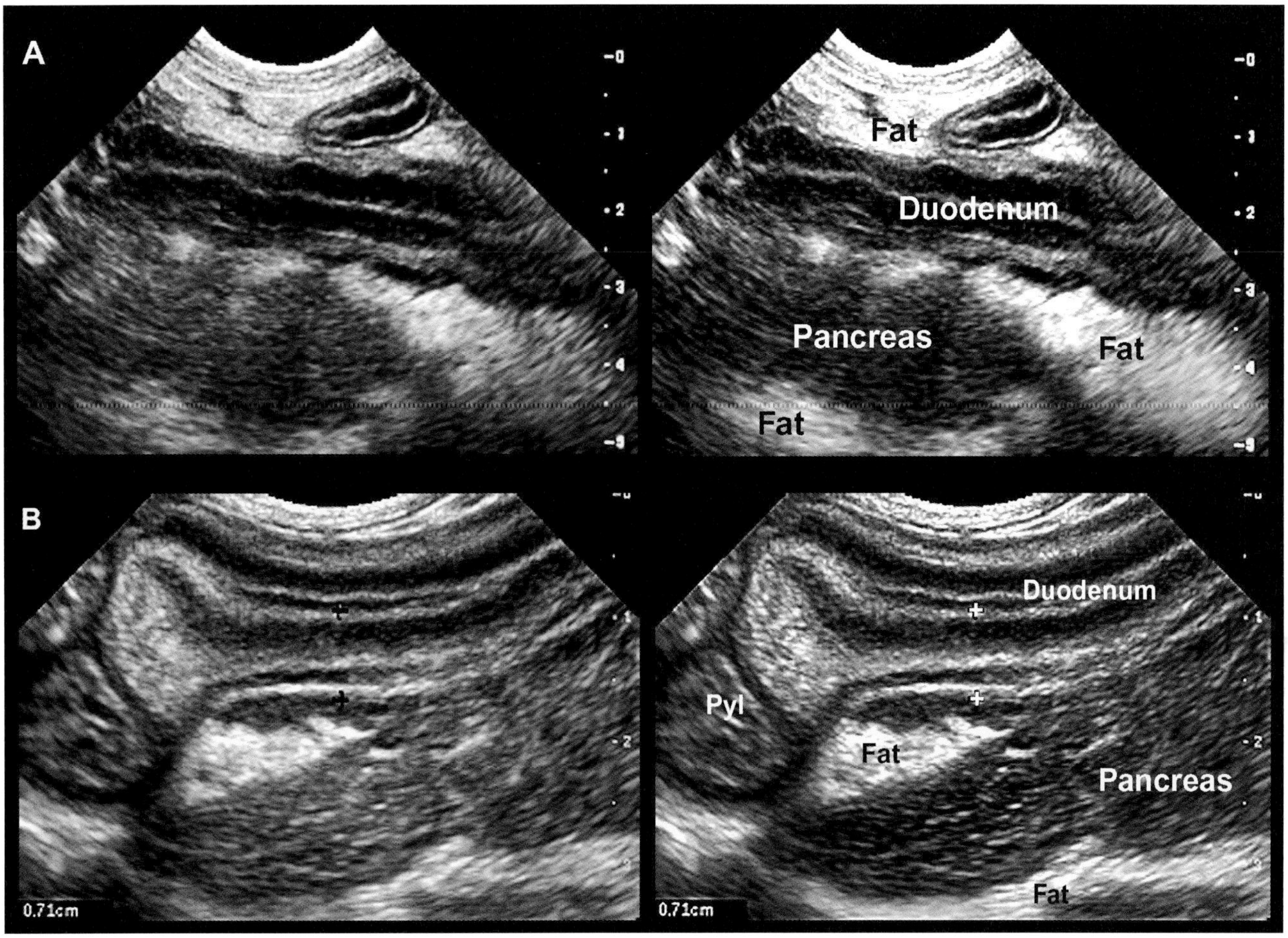

Figure 9.6. Duodenal changes associated with pancreatitis in two dogs. **A and B:** Longitudinal sonograms and corresponding schematic images of two dogs diagnosed with severe acute pancreatitis. In both, the duodenum is thickened and atonic, and the wall layering is altered. The right pancreatic limb is hypoechoic, and the surrounding fat is hyperechoic. Pyl, pylorus.

ated based on clincopathologic testing and/or sonographic abnormalities (Ferreri et al. 2003). A tissue core biopsy (under ultrasound guidance or at surgery) can be obtained to confirm the diagnosis.

In cats, the pancreatic duct can appear dilated (more than 1.3 mm) in acute pancreatitis (Wall et al. 2001) or chronic pancreatitis or even in older cats with no clinical evidence of active or chronic pancreatic disease. Pancreatic duct dilatation may also occur in association with pancreatic lithiasis (Figure 9.17E and F).

Pancreatic Nodular Hyperplasia and Neoplasia

Pancreatic nodular hyperplasia is occasionally seen in the pancreas of old dogs and cats. Well-defined hypoechoic to isoechoic nodules that can vary in size are recognized (Hecht et al. 2007) (Figure 9.18). These nodules can be confused for neoplastic disorders, such as insulinomas. They may also look similar to cystic formations, although far acoustic enhancement is not usually expected with soft-tissue nodules.

Pancreatic exocrine tumors such as adenocarcinoma arise from acinar cells or ductal epithelium. Even though these tumors are rare, they are the most common type of pancreatic neoplasia in small animals. They tend to develop in the central portion of the gland. As they grow, they may compress the common bile duct, invade the adjacent gastric and duodenal segments (Figure 9.19D), and frequently metastasize to the liver (Lamb et al. 1995). They often are poorly echogenic nodules or masses (Figure 9.18). Other

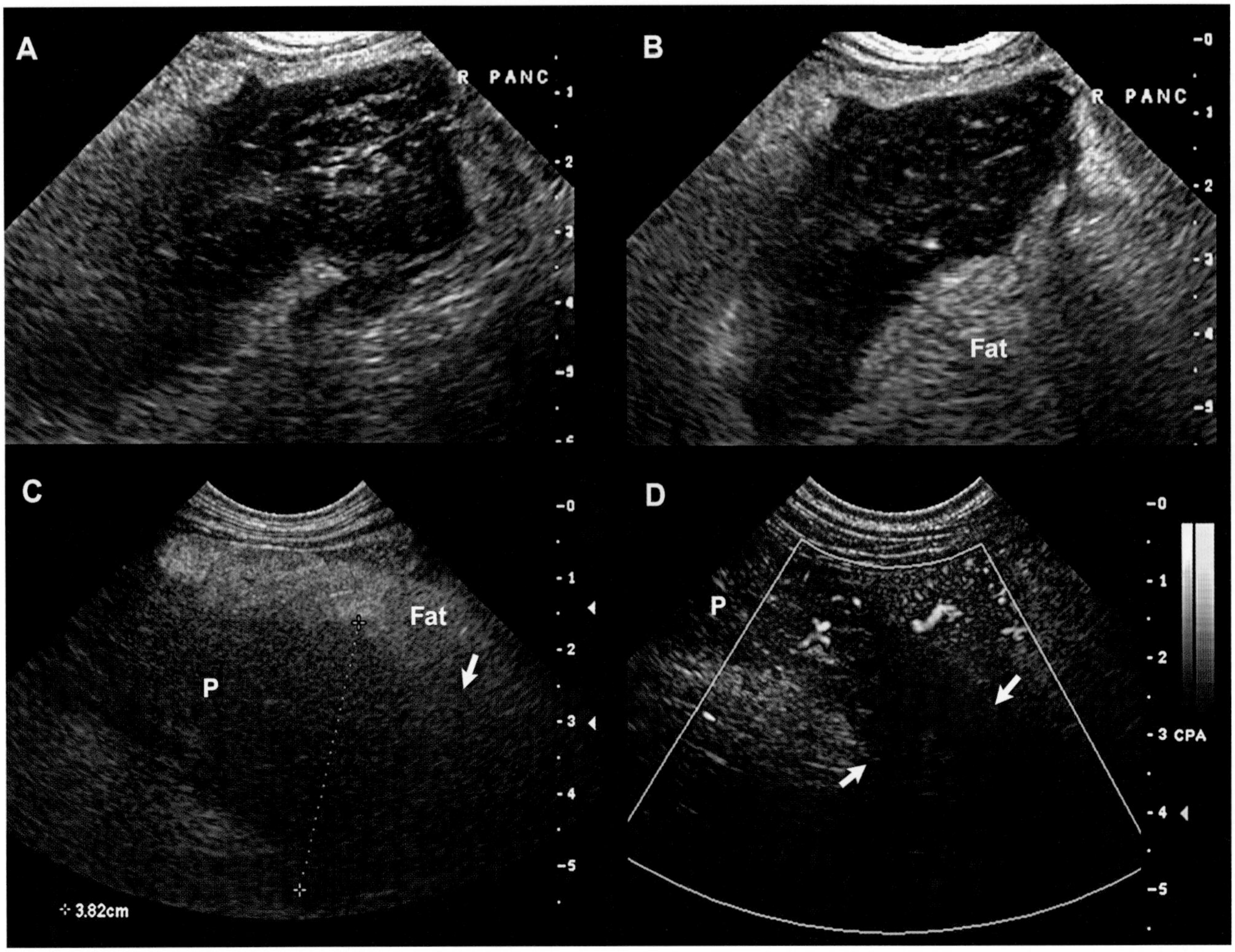

Figure 9.7. Necroticohemorrhagic pancreatitis in two dogs. **A and B:** Transverse **(A)** and longitudinal **(B)** sonograms of the thickened pancreas of an 8-year-old Labrador retriever with active suppurative pancreatitis with areas of hemorrhage and necrosis. The inhomogeneous and hypoechoic pancreas has irregular margins outlined by bright fat. **C and D:** Longitudinal sonograms of the right pancreatic limb in a 10-year-old golden retriever with severe necroticohemorrhagic pancreatitis. The pancreatic limb (P) is markedly enlarged, hypoechoic, and ill-defined, particularly in its distal extremity (arrows). Using Power Doppler **(D)** in this same region, there is no evidence of vascular flow motion, in comparison with the proximal portion of the limb. The superficial fat shows increased vascularity. Images C and D courtesy of M.A. d'Anjou.

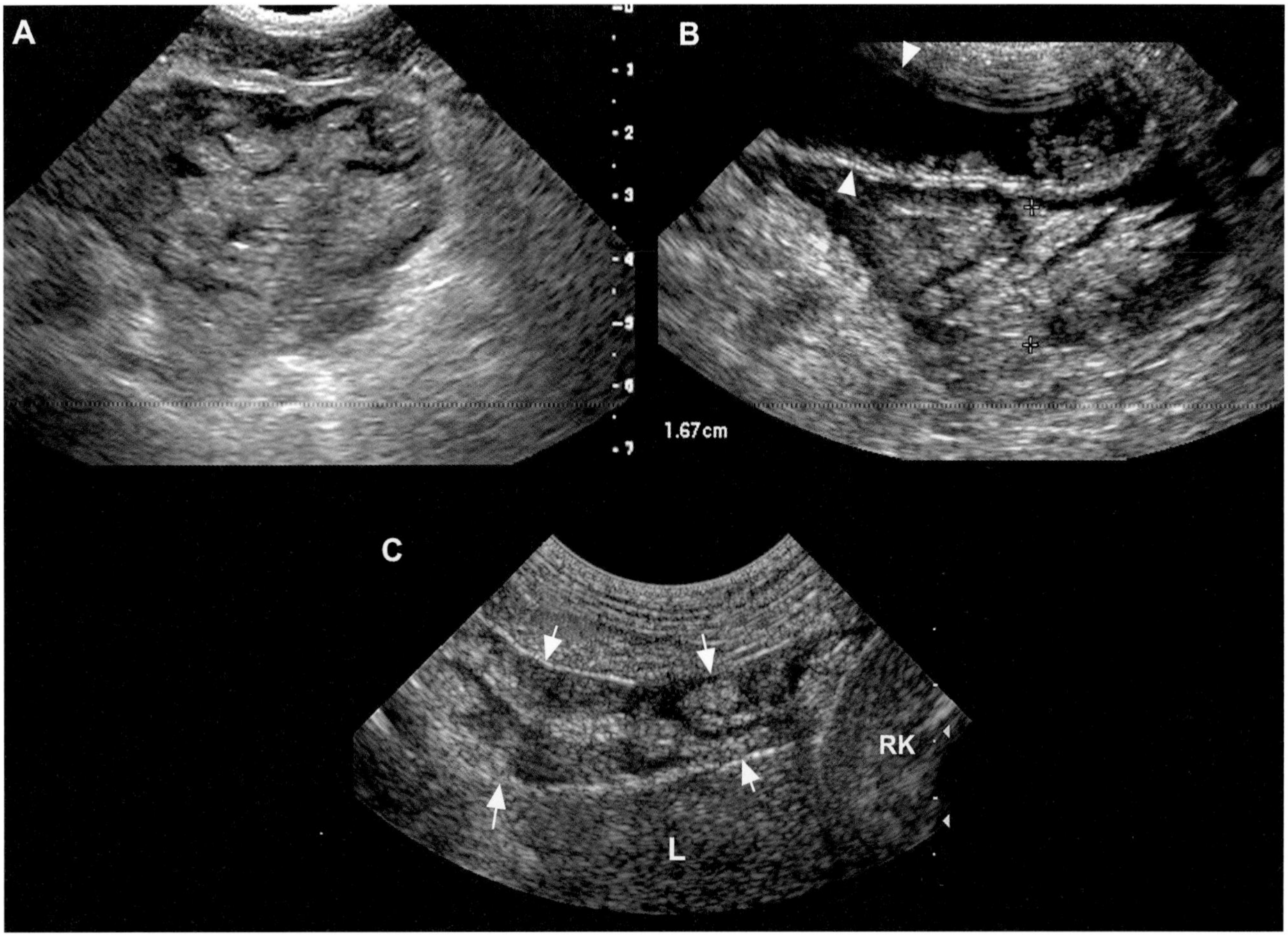

Figure 9.8. Pancreatic edema in dogs. **A:** Transverse sonogram of the edematous thickened pancreas (the same dog as in Figure 9.7A and B). The pancreas is enlarged and has anechoic stripes. The surrounding fat is hyperechoic. **B:** Longitudinal sonogram of the right pancreatic lobe of a 3-year-old Welsh corgi with pancreatitis. Hypoechoic striations are crossing the pancreas, and the contours of the pancreas are outlined by fluid. A dilated, fluid-filled segment of bowel is noted in the near field (arrowheads). **C:** Longitudinal sonographic image of the right pancreatic limb (arrows) in a small dog with acute portal hypertension following surgery for an extrahepatic portosystemic shunt. Characteristic hypoechoic to anechoic stripes noted in the pancreas are consistent with edema. These changes resolved a day later. L, liver; and RK, right kidney. Image C courtesy of M.A. d'Anjou.

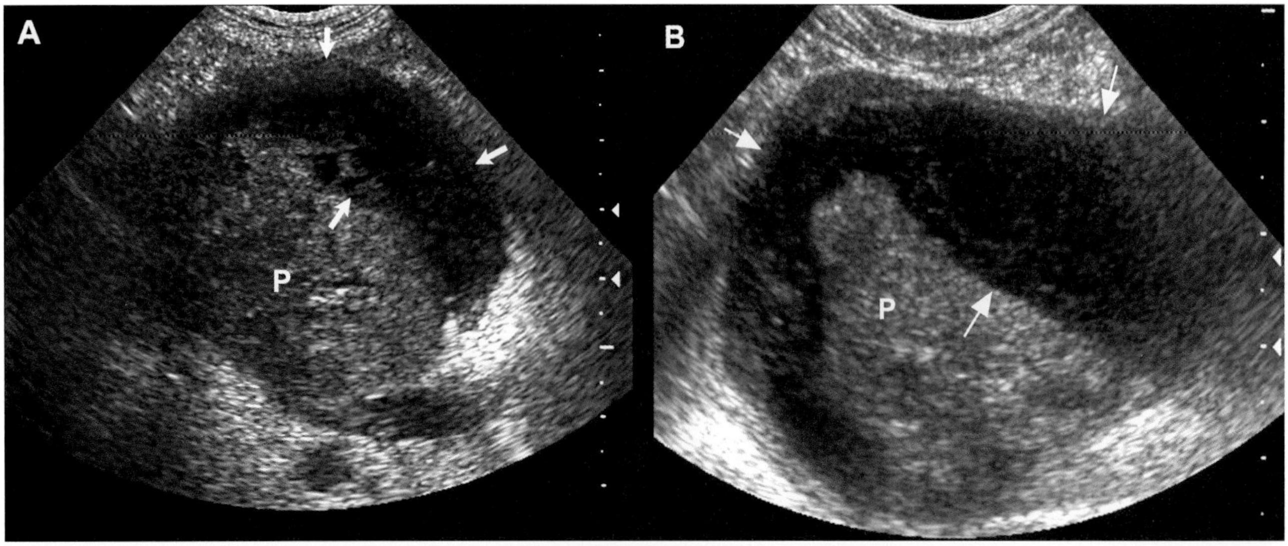

Figure 9.9. Pancreatic pseudocyst in a dog. Transverse **(A)** and longitudinal **(B)** sonograms of a large pancreatic pseudocyst associated with a severe acute pancreatitis. Part of the thickened and hypoechoic pancreas (P) is in the center of the hypoechoic to nearly anechoic lesion representing the pseudocyst (arrows). Ultrasound-guided fine-needle aspiration confirmed the diagnosis.

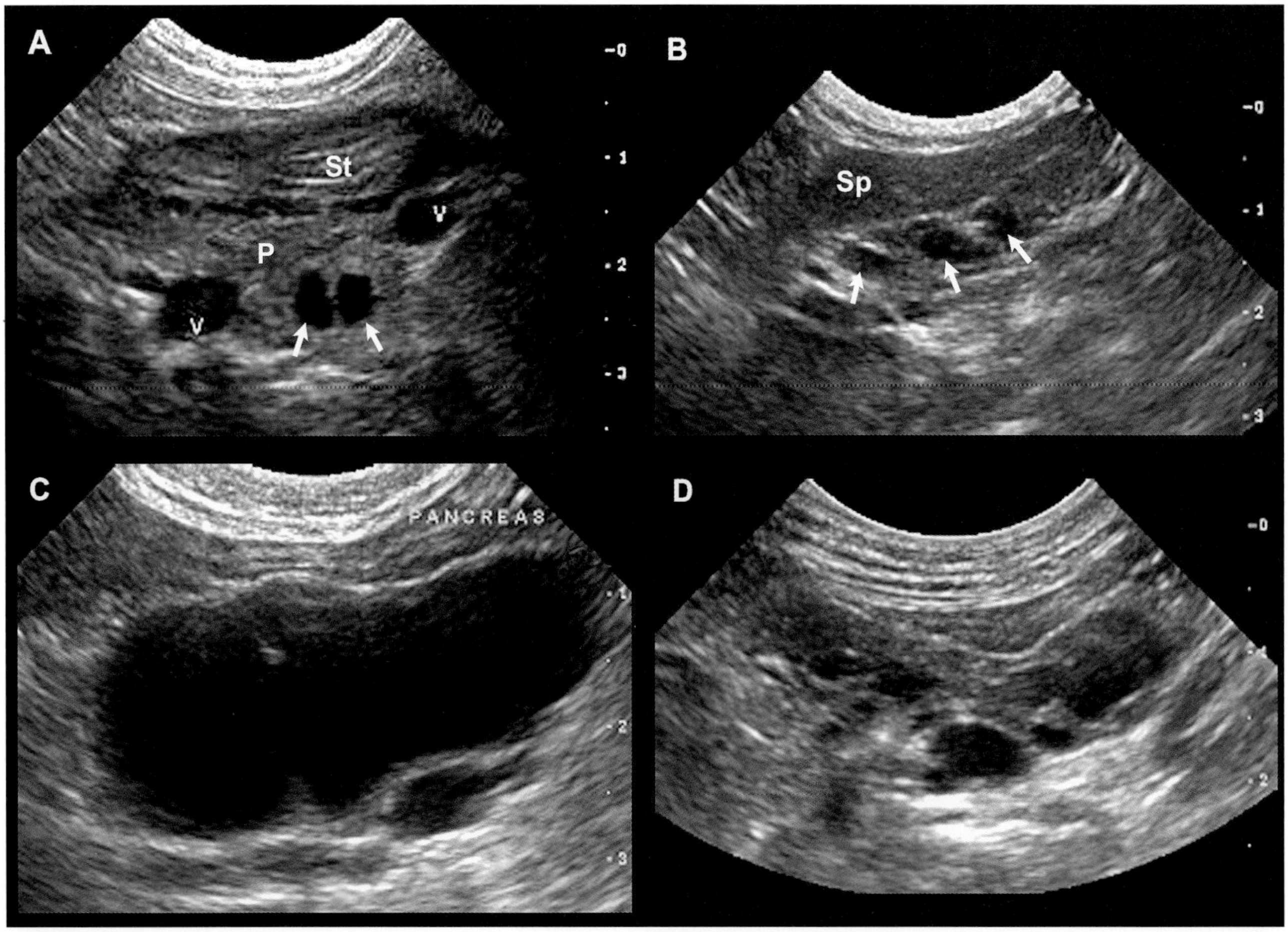

Figure 9.10. Pancreatic cysts in dogs and cats. **A:** Oblique sonogram of two small cystic lesions (arrows) in the left pancreatic lobe (P) of an 11-year-old miniature schnauzer. St, stomach; and V, adjacent vessels. **B:** Longitudinal sonogram of the distal extremity of the left pancreatic lobe of an 18-year-old cat with several cystlike changes (arrows). This cat had no clinical history of previous pancreatitis. Sp, spleen. **C:** Large pancreatic cyst on the left lobe and body of the pancreas in a 16-year-old cat. **D:** The same region after ultrasound-guided drainage of the cyst presented in Figure 9.10C.

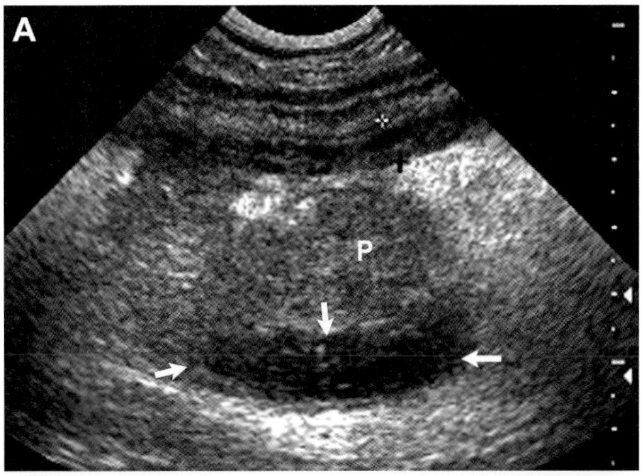

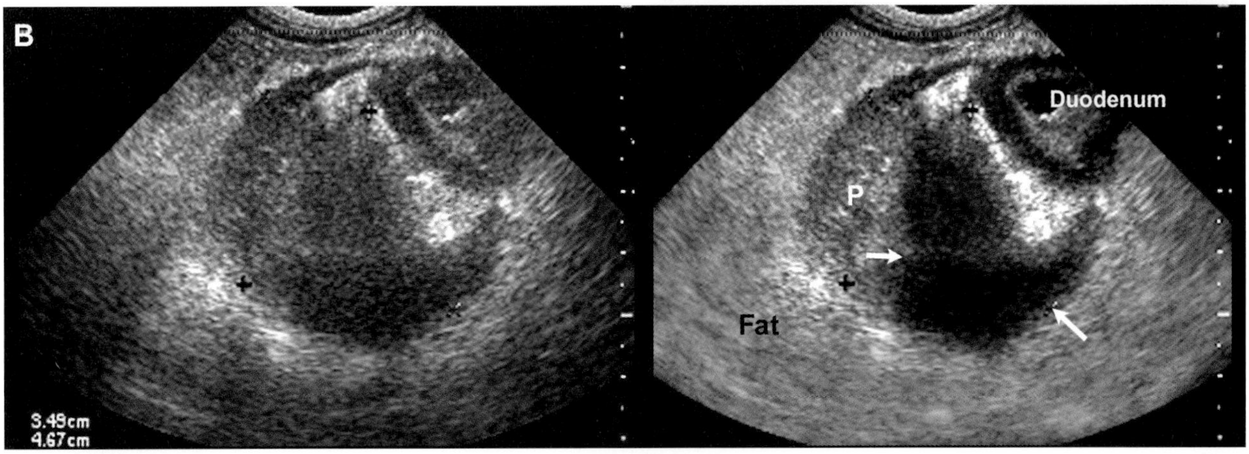

Figure 9.11. Pancreatic abscess in two dogs. **A:** Longitudinal sonogram of an ovoid discrete hypoechoic cavity (arrows) in the right pancreatic lobe (P) of a 6-year-old cocker spaniel. Notice the thickened and atonic (fluid filled) duodenum in the near field (cursors). The muscularis layer of the duodenal wall is especially prominent. Hyperechoic fat is seen around the pancreas. The cavity was confirmed by ultrasound-guided aspiration to be an abscess. **B:** Transverse sonogram and corresponding schematic sonogram of an abscess (arrows) in the right pancreatic lobe (P) of a 10-year-old Labrador crossed. The peripheral fat is hyperechoic, indicating steatitis.

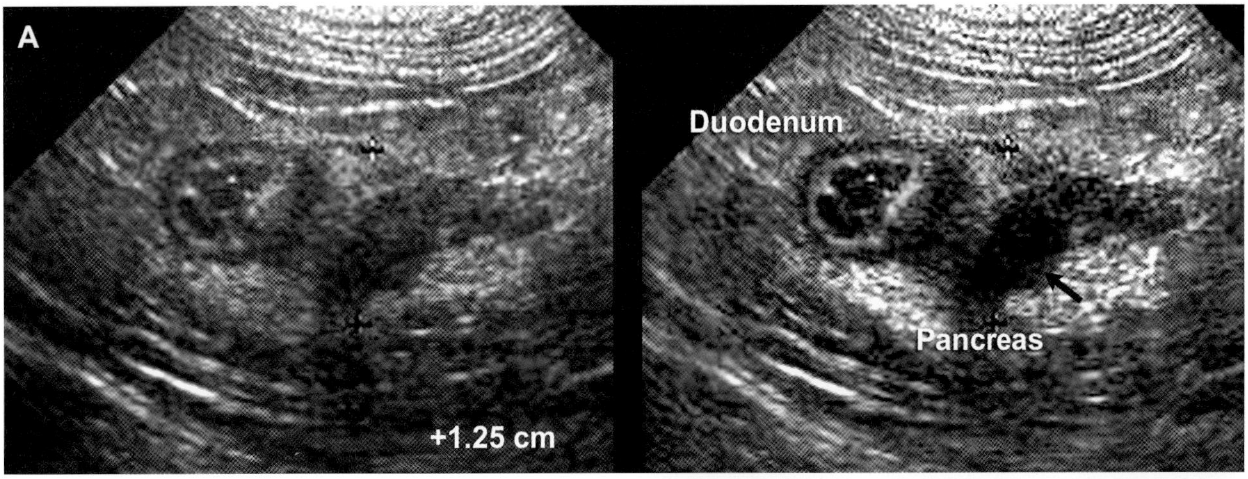

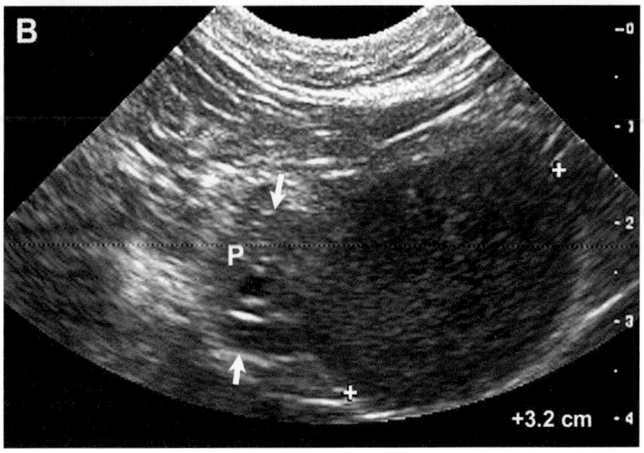

Figure 9.12. Pancreatic abscess in two cats. **A:** Sonogram and corresponding schematic image of a small hypoechoic cavity (arrow) in the cranial part of the right pancreatic lobe (between the cursors). The lesion deforms the contour of the pancreas and is outlined by focally bright fat. **B:** Large cavity containing a mildly echogenic fluid (between the cursors, +) severely deforming the right lobe of the pancreas (P, between the arrows). With gentle pressure, the echogenic fluid moved on real-time examination.

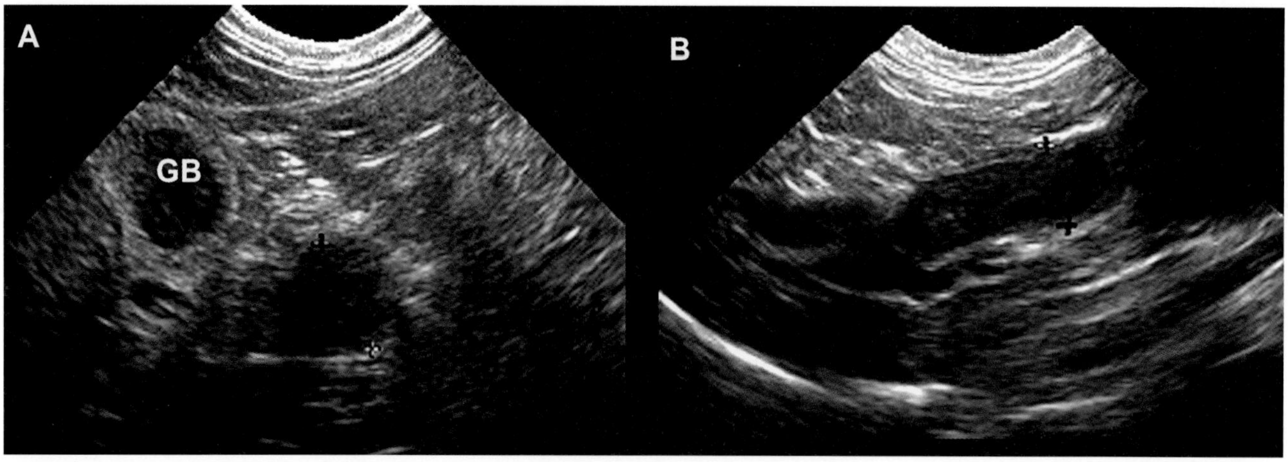

Figure 9.13. Dilated common bile duct in a cat with pancreatitis. Transverse **(A)** and longitudinal **(B)** sonograms of the common bile duct (between the cursors) in a cat with pancreatitis and pancreatic abscess (the same cat as in Figure 9.12B). The CBD is greatly distended, reaching 1.4 cm in diameter proximally **(A)** and 1.2 cm distally **(B)**. Notice that the CBD and gallbladder (GB) walls are thickened.

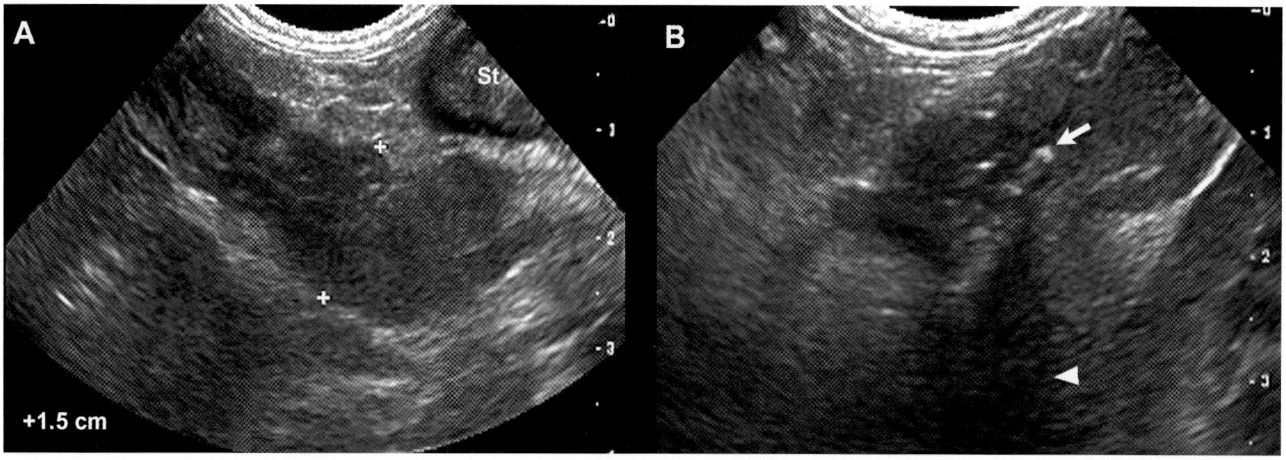

Figure 9.14. Chronic pancreatitis in two dogs. **A:** Diffuse chronic active necrotizing pancreatitis with fibrosis and regeneration in a 14-year-old shih tzu. The pancreas (cursors) is markedly irregular and mostly hypoechoic, with a few inhomogeneous areas. It is 1.5 cm thick. St, stomach. **B:** Presumptive chronic pancreatitis in an 11-year-old mixed-breed dog. Numerous hyperechoic foci are seen in the pancreas (arrow). Some of these foci are associated with shadowing (arrowhead), suggesting mineralization. The pancreas is hypoechoic, but the surrounding fat is normal.

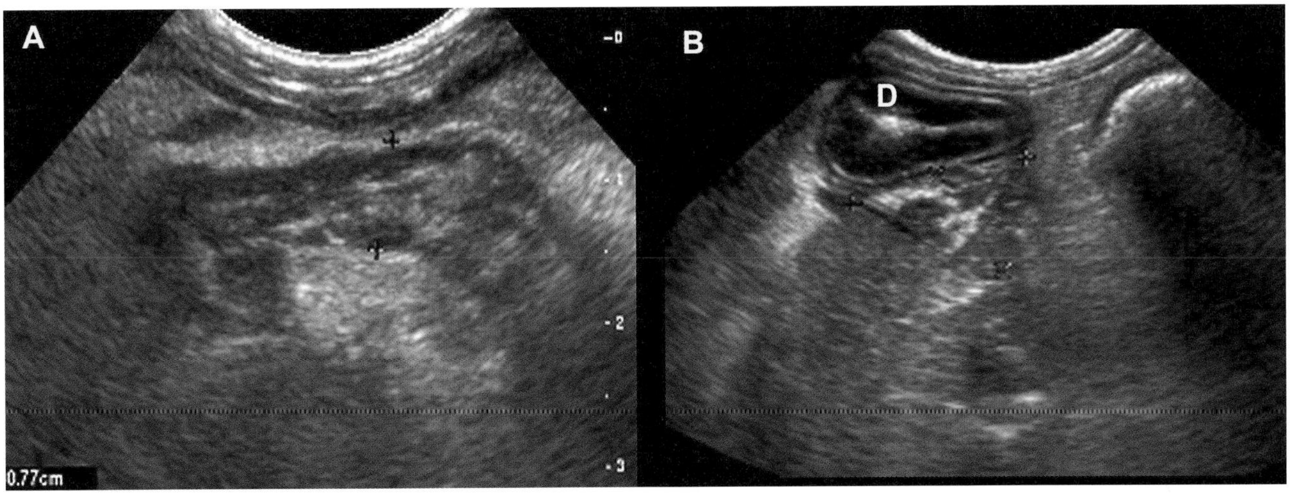

Figure 9.15. Chronic pancreatitis in an 8-year-old Australian shepherd. The sagittal **(A)** and transverse **(B)** sonograms of the right pancreatic lobe (between the cursors) show a pancreas that is within normal range for size but very inhomogeneous. D, duodenum.

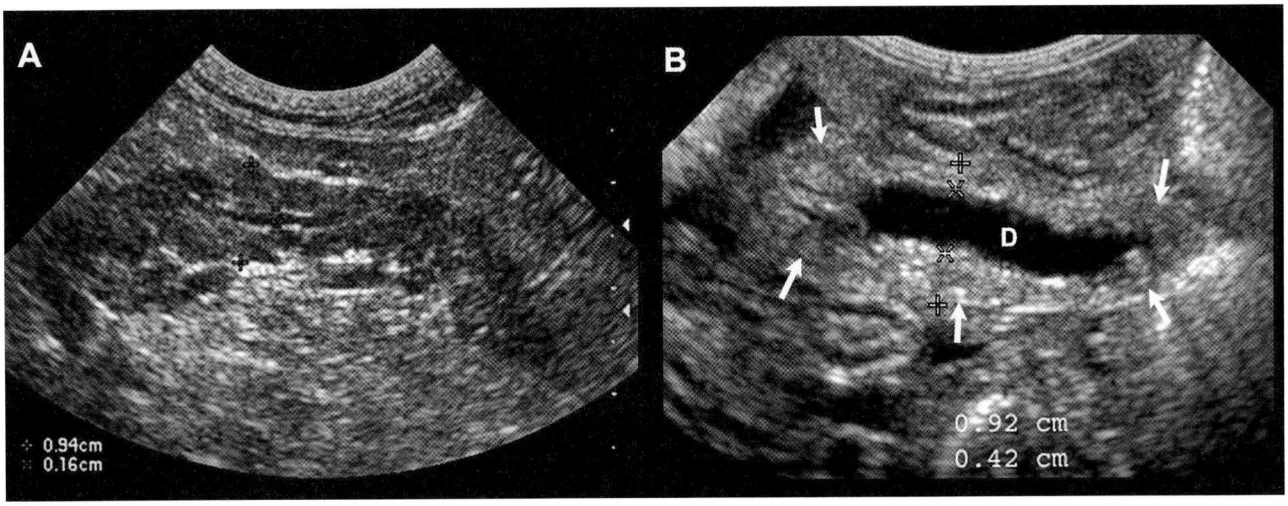

Figure 9.16. Chronic pancreatitis in two cats. **A:** Longitudinal sonographic image of the left pancreatic limb of a cat with diffuse lymphoplasmocytic pancreatitis. The pancreas is irregular and mildly hypoechoic. The central pancreatic duct appears normal. **B:** Chronic pancreatitis with pancreatic atrophy and Islet cell fibrosis in another cat. The pancreas (arrows) appears thickened (9.2 mm) and hyperechoic, but the pancreatic duct (D) is dilated (4.2 mm), counting for nearly half of the overall pancreatic lobe thickness.

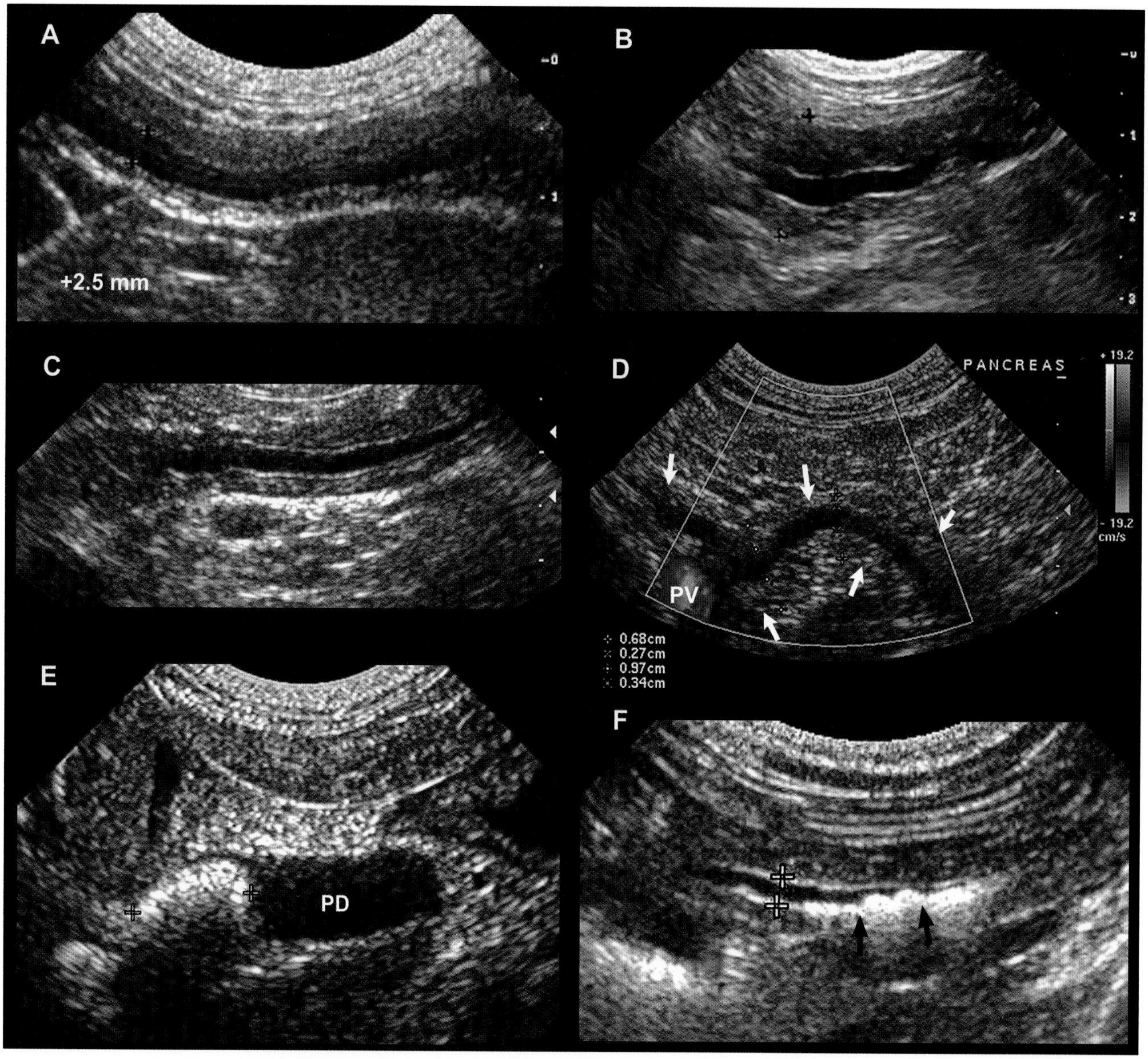

Figure 9.17. Dilated pancreatic duct (PD) in cats. **A:** Smoothly dilated, 2.5-mm-wide PD (between the cursors) in a 12-year-old cat with two concurrent pancreatic cystic lesions and hepatic disease. **B:** Dilated, 3-mm-wide PD in a 16-year-old cat with concurrent hepatitis and suspected pancreatitis. The pancreas is delineated by the cursors. **C:** Dilated and thickened, 3.5-mm-wide PD in a 14-year-old cat with hepatitis and fibrosing choledochitis. The pancreas appears normal. **D:** Dilated, 3.4-mm-wide PD (between the cursors) in an elderly cat with pancreatic atrophy. The pancreatic tissue around the PD is barely visible (arrows). Color Doppler can be useful in differentiating a PD from vessels. PV, portal vein. **E:** Large calculus (between the cursors) in this dilated, 1-cm-wide PD. **F:** Dilated PD with small intraluminal calculi and mineralized sediments.

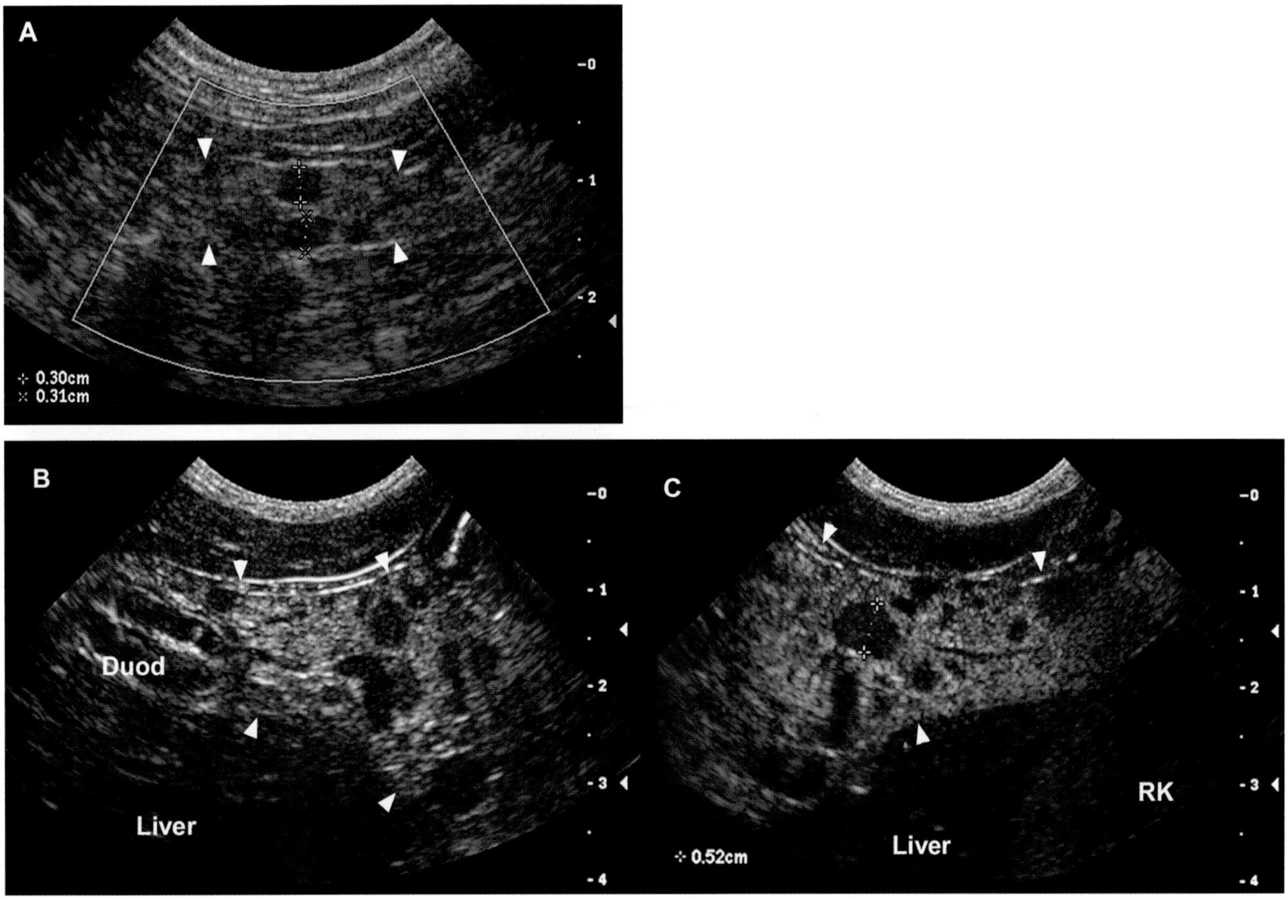

Figure 9.18. Nodular hyperplasia in a cat and a dog. **A:** Longitudinal sonographic image with color Doppler of the pancreas of a cat with chronic inflammatory bowel disease. Two well-defined 3-mm hypoechoic nodules (between the cursors) are identified in the left pancreatic limb (arrowheads). The rest of the pancreas is mildly heterogeneous. **B and C:** Transverse **(B)** and longitudinal **(C)** sonographic images of the right pancreatic limb of a small-breed dog with diabetes mellitus. Several well-defined, hypoechoic nodules of variable size and shape are seen throughout the pancreatic tissue (arrowheads), which is otherwise hyperechoic. There was no evidence of changes to the peripheral fat. Fine-needle aspiration of the pancreas revealed the presence of mild, chronic pancreatitis with nodular hyperplasia. Duod, duodenum; and RK, right kidney. Images courtesy of M.A. d'Anjou.

tumors have occasionally been encountered in the pancreas of dogs and cats: cystadenoma, metastatic carcinoma, and lymphoma (Figure 9.20).

Pancreatic endocrine tumors such as glucagonomas, insulinomas, and gastrinomas are uncommon. From that group, insulinomas are the most commonly encountered in dogs. The ultrasound detection rate varies depending on the size and distribution of the lesions, the equipment quality, and the operator's experience. The visibility of these lesions may also be affected by the presence of overlying gastrointestinal content and by body conformation (e.g., deep-chested or obese dogs). Insulinomas can present as a solitary nodule, multiple nodules, or an ill-defined area of abnormal echogenicity (Figure 9.21). The size of the pancreatic lesions varies greatly, but a majority of the lesions tend to be less or equal to 2.5 cm and poorly echogenic (Lamb et al. 1995).

Most endocrine tumors are malignant and tend to spread to the regional lymph nodes and liver. Therefore, sonographic screening of the hepatic parenchyma and regional lymph nodes is recommended to detect possible hepatic metastasis (Figure 9.22). Metastatic lymph nodes often are enlarged and hypoechoic.

Whereas pancreatic tumors usually present as a focal nodule or mass, neoplasia cannot reliably be differentiated from pancreatitis (Figure 9.23) or nodular hyperplasia.

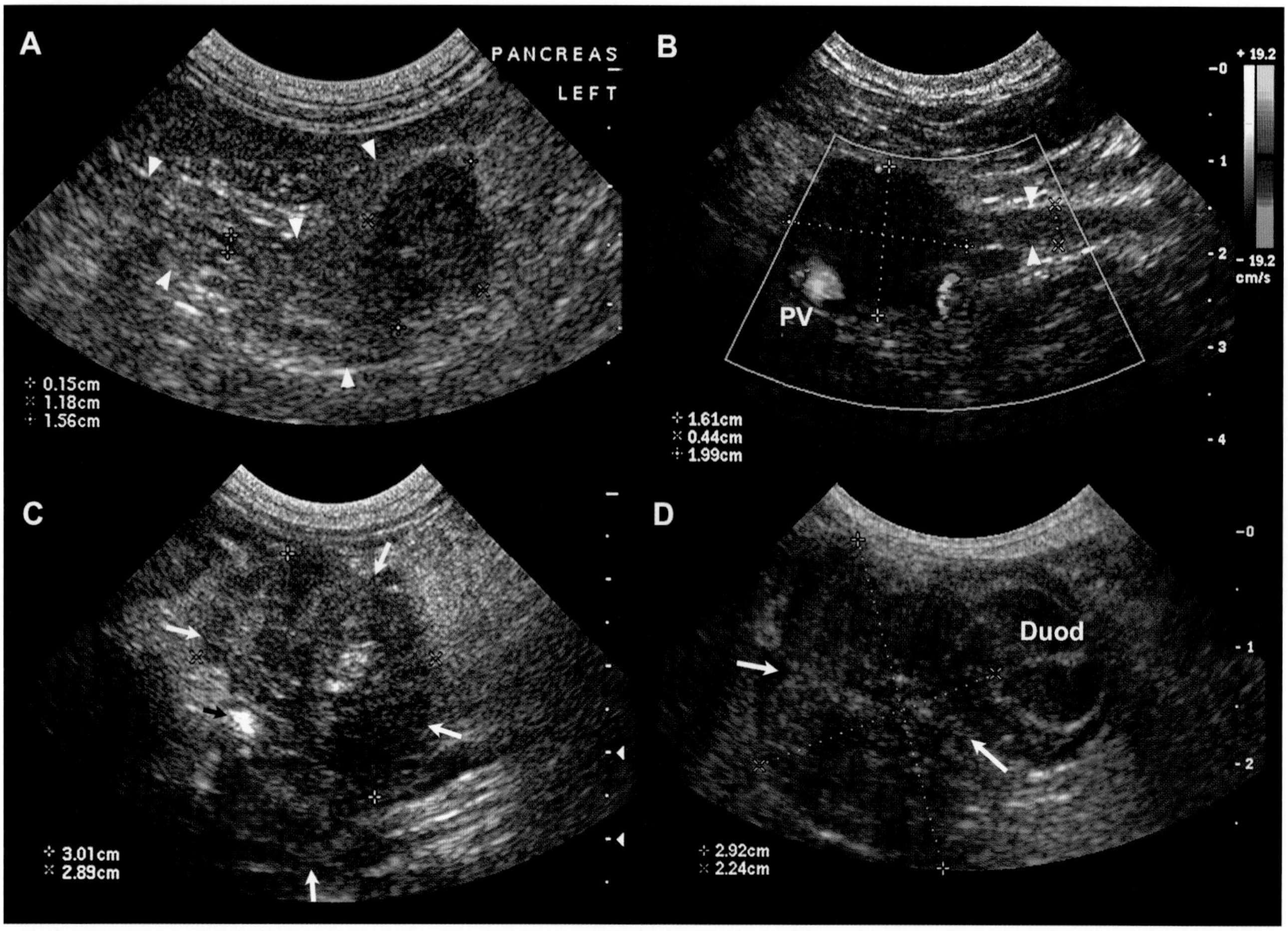

Figure 9.19. Pancreatic carcinomas in cats and dogs. **A:** Longitudinal sonographic image of the left pancreatic limb (arrowheads) in a cat. A small hypoechoic mass (1.5 cm) at the tail of this limb indicated pancreatic adenocarcinoma. **B:** Another hypoechoic mass found in the proximal portion of the left pancreatic limb of a cat. This mass is adjacent to the portal vein (PV). The rest of the left limb (arrowheads) is normal. Pancreatic adenocarcinoma was confirmed histologically. **C:** A larger mass (white arrows, 3 cm) in another cat is consistent with a poorly differentiated carcinoma. This mass is heterogeneous and has mineral foci (black arrow) associated with acoustic shadowing. **D:** Transverse sonographic view of a pancreatic mass (arrows) invading the wall of the duodenum in a dog. A poorly differentiated carcinoma was diagnosed with cytology after fine-needle aspiration. Images courtesy of M.A. d'Anjou.

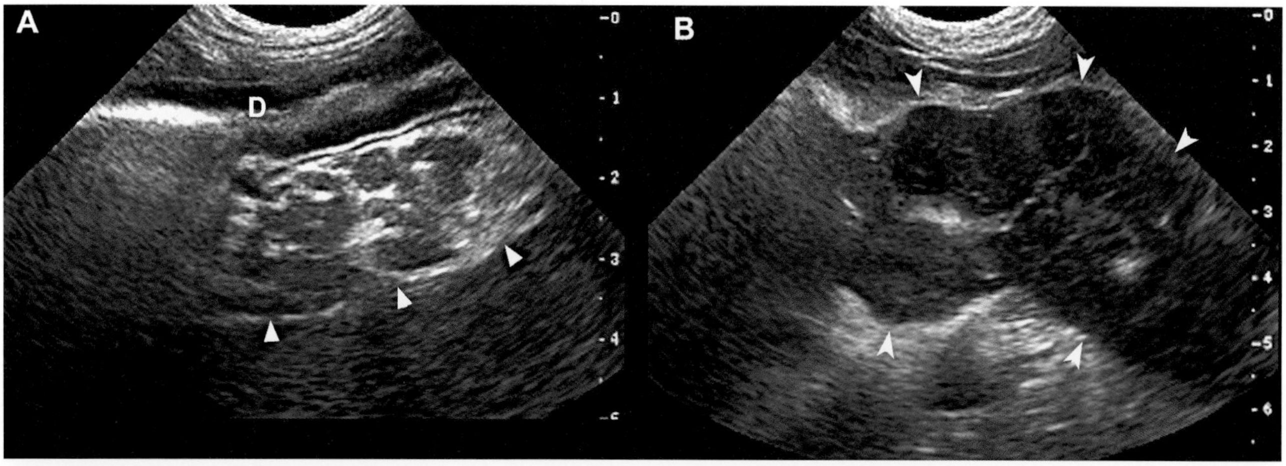

Figure 9.20. Pancreatic lymphoma in two dogs. **A:** Numerous variably sized hypoechoic nodules replace the normal echotexture of the pancreas (arrowheads) in this 4-year-old mixed-breed dog. The duodenum (D) is seen in the near field. **B:** Diffuse pancreatic enlargement (arrowheads) associated with diffuse hypoechogenicity in this 7-year-old Labrador retriever.

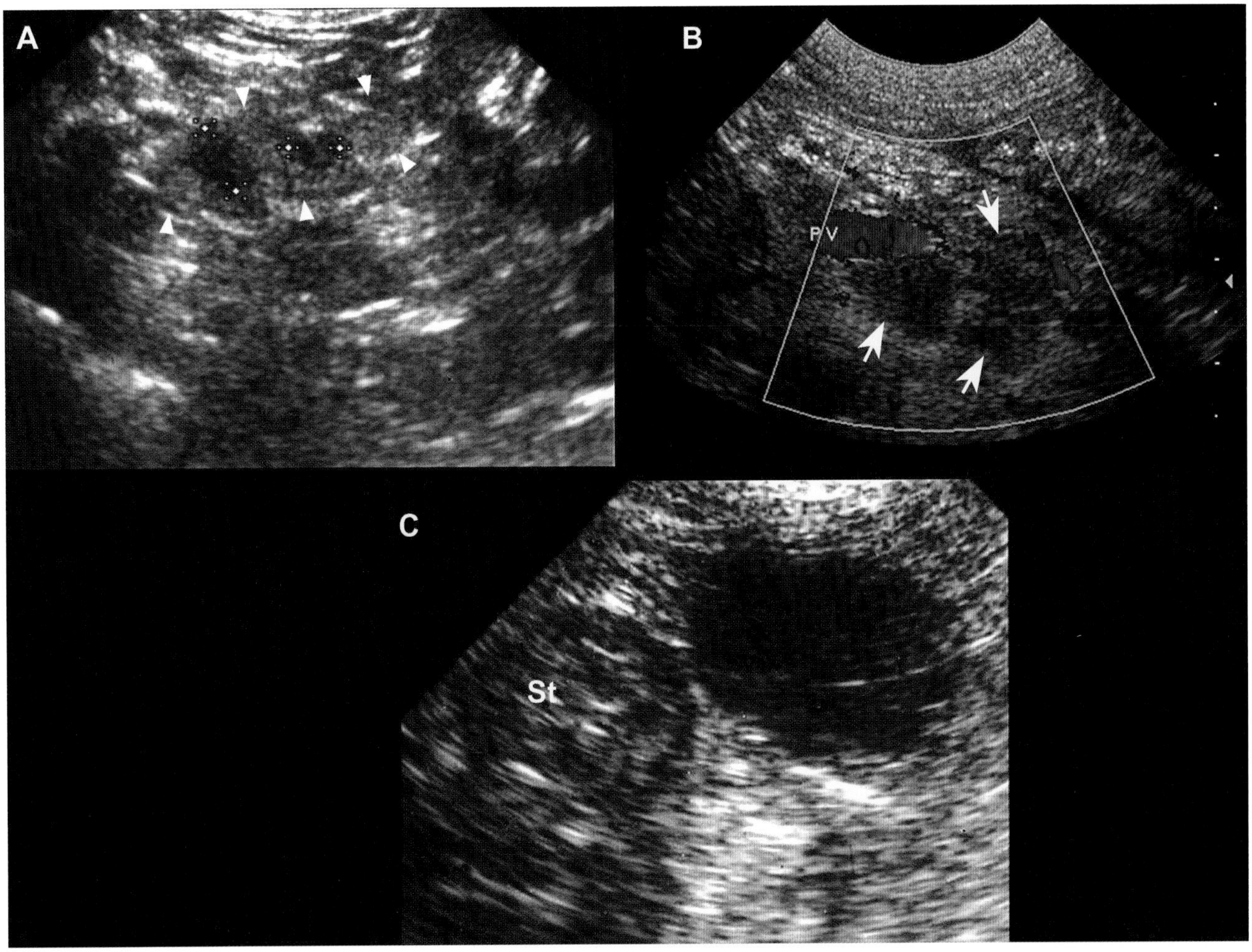

Figure 9.21. Pancreatic insulinoma in dogs. Insulinoma can appear as a single hypoechoic nodule or as several hypoechoic nodules **(A and B)** or less commonly as a hypoechoic mass **(C)**. The nodular lesions are between the cursors **(A)** and the arrows **(B)**. The pancreas is delineated by the arrowheads in **A**. In **B** is color Doppler assessment of the pancreatic region with several small hypoechoic nodules (arrows). The portal vein (PV) is ventral to the body of the pancreas. St, stomach.

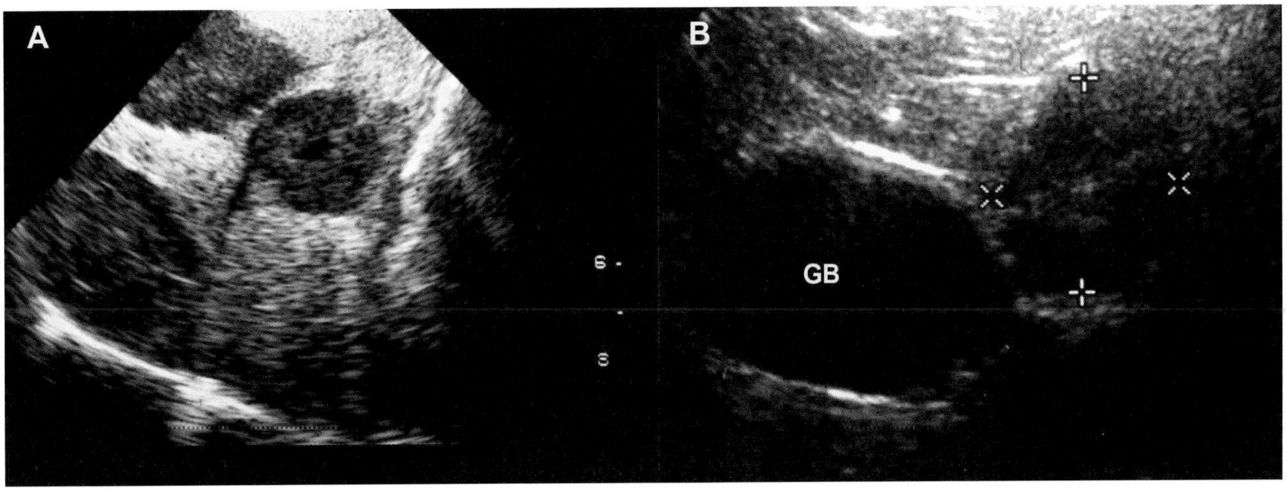

Figure 9.22. Metastatic insulinoma to the liver and lymph nodes. **A:** Multiple target-shaped nodules are present in several liver lobes. Ultrasound-guided core biopsies confirmed the diagnosis of hepatic metastases caused by insulinoma. **B:** A single large hypoechoic nodule is in the hilus of the liver, near the gallbladder (GB), which is consistent with metastatic lymphadenopathy.

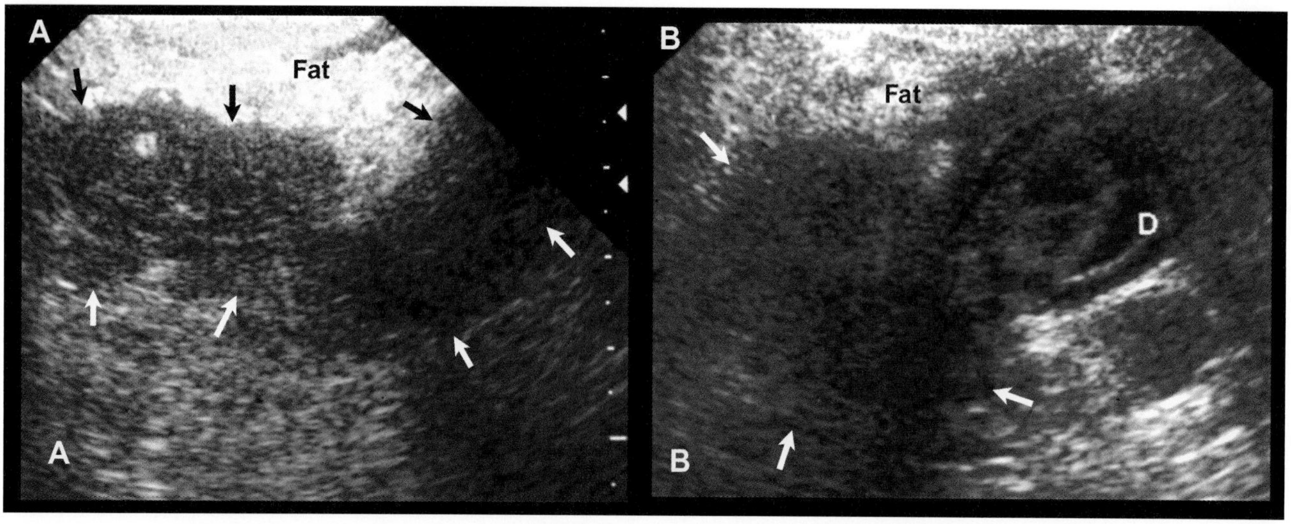

Figure 9.23. Pancreatic adenocarcinoma in a dog. Longitudinal **(A)** and transverse **(B)** sonograms of the diffusely thickened and hypoechoic pancreas (arrows) surrounded by bright fat mimics pancreatitis. The histopathologic diagnosis on surgical samples is adenocarcinoma. Tumoral infiltration can also be associated with inflammation. D, duodenum.

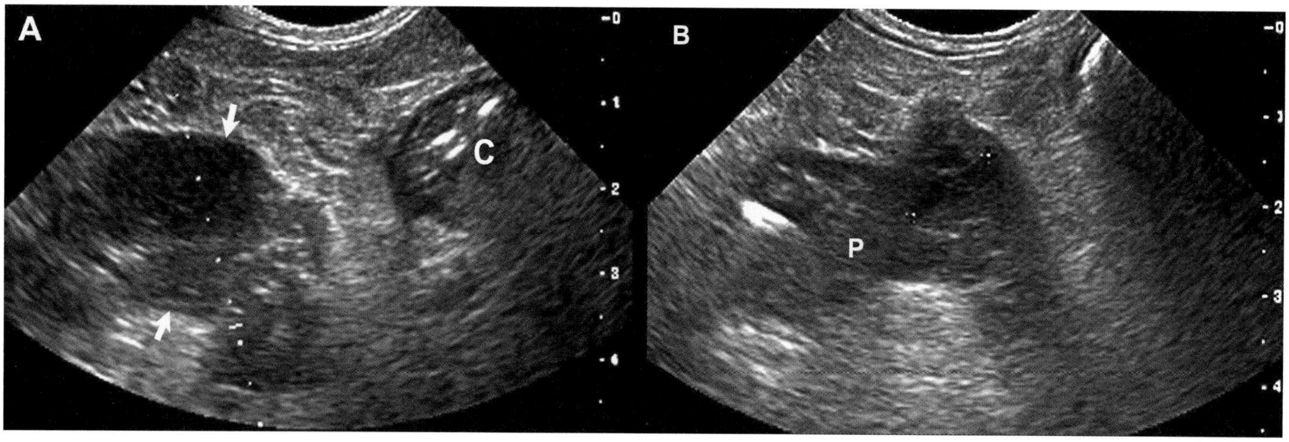

Figure 9.24. Drainage of cavitary lesion in 9-year-old Australian shepherd. **A:** A hypoechoic cavity (arrows) is present in the enflamed pancreas of this dog. The needle track is centered on the cavity. The cavity was drained, and about 10 mL of bloody purulent fluid was withdrawn. The final diagnosis was sterile abscess. C, colon. **B:** A recheck 1 week later shows a smaller and poorly defined cavity (between the cursors) in the same portion of the pancreas (P), and the dog's condition improved clinically. The peripheral fat remained hyperechoic.

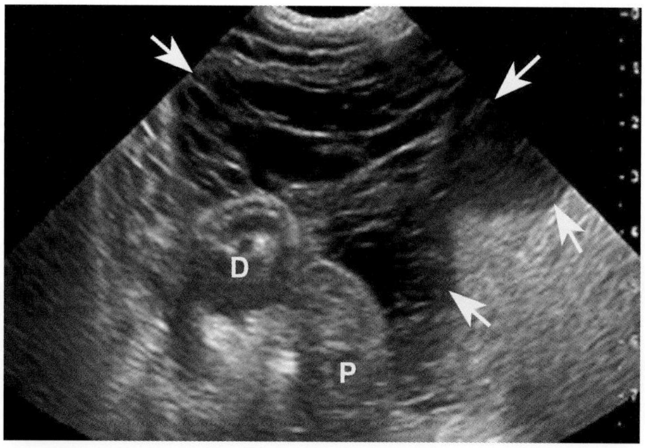

Figure 9.25. Recheck after lidocaine intraperitoneal injection in a miniature schnauzer with pancreatitis. The injection was performed to control persistent and severe pain. An extensively hypoechoic to anechoic and striated area (arrows) near the pancreas (P) and duodenum (D) most likely represents an iatrogenic hematoma.

Special Procedures

Fine-needle aspiration or core biopsy of diffuse or focal pancreatic lesions can be performed safely if adequate precautions are taken to avoid large vessels.

Fluid-filled lesions, such as pseudocysts and abscesses, can also be sampled and drained safely under ultrasound guidance (Figure 9.24). Serial ultrasound examinations are useful in monitoring resolution or progression of fluid-filled lesions or response to treatment (Figure 9.25).

References

Akol KG, Washabau RJ, Saunders HM, Hendrick MJ (1993) Acute pancreatitis in cats with hepatic lipidosis. J Vet Intern Med 7:205–209.

Edwards DF, Bauer MS, Walker MA, Pardo AD, McCracken MD, Walker TL (1990) Pancreatic masses in seven dogs following acute pancreatitis. J Am Anim Hosp Assoc 26:189–198.

Etue SM, Penninck DG, Labato MA, Pearson S, Tidwell A (2001) Ultrasonography of the normal feline pancreas and associated anatomical landmarks: A prospective study of 20 cats. Vet Radiol Ultrasound 42:330–336.

Ferreri JA, Hardam E, Kimmel SA, et al. (2003) Clinical differentiation of acute necrotizing from chronic nonsuppurative pancreatitis in cats: 63 cases (1996–2001). J Am Vet Med Assoc 223:469–474.

Hecht S, Penninck DG, Keating JH (2007) Imaging findings in pancreatic neoplasia and nodular hyperplasia in 19 cats. Vet Radiol Ultrasound 48:45–50.

Hecht S, Penninck DG, Mahony OM, King R, Rand WM (2006) Relationship of pancreatic duct dilation to age and clinical findings in cats. Vet Radiol Ultrasound 47:287–294.

Hines BL, Salisbury SK, Jakovljevic S, De Nicola DB (1996) Pancreatic pseudocyst associated with chronic-active necrotizing pancreatitis in a cat. J Am Anim Hosp Assoc 32:147–152.

Lamb CR (1999) Pancreatic edema in dogs with hypoalbuminemia and portal hypertension. J Vet Intern Med 13:498–500.

Lamb CR, Simpson KW, Boswood A, Matthewman LA (1995) Ultrasonography of pancreatic neoplasia in the dog: A retrospective review of 16 cases. Vet Rec 37:65–68.

Léveillé R, Biller DS, Shiroma JT (1996) Sonographic evaluation of the common bile duct in cats. J Vet Intern Med 10:296–299

Moon ML, Panciera DL, Ward DL, Steiner JM, Williams DA (2005) Age-related changes in the ultrasound appearance of the normal feline pancreas. Vet Radiol Ultrasound 46:138–142.

Murtaugh RJ, Herring DS, Jacobs RM, DeHoff WD (1985) Pancreatic ultrasonography in dogs with experimentally induced acute pancreatitis. Vet Radiol Ultrasound 26:27–32.

Nyland TG, Gillette NA (1982) Sonographic evaluation of experimental bile duct ligation in the dog. Vet Radiol Ultrasound 23:252–260.

Nyland TG, Mulvany MH, Strombeck DR (1983) Ultrasonic features of experimentally induced, acute pancreatitis in the dog. Vet Radiol Ultrasound 24:260–266.

Rutgers C, Herring DS, Orton EC (1985) Pancreatic pseudocyst associated with acute pancreatitis in a dog: Ultrasonographic diagnosis. J Am Anim Hosp Assoc 21:411–416.

Salisbury SK, Lantz GC, Nelson RW, Kazacos EA (1988) Pancreatic abscess in dogs: Six cases (1978–1986). J Am Vet Med Assoc 193:1104–1108.

Saunders HM (1991) Ultrasonography of the pancreas. Probl Vet Med 3:583–603.

Saunders HM, VanWinkle TJ, Drobatz K, Kimmel SE, Washabau RJ (2002) Ultrasonographic findings in cats with clinical, gross pathologic, and histologic evidence of acute pancreatic necrosis: 20 cases (1994–2001) J Am Vet Med Assoc 221:1724–1730.

VanEnkevort BA, O'Brien RT, Young KM (1999) Pancreatic pseudocysts in 4 dogs and 2 cats: Ultrasonographic and clinicopathologic findings. J Vet Intern Med 13:309–313.

Wall M, Biller DS, Schoning P, Olsen D, Moore LE (2001) Pancreatitis in a cat demonstrating pancreatic duct dilatation ultrasonographically. J Am Anim Hosp Assoc 37:49–53.

CHAPTER TEN

Kidneys and Ureters

Marc-André d'Anjou

Preparation and Scanning Technique

Prior to the ultrasonographic examination, the animal's hair must be clipped, and ultrasonic gel must be applied to its skin to optimize images of the kidneys. Animals can be scanned in dorsal, left, or right recumbency. The left kidney can usually be well visualized with a ventrolateral approach, although the presence of gas or feces in the descending colon can sometimes limit its evaluation. The right kidney is typically more difficult to image, especially in deep-chested dogs, because of its deep localization in the craniodorsal abdomen. The right ventrolateral subcostal approach is usually sufficient. However, in certain dogs, a lateral approach through the 11th or 12th intercostal space might be necessary. The visualization of the right kidney can also be affected by the presence of intestinal content, especially in the descending duodenum, ascending colon, or cecum.

Kidneys can markedly vary in depth according to an animal's body conformation. In small dogs and cats, a high-frequency sonographic probe (7.5 MHz and higher) is recommended, whereas kidneys of larger dogs usually require a probe with more penetration (5 MHz and lower). Sectorial or convex probes are considered more useful because they enable the entire kidney to be imaged. Additionally, these probes tend to have a smaller footprint, which can more easily be used intercostally.

Kidneys should be scanned from cranial to caudal and lateral to medial, in several transverse and longitudinal planes, to fully assess all portions, including the cortex, medulla, and collecting system (Figure 10.1).

Ultrasonographic Anatomy of Normal Kidneys

In many dogs, the left kidney can be evaluated through the body of the spleen, which provides a good acoustic window. The right kidney is more cranial and dorsal, particularly in dogs, and usually is in contact or close proximity with the hepatic parenchyma at the level of the caudate lobe. Both kidneys are symmetrical in size and shape in cats and dogs. Kidneys can be oval, particularly in cats, or bean shaped, which is more common in dogs. Kidneys can be measured on all planes, and volumes can be estimated. In normal cats, renal length has been reported to vary between 3.0 and 4.3 cm (Walter et al. 1987a). In dogs, absolute measurements must take into account total body weight and conformation, because great variations exist (Barr et al. 1990). A new method using a ratio between the renal length and the aorta diameter was recently proposed (Mareschal et al. 2007). This ratio is obtained by dividing the maximal renal length by the luminal diameter of the aorta. The aorta must be measured at the level of the kidneys when it is maximally distended during the cardiac cycle. The renal size should be considered reduced if the K/Ao ratio is less than 5.5 and increased when greater than 9.1.

Renal cortex, medulla, and the collecting system can be visualized with ultrasonography in dogs and cats (Konde et al. 1984; Walter et al. 1988) (Figures 10.1 and 10.2). The renal medulla is hypoechoic when compared with the cortex, which is usually hypoechoic or isoechoic to the liver and typically hypoechoic to the spleen. However, in certain dogs and several cats with normal renal function, renal cortices can be hyperechoic to the liver (Figure 10.3). In cats, the accumulation of fatty vacuoles in the renal cortex appears to contribute to its hyperechogenicity (Yeager and Anderson 1989). The medulla appears separated into several lobulated segments by the presence of linear echogenicities representing borders of the interlobar vessels and diverticuli. The medulla is nearly anechoic in certain animals and should not be confused with dilatation of the renal pelvis. The renal crest is the prolongation of the renal medulla, which is in contact with the pelvis. The walls of the arcuate arteries can be observed as paired, short, hyperechoic lines at the corticomedullary junction, which can sometimes generate an acoustic shadow and must be differentiated from mineralization (Figure 10.4). These vessels, as

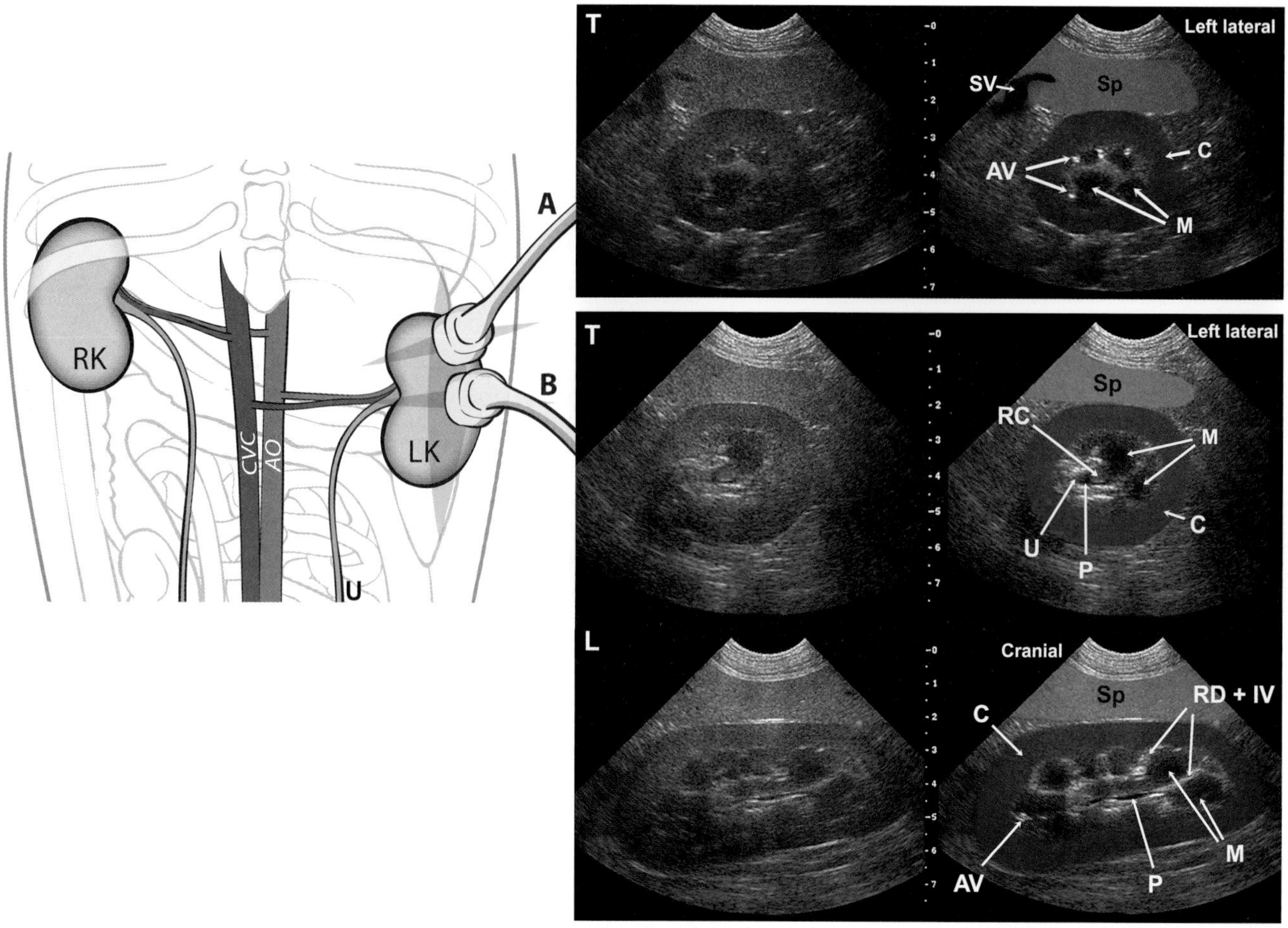

Figure 10.1. Sonographic approach and normal anatomy in the dog. In dorsal recumbency, a ventrolateral approach to the left kidney is used. The probe is moved through the kidney sequentially in transverse and longitudinal planes. AO, aorta; CVC, caudal vena cava; LK, left kidney; and RK, right kidney. **A:** Transverse **(T)** sonogram performed on the cranial pole of the left kidney. **B:** The probe is placed at the hilus region: Transverse **(T)** and longitudinal **(L)** sonograms with corresponding schematic and labeled images. AV, arcuate vessels; C, renal cortex; M, renal medulla; P, pelvis; RC, renal crest; RD + IV, renal diverticuli and interlobar vessels; Sp, spleen; SV, splenic vein; and U, ureter.

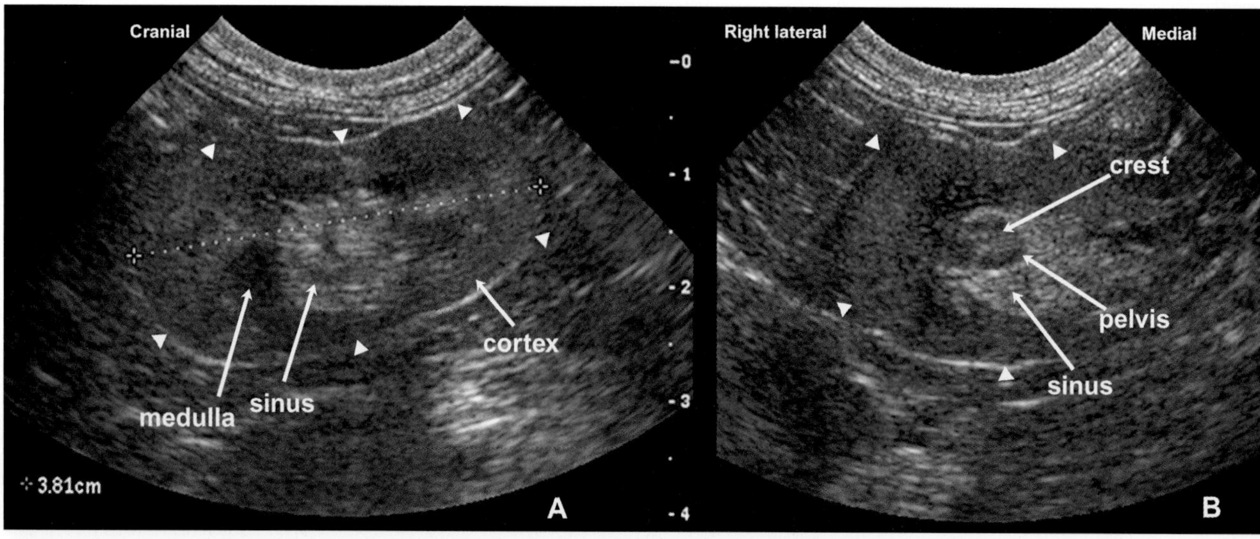

Figure 10.2. Normal feline kidney. Longitudinal **(A)** and transverse **(B)** images of the right kidney (arrowheads) in a normal cat.

well as the larger renal and intralobar vessels, can also be evaluated with color Doppler or power Doppler (Figure 10.5). The renal arteries and veins, usually single on each side, can be followed from the hilus to the aorta and caudal vena cava, respectively. These vessels must be differentiated from dilated ureters.

The renal pelvis can sometimes be visualized in normal dogs and cats, especially in animals receiving intravenous fluids or being treated with diuretics (Pugh et al. 1994). The visualization of the renal pelvis is facilitated by the use of newer high-resolution systems. The pelvic height should measure less than 2 mm (Figure 10.6). The renal diverticuli and ureter, unless distended, are not normally seen in dogs and cats. The pelvis is surrounded by the sinus, which contains fat and appears hyperechoic and is particularly prominent in obese cats.

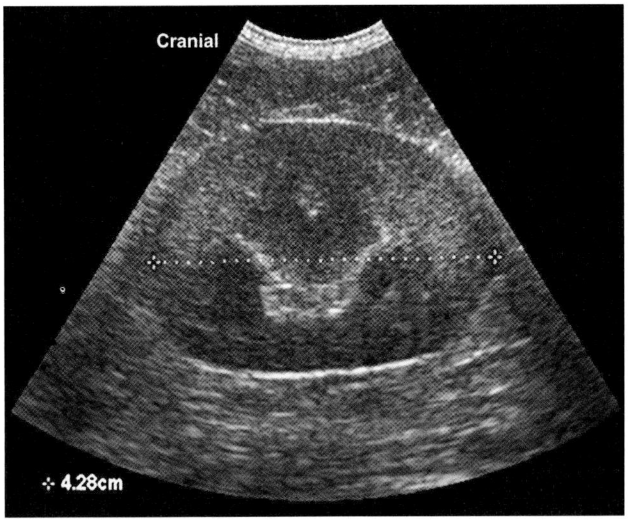

Figure 10.3. Hyperechoic kidney in a normal cat. Longitudinal image of the left kidney of a cat with normal renal function. The renal cortex appeared hyperechoic to the liver (not shown). This kidney is otherwise normal in shape, size, and contour.

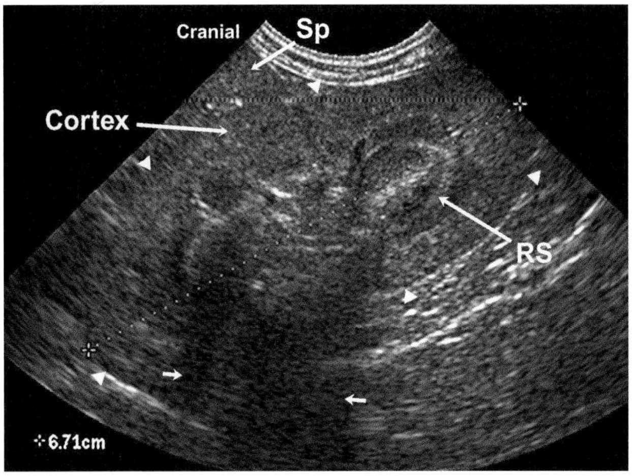

Figure 10.4. Hyperechoic kidney in a clinically normal dog. Longitudinal image of the left kidney. The renal cortex (arrowheads) is isoechoic to the adjacent spleen (Sp). A thin, hyperechoic band is also noted in the medulla, consistent with an incidental rim sign (RS). Acoustic shadowing is also observed dorsally (short arrows) because of attenuation and refraction of the ultrasound waves by normal structures such as walls of vessels and collecting system, and sinus fat. This shadowing must not be misinterpreted as a sign of nephrolithiasis.

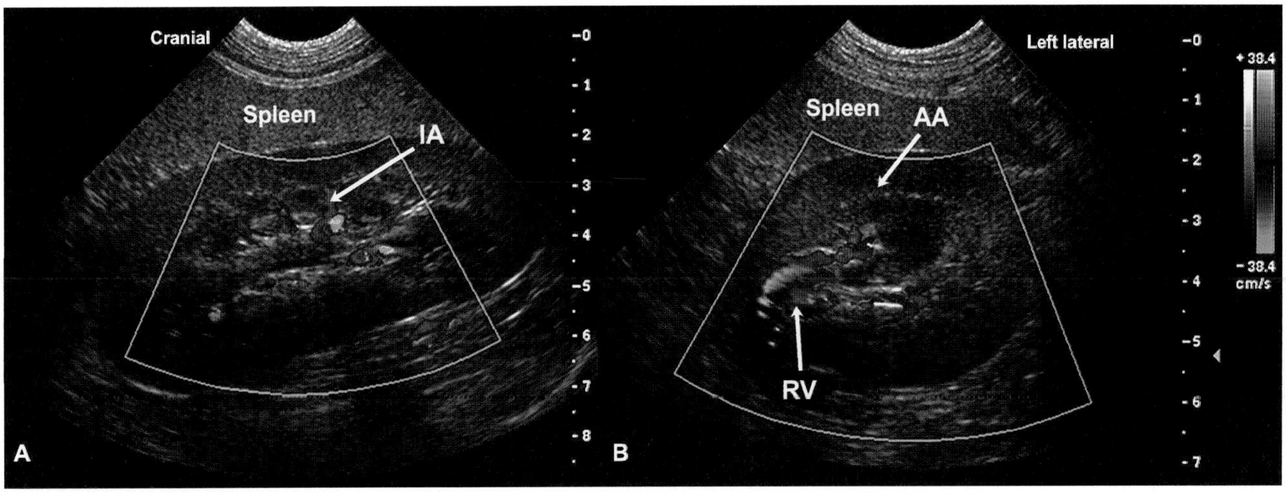

Figure 10.5. Renal vasculature with color Doppler in a normal dog. Longitudinal **(A)** and transverse **(B)** images of the left kidney. The vascular flow can be observed with color Doppler through the renal, interlobar, and arcuate vessels. AA, arcuate artery; IA, interlobar artery; and RV, renal vein.

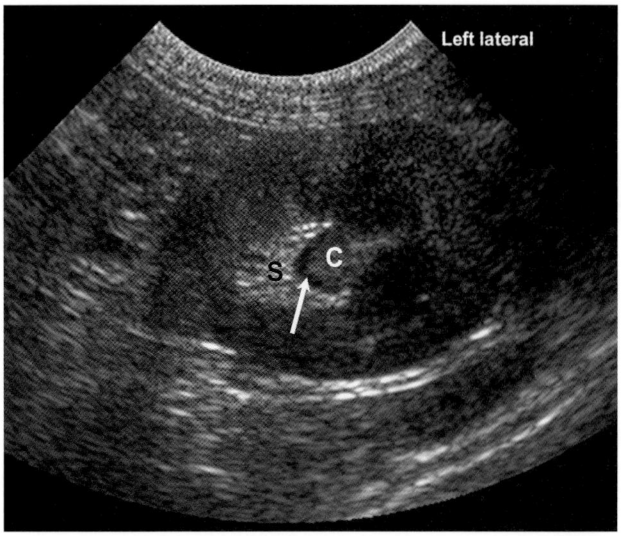

Figure 10.6. Physiological pyelectasia in a cat. On this transverse image obtained in the central portion of the left kidney, minimal distension of the renal pelvis appears as an anechoic, crescent-shaped region just medial to the renal crest (C). This pelvis is surrounded at the hilus by hyperechoic fat contained in the sinus (S). The ureter is not visible. This cat was receiving intravenous fluids.

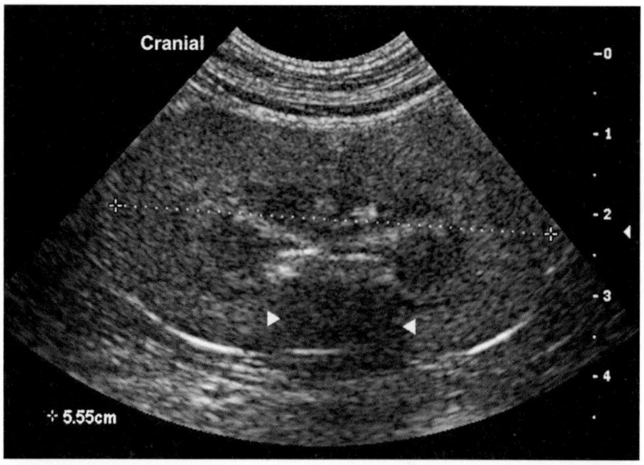

Figure 10.7. Compensatory hypertrophy. Longitudinal image of the left kidney of a cat with right renal agenesis but normal renal function. This unique kidney is enlarged but normal in shape and contour. Some acoustic shadowing is (arrowheads) caused by excessive attenuation of the ultrasound beam by the region of the sinus.

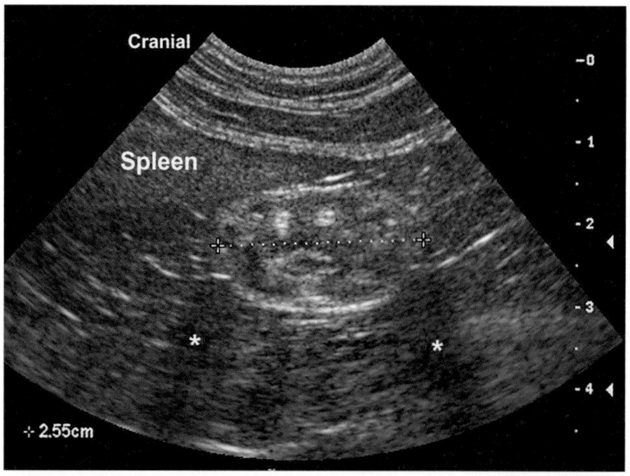

Figure 10.8. Renal dysplasia in a dog. Longitudinal image of the left kidney of a mixed-breed dog with unilateral renal dysplasia. This kidney is small and hyperechoic to the spleen. Edge shadowing is also observed (*).

Ultrasonographic Features of Renal Disorders

Congenital Renal and Ureteral Malformations

With the exception of polycystic kidney disease and ectopic ureters, congenital malformations of the upper urinary tract are rare in dogs and cats. Renal agenesis (complete absence) or hypoplasia is often associated with compensatory enlargement of the unique kidney (Figure 10.7). Renal ectopia and fusion have also been reported (Allworth and Hoffman 1999; Hecht et al. 2005). Renal dysplasia is defined as disorganized development of renal parenchyma because of anomalous differentiation. The kidneys are typically small, irregular, and hyperechoic, with reduced corticomedullary distinction, similarly to kidneys with chronic inflammatory disease (Abraham 2003) (Figure 10.8). These young dogs may be predisposed to ascending pyelonephritis, which contributes to the morphological modifications observed on ultrasound (Abraham 2003). Although renal developmental anomalies can be confirmed only with histological analysis, renal dysplasia should be suspected in a young dog with deformed kidneys and clinical renal insufficiency.

Diffuse Parenchymal Renal Diseases

Increased renal echogenicity is one of the most common findings in dogs and cats with renal insufficiency. Several renal diseases can be associated with increased cortical and/or medullary echogenicity in the acute or chronic phases of the process. Interstitial and glomerular nephritis, acute tubular nephrosis or necrosis (caused by ethylene glycol, grapes in dogs, and lily in cats), end-stage renal disease, and nephrocalcinosis can all cause renal hyperechogenicity (Walter et al. 1987; Barr et al. 1989; Adams et al. 1991; Forrest et al. 1998; Eubig et al. 2005). In some of these disease processes, the cortical echogenicity can be more specifically increased, enhancing the corticomedullary distinction. This can be dramatic in cases of acute tubular necrosis and calcium oxalate deposition caused by ethylene glycol toxicity (Figure 10.9). In other cases, both medulla and cortex can become hyperechoic, causing reduced corticomedullary border distinction (Figure 10.10). This is particularly evident in dogs and cats with chronic renal disease (Figures 10.11–10.14).

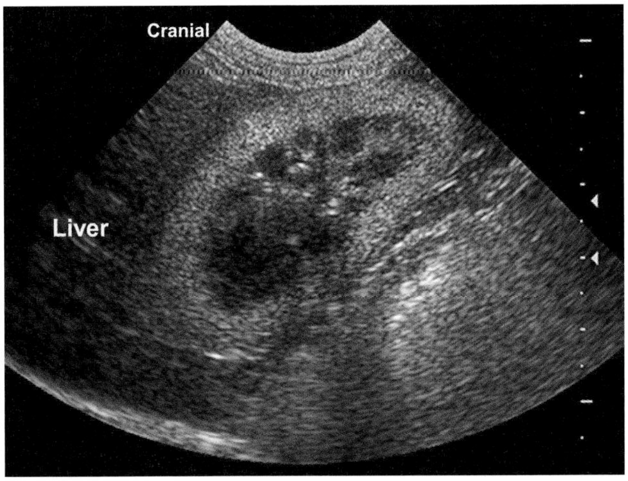

Figure 10.9. Ethylene glycol toxicity in a dog. On this longitudinal image of the right kidney, the cortex is markedly hyperechoic in comparison with the adjacent hepatic caudate lobe because of oxalate crystal deposition and tubular necrosis. The renal medulla is not affected, and the corticomedullary distinction is enhanced.

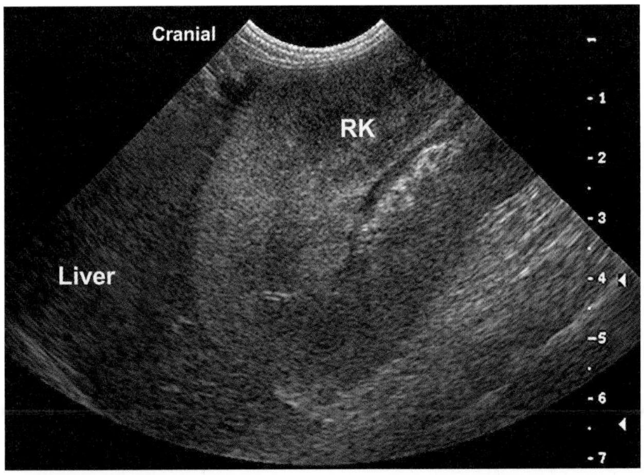

Figure 10.10. Acute interstitial nephritis caused by leptospirosis. Longitudinal image of the right cranial abdomen of a dog with acute renal insufficiency. The right kidney (RK) is enlarged and diffusely hyperechoic. This hyperechogenicity contrasts with the concurrent hypoechogenicity involving the adjacent liver, which was presumably caused by hepatitis. The renal corticomedullary distinction is significantly reduced.

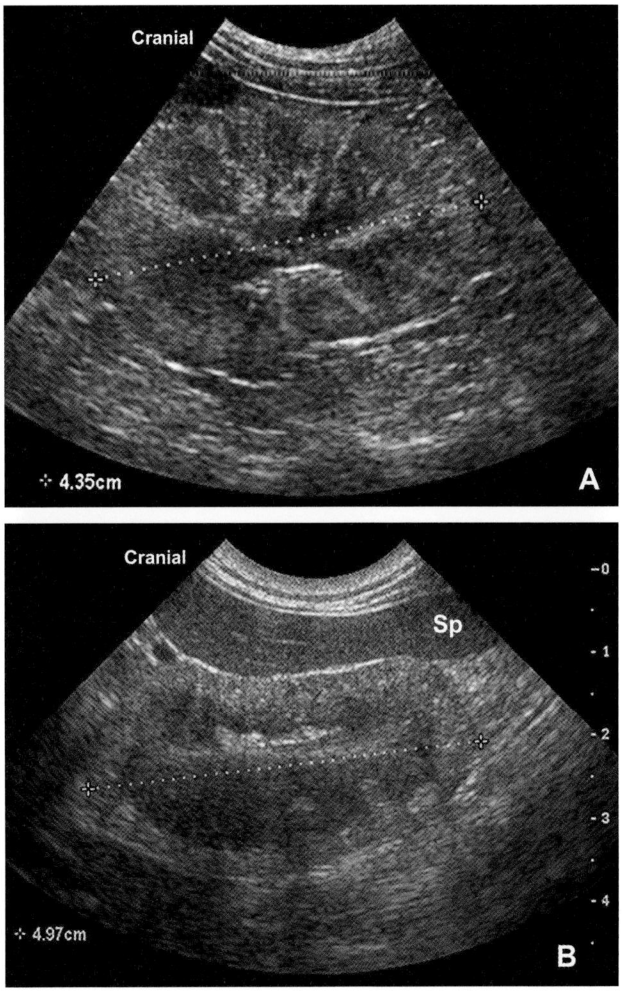

Figure 10.11. Chronic renal disease. **A: Chronic interstitial nephritis and sclerosis in a dachshund.** On this longitudinal image of the left kidney, both the cortex and medulla appear hyperechoic, heterogeneous, and poorly demarcated. The kidney is small and irregular in contour, and several hyperechoic stripes are observed, which may have been related to fibrosis and/or dystrophic mineralization observed on histopathology. **B: Nephrosclerosis.** Longitudinal image of the left kidney of a 5-year-old shar-pei with chronic renal insufficiency and proteinuria. The cortex is markedly hyperechoic, granular in echotexture, and appears thinned when compared with the medulla. The kidney is also small and mildly irregular. Nephrosclerosis was the histological diagnosis based on ultrasound-guided biopsies. Sp, spleen.

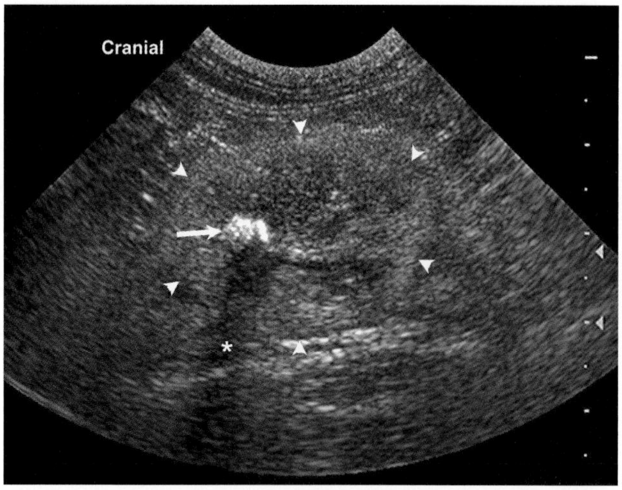

Figure 10.12. Chronic interstitial nephritis with nephrolithiasis. Longitudinal image of the left kidney in a small-breed dog. Both the cortex and medulla appear hyperechoic and poorly demarcated. This kidney is also small and irregularly shaped (arrowheads), and a hyperechoic focus (arrow) associated with acoustic shadowing (*) is present in its cranial pole. This mineral focus was confirmed to represent a nephrolith.

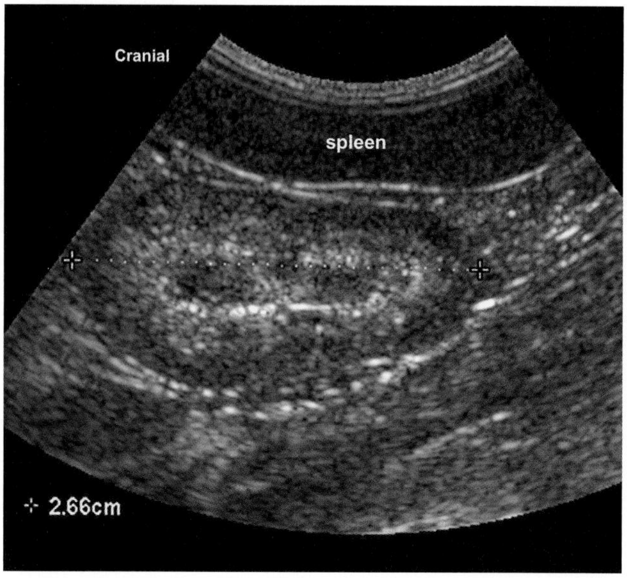

Figure 10.14. Nephrocalcinosis. Longitudinal image of the left kidney in a cat with hypercalcemia. An irregular hyperechoic band is seen involving the region of the corticomedullary junction, secondary to renal tubular calcification.

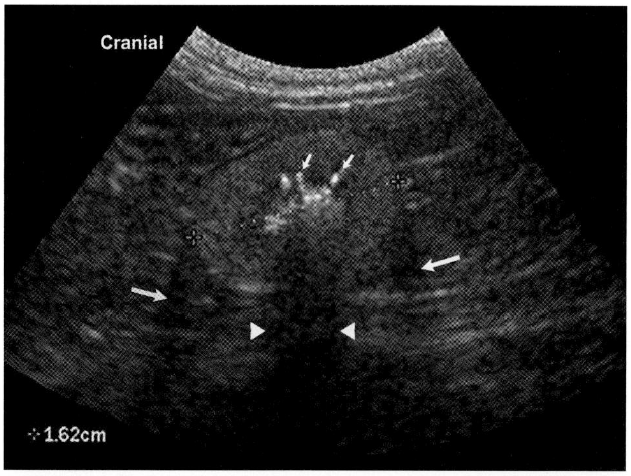

Figure 10.13. Chronic interstitial nephritis with dystrophic mineralization. Longitudinal image of the left kidney in a cat with chronic renal insufficiency. This kidney is small and hyperechoic. The corticomedullary distinction is reduced, and several linear and irregular hyperechoic foci noted in the region of the pelvis and diverticuli (short arrows) are associated with acoustic shadowing (arrowheads). These foci indicated dystrophic mineralization. Edge shadowing is also observed (long arrows).

Additionally, in several cases of parenchymal renal disease, a circumferential hyperechoic band can be found in the medulla, parallel to the corticomedullary border, consistent with mineralization, necrosis, congestion, and/or hemorrhage. This finding, known as the *medullary rim sign*, has been observed in several disease processes, such as acute tubular necrosis (ethylene glycol toxicity), nephrocalcinosis, leptospirosis, and pyogranulomatous vasculitis caused by feline infectious peritonitis, as well as in normal cats and dogs (Barr et al. 1989; Biller et al. 1992; Forrest et al. 1998; Mantis and Lamb 2000) (Figures 10.15–10.17). This hyperechoic band has been attributed to an insult to the renal tubules in the deepest portion of the medulla, which is most metabolically active and therefore more susceptible to ischemia (Biller et al. 1992). Because of their relatively high prevalence in dogs and cats, renal hyperechogenicity and medullary rim signs should not be considered as accurate indicators of renal disease; however, the possibility remains that these findings could represent sentinel signs of early renal disease or past renal insult (Mantis and Lamb 2000).

Although it can be difficult to distinguish clinically normal kidneys from acute and chronic renal disease processes, several other ultrasonographic parameters can be helpful, such as size, shape, contour, and internal architecture. Kidneys affected with chronic interstitial nephritis tend to become small, irregular, and more diffusely hyperechoic (Walter et al. 1987) (Figures 10.11–10.13). The remodeling process affecting these kidneys, which involves fibrosis, causes architectural distortions. Linear or patchy dystrophic

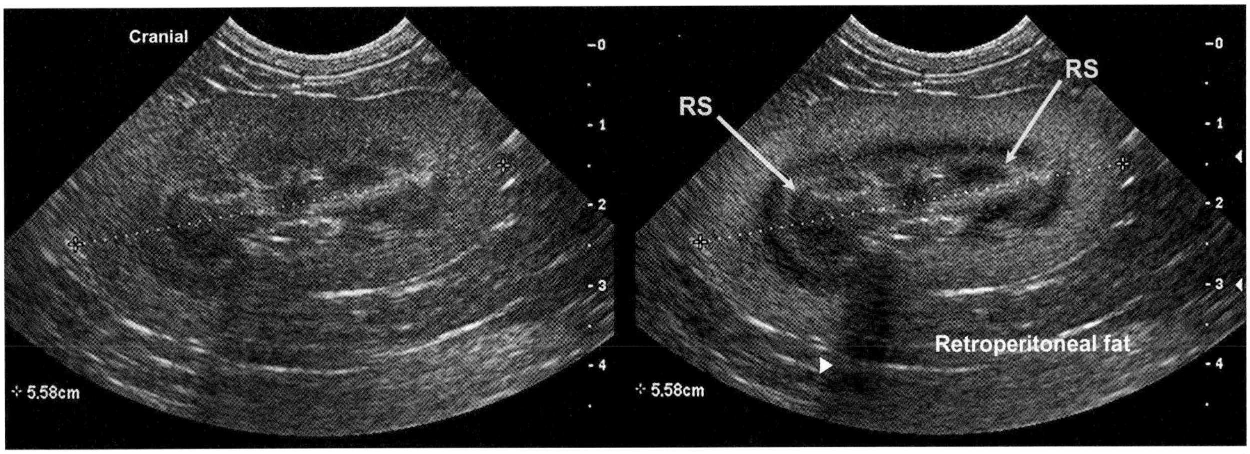

Figure 10.15. Medullary rim sign. Longitudinal ultrasonographic and schematic images of the left kidney of a dog with normal renal function. A thin hyperechoic band is noted in the deep portion of the medulla, parallel to the corticomedullary junction. This rim sign (RS) is not a sensitive or specific sign of renal disease. Additionally, the renal cortex is mildly hyperechoic and irregular, which can also be observed in dogs with normal renal function. Acoustic shadowing, probably related to normal structures, is also present deep to the renal pelvis (arrowhead).

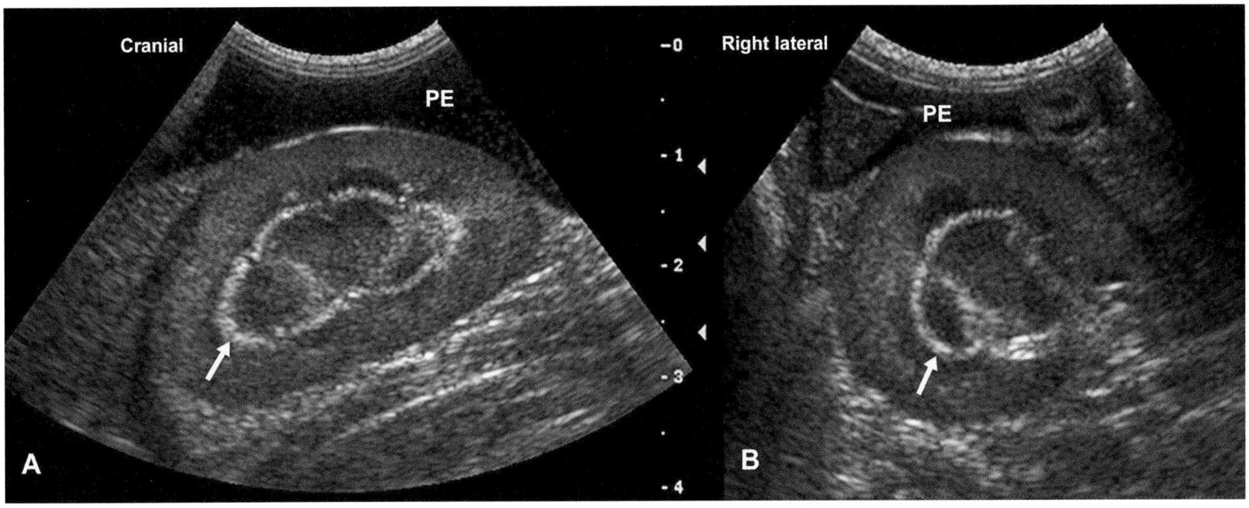

Figure 10.16. Pyogranulomatous vasculitis. Longitudinal **(A)** and transverse **(B)** images of the right kidney in a cat diagnosed with feline infectious peritonitis. A prominent hyperechoic band is in the medulla (arrow), parallel to the cortical margin, consistent with a medullary rim sign. Pronounced peritoneal effusion (PE) is also present.

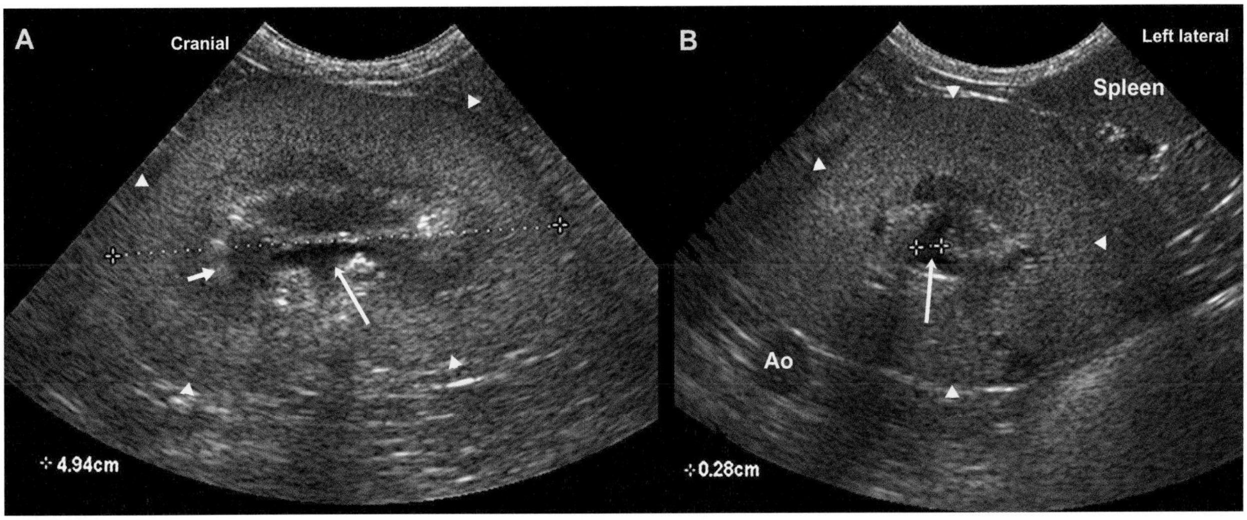

Figure 10.17. Acute leptospirosis. Longitudinal **(A)** and transverse **(B)** image of the left kidney (arrowheads) in a small-breed dog diagnosed with leptospirosis. The kidney is smoothly enlarged and hyperechoic, and the corticomedullary distinction is reduced. The renal pelvis (long arrow) is also dilated. Additionally, a medullary rim sign is present (short arrow). Ao, aorta.

mineralization can also be observed in these kidneys, especially in the region of the collecting system, where the mineralization appears as poor or well-defined hyperechoic foci that cause acoustic shadowing (Figure 10.13). These mineral foci are usually difficult to differentiate from true nephroliths, which can also accompany chronic renal diseases. Kidneys affected with acute processes, such as infectious pyelonephritis, interstitial nephritis (e.g., caused by leptospirosis), or acute tubular necrosis (e.g., caused by ethylene glycol), can become enlarged and hyperechoic, with a contour that usually remains smooth (Figures 10.9 and 10.10). Perinephric effusion can also be observed in these patients and was described particularly with leptospirosis (Forrest et al. 1998).

Protein-losing glomerular diseases, such as glomerulonephritis and renal amyloidosis, cannot be distinguished from other types of diffuse renal disorders. Affected kidneys are commonly hyperechoic and can vary in size according to the chronicity of the disease (Figure 10.18).

Renal parenchymal mineralization (nephrocalcinosis) in dogs and cats with or without hypercalcemia can cause renal diffuse cortical and/or medullary hyperechogenicity, a medullary rim sign, and/or dispersed hyperechoic foci (Figures 10.14 and 10.19).

Neoplastic processes typically cause focal or multifocal renal changes, with the exception of lymphoma in cats. With lymphoma in cats, the kidneys typically become enlarged, irregular, and hyperechoic (Figure 10.20). Other findings can include a hypoechoic halo at the periphery of the cortex, hyperechoic foci or striations throughout the medulla, pyelectasia, and hypoechoic medullary or cortical nodules or masses (Figures 10.20 and 10.21). Other tumors, such as squamous cell carcinoma, may diffusely infiltrate the kidney and markedly distort the renal architecture (Figures 10.21 and 10.22).

Focal Parenchymal Renal Disorders

Focal significant or nonsignificant renal lesions are common in dogs and cats. Renal cysts, nephroliths or dystrophic mineralization, and cortical infarcts are more common than primary or metastatic neoplasia, granulomas, and abscesses.

Renal Cavitary Lesions

Benign renal cysts typically appear as round to oval, anechoic structures with a thin, well demarcated, hyperechoic rim and may show distal acoustic enhancement (Reichle et al. 2002) (Figure 10.23). Cysts can be solitary or multifocal and vary in size. In some patients, internal echoes can be observed in association with hemorrhage or necrotic debris. Inherited polycystic kidney disease, which affects long-haired cats and Cairn terriers, can be variable in severity, can be sometimes associated with chronic interstitial nephritis, and may cause significant renal distortion (Figures 10.24

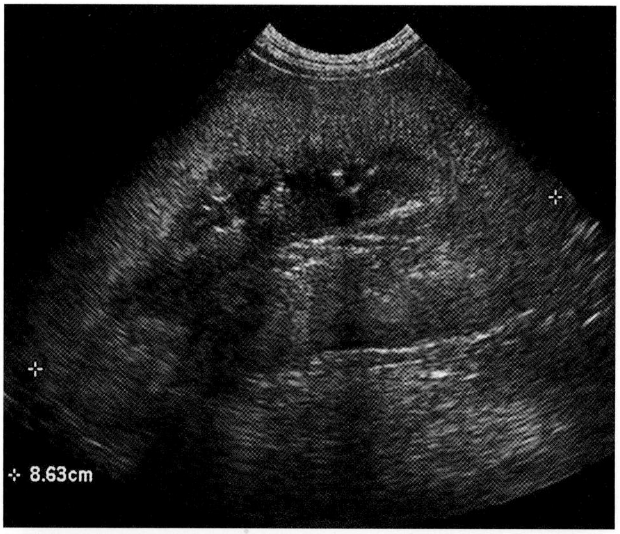

Figure 10.18. Glomerulonephritis. Longitudinal image of the left kidney (arrowheads) of a German shepherd diagnosed with bilateral glomerulonephritis. The kidney appears smoothly enlarged and hyperechoic, particularly at the level of the cortex, which also appears subjectively thickened.

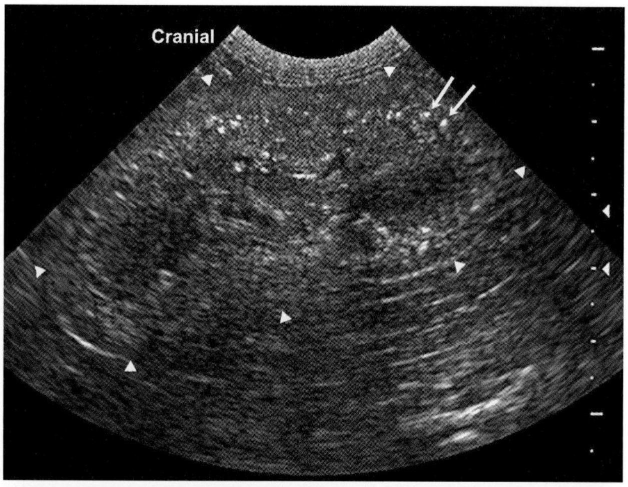

Figure 10.19. Nephrocalcinosis in a dog with hypercalcemia. On this longitudinal image, small hyperechoic foci (arrows) are seen throughout the left kidney, particularly involving the cortex, consistent with extensive renal calcification.

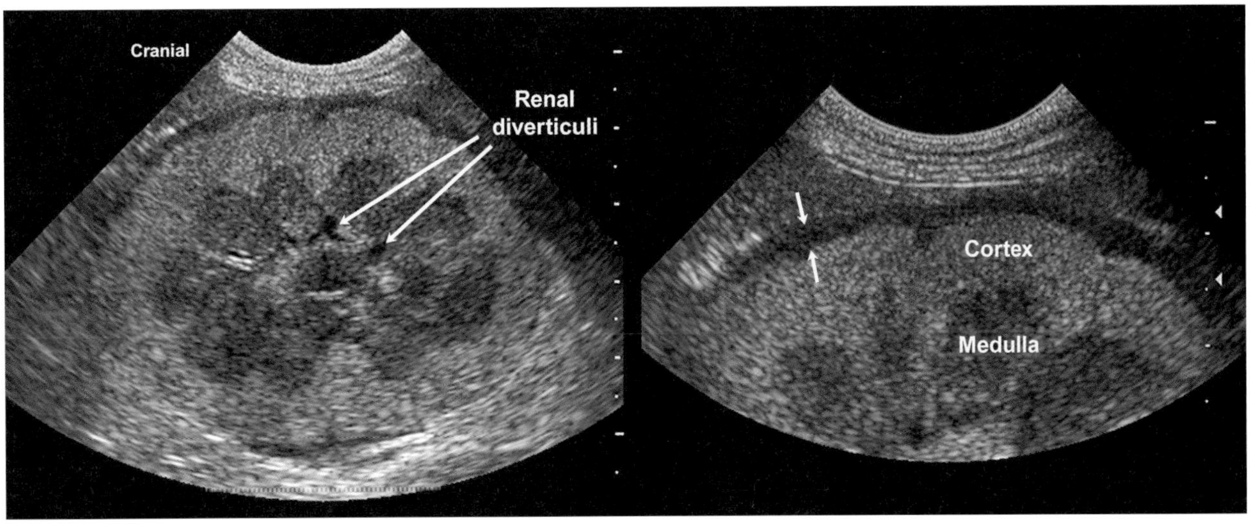

Figure 10.20. Renal lymphoma in a cat. On these longitudinal images, the left kidney is enlarged, reaching more than 6 cm in length, and moderately hyperechoic. The lobulated sections of the medulla appear prominent, and a hypoechoic halo is present at the periphery of the cortex (between the short arrows). Mild dilatation of the renal diverticuli is also apparent (long arrows). These features are commonly seen with renal lymphoma in cats.

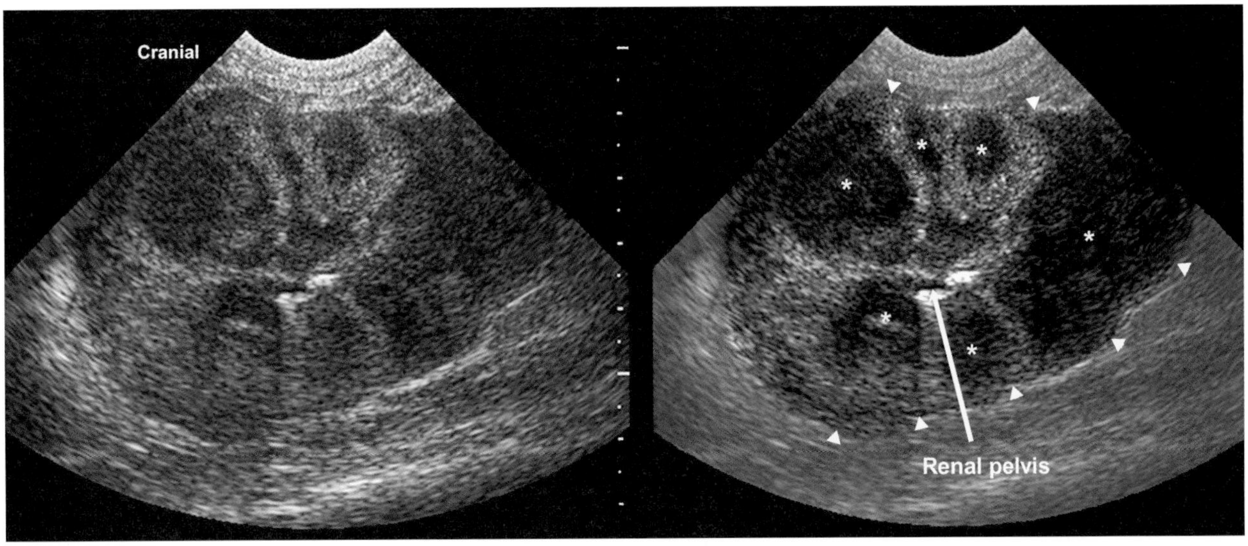

Figure 10.21. Renal lymphoma in a cat. Longitudinal ultrasonographic and schematic images of the right kidney (arrowheads) in another cat with lymphoma. The kidney is enlarged, reaching more than 8 cm in length, and markedly heterogeneous. Several ill-defined hypoechoic nodules and masses (*) are in the parenchyma, distorting its architecture. This pattern is another manifestation of lymphoma in cats and sometimes in dogs.

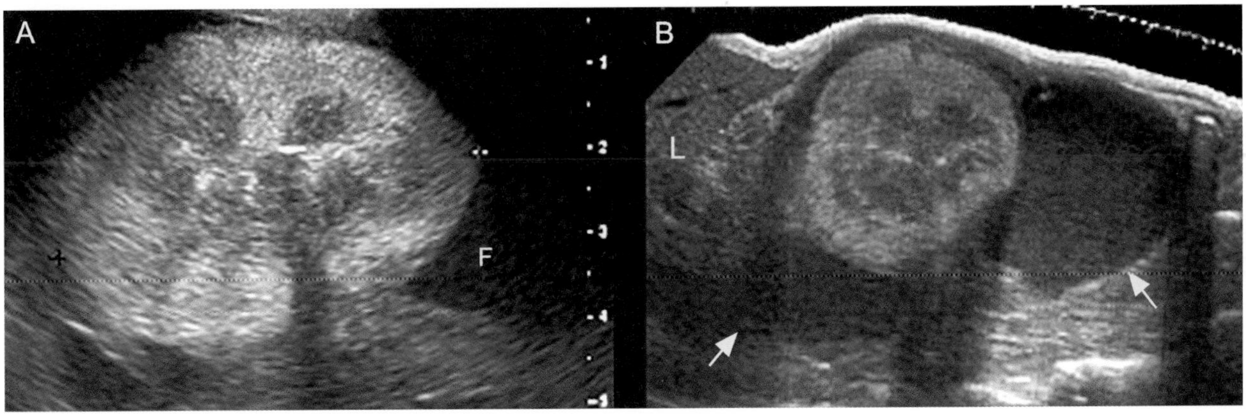

Figure 10.22. Diffuse squamous cell carcinoma in a cat. **A:** Longitudinal sonogram of the right kidney that is enlarged (5.3 cm), irregularly shaped, and diffusely increased in echogenicity. The kidney is surrounded by fluid (F). **B:** Panoramic view of the same kidney showing the subcapsular echogenic fluid distention (arrows). L, liver. Images courtesy of D. Penninck.

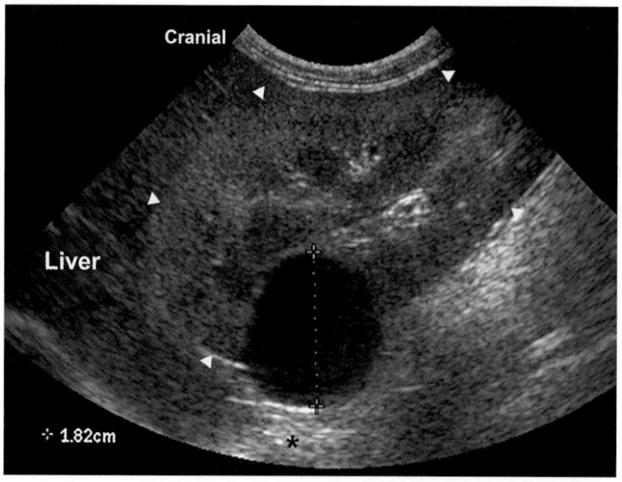

Figure 10.23. Renal cyst. Longitudinal image of the right kidney in a dog with an incidental cortical cyst, which appears as a 1.8 cm, round, well-defined, anechoic structure, associated with distal acoustic enhancement (*). The renal cortex (delineated by arrowheads) is hyperechoic to the adjacent liver, although there was no clinical evidence of renal failure.

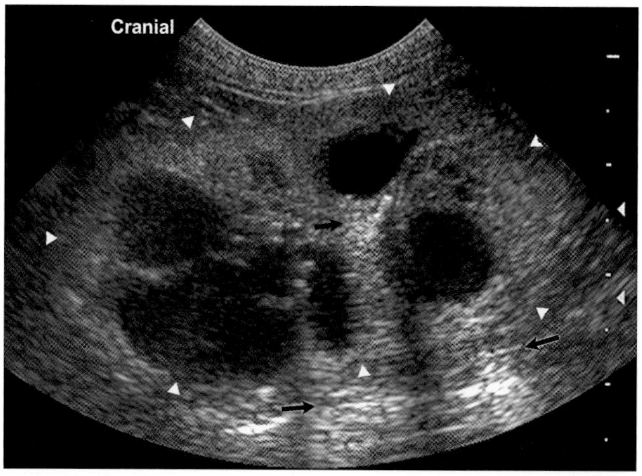

Figure 10.24. Polycystic renal disease. Longitudinal image of the left kidney of a Himalayan cat with bilateral polycystic renal disease. Several well-defined, round, anechoic structures are found throughout the renal parenchyma (delineated by arrowheads), in association with far acoustic enhancement (arrows), consistent with cavitary lesions containing a hypoattenuating fluid.

and 10.25). Most of these cysts are in the cortex or at the corticomedullary junction (Reichle et al. 2002). Renal cysts can also be secondary to chronic renal diseases in dogs and cats (Figure 10.26).

Solitary cysts, which can sometimes become relatively large, must be differentiated from solitary solid or cavitary masses, abscesses, and hematomas. Solid masses or nodules are typically associated with static

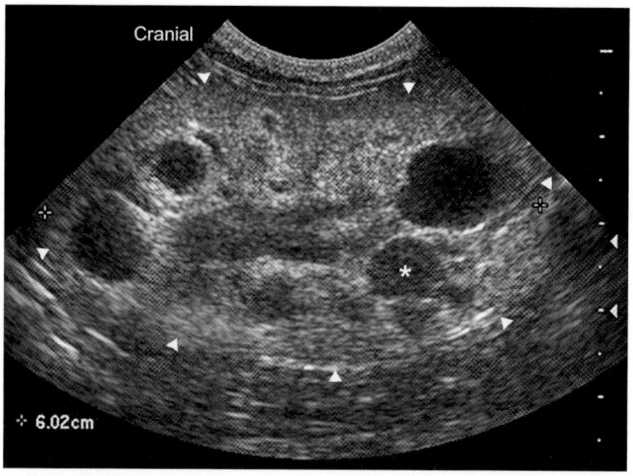

Figure 10.25. Polycystic renal disease. Longitudinal image of the left kidney in a Persian cat with bilateral polycystic renal disease. Several round hypoechoic to anechoic structures, delineated by a thin, well-defined, hyperechoic rim, are found throughout the renal parenchyma (delineated by the arrowheads). The mild echogenicity noted in some of these cysts (*) may be the result of partial volume averaging (the combination of tissue and cystic fluid in the same imaged slice) or the presence of intracystic hemorrhage or debris. This polycystic disease causes renal enlargement. The hyperechogenicity noted involving the renal parenchyma is caused by concurrent interstitial nephritis and fibrosis.

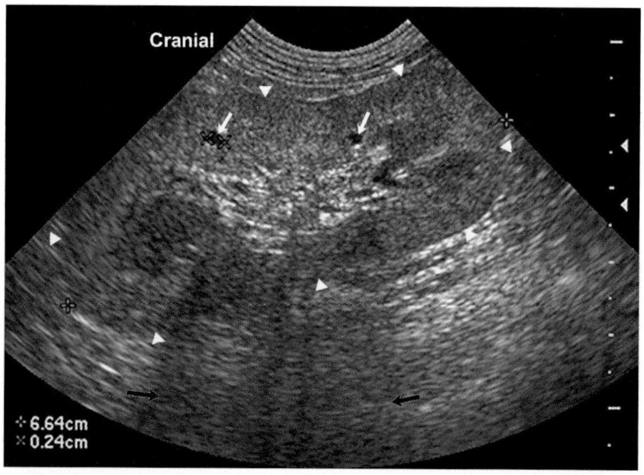

Figure 10.26. Chronic renal degeneration and cyst formation. Longitudinal image of the left kidney of an adult Labrador retriever with chronic renal insufficiency. The kidney (arrowheads) is hyperechoic, and the corticomedullary distinction is reduced. Two well-defined, circular, anechoic foci (white arrows) are noted in the region of the corticomedullary junction, consistent with degenerative cysts. The cysts are presumed to be secondary to the presence of the chronic renal disease. Incomplete acoustic shadowing is also apparent dorsally (black arrows) because of higher ultrasound beam attenuation by the structures in the peripelvic region and sinus and/or possibly because of early dystrophic mineralization.

internal echoes that can be affected by gain settings and that are usually not associated with distal acoustic enhancement. Large solid masses can also appear cavitated because of necrosis. Renal cystadenocarcinomas have been reported in German shepherds and are usually associated with dermatofibrosis (Moe and Lium 1997). With ultrasonography, a fluid-filled cavity (or cavities) typically predominates, infiltrating the kidney, with a solid-tissue component that can protrude inside the cyst(s) (Figure 10.27).

Renal abscesses can usually be differentiated from true cysts by the presence of echoes and sedimentation within the cavitary lesion and especially by a rather poorly demarcated and irregular contour (Figure 10.28). Distal enhancement may still be present if the cellular count remains relatively small.

Renal Solid-Mass Lesions

Solid-tissue proliferative diseases can appear as homogeneous or heterogeneous, hypoechoic, isoechoic or hyperechoic, regular or irregular lesions, with variably well-defined margins (Figure 10.29). This variable ultrasonographic appearance is reflected by the cell type, as well as by the variable presence and distribution of vessels, tissue necrosis, fibrosis, mineralization, and hemorrhage (Walter et al. 1987b). When large, these lesions can alter the renal internal architecture (Figure 10.30). Because their variable characteristics, renal primary or metastatic neoplastic processes cannot be easily distinguished with ultrasonography. However, lymphoma and malignant histiocytosis (histiocytic sarcoma) tend to appear as hypoechoic nodules or masses (Figure 10.31).

Other types of solitary neoplastic masses include adenocarcinomas, hemangiomas, nephroblastomas, and several types of sarcomas, including hemangiosarcoma, as well as metastases (Gasser et al. 2003) (Figures 10.30, 10.32, and 10.33). These neoplastic processes can be well defined or ill-defined and can be associated with retroperitoneal hemorrhage or completely replace normal parenchymal architecture. The absence of an identifiable kidney in the region lateral to the origin of the renal vessels might be the only sign that can help in confidently suspecting a renal mass. Other imaging tests (excretory urography, computed tomography, or magnetic resonance) can be required to confirm the origin of the mass.

Other less common solid processes, such as granulomas (fungal diseases), pyogranulomas (feline infectious peritonitis), or solid abscesses can appear similar to neoplastic processes (Figure 10.34). Hence, fine-needle aspiration or biopsy is required in most cases to achieve a precise diagnosis.

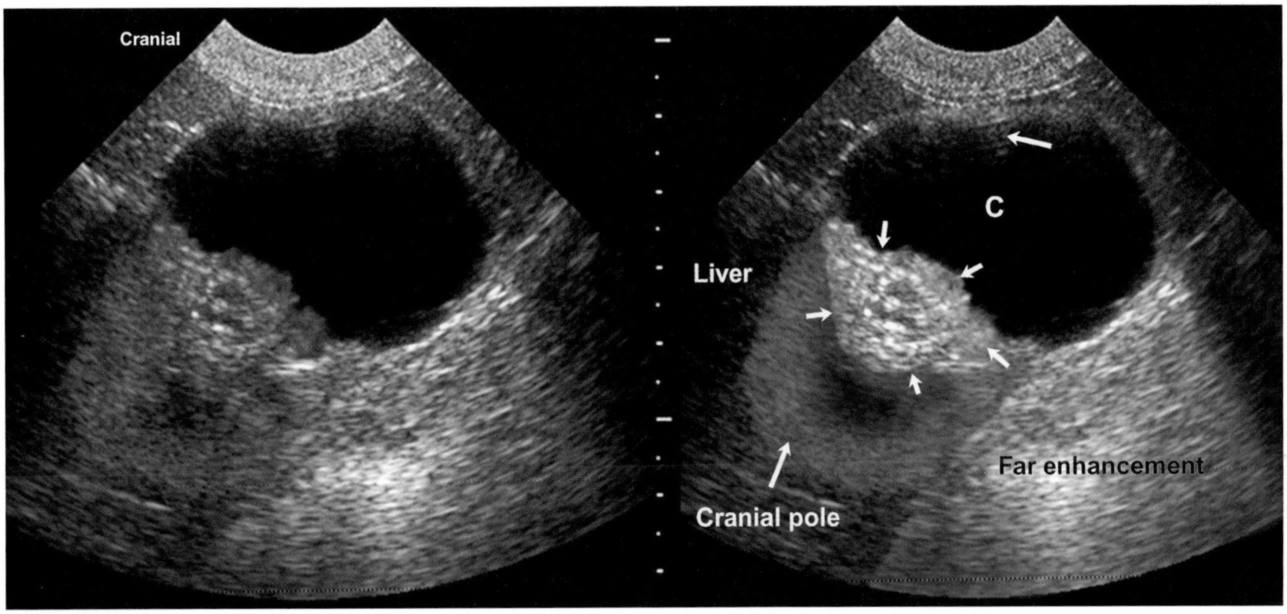

Figure 10.27. Cystadenocarcinoma. Longitudinal ultrasonographic and schematic images of the right kidney of a German shepherd with a palpable renal mass. A large anechoic cystic (C) cavitary lesion involves the caudal renal pole, in association with far acoustic enhancement. An irregular hyperechoic mass (short arrows) is noted at the cranial margin of the "cyst" in the central portion of the kidney. Artifactual hyperechoic lines are at the inner ventral margin of the cystic component of the renal mass (long arrow at the top), consistent with acoustic reverberation.

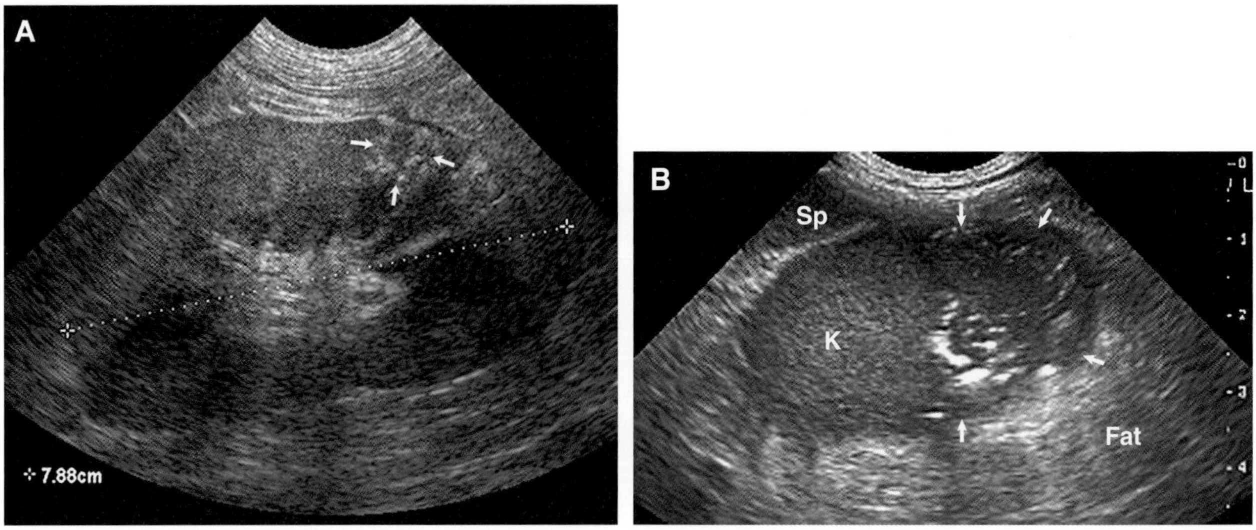

Figure 10.28. Renal abscesses. **A: Septic embolus and abscess formation.** Longitudinal image of the left kidney in a golden retriever diagnosed with bacterial septicemia. An ill-defined hyperechoic rimlike focus (arrows), with a hypoechoic center, is at the level of the renal cortex. A septic exudate was aspirated with ultrasound guidance. **B: Renal abscess caused by a wooden foreign-body perforation.** A poorly echogenic cavity (arrows) with a few bright echoes (mixture of debris and gas) involves the caudal pole of the left kidney (K). The retroperitoneal fat is hyperechoic, and a small amount of fluid is noted in the near field, adjacent to the abscess, which was confirmed at surgery. S, spleen. Image B courtesy of D. Penninck.

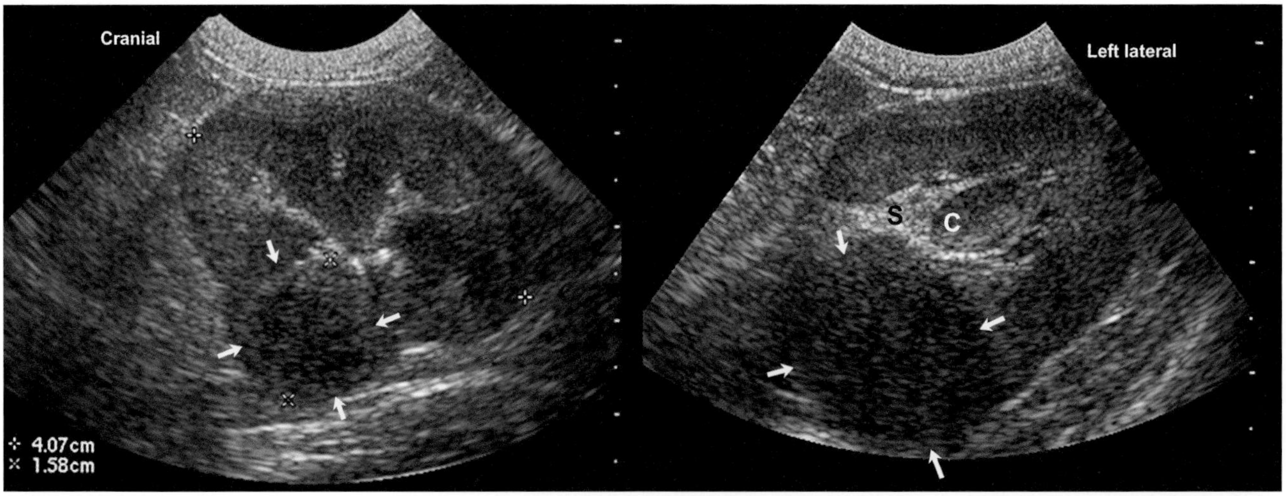

Figure 10.29. Solitary nodule. Longitudinal **(left)** and transverse **(right)** images of the left kidney in a Lhasa apso with multicentric lymphoma. A hypoechoic nodule (arrows) is in the renal cortex, adjacent to the renal sinus (S) and crest (C).

Other Focal Lesions

Mineral foci are commonly identified in kidneys of older dogs and cats because of soft-tissue mineralization or urolithiasis (Figure 10.35). Renal infarcts can also be identified as linear or wedged-shaped, well-defined lesions in the cortex, perpendicular to the capsule. Although their appearance can vary, chronic infarcts are typically hyperechoic and cause focal cortical depression (Figures 10.36 and 10.37). These chronic infarcts may also be hyperattenuating, generating an acoustic shadow. Benign renal infarcts can also look similar to septic emboli, although these tend to be more heterogeneous in appearance. Although extremely rare, gas foci can also be present within kidneys because of hematogenous or ascending infection.

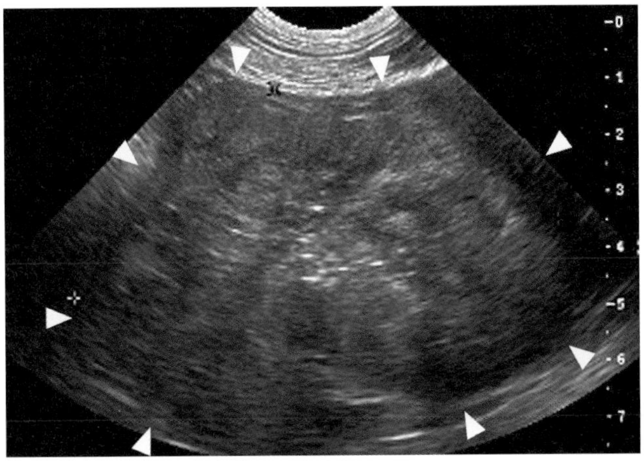

Figure 10.30. Nephroblastoma in a boxer. A large mass (arrowheads) measuring about 9 cm long entirely distorts the renal architecture. Image courtesy of D. Penninck.

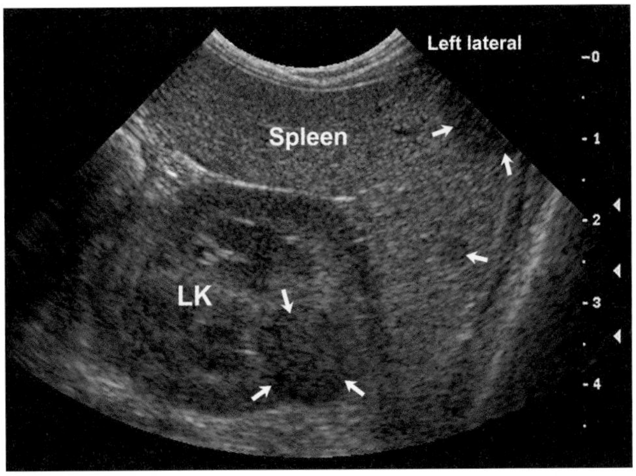

Figure 10.31. Renal and splenic nodules. Transverse image of the left kidney (LK) in a medium-sized dog. A hypoechoic nodule (arrows) involves the renal cortex, deforming its contour. This nodule was not associated with far acoustic enhancement. Similar nodules of variable size were also detected in the liver and spleen (other arrows). Tumors of round-cell origin should be considered when these lesions are found. Disseminated histiocytic sarcoma (malignant histiocytosis) was identified.

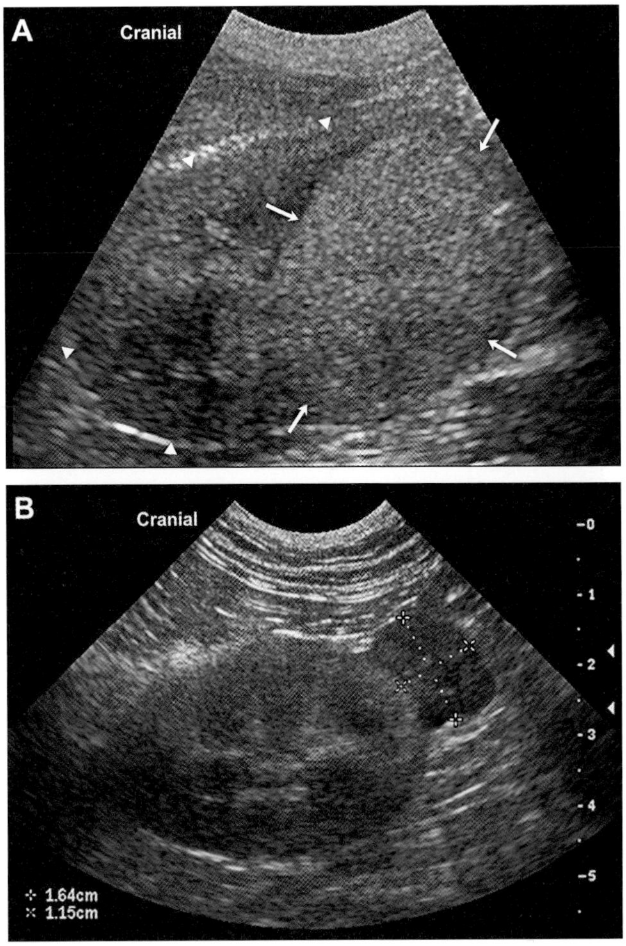

Figure 10.32. Primary and metastatic renal neoplasia. **A: Renal adenocarcinoma.** Longitudinal image of the left kidney (arrowheads) of a 6-year-old dog with chronic weight loss and anorexia. A relatively well-circumscribed hyperechoic mass (arrows) found in the caudal pole was confirmed to be a renal primary adenocarcinoma. Image courtesy of S. Hecht. **B: Metastatic carcinoma.** Longitudinal image of the left kidney of a cat in which a pulmonary mass was identified on radiographs. Tumor staging revealed a paracortical hypoechoic nodule at the caudal renal pole. A metastatic focus of bronchoalveolar carcinoma was suspected on cytological examination.

Disorders of the Collecting System

The renal pelvis and diverticuli are usually not distended in normal dogs and cats. Dilatation of the pelvis, also termed pyelectasia, is usually more apparent on transverse planes at the level of the renal hilus. It appears as an anechoic crescent at the medial margin of the renal crest (the deep portion of the medulla) (Figure 10.6). Mild dilatation of the pelvic diverticuli can sometimes be difficult to differentiate from adjacent interlobar without the use of color or power Doppler (Figure 10.38).

Pyelectasia can be observed in animals with increased diuresis (e.g., diuretic therapy or chronic renal insufficiency) and in animals with a congenital malformation (e.g., ureteral ectopia), pyelonephritis, or lower urinary obstruction (Felkei et al. 1995). The ureter can also be seen in these patients and be most

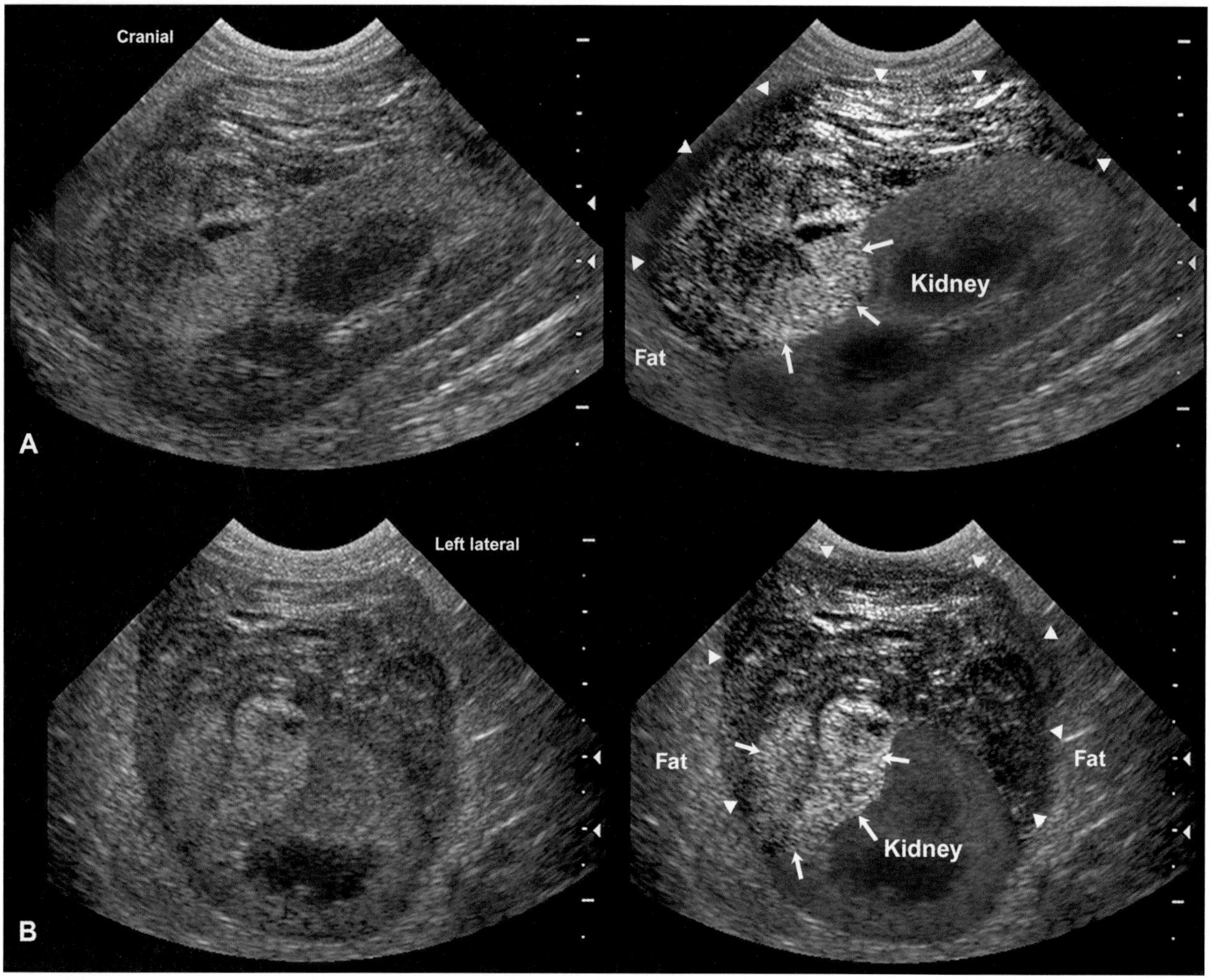

Figure 10.33. Renal hemangiosarcoma and retroperitoneal hemorrhage. Longitudinal **(A)** and transverse **(B)** ultrasonographic and schematic images of the left kidney in a large dog with suspected intra-abdominal hemorrhage. A large, ill-defined and heterogeneous mass encircles the ventral aspect of the left kidney (arrowheads). The most ventral component of this mass appears lamellate, consistent with hemorrhage. A smaller portion of this retroperitoneal mass appears more solid, uniform and hyperechoic (arrows), and appears to invade the renal cortex, consistent with a primary renal hemangiosarcoma.

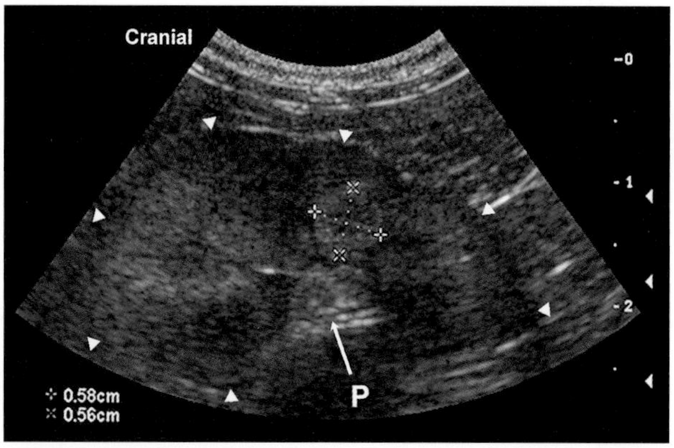

Figure 10.34. Renal pyogranuloma. Longitudinal image of the left kidney of a cat with clinically suspected infectious peritonitis. The renal architecture and contour (arrowheads) are markedly deformed, and the renal parenchyma is heterogeneous. A 0.6-cm hyperechoic nodule (cursors) is in the medulla, adjacent to the renal pelvis (P). Pyogranulomatous nephritis was diagnosed by fine-needle aspiration.

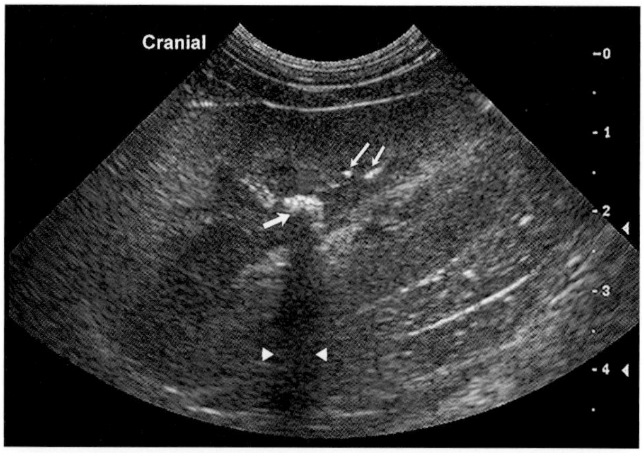

Figure 10.35. Renal mineralization. Longitudinal image of the left kidney of a clinically normal dog. Several foci of mineralization (arrows) are in the region of the collecting system, the largest being associated with acoustic shadowing (arrowheads). These mineral foci may represent nephroliths and/or dystrophic mineralization.

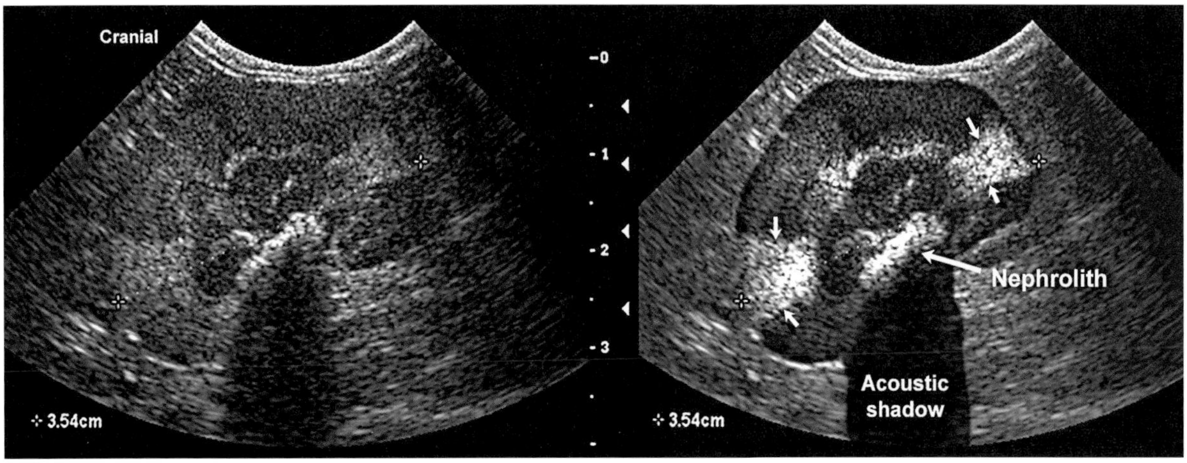

Figure 10.36. Cortical infarcts and pelvic nephrolith. Longitudinal ultrasonographic and schematic images of the right kidney of a cat with chronic urolithiasis but normal renal function. Triangular shaped hyperechoic foci are noted in the cranial and caudal renal poles, consistent with incidental infarcts (arrows). A large nephrolith in the region of the pelvis is not associated with outflow obstruction.

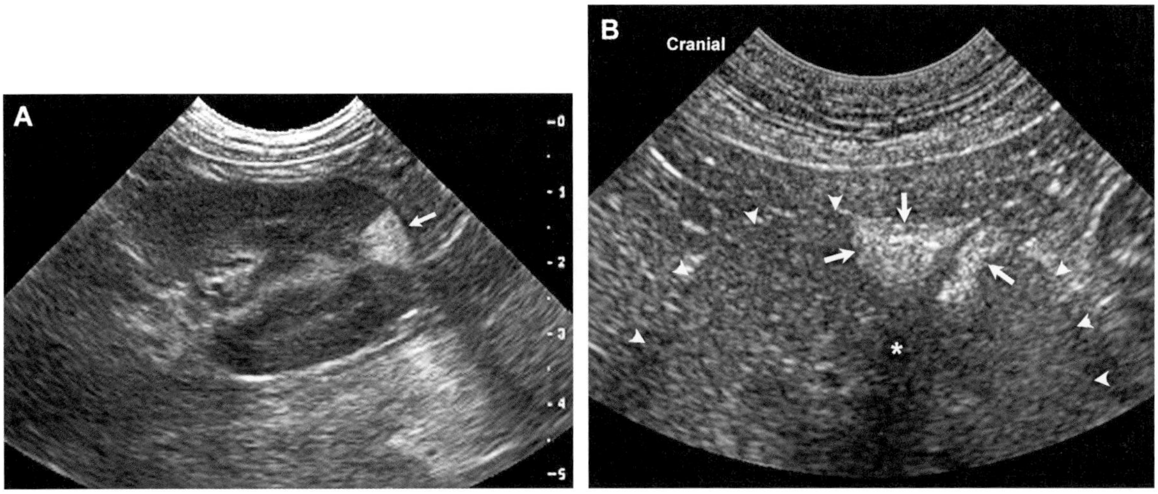

Figure 10.37. Chronic renal infarcts. **A:** Chronic infarct (arrow) on the caudal pole of the left kidney in a dog with normal renal function. Image courtesy of D. Penninck. **B:** Close-up longitudinal image of the left kidney (arrowheads) in a cat with normal renal function. At the periphery of the kidney are triangular-shaped hyperechoic foci (arrows) that are associated with focal cortical depression, consistent with chronic renal infarction. Acoustic shadowing was observed deep to the largest infarct (*), likely because of the presence of hyperattenuating fibrosis and possibly mineralization.

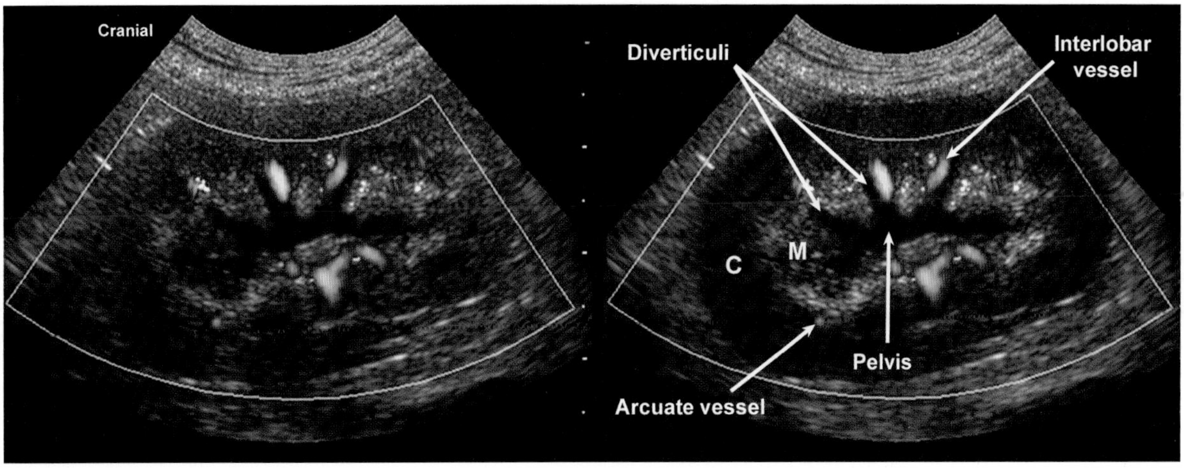

Figure 10.38. Dilated diverticuli in a cat with chronic pyelonephritis. Sagittal ultrasonographic and schematic images of the left kidney. The renal pelvis is distended, as well as the diverticuli, which appear distinct from the interlobar vessels on power Doppler. The medulla (M) is hyperechoic to the cortex (C) because of nephrocalcinosis.

easily identified on transverse planes at the level of the hilus, central to the renal vessels (Figure 10.39). Table 10.1 lists causes of pyelectasia and hydronephrosis in dogs and cats.

When pyelectasia is more pronounced or if hydronephrosis develops because of urinary flow obstruction, renal diverticuli appear as rounded, anechoic fingerlike projections that connect with the renal pelvis (Figures 10.40–10.42). Markedly dilated diverticuli and pelvis must be differentiated from renal cysts or sections of the medulla. The presence of protein or cells (pus or hemorrhage) may increase the urine echogenicity and even be associated with sedimentation, such as sometimes seen in cases of pyelonephritis (Figures 10.40 and 10.43).

With chronic pyelonephritis, in addition to parenchymal changes, the pelvis and diverticuli can become distorted and show a hyperechoic rim because of fibrous tissue remodeling (Figure 10.44). However, it must be pointed out that the renal pelvis may remain normal in mild or early pyelonephritis (Neuwirth et al. 1993).

As opposed to pyelectasia, hydronephrosis is considered to be consecutive to an obstructive disease (Pugh et al. 1994), such as that caused by the migration of a nephrolith or caused by an infiltrating process involving the pelvis, the ureter, or more commonly the ureterovesicular junction. In cases of chronic obstruction, progressive distension of the renal pelvis and diverticuli can cause marked parenchymal atrophy (Figures 10.45–10.47).

Ureteral distension, also termed hydroureter, is usually observed in combination with hydronephrosis in cases of urine flow obstruction. Distended ureters,

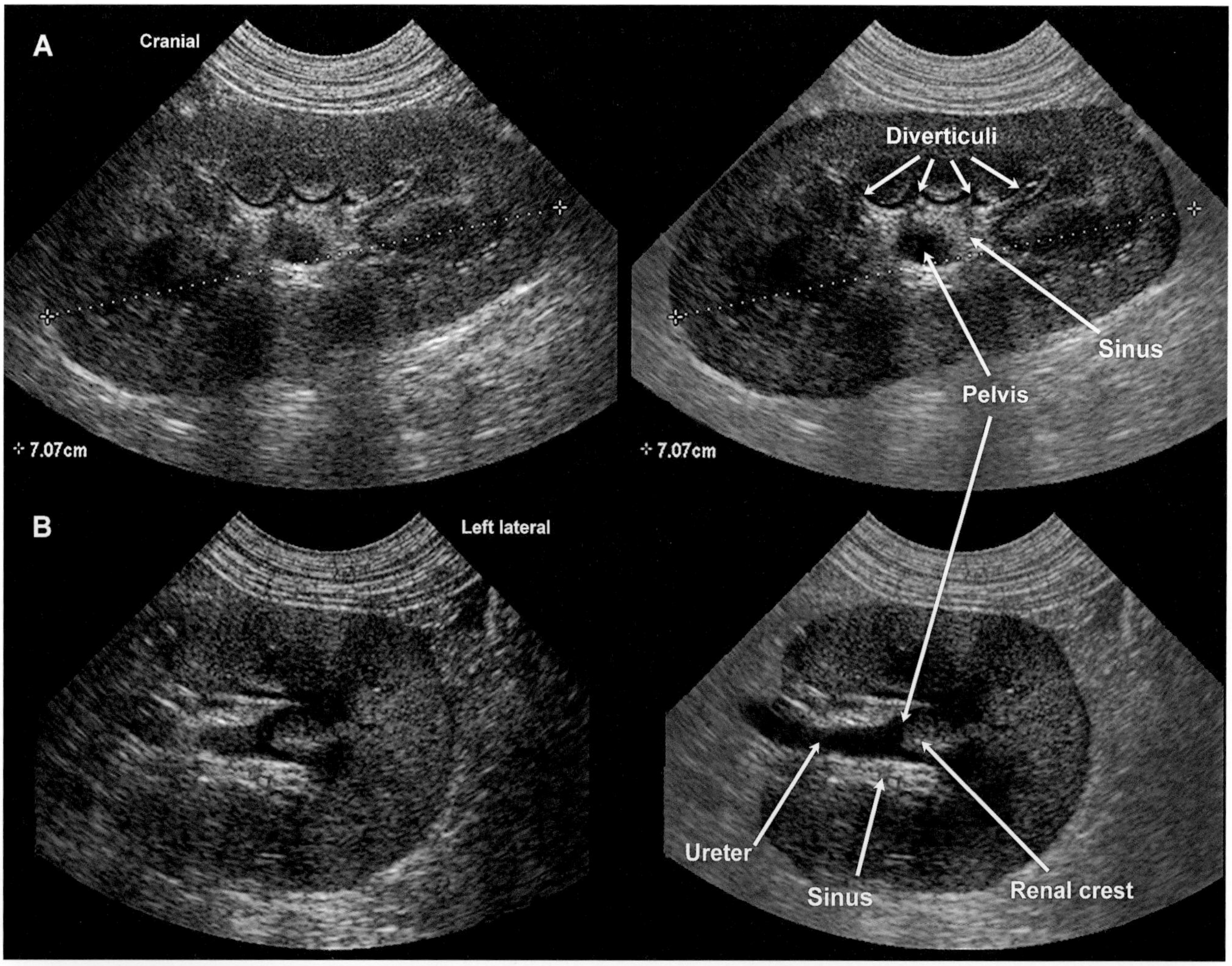

Figure 10.39. Mild hydronephrosis. Longitudinal **(A)** and transverse **(B)** ultrasonographic and schematic images of the left kidney of a dog with urethral obstruction. The proximal ureter, pelvis, and diverticuli appear mildly distended because of outflow obstruction. The proximal ureter is better identified on the transverse image.

Table 10.1.
Differential diagnosis for pyelectasia and hydronephrosis in small animals

Pyelectasia	Hydronephrosis
Intravenous fluid therapy	Lower urinary-tract obstruction
Diuretic therapy	Pelvic or ureteral obstruction: a stone, an infiltrative mass at the bladder trigone, a stricture, or a retroperitoneal mass
Increased diuresis caused by renal insufficiency	Congenital malformation
Distended bladder	
Pyelonephritis or ureteritis	
Ectopic ureter or another congenital malformation	

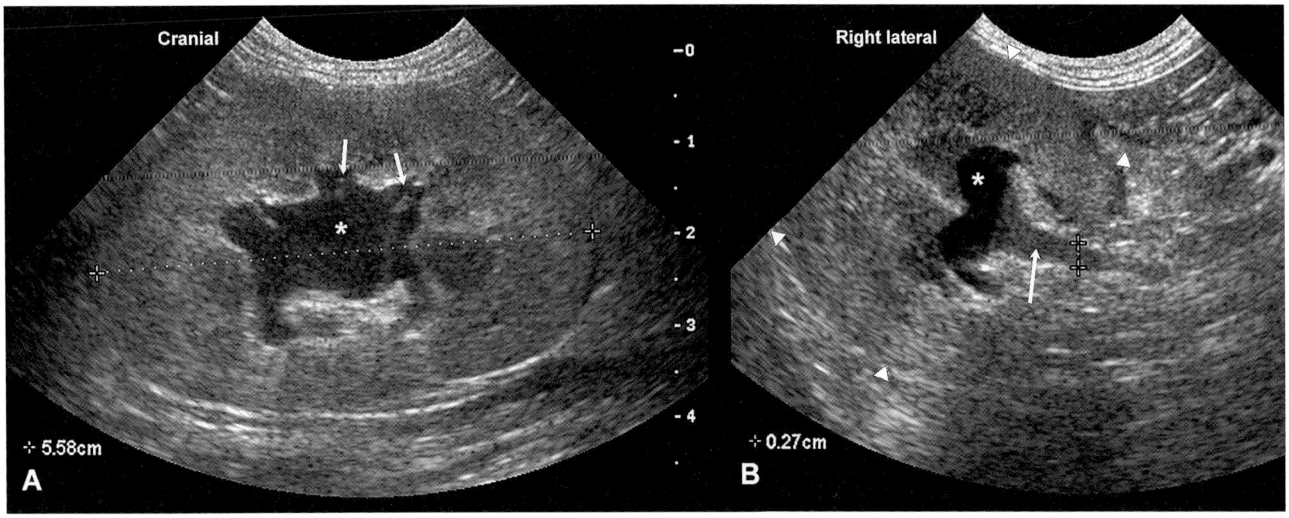

Figure 10.40. Moderate hydronephrosis. Longitudinal **(A)** and transverse **(B)** ultrasonographic images of the right kidney of a small-breed dog with acute renal failure and abdominal pain. The kidney (arrowheads) is enlarged and hyperechoic, and the corticomedullary distinction is attenuated. The renal pelvis (*) and diverticuli (short arrows) are moderately dilated. The proximal ureter is also mildly dilated and contains highly echogenic urine (long arrow), consistent with pus. These signs were caused by ascending urinary infection. Note the sharp, oblique line of cellular sediment in the pelvis on the transverse view, which was parallel to the exam table.

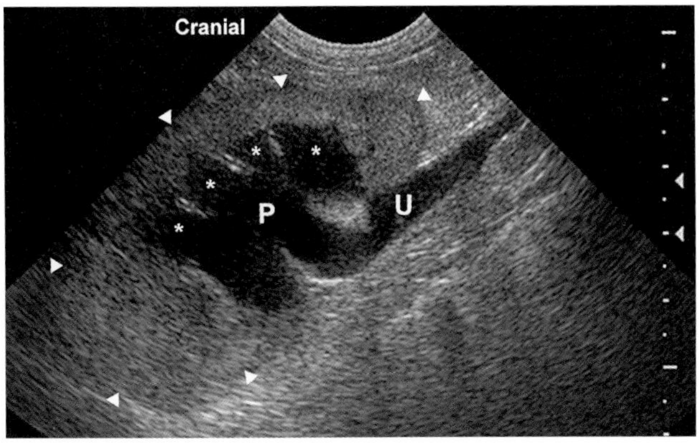

Figure 10.41. Obstructive hydronephrosis. Longitudinal image of the right kidney (arrowheads) in a dog with ureteral obstruction caused by a ureterolith. The distended pelvic diverticuli (*) are rounded and partially separated by hyperechoic septa that contain interlobar arteries and veins. The distended proximal ureter (U) is also apparent, communicating with the pelvis (P).

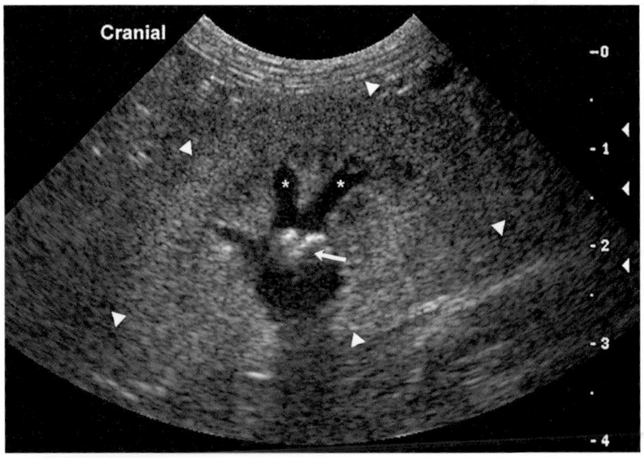

Figure 10.42. Chronic pyelonephritis and nephroliths. Longitudinal image of the left kidney of a cat with renal failure and abdominal pain. The kidney (outlined by arrowheads) is hyperechoic and irregular, and its pelvis and diverticuli (*) are distended and deformed, appearing as hypoechoic fingerlike projections. Irregular hyperechoic and hyperattenuating foci (arrow) are in the center of the pelvis, consistent with small nephroliths. The corticomedullary junction is indistinct. These signs were caused by chronic pyelonephritis in association with urolithiasis.

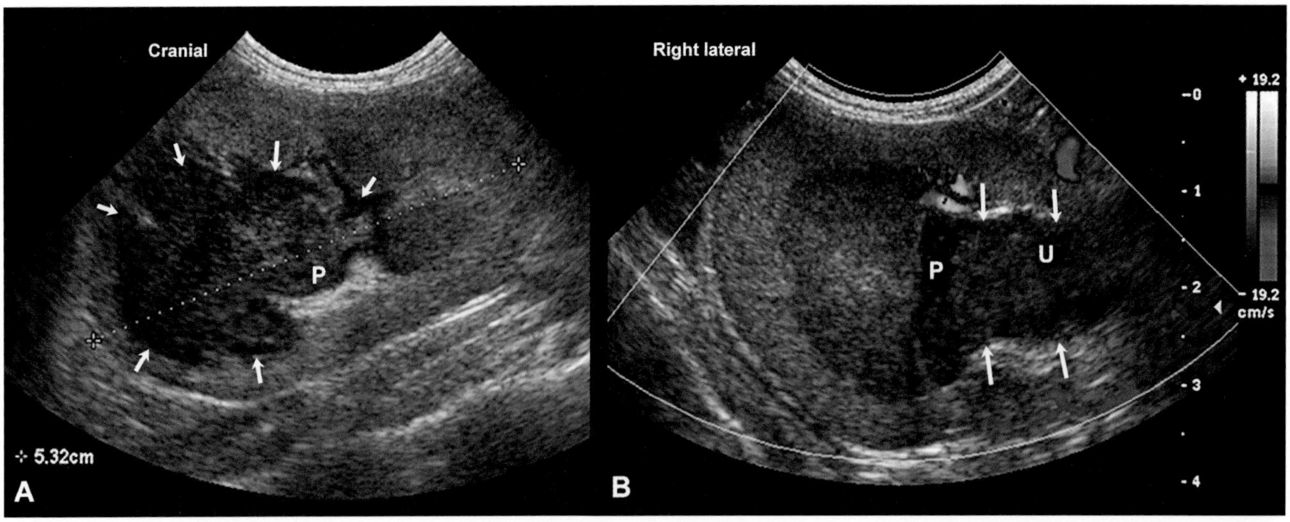

Figure 10.43. Pyonephrosis and ureteral abscess. Longitudinal **(A)** and transverse **(B)** images of the right kidney of a dog with fever and abdominal pain. The renal pelvis (P) and diverticuli are asymmetrically dilated in the cranial pole of the kidney (arrows). The proximal portion of the ureter (U) is also distended. These portions of the collecting system contain echogenic material diagnosed as pus by means of ultrasound-guided pyelocentesis.

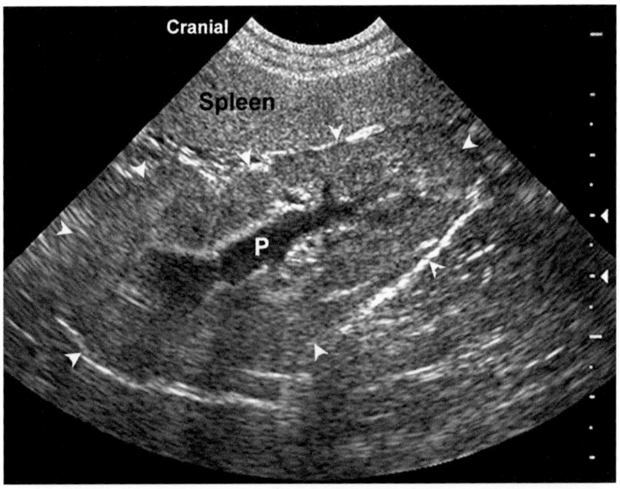

Figure 10.44. Severe chronic pyelonephritis. Longitudinal image of the left kidney in a large-breed dog with chronic renal insufficiency and recurrent cystitis. The kidney is markedly irregular (arrowheads) and diffusely hyperechoic, appearing isoechoic to the spleen. The hypoechoic pelvis (P) is moderately distended and irregular, and its contour is hyperechoic.

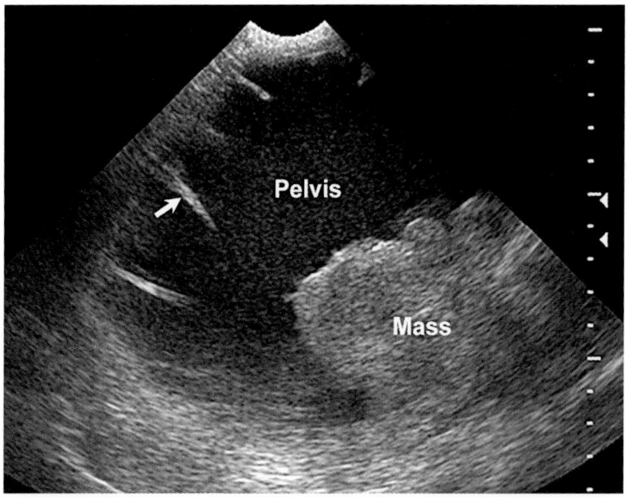

Figure 10.45. Severe hydronephrosis. Longitudinal image of the left kidney in a dog with severe renomegaly diagnosed on radiographs. The kidney appears as a fluid-filled cavity with peripheral hyperechoic bands consistent with interdiverticular septa (arrow). A large, irregular, hyperechoic mass at the level of the renal hilus is invading the renal pelvis and ureter and causing the hydronephrosis. Surgical resection confirmed the presence of a soft-tissue sarcoma.

which can become markedly enlarged and tortuous with long-standing obstructions, can usually be followed caudally to the level of the obstruction. Color or Power Doppler can be useful in differentiating an abdominal vessel from a distended ureter (Figure 10.48). Migrated uroliths appear as hyperechoic structures that are usually associated with acoustic shadowing (Figure 10.49). With complete obstruction, the ureter appears dilated cranially and abruptly blunted caudally at the level of the urolith. Several migrating uroliths may be present, justifying a detailed examination of the entire region of each ureter, up to the level

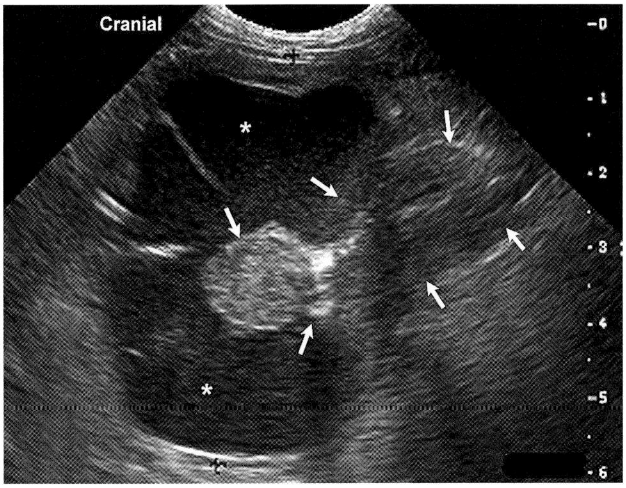

Figure 10.46. Hemangiosarcoma in a dachshund. The mass (arrows) is centered on the pelvis and is responsible for the severe hydronephrosis affecting the right kidney. The renal diverticuli are markedly dilated (*) and contain echogenic fluid, particularly in the dependent portion, consistent with hemorrhage. Image courtesy of D. Penninck.

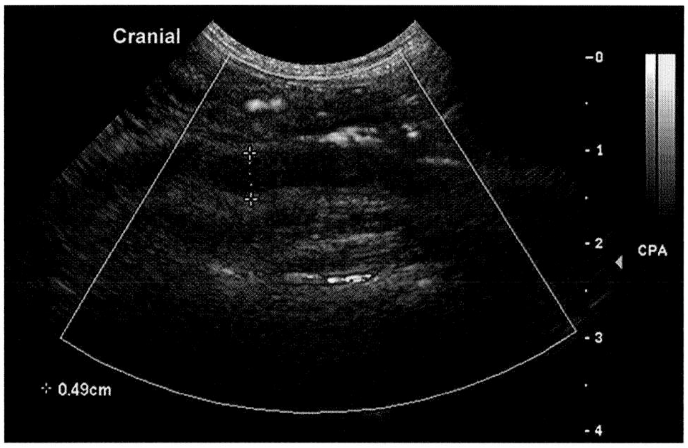

Figure 10.48. Hydroureter. Longitudinal image obtained with Power Doppler in the left midabdomen of a young female dog with urinary incontinence. A 0.5-cm-wide hypoechoic tubular structure can be seen coursing from the renal pelvis to the caudal abdomen, consistent with a dilated ureter. No flow is present. This ureter terminated in the vagina rather than in the urinary bladder, indicating ectopia.

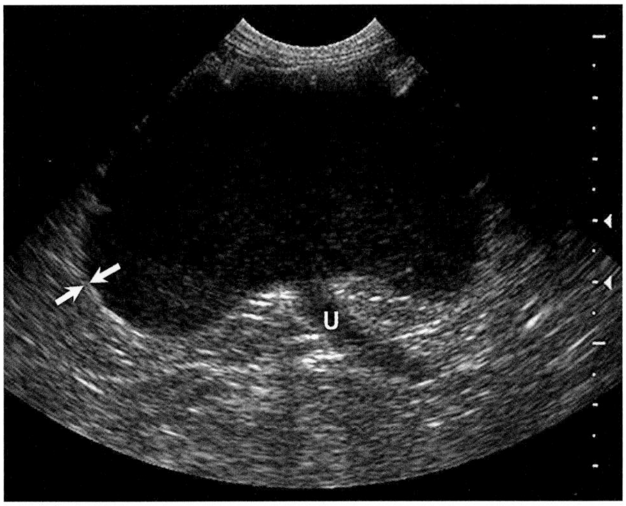

Figure 10.47. Severe hydronephrosis. Longitudinal image of the left kidney in a cat with severe renomegaly. The kidney is completely replaced by hypoechoic fluid, with a rim of parenchyma remaining that is only a few millimeters thick (arrows). Hydroureter is also identified (U). Inadvertent ligation of the distal ureter, secondary to a previous ovariohysterectomy, was identified during exploratory surgery.

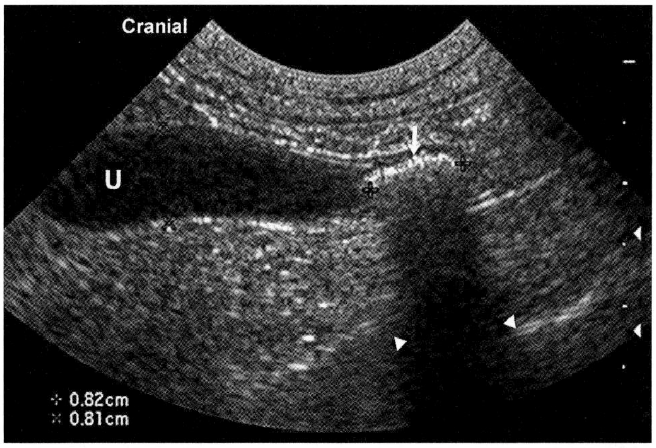

Figure 10.49. Hydroureter. Longitudinal image obtained along the midportion of the right ureter (u) in a dog with hydronephrosis. An ovoid 0.8-cm-wide hyperechoic structure (arrow) found in the lumen of the ureter is associated with a strong acoustic shadow (arrowheads), with proximal luminal dilatation, indicating an obstructive urolith. U, ureter.

of the bladder. The identification of small uroliths can be limited by the presence of overlying gastrointestinal structures, such as the descending colon, or by the lack of significant ureteral distension (Kyles et al. 2005) (Figure 10.50). When combining radiography and ultrasonography, the sensitivity to detect urolithiasis in cats has been reported to reach 90% (Kyles et al. 2005).

Although neoplastic processes infiltrating the bladder trigone and/or ureter are more commonly responsible for ureteral obstruction (Figures 10.51 and 10.52), especially in dogs, other retroperitoneal processes, such as soft-tissue sarcomas, abscesses, or granulomas, can also compress and/or infiltrate the ureter.

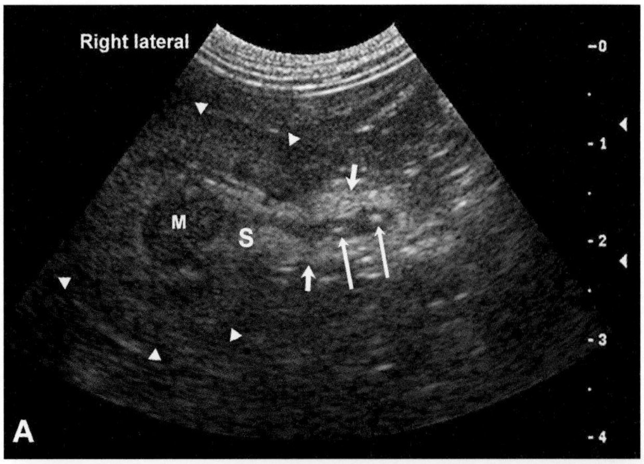

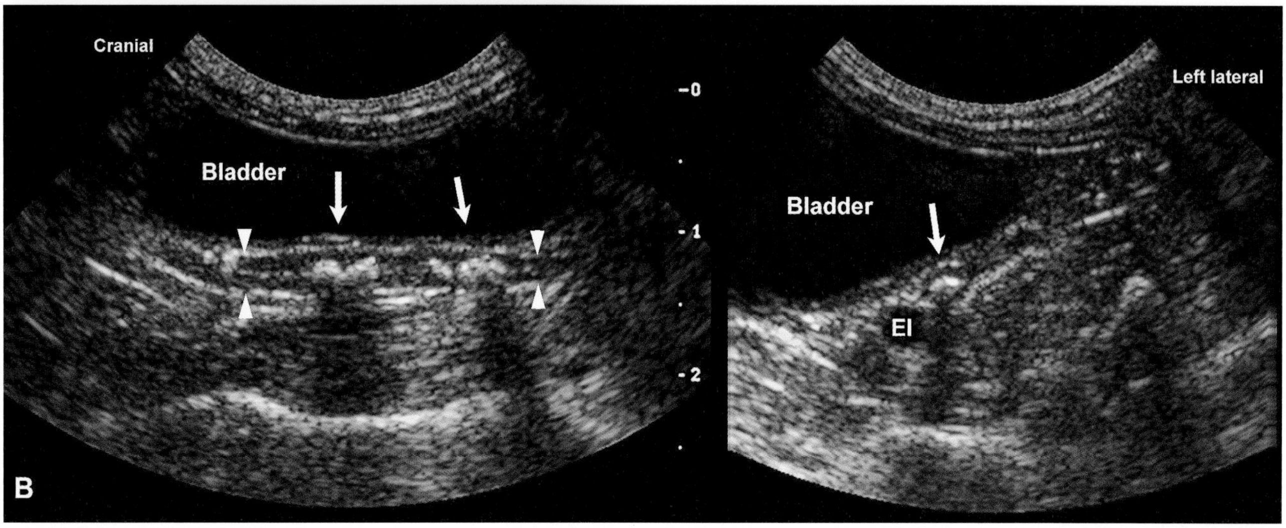

Figure 10.50. Nonobstructive uroliths in two cats. **A:** Transverse image obtained at the level of the right renal hilus of a cat with abdominal pain. Two small hyperechoic foci in the center of the ureter (long arrows) are associated with peripheral fat hyperechogenicity (short arrows), suggesting ureteritis. There is no evidence of ureteral outflow obstruction. On the follow-up exam, these small uroliths were found in the urinary bladder. M, medulla; and S, sinus. **B:** Longitudinal **(left)** and transverse **(right)** images of the distal right ureter of a cat with a chronic history of urolithiasis. Several hyperechoic foci (arrows) are found in the ureter (arrowheads) of this cat without evidence of hydroureter or hydronephrosis. Acoustic shadows are noted in the far field. Some of these calculi were eventually found in the bladder. The ureteral wall is mildly thickened due to edema and/or inflammation. EI, external iliac vessel.

Ureteral obstruction can also be caused by a blood clot, an inflammatory stricture, or a small infiltrative mass, which can be more challenging to diagnose and differentiate. Other imaging tests, such as excretory urography, which can be combined with computed tomography, can be required in patients in which a clear diagnosis cannot be made by using ultrasonography.

Unilateral or bilateral congenital ectopic ureters, which are more common in female dogs, can sometimes be identified and followed to their termination site (the urethra, most commonly, or the vagina or the colon) (Figure 10.53). These ureters are often distended because of partial obstruction at the site of termination or intramural tunneling, ileus, and/or ascending infection. Hydronephrosis can also be present, especially when there is marked hydroureter. With B-mode or with color or power Doppler ultrasonography, an intravesical urine jet can sometimes be observed adjacent to the ureterovesical junction (Lamb and Gregory 1998). The visualization of this ureteral jet can be facilitated by administering a diuretic after withholding water for several hours. A jet of diluted urine can be more easily observed within a bladder filled with more

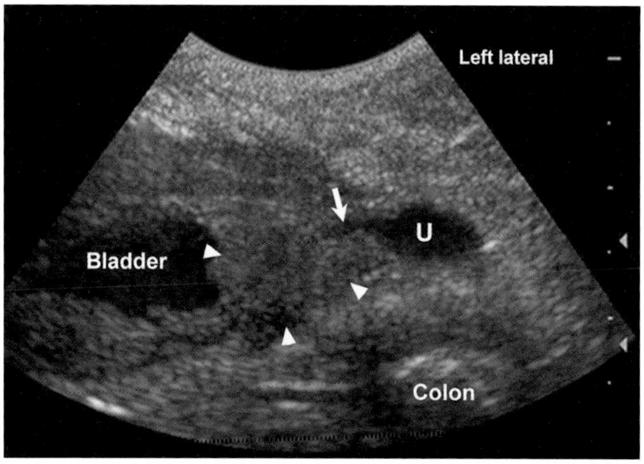

Figure 10.51. Infiltrative bladder mass and hydroureter. Transverse image obtained at the level of the neck of the urinary bladder in a female dog with chronic hematuria. An irregular and poorly defined transmural mass involves the region of the right ureterovesicular junction (arrowheads). The distal portion of the right ureter is dilated (U) by the stenosis (arrow).

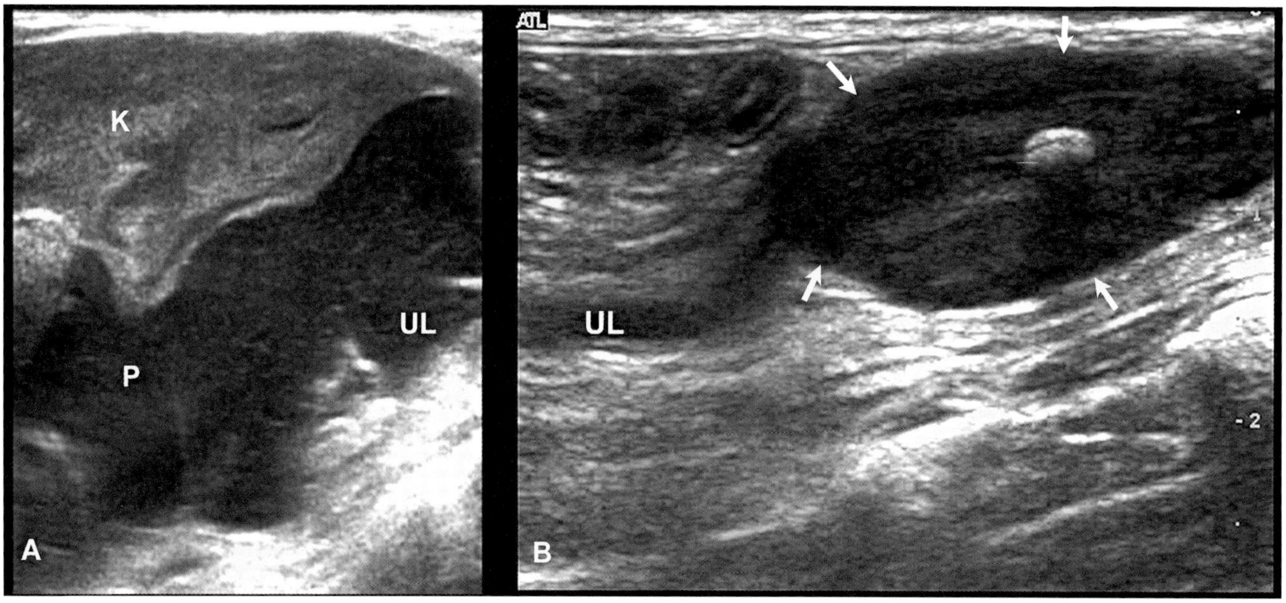

Figure 10.52. Infiltrative ureteral lymphoma. Longitudinal images obtained at the level of the right kidney **(A)** and midright ureter **(B)** in a cat. The kidney (K) is deformed, and the corticomedullary distinction is significantly reduced. The renal pelvis (P) and proximal ureter (UL) are dilated. An oval, hypoechoic, uniform mass (arrows) is found at the level of the right ureter. The ureteral lumen (UL) is dilated cranially. A 3-mm hyperechoic structure in the center of this mass is associated with partial acoustic shadowing and consistent with a concurrent urolith, obstructed at the level of by the infiltrative mass. Histopathology revealed the presence of an unusual lymphoma infiltrating the kidney and ureter. Images courtesy of D. Penninck.

concentrated urine. However, the visualization of a urine jet into the bladder lumen cannot exclude the possibility of tunneling ectopic ureters with multiple fenestrations.

Ureterocele is another congenital ureteral malformation, which can sometimes be associated with ectopia (Stiffler et al. 2002). An intravesical ureterocele is characterized by a focal cystic dilatation of the distal submucosal portion of the ureter that protrudes into the bladder lumen (Figure 11.35). A thin-walled, round structure containing anechoic fluid can be observed within the neck of the bladder by means of ultrasonography (Stiffler et al. 2002). Ectopic ureterocele involves the distal portion of an ectopic ureter.

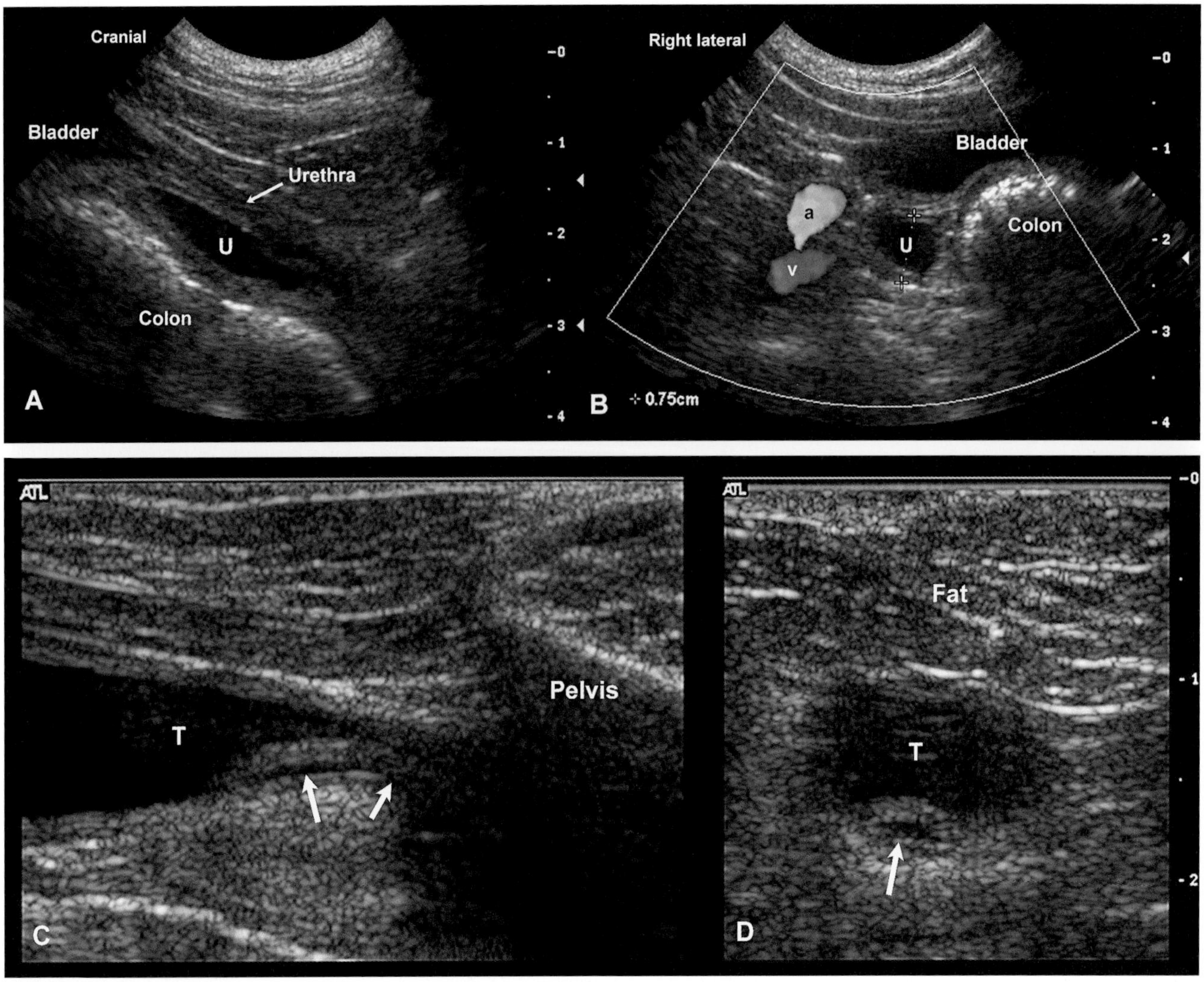

Figure 10.53. Ectopic ureters. **A and B:** Longitudinal **(A)** and transverse **(B)** images obtained in the region of the bladder trigone, in which a tubular structure filled with an anechoic fluid (U) extends beyond the ureterovesicular junction, along the distal colon. There is no flow on color Doppler, as opposed to the external iliac artery (a) and vein (v), which supports a diagnosis of ureteral ectopia. Excretory urography confirmed a termination into the distal portion of the urethra. **C and D:** Longitudinal **(C)** and transverse **(D)** images of the bladder trigone (T) in a young female dog with urinary incontinence. A fluid-filled tubular structure (arrows) consistent with a distal ureter extends through the wall of the bladder, on the dorsal midline, beyond the ureteral papilla. Because of the shadow created by the pelvis, the termination of this ureter could not be determined with ultrasonography. An intramural (tunneling) ectopic ureter terminating into the urethra was confirmed at surgery.

Disorders of the Perinephric Retroperitoneal Space

Several types of fluid can accumulate in the retroperitoneal space at the periphery of the kidneys. Retroperitoneal transudate, which can be seen with several types of renal disease, appears as linear or triangular to oval-shaped, anechoic to hypoechoic foci at the periphery of the renal cortex (Figure 10.54). These changes can also be found with the accumulation of urine or blood, usually following trauma to the kidney and/or ureter (Figure 10.55). Although the effusion can be confirmed and characterized with ultrasonography and fine-needle aspiration, the rupture cannot be easily localized and usually requires other imaging tools, such as excretory urography.

Exudates and acute hemorrhage tend to be more echogenic because of their higher cell count. In cases

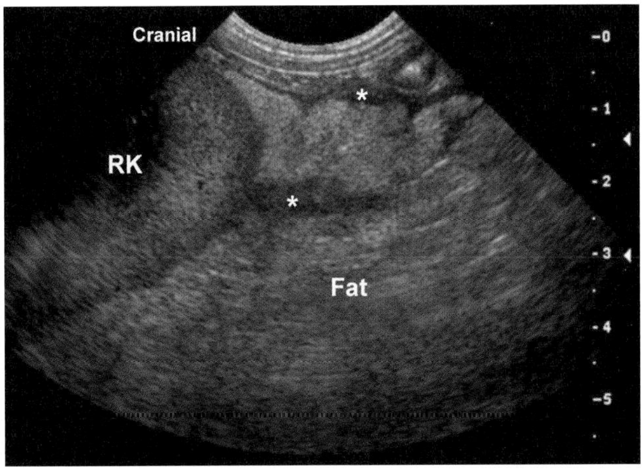

Figure 10.54. Retroperitoneal effusion. Longitudinal image obtained in the region just caudal to the right kidney (RK) of a dog with acute renal insufficiency caused by leptospirosis. Irregular linear hypoechoic regions (*) are within the retroperitoneal space, caudal to the renal cortex, consistent with transudation. The fat appears mildly hyperechoic, which was attributed to edema.

of inflammatory processes involving the retroperitoneal space, the retroperitoneal fat typically becomes hyperechoic and hyperattenuating. These changes are common with acute pyelonephritis and ureteritis (Figure 10.56).

Perinephric pseudocysts, which have been more commonly reported in cats, appear as an accumulation of fluid, usually anechoic, around one or both kidneys, and most commonly between the capsule and the renal cortex (Ochoa et al. 1999; Beck et al. 2000) (Figure 10.57). These pseudocysts typically encircle the kidneys, although they can be focal (Miles and Jergens 1992). According to a report on 26 cats, subcapsular perirenal pseudocysts are formed by accumulation of a transudate between the capsule and parenchyma of the kidney, because of underlying parenchymal disease, and may contribute to abdominal discomfort (Beck et al. 2000). Urine may also be contained in these pseudocysts (Ochoa et al. 1999).

Urinomas, described as an encapsulated accumulation of urine caused by traumatic extravasation (Figure 10.55), can appear similar to pseudocysts. Fine-needle aspiration can be helpful in confirming the nature of the perirenal fluid.

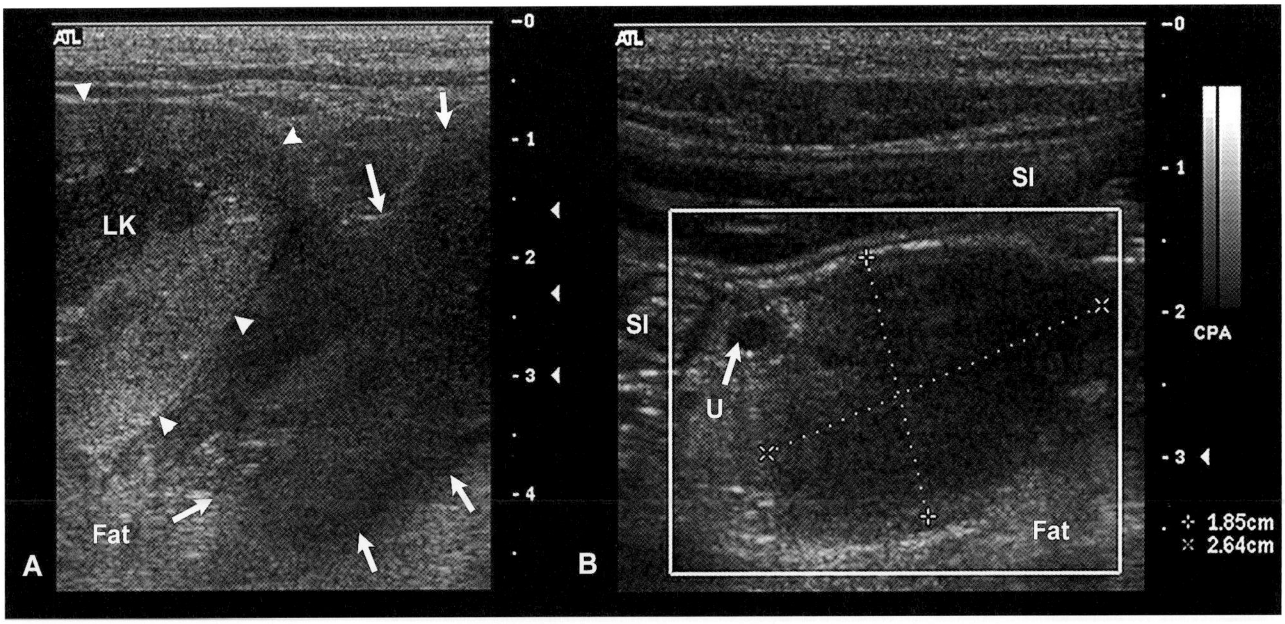

Figure 10.55. Ureteral rupture, retroperitoneal urinoma, and abscess. Longitudinal **(A)** and transverse **(B)** ultrasound images obtained with a linear transducer at the caudal aspect of the left kidney (LK, arrowheads). A poorly defined accumulation of hypoechoic fluid (arrows) is in the retroperitoneal space, caudal to the kidney **(A)** and lateral to the left ureter (U) **(B)**. The retroperitoneal fat is hyperechoic. In **B**, power Doppler is used to differentiate the mildly dilated ureter from an abdominal vessel. The paraureteral fluid collection was sampled with ultrasound guidance, and urine and pus were identified. SI, small intestine.

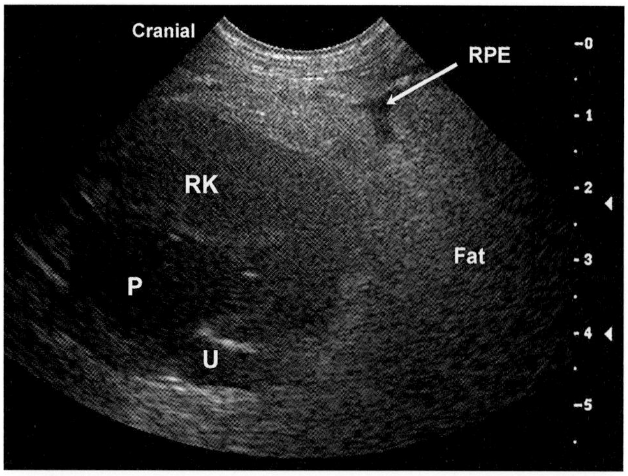

Figure 10.56. Retroperitoneal steatitis. Longitudinal image obtained in the region of the caudal pole of the right kidney (RK) of a cat with hydronephrosis and severe pyelonephritis. The renal pelvis (P) and proximal ureter (U) are distended, and the surrounding fat is hyperechoic and markedly hyperattenuating. The renal contour is consequently poorly defined. A small amount of retroperitoneal effusion (RPE) is also present. Fine-needle aspiration confirmed the presence of sterile retroperitoneal steatitis.

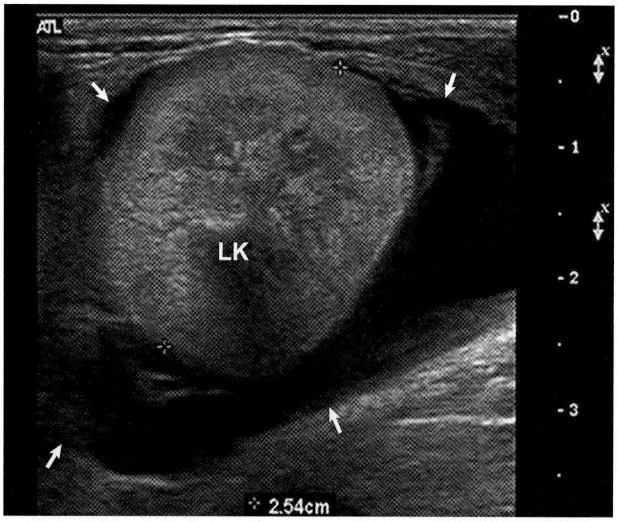

Figure 10.57. Perinephric pseudocyst. Longitudinal image of the left kidney (LK) of a cat with chronic renal insufficiency. The kidney is small (2.54 cm), deformed, irregular, and diffusely hyperechoic because of chronic interstitial nephritis. The kidney is contained in a large anechoic cystlike cavity (arrows), consistent with a perinephric pseudocyst. Image courtesy of J. Sutherland-Smith.

Interventional Procedures

Ultrasound-guided fine-needle aspiration and biopsy have become routine procedures complementing renal ultrasonography. The choice of needle size (gauge)

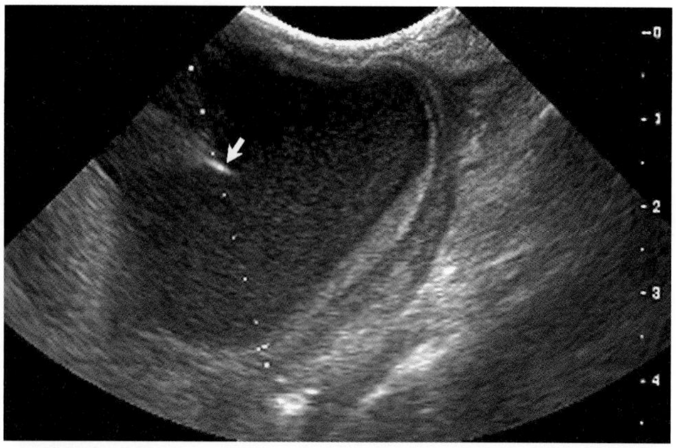

Figure 10.58. Ultrasound-guided aspiration. A fine-needle aspiration is performed on a perirenal pseudocyst (the same cat as in Figure 10.22). The needle tip (arrow) is in the fluid-filled cavity. Image courtesy of D. Penninck.

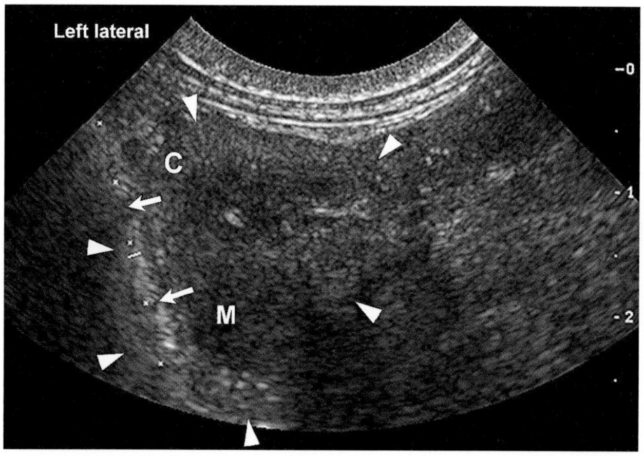

Figure 10.59. Ultrasound-guided renal biopsy. A biopsy is performed through the lateral cortex (C) of the left kidney (arrowheads) of a shar-pei (the same as in Figure 10.11B). The hyperechoic needle (arrows) is seen along the biopsy-guided tract (dotted line), avoiding the medulla (M).

and length depends on the size, vascularity, and depth of the targeted tissue. Usually, 20- to 22-gauge needles are used for fine-needle aspiration, and 14- to 20-gauge needles are used for automated core biopsy (Figures 10.58 and 10.59). Fine-needle aspiration can usually be performed with the animal under minimal sedation, whereas biopsy usually requires general anesthesia. Neoplastic processes, such as lymphoma, are usually diagnosed on a cytological specimen obtained with fine-needle aspiration, although a more confident diagnosis can sometimes require a biopsy. When inflammatory processes are suspected, biopsy is generally recommended because it enables a better discrimination between processes. Complications

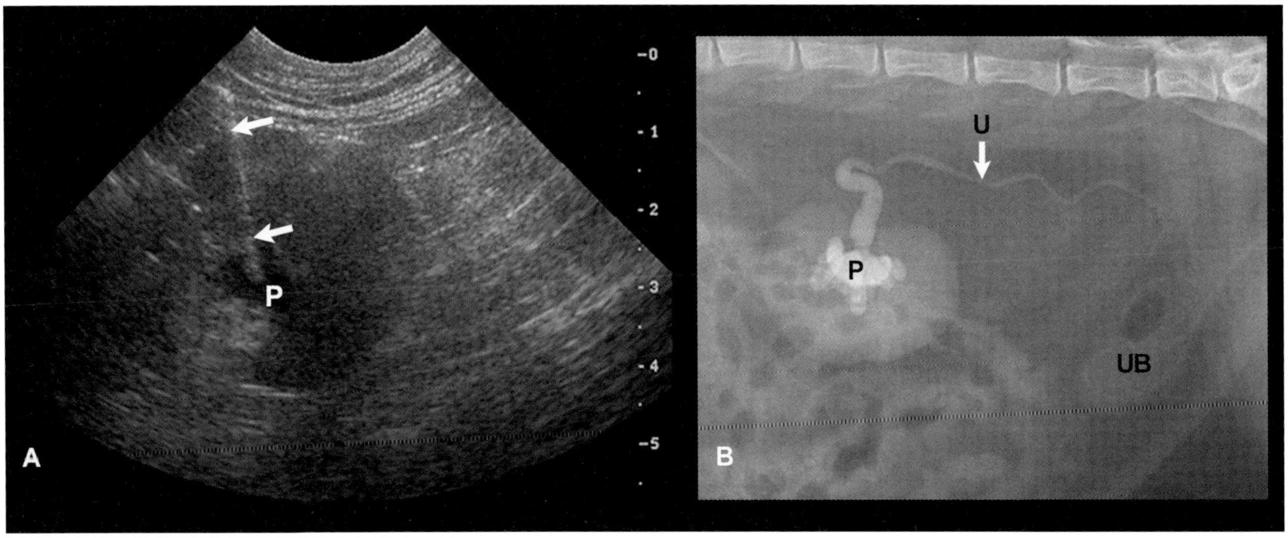

Figure 10.60. Ultrasound-guided pyelocentesis and pyelography. **A:** Transverse ultrasound image of the left kidney in cat with acute renal failure and anuria. The right kidney was previously removed for a suspected tumor. A 21-gauge 1.5-inch-long needle (arrows) was inserted into the renal pelvis (P) for urine collection. This was followed by the injection of 5 mL of iopamidol (300 mg iodine/mL). **B:** On a lateral radiograph of the caudal abdomen obtained 10 min later, opacification of the pelvis and ureter (U) is observed. A urinary catheter and an oval gas bubble are visible in the bladder. Ureteral obstruction is indicated by the lack of contrast medium reaching the distal ureter and urinary bladder (UB). An obstructive clot was identified in the distal ureter at surgery.

associated with ultrasound-guided biopsy have been reported to vary between 9% in dogs and 15% in cats, and most commonly have included hemorrhage (Vaden et al. 2005). Older dogs and severely azotemic dogs were at higher risk for complications (Vaden et al. 2005). Larger-gauge needles (14 or 16 gauge) are associated with higher-quality specimens (i.e., with larger number of glomeruli), but also with greater likelihood of hemorrhage (Rawlings et al. 2003).

Fine-needle drainage of cavitary lesions, such as cysts or abscesses, can also be performed as a diagnostic and/or therapeutic procedure (Figure 10.58). In place of excretory urography, fine-needle aspiration of a distended pelvis (pyelocenthesis) can be performed and followed by intrapelvic injection of iodine-based contrast medium (Rivers et al. 1997) (Figure 10.60). After a 22-gauge spinal needle with a 45° angle is inserted through the great curvature of the kidney, a volume of contrast medium equal to one-half of the aspirated volume of urine is injected with ultrasound guidance prior to radiographic exposure. By allowing a higher concentration of contrast medium to reach the pelvis and ureter in cases of renal failure, their shape and content can be better defined. Additionally, the risk of contrast medium-induced nephropathy can be lowered in animals with compromised renal function. Antegrade pyelography can be a useful alternative in the diagnosis and localization of ureteral obstructions in azotemic cats (Adin et al. 2003). Complications are considered rare. As with renal aspiration or biopsy, hematuria can occur.

Some dogs and cats can benefit from drainage of large renal cysts or pseudocysts (Ochoa et al. 1999). Therapeutic drainage and lavage of the renal pelvis can also help to remove obstructive pus in dogs with pyonephrosis (Szatmari et al. 2001).

References

Abraham LA, Beck C, Slocombe RF (2003) Renal dysplasia and urinary tract infection in a Bull Mastiff puppy. Aust Vet J 81:336–339.

Adams WH, Toal RL, Breider MA (1991) Ultrasonographic findings in dogs and cats with oxalate nephrosis attributable to ethylene glycol intoxication: 15 cases (1984–1988). J Am Vet Med Assoc 199:492–496.

Adin CA, Herrgesell EJ, Nyland TG, et al. (2003) Antegrade pyelography for suspected ureteral obstruction in cats: 11 cats (1995–2001). J Am Vet Med Assoc 222:1576–1581.

Allworth MS, Hoffman KL (1999) Crossed renal ectopia with fusion in a cat. Vet Radiol Ultrasound 40:357–360.

Barr FJ, Holt PE, Gibbs C (1990) Ultrasonographic measurements of normal renal parameters. J Small Anim Pract 31:180–184.

Barr FJ, Petteson MW, Lucke VM, Gibbs C (1989) Hypercalcemic nephropathy in three dogs: Sonographic appearance. Vet Radiology Ultrasound 30:169–173.

Beck JA, Bellenger CR, Lamb WA, et al. (2000) Perirenal pseudocysts in 26 cats. Aust Vet J 78:166–171.

Biller DS, Bradley GA, Partington BP (1992) Renal medullary rim sign: Ultrasonographic evidence of renal disease. Vet Radiol Ultrasound 33:286–290.

Eubig PA, Brady MS, Gwaltney-Brant SM, Khan SA, Mazzaferro EM, Morrow CM (2005) Acute renal failure in dogs after the ingestion of grapes or raisins: A retrospective evaluation of 43 dogs (1992–2002). J Vet Intern Med 19:663–674.

Felki C, Voros Fenyves B (1995) Lesions of the renal pelvis and proximal ureter in various nephro-urological conditions: An ultrasonographic study. Vet Radiol Ultrasound 36:397–401.

Forrest LJ, O'Brien RT, Tremelling MS, Steinberg H, Cooley AJ, Kerlin RL (1998) Sonographic renal findings in 20 dogs with leptospirosis. Vet Radiol Ultrasound 39:337–340.

Gasser AM, Bush WW, Smith SS, Walton R (2003) Extradural spinal, bone marrow, and renal nephroblastoma. J Am Anim Hosp Assoc 39:80–85.

Hecht S, McCarthy RJ, Tidwell AS (2005) What is your diagnosis? Ectopic kidney. J Am Vet Med Assoc 227: 223–224.

Konde LJ, Wrigley RH, Park RD, Lebel JL (1984) Ultrasonographic anatomy of the normal canine kidney. Vet Radiol 25:173–178.

Kyles AE, Hardie EM, Wooden BG, et al. (2005) Clinical, clinicopathologic, radiographic, and ultrasonographic abnormalities in cats with ureteral calculi: 163 cases (1984–2002). J Am Vet Med Assoc 226:932–936.

Lamb CR, Gregory SP (1998) Ultrasonographic findings in 14 dogs with ectopic ureter. Vet Radiol Ultrasound 39:218–223.

Mantis P, Lamb CR (2000) Most dogs with medullary rim sign on ultrasonography have no demonstrable renal dysfunction. Vet Radiol Ultrasound 41:164–166.

Mareschal A, d'Anjou MA, Moreau M, Alexander K, Beauregard G (2007) Ultrasonographic measurement of kidney-to-aorta ratio as a method os estimating renal size in dogs. Vet Radiol Ultrasound 48(5):434–438.

Miles KG, Jergens AE (1992) Unilateral perinephric pseudocyst of undetermined origin in a dog. Vet Radiol Ultrasound 33:277–281.

Moe L, Lium B (1997) Hereditary multifocal renal cystadenocarcinomas and nodular dermatofibrosis in 51 German shepherd dogs. J Small Anim Pract 38:498–505.

Neuwirth L, Mahaffey M, Crowell W, et al. (1993) Comparison of excretory urography and ultrasonography for detection of experimentally induced pyelonephritis in dogs. Am J Vet Res 54:660–669.

Ochoa VB, DiBartola SP, Chew DJ, Westropp J, Carothers M, Biller D (1999) Perinephric pseudocysts in the cat: A retrospective study and review of the literature. J Vet Intern Med 13:47–55.

Pugh CR, Schelling CG, Moreau RE, Golden D (1994) Iatrogenic renal pyelectasia in the dog. Vet Radiol Ultrasound 35:50–51.

Rawlings CA, Diamond H, Howerth EW, Neuwirth L, Canalis C (2003) Diagnostic quality of percutaneous kidney biopsy specimens obtained with laparoscopy versus ultrasound guidance in dogs. J Am Vet Med Assoc 223:317–321.

Reichle JK, DiBartola SP, Léveillé R (2002) Renal ultrasonographic and computed tomographic appearance, volume, and function of cats with autosomal dominant polycystic kidney disease. Vet Radiol Ultrasound 43:368–373.

Rivers BJ, Walter PA, Polzin DJ (1997) Ultrasonographic-guided, percutaneous antegrade pyelography: Technique and clinical application in the dog and cat. J Am Anim Hosp Assoc 33:61–68.

Stiffler KS, Stevenson MAM, Mahaffey MB, Howerth EW, Barsanti JA (2002) Intravesical ureterocele with concurrent renal dysfunction in a dog: A case report and proposed classification system. J Am Anim Hosp Assoc 38:33–39.

Szatmari V, Osi Z, Manczur F (2001) Ultrasound-guided percutaneous drainage for treatment of pyonephrosis in two dogs. J Am Vet Med Assoc 218:1796–1799.

Vaden SL, Levine JF, Lees GE, Groman RP, Grauer GF, Forrester SD (2005) Renal biopsy: A retrospective study of methods and complications in 283 dogs and 65 cats. J Vet Intern Med 19:794–801.

Walter PA, Feeney DA, Johnston GR, Fletcher TF (1987a) Feline renal ultrasonography: Quantitative analyses of imaged anatomy. Am J Vet Res 48:596–599.

Walter PA, Feeney Da, Johnston GR, O'Leary TP (1987b) Ultrasonographic evaluation of renal parenchymal diseases in dogs: 32 cases (1981–1986). J Am Vet med Assoc 191:999–1007.

Walter PA, Johnston GR, Feeney DA, O'Brien TD (1988) Applications of ultrasonography in the diagnosis of parenchymal kidney disease in cats: 24 cases (1981–1986). J Am Vet Med Assoc 192:92–98.

Yeager AE, Anderson WI (1989) Study of association between histologic features and echogenicity of architecturally normal cat kidneys. Am J Vet Res 50:860–863.

CHAPTER ELEVEN

Bladder and Urethra

James Sutherland-Smith

Preparation and Scanning Technique

The ventral abdominal hair is clipped to the level of the pubic bone, and ultrasonic gel is applied to the skin. A transabdominal approach with the animal in dorsal recumbency is preferred, but left or right lateral recumbency or a standing position may be used in confirming the presence of intraluminal sediment or calculi, which will fall toward the gravity-dependent wall. If the penile urethra is to be imaged, then hair may be clipped from the perineum and the region cranial to the scrotum.

A real-time medium- to high-frequency (5 to 7.5 MHz or higher) convex, linear, or vector transducer is recommended. A microconvex transducer with a small contact area has the advantage of being easier to point toward the intrapelvic structures. Two complementary transverse and longitudinal planes are used to fully assess the bladder and urethra (Figure 11.1).

The best ultrasound images of the bladder are obtained when it is moderately distended (Figure 11.2). If the bladder is empty and pathology is suspected, it is advisable either to rescan the bladder after waiting for it to refill naturally, to place a urinary catheter and fill the bladder with sterile isotonic (0.9%) saline, or to administer intravenous furosemide.

Ultrasonographic Anatomy of the Normal Urinary Bladder and Urethra

The bladder is within the caudoventral abdomen, and the urethra extends into the pelvic canal. The descending colon, aorta, and caudal vena cava are dorsal to the urinary bladder. These vessels can be identified by their location and by using color Doppler.

Air within the colon cause a mirror-image artifact of the wrinary bladder (Figure 11.3). In intact females, the uterine body is between the urinary bladder and the colon.

The four histological bladder wall layers are the mucosa (hypoechoic), submucosa (hyperechoic), muscularis (hypoechoic), and serosa (hyperechoic). However, these layers are difficult to define sonographically compared with the gastrointestinal tract. The bladder wall thickness decreases as the urinary bladder volume increases (Figure 11.4). The normal bladder wall thickness increases up to 1 mm with increasing body weight in dogs (Geisse et al. 1997) (Table 11.1). The normal range of bladder wall thickness in cats is between 1.3 and 1.7 mm (Finn-Bodner 1995).

The trigone of the bladder is not clearly delineated from the remainder of the bladder wall. The ureters are not seen entering the urinary bladder unless they are dilated. Ureteral papilla may be seen extending from the dorsal wall and should not be confused for abnormal focal wall thickening (Figure 11.5).

Ureteral jets may be seen emerging from the dorsal bladder wall at the trigone. They appear as a burst of hyperechoic speckles on B-mode ultrasound or a pulse of positive (red) signal on color flow Doppler (Figure 11.6). The visualization of ureteral jets is variable because it requires a difference in the specific gravity between the urine in the bladder and the urine exiting the ureter.

The normal urine within the urinary bladder is anechoic. However, echogenic urine is not specific for urinary tract disease, and a urinalysis can assist in determining its significance. Additionally, images of the urinary bladder are prone to side-lobe and grating-lobe artifacts that can create the appearance of pseudosludge (Figure 11.7). Adjustment of the gain (Figure 11.8) and use of harmonic ultrasound help to reduce the formation of these sometimes confusing echoes.

Retrograde positive-contrast urethrography remains the preferred modality for assessing the entire urethra. Ultrasound is a useful and complementary modality for part of the accessible urethra. The urethra extends caudally from the bladder into the pelvic canal (Figure 11.9).

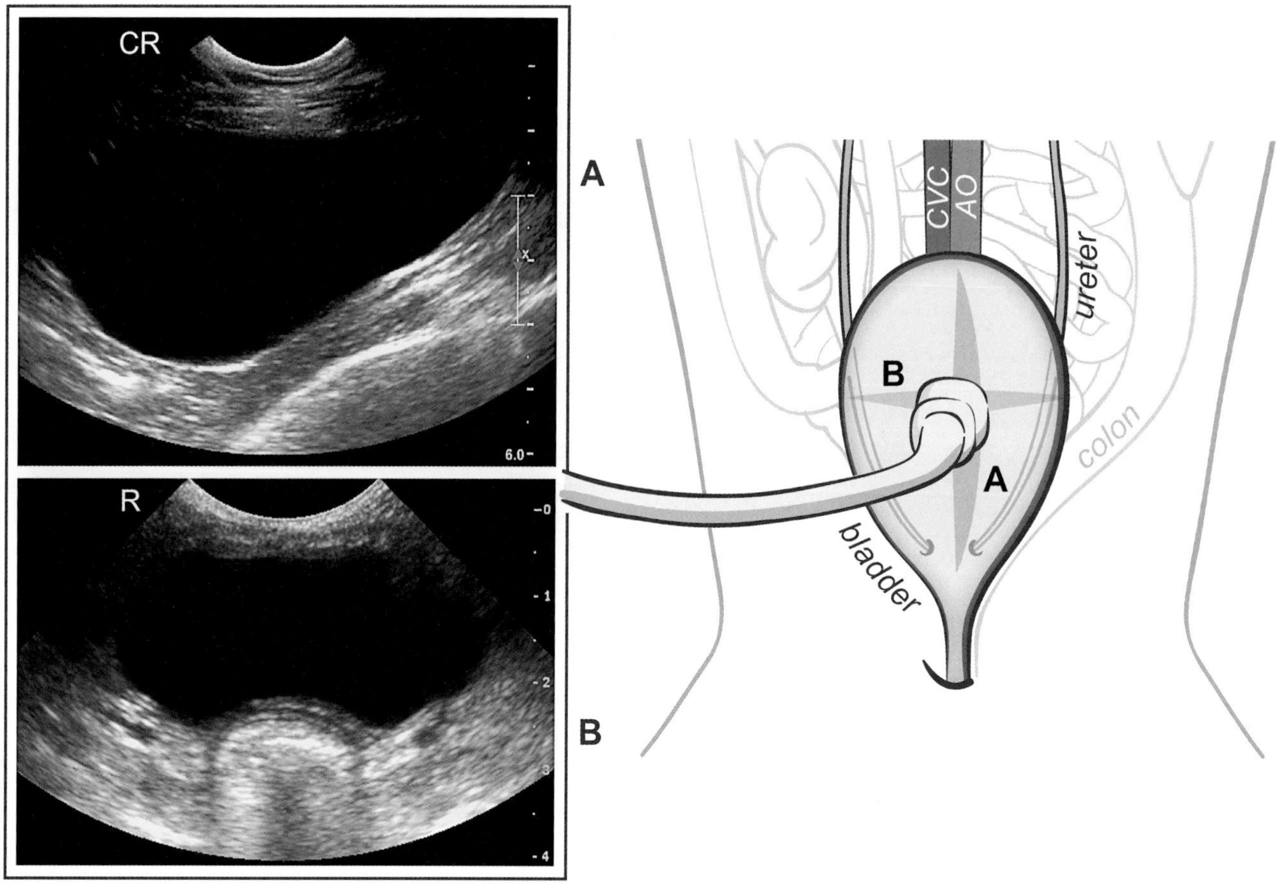

Figure 11.1. Composite image of the urinary bladder and adjacent anatomical structures in a dog. The schematic diagram on the right shows the position of the urinary bladder, the dorsally located colon, aorta, and caudal vena cava, as well as transducer positions for the standard longitudinal and transverse imaging planes. **A:** A longitudinal sonogram of the urinary bladder filled with normal anechoic urine. **B:** A transverse sonogram of the urinary bladder. The colon is located dorsally in the far field and is causing mild indentation of the dorsal bladder wall. AO, aorta; CR, cranial; CVC, caudal vena cava; and R, right.

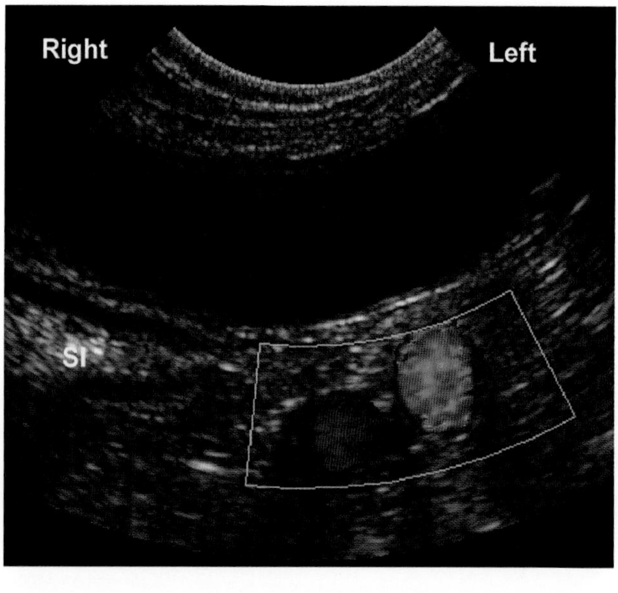

Figure 11.2. Normal bladder and main vessels in a dog. Color flow Doppler transverse sonogram of the urinary bladder and the dorsally located aorta (red) and caudal vena cava (blue), to the left of an intestinal loop (SI).

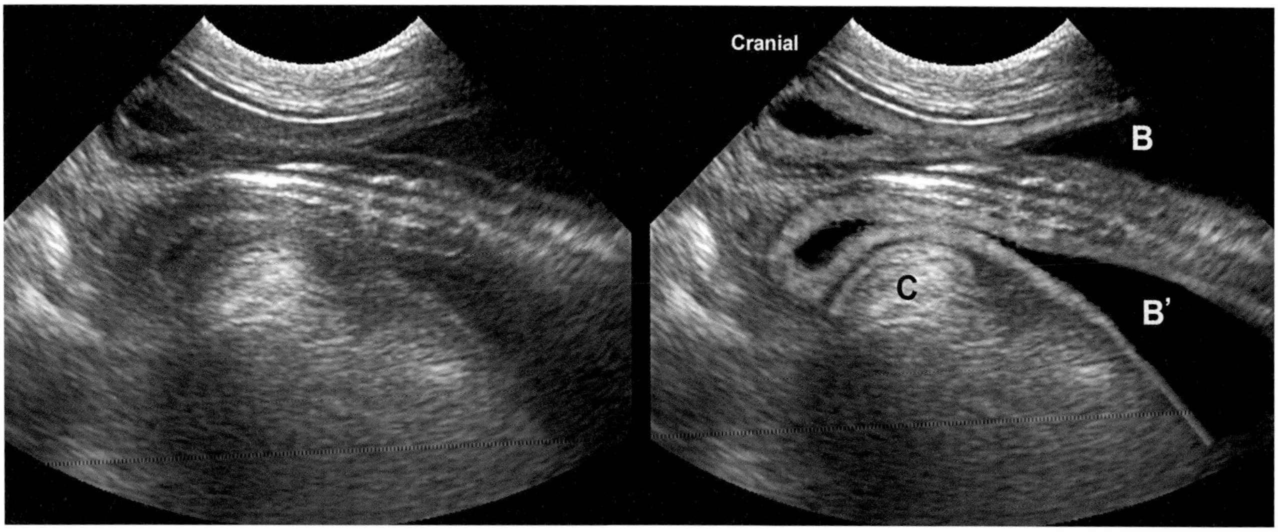

Figure 11.3. Mirror-image artifact in a dog. **Left:** Longitudinal sonogram of the urinary bladder with a mirror-image artifact caused by errors in position of echoes reflected from the ventral colon wall–colon luminal gas interface. **Right:** The corresponding labeled schematic representation. B, bladder; B′, mirror image of the bladder; and C, colon.

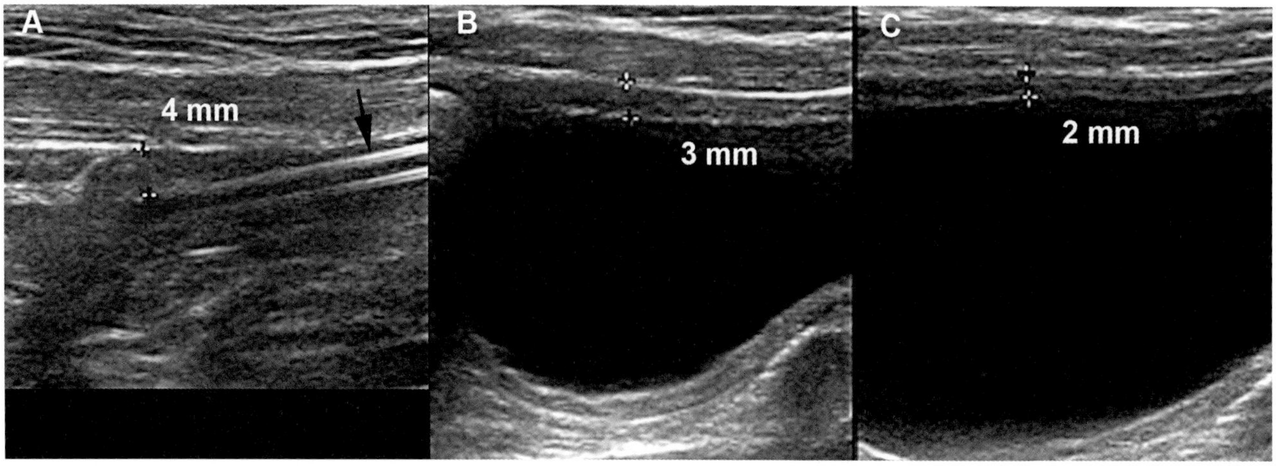

Figure 11.4. Normal bladder thickness and distension in a normal 30-kg dog. A series of longitudinal ultrasound images of the urinary bladder with different volumes of sterile saline infused into the bladder lumen. **A:** Longitudinal sonogram of an empty urinary bladder with an indwelling red-rubber urinary catheter (arrow). The urinary bladder wall thickness is 4 mm. **B:** A total of 60 mL (2 mL/kg) of saline is infused, and the bladder wall thickness now is 3 mm. **C:** With a total volume of 120 mL (4 mL/kg), the bladder wall thickness is 2 mm.

Table 11.1.
Variation in bladder wall thickness with changes in intraluminal volume in dogs

Degree of Bladder Distension	Mean Thickness (mm)	Standard Deviation (mm)
Minimal (0.5 mL/kg)	2.3	0.43
Mild (2 mL/kg)	1.6	0.29
Moderate (4 mL/kg)	1.4	0.28

Adapted from Geisse et al. (1997).

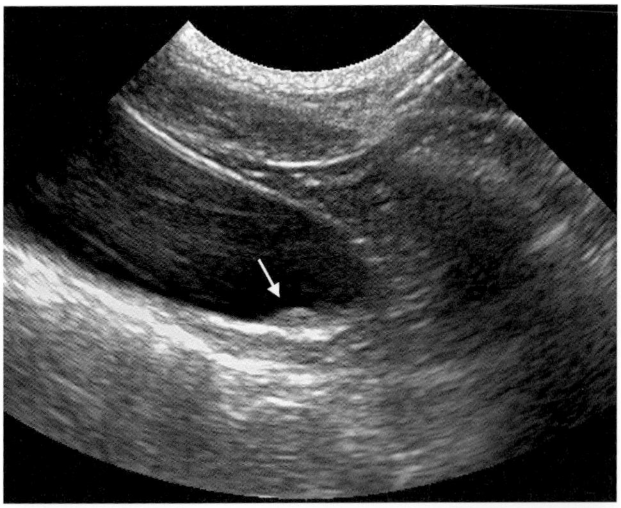

Figure 11.5. Normal ureteral papillae in a dog. Longitudinal sonogram of the trigone of the urinary bladder. There is a smooth, broad-based echogenic protuberance at (arrow) the dorsocaudal aspect of the urinary bladder. These protuberances are seen bilaterally and are visible ureteral papillae.

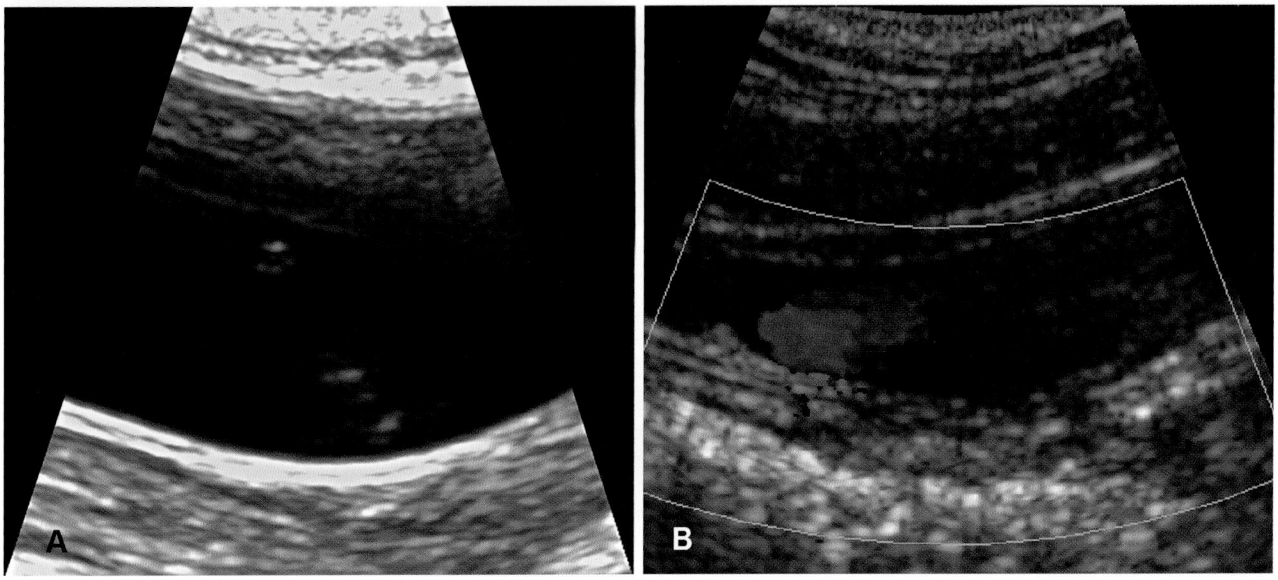

Figure 11.6. Ureteral jet in a dog. **A:** Longitudinal sonogram of a ureteral jet seen using B-mode ultrasound. Although best appreciated in real time, a fountain-like collection of echoes is seen in the otherwise anechoic urine. **B:** Transverse color flow Doppler sonogram of a ureteral jet. The use of color flow Doppler can aid the detection of ureteral jets. The red indicates flow toward the transducer.

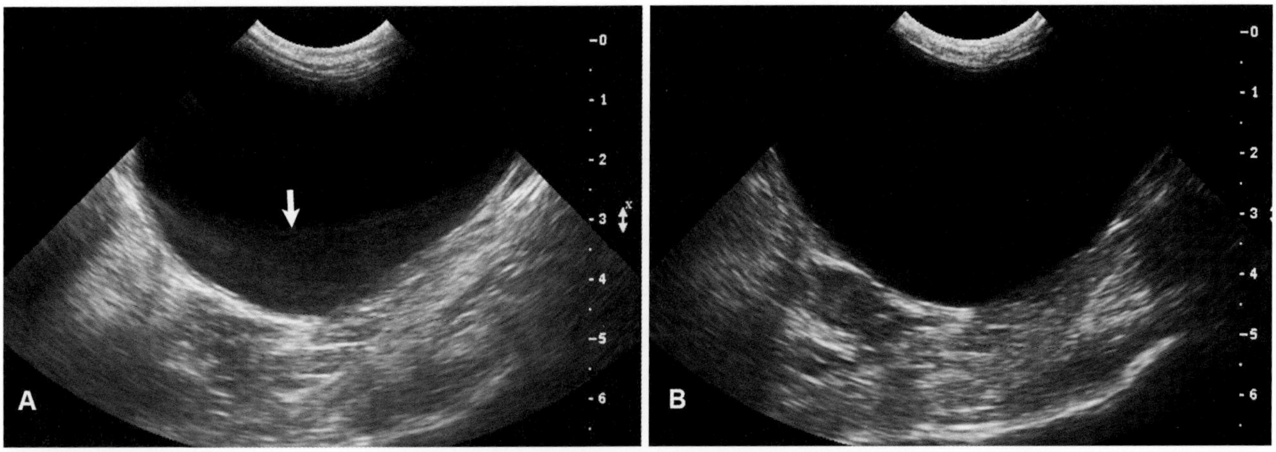

Figure 11.7. Pseudosludge and side-lobe artifacts. **A:** Longitudinal sonogram of the urinary bladder illustrating pseudosludge (arrow) caused by side-lobe and grating-lobe artifacts. These echoes are caused by reflections at the margins of the bladder wall. Scanning with the animal standing may help in confirming this artifact. True sediment should fall to the dependent wall and typically shows a straight linear border (see Figure 11.28A). **B:** Longitudinal sonogram of the same urinary bladder. The time-gain compensation has been adjusted to reduce the appearance of the pseudosludge artifact.

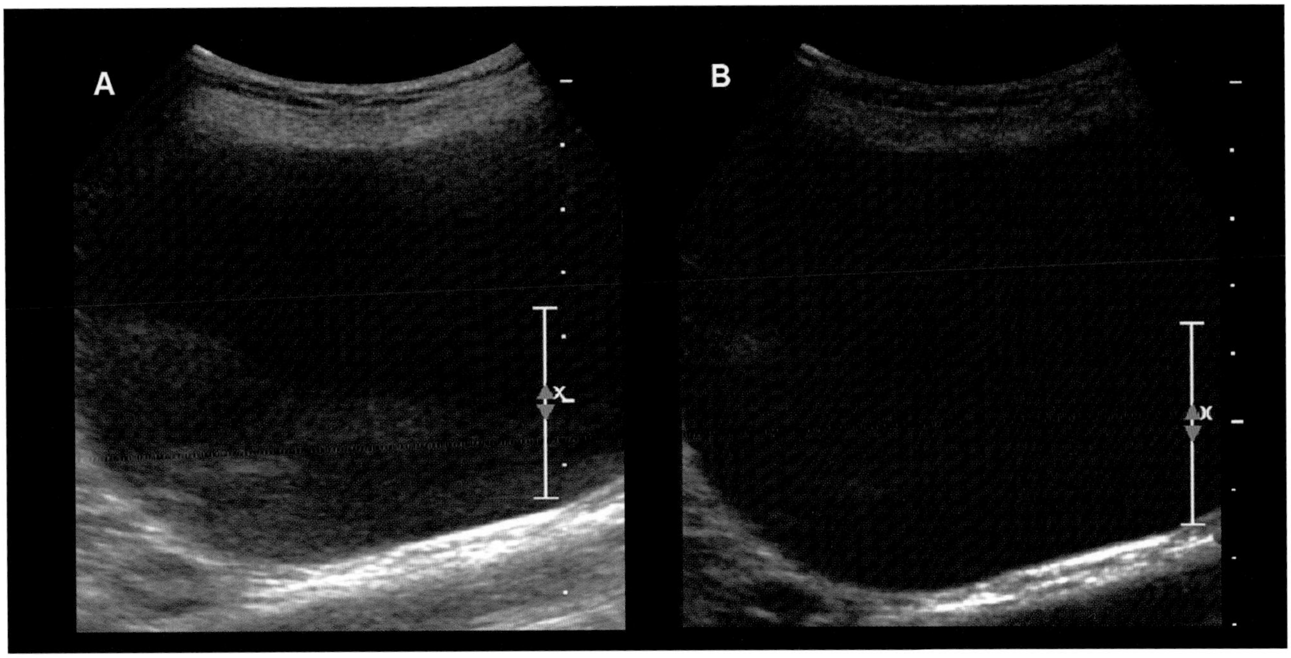

Figure 11.8. Duplex (A) and harmonic (B) longitudinal sonogram of a urinary bladder and pseudosludge in a dog. Harmonic ultrasound **(B)** reduces both the near-field and the far-field artifacts.

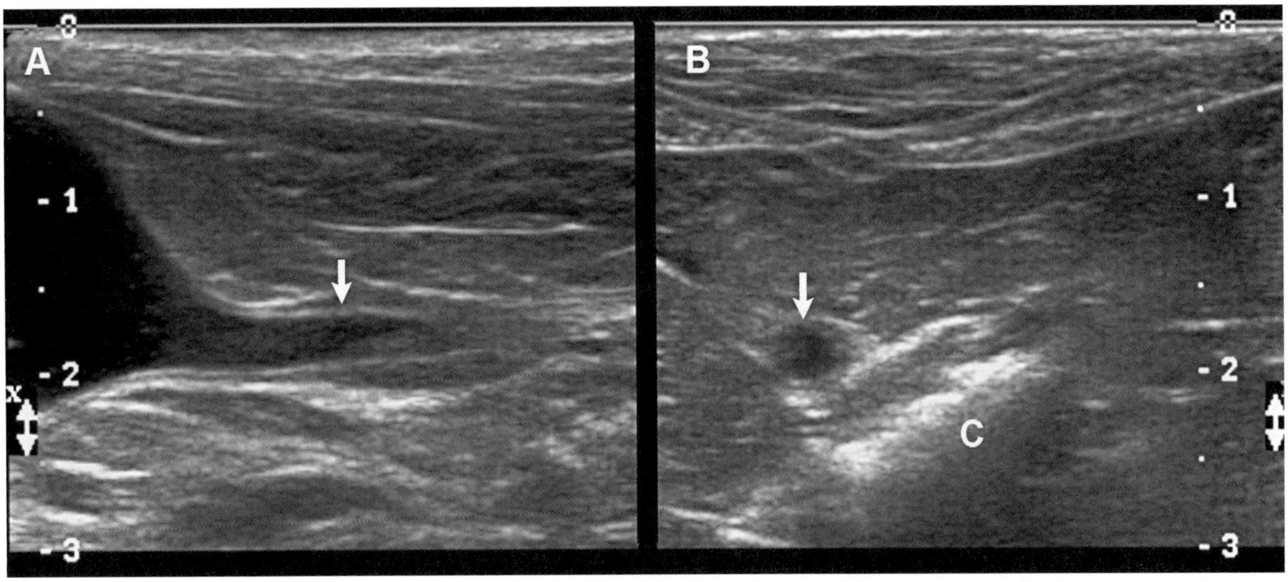

Figure 11.9. Normal urethra in a male dog. Duplex sonogram of the proximal urethra (arrow) in longitudinal **(A)** and transverse **(B)** planes. The descending colon (C) is seen in the far field in **B**.

In dogs, the prostate surrounds the proximal urethra. Shadowing from the pubis obscures the caudal intrapelvic portion of the urethra. The proximal penile urethra is located within the corpus spongiosum between the corpus cavernosum dorsally and the bulbospongiosus and retractor penis muscles ventrally (Figure 11.10A). The distal penile urethra is located within the urethral groove of the os penis dorsally and the bulbus glandis ventrally (Figure 11.10B). The urethral lumen is not normally seen unless there is urinary bladder distension, in which case urethral obstruction should be considered. The urethral wall is composed of the same histological layers as the urinary bladder. These layers are not readily resolved when normal.

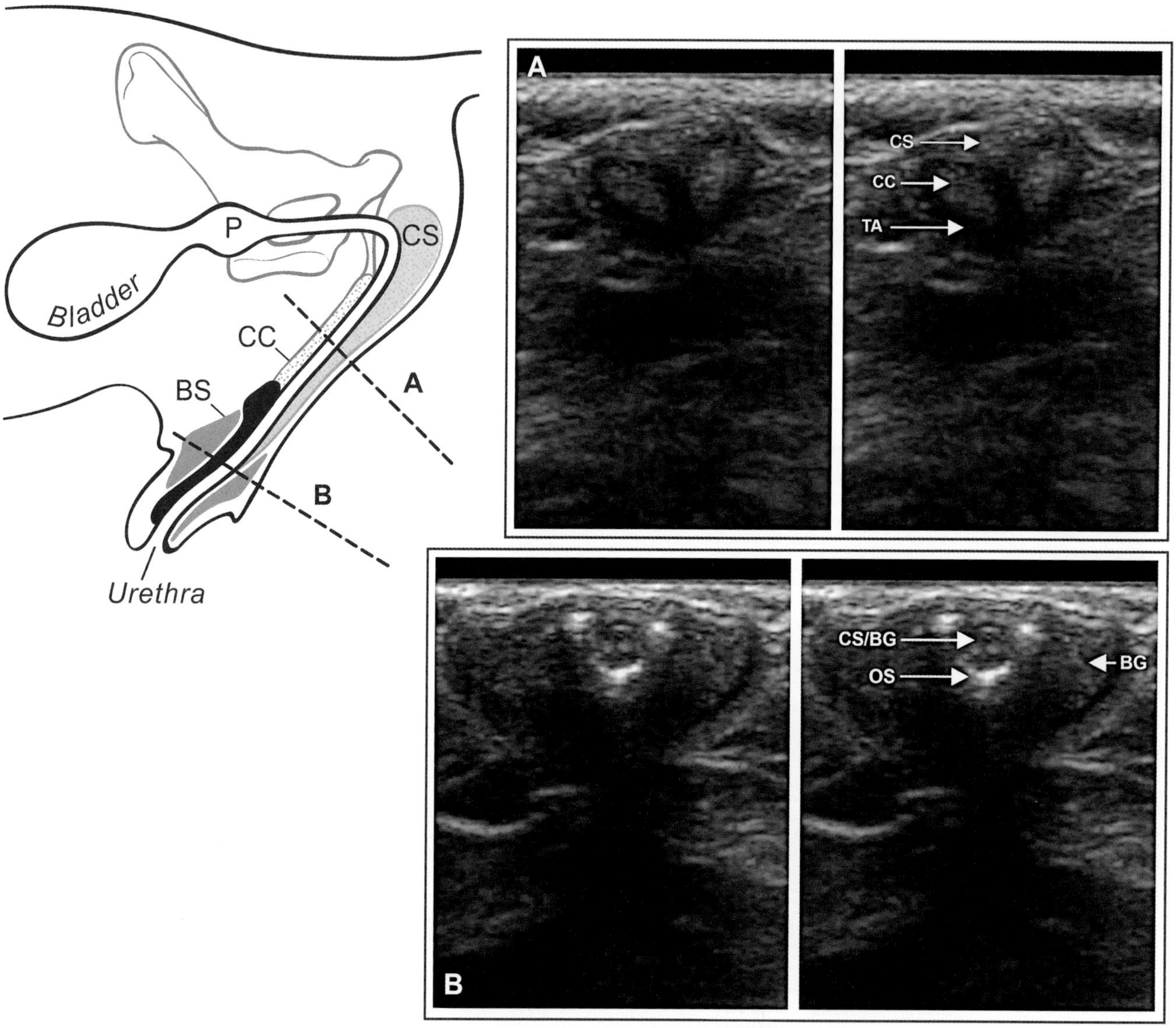

Figure 11.10. Normal penile urethra in a dog. On the left, an illustration of the anatomical structures near the urethra are presented. The dotted lines (**A**, **B**) correspond to the transverse planes seen on the sonograms on the right. P, prostate. **A:** Transverse sonogram (with and without labels) of the midpenile urethra at a level just cranial to the scrotum. The urethra cannot be delineated but is located within the corpus spongiosum (CS). CC, corpus cavernosum; and TA, tunica albuginea. **B:** Transverse sonogram (with and without labels) of the distal penile urethra at the level of the os penis (OS), which is seen as a hyperechoic U-shaped structure with distal shadow. The urethra is located within the anastomosing tissue of the corpus spongiosum and bulbus glandis (CS/BG). The bulbus glandis (BG) forms the bulk of the tissue surrounding the os penis.

Ultrasonographic Features of Bladder and Urethral Disorders

Cystitis

Cystitis most commonly causes extensive irregular hypoechoic thickening of the urinary bladder wall. This thickening is usually greatest at the cranioventral aspect of the urinary bladder (Figures 11.11 and 11.12).

The bladder wall changes can be associated with other findings, such as cystic calculi or blood clots. Polypoid cystitis is an uncommon form of cystitis reported in dogs. It can present as a hyperechoic polypoid to pedunculated mass or masses projecting into the lumen, as well as diffuse bladder wall thickening in some cases (Martinez et al. 2003) (Figure 11.13A and B). These masses occur most commonly in the cranioventral aspect of the urinary bladder (Martinez et al. 2003). Polypoid cystitis can have a similar ultrasonographic appearance to bladder wall neoplasia, and a biopsy is recommended.

Emphysematous cystitis is characterized by gas-forming bacteria such as *Escherichia coli*, *Aerobacter aerogenes*, *Proteus mirabilis*, and *Clostridium* sp. within the bladder wall and is seen most commonly in diabetic animals with glucosuria. The sonographic appearance is multifocal irregular hyperechoic interfaces with distal reverberation artifact (Petite et al. 2006) (Figure 11.14). By using alternative patient positions, free luminal gas (often seen in catheterized patients) can be distinguished from emphysematous cystitis. The free luminal gas will move with patient position, whereas the bladder wall gas will remain in the same location.

Neoplasia

Transitional cell carcinoma is the most common neoplasm of the urinary bladder. Transitional cell carcinoma is typically an irregular bladder wall mass with a broad-based attachment projecting into the urinary bladder lumen. The echogenicity is often mixed and has an overall appearance that can be hyperechoic, isoechoic, or hypoechoic compared with the bladder wall. The masses are most commonly in the bladder neck (trigone) region and dorsal bladder wall (Leveille et al. 1992) (Figures 11.5–11.18). Because of the location of the ureteral papilla in this region, unilateral or bilateral hydroureter may be encountered. It is common for the mass to extend into the proximal urethra. Dogs with transitional cell carcinoma may have concurrent cystitis, urethritis, calculi, and/or blood clots.

A wide variety of other bladder tumor types are possible, including epithelial (squamous cell

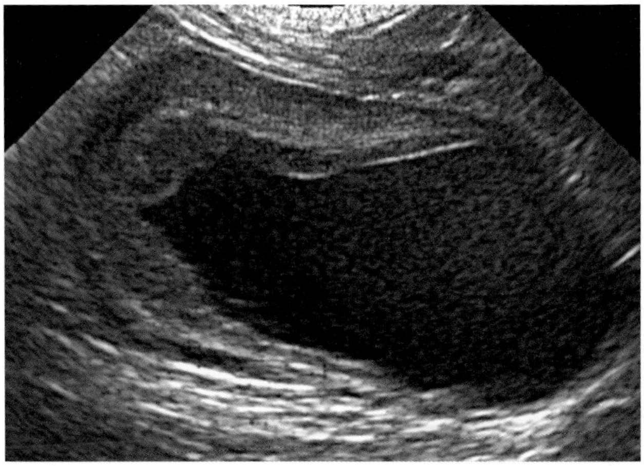

Figure 11.11. Cystitis in a dog. Longitudinal sonogram of the urinary bladder showing moderate hypoechoic cranial thickening of the body and apex of the urinary bladder wall. This finding is most consistent with cystitis. The urine from the dog cultured positive for *Escherichia coli* on multiple occasions.

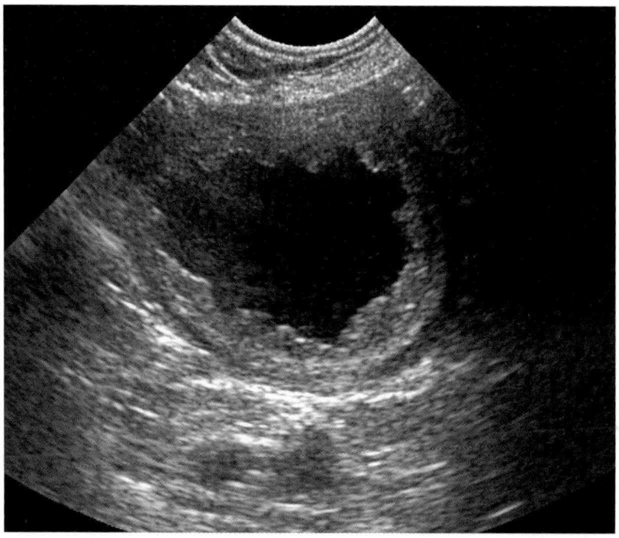

Figure 11.12. Cystitis in a dog. Transverse sonogram of the urinary bladder showing moderate, diffuse, hypoechoic, and irregular thickening of the bladder wall. This finding is consistent with cystitis. The urinalysis showed 3+ bacteria, and it cultured positive for *Escherichia coli.*

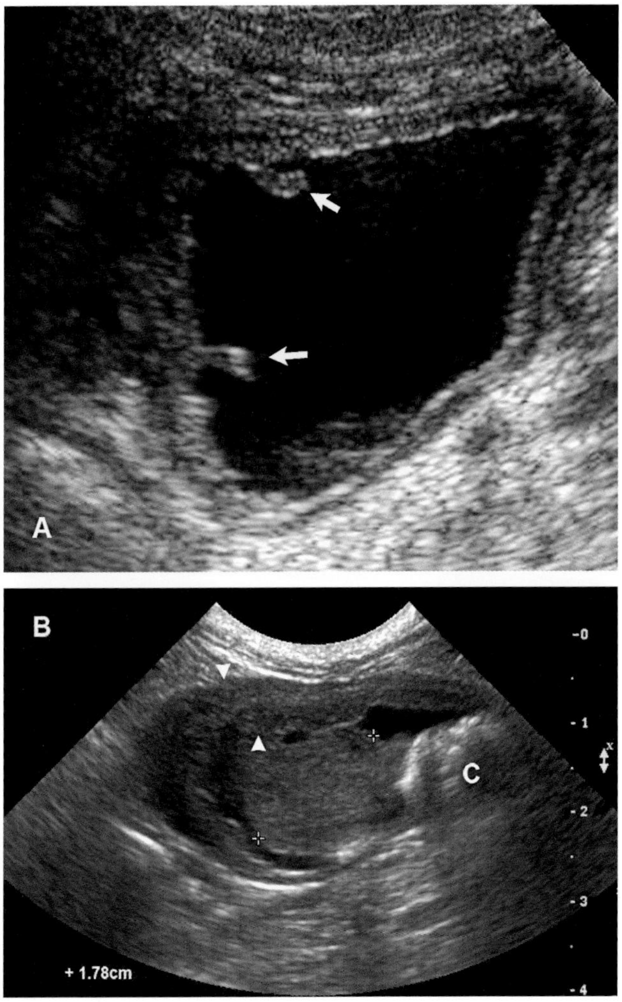

Figure 11.13. Polypoid cystitis in two dogs. **A:** Transverse sonogram of the urinary bladder with two small pedunculated masses (arrows) extending from the right bladder wall into the bladder lumen. The bladder wall thickness is within normal limits. **B:** Longitudinal sonogram of a different dog with a single broad based mass, thickening of the bladder wall (arrowheads) and shadowing calculi dorsally and caudally (C). Histopathology following surgical excisional biopsy revealed a mucosal polyp.

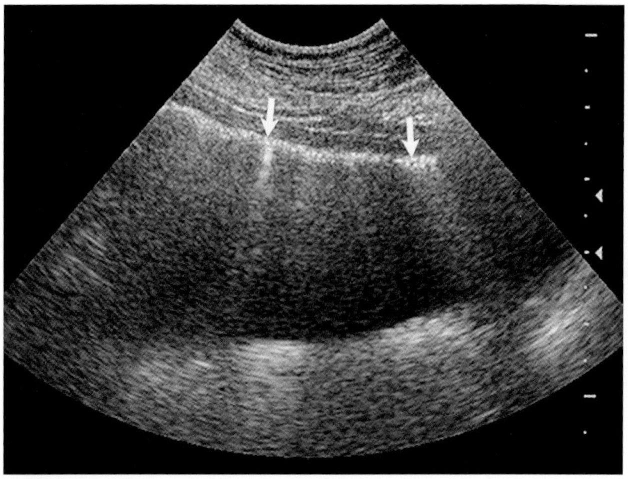

Figure 11.14. Emphysematous cystitis in a dog. Longitudinal sonogram of the urinary bladder showing a hyperechoic interface in the ventral bladder wall with reverberation (arrows), consistent with emphysematous cystitis. The urine cultured positive for *Escherichia coli*.

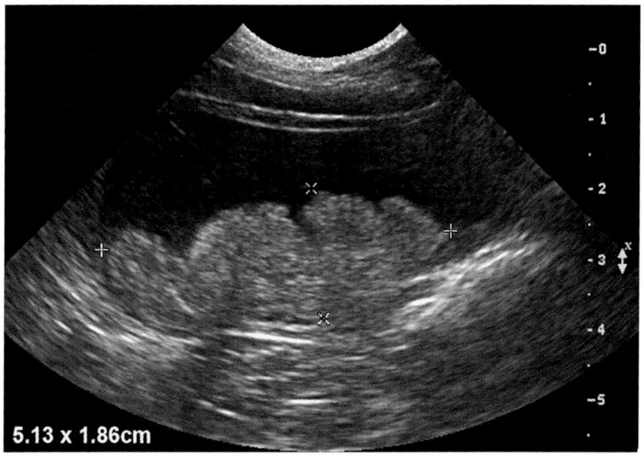

Figure 11.15. Bladder tumor in a dog. Longitudinal sonogram of a broad-based hyperechoic mass associated with the craniodorsal bladder wall, consistent with transitional cell carcinoma.

carcinoma) and mesenchymal tumors (botryoid rhabdomyosarcoma, chemodectoma, leiomyosarcoma, leiomyoma, fibroma, fibrosarcoma, hemangioma, hemangiosarcoma, lymphoma [Benigni et al. 2006], and mast cell tumor) (Figures 11.19–11.22). Ultrasonographic differentiation of tumor type and differentiation from nonneoplastic disease is often impossible without a biopsy. However, a mass with a smooth luminal surface is more likely to have a mesenchymal origin. Uncommonly, bladder tumors can diffusely invade the bladder wall (Figure 11.22B).

The most common urethral neoplasms in dogs include transitional cell carcinoma, squamous cell carcinoma, and adenocarcinoma. Proximal urethral neoplasms are often caused by local spread of bladder or prostatic neoplasms. Urethral transitional cell carcinoma has a markedly hyperechoic nonshadowing mucosal line and may be associated with hypoechoic

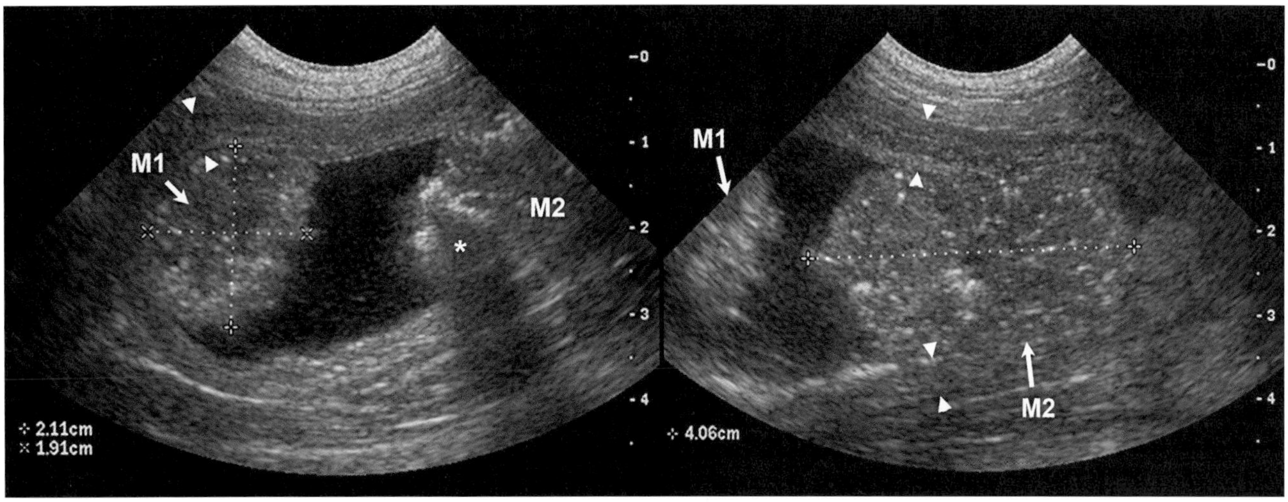

Figure 11.16. Bladder tumor in a 10-year-old female dog with hematuria. Longitudinal sonograms of the bladder. Two distinct hyperechoic masses are in the bladder lumen (M1 and M2), showing hyperechoic speckles and larger shadowing (*) foci consistent with mineralization. Both of these masses are attached to the bladder walls (arrowheads). Suction biopsies revealed transitional cell carcinomas. Images courtesy of M.A. d'Anjou.

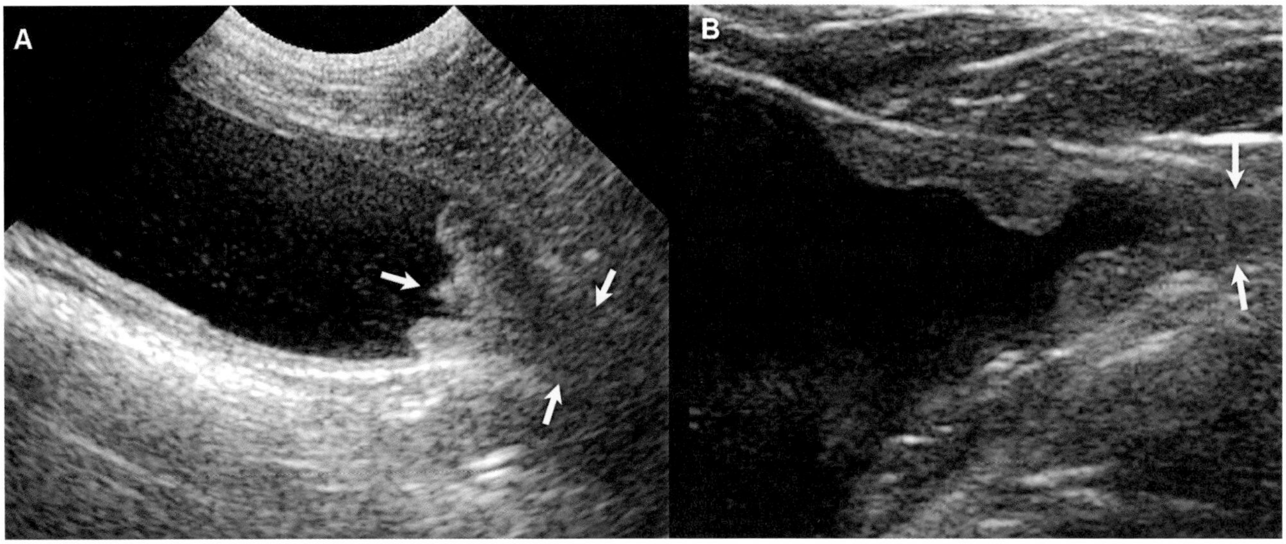

Figure 11.17. Bladder tumor in two dogs. Longitudinal sonograms of the urinary bladder of the dogs **(A and B)** with confirmed transitional cell carcinoma. In each dog, a lobulated mass occupies the bladder neck and extends into the urethra (arrows). A suction biopsy was used to confirm the diagnosis.

Figure 11.18. Bladder neck and urethral transitional cell carcinoma in a castrated male dog. Longitudinal sonogram of the bladder neck and proximal urethra. There is an irregular tissue projection into the bladder lumen, at the level of the trigone (T). The proximal urethra is also thickened (arrows), and the prostate is enlarged (arrowheads). A suction biopsy confirmed transitional cell carcinoma. Image courtesy of M.A. d'Anjou.

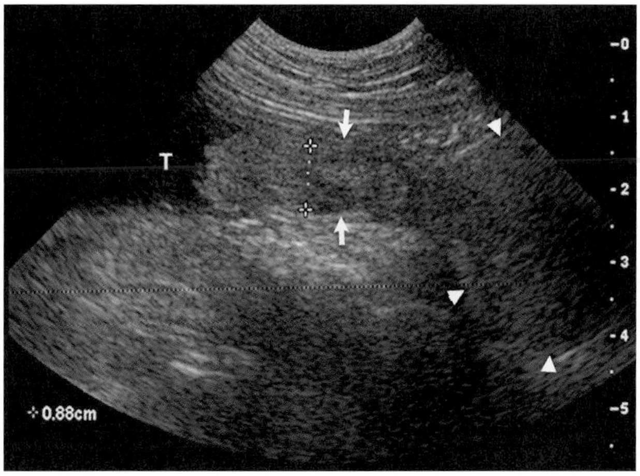

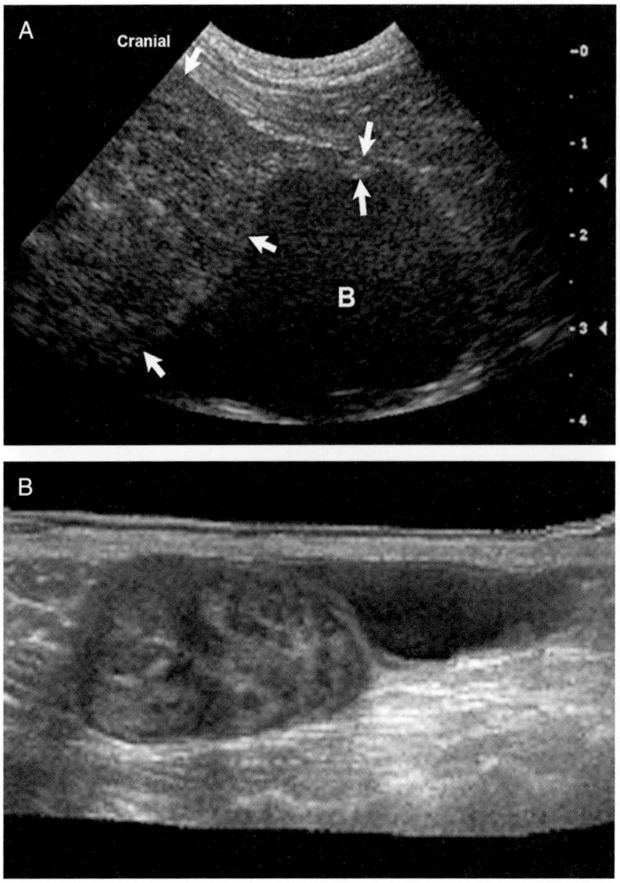

Figure 11.19. Bladder leiomyosarcoma in a dog. **A:** Sagittal sonogram of a large bladder wall leiomyosarcoma. A heterogeneous, broad-based mass (arrows) is invading the wall at the apex and body, deforming the shape of the bladder and protruding into its lumen (B). **B:** Longitudinal panoramic sonogram of another large echogenic mass deforming the contour of the bladder. The mass was diagnosed as low-grade leiomyosarcoma.

thickening of the urethral wall (Figure 11.23) (Hanson and Tidwell 1996). Squamous cell carcinoma is most commonly associated with the distal urethra. Other types of neoplastic processes can compress or invade the urethra along its path (Figure 11.24).

Enlargement of the medial iliac, hypogastric, sacral, or superficial inguinal lymph nodes is not specific to bladder or urethral disease, but they should be located and measured to aid the staging of a suspected neoplastic disease.

Calculi

High-frequency bladder ultrasound may have a similar accuracy as radiographic contrast procedures in calculi

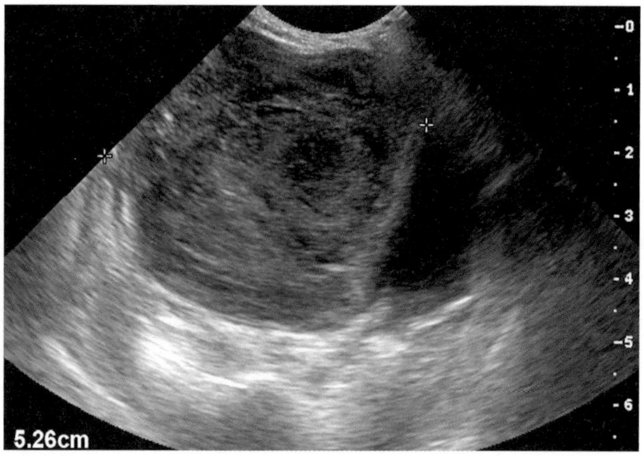

Figure 11.20. Bladder tumor (hemangiosarcoma) in a dog. Transverse sonogram of a large cavitated mass associated with the right bladder wall. Given the cavitated appearance, a hematoma was suspected. At surgery, the highly vascular bladder mass was considered unresectable and was biopsied. The histopathologic diagnosis was hemangiosarcoma.

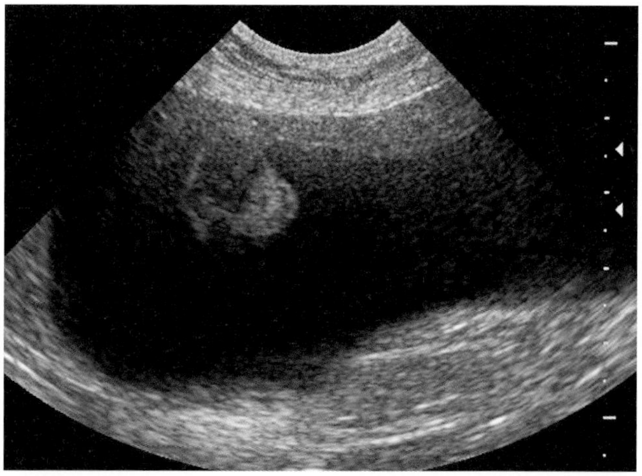

Figure 11.21. Bladder tumor (mast cell tumor) in a dog. Longitudinal sonogram of a urinary bladder with a highly vascular, pedunculated, mixed-echogenicity mass originating from the cranioventral bladder wall. Cytology of the mass with special stains was consistent with a mast cell neoplasm.

detection (Weichselbaum et al. 1999). Cystic or urethral calculi are usually mobile and collect in the dependent portion of the lumen. They are usually spherical, with a hyperechoic curvilinear interface. However, they can be a variety of sizes and shapes. A distal shadow is only variably present and is more likely seen with a higher transducer frequency and

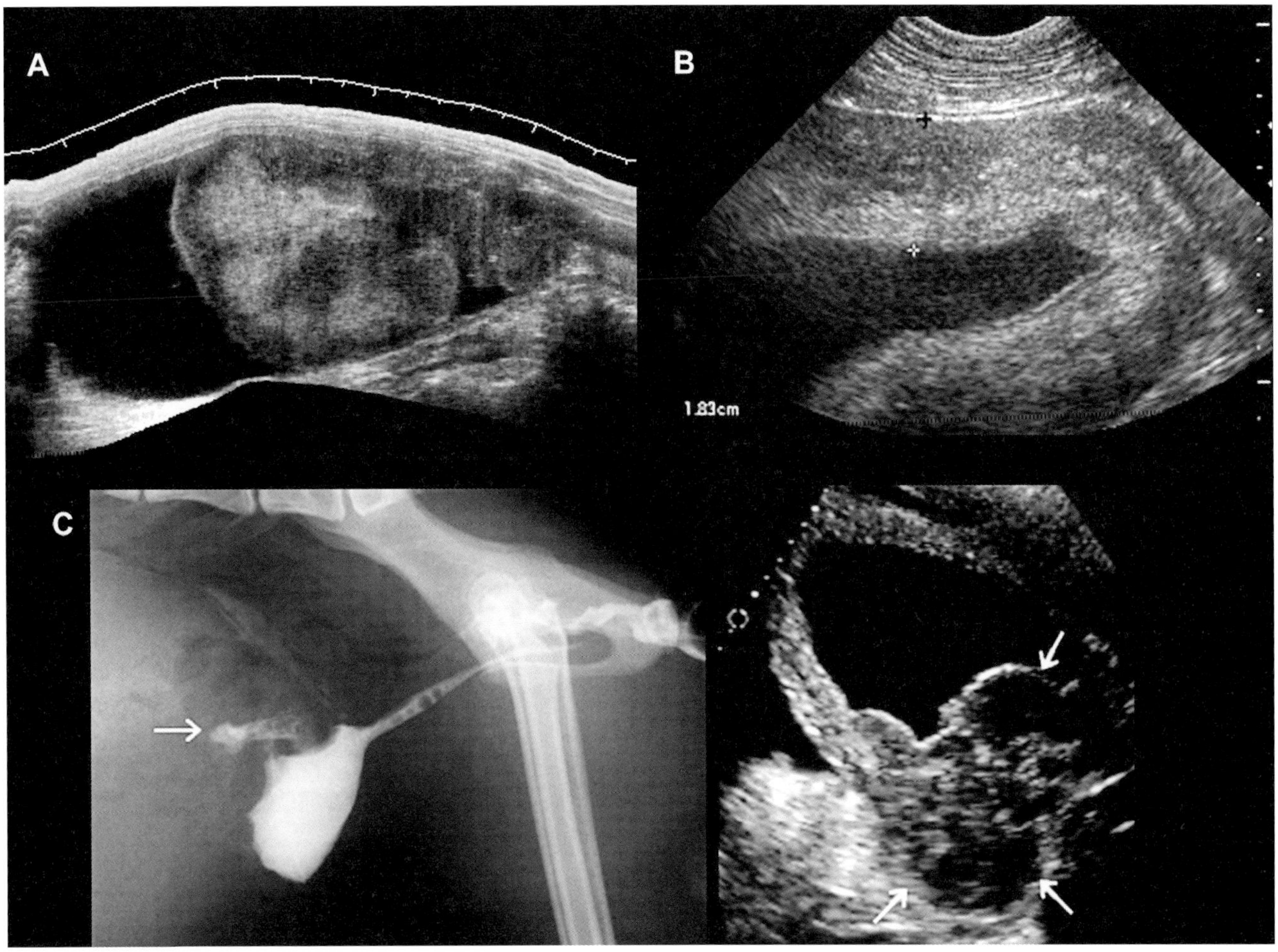

Figure 11.22. Extensive bladder tumors in two dogs and a cat. **A:** Panoramic longitudinal sonogram of a large caudal bladder mass involving the trigone of a dog. The histopathology obtained at necropsy revealed a poorly differentiated carcinoma. **B:** Longitudinal sonogram of the bladder of a 6-year-old Labrador retriever with diffuse carcinomatous infiltration of the wall. **C:** Retrograde vaginourethrocystogram **(left)** and longitudinal sonogram **(right)** of the bladder of a 1-year-old cat with urinary incontinence and hematuria. In the contrast study, the dorsal bladder wall is thick, and there is extravasation of contrast medium into the peritoneal cavity (arrow). In the sonogram, a large heterogeneous, multilobulated mass (arrows) at the trigone protruded into the peritoneal cavity through the serosa. Image C reprinted with permission from Benigni et al. (2006).

with calculi of a greater thickness (Figures 11.25 and 11.26). A reverberation artifact may also occur distal to cystic calculi. The presence or absence of these artifacts does not correlate with the composition of the calculus (Weichselbaum et al. 2000). Although the appearance is nonspecific, crystalluria may be seen as a collection of swirling moderate-intensity intraluminal echoes. A collection of small calculi or mineralized sediment may generate a linear interface (Figures 11.27 and 11.28). This sediment usually suspends with gentle agitation of the urinary bladder.

Although the urethra cannot be evaluated completely with ultrasound, urethral calculi may be identified, particularly proximal to the os penis (Figure 11.29). Enlargement of the urinary bladder with dilation of the urethral lumen is supportive of urethral obstruction (Figure 11.30).

The descending colon can indent and appear confluent with the dorsal wall of the urinary bladder. The hyperechoic interface and shadowing artifact generated by the colon can mimic cystic calculi (Figure 11.31). Rotation of the transducer into the longitudinal plane will reveal the colon as a linear interface running the length of the image, whereas the calculi should remain approximately spherical. Additionally, repositioning the animal into a standing or lateral position

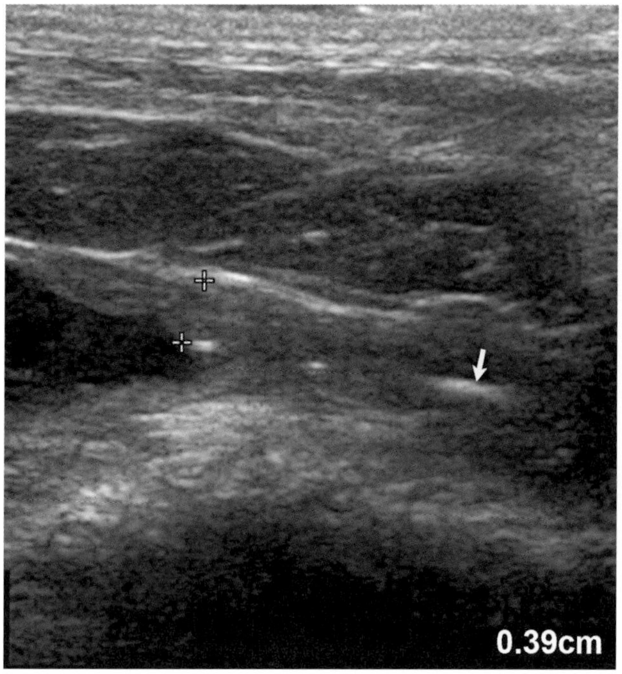

Figure 11.23. Bladder neck and urethral tumor (transitional cell carcinoma) in a dog. Longitudinal sonogram of trigone and urethra. The urethral wall is thickened, with a linear hyperechoic lining at the luminal margin (arrow). Wall thickening is also present at the bladder trigone. The histopathologic diagnosis was transitional cell carcinoma.

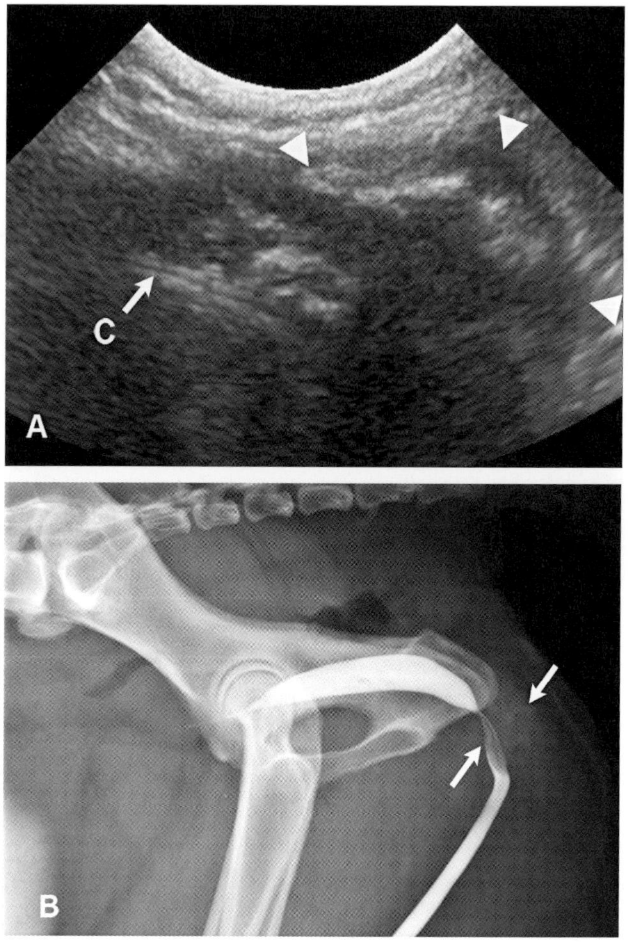

Figure 11.24. Urethral tumor (osteosarcoma) in a dog. **A:** Longitudinal sonogram of the caudal membranous urethra, which contains an indwelling catheter (arrow C). A hyperechoic shadowing mass (arrowheads) is caudodorsal to the urethra. **B:** Positive-contrast retrograde urethrogram showing a mineral opacity mass (arrows) causing marked attenuation of the urethral contrast. The histopathologic diagnosis from an ultrasound-guided microcore biopsy was osteosarcoma.

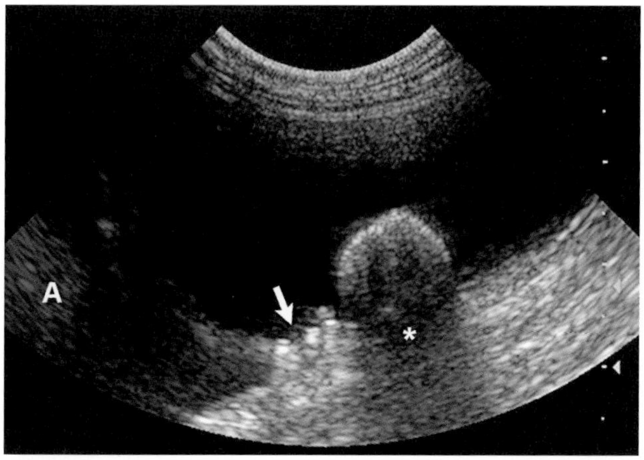

Figure 11.25. Cystic calculus in a dog. Longitudinal sonogram of the urinary bladder, which contains a spherical hyperechoic interface with distal shadowing (*), consistent with a cystic calculus. Additionally, several smaller hyperechoic interfaces are noted just cranially (arrow), also consistent with calculi, although not causing acoustic shadowing, because of their smaller size. Side-lobe artifacts are in the apical portion of the bladder (A).

should cause any calculi to fall to the dependent wall, whereas the colon remains in a dorsal location.

Intraluminal Blood Clots and Mural Hemorrhage

Blood clots and mural hemorrhage may be caused by bladder trauma, cystitis, a generalized bleeding disorder, or neoplasia. Blood within the urinary bladder lumen or wall can have a variable appearance and can mimic exuberant inflammatory disease or neoplasia. Intraluminal clots are generally hyperechoic and range

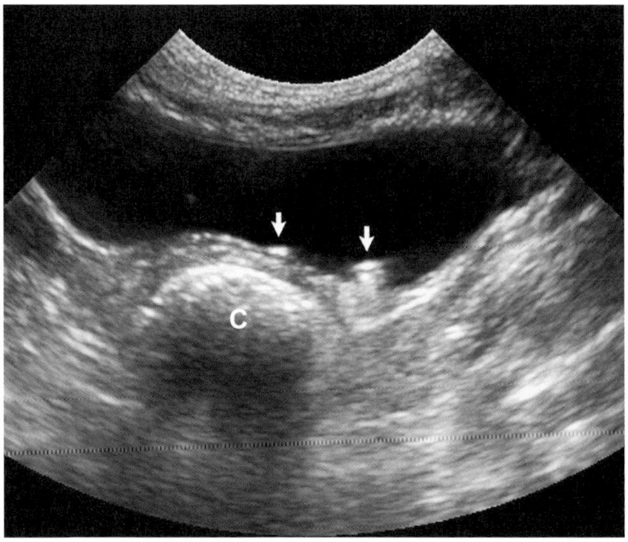

Figure 11.26. Cystic calculi in a dog. Transverse sonogram of the urinary bladder showing two small hyperechoic structures associated with the ventral bladder wall (arrows) that are thought to represent small cystic calculi. Urinalysis revealed calcium oxalate crystalluria. The colon (C) is associated with acoustic shadowing.

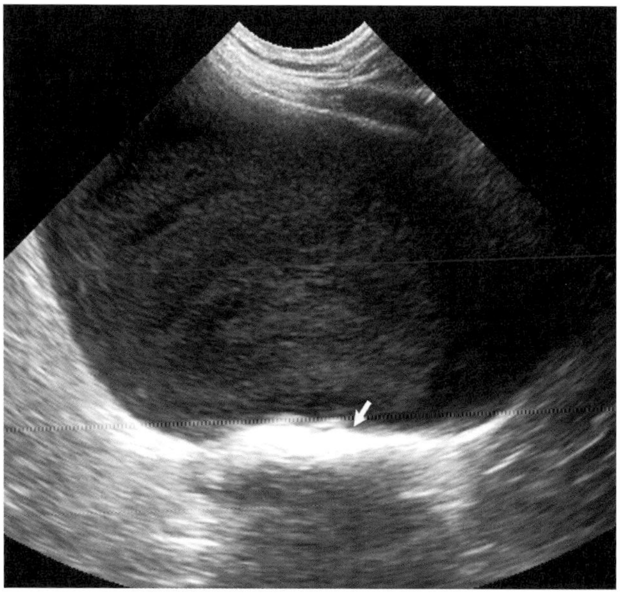

Figure 11.27. Bladder sediments in a dog. Transverse sonogram of diffusely echogenic urine and a collection of hyperechoic material (arrow) on the dependent bladder wall with distal shadowing. The urinalysis showed 3+ amorphous crystalluria.

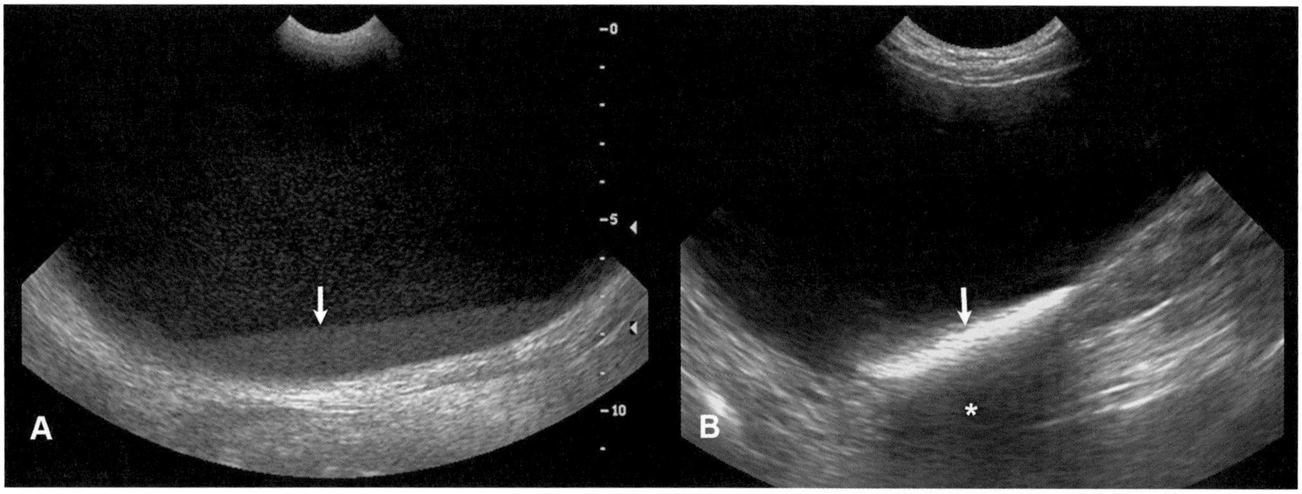

Figure 11.28. Cystic calculi and sediment in two dogs. Sedimentation in the dependent portion of the urinary bladder. **A:** Pyuria appears as nonshadowing, moderately echogenic sludge that progressively sediments during the exam. A straight horizontal border is seen (arrow). **B:** A mineral sediment, such as seen with crystalluria, is more hyperechoic and typically associated with acoustic shadowing (*). The dog was diagnosed and treated for a portoazygous shunt. Image A courtesy of M.A. d'Anjou.

from thin linear structures to large round masses (Figures 11.32–11.34).

Mural hemorrhage causes diffuse uniform wall thickening (O'Brien and Wood 1998). The absence of color flow Doppler signal can help differentiate a blood clot from a neoplastic mass. The mobility of these intraluminal structures may also be demonstrated with repositioning of the patient. Recheck examinations will help differentiate neoplastic or inflammatory mural disease because thickening secondary to sys-

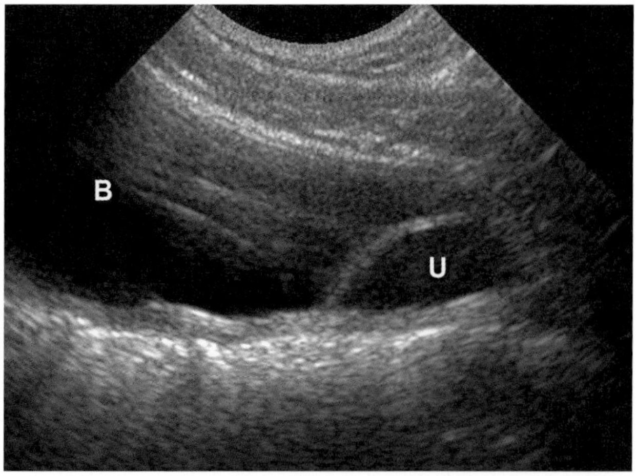

Figure 11.35. Ureterocele in a dog. Longitudinal sonogram of the urinary bladder (B) with a thin-walled cystic outpouching of the left ureter (U). The cystic structure contains anechoic fluid and is consistent with a ureterocele. Image courtesy of C. Warman, Veterinary Specialist Group, Auckland, New Zealand.

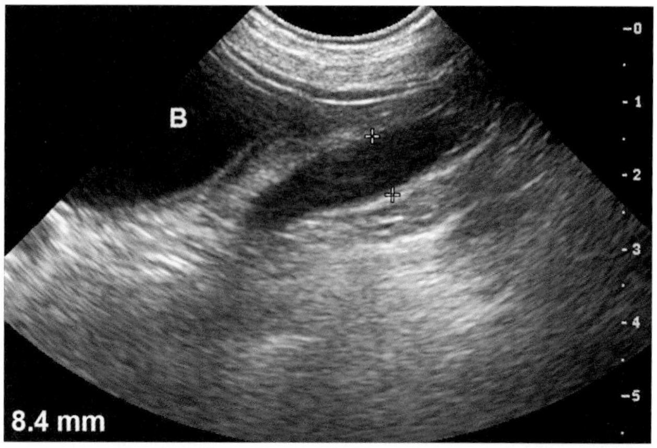

Figure 11.36. Ectopic ureter. Longitudinal sonogram of a dilated ureter (8.4 mm-cursors), which was followed from the left kidney and courses caudal to bladder neck (B), consistent with an ectopic ureter.

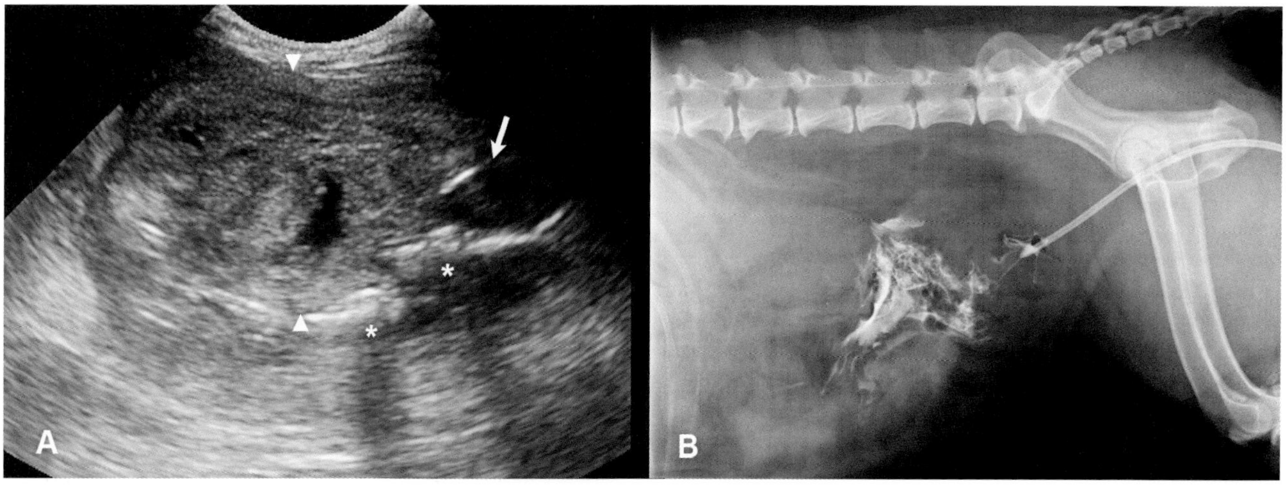

Figure 11.37. Sonogram and contrast radiographic study of a ruptured urinary bladder in a dog. **A.** Longitudinal sonogram. The indwelling, saline-filled Foley catheter can be seen caudally (arrow). There is marked thickening of the bladder wall (arrowheads) and a loss of visualization of the bladder lumen. Abdominal effusion is also noted. Because of the suspicion of bladder rupture, a positive-contrast cystogram was performed. Hyperechoic foci are noted in the dorsally displaced bladder lumen, associated with acoustic shadowing (*), consistent with calculi. **B:** Lateral radiograph of the caudal abdomen following a retrograde positive-contrast cystogram. Contrast is free within the peritoneal space. At surgery, the bladder rupture and hematoma were identified.

A vesicourachal diverticulum is a fluid-filled structure that extends as a convex outpouching of the bladder lumen, usually with a thin wall, although it can become thick and irregular in cases of chronic cystitis. These diverticuli can vary in size and are typically in cranioventral aspect of the urinary bladder wall. Diverticulum may also occur at other locations because of trauma or cystitis.

Trauma

A positive-contrast retrograde cystourethrogram is the preferred method of diagnosing rupture of the urethra or urinary bladder. On ultrasound, the ruptured urinary bladder wall is thickened (Figure 11.37), and there is abdominal effusion of echogenicity that depends on urine cellularity. Calculi or other debris can also accumulate in the peritoneal cavity. A hypoechoic bladder wall defect or tract may be seen occasionally.

This should be distinguished from a refraction artifact associated with the cranial aspect of the urinary bladder when abdominal effusion is present. The interpretation of the artifact is aided by a concurrent edge shadow and absence of bladder wall thickening (Figure 11.38).

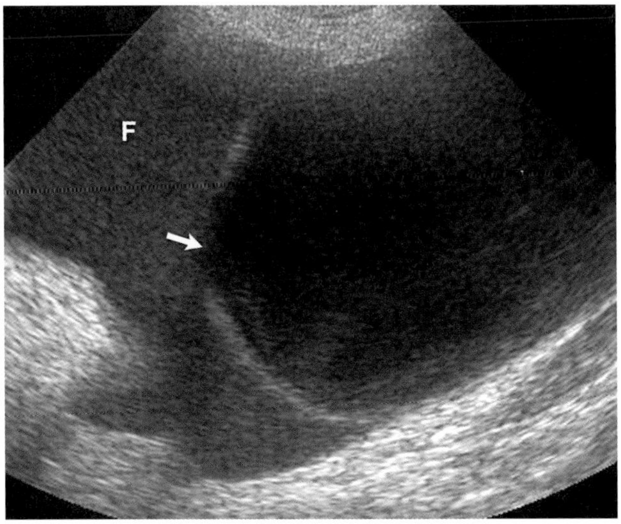

Figure 11.38. Refraction artifact versus bladder rupture in a dog. Longitudinal sonogram of the bladder containing anechoic urine surrounded by echogenic abdominal effusion (F). The refraction artifact at the cranial aspect of the bladder mimics bladder wall rupture (arrow), but no bladder wall rupture is present.

Special Procedures

Cystocentesis

Once sufficient bladder distension is determined by ultrasonography, a guided cystocentesis can be performed. The skin can be prepared with an alcohol-soaked swab. A 22-gauge, 1- or 1.5-inch needle attached to a 5-mL syringe is used. The needle is placed just cranial to the transducer while trying to keep the needle aligned with the plane of the ultrasound beam. The needle appears as a fine linear hyperechoic interface that often causes distal reverberation or shadowing artifacts (Figure 11.39).

Suction Biopsy

Cystoscopic biopsy and ultrasound-guided suction biopsy are the preferred methods of confirming bladder or urethral neoplasia. Percutaneous fine-needle aspiration of suspected transitional cell carcinoma in the bladder is not recommended because the technique can lead to regional spread of the tumor along the needle tract.

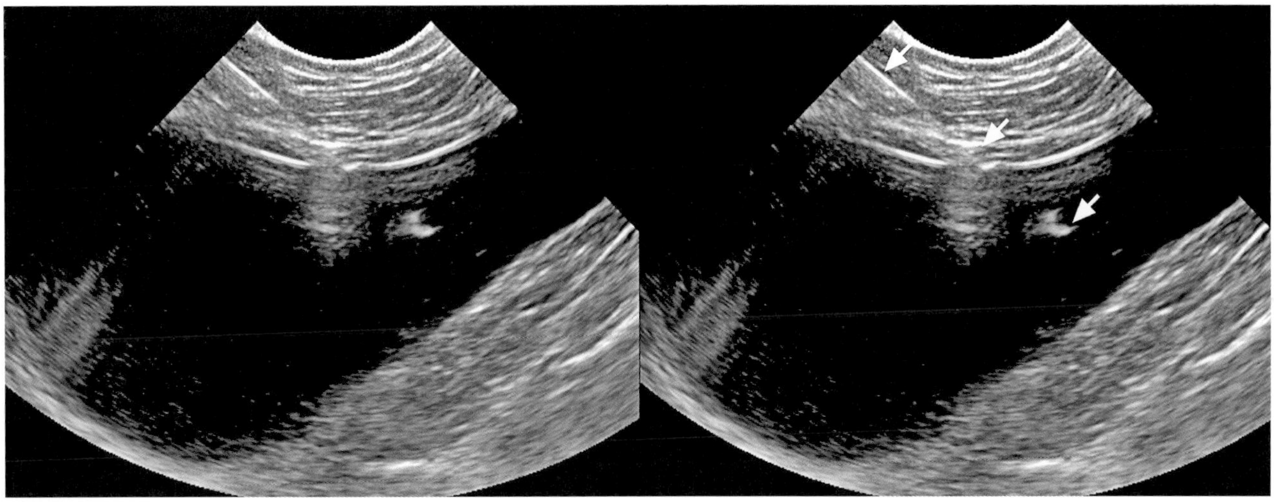

Figure 11.39. Cystocentesis in a dog. Longitudinal sonogram of the urinary bladder during cystocentesis (with and without labels). The fine hyperechoic line created by the needle and the hyperechoic needle tip within the lumen are visualized (arrows).

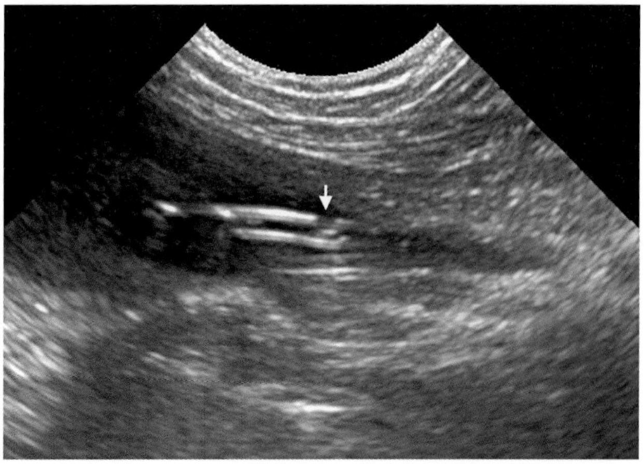

Figure 11.40. Suction biopsy in a dog. Longitudinal sonogram of the urinary bladder and an indwelling red-rubber catheter during a suction biopsy. The catheter walls are hyperechoic and the lumen hypoechoic. A small defect in the catheter wall (arrow) corresponds to one of the side holes in the catheter, which can be guided into the desired location of the biopsy.

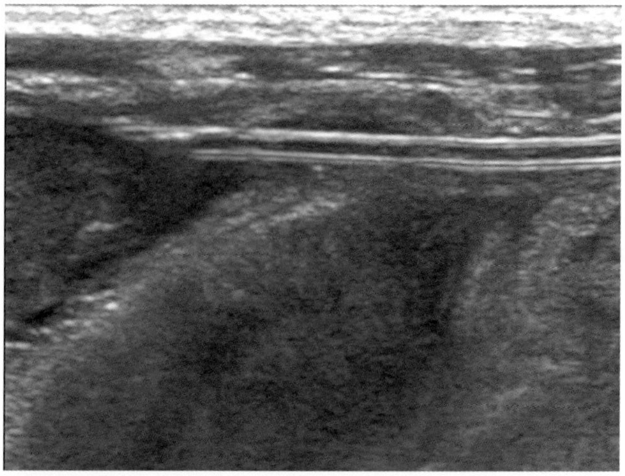

Figure 11.41. Suction biopsy in a cat. Longitudinal sonogram of the trigone of the bladder during a suction biopsy. The two parallel hyperechoic lines are the walls of the catheter. Ultrasound guidance directed the catheter in contact with the bladder mass.

The suction biopsy is performed under heavy sedation (propofol) or general anesthesia. An appropriately sized red-rubber catheter with side holes is connected to a 20-mL syringe and is placed aseptically into the urinary bladder. The urinary bladder (if empty) is filled with a small volume of sterile saline to provide an acoustic window and better delineate the abnormal tissue to sample. Only a small volume is required because the bladder wall collapsing around the catheter aids the aspiration of the targeted tissue rather than urine. The catheter tip is visualized within the urinary bladder as a pair of parallel hyperechoic lines with a hypoechoic lumen, and the side holes of the catheter can also be identified as discrete hypoechoic defects (Figures 11.40 and 11.41) The catheter tip can then be positioned adjacent to the bladder mass or wall thickening to be biopsied. High-frequency ultrasound may enable more specific placement by visualization of the catheter holes.

The syringe plunger is pulled back. If urine is obtained, then the catheter is rotated to reposition the side hole adjacent to the tissue of interest. Once negative pressure can be maintained, the pressure is applied and released 3–4 times, collecting tissue from the adjacent mucosa. Suction is applied and held, with the aim being to adhere the catheter to the mass. The urinary catheter is abruptly withdrawn 4–6 cm from the bladder while the suction is held, with the aim of pulling a larger fragment of tissue from the mass. The contents of the catheter are then emptied into formalin or smeared on a slide for cytology. If the procedure is repeated, a new red-rubber catheter is used. Intravesicular hemorrhage is a potential complication of this procedure (Lamb et al. 1996).

References

Benigni L, Lamb CR, Corzo-Menendez N, Holloway A, Eastwood JM (2006) Lymphoma affecting the urinary bladder in three dogs and a cat. Vet Radiol Ultrasound 47:592–596.

Finn-Bodner ST (1995) The urinary bladder. In: Cartee RE, Selcer BA, Hudson JA, et al., eds. Practical Veterinary Ultrasound. Philadelphia: Lea and Febiger, pp 210–235.

Geisse AL, Lowry JE, Schaeffer DJ, Smith CW (1997) Sonographic evaluation of urinary bladder wall thickness in normal dogs. Vet Radiol Ultrasound 38:132–137.

Hanson JA, Tidwell AS (1996) Ultrasonographic appearance of urethral transitional cell carcinoma in ten dogs. Vet Radiol Ultrasound 37:293–299.

Lamb CR, Trower ND, Gregory SP (1996) Ultrasound-guided catheter biopsy of the lower urinary tract: Technique and results in 12 dogs. J Small Anim Pract 37:413–416.

Leveille R, Biller DS, Partington BP, Miyabayashi T (1992) Sonographic investigation of transitional cell carcinoma of the urinary bladder in small animals. Vet Radiol Ultrasound 33:103–107.

Martinez I, Mattoon JS, Eaton KA, Chew DJ, DiBartola SP (2003) Polypoid cystitis in 17 dogs (1978–2001). J Vet Intern Med 17:499–509.

O'Brien RT, Wood EF (1998) Urinary bladder mural hemorrhage associated with systemic bleeding disorders in three dogs. Vet Radiol Ultrasound 39:354–356.

Petite A, Busoni V, Heinen MP, Billen F, Snaps F (2006) Radiographic and ultrasonographic findings of emphysematous cystitis in four nondiabetic female dogs. Vet Radiol Ultrasound 47:90–93.

Weichselbaum RC, Feeney DA, Jessen CR, Osborne CA, Dreytser V, Holte J (1999) Urocystolith detection: Comparison of survey, contrast radiographic and ultrasonographic techniques in an in vitro bladder phantom. Vet Radiol Ultrasound 40:386–400.

Weichselbaum RC, Feeney DA, Jessen CR, Osborne CA, Dreytser V, Holte J (2000) Relevance of sonographic artifacts observed during in vitro characterization of urocystolith mineral composition. Vet Radiol Ultrasound 41:438–446.

CHAPTER TWELVE

Adrenal Glands

John Graham

Preparation and Scanning Technique

The adrenal glands are small, paired structures located in the craniodorsal abdomen, medial to the ipsilateral kidney and adjacent to the aorta (left) and caudal vena cava (right). The cells of the adrenal cortex produce cortisol and other corticoids, aldosterone, androgens, estrogens, and progestins whereas the chromaffin cells of the medulla produce catecholamines (Feldman and Nelson 2004). The adrenal glands are a key component of the endocrine system, and their deranged function can produce a wide range of clinical signs, which may be vague or nonspecific. The ultrasonographic evaluation of the adrenal glands is technically challenging, but assessment of the glands is now considered part of a complete abdominal scan in both dogs and cats. Although the glands are small, a competent sonographer using good-quality equipment can identify both glands in most patients. For a lateral approach, the hair coat should be clipped from the lateral abdomen to the level of the transverse processes of the lumbar spine and over the last few intercostal spaces on the right. Evaluation of the adrenal glands is facilitated by the use of high-frequency linear or sector probes and a sound knowledge of normal anatomy. Sedation may be helpful in evaluating agitated, aggressive, or painful patients, and in obese patients because it relaxes the abdomen and allows the operator to apply pressure with less patient discomfort. For most dogs, a 7-Mhz or 10-Mhz sector transducer is the best choice to evaluate the adrenals. A linear transducer may be used to evaluate the left adrenal gland in many dogs and both glands in many cats. However, the large contact footprint and narrow field of view of such probes are unsuitable for evaluating the right adrenal gland in most dogs.

Sonography of the Normal Adrenal Glands

In Dogs

The normal left adrenal gland is hypoechoic to the surrounding fat, is well defined, and has an elongated bilobed shape, frequently described as resembling a peanut (Figure 12.1A and C). When using a high-frequency transducer, a thin hyperechoic line, which runs parallel to the capsule, may be seen, representing the junction between cortex and medulla (Figure 12.1C). The right adrenal gland may appear wedge shaped in some dogs (Figure 12.1D), but in most it has an elongated ovoid shape (Figure 12.1B), usually without the pronounced waist seen in the left adrenal gland. The right adrenal gland is also hypoechoic in comparison to the surrounding fat and may exhibit a thin hyperechoic band separating cortex and medulla.

The adrenal glands are located in the retroperitoneal space, medial to the ipsilateral kidney. The left adrenal gland is located along the lateral aspect of the abdominal aorta, just cranial to the origin of the left renal artery. The left phrenicoabdominal artery and vein pass dorsal and ventral, respectively, to the midbody of the gland. The right adrenal gland is located close to caudal vena cava, lying between lateral and dorsal to this vessel, just cranial to the right renal artery and right renal vein. The right phrenicoabdominal artery and vein pass dorsal and ventral to the gland, as on the left. The adrenal glands may be scanned from the ventral abdomen, but interference from gas and ingesta within the gastrointestinal tract makes this approach more difficult. When scanning patients in dorsal recumbency, it may be helpful to tilt them toward or away from the operator to enable one to place the probe further dorsal. The author prefers to scan the

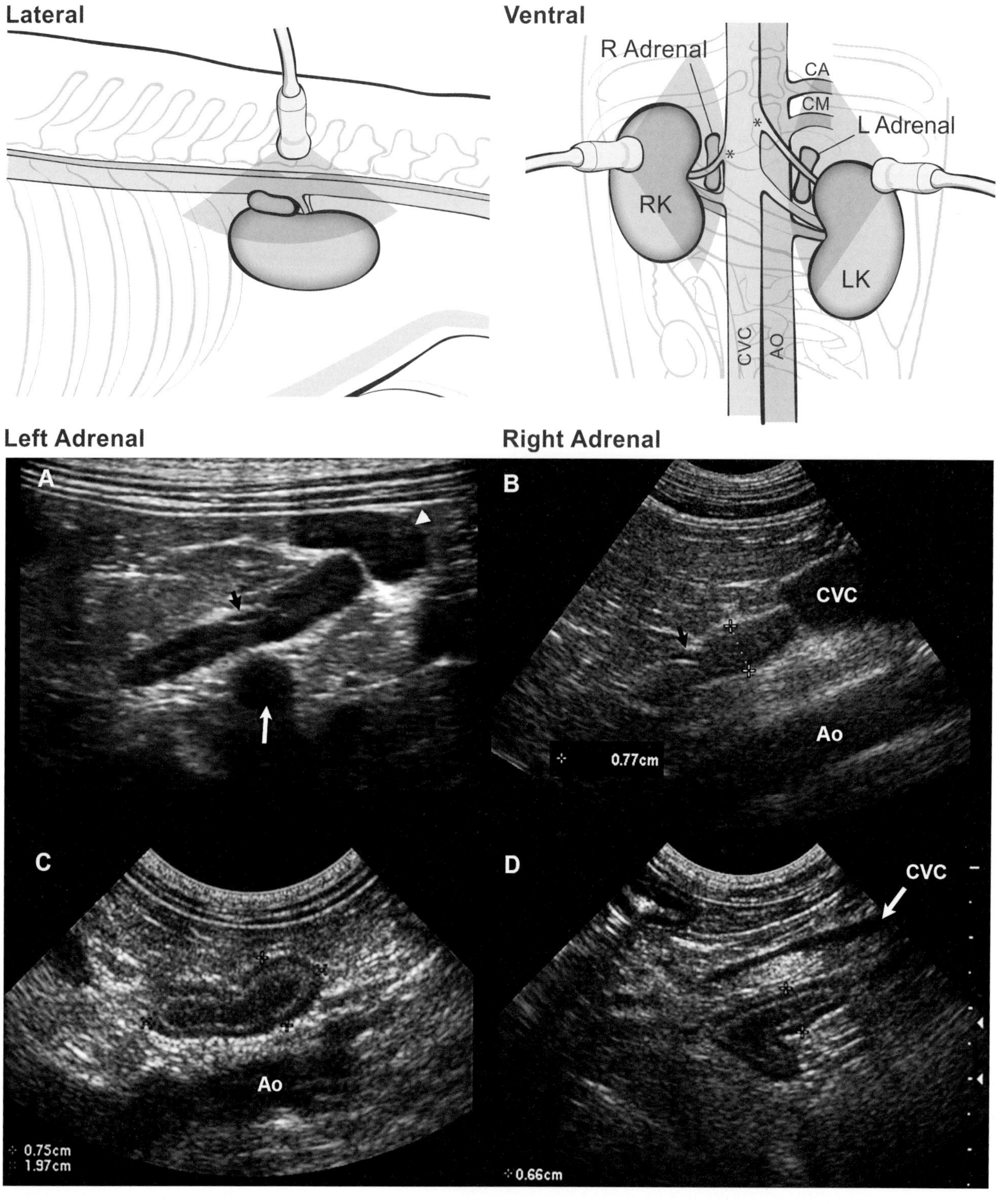

Figure 12.1. Normal adrenal glands in dogs. The two schematic drawings on **top** illustrate the localization of the adrenal glands in a dog placed on lateral recumbency **(left)** and on dorsal recumbency (ventral approach: **top right**). AO, aorta; CA, celiac artery; CM, cranial mesenteric; CVC, caudal vena cava; LK, left kidney; and RK, right kidney. **A:** Dorsal plane image of a normal canine left adrenal gland. Note the elongated bilobed shape with a portion of a phrenicoabdominal vessel in cross section within the ventral groove (black arrow). The anechoic structure caudal and lateral to the gland is the left renal vein (arrowhead), whereas the cranial mesenteric artery (white arrow) lies deep to the midbody of the adrenal gland. **B:** Sagittal plane image of a normal canine right adrenal gland. The gland is fusiform and is parallel to the aorta (Ao) in the far field. It is also closely apposed to the caudal vena cava (CVC), which runs medially and somewhat parallel to the gland. Hyperechoic borders of the phrenicoabdominal vein are noted at the mid-ventromedial aspect of the gland (black arrow) **C and D:** Sagittal plane images of normal left **(C)** and right **(D)** adrenal glands. A well-defined hyperechoic rim is at the corticomedullary junction. The left gland is slightly oblique in regard to the aorta (Ao), located dorsally, and has a characteristic peanut shape, and the right gland appears as an arrowhead cranially. The caudal vena cava (CVC) is compressed in the near field. Images B–D courtesy of M.A. d'Anjou.

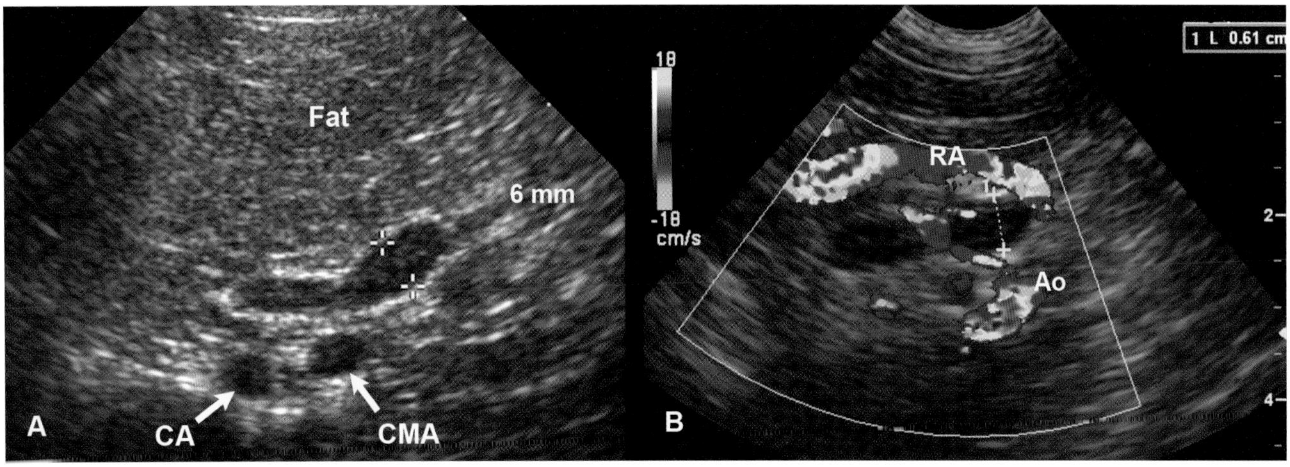

Figure 12.2. Anatomical landmarks for the left adrenal gland in dogs. **A:** Dorsal plane image of a normal canine left adrenal gland. The cranial pole of the gland is located just ventral to the celiac (CA) and cranial mesenteric (CMA) arteries. **B:** Dorsal plane image of a normal canine left adrenal gland with color flow Doppler. The left renal artery (RA) originates caudal to the left adrenal gland and courses cranially around it. The aorta (Ao) is located just dorsal to the gland and to cross-sectional views of the celiac and cranial mesenteric arteries. The thin vessel, with arterial flow, which originates from the aorta and crosses the midbody of the adrenal gland, is the left phrenicoabdominal artery. The layered pattern of colors noted in several arteries is caused by aliasing and does not truly indicate flow reversal.

adrenals by using a lateral approach. When scanning patients in lateral recumbency, the probe is placed on the upper side of the abdomen as far dorsal as possible, just ventral to the lumbar transverse processes, to minimize interference from interposed gas in the small intestine and colon.

The initial approach to the left adrenal gland is to scan the area medial to the left kidney and lateral to the abdominal aorta. For the right adrenal gland, area medial to the right kidney and lateral to dorsal to the caudal vena cava is scanned. This technique may be successful in many patients. However, the position of the adrenal glands varies in relation to the kidneys. The left kidney in particular may rotate and drop when a dog is placed in right lateral recumbency. If this initial approach fails, the glands can be more reliably located by using vascular landmarks in either lateral or dorsal recumbency (Spaulding 1997) (Figure 12.2).

To identify the left adrenal gland, the probe is placed on the left abdominal wall, just ventral to the lumbar transverse processes and approximately halfway between the last rib and the iliac crest. A dorsal plane image is obtained, and the ultrasound beam is fanned ventral and dorsal until the aorta is found. The probe is then rotated until a longitudinal image of the aorta is obtained. One then follows the aorta cranial to the origin of the left renal artery, which usually originates from the lateral aspect of the aorta and courses a short distance laterally before making a sharp turn cranially. From this point, one scans further cranially, fanning the beam dorsally and ventrally. A short distance cranially to the left renal artery, the celiac artery cranially and the cranial mesenteric artery caudally arise from the aorta. As one fans the beam ventrally from the aorta, these arteries appear as two well-defined, circular, hypoechoic or anechoic pulsing structures (Figure 12.2). The left adrenal gland is ventrolateral or lateral to the aorta, cranial to the left renal artery and vein, and at the level or immediately caudal to the origin of the cranial mesenteric artery (Figures 12.1 and 12.2). Once these vessels are identified, the beam is fanned ventral to dorsal and back again through this area until the adrenal gland is found. In thin animals, the gland is closely apposed to the aorta. As the quantity of body fat increases, it is laid down around the adrenal gland, increasing separation from the aorta, but also providing contrast and making the gland more prominent. The long axis of the left adrenal gland may be slightly tilted in comparison with the long axis of the aorta, and the probe may need to be rotated until the length of the left adrenal gland is maximized. The phrenicoabdominal vein may be seen as two fine, hyperechoic parallel lines obliquely crossing the midbody of the adrenal gland (Figure 12.1A). The phrenicoabdominal vessels may be quite small and not seen on B-mode images, but blood flow can usually be seen with color Doppler examination (Figure 12.2B).

To identify the right adrenal gland, the probe is placed in the right paralumbar fossa just ventral to the transverse processes. The beam is fanned dorsal and ventral until the caudal vena cava is identified. A common error is to apply too much pressure to the abdominal wall, which collapses the caudal vena cava and prevents its identification. The caudal vena cava may appear to pulse because of referred motion from the adjacent aorta, but may be distinguished from the aorta by applying mild or moderate pressure, which will cause the vessel to collapse (Figures 12.1D and 12.3). Alternatively, color or pulsed Doppler interrogation reveals craniad, low-velocity venous flow within the vena cava. The vena cava and aorta are close together in the midabdomen, and in some dogs both vessels can be seen in the same scan plane. The vena cava is followed cranially, which usually requires the probe be placed caudal to the last rib and angled cranially. In the cranial abdomen, the aorta and caudal vena cava separate. The beam is fanned ventral and dorsal through the caudal vena cava until the cranial mesenteric and celiac arteries are identified. The appearance of these vessels is identical to that seen from the left side of the abdomen: They appear as two round hypoechoic or anechoic structures just ventral to the aorta and medial to the caudal vena cava. The right adrenal gland is located between dorsal and dorsolateral to the caudal vena cava, at approximately the level of the cranial mesenteric and celiac arteries. In almost all dogs, the right adrenal gland is closely apposed to the caudal vena cava and may be difficult to distinguish in a dorsal plane image because of volume averaging. Obtaining a transverse or frontal plane image through the caudal vena cava may be helpful in identifying the gland (Figure 12.3). It may be necessary to place the probe in one of the last two or three intercostal spaces if the gland cannot be imaged by angling the probe cranially from a position caudal to the last rib. This approach works better in small dogs because pressure cannot be used to bring the gland closer to the probe.

A wide range of normal adrenal sizes has been reported in dogs. The left adrenal gland is 3–16 mm in maximum diameter and 10–50 mm long. The right adrenal gland is up to 3–14 mm in maximum diameter and 10–39 mm long (Barthez et al. 1995; Grooters et al. 1995; Hoerauf and Reusch 1996; Douglass et al. 1997). There appears to be a poor correlation between body weight and maximum adrenal diameter and better correlation between adrenal length and body size. The broad range of reported sizes reflects that patients selected for inclusion were described as normal, young, old, healthy, or not showing signs of any endocrine disease, and these studies may have included dogs with subclinical or nonfunctional adrenal lesions. The maximum diameter of the adrenal gland at the caudal pole seems to be the most reliable measure of adrenal size, and a measurement of 7.4 mm as the maximum normal measurement appears to offer a reasonable combination of sensitivity and specificity (Barthez et al. 1998).

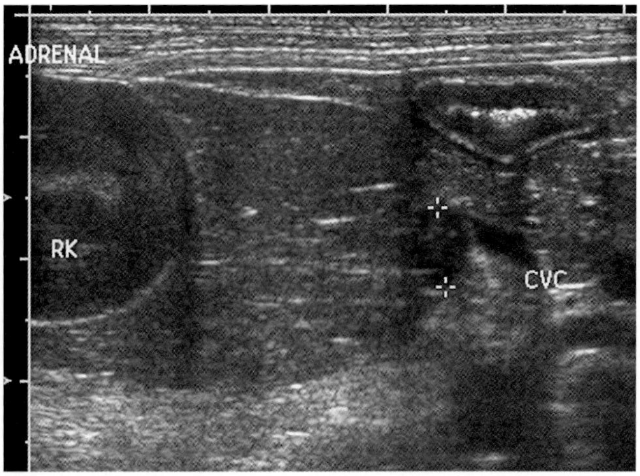

Figure 12.3. Normal canine right adrenal gland. Transverse plane image of the gland (between the cursors), and the caudal vena cava, in the right cranial abdomen. The adrenal gland is closely apposed to the dorsolateral border of the caudal vena cava (CVC). Note how the shape of the caudal vena cava is rhomboidal, a result of partial collapse caused by pressure applied by the sonographer. Fat is present between the right kidney (RK) and the adrenal.

In Cats

The adrenal glands in cats are found by using a similar approach to that employed in dogs. In most cats, scanning the area medial to the kidney and adjacent to the aorta or caudal vena cava is sufficient to identify the adrenal glands. The same vascular landmarks as used in dogs can also be used to find the feline adrenal glands. The feline adrenal gland is short, ovoid or cylindrical, and hypoechoic (Cartee et al. 1993) (Figure 12.4). With high-frequency transducers, one can sometimes distinguish between cortex and medulla. In normal cats, both adrenal glands are 10–11 mm long, and the maximum diameter of both glands is 4.3 ± 0.3 mm.

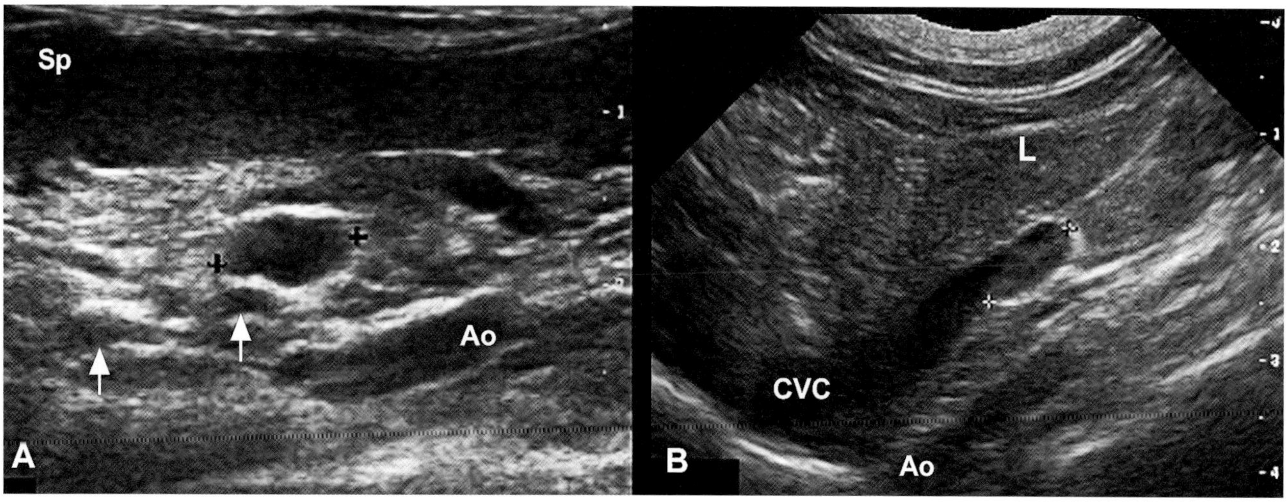

Figure 12.4. Normal adrenal glands in cats. **A:** Sagittal plane image of a normal feline left adrenal gland. The gland is ovoid (between the cursors, 9.5 mm). The celiac (left arrow) and cranial mesenteric (right arrow) arteries are seen medial to the gland. Ao, aorta; and Sp, spleen. **B:** Sagittal plane image of a normal feline right adrenal gland. The gland appears as an ovoid hypoechoic structure (between the cursors, 1 cm), and the medulla is slightly more echogenic than the cortex (L, liver). The caudal vena cava (CVC) and aorta (Ao) are in the same plane. Images courtesy of D. Penninck.

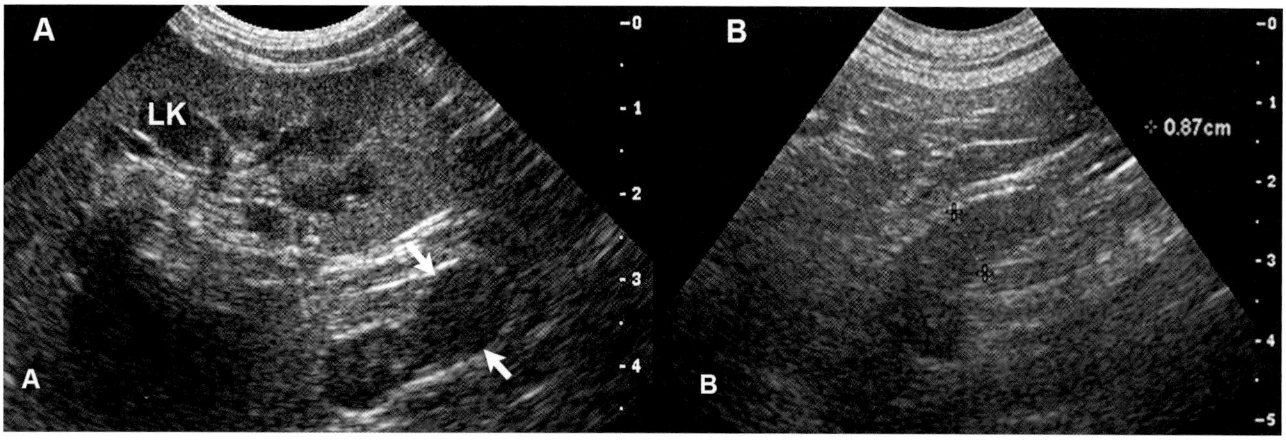

Figure 12.5. Pituitary dependent adrenal hyperplasia in two dogs. **A:** Dorsal plane image of a left adrenal gland. The gland is uniformly enlarged (the caudal pole [arrows] is approximately 10 mm wide), but retains a normal shape. There was similar enlargement of the right adrenal gland. This finding is consistent with pituitary-dependent hyperadrenocorticism. The left kidney (LK) is in the near field. **B:** Sagittal plane image of the right adrenal gland in another dog with pituitary-dependent hyperadrenocorticism. This gland is smoothly enlarged. The left gland was within normal limits for size (7 mm thick).

Sonographic Findings in Adrenal Disorders

Cushing's Syndrome

Cushing's syndrome or hyperadrenocorticism is one of the most common endocrinopathies in dogs. Ultrasound is frequently used as part of the medical database of suspected cases (Behrend et al. 2002). However, it must be remembered that, although ultrasound may provide useful data, it cannot be used alone in diagnosing hyperadrenocorticism. Pituitary-dependent hyperadrenocorticism (PDH) accounts for approximately 80% of dogs with hyperadrenocorticism. If a patient's history, clinical signs, and laboratory test results support a diagnosis of hyperadrenocorticism, PDH should be suspected if both adrenal glands appear symmetrically enlarged (often described as plump) (Barthez et al. 1998; Feldman and Nelson 2004) (Figures 12.5 and 12.6).

Unfortunately, the adrenal glands may measure within the normal range (less than 7.4 mm) in some

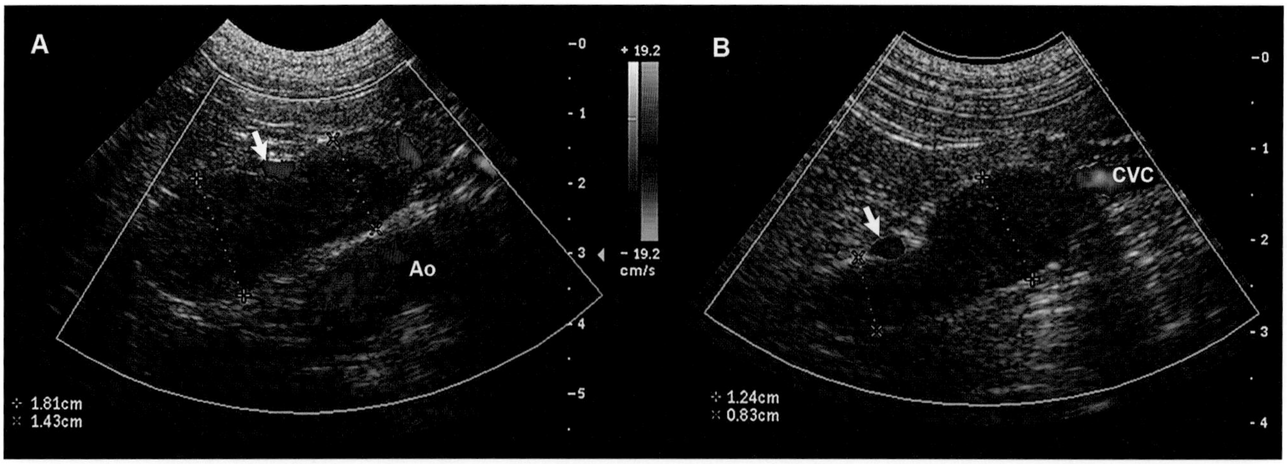

Figure 12.6. Pituitary-dependent adrenal hyperplasia in a dog. Color Doppler images obtained in a dog with a pituitary tumor and signs of hyperadrenocorticism. Both adrenals are enlarged, which is more evident on the left side **(A)**. The caudal pole of the right gland **(B)** is thicker than the cranial pole. The left adrenal gland **(A)** is mildly inhomogeneous. Phrenicoabdominal vessels are seen at the ventromedial aspect of each gland (arrows). Other vascular landmarks, such as the aorta (Ao) and the caudal vena cava (CVC), are also in the scanned field. Images courtesy of M.A. d'Anjou.

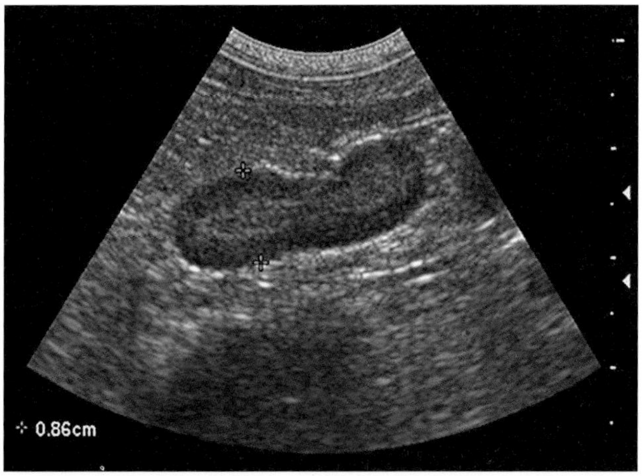

Figure 12.7. Rounded adrenal gland in a dog with a chronic, nonendocrinian disorder. Dorsal oblique image of the left adrenal gland in a small-breed dog with a chronic disease, but without evidence of hyperadrenocorticism. The gland is rounded. Note the hyperechoic medulla in comparison to the cortex. Images courtesy of M.A. d'Anjou.

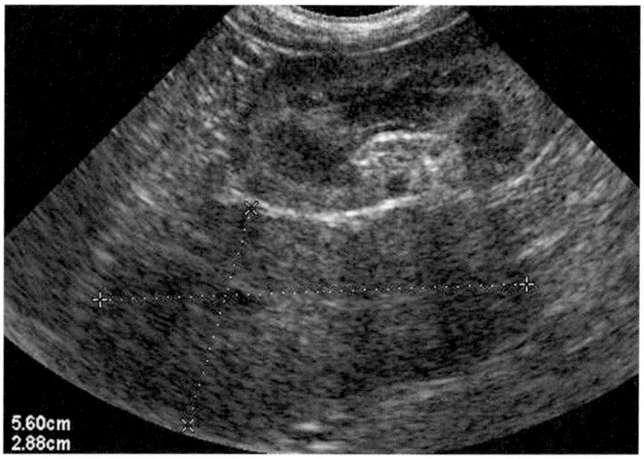

Figure 12.8. Primary adrenal hyperadrenocorticism in a dog. Dorsal plane image obtained in the left craniodorsal abdomen. A large bilobed mass is medial and cranial to the kidney (between the cursors). The mass has a mottled echotexture and is well defined. The right adrenal gland was not identified, and these findings are consistent with primary unilateral adrenal hyperadrenocorticism.

cases of PDH or may demonstrate unilateral or asymmetrical enlargement (Barthez et al. 1995). As already mentioned, some healthy dogs have adrenal glands that exceed 7.4 mm in maximal diameter. Some dogs with chronic nonendocrine disease may also exhibit mild symmetrical adrenal enlargement (Figure 12.7).

Adrenal tumor hyperadrenocorticism (ATH) caused by functional adrenocortical tumors accounts for approximately 20% of dogs with naturally occurring hyperadrenocorticism. In dogs with compatible clinical signs and clinicopathologic findings, ATH should be considered if one adrenal gland is enlarged, contains a nodule, or has been effaced by a mass and the contralateral gland is small or not seen, suggesting that it has been suppressed (Figure 12.8). However, in some cases, the functional tumor may be small and is not detected by ultrasonography. Further confounding the diagnosis, there are reports of dogs with tumors of both the pituitary gland and the adrenal cortex, as well as bilateral primary adrenal neoplasia (Greco et al. 1999). In dogs with hyperadrenocorticism caused by

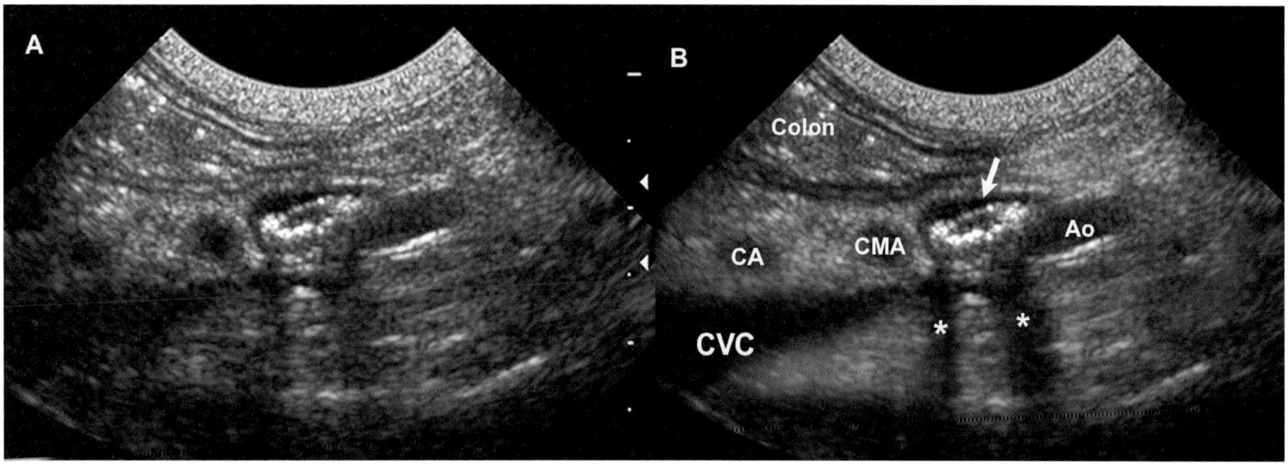

Figure 12.9. Incidental adrenal mineralization in an old cat. Sagittal ultrasound **(A)** and schematic **(B)** images of the right adrenal gland on which hyperechoic foci are seen in association with acoustic shadowing (*), but without evidence of adrenomegaly. These changes were also apparent on the left side. Vascular landmarks are noted. Ao, aorta; CA, celiac artery; CMA, cranial mesenteric artery; and CVC, caudal vena cava. Images courtesy of M.A. d'Anjou.

exogenous steroid administration, the adrenal glands may appear small or may not be seen.

In contrast to dogs, adrenal disease is uncommon in cats. Adrenal mineralization is common in older cats and should not be considered a sign of neoplasia (Figure 12.9). Feline Cushing's syndrome is uncommon, but ultrasonography may be helpful in determining whether the disease is pituitary dependent or caused by a functional adrenal cortical tumor. The criteria are similar to those in dogs and, based on the limited data available, may be more reliable (Watson and Herrtage 1998; Feldman and Nelson 2004). Bilateral adrenal enlargement suggests PDH, whereas a unilateral nodule or mass suggests ATH. However, as in dogs, some cats with PDH had normal adrenal glands while one cat with ATH had bilateral adrenal enlargement.

Addison's Disease

A diagnosis of Addison's disease cannot be made based on ultrasonographic findings alone. However, a study showed measurable reduction in thickness (range for left adrenal gland, 2.2 to 3.0 mm, and for right adrenal gland, 2.2 to 3.4 mm) and length (range for left adrenal gland, 10.0 to 19.7 mm, and for right adrenal gland, 9.5 to 18.8 mm) of affected adrenal glands compared to the normal dogs (Hoerauf and Reusch 1999). Therefore, in a patient with consistent clinical and laboratory findings, the detection of small adrenal glands or failure to detect the glands, despite a technically adequate study, can be considered circumstantial evidence supporting a diagnosis of hypoadrenocorticism (Figure 12.10).

Adrenal Nodules and Masses

The differential diagnosis for adrenal nodules and masses includes cortical adenoma, cortical adenocarcinoma, pheochromocytoma, metastasis, and hyperplasia. Cortical tumors may or may not be functional, and there may be no signs of hyperadrenocorticism. The sonographic appearance of these lesions is nonspecific (Figure 12.11). Clinical signs of pheochromocytomas are often vague, nonspecific, or intermittent (Feldman and Nelson 2004), and their sonographic features are nonspecific (Figures 12.12 and 12.13). Nodules and masses vary in size and echogenicity. However, if the nodules exceeds 2 cm, benign or malignant neoplasia is more likely, and if the lesion exceeds 4 cm, malignant neoplasia is more likely (Besso et al. 1997). However, both benign neoplasms and hyperplasia may produce quite large lesions. The most reliable sign of malignancy is evidence of invasion of local tissues and structures, which can occur with adrenocortical carcinomas and pheochromocytomas (Platt et al. 1998).

These tumors may invade the adjacent kidney or musculature and extend to involve the vertebrae and cause neurological signs. Locally invasive lesions may be recognized sonographically especially if they distort the kidney (Figure 12.13).

Invasion of the caudal vena cava and formation of a thrombus within its lumen may occur with malignancies of the right adrenal gland (Figures 12.14–12.16).

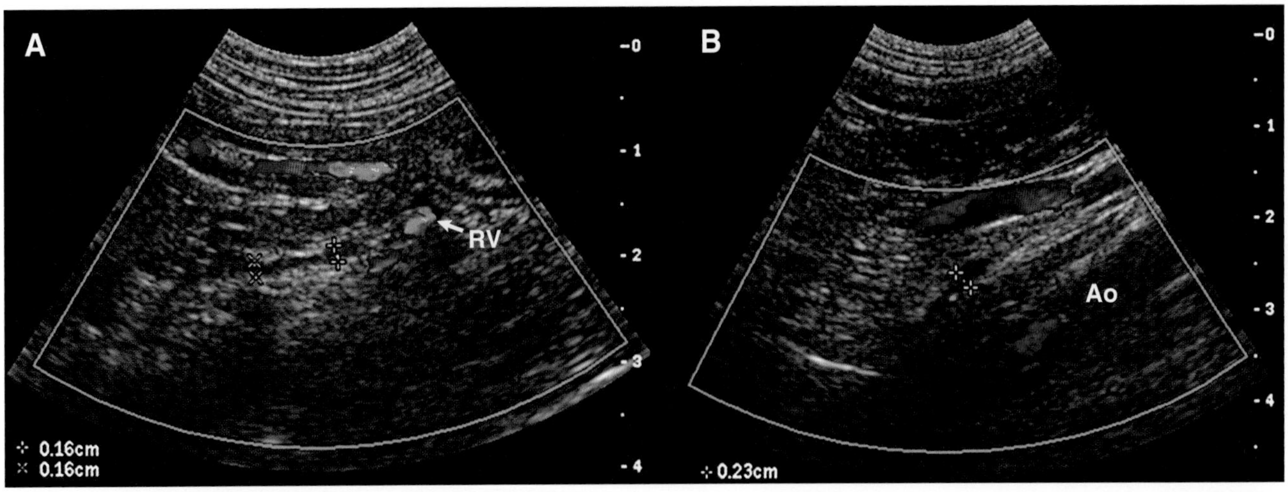

Figure 12.10. Addison's disease in a dog. Sagittal ultrasound images of the left **(A)** and right **(B)** adrenal glands in a dog with hypoadrenocorticism. Both glands are significantly reduced in diameter (between the cursors). Ao, aorta; and RV, left renal vein. Images courtesy of M.A. d'Anjou.

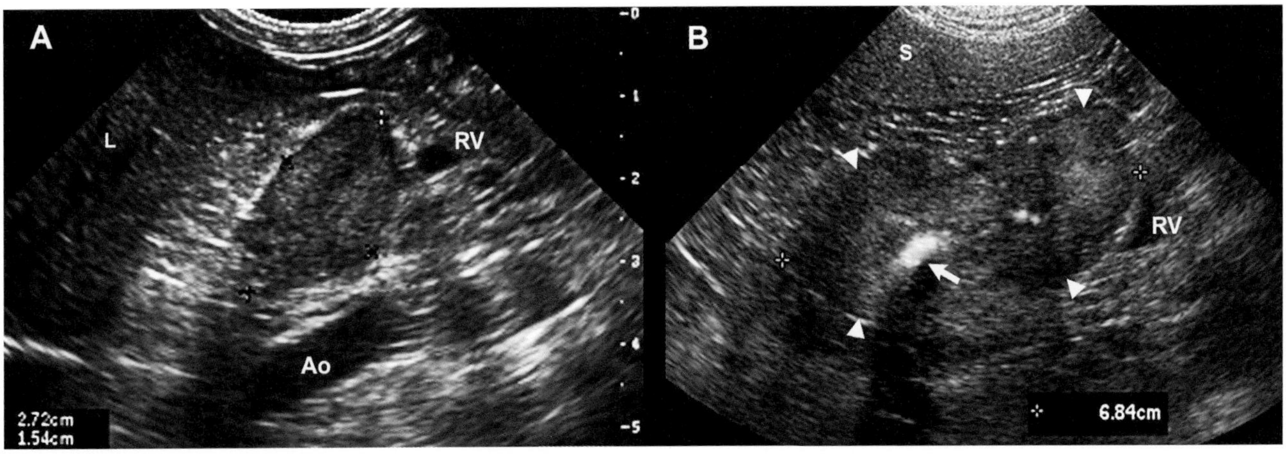

Figure 12.11. Adrenal tumors in two dogs. **A:** Sagittal sonogram of a pheochromocytoma of the right adrenal gland in a 9-year-old Chihuahua crossed. The mass is homogeneously echogenic and appears dorsal to the aorta (Ao) and just cranial to the left renal vein (RV). L, liver. **B:** Transverse sonogram of an adenocarcinoma of the left adrenal gland in an 11-year-old large-breed dog. A large, irregular, inhomogeneous mass (arrowheads) has replaced the left adrenal gland. This mass contains amorphous mineralization, as seen as shadowing hyperechoic foci (arrow), which is more typical of this malignant process. In both lesions, there was no sonographic evidence of vascular invasion, although caudal displacement and compression of the left renal vein (RV) is seen in **B**. S, spleen. Images courtesy of D. Penninck and M.A. d'Anjou.

Other local vessels may also be invaded, such as the renal veins, adrenal veins, and phrenicoabdominal vessels. Vascular invasion by malignant adrenal neoplasms is detected more commonly by histopathology and necropsy than by ultrasound, because the affected vessels may be quite small and below the limit of ultrasound resolution (Besso et al. 1997; Feldman and Nelson 2004). The presence of a venous thrombus adjacent to an adrenal mass is highly suggestive of malignancy.

Hyperadrenocorticism may cause a hypercoagulable state and, in this condition, aortic thrombus can be detected. Aortic thrombosis caused by tumor invasion has not been reported (Besso et al. 1997). Hyperechoic foci with distal acoustic shadowing, representing mineralization, have been reported more commonly with adrenocortical tumors, but may occur in medullary tumors and with benign lesions (Figure 12.11). The shape of the adrenal lesion may offer some circumstantial evidence as to type. If the gland retains a normal shape, hyperplasia is considered more likely. Discrete, well-defined nodules suggests benign neoplasia, whereas amorphous or irregularly shaped masses suggest malignancy (Besso et al. 1997).

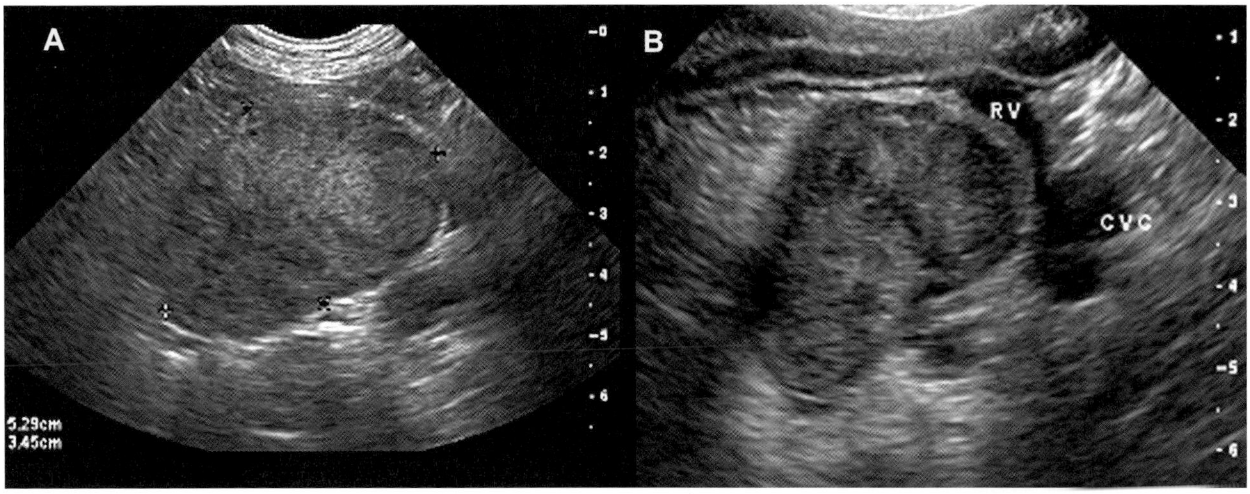

Figure 12.12. Adrenal pheochromocytomas in two dogs. **A:** Sagittal sonogram of a pheochromocytoma in the 8-year-old boxer crossed. A large mass is medial to the left kidney, but not invading the adjacent vessels. **B:** Sagittal sonogram of a pheochromocytoma in the 15-year-old golden retriever. The mass is adjacent to right renal vein (RV) and caudal vena cava (CVC), but not invading them, as confirmed during surgery. Images courtesy of D. Penninck.

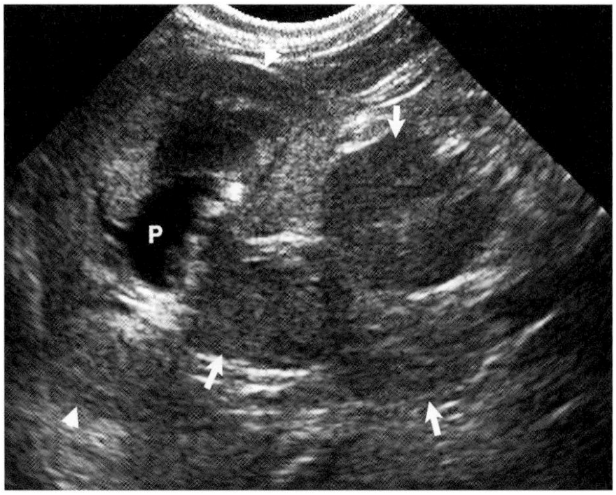

Figure 12.13. Invasive pheochromocytoma in a dog. Dorsal plane image obtained in the right craniodorsal abdomen. The right kidney is in the near field (arrowheads), and the renal pelvis (P) is moderately dilated. A bilobed, hypoechoic mass (arrows) is present medial to the right kidney and extends into the hilus of the kidney. The pelvic dilation suggests partial obstruction of the ureter by invasion or encasement by the mass. The mass was found to be a pheochromocytoma.

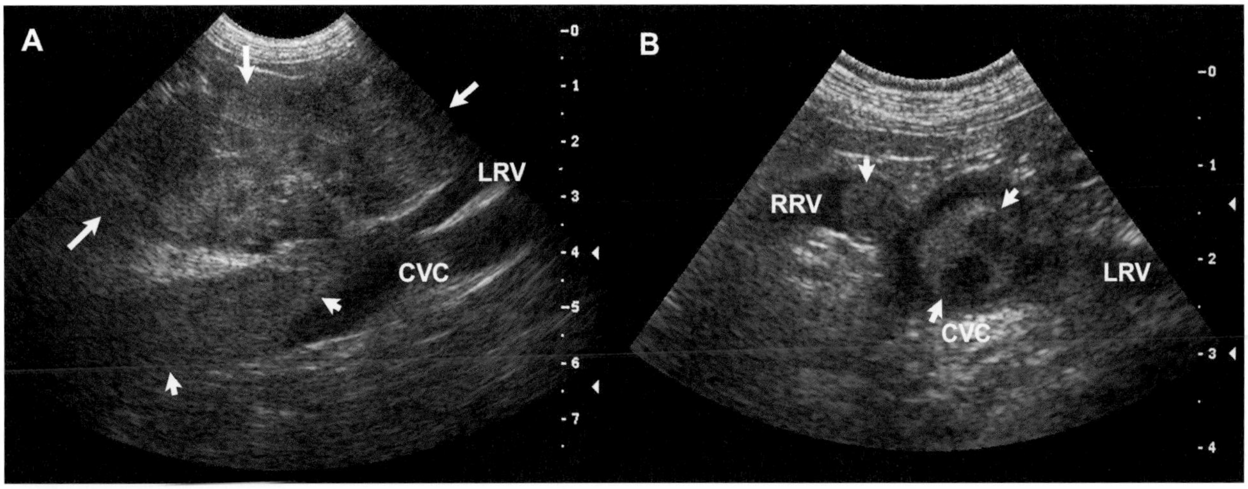

Figure 12.14. Adrenocortical carcinoma and venous thrombosis in a dog. Sagittal **(A)** and transverse **(B)** plane images obtained in the left midabdomen of a dog with peritoneal effusion and pelvic limb swelling. A large, irregular, inhomogeneous mass (arrowheads) is ventral to the caudal vena cava (CVC), displacing the left renal vein caudally (LRV). A moderately echogenic structure, with hypoechoic portions **(B)**, is found in the lumen of the CVC, protruding into the right renal vein (RRV), consistent with thrombosis (arrows). At surgery, there was no evidence of vascular invasion by the mass, although this was initially suspected. Images courtesy of M.A. d'Anjou.

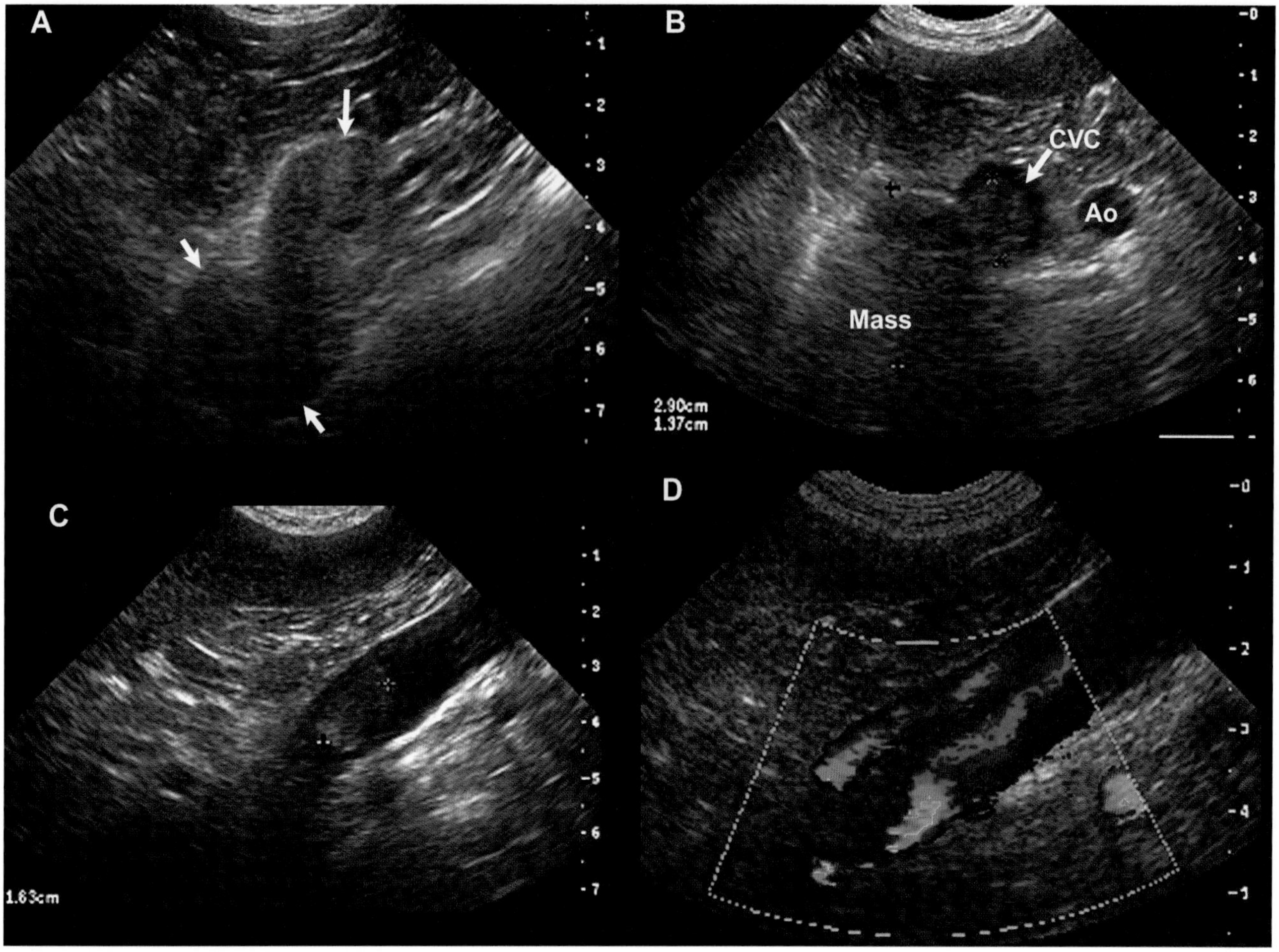

Figure 12.15. Large pheochromocytoma and venous thrombosis in a 12-year-old mixed-breed dog. **A:** Sagittal sonogram of a large pheochromocytoma (arrows) of the right adrenal gland. **B:** A transverse sonogram of the mass and the invaded caudal vena cava (CVC), which appears significantly larger than the adjacent aorta (Ao). **C:** The echogenic thrombus is well seen in the lumen of the vessel. **D:** The color Doppler assessment outlines the caudal margin of the thrombus. The vascular invasion was confirmed at surgery. Images courtesy of D. Penninck.

Adrenal nodules and small masses have become more common incidental findings as operator experience has increased and machine quality has improved. These are sometimes referred to as "incidentalomas" (Figure 12.17) and leave clinicians with the dilemma of how far the diagnosis should be pursued. Many of these lesions cause no clinical signs, and a diagnosis is never confirmed. Reported diagnoses include normal tissue, nonfunctional cortical tumors, granulomas, adrenal cysts, myelolipoma, hemorrhage, metastatic tumor, and pheochromocytoma (Feldman and Nelson 2004). The medical history and clinical signs should be reviewed for evidence of endocrine disease. Clinicopathologic tests are indicated if any such signs are identified. Larger masses or nodules (greater than 2 cm) are more likely to be neoplastic, so surgical removal should be considered. However, many of these patients have serious concurrent illnesses and may be quite aged, so such an aggressive approach may not be indicated or acceptable to the owner. If there is no evidence of endocrine disease or sonographic evidence of invasiveness, serial ultrasound examinations at 1- to 3-month intervals can be used to monitor for enlargement or progression of the lesion. If there is evidence of progression, surgical excision may be prudent.

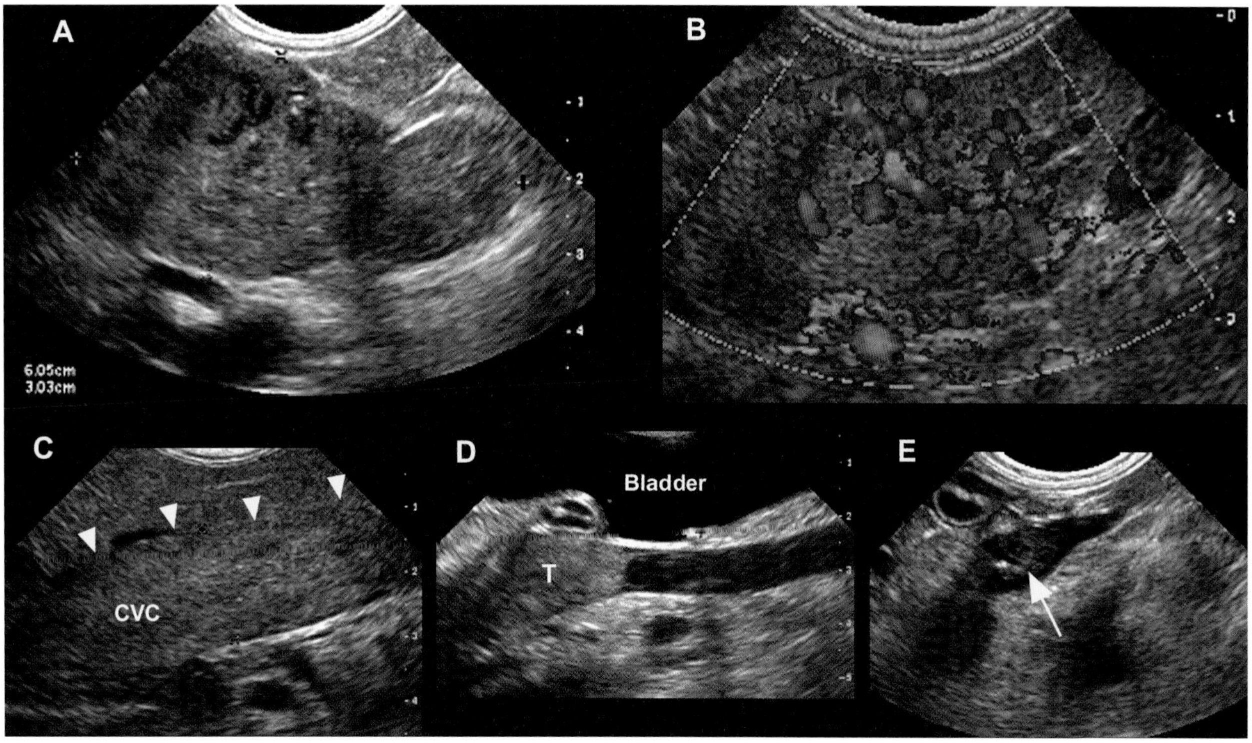

Figure 12.16. Invasive adrenal tumor in an 11-year-old schnauzer. **A:** Sagittal sonogram of a large invasive tumor of the left adrenal gland. **B:** On color Doppler evaluation, the mass appears highly vascular. **C:** An extensive thrombus is within the caudal vena cava (CVC) outlined by white arrowheads. **D:** The thrombus (T) extends caudally up to the level of the bladder. **E:** Inhomogeneous, echogenic thrombus (arrow) is also seen invading the renal vein. The small bright focus within the thrombus most likely represents mineralization. The highly vascular mass and dependent thrombus could not be successfully resected at surgery. Images courtesy of D. Penninck.

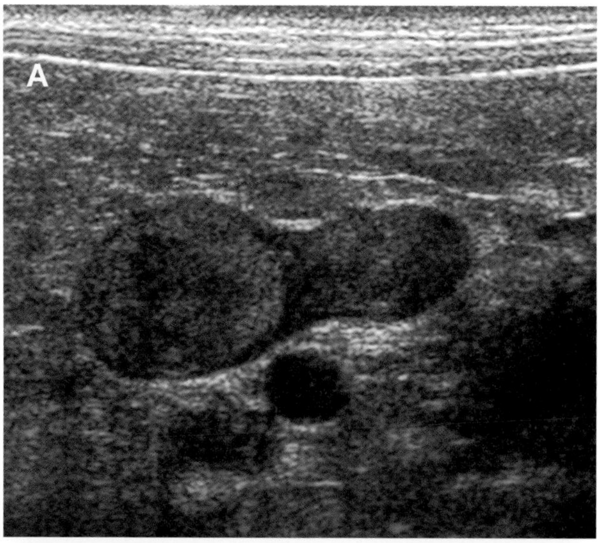

Figure 12.17. Incidental adrenal nodules in two dogs. **A:** Dorsal plane image of a left adrenal gland. A well-defined, inhomogeneous, hyperechoic nodule is in the cranial pole of the adrenal gland. The nodule was an incidental finding and remained unchanged on serial examinations. Anechoic cross sections of the celiac and cranial mesenteric arteries are seen dorsally. **B:** Sagittal sonogram of both adrenal glands of a 15-year-old Siberian husky with incidental bilateral changes in echogenicity and shape (arrows). These changes remained unchanged on serial examinations. Images courtesy of D. Penninck.

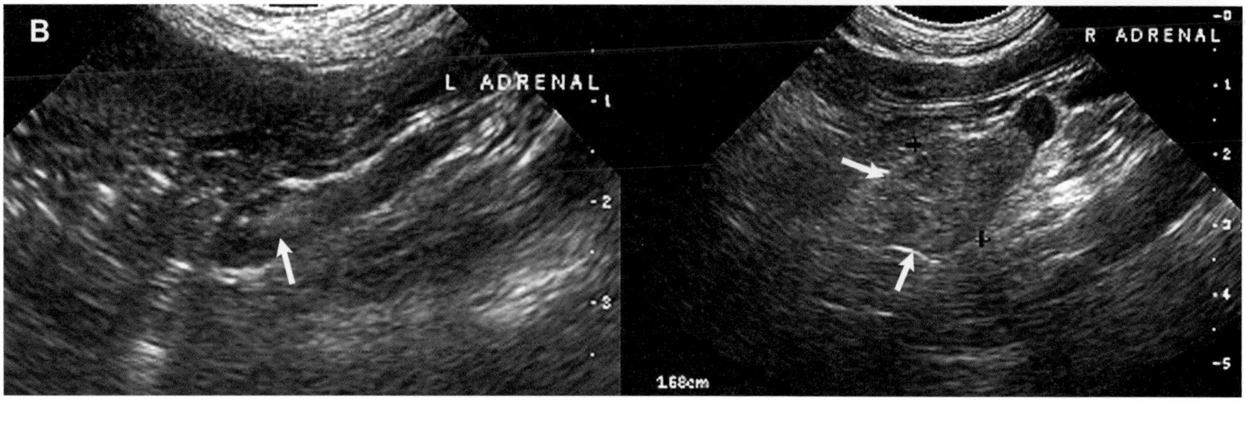

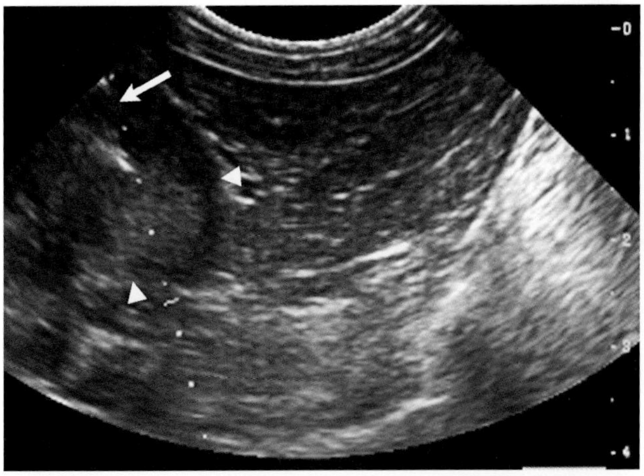

Figure 12.18. Fine-needle aspiration using a 22-gauge spinal needle (arrow) was performed on this adrenal mass (arrowheads) in a dog. No complication was encountered during the procedure. The final diagnosis was adrenocortical adenocarcinoma.

Interventional Procedures

Fine-needle aspiration or biopsy of adrenal nodules or masses may be attempted (Figure 12.18) and is routinely performed in human patients. However, in dogs these tests are of equivocal value and are not without risk. It may be difficult to distinguish hyperplasia and benign and malignant adrenocortical tumors based on cytologic criteria. Attempted fine-needle aspiration or biopsy of a pheochromocytoma may cause uncontrollable hemorrhage or paroxysmal hypertension.

References

Barthez PY, Nyland TG, Feldman EC (1995) Ultrasonographic evaluation of adrenal glands in dogs. J Am Vet Med Assoc 207:1180–1183.

Barthez PY, Nyland TG, Feldman EC (1998) Ultrasonography of the adrenal glands in the dog, cat, and ferret. Vet Clin North Am Small Anim Pract 28:869–885.

Behrend EN, Kemppainen RJ, Clark TP, Salman MD, Peterson ME (2002) Diagnosis of hyperadrenocorticism in dogs: A survey of internists and dermatologists. J Am Vet Med Assoc 220:1643–1649.

Besso JG, Penninck DG, Gliatto JM (1997) Retrospective ultrasonographic evaluation of adrenal lesions in 26 dogs. Vet Radiol Ultrasound 38:448–455.

Cartee RE, Finn-Bodner ST, Gray BW (1993) Ultrasound examination of the feline adrenal gland. J Diagn Med Sonogr 9:327–330.

Douglass JP, Berry CR, James S (1997) Ultrasonographic adrenal gland measurements in dogs without evidence of adrenal disease. Vet Radiol Ultrasound 38:124–130.

Feldman EC, Nelson RW (2004) The adrenal gland. In: Feldman EC, Nelson RW, eds. Canine and Feline Endocrinology and Reproduction, 3rd edition. St Louis: WB Saunders, pp 394–439.

Greco DS, Peterson ME, Davidson AP, Feldman EC, Komurek K (1999) Concurrent pituitary and adrenal tumors in dogs with hyperadrenocorticism: 17 cases (1978–1995). J Am Vet Med Assoc 214:1349–1353.

Grooters AM, Biller DS, Merryman J (1995) Ultrasonographic parameters of normal canine adrenal glands: Comparison to necropsy findings. Vet Radiol Ultrasound 36:126–130.

Hoerauf A, Reusch C (1996) Ultrasonographic evaluation of the adrenal glands in healthy dogs, dogs with Cushing's disease due to functional adrenal tumors and dogs with Addison's disease [Abstract]. Vet Radiol Ultrasound 37:488.

Hoerauf A, Reusch C (1999) Ultrasonographic evaluation of the adrenal glands in six dogs with hypoadrenocorticism. J Am Anim Hosp Assoc 35:214–218.

Platt SR, Sheppard BJ, Graham J, Uhl EW, Meeks J, Clemmons RM (1998) Pheochromocytoma in the vertebral canal of two dogs. J Am Anim Hosp Assoc 34:365–371.

Spaulding KA (1997) A review of sonographic identification of abdominal blood vessels and juxtavascular organs. Vet Radiol Ultrasound 38:4–23.

Watson PJ, Herrtage ME (1998) Hyperadrenocorticism in six cats. J Small Anim Pract 39:175–184.

CHAPTER THIRTEEN

Female Reproductive Tract

Silke Hecht

Examination Technique

The ovaries and the uterus are the only female reproductive organs routinely visualized by means of ultrasonography. The normal uterine tubes are usually too small to be seen, and the vulva and vagina are difficult to image transabdominally because of their intrapelvic location. Mammary glands are infrequently examined.

Indications for ultrasonographic examination of the female reproductive tract include pregnancy diagnosis, assessment of normal fetal development and viability, vaginal discharge, clinical signs compatible with hormonal imbalances suggesting ovarian dysfunction, and abdominal mass lesions in intact queens and bitches. Indications for ultrasonographic examination of the mammary glands include abnormal findings on palpation (swelling, pain, and heat) and a need to assess the extent of mammary gland neoplasia.

The examination is performed with the animal in dorsal recumbency (Figure 13.1). An approach in lateral recumbency may prove useful in the examination of the ovaries. A 5-MHz transducer is usually sufficient to visualize an enlarged fluid-filled uterus, fetal structures, or abdominal mass lesions; however, a 7.5- or 10-MHz transducer provides better detail in the examination of smaller structures and is recommended for most indications. For the examination of the mammary glands, a high-resolution transducer (7.5 MHz or higher) is recommended.

Ovaries

Normal Sonographic Anatomy

The ovaries are located caudally, and often laterally, to the caudal poles of the kidneys, which are used as landmarks for their identification. They are oval and measure approximately 2 cm long in dogs and less than 1 cm long in cats. The appearance of the ovary varies during the estrus cycle (Table 13.1 and Figures 13.2–13.5). Although ultrasonographic changes during the ovarian cycle have been well studied in dogs, the exact time of ovulation cannot be predicted (Yeager and Concannon 1995; Silva et al. 1996).

Ovarian Disorders

Ovarian diseases are uncommon in dogs and very rare in cats. In many cases, a presumptive diagnosis of an ovarian abnormality is made based on clinical findings, and ultrasonography is used to confirm the suspicion rather than serving as the primary means of diagnosis (England et al. 2003).

Ovarian cysts appear as anechoic, well-circumscribed, and thin-walled structures with distal enhancement (Figures 13.6 and 13.7). Hormonally inactive cysts arising from the ovarian bursa and hormone-producing follicular and luteinizing cysts cannot be differentiated through ultrasonography. Large follicles and corpora lutea may be confused with ovarian cysts, and the finding of fluid-filled structures associated with the ovary has to be interpreted in light of the clinical presentation.

Ovarian tumors (epithelial tumors, sex-cord stromal tumors, and germ-cell tumors), which appear as nodules or masses of variable size and echogenicity, may have a cystic or mineral component (Figures 13.8 and 13.9). Tumor types cannot be differentiated ultrasonographically, although teratomas and teratocarcinomas have the tendency to become very large and contain bone or mineral. The origin of an ovarian mass can be difficult to determine when the enlarging organ changes position and moves ventrally from its original location (Diez-Bru et al. 1998). Common concurrent findings include ascites, pyometra, and cystic endometrial hyperplasia.

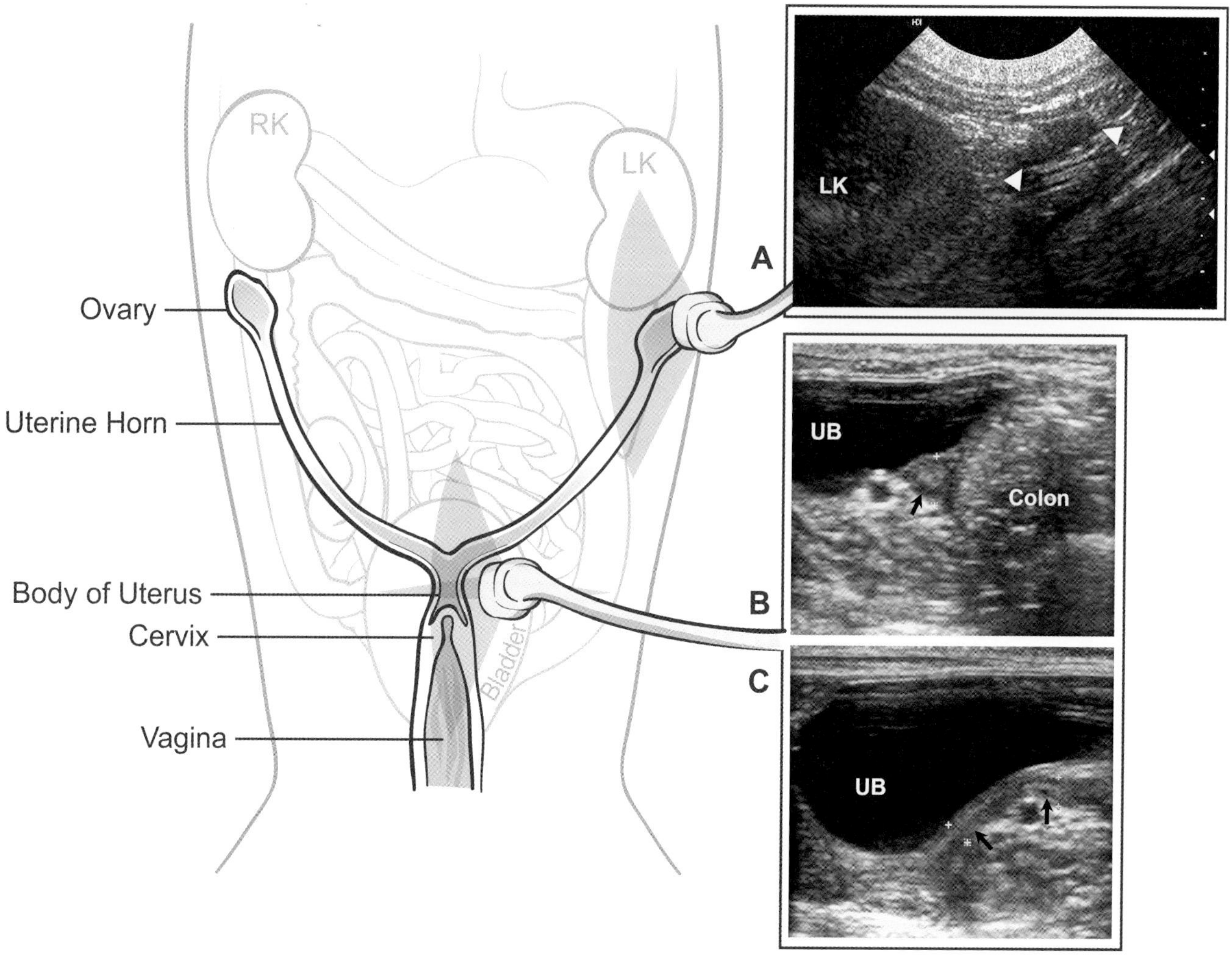

Figure 13.1. Normal female reproductive tract. On the **left** is a schematic representation of the anatomy of the female reproductive tract. The ovaries are located caudally and often laterally to the kidneys. The cervix and body of the uterus are located dorsally to the urinary bladder. The uterine horns extend craniolaterally from the uterine body and are usually not easily visible in a normal dog. **A:** Sagittal image of a normal left canine ovary (arrowheads). The left kidney (LK) is used as a landmark, and the ovary is identified as an ovoid soft-tissue structure of medium echogenicity caudal to the caudal pole. **B and C:** Transverse **(B)** and sagittal **(C)** images of the normal canine uterus. On the transverse image, the uterus (black arrow) is identified as a circular structure between the urinary bladder (UB) and colon, which are used as landmarks. On the sagittal image, the uterus (black arrows) is seen as a tubular structure of medium echogenicity dorsal to the urinary bladder (UB).

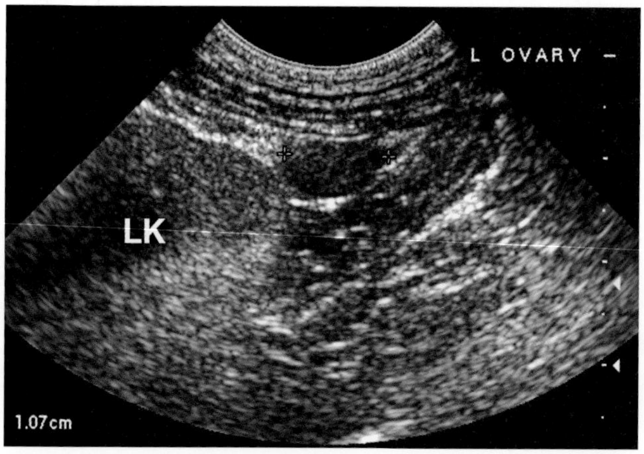

Figure 13.2. Normal ovary during anestrus. Sagittal image of the left ovary (between the cursors) in a 6-year-old Labrador retriever during anestrus. The ovary is smoothly marginated, and slightly hypoechoic to the adjacent left renal cortex (LK), without evidence of follicles or corpora lutea.

Table 13.1.
Ultrasonographic appearance of canine ovaries throughout the estrus cycle

Time of the Estrus Cycle	Appearance of the Ovary
Anestrus and early proestrus	Small (mean length, 1.2 cm) Oval shape with a smooth contour Uniform echogenicity (no follicles, CLs,[a] or other structures)
Proestrus	Size gradually increases; becomes a plumper oval shape; contour usually remains smooth. Follicles appear as round or oval-shaped anechoic fluid cavities with a thin wall or no apparent wall. Mean follicle number four (range, 0–10). Follicle diameter is breed dependent. On the day prior to ovulation, mean diameter reaches from 5 mm in beagles to 8 mm in retrievers. The maximum diameter of preovulatory follicles may be as large as 11 mm.
Day of ovulation	Follicle number usually decreases to 0–2 follicles per ovary. The remaining follicles tend to decrease in diameter, but the ovary maintains its size. Contour may appear bumpy. Solid, hypoechoic CLs may appear. A scant amount of fluid is occasionally detected adjacent to the ovary.
Estrus	Maximum ovarian size is reached 5–6 days after ovulation (300%–400% of anestrus volume). The contour is bumpy. Fluid-filled CLs have anechoic centers. There is a mean of three fluid-filled CLs per ovary. May be indistinguishable from follicles. Tend to be several millimeters larger, thicker walled, and more variable in shape than follicles. Solid CLs are 5–9 mm in diameter.
Diestrus	The contour is bumpy. Fluid-filled CLs gradually decrease in size and increase in echogenicity to become 6-mm solid CLs between 10 and 14 days after ovulation. Ovarian size decreases somewhat (200%–300% of anestrus volume) as fluid-filled CLs regress. Solid CLs persist through most of diestrus.

[a]CL, corpus luteum.
Reprinted from Yeager and Concannon (1995), with permission.

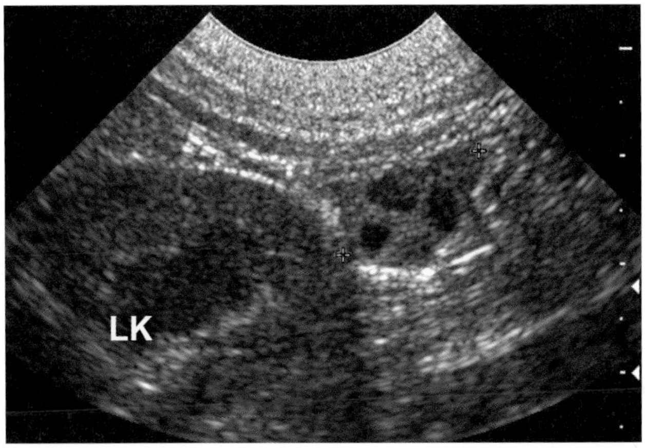

Figure 13.3. Normal ovary during anestrus. Sagittal image of the left ovary (between the cursors) in a 6-year-old Labrador retriever during late proestrus or early estrus. The three circular anechoic follicles within the ovary are associated with far enhancement. LK, left kidney.

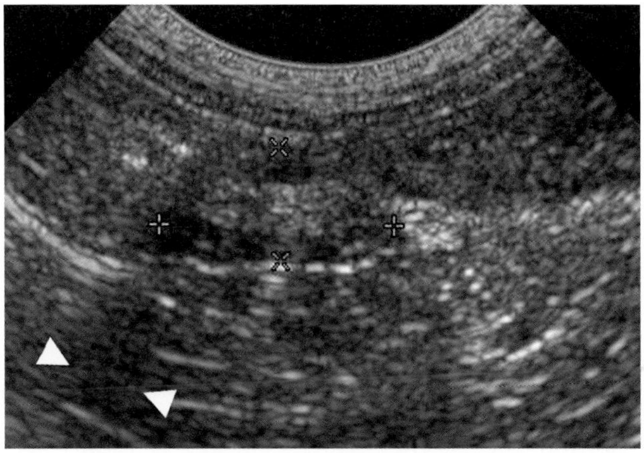

Figure 13.4. Normal ovary during diestrus. Sagittal image of the left ovary (between the cursors) in an 8-year-old shih tzu during diestrus. Several small circular hypoechoic corpora lutea are associated with the ovary. A hypoechoic linear band extending distally from the cranial pole of the ovary is consistent with edge shadowing artifact (arrowheads).

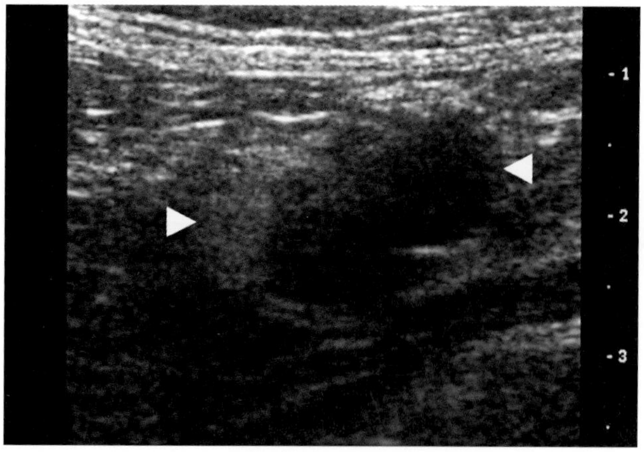

Figure 13.5. Normal ovary during pregnancy. Sagittal image of the left ovary (between the arrowheads) in a pregnant 4-year-old pointer. Two large hypoechoic corpora lutea cause a lumpy organ contour.

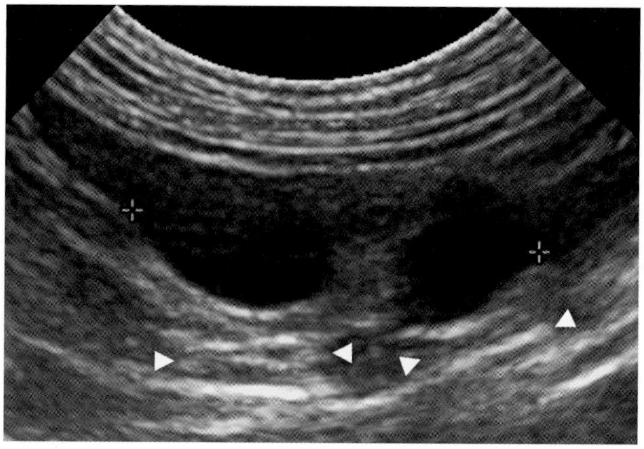

Figure 13.6. Ovarian cysts in a dog. The right ovary (between the cursors) is 2.2 cm long, and two thin-walled anechoic circular structures are associated with the cranial and the caudal poles, respectively. The cysts are characterized by distal enhancement (arrowheads).

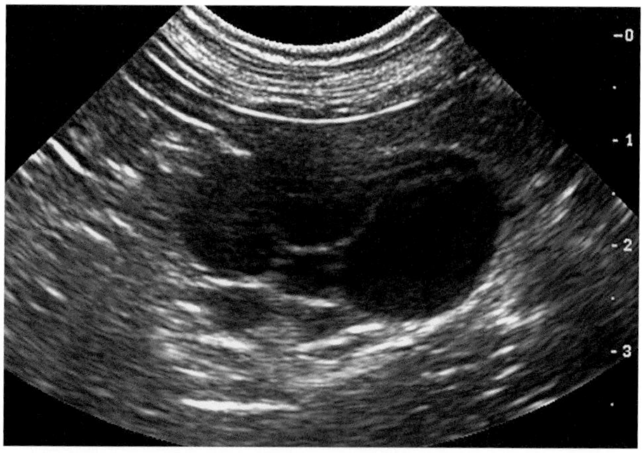

Figure 13.7. Cystic ovary in a 15-year-old vizsla. Multiple thin-walled anechoic structures are associated with the left ovary. Normal ovarian parenchyma cannot be identified.

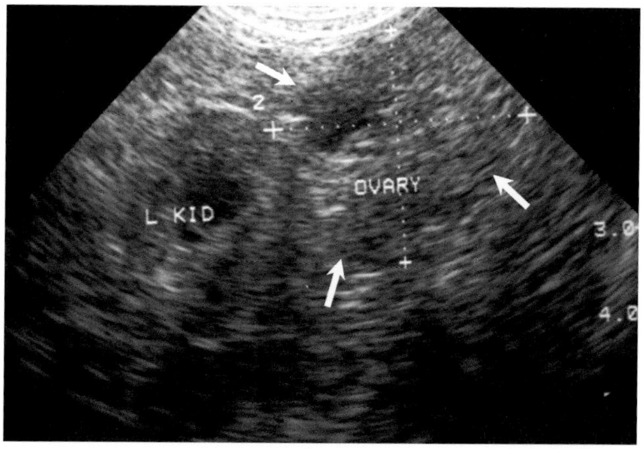

Figure 13.8. Ovarian adenocarcinoma in a dog. A 2.8 × 3.1-cm irregularly marginated and mixed echogenic mass (arrows) is caudal to the left kidney (L KID).

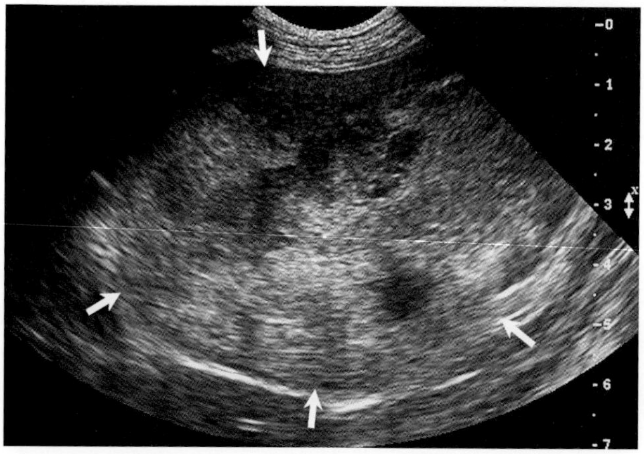

Figure 13.9. Sex-cord stromal tumor arising from residual ovarian tissue in a spayed 9-year-old Labrador retriever. A large inhomogeneous and mixed echogenic mass (arrows) is associated with the midabdomen.

Uterus

Normal Sonographic Anatomy

The normal nongravid uterus is inconspicuous, often difficult to identify in dogs, and usually not seen in cats. It is best identified in the caudal abdomen, where it appears as a tubular structure between the urinary bladder (ventral) and the descending colon (dorsal) (Figure 13.1). Its size and appearance depend on the size of the animal, previous pregnancies, and stage of the estrus cycle (Table 13.2 and Figures 13.10 and 13.11). After identification of the cervix or the uterine body, the uterus is traced cranially to the level of the bifurcation and the uterine horns. An alternative approach is the identification of the uterine horns close to the ovaries; however, their small diameter at this location hinders identification. Even if the uterine body and the cervix are seen in a nongravid animal, the uterine horns may not be visible because of their small size and surrounding intestinal segments. The lack of identifiable wall layers helps in differentiating uterine horns from intestinal loops.

In spayed dogs, the uterine stump is usually inconspicuous and may be visible as a blind-ending tubular structure between urinary bladder and colon (Figure 13.12).

Table 13.2.
Ultrasonographic appearance of the canine uterus during the estrus cycle

Time	Appearance of the Uterus
Late diestrus and anestrus	Uniformly hypoechoic Neither layered wall nor luminal echo 3–8 mm in diameter Difficult to detect Vagina and cervix difficult to distinguish from the uterine body
Proestrus, estrus, metestrus, and early diestrus	1-mm hyperechoic luminal echo and hypoechoic inner layer of uterine wall variably present Relatively easy to detect 1–3 mm larger in diameter in comparison with anestrus Focal enlargement of cervix with "bull's eye" appearance in cross section because of multiple layers

Data from Yeager and Concannon (1995).

Pregnancy

Normal Pregnancy

Ultrasonography is a reliable method for diagnosing pregnancy in small animals. Inconsistency exists in the literature regarding the time of the earliest definitive diagnosis, partially because it is difficult to determine the time of conception in dogs. The improved image detail provided by more recent ultrasound systems could contribute to earlier diagnosis.

The most commonly used definition of gestational age is the number of days after luteinizing hormone (LH) peak in dogs and the number of days after breeding in cats (Mattoon and Nyland 1995). According to

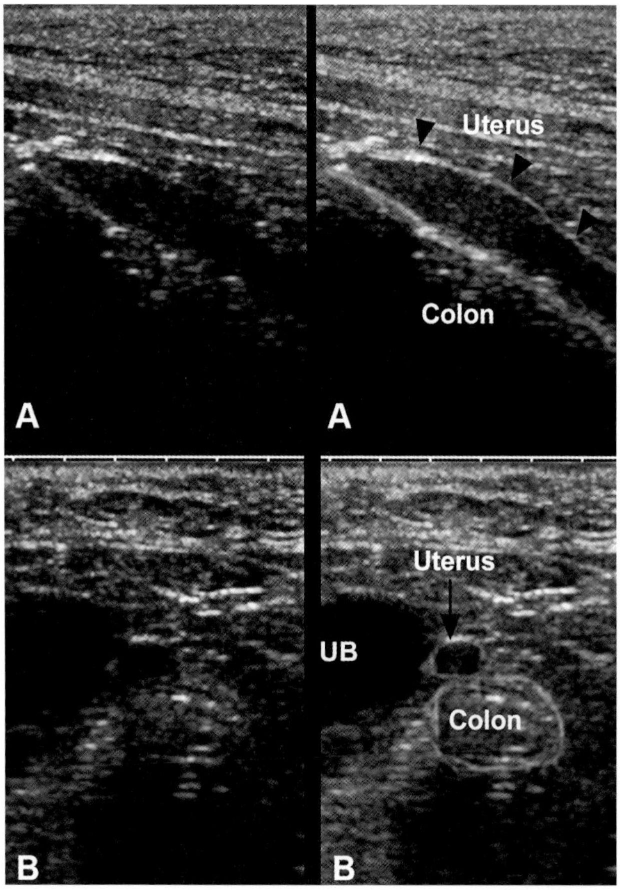

Figure 13.10. Normal anestrus uterus in a 6-year-old Scottish terrier. **A:** On the sagittal image, the uterus (arrowheads) is a tubular, homogeneous structure of medium echogenicity dorsal to the colon, which is characterized by a hyperechoic interface and distal dirty shadowing. The transition between the cervix and the uterine body is inconspicuous. The urinary bladder is not visible on this image. **B:** On the transverse image, the uterus (arrow) appears as a round, homogeneous structure dorsal to the colon and to the left of the urinary bladder (UB).

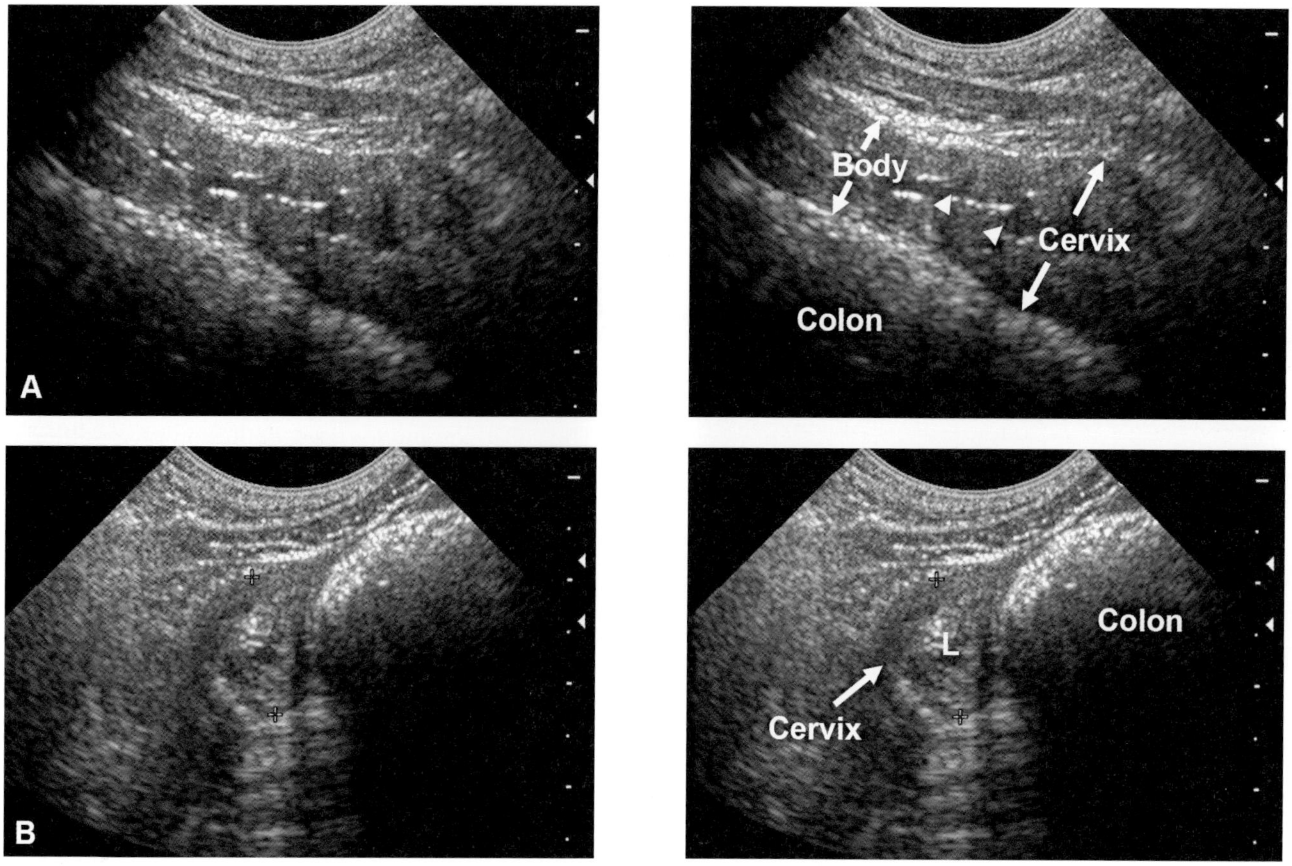

Figure 13.11. Normal late-proestrus or early-estrus uterus in a 6-year-old Labrador retriever (the same dog as in Figure 13.3). **A:** Sagittal image of cervix and body of the uterus. The uterine wall is thicker than during anestrus. Hyperechoic luminal echoes and a small volume of intraluminal fluid are present (arrowheads). The diameter of the cervix is larger than the diameter of the uterine body. **B:** Transverse image of the cervix (between the cursors). The cervix is thick walled, with hyperechoic and hypoechoic echoes within the lumen (L). The uterus appears lateral to the descending colon.

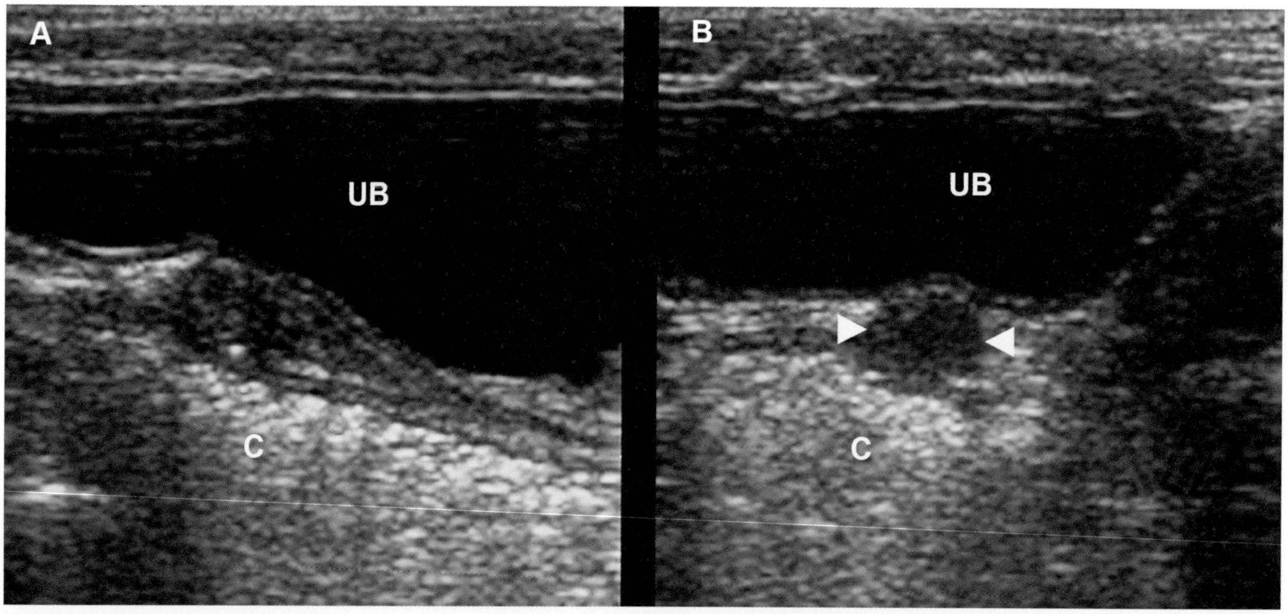

Figure 13.12. Uterine stump in a healthy 12-year-old mixed-breed dog. **A:** Sagittal image. The uterine stump) appears as tubular structure between the urinary bladder (UB) and the colon (C). **B:** Transverse image. The uterine stump (between the arrowheads) appears as a circular hypoechoic structure between the urinary bladder (UB) and the colon (C).

these definitions, the length of normal pregnancy is 65 ± 1 day for dogs and 61 days for cats. A practical problem is that information on hormone assays is often unavailable to animal owners and ultrasonographers. If the time of breeding is known, pregnancy can usually be ruled out 30–33 days after the last breeding in dogs and 15–20 days after the last breeding in cats, based on a negative ultrasonographic examination.

Ultrasonography is useful in monitoring normal embryonic and fetal development (Yeager et al. 1992; Zambelli et al. 2002) (Figures 13.13–13.18). The first reliable ultrasonographic indicator of pregnancy is the detection of gestational chambers, which appear as small, thin walled anechoic structures associated with the uterus. The embryo can be discerned at days 23–25 in dogs and at days 16–18 in cats. The fetus develops rapidly after day 30, enabling the identification of internal organs. A summary of ultrasonographic findings at different stages of pregnancy is presented in Table 13.3. Formulas have been developed and published to determine gestational age and predict time of parturition based on measurements of fetal dimensions (Beck et al. 1990; England et al. 1990; Yeager et al. 1992; Mattoon and Nyland 1995) (Table 13.4). Using these parameters, time of parturition can be predicted with an accuracy of ±2–3 days (England et al. 2003). Ultrasonographic determination of litter size is not reliable (Toal et al. 1986).

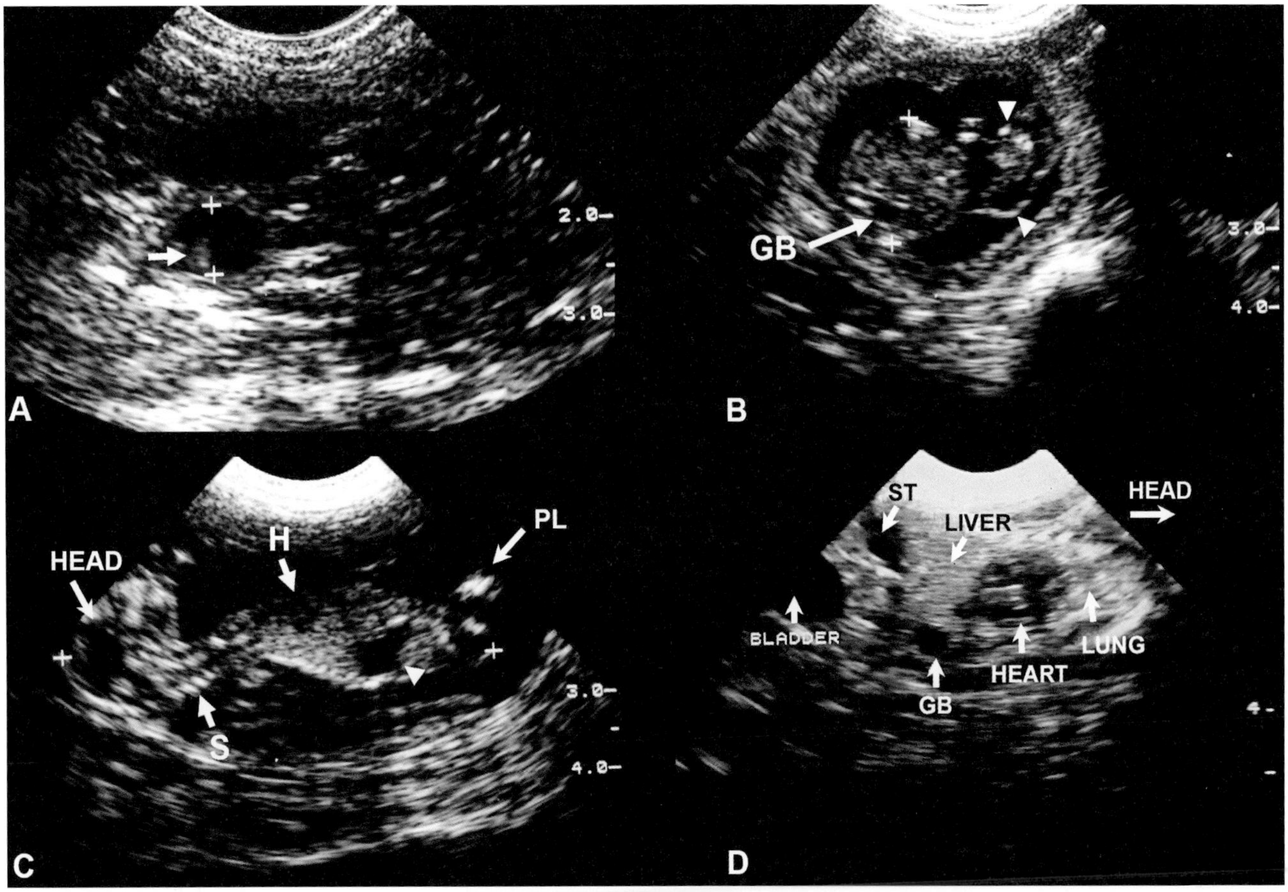

Figure 13.13. Progression of normal pregnancy in a domestic shorthair cat. **A: Day 16.** The embryo (arrow) is directly attached to the wall of the circular, fluid-filled gestational sac in the far field (between the cursors). A second fluid-filled gestational sac is in the near field. **B: Day 39.** Transverse image of the fetus (between the cursors). Hepatic parenchyma and gallbladder (GB) are visible. Linear echogenic material adjacent to the fetus is consistent with yolk-sac membrane (arrowheads). **C: Day 39.** Sagittal image of the fetus (between the cursors). The head is to the left and the pelvic limbs (PL) to the right of the image. The spine (S) is visible, the heart (H) is surrounded by hyperechoic lung, and the anechoic structure caudal to the diaphragm is consistent with a fluid-filled stomach (arrowhead). **D: Day 60.** Sagittal image of the fetal thorax and cranial abdomen. The heart is surrounded by hyperechoic pulmonary parenchyma. Gallbladder (GB), stomach (ST), and urinary bladder appear as circular anechoic structures in the abdomen.

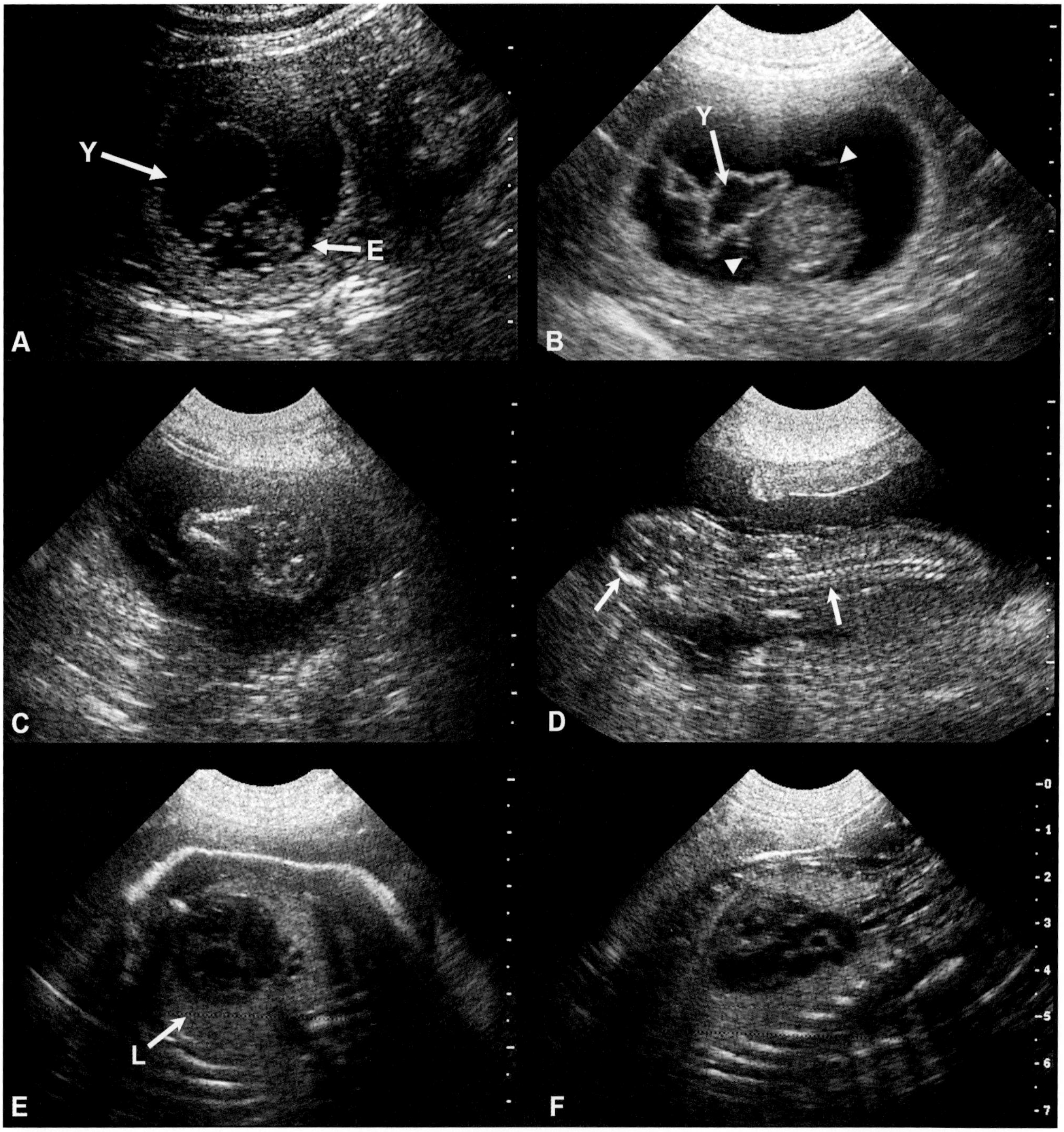

Figure 13.14. Progression of normal pregnancy in a 4-year-old Labrador retriever. The dog was bred twice during the last estrus. Initially, several embryos were identified, most of which were resorbed. One healthy puppy was delivered by cesarean section 62 days after last breeding. The results of hormone assays are not available. **A: Day 28 after last breeding.** An embryo (E) is visible in the fluid-filled gestational sac. A flickering heartbeat was observed on real-time examination. The yolk sac (Y) is the fluid-filled structure adjacent to the fetus. **B: Day 35.** Transverse image of the fetus. The surrounding allantoic membrane is indicated by arrowheads. The yolk sac (Y) is the folded fluid-filled structure adjacent to the fetus. **C: Day 42.** Dorsal plane image of the fetal head. The mandible is to the left on the image, and the cranium and brain are to the right. **D: Day 42.** Dorsal plane image of the fetal body. Skull (to the left of the image) and vertebral column are clearly visible (arrows). **E: Day 60.** Transverse image of the fetal thorax. The heart is clearly visible and is surrounded by hyperechoic lung (L). **F: Day 60.** Sagittal image of the fetal thorax. Cardiac chambers and large vessels are clearly visible. The surrounding lung is hyperechoic.

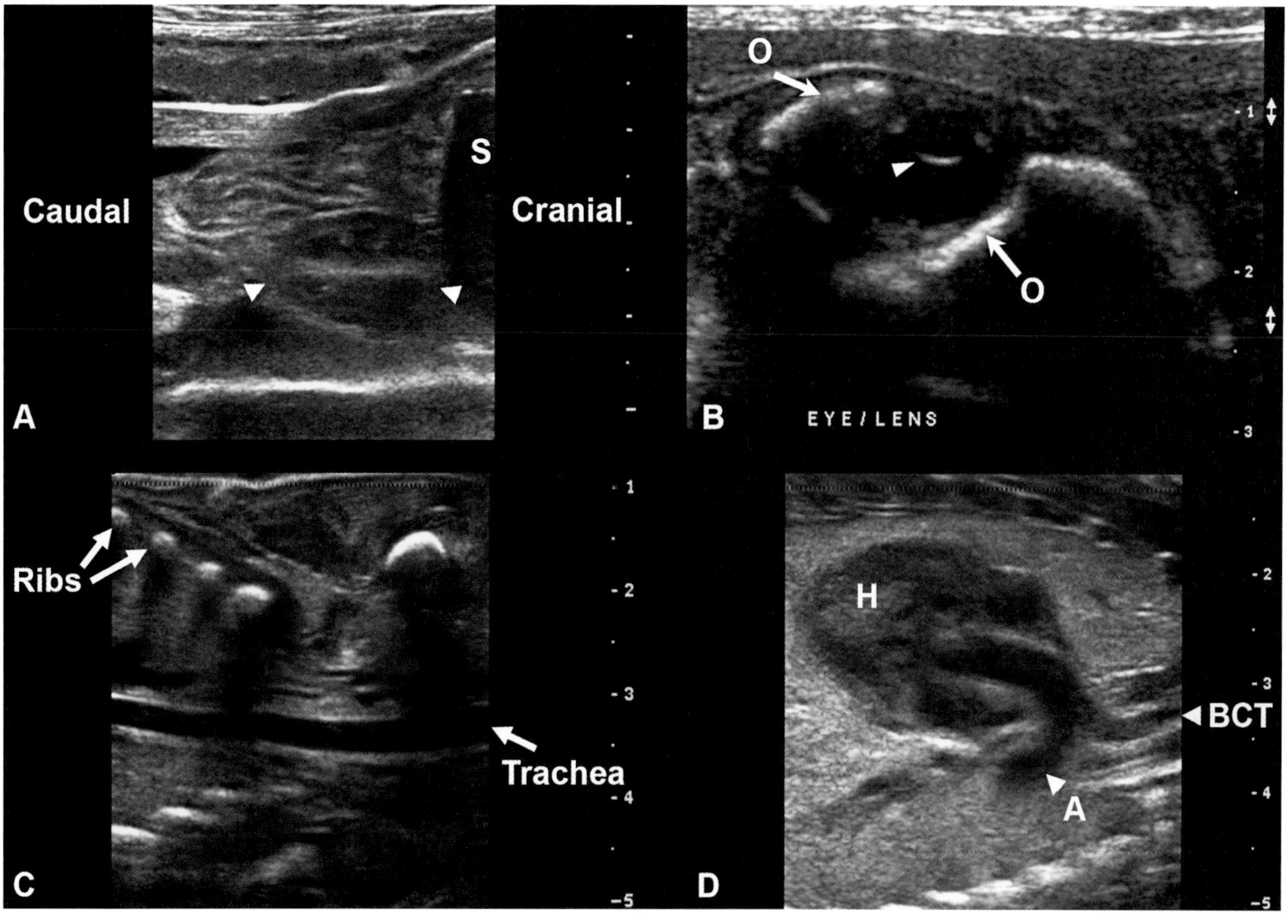

Figure 13.15. Normal late-term pregnancy in a 4-year-old pointer. Ultrasonographic examination was performed 2 months after last breeding. The dog had four healthy puppies delivered by cesarean section 2 days after the ultrasonographic examination. **A: Sagittal image of the fetal abdomen.** The left kidney (arrowheads), with distinct cortex and medulla, is caudal to the fluid-filled stomach (S). Tubular intestinal segments are in the near field. **B: Sagittal image of the fetal eye,** which appears as a circular anechoic structure within a hyperechoic osseous orbit (O). The posterior capsule of the lens is clearly seen (arrowhead). **C: Dorsal image of fetal caudal neck and cranial thorax.** The trachea is tubular and fluid filled. The ribs are characterized by small curvilinear bright interfaces associated with strong shadows. **D: Sagittal image of the thorax.** The aortic arch and proximal aorta (A) are well visualized, originating from the heart (H) in the near field. The aortic arch gives off the brachiocephalic trunk (BCT).

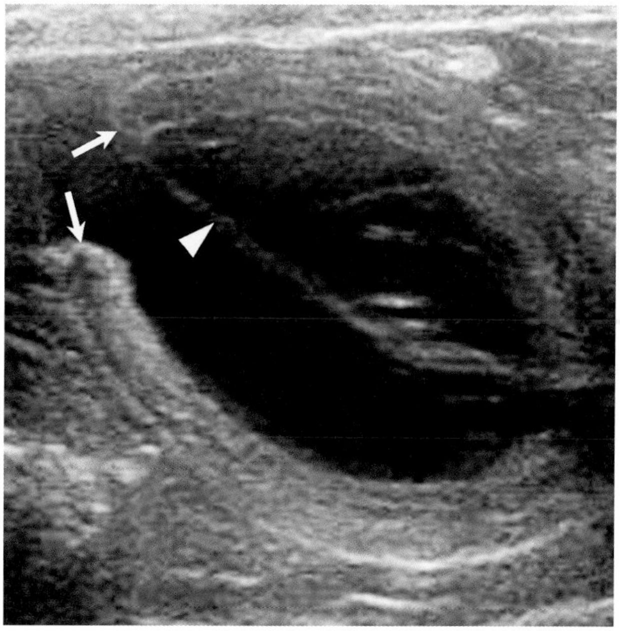

Figure 13.16. Sonogram of a 25-day-old canine fetus. The zonular placenta is distinctly identified (arrows). The arrowhead points to a thin membrane probably representing either part of the allantoic membrane or the yolk sac. Image courtesy of D. Penninck.

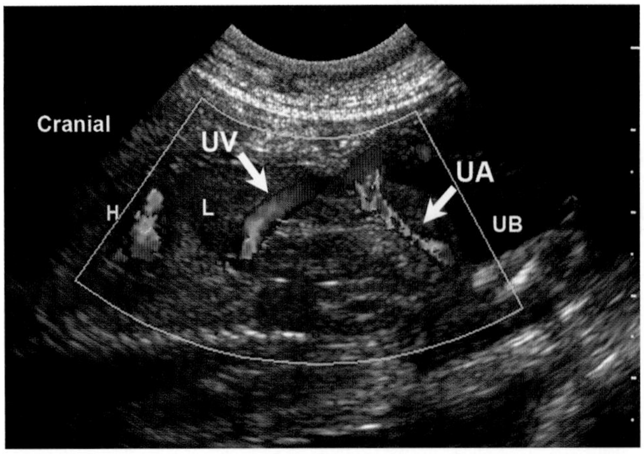

Figure 13.17. Normal fetal circulation. The head of the fetus is to the left of the image. The umbilical vein (UV) and umbilical artery (UA) extend cranially to the liver (L) and caudally to the cranial aspect of the fluid-filled urinary bladder (UB), respectively. The heart (H) is visible cranial to the diaphragm. The heterogeneous color pattern observed in the umbilical artery is caused by aliasing, a Doppler artifact that results when pulse-repetition frequency is too low in regard to a high-velocity blood flow.

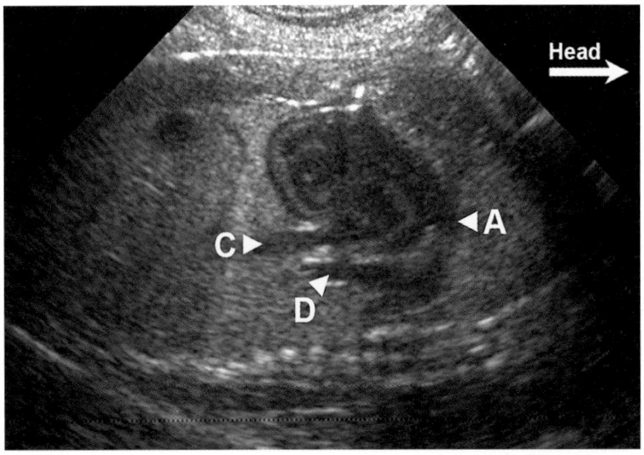

Figure 13.18. Normal fetal circulation. The head of the fetus is to the right of the image. The caudal vena cava (C) and the aorta (A) enter and leave the right and left heart, respectively. The aorta gives off the ductus arteriosus (D).

Normal Postpartum Uterus

Ultrasonographic changes during normal involution of the postpartum uterus have been described. Uterine wall thickness and volume of intraluminal fluid decrease, and the uterus becomes less conspicuous over time. Uterine involution usually takes 3–4 weeks in dogs and 24 days in cats (Pharr and Post 1992; Ferretti et al. 2000).

Table 13.3.
Ultrasonographic diagnosis of pregnancy

Ultrasonographic Findings	Dog (Days After LH[a] Surge)	Cat (Days After Breeding)
Gestational chamber	20	10
Placental layers of uterine wall	22–24	15–17
Embryo and heartbeat	23–25	16–18
Fetal movement	34–36	30–34
Skeleton	33–39	30–33
Bladder and stomach	35–39	29–32
Liver (hypoechoic) and lung (hyperechoic)	38–42	29–32

[a]LH, luteinizing hormone.
Data from Yeager et al. (1992) and Zambelli et al. (2002).

Table 13.4.
Formulas to predict gestational age and days before parturition in dogs and cats[a]

Gestational age in dogs (±3 days)
- Less than 40 days
  - GA = (6 × GSD) + 20
  - GA = (3 × CRL) + 27
- More than 40 days
  - GA = (15× HD) + 20
  - GA = (7 × BD) + 29
  - GA = (6 × HD) + (3 × BD) + 30

Days before parturition in dogs
- DBP = 65 − GA

Gestational age in cats (±2 days)
- Greater than 40 days
  - GA = 25 × HD + 3
  - GA = 11 × BD + 21

Days before parturition in cats
- DBP = 61 − GA

[a]Gestational age (GA) is based on days after luteinizing hormone (LH) surge in dogs and days after breeding in cats. Gestational sac diameter (GSD), crown-rump length (CRL), head diameter (HD), and body diameter (BD) measurements are in centimeters. Days before parturition (DBP) is based on 65 ± 1 days after LH surge in dogs and 61 days after breeding in cats.

Data modified and adapted from England et al. (1990), Yeager et al. (1992), and Beck et al. 1990.

Reprinted from Mattoon and Nyland (1995), with permission from Elsevier.

Sonography of Abnormal Pregnancy

The most common abnormalities of pregnancy in dogs and cats are resorption (embryonic death before 25 days) and abortion (fetal death after 35 days). Embryonic resorption manifests as loss of the normal anechoic gestational chamber, with accumulation of

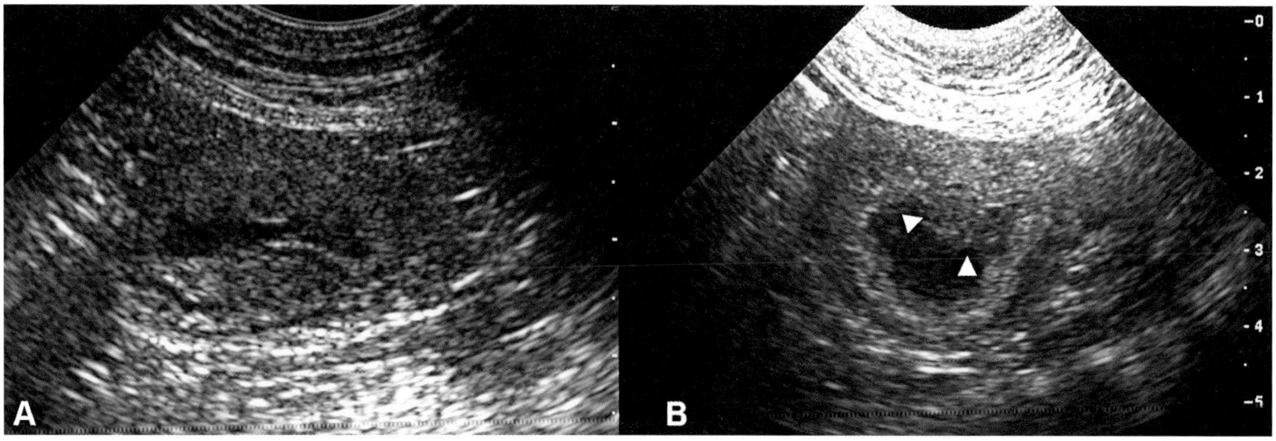

Figure 13.19. Embryonic resorption in a 4-year-old Labrador retriever (the same dog as in Figure 13.14). **A: Day 28 after the last breeding.** Transverse image of a collapsed thick-walled gestational chamber, which contains a small amount of echogenic fluid. The embryo is no longer identified. The appearance of the gestational chamber suggests that embryonic death occurred several days prior to the ultrasonographic examination. **B: Day 35 after the last breeding.** Embryonic death was more recent in respect to the ultrasonographic examination than in **A**. Transverse image of a thick-walled gestational chamber, which is filled with echogenic fluid. The embryonic remnant is indistinctly visible (arrowheads). The gestational chamber has not yet collapsed.

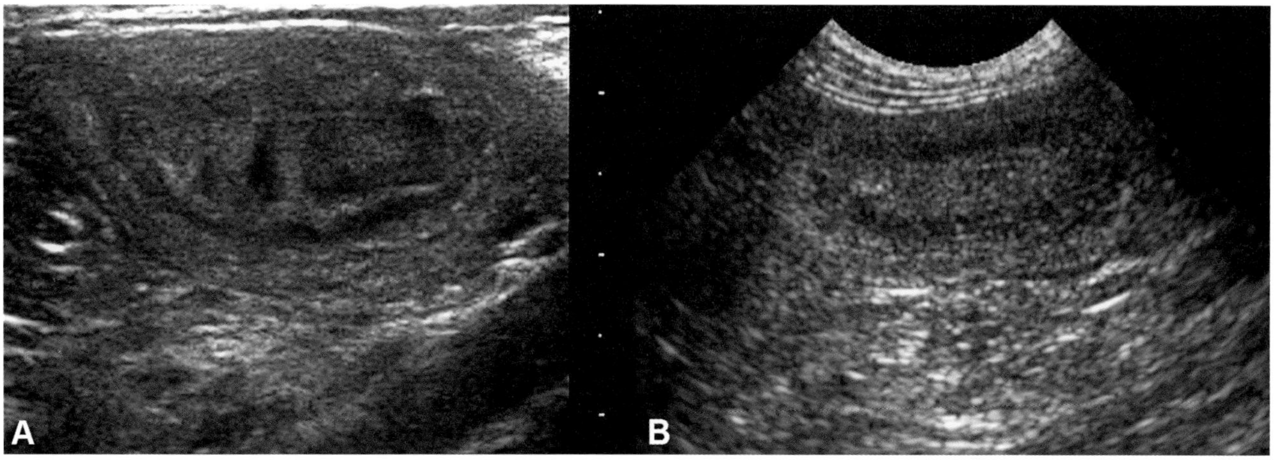

Figure 13.20. Embryonic resorption in a 4-year-old pointer. (the same dog as in Figure 13.15). **A:** Ultrasonographic examination 23 days after the last breeding. A thick-walled gestational chamber is filled with echogenic material and fluid. Embryonic structures are not visible. **B:** Ultrasonographic examination 1 month after the last breeding. The gestational chamber has collapsed.

echogenic material within the lumen, loss of embryonic heartbeat, embryonic disintegration, and ultimately collapse of the gestational chamber with thickening of the uterine wall (England 1998) (Figures 13.19 and 13.20).

Signs of fetal death include absence of heartbeat and fetal movement, abnormal fetal posture, reduced volume and increased echogenicity of fetal fluid, accumulation of gas within fetus or uterus, and fetal disintegration (England et al. 2003) (Figure 13.21). Failure of implantation of the conceptus, small size or underdevelopment of the conceptus for true gestational age, and abnormal location of the conceptus within the uterus can usually not be diagnosed (England 1998). Ultrasonography is of particular value in assessing fetal viability and distress. Normal fetal heart rate has

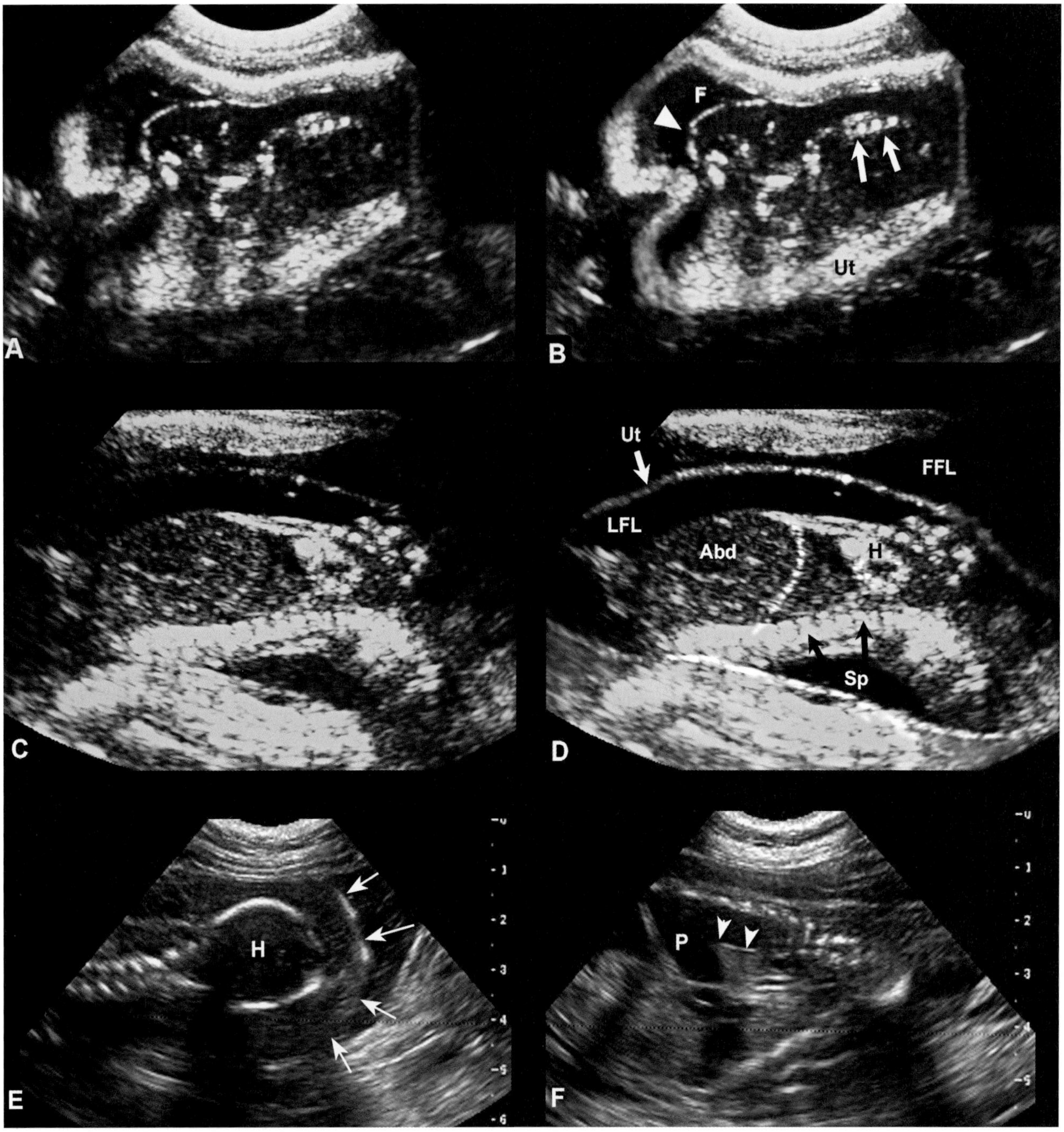

Figure 13.21. Fetal abnormalities. Ultrasonographic **(left)** and schematic **(right)** images of a feline dead fetus. **A:** The transverse image of the fetus is small, the skull bones are collapsed (arrowhead), and only a small amount of echogenic fluid (F) is seen adjacent to the fetus. Normal fetal anatomy (skeleton and organs) is not recognized because of fetal disintegration. In **B** (schematic image of **A**), the small arrows indicate bones or mineral foci within the dead fetus. The nature of the changes and the small size of the fetus in comparison to a near-term fetus (see **C and D**) suggest that this fetus died several days prior to the ultrasonographic examination. Ut, wall of the uterus and/or placenta. **C and D**: Sagittal image of a dead, near-term fetus in the same cat. There is normal fetal anatomy, but a heartbeat was not detected on ultrasonographic examination. The diaphragm is a fine echogenic curvilinear line. Spine (Sp), abdominal structures (Abd), and heart (H) with adjacent hypoechoic lung are clearly seen. Anechoic intraluminal uterine fluid (LFL) is present. A small amount of abdominal effusion (FFL) is seen in the near field. The appearance of the fetus indicates that death has occurred recently. **E and F:** Anasarca in a Chinook dog. The affected fetus was surrounded by contained fluid (arrows in **E**) best seen here around the head (H) and neck. A moderate pleural effusion (P) associated with retracted echogenic lungs (arrowheads) is noted in **F**.

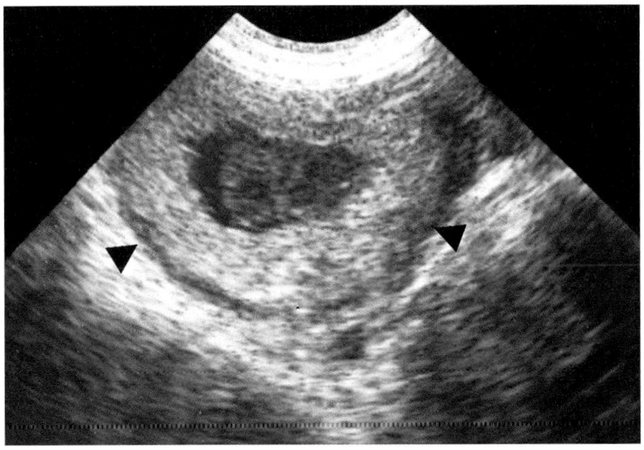

Figure 13.22. Uterine torsion in a pregnant cat. Transverse sonogram of the uterine horn (arrowheads) that is thickened, hyperechoic, and contains material of soft-tissue echogenicity. Fetal structures cannot be discerned.

been reported to be twice that of maternal heart rate and is a reliable indicator of fetal viability. Bradycardia is the normal response of a fetus to hypoxia and is an important parameter in identifying in dystocia.

Although a large number of congenital defects can occur in dogs and cats, these defects are very rarely diagnosed in utero. Examples of fetal abnormalities that can be detected by means of ultrasonography include hydrocephalus, fetal pleural effusion, and hydrops fetalis or anasarca (Allen et al. 1989). Only a few other pregnancy disorders have been reported in small animals. Uterine torsion is a potentially life-threatening condition that is characterized by infarction of the affected uterine segment, with subsequent wall thickening, increased echogenicity of uterine wall and fetal fluids, and fetal death (Figure 13.22).

Uterine Diseases

Fluid within the uterus is easily visualized by means of ultrasonography. Echogenicity of the luminal contents is variable. Although hydrometra and mucometra are usually characterized by anechoic luminal fluid, and pyometra and hemometra tend to show echogenic luminal contents, ultrasonographic differentiation of these entities is often not possible (Figures 13.23–3.26). Concurrent uterine wall thickening, endometrial cysts, and polyps are common. Uterine stump pyometra manifests as a fluid-filled, blind-ending pouch between the urinary bladder and descending colon (Figure 13.27).

Cystic endometrial hyperplasia causes thickening of the endometrium, with cystic lesions embedded in the uterine wall because of proliferation of endometrial glands (Voges and Neuwirth 1996) (Figure 13.28). The hyperplasia is commonly associated with fluid accumulation within the uterine lumen and may precede the development of mucometra or pyometra (Figure 13.29) or be associated with endometritis.

Neoplasms of the uterus or the uterine stump, such as polyps, leiomyomas, leiomyosarcomas, or adenocarcinomas, are rare (Klein 1996). They appear as nodules or masses of variable shape, size, and echogenicity and may be associated with fluid accumulation within the uterine lumen (Figures 13.30–13.32). Vaginal masses can be visualized when they become large enough to extend from the pelvic canal into the abdomen (Figure 13.33). Uterine stump granulomas manifest as mass lesions of variable echogenicity between the bladder and colon (Figure 13.34). Differentiation of neoplastic from nonneoplastic uterine or vaginal mass lesions and ultrasonographic distinction among different tumor types is not possible.

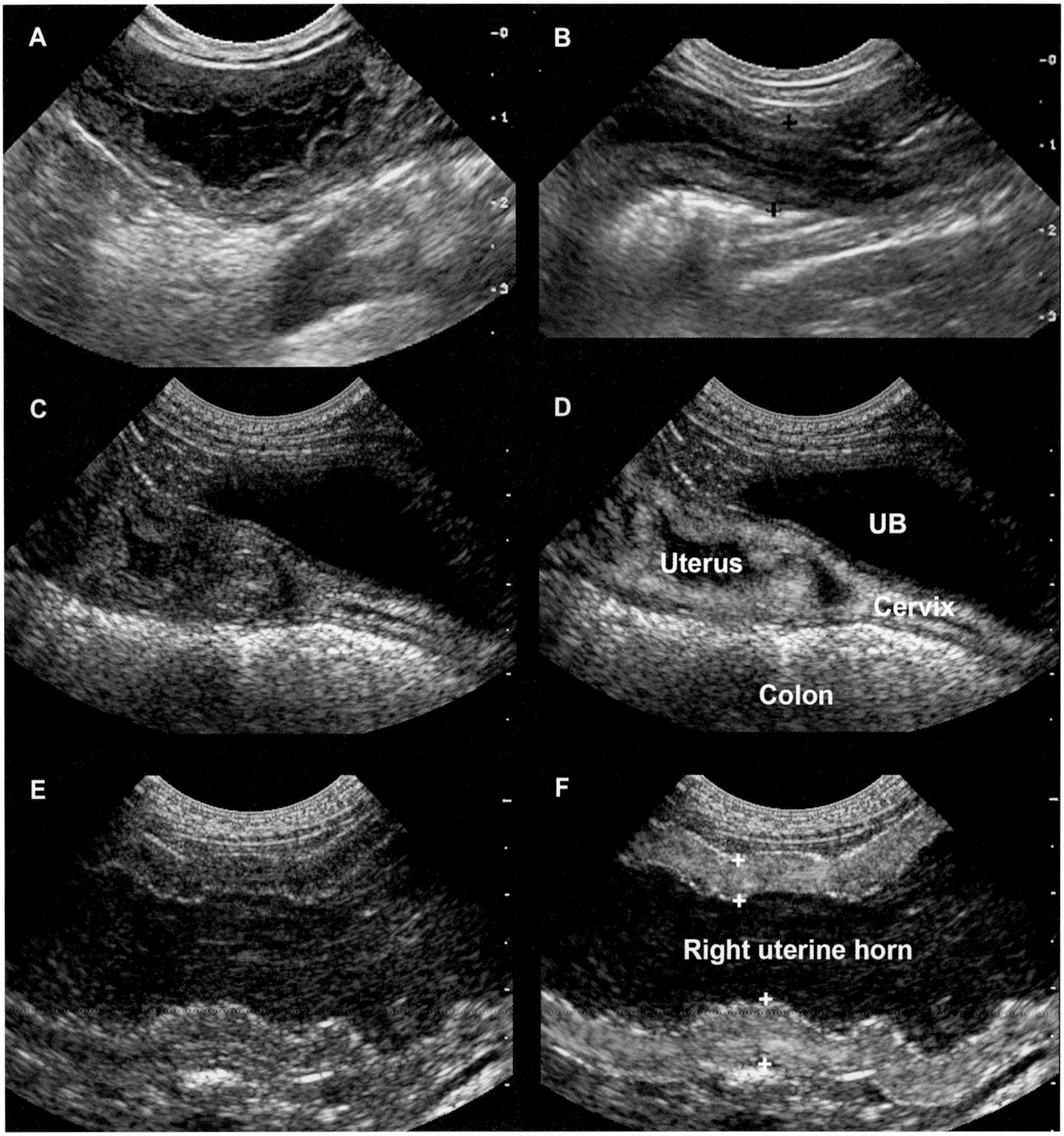

Figure 13.23. Endometritis and pyometra in dogs. **A and B:** Endometritis and cystic endometrial hyperplasia in a 1-year-old German shepherd. Sagittal sonograms of a thickened uterine horn **(A)** and body **(B)** containing a small amount of anechoic fluid. Notice the irregular margins of the uterus. Images courtesy of D. Penninck. **C–F:** Pyometra in an 8-year-old shih tzu. Ultrasonographic **(C)** and schematic **(D)** images of the cervix and body of the uterus. The cervix is closed. The uterus is thick walled and distended with echogenic material. The uterus appears between the descending colon containing gas, dorsally, and the urinary bladder (UB), ventrally. Ultrasonographic **(E)** and schematic **(F)** images of the right uterine horn showing a thickened wall (between the cursors, 0.5–0.8 cm). The lumen of the uterus contains echogenic fluid.

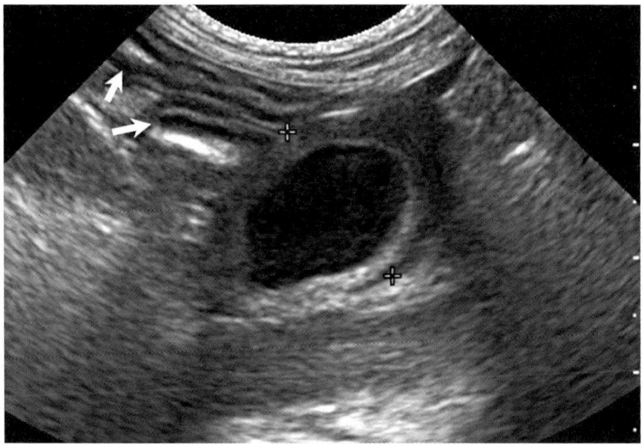

Figure 13.24. Pyometra in a dog. Transverse image of the left uterine horn (between the cursors) in an 11-year-old whippet. The uterus is thick walled (approximately 3 mm) and contains anechoic fluid. The uterine wall does not show wall layers, enabling differentiation from adjacent small intestinal segments (arrows).

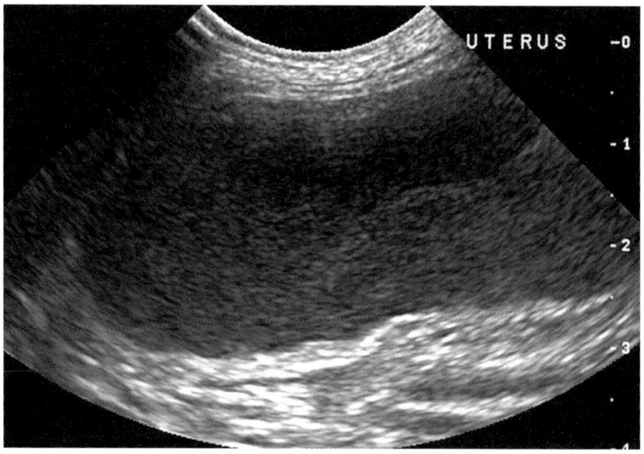

Figure 13.25. Pyometra in an 11-year-old Shiba Inu. The uterus is distended with fluid. The echogenicity of the fluid in the far field is higher than in the near field, indicating settling of particles (cells) in the dependent portion of the uterus.

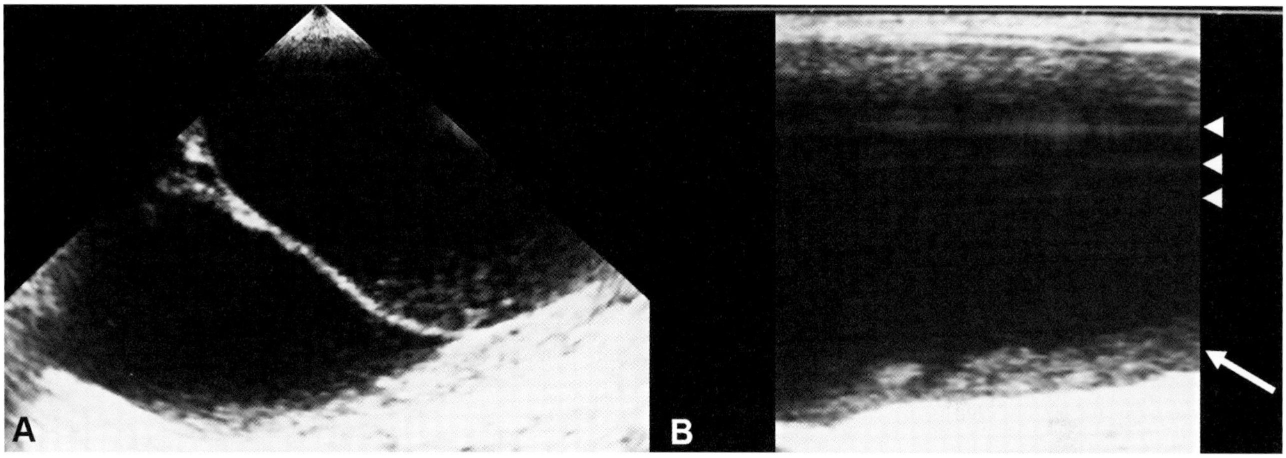

Figure 13.26. Hydrometra in a 13-year-old cat. **A:** Transverse image of the uterine horns, which are distended with anechoic fluid and measure up to 3 cm in diameter. **B:** Sagittal image of one of the fluid-distended uterine horns. There is irregularity of the uterine wall in the far field (arrow). Linear hyperechoic lines projected on the lumen are consistent with reverberation artifact (arrowheads).

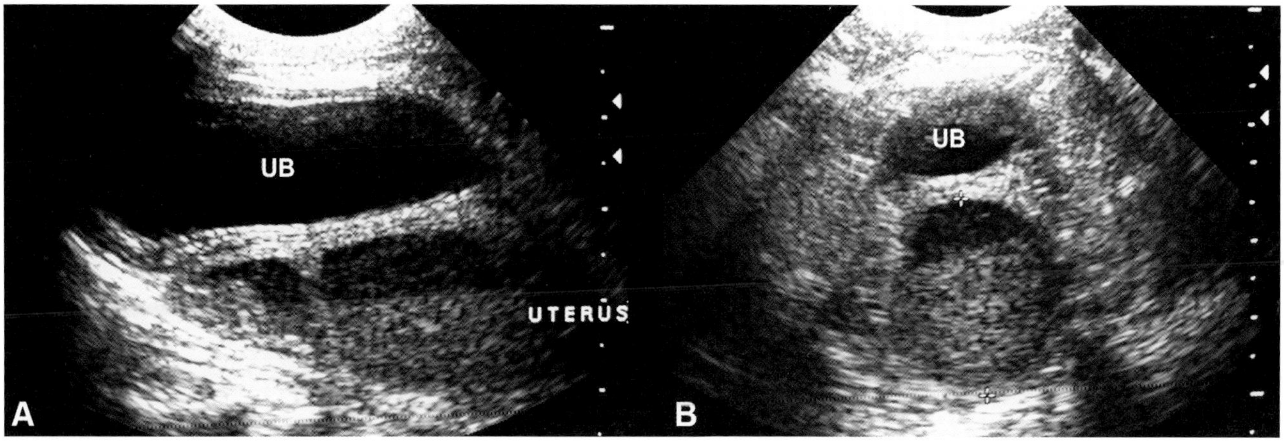

Figure 13.27. Uterine stump pyometra in a dog. Sagittal **(A)** and transverse **(B)** images of the uterus of a dog that previously had a hysterectomy. The uterine stump appears as blind-ending pouch dorsal to the urinary bladder (UB). The luminal fluid in the far field is more echogenic than in the near field, consistent with settling of solid particles (cells) in the dependent portion.

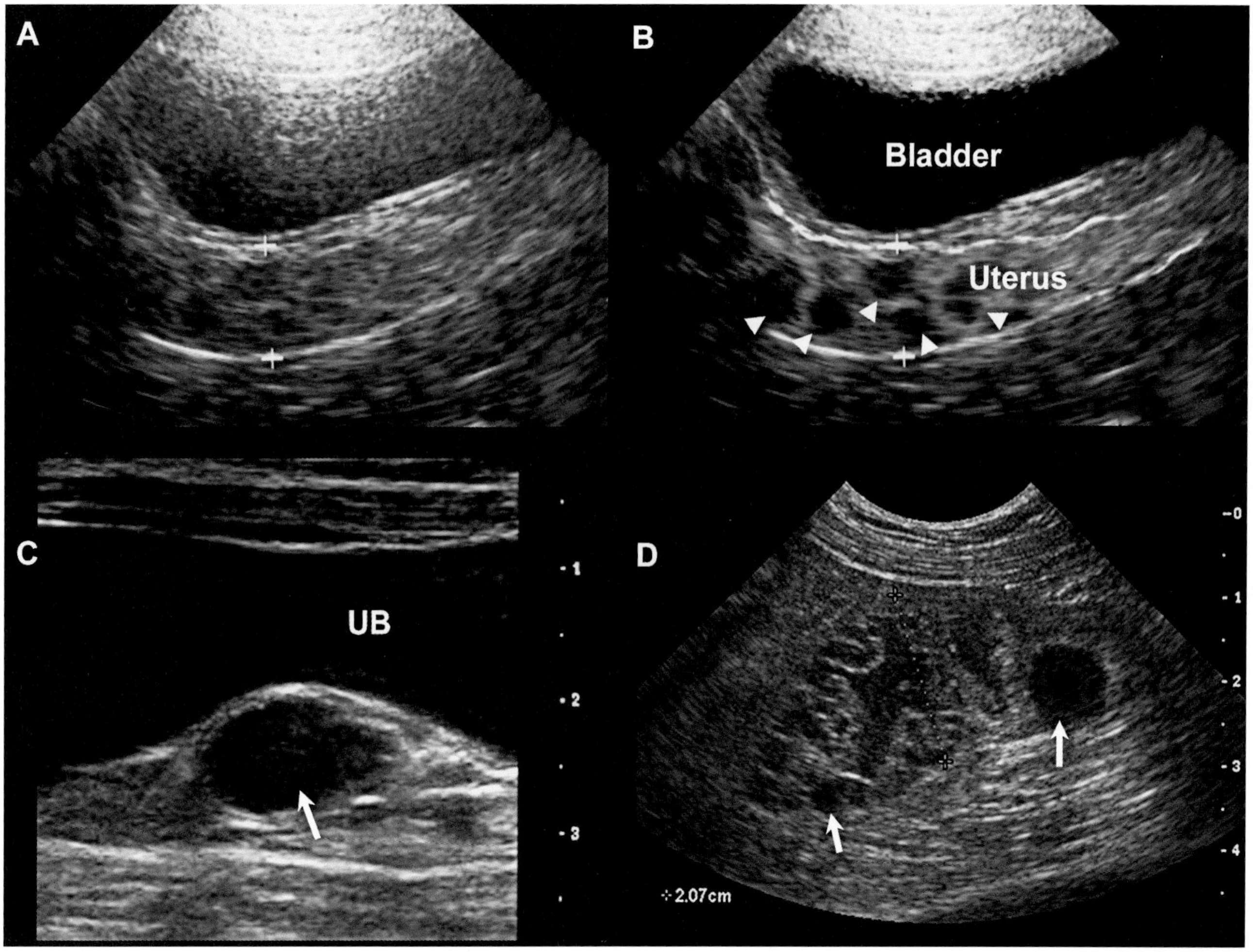

Figure 13.28. Cystic endometrial hyperplasia in dogs. **A and B:** Ultrasonographic and schematic images of the uterus in a dog with endometrial cystic hyperplasia. The uterus is thickened, and multiple circular hypoechoic and anechoic structures are embedded in the uterine wall, consistent with cysts (arrowheads). **C:** Cystic endometrial hyperplasia in a 1-year-old spayed sheltie with remnant ovarian tissue. A lobulated cystic structure (arrow) confined to the uterine stump is present dorsal to the urinary bladder (UB). Image courtesy of D. Penninck. **D:** Ultrasound image of a segment of an enlarged uterine horn (between the cursors) in an intact female dog with a history of chronic vulvar discharge. The uterine wall is thickened and irregular, and several anechoic to hypoechoic cysts (arrows) are identified. Image courtesy of M.A. d'Anjou.

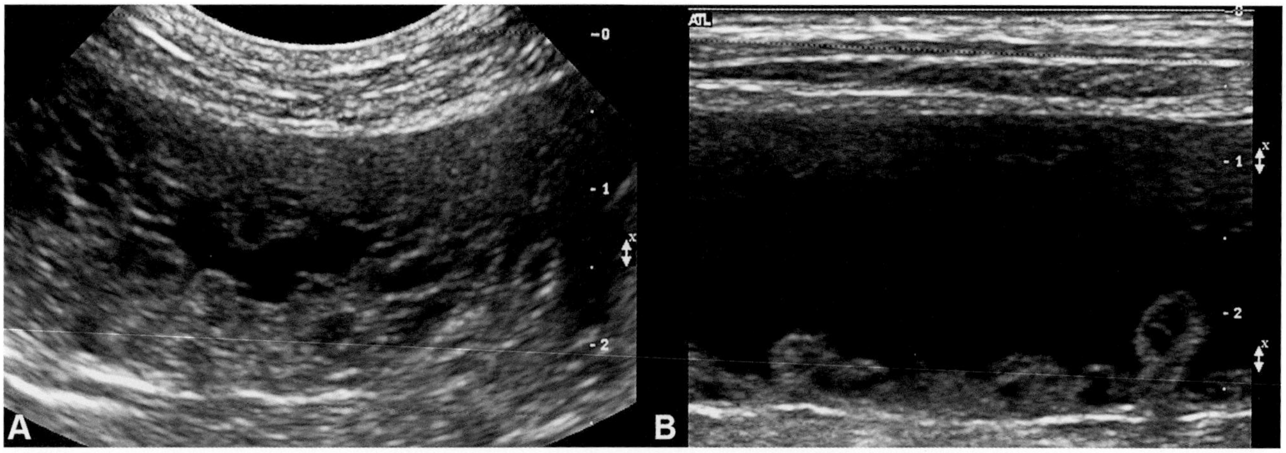

Figure 13.29. Presumptive cystic endometrial hyperplasia and mucometra in a 5-year-old briard. Sagittal images of different areas of the left uterine horn obtained with a curvilinear **(A)** and a linear **(B)** transducer. The uterus is filled with anechoic fluid and thick walled, with multiple anechoic cysts embedded in the uterine wall.

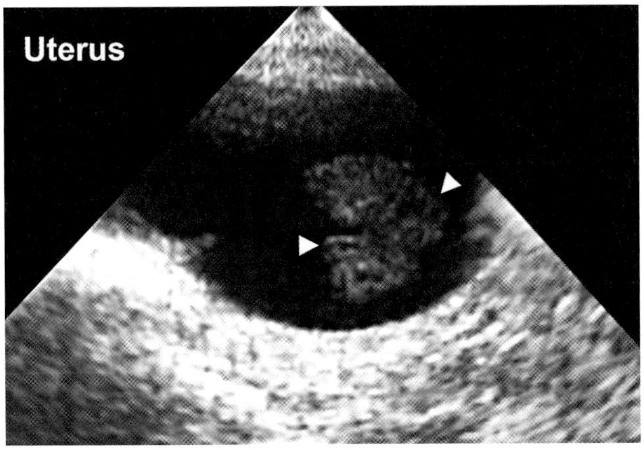

Figure 13.30. Uterine polyp and hydrometra in a 13-year-old cat. (the same cat as in Figure 13.28). The transverse image of the uterus shows a lobulated soft-tissue structure of 1-cm diameter surrounded by anechoic fluid (arrowheads).

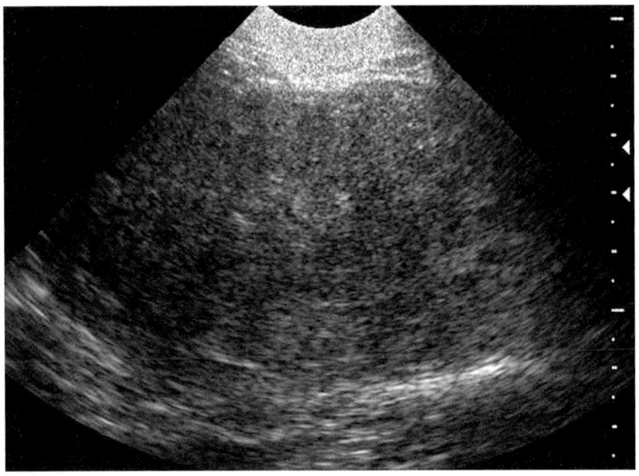

Figure 13.31. Uterine stump adenocarcinoma in a 16-year old mixed-breed dog. A mixed echogenic mass of more than 7-cm diameter is associated with the caudal abdomen.

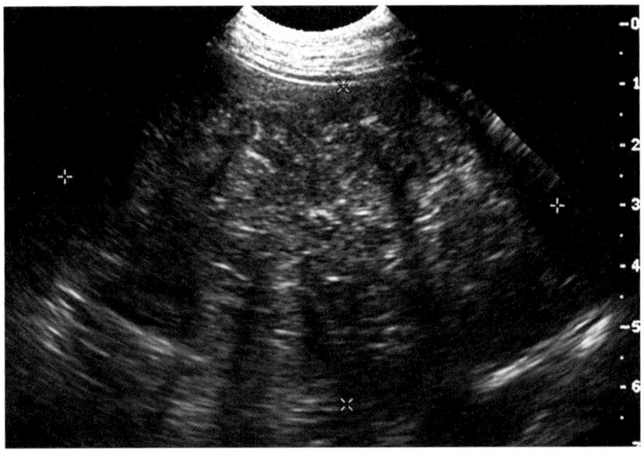

Figure 13.32. Uterine leiomyoma in an 8-year-old Rottweiler. A mixed echogenic mass (between the cursors) is associated with the caudal abdomen, which measures 8.3 × 5.2 cm in maximum diameter.

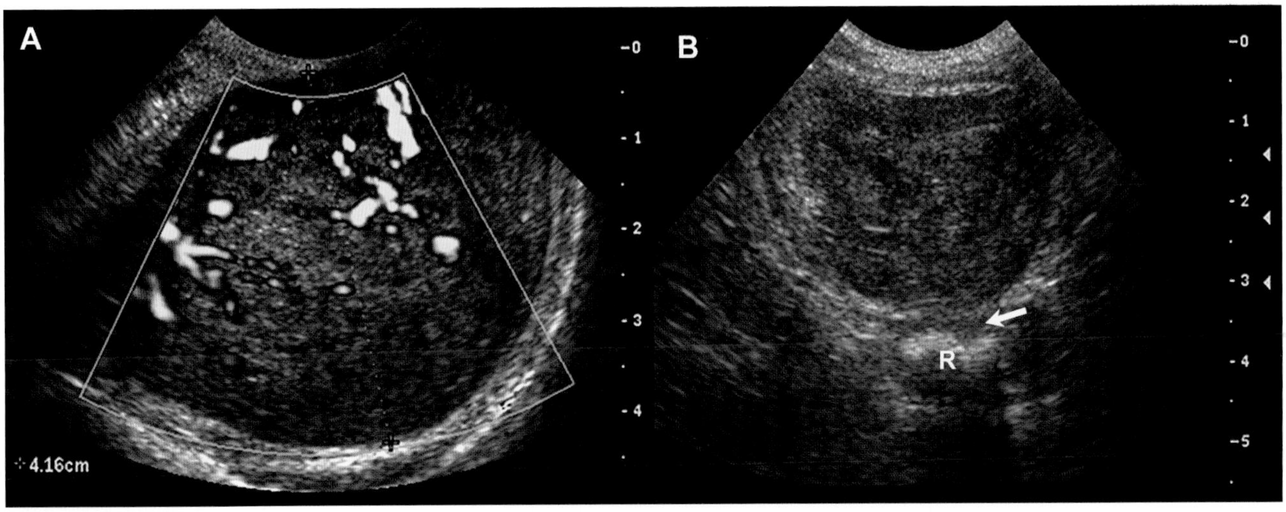

Figure 13.33. Vaginal leiomyoma. Power Doppler **(A)** and B-mode **(B)** ultrasound images of a prolapsing mass in the vagina of a 10-year-old American Eskimo female dog. A prominent vascular pattern is seen throughout the mass, which is also heterogeneous. This mass causes dorsal displacement of the rectum (R), but without evidence of wall invasion (arrow). Images courtesy of M.A. d'Anjou.

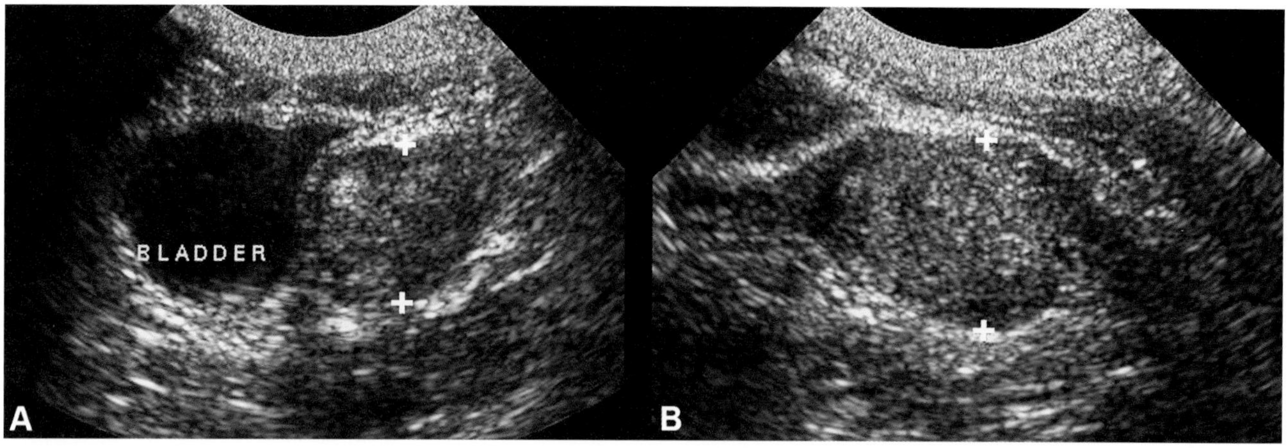

Figure 13.34. Uterine granulomas in a cat. Transverse **(A)** and sagittal **(B)** images of a uterine stump granuloma in a 13-year-old cat. There is a 1.5-cm homogeneous mass lesion of medium echogenicity (between the cursors) dorsal and to the left of the urinary bladder.

Mammary Glands

Sonography of Normal Mammary Glands

The appearance of the mammary glands changes under hormonal influences (late-term pregnancy and lactation). Normal mammary tissue in nonlactating dogs is coarse and hypoechoic (Figure 13.35). In lactating bitches, mammary tissue is more prominent, large vessels enter the glands, and milk-filled ducts are encountered (Figure 13.36).

Sonography of Abnormal Mammary Glands

Abnormalities of the mammary glands include neoplasia, cysts, and inflammation. Mammary tumors appear ultrasonographically as irregular, mixed echogenic mass lesions of variable size (Figures 13.37 and 13.38). Benign and malignant mammary tumors cannot be differentiated based on their ultrasonographic appearance. Since metastases are common in malignant tumors, the axillary and/or inguinal lymph nodes should be examined for enlargement and abnormal echotexture. Mastitis manifests as swelling and hypoechogenicity of the mammary tissue, with abscessation in severe cases.

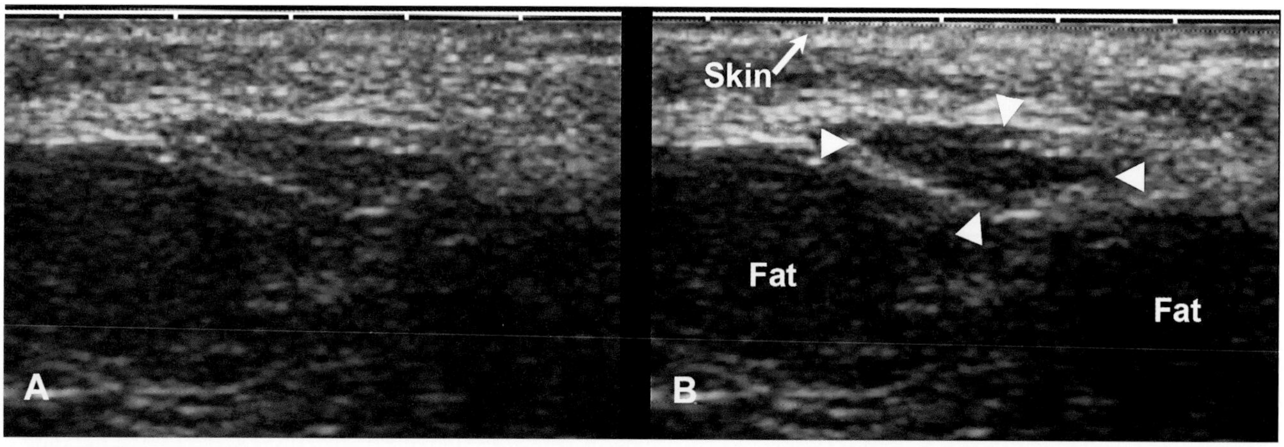

Figure 13.35. Inactive mammary tissue in an anestrus 7-year-old nulliparous beagle. Ultrasonographic and schematic images on which the mammary gland (arrowheads) is inconspicuous, small (1.0 × 0.5 cm), and of similar echogenicity and texture as adjacent subcutaneous fat.

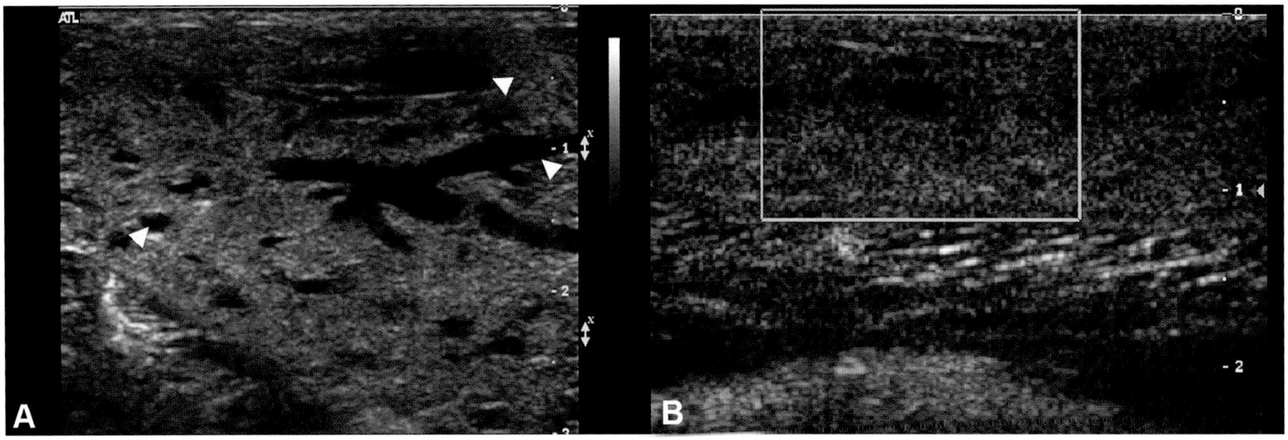

Figure 13.36. Active mammary tissue in a 4-year-old dog 2 days prior to parturition. **A:** The mammary tissue measures up to 3 cm in thickness, is of medium echogenicity, and contains numerous tubular milk-filled ducts (arrowheads). **B:** On color Doppler examination, the mammary tissue is well vascularized. No color signal is detected in the ducts.

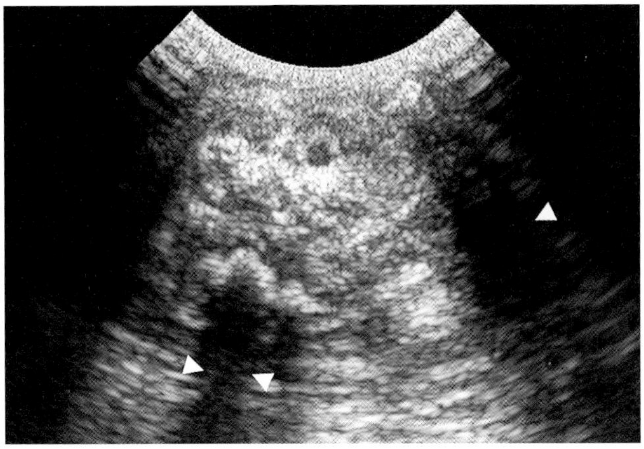

Figure 13.37. Mixed mammary tumor in a 6-year-old Rottweiler. An approximately 3-cm heterogeneous mass is associated with a mammary gland. Strong distal acoustic shadowing (arrowheads) indicates mineralization.

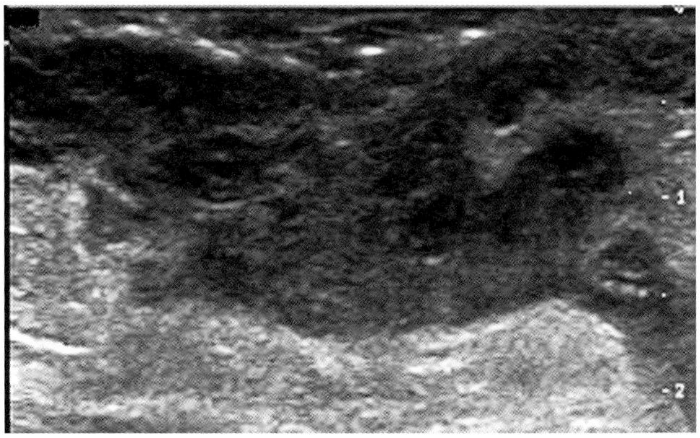

Figure 13.38. Ulcerated and extensive mammary carcinoma invading most of the right middle to caudal mammary chain in a 14-year-old cat. The mass is mostly hypoechoic and has irregular margins. Image courtesy of D. Penninck.

Interventional Procedures

Depending on size and location, fine-needle aspiration or biopsy of mass lesions associated with the ovary or the uterus can be performed under ultrasound guidance following the same principles and precautions as in other organ systems. Because of the risk of leakage into the peritoneal cavity, uterine fluid is usually not aspirated. Amniocentesis is not a routine procedure in the assessment of pregnant dogs or cats.

References

Allen WE, England GCW, White KB (1989) Hydrops foetalis diagnosed by real time ultrasonography in a bichon frisé bitch. J Small Anim Pract 30:465–467.

Beck KA, Baldwin CJ, Bosu WTK (1990) Ultrasound prediction of parturition in the queen. Vet Radiol Ultrasound 31:32–35.

Diez-Bru N, Garcia-Real I, Martinez EM, Rollan E, Mayenco A, Llorens P (1998) Ultrasonographic appearance of ovarian tumors in 10 dogs. Vet Radiol Ultrasound 39:226–233.

England GCW (1998) Ultrasonographic assessment of abnormal pregnancy. Vet Clin North Am Small Anim Pract 28:849–868.

England GCW, Allen WE, Porter DJ (1990) Studies on canine pregnancy using B-mode ultrasound: Development of the conceptus and determination of gestational age. J Small Anim Pract 31:324–329.

England GCW, Yeager AE, Concannon PW (2003) Ultrasound imaging of the reproductive tract of the bitch. In: Concannon PW, England GCW, Verstegen JP, Linde-Forsberg C, eds. Recent Advances in Small Animal Reproduction. Ithaca, NY: International Veterinary Information Service.

Ferretti LM, Newell SM, Graham JP, Roberts GD (2000) Radiographic and ultrasonographic evaluation of the normal feline postpartum uterus. Vet Radiol Ultrasound 41:287–291.

Klein MK (1996) Tumors of the female reproductive system. In: Withrow SJ, MacEwen EG, eds. Small Animal Clinical Oncology. Philadelphia: WB Saunders, pp. 347–355.

Mattoon JS, Nyland TG (1995) Ovaries and uterus. In: Nyland TG, Mattoon JS, eds. Small Animal Diagnostic Ultrasound. Philadelphia: WB Saunders, pp. 231–249.

Pharr JW, Post K (1992) Ultrasonography and radiography of the canine postpartum uterus. Vet Radiol Ultrasound 33:35–40.

Silva LDM, Onclin K, Verstegen JP (1996) Assessment of ovarian changes around ovulation in bitches by ultrasonography, laparoscopy and hormonal assays. Vet Radiol Ultrasound 37:313–320.

Toal RL, Walker MA, Henry GA (1986) A comparison of real-time ultrasound, palpation and radiography in pregnancy detection and litter size determination in the bitch. Vet Radiol Ultrasound 27:102–108.

Voges AK, Neuwirth L (1996) Ultrasound diagnosis: Cystic uterine hyperplasia. Vet Radiol Ultrasound 37: 131–132.

Yeager AE, Concannon PW (1995) Ultrasonography of the reproductive tract of the female dog and cat. In: Bonagura JD, ed. Kirk's Current Veterinary Therapy XII. Philadelphia: WB Saunders, pp. 1040–1052.

Yeager AE, Mohammed HO, Meyers-Wallen V, Vannerson L, Concannon PW (1992) Ultrasonographic appearance of the uterus, placenta, fetus, and fetal membranes throughout accurately timed pregnancy in beagles. Am J Vet Res 53:342–351.

Zambelli D, Caneppele B, Bassi S, Paladini C (2002) Ultrasound aspects of fetal and extrafetal structures in pregnant cats. J Feline Med Surg 4:95–106.

CHAPTER FOURTEEN

MALE REPRODUCTIVE TRACT

Silke Hecht

PREPARATION AND SCANNING PROCEDURE

Ultrasonographic examination of male reproductive organs is commonly performed in dogs but rarely in cats. Examination technique, normal findings, and disorders of the male reproductive tract described in this chapter relate to dogs.

Indications for examination of the male reproductive tract include andrologic evaluation of breeding dogs; identification of retained testicles; difficulties or abnormalities in urination or defecation; abdominal, scrotal, and penile pain or discomfort; caudal abdominal mass lesions; perineal hernia; clinical signs compatible with hormonal imbalances (hyperestrogenism); scrotal or penile trauma; and palpable scrotal abnormalities.

The prostate is examined transabdominally after routine clipping and application of contact gel. The dog is usually positioned in dorsal recumbency. A rectal examination technique has been described (Zohil and Castellano 1995), but is not used routinely. A 5.0-MHz transducer may be sufficient to identify gross prostatic abnormalities such as paraprostatic cysts or prostatic abscesses; however, a 7.5- or 10-MHz transducer provides better detail and is recommended for most indications. The prostate is located in the caudal abdomen or cranial pelvic canal. It is identified caudal to the urinary bladder and ventral to the distal descending colon and rectum. Examination is performed in transverse and sagittal planes (Figure 14.1). Instillation of saline into the urinary bladder may improve the acoustic window (Feeney et al. 1989; Johnston et al. 1991b). In some dogs, especially in neutered dogs with an empty or intrapelvic bladder, ultrasonographic identification of the prostate may be challenging. In these cases, a concurrent digital rectal examination can be performed to identify the prostate and direct it toward the ultrasound transducer.

The testicles should be examined with a high-frequency transducer (at least 7.5 MHz). The author prefers a linear transducer with broad contact area and good resolution in the near field over a sector or curvilinear transducer. Use of a standoff pad is recommended by some examiners. Clipping of the scrotum is usually unnecessary. Ultrasound gel is preferred as a contact medium over alcohol because of the risk of scrotal irritation. The testicles are scanned in at least two planes (sagittal and transverse) (Figure 14.2).

The penis is occasionally examined to identify urethral abnormalities or to assess integrity of the os penis. Dependent on the examiner's preference, a linear or curvilinear high-frequency transducer (7.5 MHz or higher) may be used. The examination is started at the level of the os penis and is continued proximally to the level of the ischium. Evaluation of the penile urethra may be enhanced by instillation of saline by using a balloon-type catheter inserted into the distal penile urethra.

PROSTATE

Normal Sonographic Anatomy of the Prostate

Location, size, and appearance of the prostate vary with age, previous disease, and status (intact versus neutered) (Feeney et al. 1989; Johnston et al. 1991b). In intact dogs, the prostate is of medium echogenicity and homogeneous, with a fine to medium coarse echotexture and smooth margins (Mattoon and Nyland 2002). On sagittal image, the shape is rounded to ovoid. On transverse image, the two prostatic lobes are symmetrical. The vertical raphe and prostatic urethra with surrounding urethralis muscle are generally visible as a hypoechoic area between both lobes (Figures 14.1 and 14.3). The urethral structures may be associated with edge shadowing on transverse planes, which should not be misinterpreted as a lesion. In intact males, age-related changes in ultrasonographic appearance of the prostate include increase in size and echogenicity (Figures 14.1 and 14.4). Prostatic cysts are a common incidental finding in older dogs (Ruel et al. 1998; Mattoon and Nyland 2002). Prostatic size in intact dogs is significantly correlated with age and body weight (Ruel et al. 1998; Atalan et al. 1999) (Table 14.1). In neutered dogs, the prostate is small, inconspicuous, hypoechoic, and homogeneous. The two lobes can usually not be distinguished (Figure 14.5A

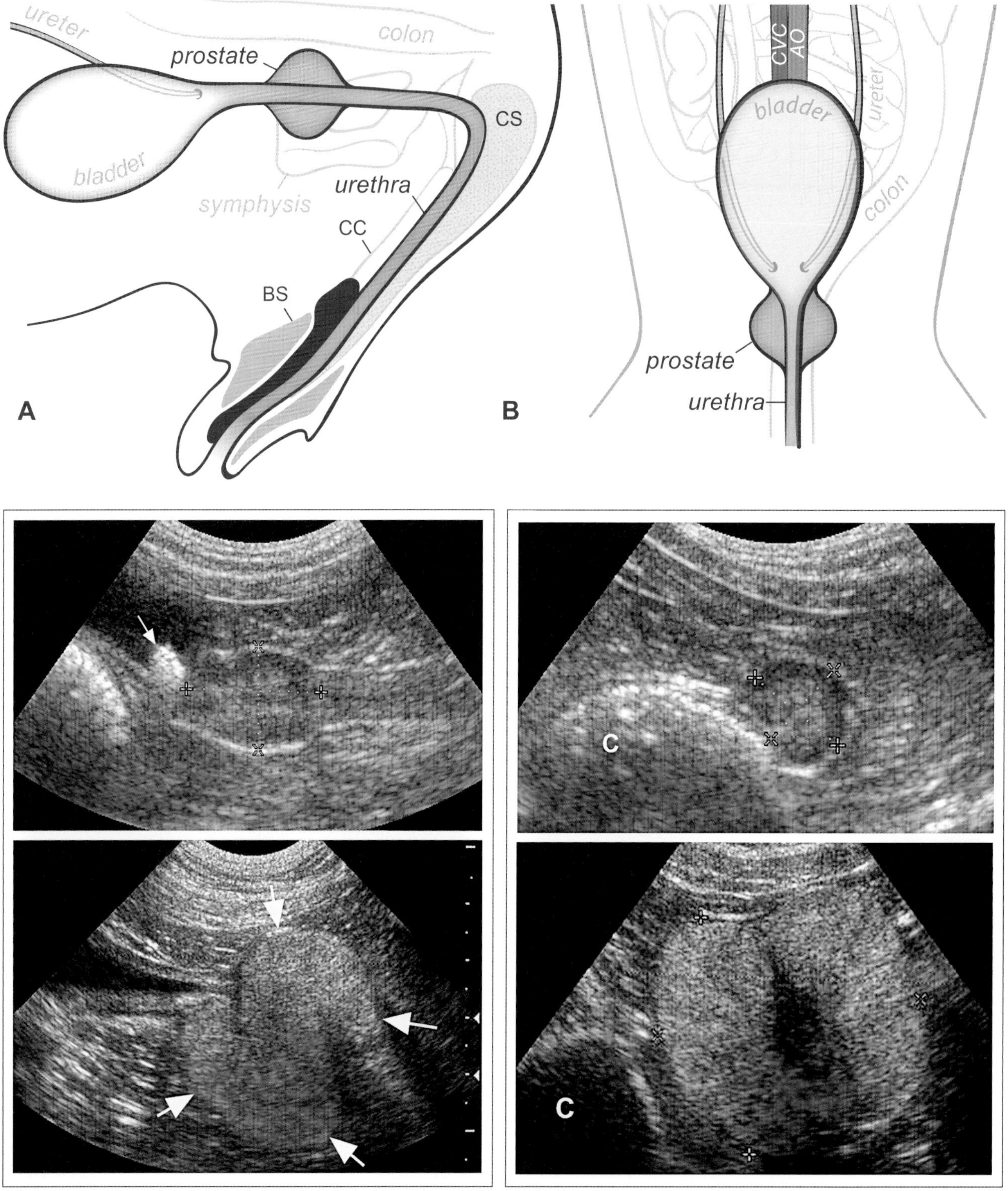

Figure 14.1. Normal anatomy of the canine prostate. On the **top** are illustrations (**A**, longitudinal; and **B**, transverse) of the prostate and the surrounding structures in an adult male dog. BS, bulbus glandis; CC, corpus cavernosum; and CS, corpus spongiosum. The sonograms on the **top** are sagittal **(left)** and transverse **(right)** images of a castrated dog. The sonograms at the **bottom** are sagittal **(left)** and transverse **(right)** images of an intact male (a 5-year-old intact golden retriever). C, colon. On the **bottom left** image, the arrows delineate the prostate. On the **top left** sonogram, the arrow points to a small cystic calculus in the bladder neck. Images courtesy of M.A. d'Anjou and D. Penninck.

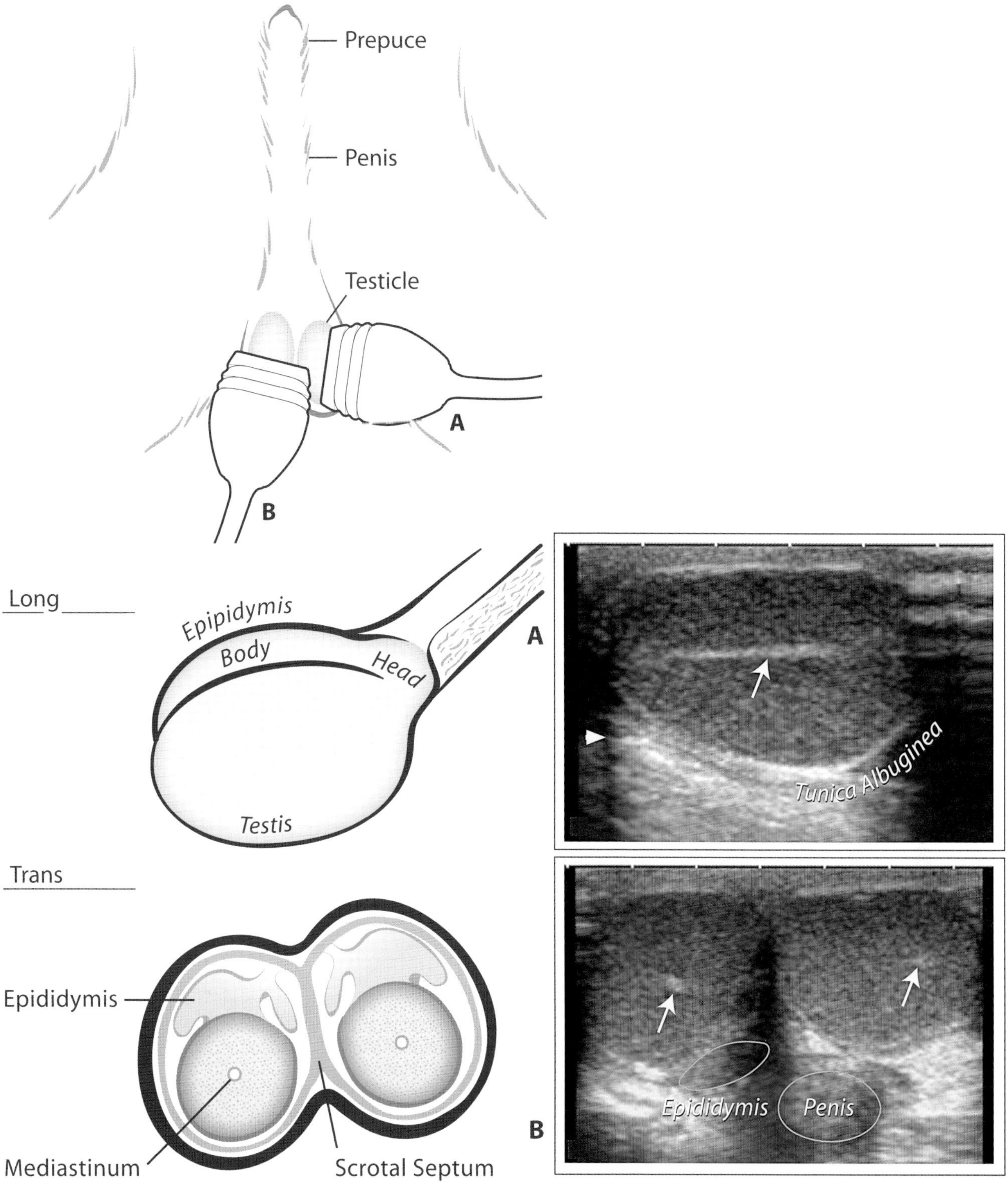

Figure 14.2. Scanning technique and normal sonographic anatomy of the testicle in an adult dog. On the top of the figure, there is a schematic representation of the position of the probe on the testicles, **A** and **B** corresponding to the images below. **A: Sagittal image of the right testicle.** The testicle is oval, of medium echogenicity, and of fine and homogeneous echotexture. The tunica albuginea is smooth, thin, and hyperechoic. The mediastinum testis is seen as a central linear hyperechoic band. The epididymis is not visualized. Edge shadowing occurs at the cranial pole of the testicle (arrowhead). **B: Transverse image of the testicles.** The testicles are round and of medium echogenicity. The mediastinum testis is seen as a central or slightly eccentric hyperechoic focus in the right and left testicles, respectively. Part of epididymal bodies is visualized dorsal to the testicles. The ovoid structure dorsal to the testicles represents part of the penis.

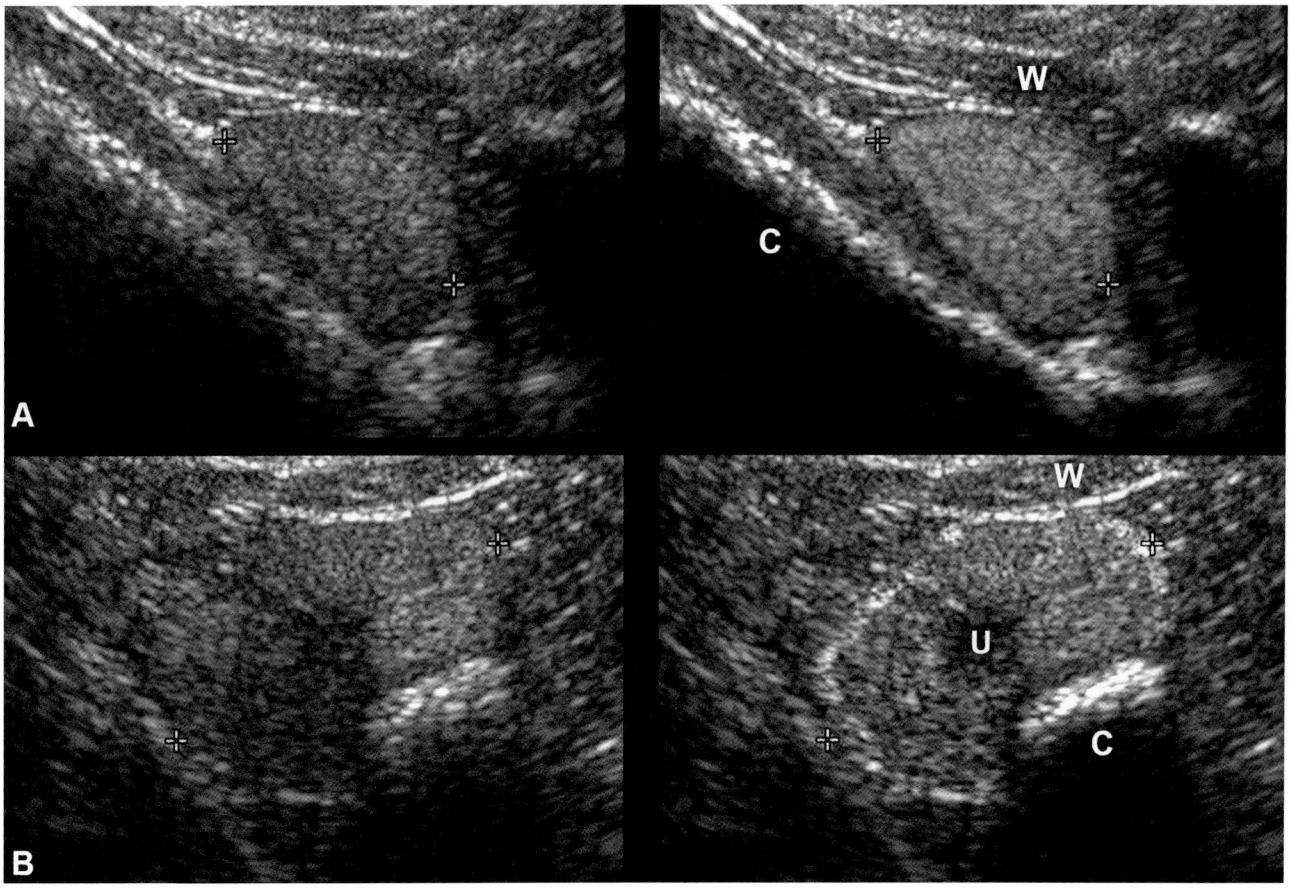

Figure 14.3. Normal prostate in a 1-year-old intact Boston terrier. **A: Sagittal image.** The prostate appears as an ovoid, homogeneous structure of medium echogenicity dorsal to the abdominal wall (W) and ventral to the colon (C). The irregular, hyperechoic interface that casts a strong shadow in the colon is caused by the presence of feces. The urinary bladder is not visible in this image. Caudal and ventral to the prostate, the hyperechoic interface of the pubis marks the pelvic inlet. The shadow caused by the pubis represents a limiting factor when assessing the structures contained in the pelvis canal. **B: Transverse image.** The prostate is bilobed and appears oblique because of the angulation of the probe. The lobes are symmetrical and homogeneous. The central prostatic urethra and urethralis muscle (U) are hypoechoic. The colon is dorsal to the prostate. C, colon; and W, wall.

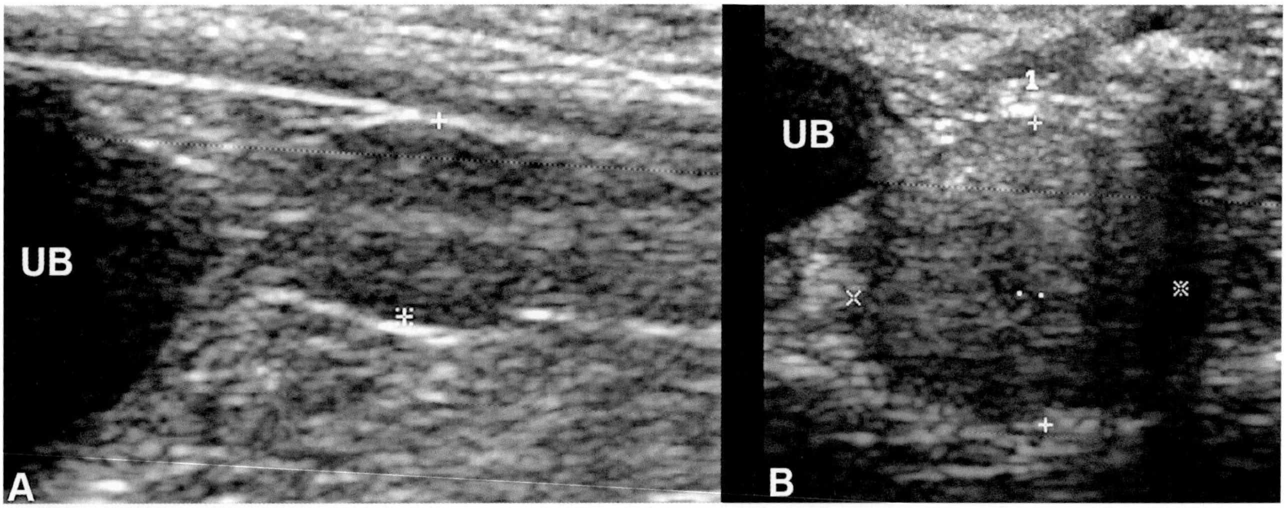

Figure 14.4. Comparison of the prostate in two small-breed intact dogs with age-related changes of the normal canine prostate. **A:** Sagittal image of the prostate in a 3-month-old shih tzu. The prostate (between the cursors) is ovoid, hypoechoic, and small (5 mm high). The urinary bladder (UB) is noted cranial to the prostate. **B:** Sagittal image of the prostate in a 9-year-old toy poodle. The prostate (between the cursors) is rounded, of medium echogenicity, and 1.8 cm high. UB, urinary bladder.

Table 14.1.
Prostatic dimensions in healthy intact dogs and correlation to age and body weight

	Ruel et al. 1998	Atalan et al. 1999
Length (cm)	1.7–6.9	1.8–5.0
Height (on transverse image) (cm)	1.3–4.7	1.4–3.6
Width (cm)	1.8–6.9	1.4–4.3
Volume (cm^3)	2.3–80.0	8.1–28.2
Correlation between prostatic length (L [cm]), age (A [years]), and body weight (BW [kg])	$L = (0.055 \times BW) + (0.143 \times A) + 3.31$	
Correlation between prostatic height (H [cm]), age (A [years]), and body weight (BW [kg])	$H = (0.044 \times BW) + (0.083 \times A) + 2.25$	
Correlation between prostatic width (W [cm]), age (A [years]), and body weight (BW [kg])	$W = (0.047 \times BW) + (0.089 \times A) + 3.45$	
Correlation between prostatic volume (V [cm^3]), age (A [years]), and body weight (BW [kg])	$V = (0.867 \times BW) + (1.885 \times A) + 15.88$	$V = 8.48 + (0.238 \times BW)$ $V = 9.79 + (0.871 \times A)$

Adapted from Ruel et al. (1998) and Atalan et al. (1999).

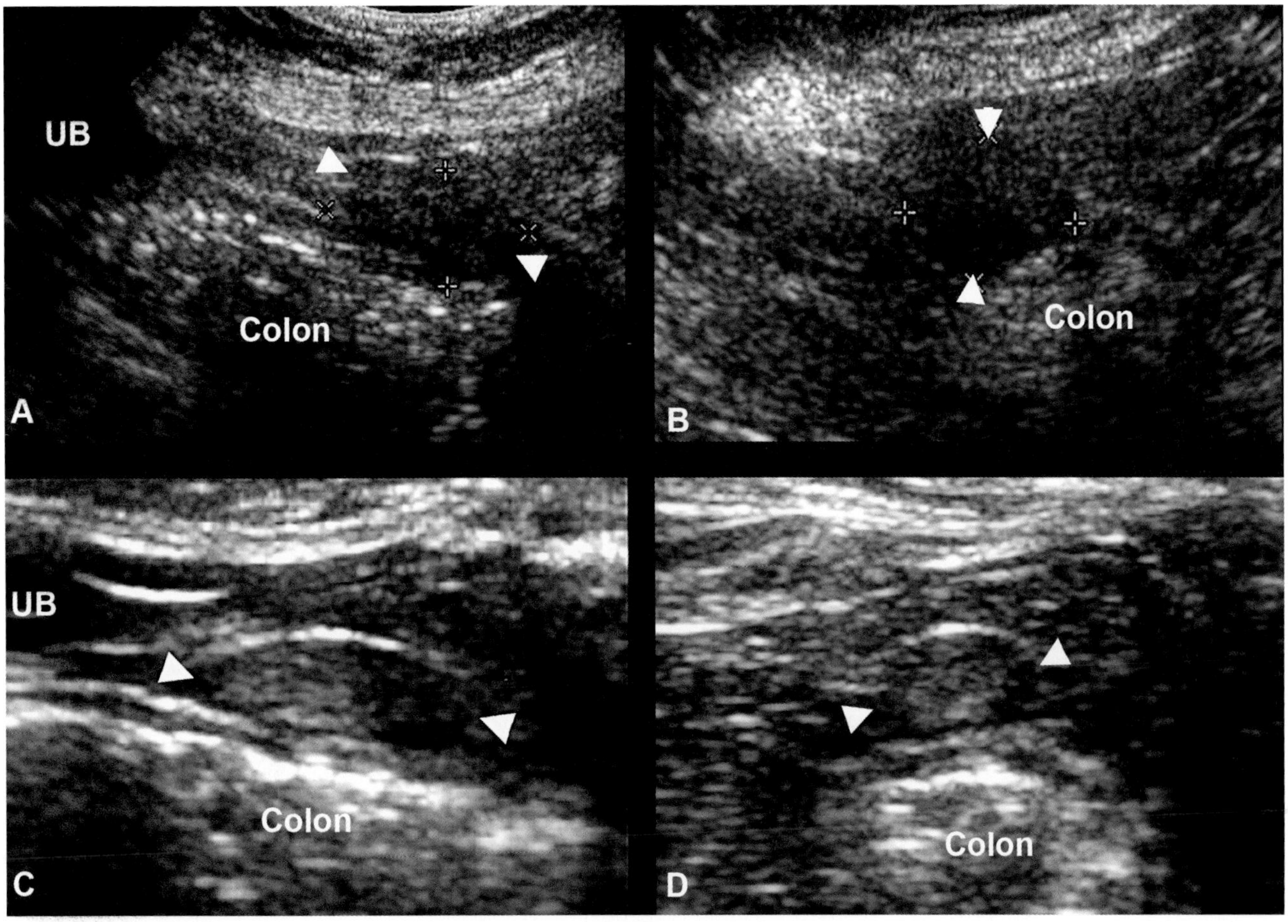

Figure 14.5. Normal prostate in two neutered dogs. **A and B:** Sagittal **(A)** and transverse **(B)** images of a normal prostate in a 7-year-old, neutered, mixed-breed dog. The prostate (between the cursors and arrowheads) is caudal to the neck of the urinary bladder (UB) and ventral to the colon. It is small, inconspicuous, and oval in sagittal view, rounded in transverse view, and homogeneously hypoechoic. **C and D:** Sagittal **(C)** and transverse **(D)** images of a normal prostate in an 8-year-old neutered Pomeranian. The prostate (arrowheads) is small, elongated in sagittal view, rounded in transverse view, and of medium echogenicity.

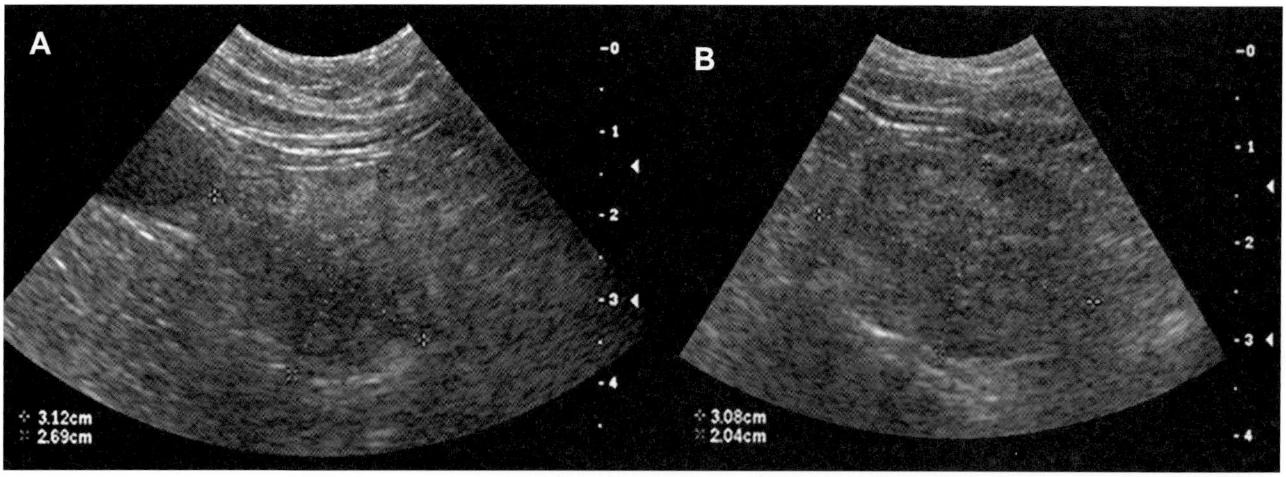

Figure 14.6. Prostatic remodeling in an old dog with late neutering. Sagittal **(A)** and transverse **(B)** planes of the prostate of a 10-year-old dog neutered at the age of 8 years. The prostate (between the cursors) is enlarged compared with that in Figure 14.4 and appears heterogeneous. Biopsies revealed the presence of normal prostatic tissue with fibrosis and small residual cysts. Some of these changes may be attributed to previous prostatitis. The images appeared similar on follow-up exams. Images courtesy of M.A. d'Anjou.

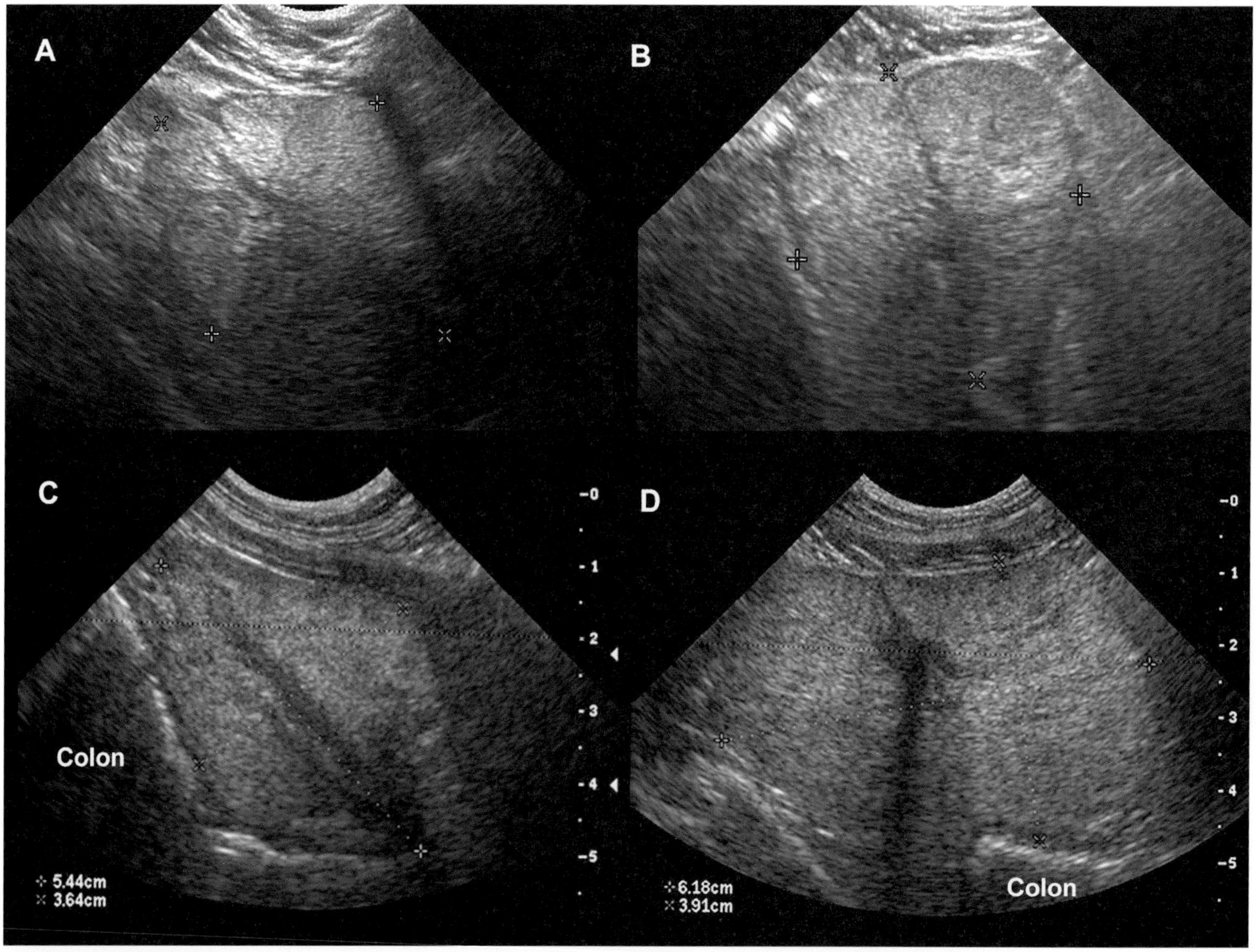

Figure 14.7. Benign prostatic hyperplasia in two dogs. **A and B:** Sagittal **(A)** and transverse **(B)** images of the prostate in a 9-year-old German shorthair pointer with benign prostatic hyperplasia. The prostate (between the cursors) is enlarged (5.8 × 4.6 × 4.0 cm). The prostatic parenchyma is mostly hyperechoic and slightly inhomogeneous. The prostatic lobes are symmetrical on transverse view. **C and D:** Sagittal **(A)** and transverse **(B)** images of the prostate of a 6-year-old Rottweiler in which similar signs are observed. An edge shadow noted on the transverse plane is caused by the presence of the round, central urethra. Images C and D courtesy of M.A. d'Anjou.

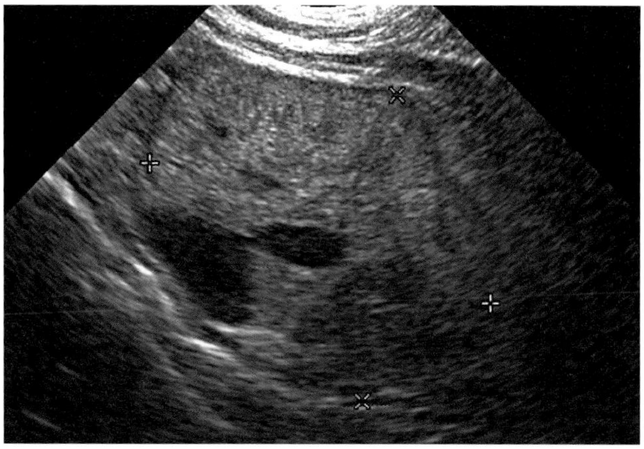

Figure 14.8. Benign prostatic hyperplasia and intraprostatic cysts in a 10-year-old husky. Sagittal image of the prostate shows prostatic enlargement (5.3×4.4 cm), inhomogeneity of the parenchyma, and multiple anechoic areas consistent with prostatic cysts.

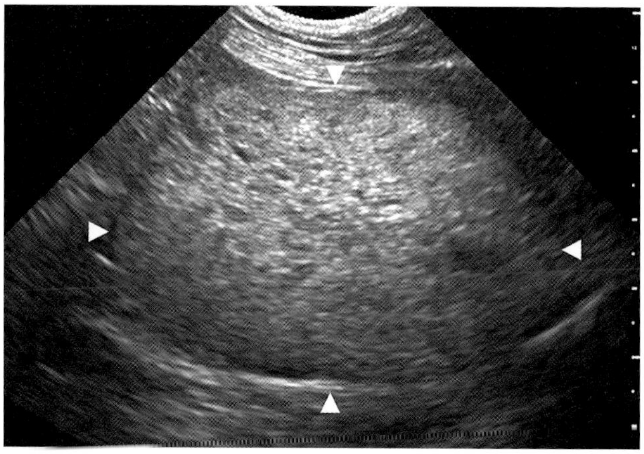

Figure 14.9. Benign cystic prostatic hyperplasia in a 10-year-old golden retriever. Parasagittal image (arrowheads) shows prostatic enlargement (7.2 × 4.2 cm) and generalized hyperechogenicity of the parenchyma, with numerous interspersed hypoechoic foci consistent with small cysts.

and B). Incidental parenchymal inhomogeneities may occasionally be observed in the prostate of older castrated dogs (Figure 14.6).

Sonographic Findings in Prostatic Abnormalities

Benign prostatic hyperplasia (BPH), bacterial prostatitis, paraprostatic cysts, and prostatic neoplasia are the most common prostatic disorders in dogs. Prostatic cysts are a common incidental finding or may be seen in association with BPH and other prostatic diseases. Prostatic abscesses may develop as a complication of bacterial prostatitis and/or infected cysts.

BPH is a spontaneous condition in older dogs and is a common incidental finding. The prostate is enlarged, of normal to increased echogenicity, and of homogeneous or inhomogeneous echotexture (Figure 14.7). On transverse image, the two lobes are usually symmetrical, although asymmetrical enlargement may occur. Intraprostatic cysts are common and manifest as circular to irregularly shaped anechoic areas of variable size (Figures 14.8 and 14.9).

Acute and chronic infections occur in the canine prostate, usually secondary to ascent of urethral bacteria into a gland with BPH (Johnston et al. 2000). The prostate may be of normal size or enlarged. Echogenicity and echotexture of the prostatic parenchyma are variable, ranging from normal to heterogeneous. Although changes in echogenicity and echotexture tend to be more severe than those seen in BPH, ultrasonographic differentiation of these conditions is often not possible, and prostatitis in many cases complicates preexisting BPH (Figure 14.10). In some cases of acute prostatitis, hyperechoic fat or a scant volume effusion may be detected adjacent to the prostate (Figure 14.11). Prostatic abscesses can develop subsequent to prostatitis and may appear similar to prostatic cysts (Figures 14.12 and 14.13). Other ultrasonographic findings in prostatic abscessation include development of a thick wall around the abscess cavity, intracavitary accumulation of echogenic fluid, gas inclusions in case of infection with gas-producing bacteria, and septation (Figure 14.14). Dystrophic mineralization may be encountered in chronic prostatitis (Figure 14.12).

Fungal prostatitis is rare, causes variable ultrasonographic changes, and may mimic prostatic neoplasia (Figure 14.15).

Paraprostatic cysts are fluid-filled remnants of the müllerian duct system that occur predominantly in older large-breed dogs (Stowater and Lamb 1989). Unlike true intraprostatic cysts, paraprostatic cysts are located in the vicinity of the prostate, but may communicate with intraprostatic cavitations. The cyst wall is of variable thickness (Figures 14.16 and 14.17).

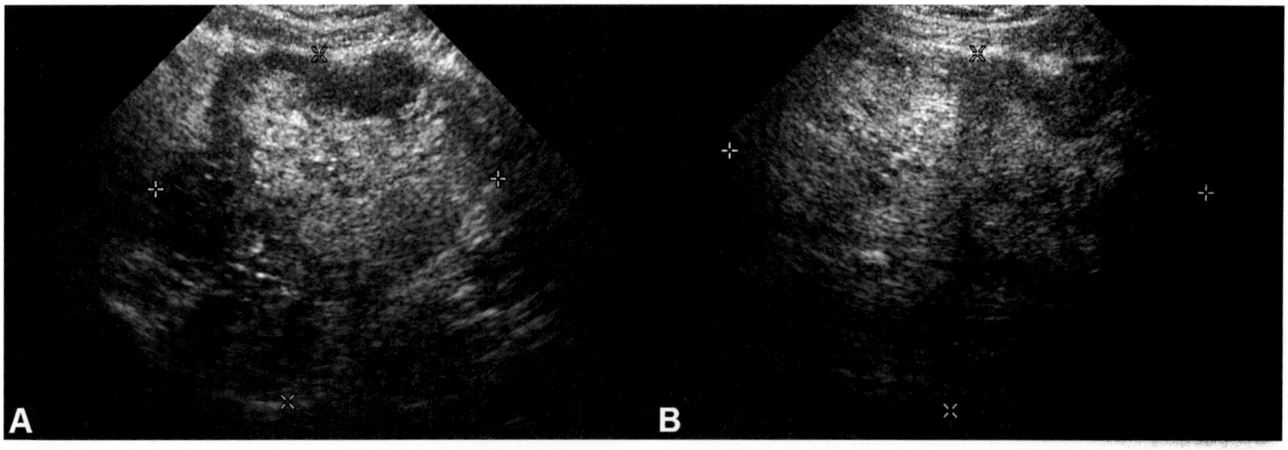

Figure 14.10. Benign prostatic hyperplasia and chronic lymphoplasmacytic prostatitis in an 11-year old mixed-breed dog. Sagittal **(A)** and transverse **(B)** images of the prostate (between the cursors), which is enlarged (5.9 × 5.7 × 8.0 cm), inhomogeneous, with an irregular contour and mixed echogenicity.

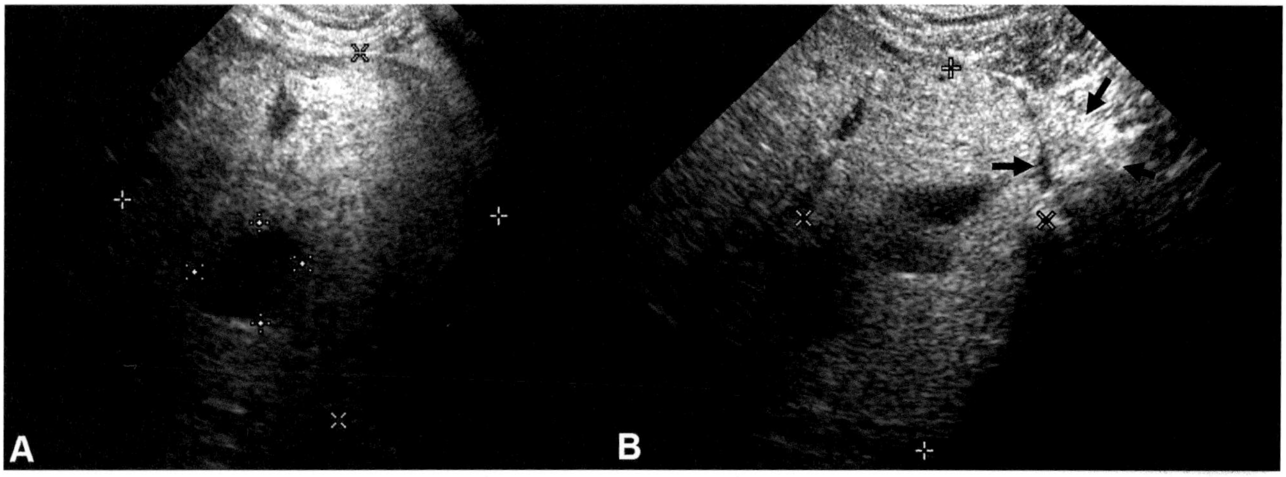

Figure 14.11. Acute prostatitis, benign prostatic hyperplasia, and intraprostatic cysts in an 8-year-old German shepherd. The diagnosis of prostatitis was based on clinical and ultrasonographic findings. No infectious organisms were seen on aspirates of one of the prostatic cysts. **A:** Sagittal image of the prostate. The prostate (between the cursors) is enlarged (6.4 × 6.0 cm), hyperechoic, and has multiple round to oval, hypoechoic to anechoic cavitations of up to 1.8-cm diameter. **B:** Transverse image of the left lobe of the prostate (between the cursors) and the paraprostatic tissues. The right lobe of the prostate is not completely included in the field of view. A small volume of abdominal effusion and strongly hyperechoic fat is adjacent to the prostate (arrows), suggesting a component of prostatic inflammation with secondary steatitis.

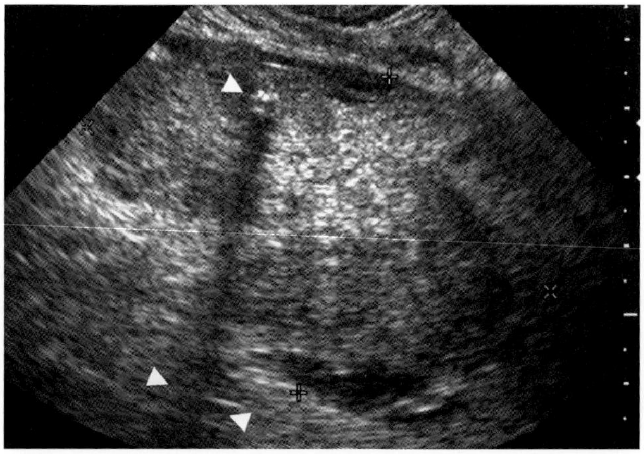

Figure 14.12. Severe, diffuse chronic-active, suppurative prostatitis with multifocal necrosis, abscessation, and interstitial hemorrhage in a 9-year-old mixed-breed dog. Sagittal sonogram of the prostate (between the cursors), which is enlarged (7.5 × 4.8 cm), irregular in contour, and mixed in echogenicity, with multiple irregularly marginated anechoic areas consistent with abscesses. Parenchymal mineralization is seen as strongly hyperechoic focus with distal shadowing (arrowheads).

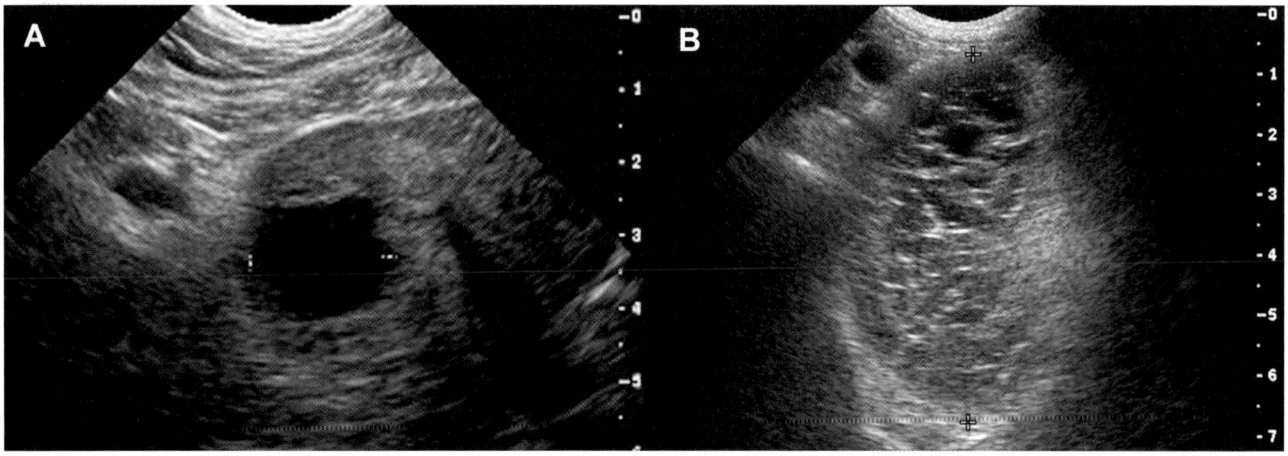

Figure 14.13. Prostatic abscesses in two dogs. **A: Septic abscess.** Transverse sonogram centered on the right lobe of the prostate of a 3-year-old Border collie. A well-defined anechoic cavity (between the cursors) is present. The volume of the lesion is estimated at 3.9 mL. **B: Sterile prostatic abscess in an 8-year-old boxer.** Transverse image shows a lacy hypoechoic to anechoic septated lesion of more than 6-cm maximum diameter associated with the right lobe (between the cursors).

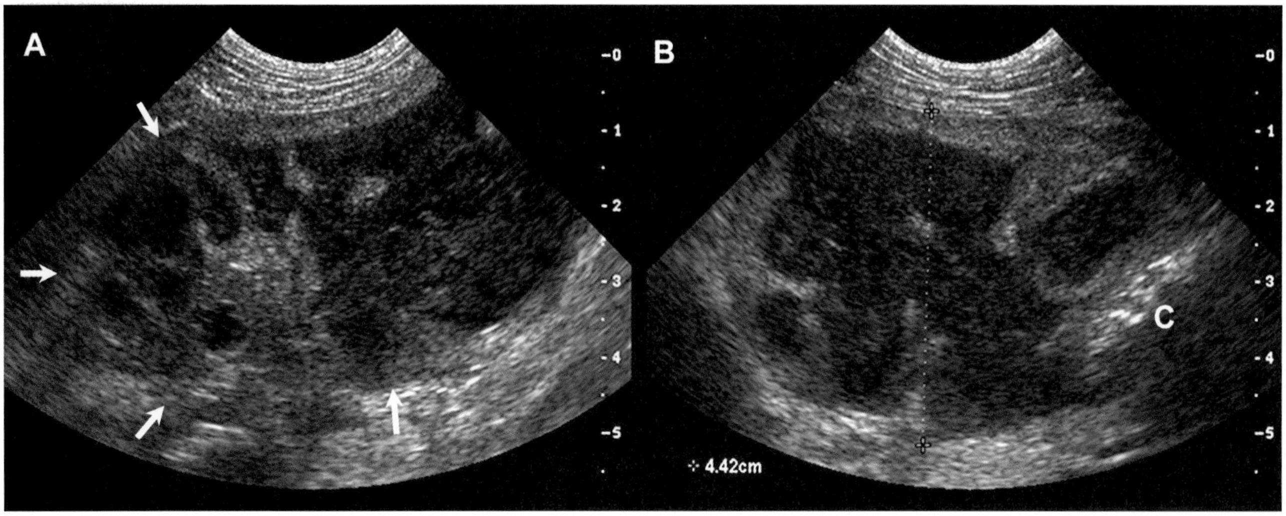

Figure 14.14. Septic prostatitis in a dog. Sagittal **(A)** and transverse **(B)** images of the prostate of an intact male dog with signs of abdominal pain and fever. The prostate is markedly enlarged and deformed (arrows) because of multiple hypoechoic cavitary lesions, the largest reaching 4.4 cm. Ultrasound-guided aspirations of these cavitations revealed the presence of neutrophils with bacteria. C, descending colon. Images courtesy of M.A. d'Anjou.

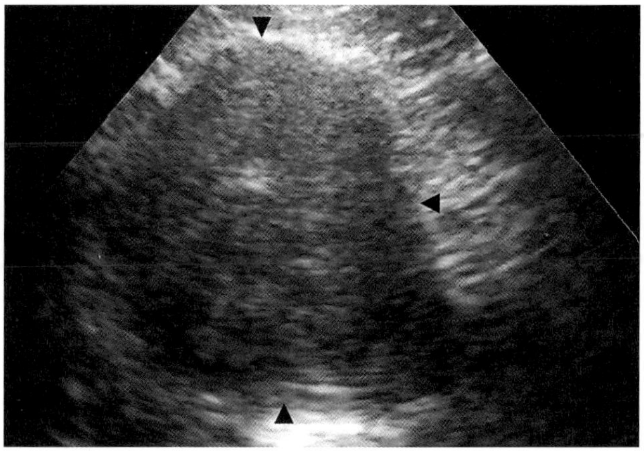

Figure 14.15. Fungal prostatitis (blastomycosis) in an 8-year-old cocker spaniel. The transverse image shows an enlarged, irregularly marginated, inhomogeneously hypoechoic prostate (arrowheads) with surrounding hyperechoic fat. Enlarged medial iliac lymph nodes were also seen (not shown).

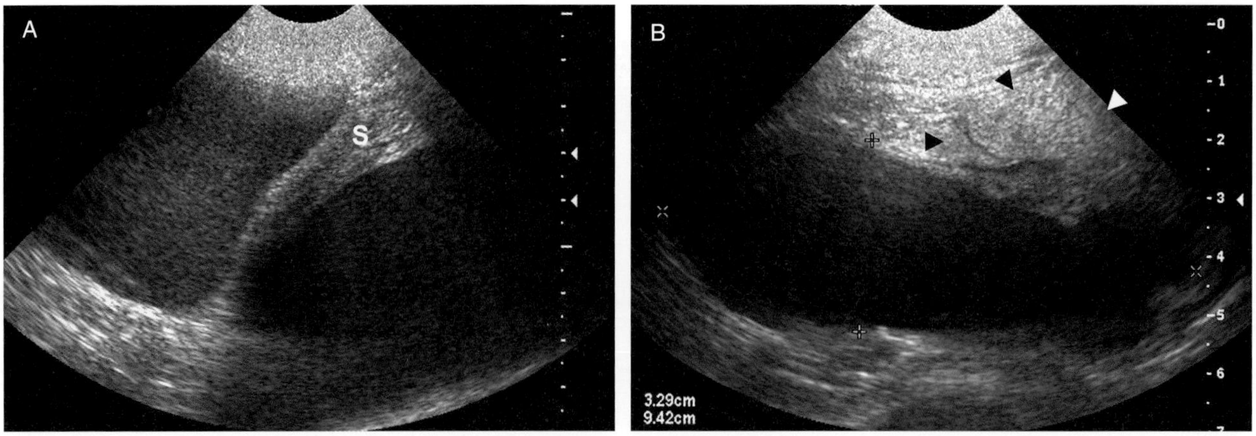

Figure 14.16. **A: Paraprostatic cyst in a 4–year-old cryptorchid Labrador retriever.** The transverse image was acquired at the level of the midabdomen. The fluid-filled structures were separate from the urinary bladder (not shown). A thick echogenic septum (S) separates a compartment filled with very echogenic fluid (left) from a compartment with less echogenic fluid (right). **B: Paraprostatic cyst in a middle-aged dog.** The cyst (between the cursors) is seen as tubular anechoic structure without a discernible wall extending cranially from the dorsal aspect of the hyperechoic prostate (arrowheads).

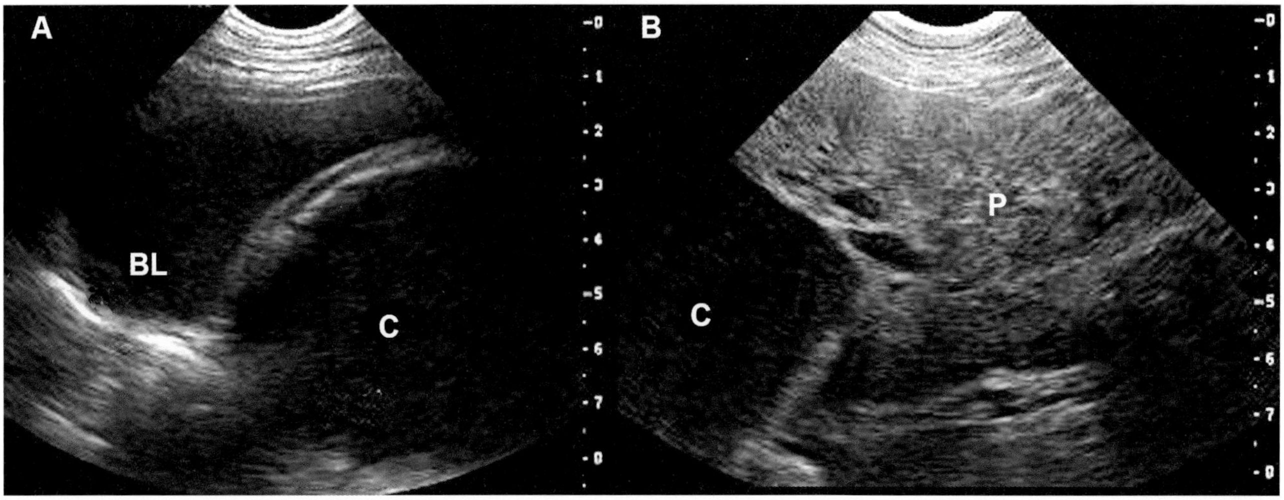

Figure 14.17. Paraprostatic cysts associated with acute prostatitis in an 8-year-old boxer. **A:** The main cyst (C) is dorsal to the bladder (BL). **B:** The prostate (P) is moderately enlarged and contains several smaller parenchymal cysts. The main large cyst (C) appears to originate from the right lobe.

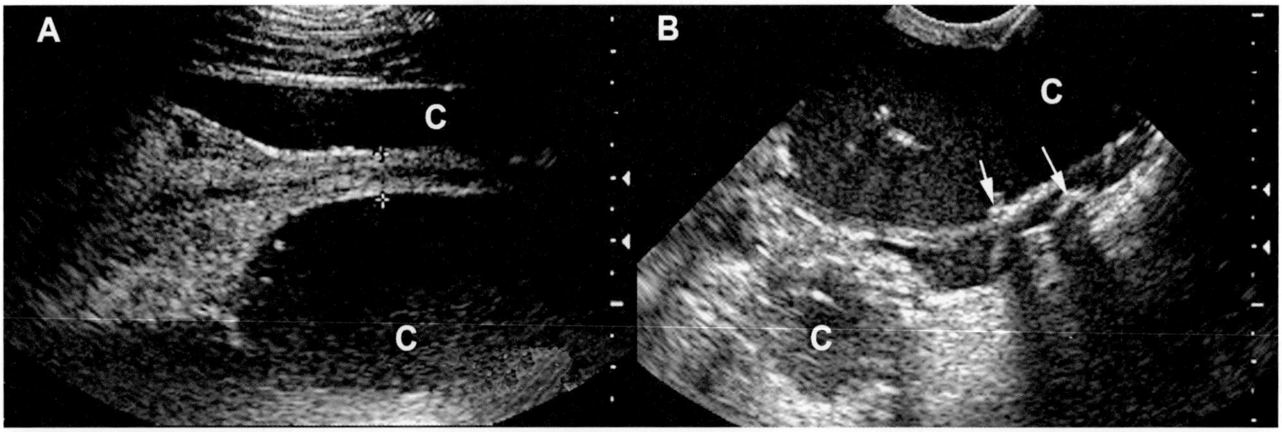

Figure 14.18. Complex paraprostatic cysts associated with suppurative prostatitis in a German shepherd. Numerous cysts (C) are in the midabdomen and caudal abdomen. **A:** The cystic wall is thickened (between the cursors). **B:** Some cysts (C) are filled with echogenic debris, and mineralized foci (arrows) are noted, as well.

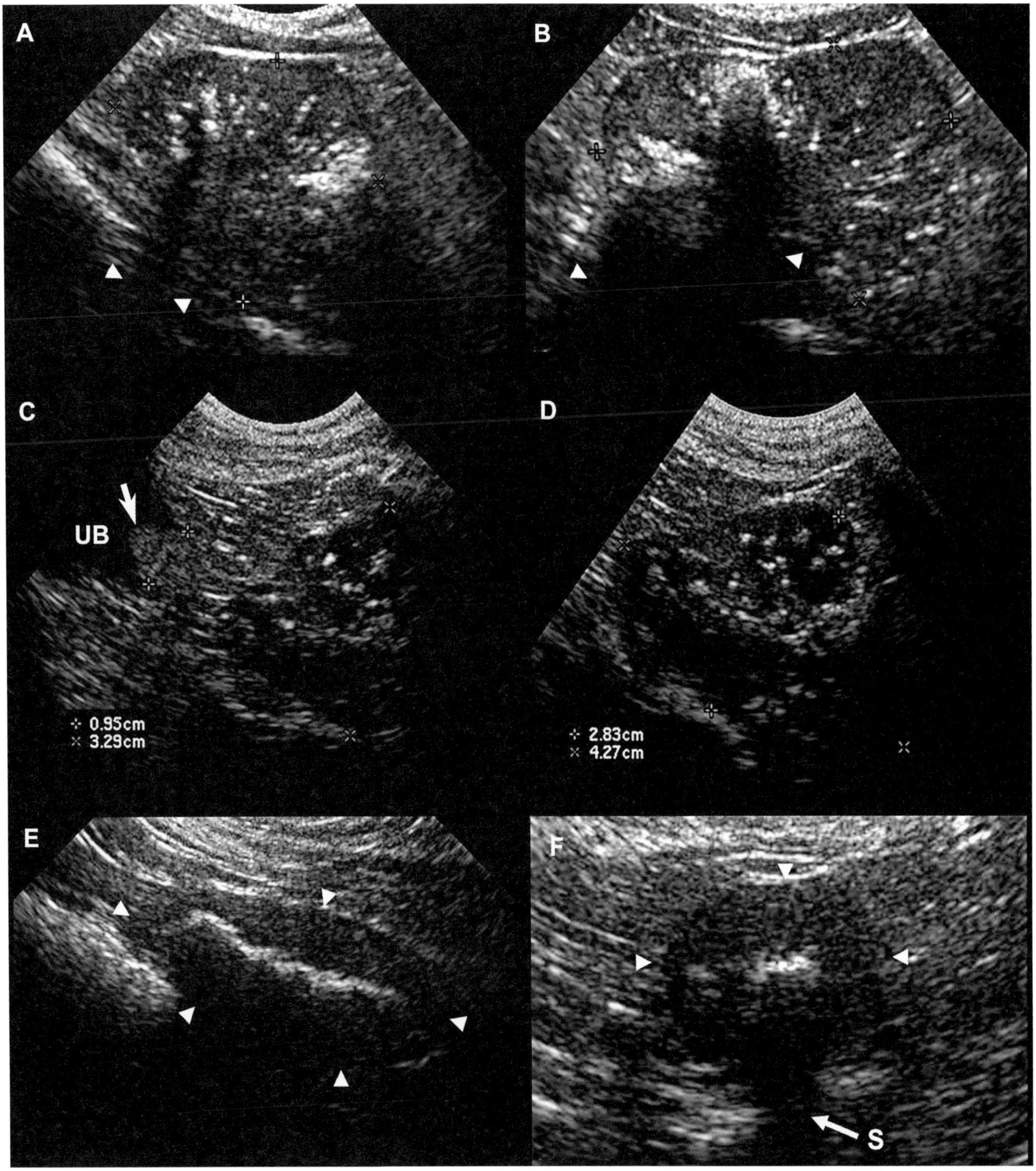

Figure 14.19. Prostatic adenocarcinoma and transitional cell carcinoma in three dogs. **A and B:** Sagittal **(A)** and transverse **(B)** images of a prostatic adenocarcinoma in an older, neutered, mixed-breed dog. The prostate (between the cursors) is large for a neutered dog, inhomogeneous, and has irregular margins. Prostatic parenchyma is of mixed echogenicity. Multiple strongly hyperechoic areas with distal shadowing (arrowheads) are consistent with mineralization. **C and D:** Sagittal **(C)** and transverse **(D)** images of a prostatic adenocarcinoma in an older, neutered, large-breed dog. The prostate is enlarged, irregular, and relatively hypoechoic, with several small hyperechoic foci. A protuberance (arrow) is also seen projecting into the urinary bladder (UB) secondary to tumor invasion. Images C and D courtesy of M.A. d'Anjou. **E and F:** Sagittal **(E)** and transverse **(F)** images of transitional cell carcinoma, probably originating from the prostatic urethra, in a 12-year-old, neutered Labrador retriever. The prostate (arrowheads) has retained an normal shape, but is large for a neutered dog. Prostatic parenchyma is hypoechoic. The centrally located, strongly hyperechoic line with distal acoustic shadowing (arrow, S) is consistent with urethral mineralization.

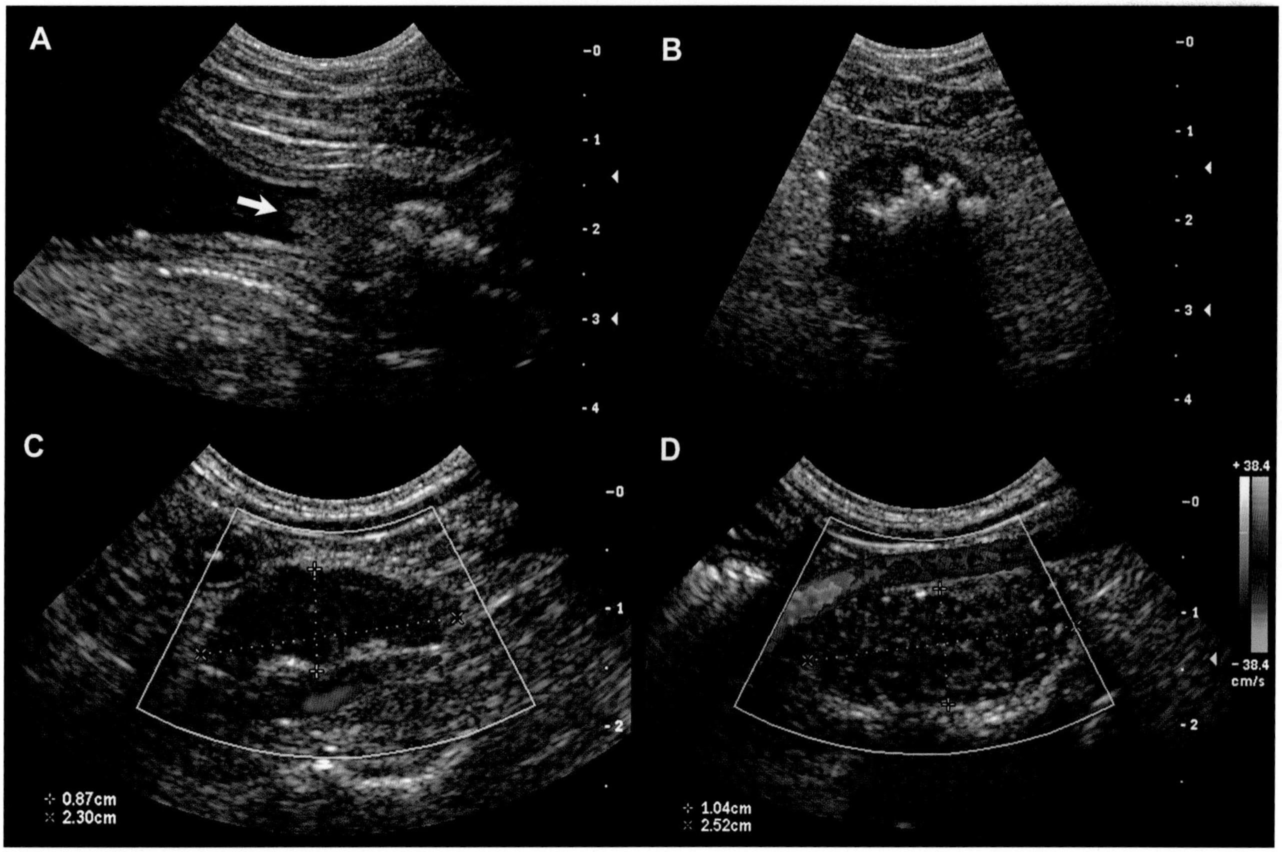

Figure 14.20. Transitional cell carcinoma and regional lymphadenopathy in an old, neutered dog with hematuria and dysuria. Sagittal **(A)** and transverse **(B)** images of the bladder neck and prostate. Strongly shadowing hyperechoic foci are in the prostate, and a soft-tissue projection is in the bladder lumen (arrow). Sagittal images of right medial iliac **(C)** and hypogastric **(D)** lymph nodes, which appear enlarged and irregular. The medial iliac node **(C)** is relatively uniform and nearly anechoic in comparison with the hypogastric **(D)** node that is heterogeneous and course in echotexture. These lymph nodes are adjacent to the external and internal iliac vessels, respectively. Images courtesy of M.A. d'Anjou.

Paraprostatic cysts contain anechoic to echogenic fluid, can become very large, may contain internal septa, and may be mineralized (Figure 14.18). Sometimes it is difficult to differentiate paraprostatic cysts from the urinary bladder. In these cases, catheterization of the urinary bladder with evacuation of urine or infusion of saline is useful in differentiating urinary bladder from paraprostatic cysts.

Ultrasonographic findings in prostatic neoplasia are variable. Adenocarcinoma is the most common tumor type. Other tumor types include undifferentiated carcinoma, squamous cell carcinoma, transitional cell carcinoma, lymphoma, and hemangiosarcoma (Winter et al. 2006). Bladder or urethral transitional cell carcinoma can extend into the prostatic parenchyma. In contrast to other prostatic disorders, neutered dogs are as commonly affected as intact dogs (Bell et al. 1991). Typically, the prostate is enlarged and irregular, with a hypoechoic to heterogeneous echotexture (Figures 14.19 and 14.20). On transverse view, the prostatic lobes are usually asymmetrical (Figures 14.19 and 14.21). Mineralization of the prostatic parenchyma is

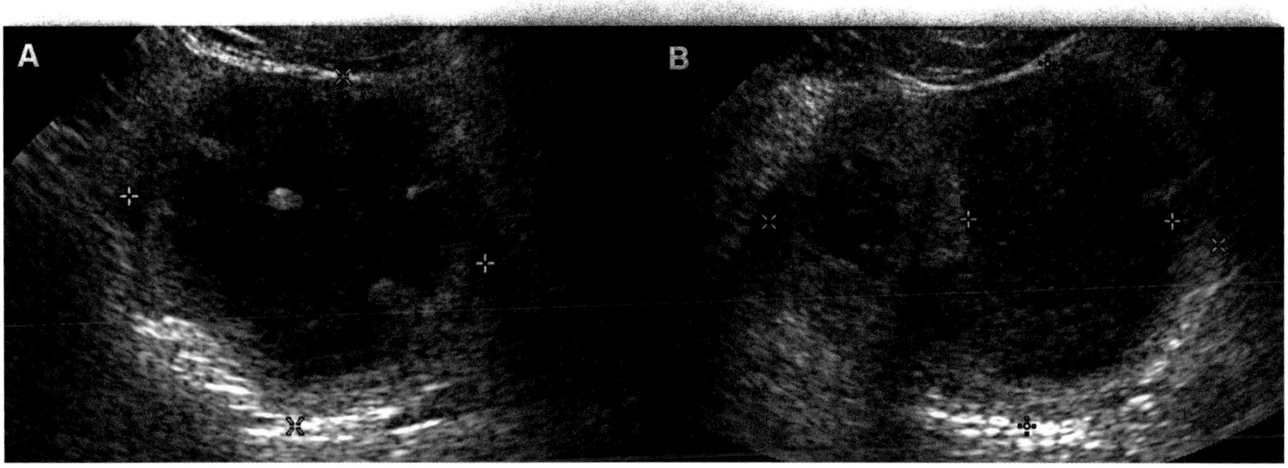

Figure 14.21. Prostatic hemangiosarcoma in a 10-year-old, neutered greyhound. **A:** Sagittal image. The prostate (between the cursors) is enlarged with echogenic margins and a central hypoechoic to anechoic area. **B:** Transverse image. There is asymmetry and inhomogeneity of the prostatic lobes. The prostate (between the cursors) is of mixed echogenicity, with hypoechoic to anechoic cavitary areas.

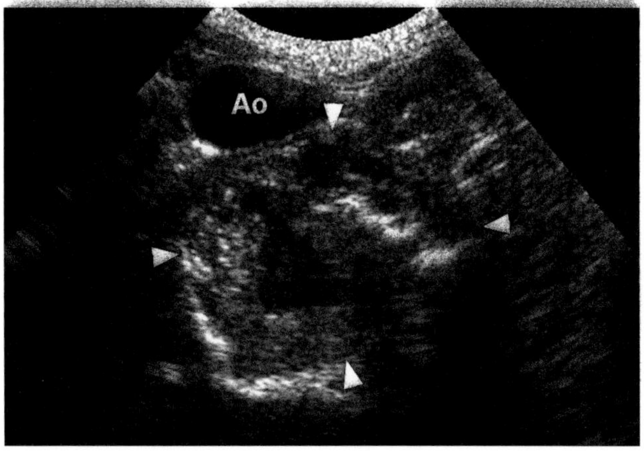

Figure 14.22. Metastatic lymphadenopathy secondary to prostatic adenocarcinoma in an older, neutered, mixed-breed dog (the same dog as in Figure 14.18A and B). On this transverse image, the right medial iliac lymph node (arrowheads) is enlarged and irregular in shape and margination. Multiple hypoechoic to anechoic areas indicate cavitation, and multifocal strongly hyperechoic foci with acoustic shadowing are compatible with mineralization. The aorta (Ao) is visualized as an anechoic circular structure in the near field.

often seen, and metastases to medial iliac or hypogastric lymph nodes are common (Figures 14.20 and 14.22). The surrounding fat may also become hyperechoic, and irregular bony proliferation of the ventral margin of the vertebral bodies of the caudal lumbar vertebrae may be seen, consistent with bone metastases. Other occasional findings in prostatic neoplasia are urethral obstruction, bladder wall thickening, or ureteral obstruction with hydroureter and hydronephrosis if the mass is invading the trigone.

TESTICLES

Normal Sonographic Anatomy of the Testicles

Normal testicles are of medium echogenicity and have a fine, homogeneous echotexture (Pugh et al. 1990). The testicular border is characterized by a thin, smooth and hyperechoic tunica albuginea. On sagittal image, a central hyperechoic line is visible that represents the mediastinum testis (Figure 14.2A). On transverse view, the mediastinum testis appears as a centrally located hyperechoic focus (Figure 14.2B). In very young dogs, the testicles are small but homogeneous, and the mediastinum can be identified (Figure 14.23). In older dogs, small hyperechoic foci representing testicular septa are occasionally visible. Testicular size is directly related to body weight (Hecht 2001; Hecht et al. 2003) (Table 14.2).

The head and tail of the epididymis are located at the cranial and caudal poles of the testicle, respectively, and the body is found dorsal to the testicle. In comparison with testicular parenchyma, epididymal parts are hypoechoic and of coarse echotexture (Figure 14.24A–C). Examination of the entire epididymis in one plane is usually not possible because of its location and course, and requires repositioning of the ultrasound probe and examination in at least two planes. The spermatic cord can be followed from the head of the epididymis to the inguinal ring and is characterized by the large tortuous anechoic venous structures of the pampiniform plexus. This plexus presents a prominent and complex flow pattern on color Doppler or power Doppler (Figure 14.24D).

Sonographic Findings in Testicular Abnormalities

Testicular disorders include cryptorchidism, testicular neoplasia, inflammatory disorders (orchitis and epididymitis), testicular or epididymal cysts, torsion, infarction, atrophy, and trauma. Other disease processes affecting the scrotum include accumulation of

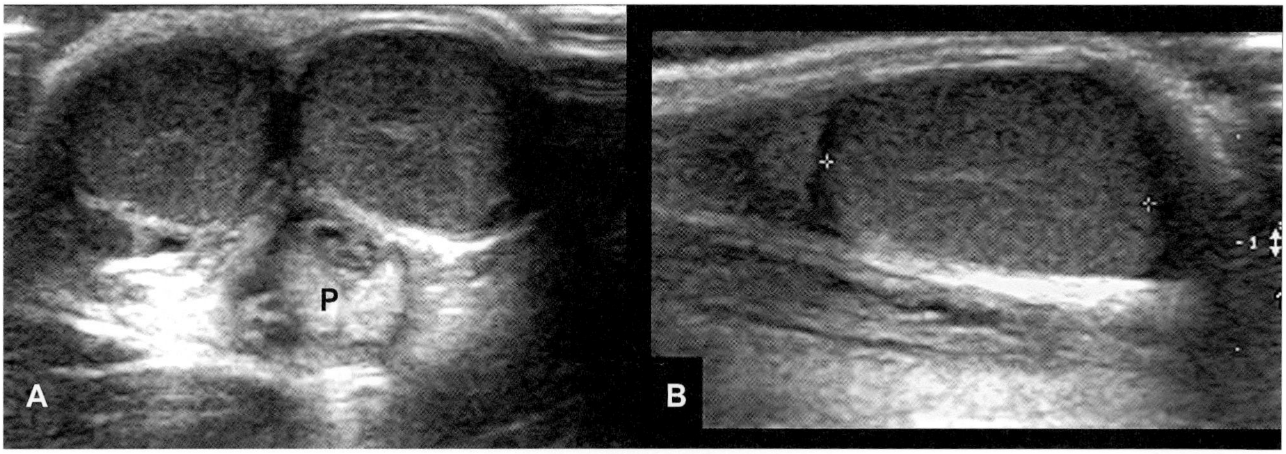

Figure 14.23. Testicles in a 3-month-old pointer. The testicles (between the cursors) are small (less than 2 cm long), ovoid, and homogeneous. **A:** Transverse sonogram of both testicles. Part of the penis (P) is dorsal to the testicles. **B:** Sagittal sonogram of the left testis. The mediastinum testis is seen. The epididymis is on the left of the image. Images courtesy of D. Penninck.

Table 14.2.
Testicular dimensions in healthy intact dogs and correlation to body weight

Body Weight (kg)	Length (cm)	Width (cm)	Height (cm)	Mediastinal Width (cm)
1–10	1.5–3.3	1.0–2.2	0.8–1.6	0.1–0.2
11–20	2.0–3.9	1.4–3.2	1.3–2.2	0.1–0.2
21–30	3.0–4.0	1.5–3.6	1.5–2.4	0.1–0.3
31–40	2.6 to >4.0[a]	1.7–3.7	1.6–3.2	0.1–0.3
>40	3.4 to >4.0[a]	2.6–3.8	1.6–3.0	0.1–0.3

[a]The transducer field of view was limited to 4 cm, and accurate measurements were not possible beyond that point.
Adapted from Hecht (2001).

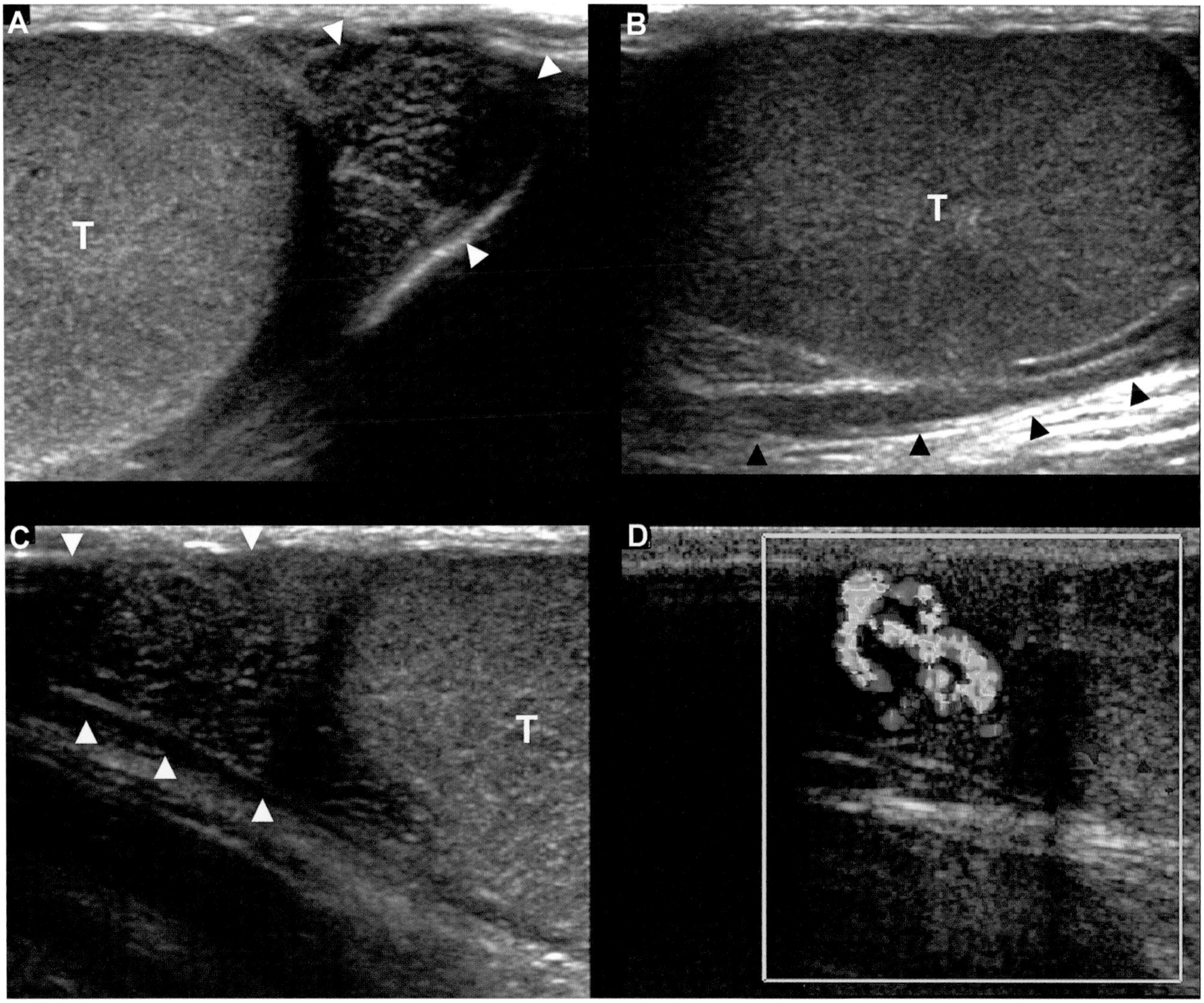

Figure 14.24. Normal epididymis and pampiniform plexus in a 9-year-old mixed-breed dog. **A:** Sagittal image of the epididymal tail (arrowheads). It is caudal to the testicle (T), hypoechoic, and of coarse echotexture. **B:** Parasagittal image of the testicle demonstrating the tubular body of the epididymis (arrowheads) dorsolateral to the testicle (T). **C:** Sagittal image of the epididymal head and adjacent part of the spermatic cord (arrowheads), which appear hypoechoic and coarse in comparison with the cranial pole of the testicle (T). **D:** Sagittal color Doppler image of part of the spermatic cord. Tortuous vessels of the pampiniform plexus show the color flow signal.

fluid (hydrocele or hematocele) and scrotal hernia. The accuracy in diagnosis of testicular and/or scrotal disorders in dogs is high (Hecht 2001; Hecht et al. 2003).

Cryptorchid testicles are usually small and hypoechoic, but have normal architecture with a central hyperechoic mediastinum (Figures 14.25 and 14.26). They can be found anywhere between the caudal pole of the kidneys to the inguinal area. If the mediastinum testis is not developed, identification of an undescended testicle may be difficult (Figure 14.27). Sensitivity of ultrasonography in the identification of inguinal or abdominal cryptorchid testicles in dogs is high (Hecht 2001), but is likely facilitated by the use of high-resolution ultrasound systems.

Occasionally, the gubernaculum testis is visualized. It appears as tubular structure extending from the caudal pole of the retained testicle to the inguinal ring (Figure 14.28). Abdominally and inguinally located testicles are predisposed to neoplastic transformation and can reach considerable size in this instance.

Testicular tumors are common. Leydig and interstitial cell tumors are frequent incidental findings in descended testicles in older dogs and may occur bilaterally. They are usually benign. Seminomas and Sertoli

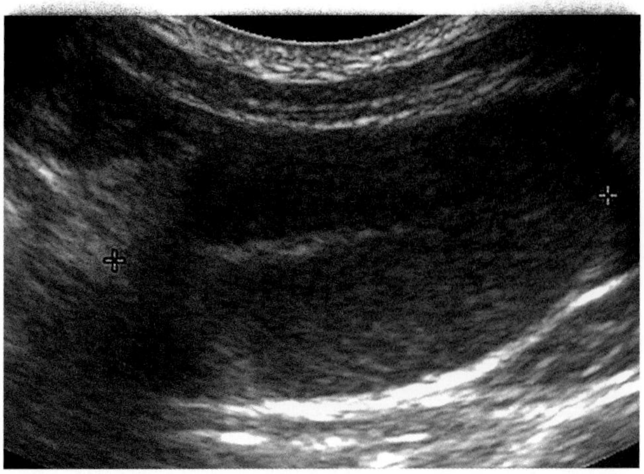

Figure 14.25. Abdominal cryptorchidism in a 1-year-old golden retriever. The left testicle (between the cursors) is intra-abdominal, small (3.1 cm long), hypoechoic, and of normal architecture.

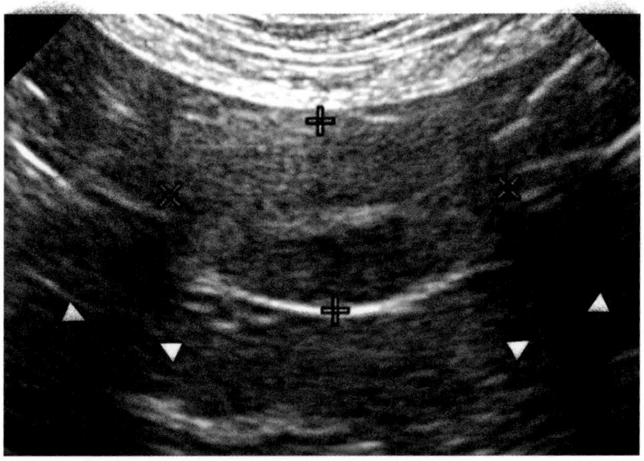

Figure 14.26. Abdominal cryptorchidism in a 10-year-old golden retriever. The left testicle (between the cursors) is intra-abdominal, small (2.6 cm long), and of normal architecture. Linear hypoechoic areas emanating from the cranial and caudal poles are consistent with edge-shadowing artifacts (arrowheads).

cell tumors can affect cryptorchid and descended testicles. These tumors have the potential for hormone production and metastases. Other tumor types are extremely rare. Testicular tumors in cryptorchid testicles tend to exhibit more malignant behavior than in descended testicles and occur in younger animals.

Ultrasonographic findings in testicular tumors range from circumscribed small nodules to large complex masses with disruption of normal testicular anatomy (Johnston et al. 1991a) (Figures 14.29–14.32). Different tumor types cannot be distinguished ultrasonographically (Pugh and Konde 1991; Hecht et al. 2003).

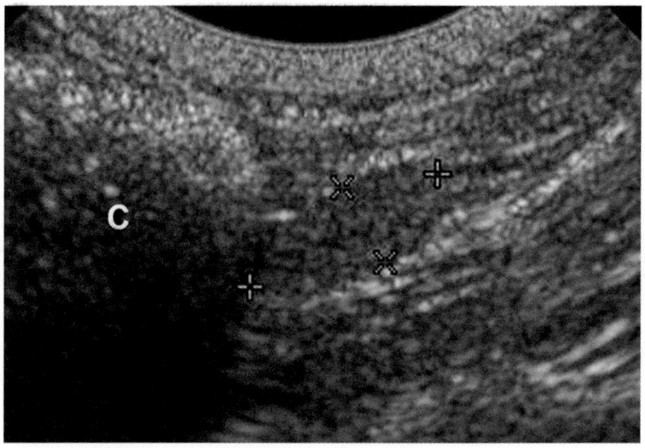

Figure 14.27. Abdominal cryptorchidism in a 7-month-old Boston terrier. The testicle (between the cursors) is adjacent to the descending colon (C). It is inconspicuous, homogeneous, and 1.0 × 0.4 cm. The mediastinum testis is not visible.

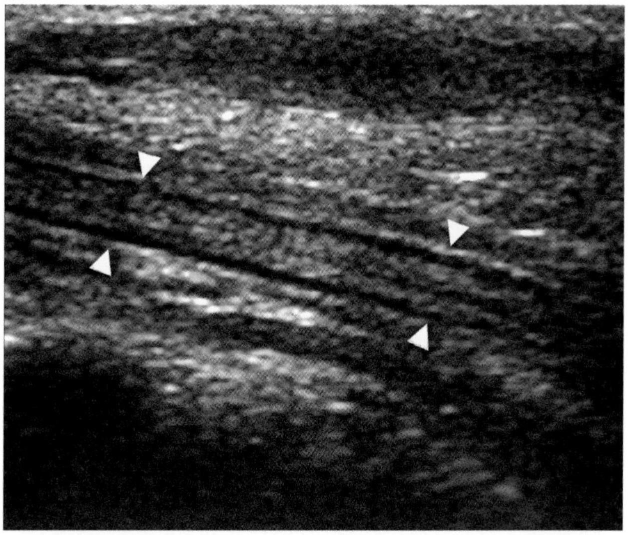

Figure 14.28. Prominent gubernaculum testis in a cryptorchid 5-month old mastiff. The gubernaculum (arrowheads) appears as tubular structure of 3-mm diameter and was seen extending from the caudal pole of the intra-abdominal right testicle to the inguinal ring.

Concurrent prostatic changes such as benign prostatic hyperplasia or squamous metaplasia are common, especially in hormone-producing tumors. In case of metastatic neoplasia, enlarged medial iliac lymph nodes may be seen.

Orchitis and epididymitis may occur subsequent to hematogenous spread of infectious organisms, may result from urinary tract or prostatic inflammation, or may be caused by scrotal trauma. Inflammatory scrotal disorders exhibit variable ultrasonographic

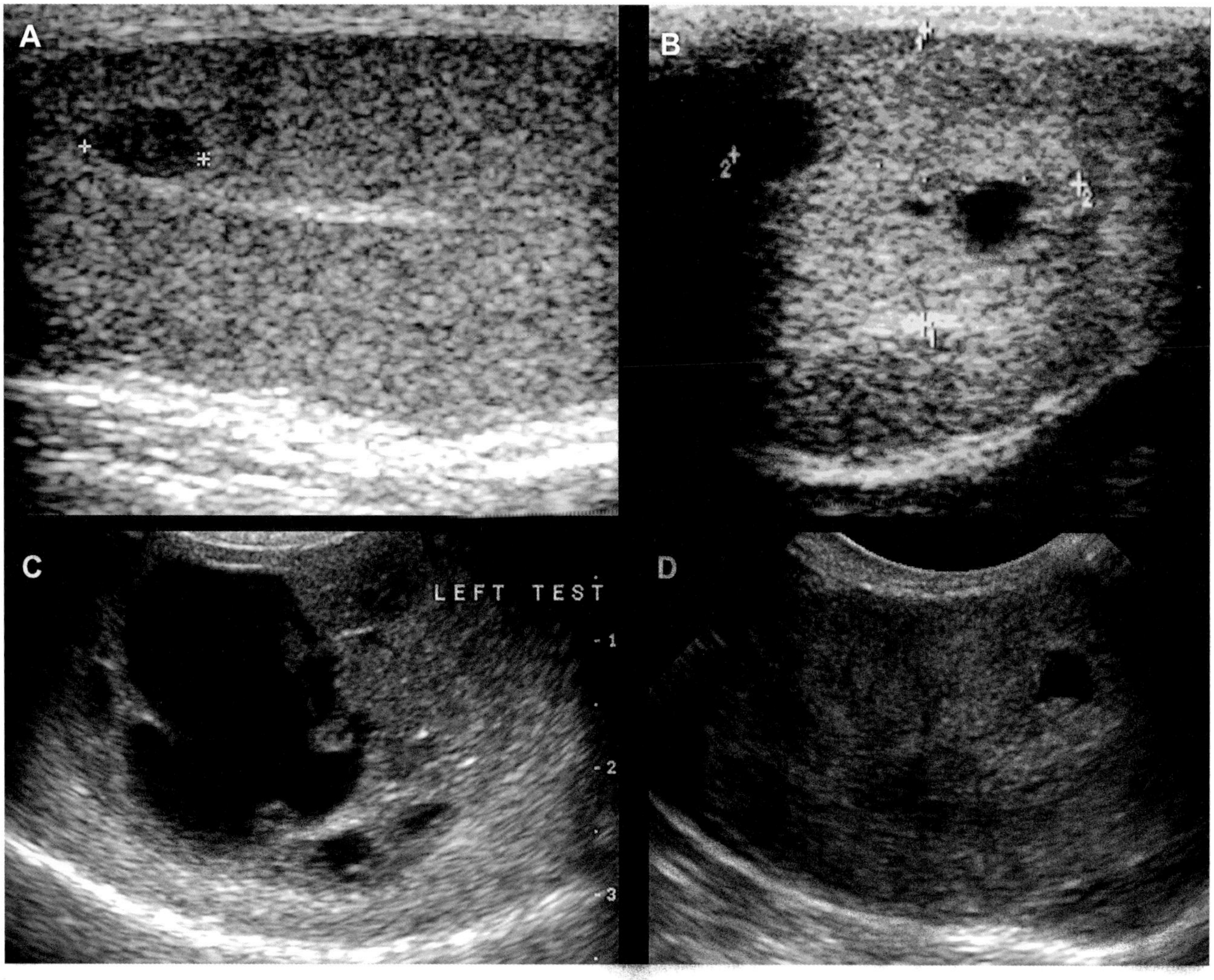

Figure 14.29. Leydig cell tumor in four dogs. **A:** Sagittal image of the left testicle in a 15-year-old Labrador retriever. A hypoechoic nodule of 5-mm diameter (between the cursors) is associated with the testicular parenchyma adjacent to the linear hyperechoic mediastinum testis. **B:** Transverse image of the right testicle in a 6-year-old boxer. A 2.4 × 2.0-cm nodule (between the cursors) is slightly hyperechoic to surrounding normal testicular parenchyma and has two small anechoic foci. **C:** Sagittal image of the left testicle in a 10-year-old golden retriever. The testicular parenchyma has been largely replaced by an approximately 3-cm, mixed echogenic and cavitary mass. **D:** Sagittal image of the left testicle in a 13-year-old sheltie. The testicular parenchyma is of mixed echogenicity, the testicle has an irregular margin, and the mediastinum testis is not visible.

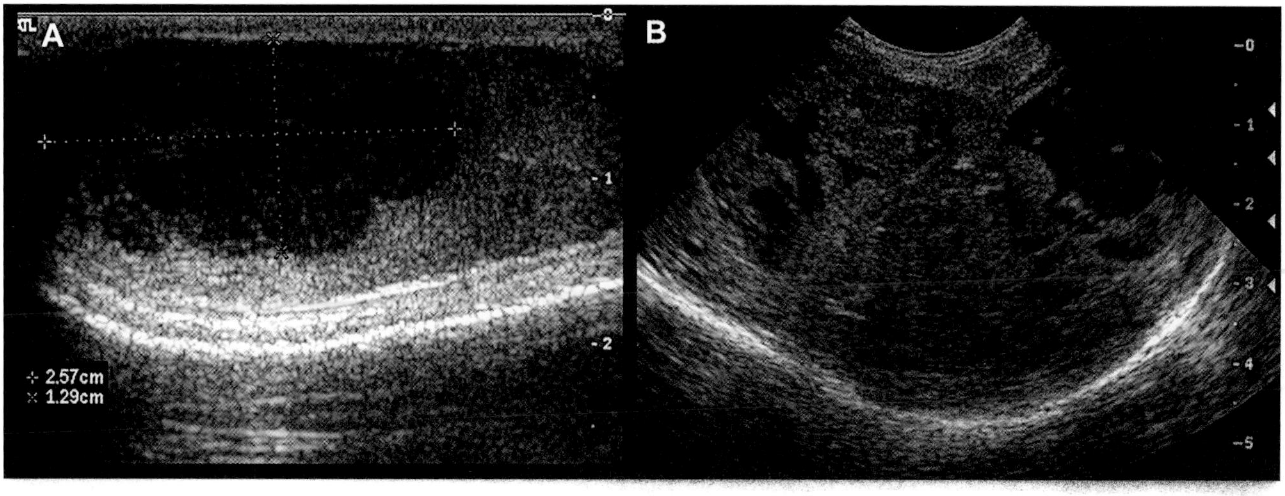

Figure 14.30. Seminoma in two dogs. **A:** Sagittal image of the left testicle in a 8-year-old large-breed dog. An irregular, but well-defined, hypoechoic nodule measuring 2.6 × 1.3 cm is in the testicle (between the cursors). **B:** Sagittal image of the left testicle in a 10-year-old Labrador retriever with an enlarged, endured scrotum. The testicular parenchyma is completely replaced by an inhomogeneous mass with several irregular cavitations containing anechoic to echogenic fluid. Images courtesy of M.A. d'Anjou.

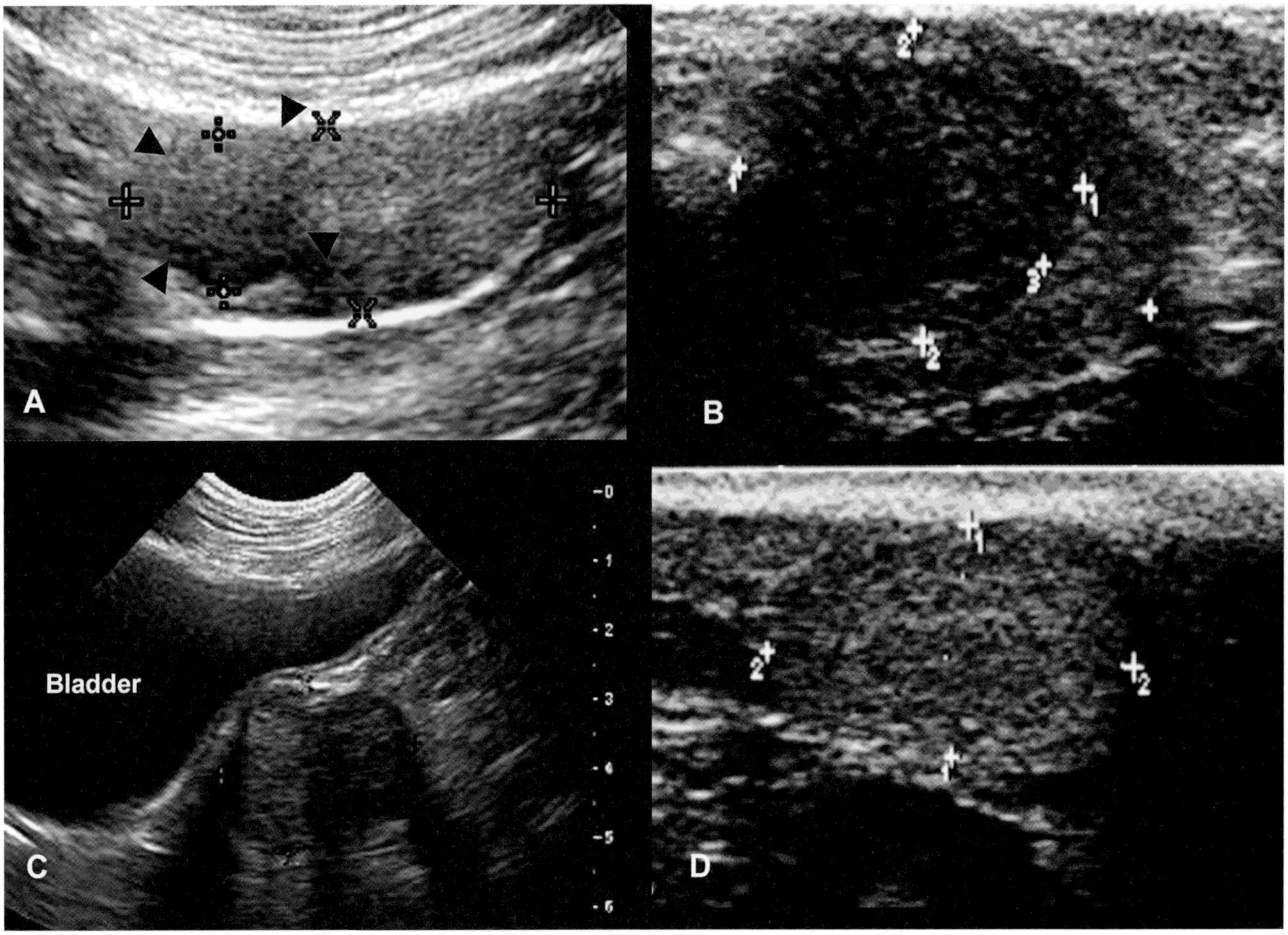

Figure 14.31. Sertoli cell tumor in four dogs. **A:** Sagittal image of the right abdominal cryptorchid testicle (between the cursors) in a 10-year-old golden retriever. The testicle is small (2.8 × 1.2 cm). A hypoechoic nodule of 1.0-cm diameter (arrowheads) is associated with the cranial pole of the testicle. **B:** Transverse image of the right inguinal cryptorchid testicle in an 8-year-old mixed-breed dog. A 1.9 × 1.8-cm hypoechoic nodule (between the cursors) is associated with the testicle. **C:** Sertoli cell tumor of a retained right testicle in an 8-year-old boxer. An echogenic mass of approximately 2.5-cm-diameter dorsal to the bladder is associated with strong edge shadows. **D:** Sagittal image of the left testicle in a 12-year-old West Highland white terrier. The testicle is within the scrotum and of normal size and shape. The testicular parenchyma is of mixed echogenicity, and the mediastinum testis is not visible.

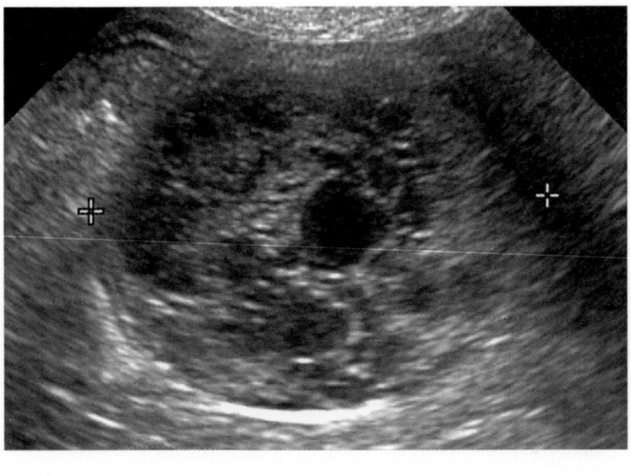

Figure 14.32. Mixed testicular tumors in a 13-year-old sheltie. Mixed tumor (seminoma and Sertoli cell tumor) in an abdominal cryptorchid testicle. The enlarged (4.5 cm), mixed echogenic testicle (between the cursors) has multiple anechoic areas.

characteristics, ranging from diffuse echogenicity changes of testicle and/or epididymis to complex masses and anechoic areas subsequent to abscess formation (Pugh and Konde 1991; Hecht et al. 2003; Ober et al. 2004) (Figures 14.33–14.36). Fluid may accumulate within the scrotum or the scrotum may thicken. Whereas testicular and epididymal size increase in acute inflammation, they decrease in chronic cases.

Testicular or epididymal cysts are occasional incidental findings. They appear as anechoic, well-circumscribed, rounded areas, often with distal acoustic enhancement (Figures 14.37 and 14.38).

Testicular torsion most commonly affects retained neoplastic testicles. In this instance, the ultrasonographic examination shows an abdominal mass of variable size and echogenicity, with decreased or absent blood flow on color Doppler examination (Miyabashi et al. 1990; Hecht 2001) (Figure 14.39). Intra-abdominal and intrascrotal torsion of nonneoplastic testicles and vascular compromise of other etiology of the testicle (infarction or space-occupying lesions within the inguinal ring) are rare (Hecht et al. 2004) (Figures 14.40 and 14.41). Dependent on the degree and duration of vascular occlusion, the affected testicle may appear hyperechoic or hypoechoic, increased, or normal or decreased in size, with initially normal architecture. Concurrent abdominal or scrotal effusion is common, especially in acute cases.

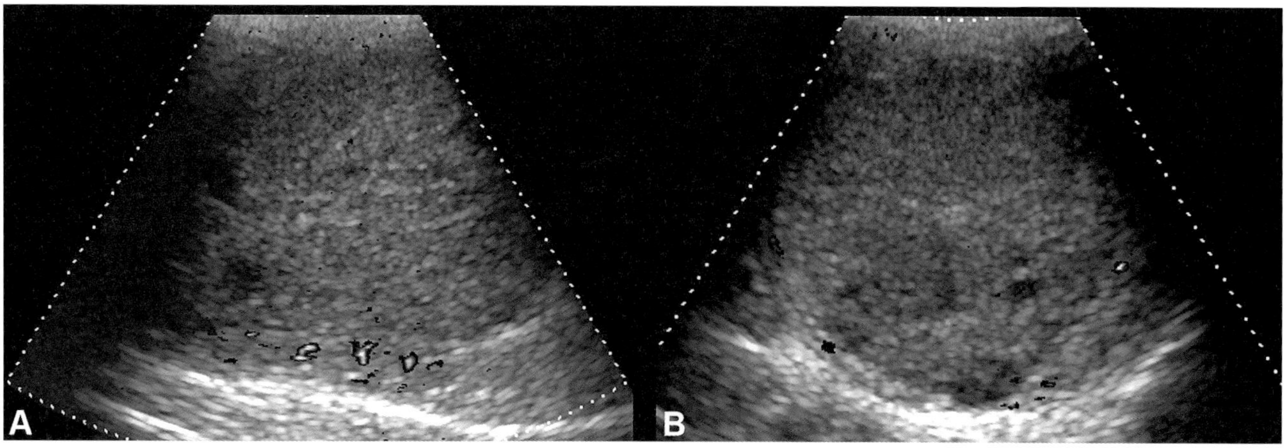

Figure 14.33. Severe, subacute, necrotizing and suppurative orchitis and epididymitis of undetermined etiology in a 3-year-old golden retriever. Sagittal **(A)** and transverse **(B)** images of the left testicle show that the testicle is enlarged and heterogeneous, with disruption of normal architecture. On color Doppler examination, blood flow was reduced compared with the normal right testicle (not shown).

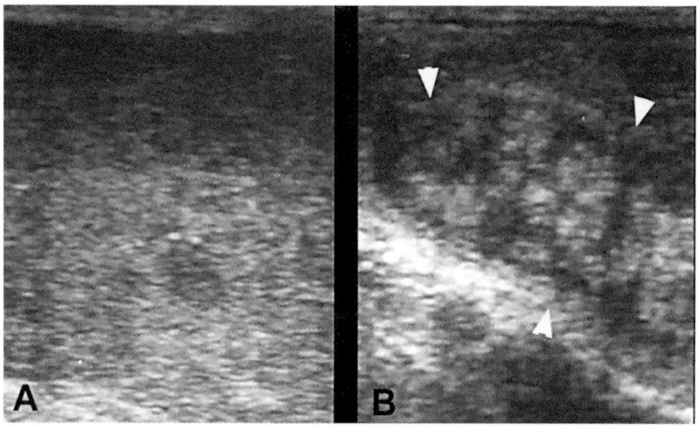

Figure 14.34. Fungal orchitis and epididymitis (blastomycosis) in a 3-year-old Walker hound. Sagittal images of the right testicle **(A)** and head of the epididymis **(B)** show testicular and epididymal (arrowheads) enlargement and inhomogeneity.

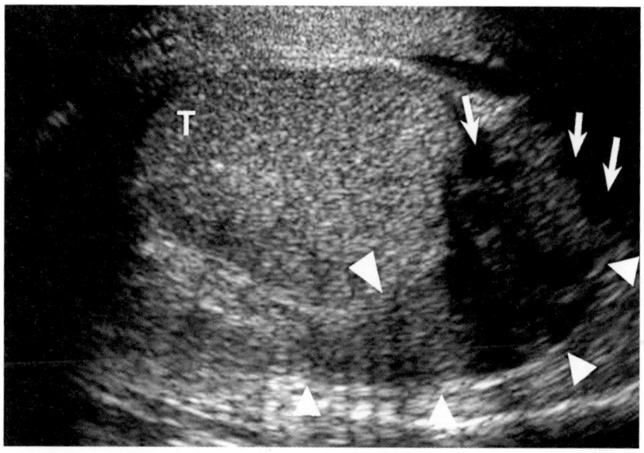

Figure 14.35. Epididymitis in a 9-year-old Labrador retriever. In the parasagittal image of the left testicle, the epididymis (arrowheads) is larger than usual and of mixed echogenicity. Several anechoic areas are in the tail of the epididymis (arrows). The testicle (T) is within normal limits for size and echotexture.

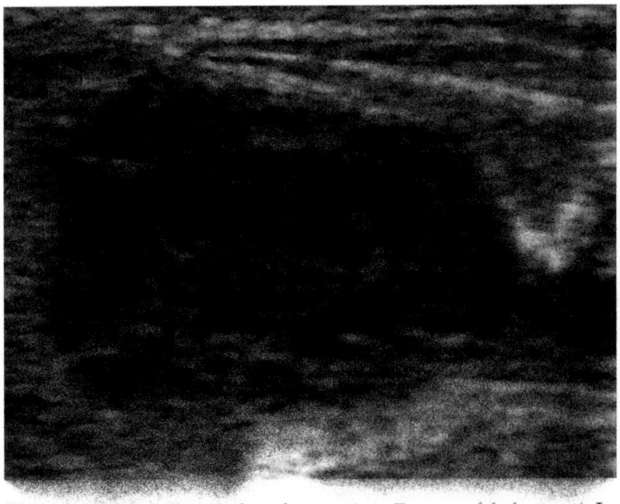

Figure 14.36. Testicular abscess in a 7-year-old shar-pei. In the sagittal image of the right testicle is an approximately 2-cm, inhomogeneous hypoechoic to anechoic mass. Normal testicular parenchyma is not visible.

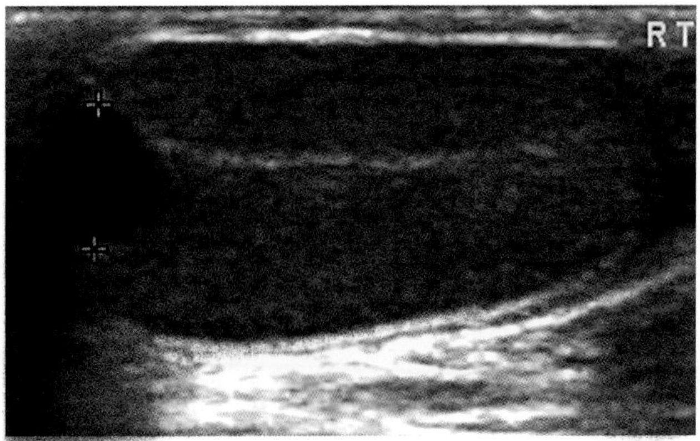

Figure 14.37. Cyst associated with the cranial pole of the right testicle in a 7-year-old Yorkshire terrier. A round anechoic structure of 5-mm diameter (between the cursors) is associated with the testicular parenchyma.

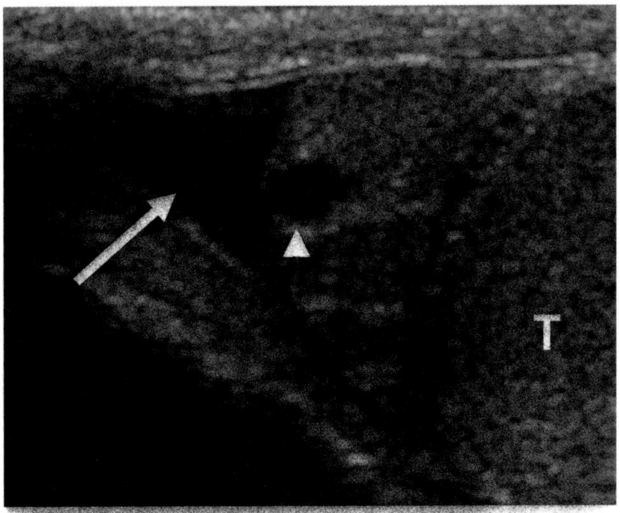

Figure 14.38. Epididymal cyst and mild hydrocele in a 7-year-old mixed-breed dog. An anechoic structure of approximately 3-mm diameter is associated with the head of the epididymis (arrowhead), just cranial to the testicle (T). The triangular anechoic area cranial to the head of the epididymis is consistent with a small volume of intrascrotal fluid (arrow).

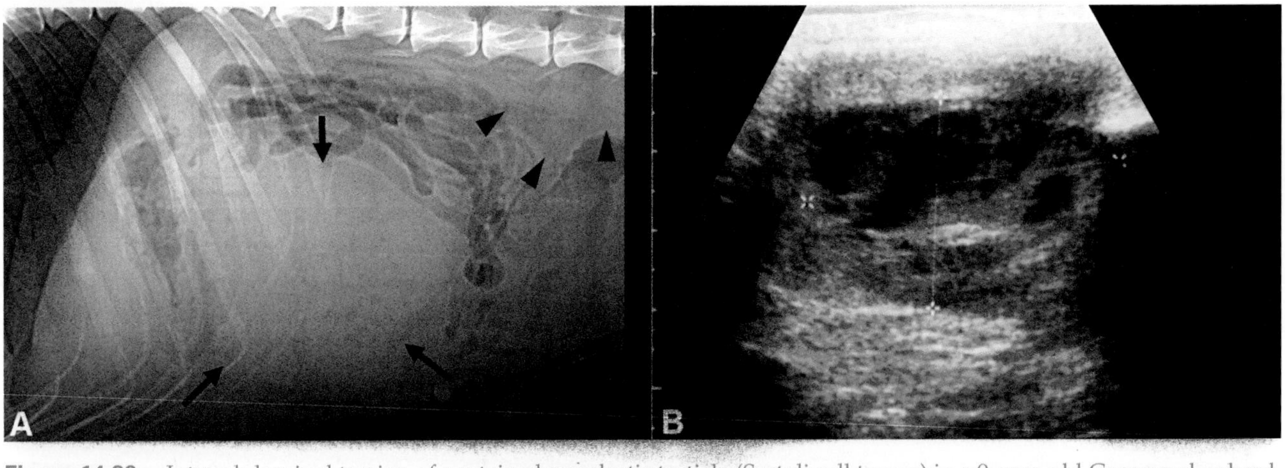

Figure 14.39. Intra-abdominal torsion of a retained neoplastic testicle (Sertoli cell tumor) in a 9-year-old German shepherd. **A:** The lateral abdominal radiograph shows a lobulated soft-tissue mass of more than 20 cm in diameter associated with the cranial ventral abdomen (arrows). Enlarged sublumbar lymph nodes (arrowheads) are consistent with metastatic disease. Prominent mammillae are noted, consistent with feminization caused by hormone-producing tumor. **B:** The ultrasonographic image shows a mixed echogenic mass (only shown in part).

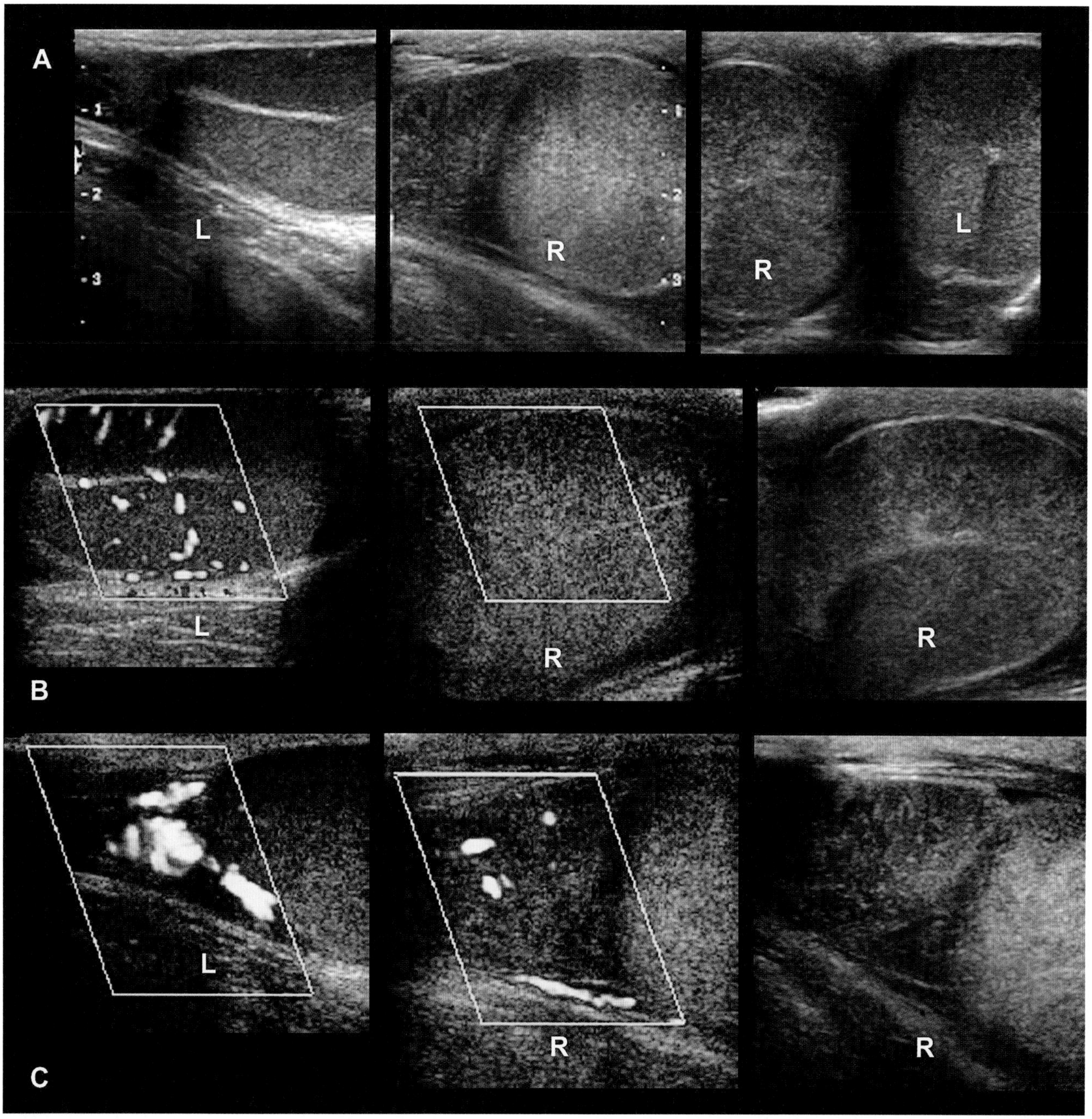

Figure 14.40. Testicular torsion in a 1-year-old Border collie. The left testis (L) is normal, whereas the right testicle (R) has hemorrhage and numerous thrombi, compatible with torsion and underlying orchitis and epididymitis. **A:** The left and right testicles are imaged side by side. There is a significant difference in size. The right testicle and epididymis are larger than the left. **B:** Comparative color Doppler signal between the left (normal) and the right testis (no flow). **C:** Comparative color Doppler signal between the left (normal) and the right epididymis (poor flow).

Testicular atrophy may have a number of causes, such as thermal insult (e.g., in cryptorchid testicles), previous orchitis, hormonal influences, or vascular compromise. Atrophic testicles are small and hypoechoic, but maintain their normal architecture (Figures 14.42 and 14.43; see also Figures 14.26 and 14.27).

Whereas ultrasonography plays a major role in assessing human patients with scrotal trauma, it is rarely performed for this indication in dogs. Findings in scrotal trauma include scrotal hematoma, hematocele, scrotal contusion, intratesticular hematoma, and testicular rupture. Scrotal hematomas with accumulation of blood within scrotal soft tissues manifest as

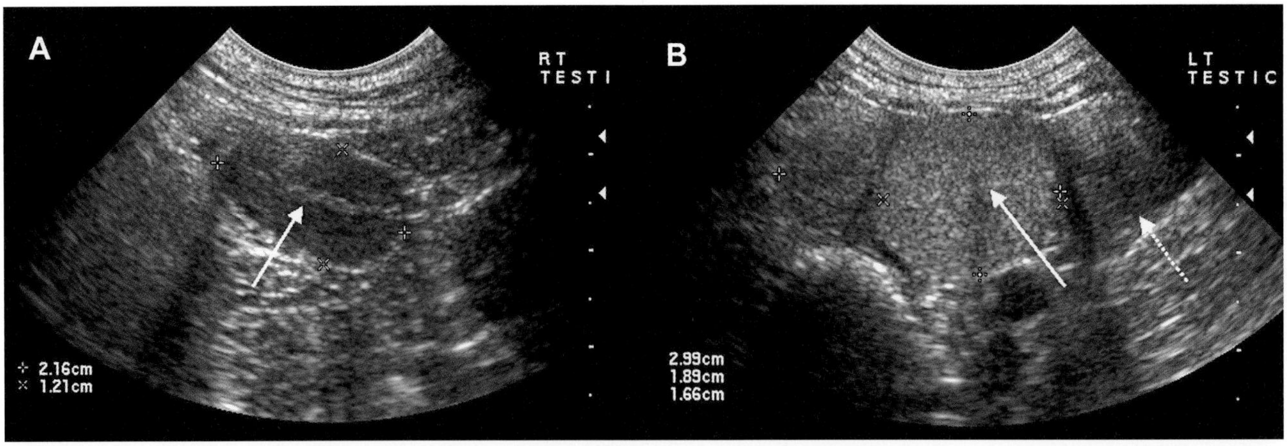

Figure 14.41. Torsion of a nonneoplastic testicle in a 6-month-old, bilaterally cryptorchid boxer. **A:** Sagittal ultrasonographic image of the right intra-abdominal atrophic testicle (between the cursors). The mediastinum testis (arrow) is within the hypoechoic testicle. **B:** Sagittal ultrasonographic image of the left intra-abdominal testicle. The testicle appears globoid rather than oval and hyperechoic compared with the right. The mediastinum testis (solid arrow) is barely recognizable. Two additional round structures are seen adjacent to the testicle and are relatively hypoechoic. They represent the enlarged head and tail (broken arrow) of the epididymis. Reprinted with permission from Hecht et al. (2004).

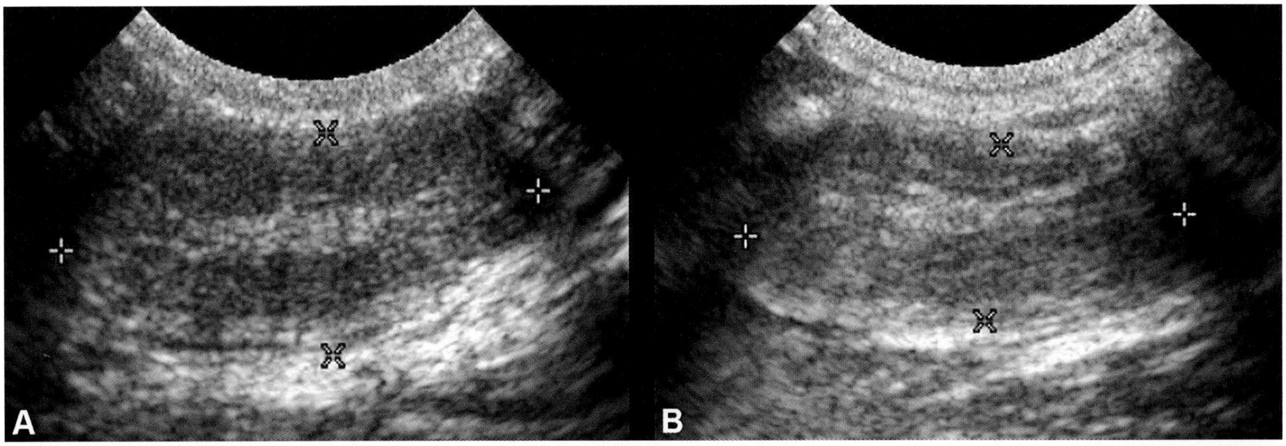

Figure 14.42. Testicular atrophy in an 8-year-old, bilaterally cryptorchid German shepherd. On sagittal image, the right testicle **(A)** and the left testicle **(B)** are small (3cm long [between the cursors]) and hypoechoic.

space-occupying lesions of variable echogenicity that displace the testicle and epididymis (Figure 14.44). In hematocele, there is intrascrotal fluid accumulation of variable echogenicity. Testicular contusion and hematoma appear as diffuse echogenic changes of testicular parenchyma or mass lesions of variable echogenicity. Differentiation from testicular lesions of inflammatory or neoplastic etiology is mainly based on medical history rather than ultrasonographic characteristics. Inhomogeneous echotexture of the testicular parenchyma with loss of contour definition indicates testicular rupture.

Hydrocele manifests as anechoic to echogenic material adjacent to the testicles. The condition is rare in dogs. It may be an occasional incidental finding, but is more commonly found secondary to a variety of scrotal disorders (e.g., orchitis and testicular torsion). It may also occur secondary to ascites when abdominal fluid descends through the inguinal ring (Figure 14.45).

In inguinal or scrotal hernia, abnormal contents (e.g., bowel loops or mesenteric fat) may be found within the inguinal ring or scrotum. Concurrent findings include hydrocele and testicular congestion or infarction.

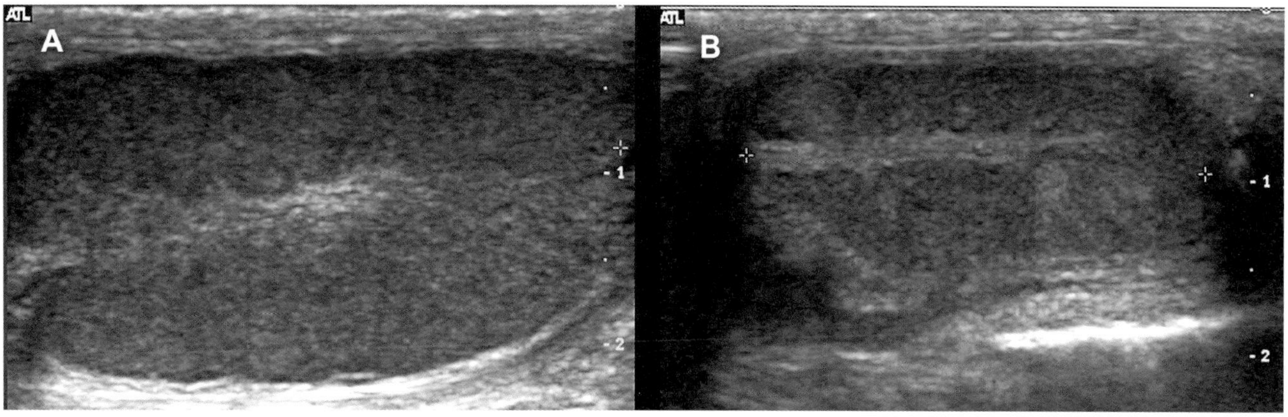

Figure 14.43. Testicular atrophy of unknown etiology in a 12-year-old Doberman. **A:** Sagittal image of normal right testicle. The testicle measures 3.8 cm long (between the cursors), is of normal medium echogenicity, homogeneous, with centrally located linear hyperechoic mediastinum testis. **B:** Sagittal image of atrophic left testicle. The testicle is smaller than the right (2.7 cm long [between the cursors]), hypoechoic, and slightly inhomogeneous. Centrally located mediastinum testis is unremarkable.

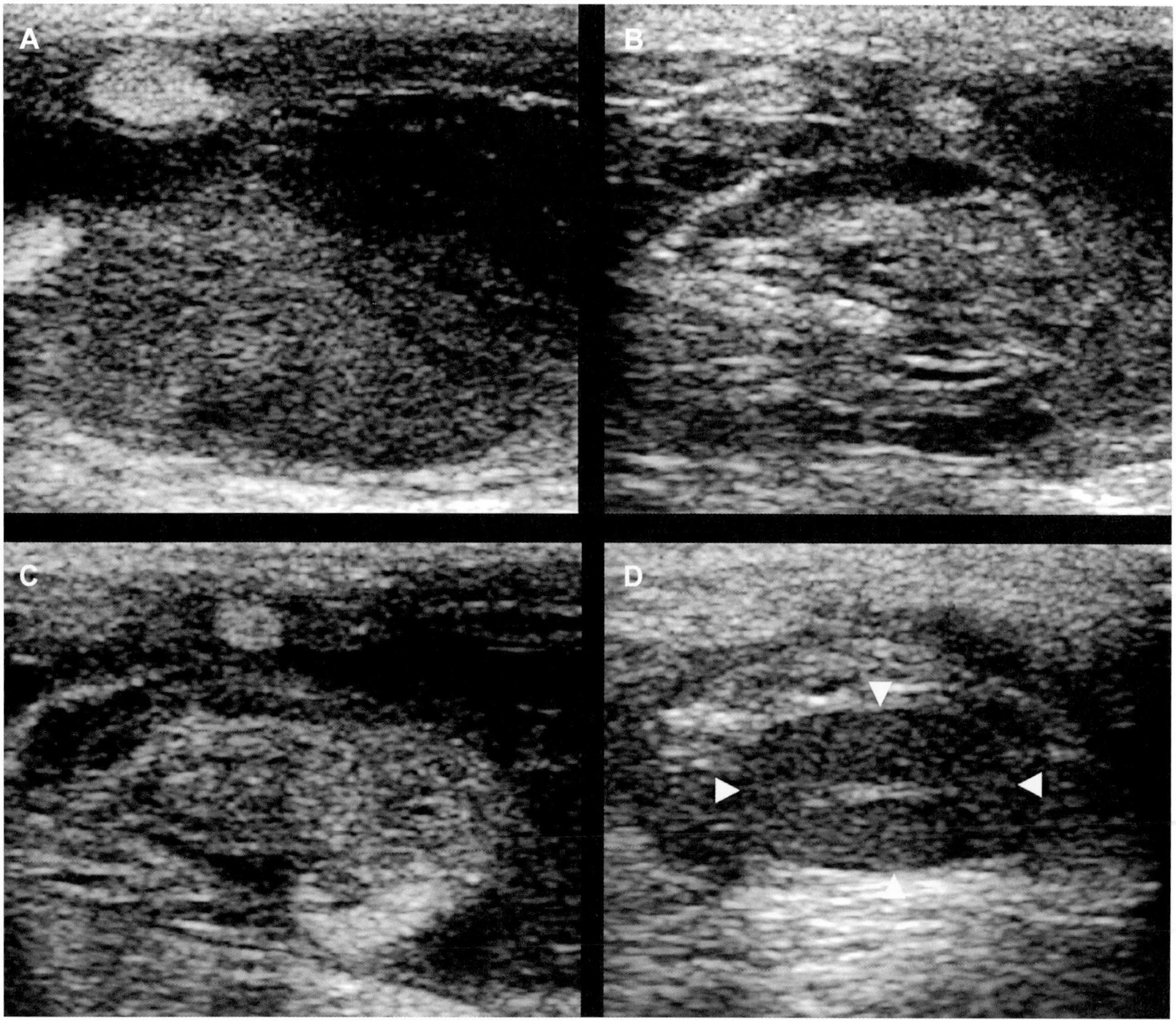

Figure 14.44. Blunt scrotal trauma in a 5-month-old dog. **A–C:** The scrotum is enlarged and filled with material of mixed echogenicity, representing a hematoma at varying stages of organization. **D:** The left testicle (arrowheads) is displaced and surrounded by material of mixed echogenicity.

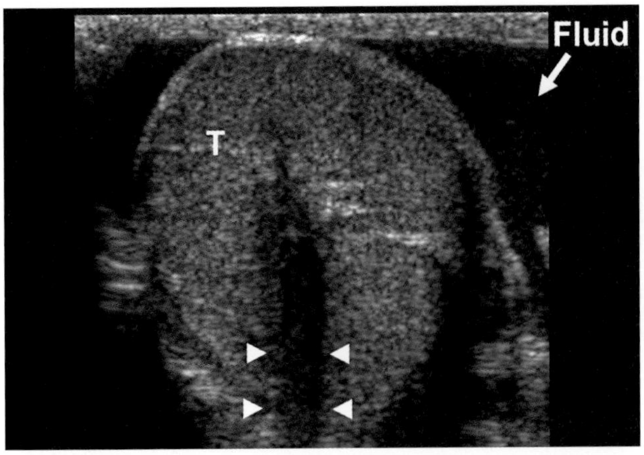

Figure 14.45. Transverse image of the right hemiscrotum in a 9-year-old dog with ascites and subsequent hydrocele. The testicle (T) is surrounded by anechoic fluid. Acoustic shadowing (arrowheads) is observed distal to the centrally located mediastinum testis.

Penis

Normal Sonographic Anatomy of the Penis

At the level of the distal penis, the smooth, hyperechoic interface of the os penis is surrounded by penile soft tissues (glans penis) and prepuce. The urethra is located within a V-shaped ventral groove in the os penis and is usually not visible unless distended (Figure 14.46). Proximal to the osseous part, penile soft tissues (corpus cavernosum, corpus spongiosum, and muscles of the penis) are of medium echogenicity and inconspicuous.

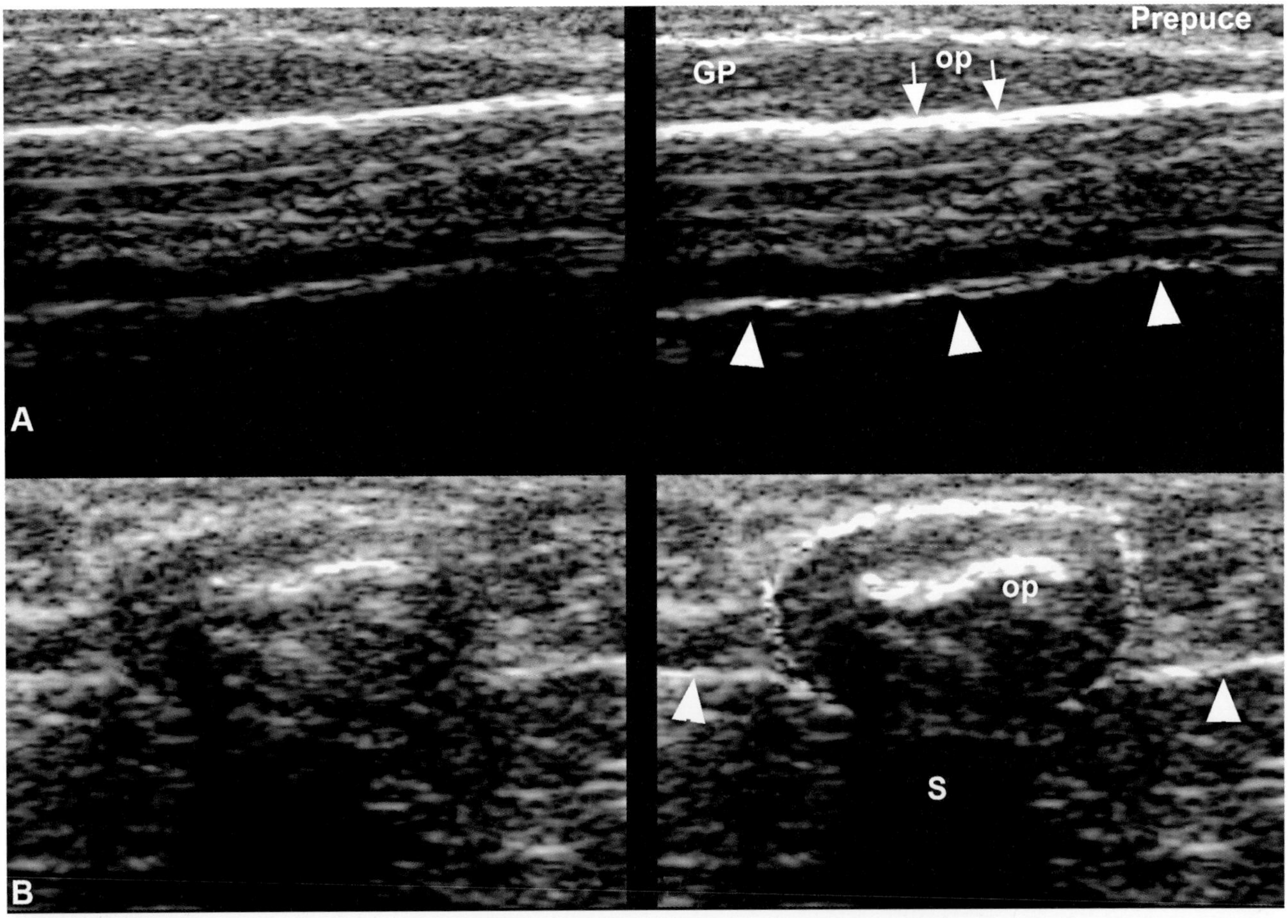

Figure 14.46. Normal canine penis. Sagittal **(A)** and transverse **(B)** sonographic and schematic images of the penis in a 6-year-old, neutered, mixed-breed dog. On sagittal view **(A)**, prepuce and part of the glans penis (GP) are in the near field ventral to the linear strongly hyperechoic interface of the os penis (op outlined by arrows). In the far field, penile soft tissues and the abdominal wall (arrowheads) are visible. On transverse view **(B)**, the hyperechoic os penis (op) is characterized by distal shadowing (S). Differentiation of surrounding penile soft tissues is not possible on this image. The urethra is not visible. Shadowing (S) is noted distal to the os penis. Surrounding penile soft tissues are symmetrical.

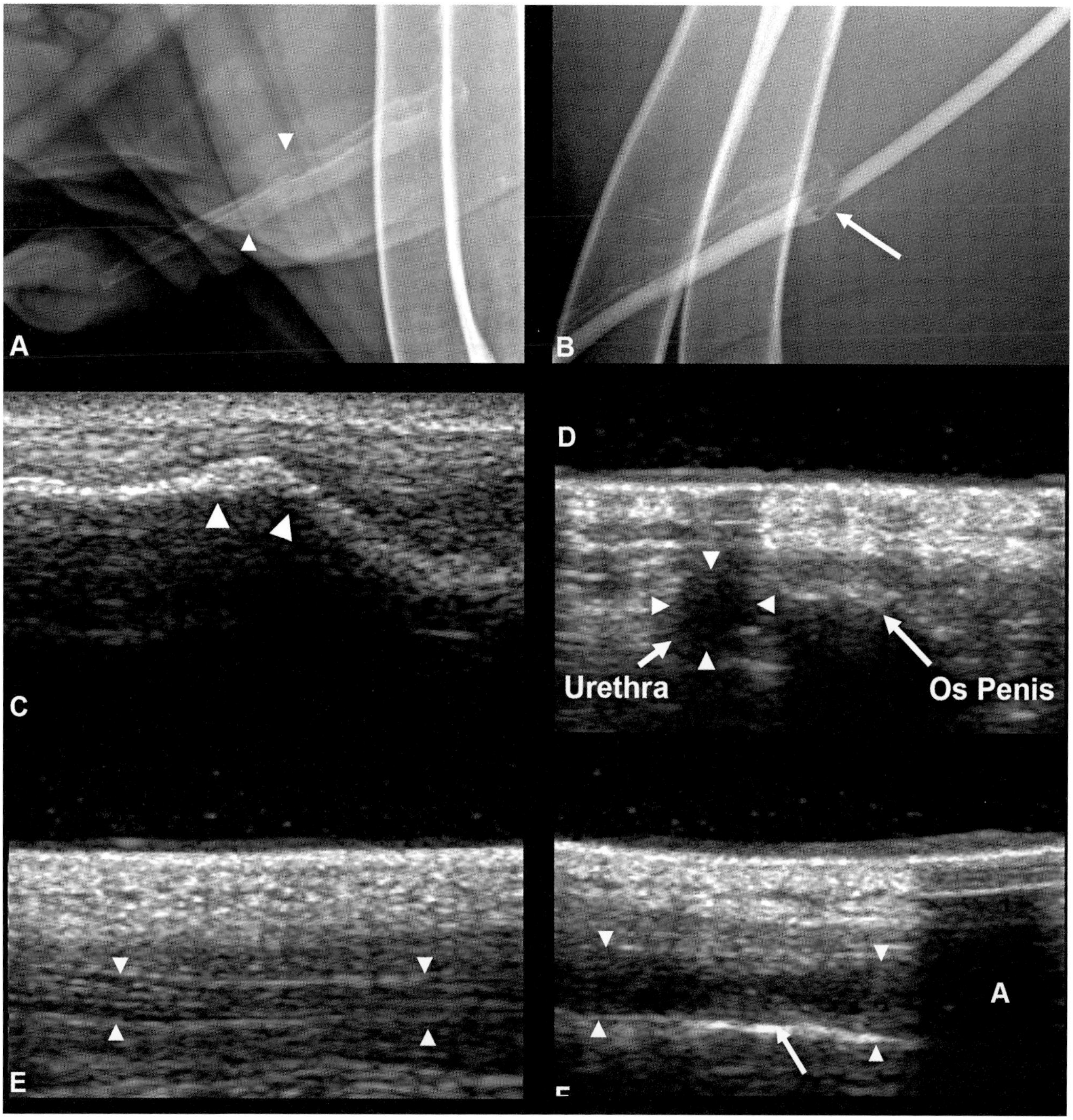

Figure 14.47. Healed fracture of the os penis and mural urethral lesion (urethritis) in a 6-year-old mastiff with dysuria. **A:** The lateral radiograph shows irregularity of penile contour at the midbody of os penis (arrowheads), consistent with previous fracture. **B:** Urethrogram demonstrating a filling defect associated with the prostatic urethra at the most caudal level of the os penis (arrow). **C:** Sagittal ultrasonographic image of the midbody of the os penis. There is an irregular contour to the hyperechoic interface of the os penis at the previous fracture site (arrowheads). **D:** Transverse image of the penis during instillation of saline to facilitate urethral identification. The os penis is characterized by its irregular hyperechoic surface and distal shadowing. The fluid-distended urethra is visible as an anechoic circular structure (arrowheads) lateral to the os penis. The unusual urethral position was attributed to previous trauma. The anechoic area in the near field represents part of the standoff pad. **E:** Sagittal image of the urethra, which appears as an inconspicuous tubular structure (arrowheads). The anechoic area in the near field represents part of the standoff pad. **F:** Sagittal image of the urethra during instillation of saline. The urethra (arrowheads) is fluid filled. The filling defect identified during the urethrogram manifests as urethral wall thickening and irregularity (arrow). The hypoechoic area to the right of the **A** is artifactual because of poor transducer-to-skin contact. The anechoic area in the near field represents part of the standoff pad.

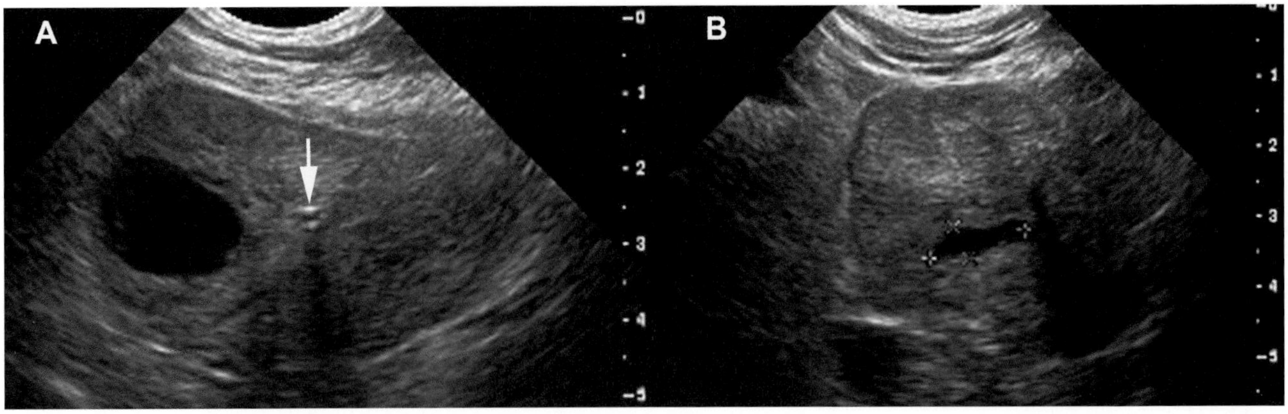

Figure 14.48. Drainage of prostatic abscess in a 3-year-old Border collie. **A:** Transverse sonogram of the prostate with right lobe abscess. The arrow points to the urethral catheter placed to better identify and avoid the urethra during the procedure. **B:** Transverse sonogram of the prostate after drainage. The abscess cavity is nearly collapsed.

Sonographic Findings in Penile Abnormalities

Common abnormalities of the penis warranting ultrasonographic examination include urethral calculi, fracture or neoplasia of the os penis, or urethral lesions such as tumor or stricture. Lesions of the os penis cause discontinuity of its osseous contour (Figure 14.47). Concurrent soft-tissue changes may be encountered, especially in acute trauma. Urethrography remains the imaging modality of choice for assessing urethral patency and integrity.

Interventional Procedures

Percutaneous fine-needle aspiration or biopsy of the prostate is easily performed. The same principles and precautions used in other interventional procedures apply. To avoid urethral injury during the procedure, a urinary catheter should be placed to facilitate identification of the prostatic urethra. In cases of suspected prostatic neoplasia, sampling by means of traumatic catheterization or prostatic massage should be given preference because of the risk of implantation of metastases along the needle tract after percutaneous aspiration (Nyland et al. 2002).

Percutaneous drainage of prostatic abscesses and in situ injection of antibiotics is a valid alternative method to surgical intervention, especially in immunocompromised patients (Boland et al. 2003) (Figure 14.48). Percutaneous drainage of paraprostatic cysts can be performed to temporarily relieve patient discomfort. However, recurrent filling usually warrants surgery at a later stage.

Fine-needle aspiration or biopsy of intra-abdominal testicular tumors is commonly performed, following the same principles and precautions as in biopsies of other abdominal organs. Fine-needle aspiration of intrascrotal testicles is infrequently performed in veterinary medicine. However, the procedure has a high accuracy in the diagnosis of testicular neoplasms, with a low risk of adverse effects (Dorsch et al. 2006).

References

Atalan G, Holt PE, Barr FJ (1999) Ultrasonographic estimation of prostate size in normal dogs and relationship to bodyweight and age. J Small Anim Pract 40:119–122.

Boland LE, Hardie RJ, Gregory SP, Lamb CR (2003) Ultrasound-guided percutaneous drainage as the primary treatment for prostatic abscesses and cysts in dogs. J Am Anim Hosp Assoc 39:151–159.

Dorsch R, Majzoub M, Hecht S, Hartmann K, Hirschberger J (2006) Diagnostische Wertigkeit der Hodenzytologie beim Hund. Tieraerztl Prax 34:91–98.

Feeney DA, Johnston GR, Klausner JS, Bell FJ (1989) Canine prostatic ultrasonography: 1989. Semin Vet Med Surg (Small Anim) 4:44–57.

Hecht S (2001) Sonographische Diagnostik des Skrotalinhaltes beim Hund unter besonderer Beruecksichtigung testikulaerer Neoplasien [PhD thesis]. Munich: Chirurgische Tierklinik, Ludwig-Maximilians University.

Hecht S, King R, Tidwell AS, Gorman SC (2004) Ultrasound diagnosis: Intra-abdominal torsion of a non-neoplastic testicle in a cryptorchid dog. Vet Radiol Ultrasound 45:58–61.

Hecht S, Matiasek K, Koestlin R (2003) Die sonographische Untersuchung des Skrotalinhaltes beim Hund unter besonderer Beruecksichtigung testikulaerer Neoplasien. Tieraerztl Prax 31:199–210.

Johnston GR, Feeney DA, Johnston SD, O'Brien TD (1991a) Ultrasonographic features of testicular neoplasia in dogs: 16 cases (1980–1988). J Am Vet Med Assoc 198:1779–1784.

Johnston GR, Feeney DA, Rivers B, Walter PA (1991b) Diagnostic imaging of the male canine reproductive organs: Methods and limitations. Vet Clin North Am Small Anim Pract 21:553–589.

Johnston SD, Kamolpatana K, Root-Kustritz MV, Johnston GR (2000) Prostatic disorders in the dog. Anim Reprod Sci 60–61:405–415.

Mattoon JS, Nyland TG (2002) Prostate and testes. In: Nyland TG, Mattoon JS, eds. Small Animal Diagnostic Ultrasound. Philadelphia: WB Saunders, pp. 250–266.

Miyabashi T, Biller DS, Cooley AJ (1990) Ultrasonographic appearance of torsion of a testicular seminoma in a cryptorchid dog. J Small Anim Pract 31:401–403.

Nyland TG, Wallack ST, Wisner ER (2002) Needle-tract implantation following US-guided fine-needle aspiration biopsy of transitional cell carcinoma of the bladder, urethra, and prostate. Vet Radiol Ultrasound 43:50–53.

Ober CP, Spaulding K, Breitschwerdt EB, Malarkey DE, Hegarty BC (2004) Orchitis in two dogs with Rocky Mountain spotted fever. Vet Radiol Ultrasound 45:458–465.

Pugh CR, Konde LJ (1991) Sonographic evaluation of canine testicular and scrotal abnormalities: A review of 26 case histories. Vet Radiol Ultrasound 32:243–250.

Pugh CR, Konde LJ, Park RD (1990) Testicular ultrasound in the normal dog. Vet Radiol Ultrasound 31:195–199.

Ruel Y, Barthez PY, Mailles A, Begon D (1998) Ultrasonographic evaluation of the prostate in healthy intact dogs. Vet Radiol Ultrasound 39:212–216.

Stowater JL, Lamb CR (1989) Ultrasonographic features of paraprostatic cysts in nine dogs. Vet Radiol Ultrasound 30:232–239.

Winter MD, Locke JE, Penninck DG (2006) Imaging diagnosis: Urinary obstruction secondary to prostatic lymphoma in a young dog. Vet Radiol Ultrasound 47:597–601.

Zohil AM, Castellano C (1995) Prepubic and transrectal ultrasonography of the canine prostate: A comparative study. Vet Radiol Ultrasound 36:393–396.

CHAPTER FIFTEEN

Abdominal Cavity, Lymph Nodes, and Great Vessels

Marc-André d'Anjou

Preparation and Scanning Technique

To have access to all portions of the abdominal cavity of dogs and cats, hair must be clipped ventrally and laterally between the costal arch and caudal margin of the abdomen. Clipping may be extended more cranially in deep-chested dogs to better visualize the subcostal region. After the application of acoustic gel, the animal can be scanned in dorsal, left, or right recumbency. Some disorders of the peritoneal space, such as effusion or free air, respond to gravity and may require repositioning the animal to reach a diagnosis.

Ultrasonographic probes must be selected according to the size of the animal and the depth of the evaluated region(s). A high-frequency probe (7.5 MHz and higher) is recommended in cats and in small dogs or if superficial structures are examined, whereas probes with more penetration (5.0–7.5 MHz and lower) are generally indicated in larger dogs. Disorders affecting the attenuation of the ultrasound beam may also influence the probe selection. For example, peritoneal transudation is associated with reduced sound attenuation, as opposed to inflammatory or neoplastic processes involving the omentum that typically produce increased ultrasound attenuation. In these instances, probes with a higher or lower frequency, respectively, may improve image quality. Sectorial or convex probes are preferred because they can reach all portions of the abdomen, including the subcostal region, as opposed to linear probes, which have a larger footprint. Doppler evaluation of abdominal vascular structures requires the use of dedicated probes and software.

Ultrasonographic Anatomy of the Normal Peritoneal Cavity, Fat, Vessels, and Lymph Nodes

The peritoneum is composed of a thin serous membrane that is divided into parietal and visceral components. The peritoneal cavity is a potential space located between these two layers that contains only a small volume of fluid that serves as a lubricant. However, this amount of fluid is usually not detectable with ultrasound. The peritoneum appears as a smooth hyperechoic interface that is better appreciated when a moderate volume of ascites is present. A variable amount of fat is present, mainly in the falciform ligament, omentum, mesentery, and retroperitoneum. The fat appears coarse in echotexture and relatively isoechoic to the liver. The mesentery contains vessels and lymph nodes that can be visualized in most patients.

A thorough knowledge of vascular anatomy and hemodynamics is necessary to facilitate the identification and assessment of abdominal vessels (Evans 1993a, 1993b; Spaulding 1997; Finnn-Bodner and Hudson 1998; Szatmari et al. 2001).

A schematic illustration of the principal vessels in the abdomen, as well as major lymph nodes, of dogs and cats is presented in Figure 15.1. Although the arterial flow of all structures is supplied by the abdominal aorta, the venous flow is separated between the portal system and the systemic circulation (see the Extrahepatic Portal Vasculature section in Chapter 6). In comparison with the portal system, a limited number of

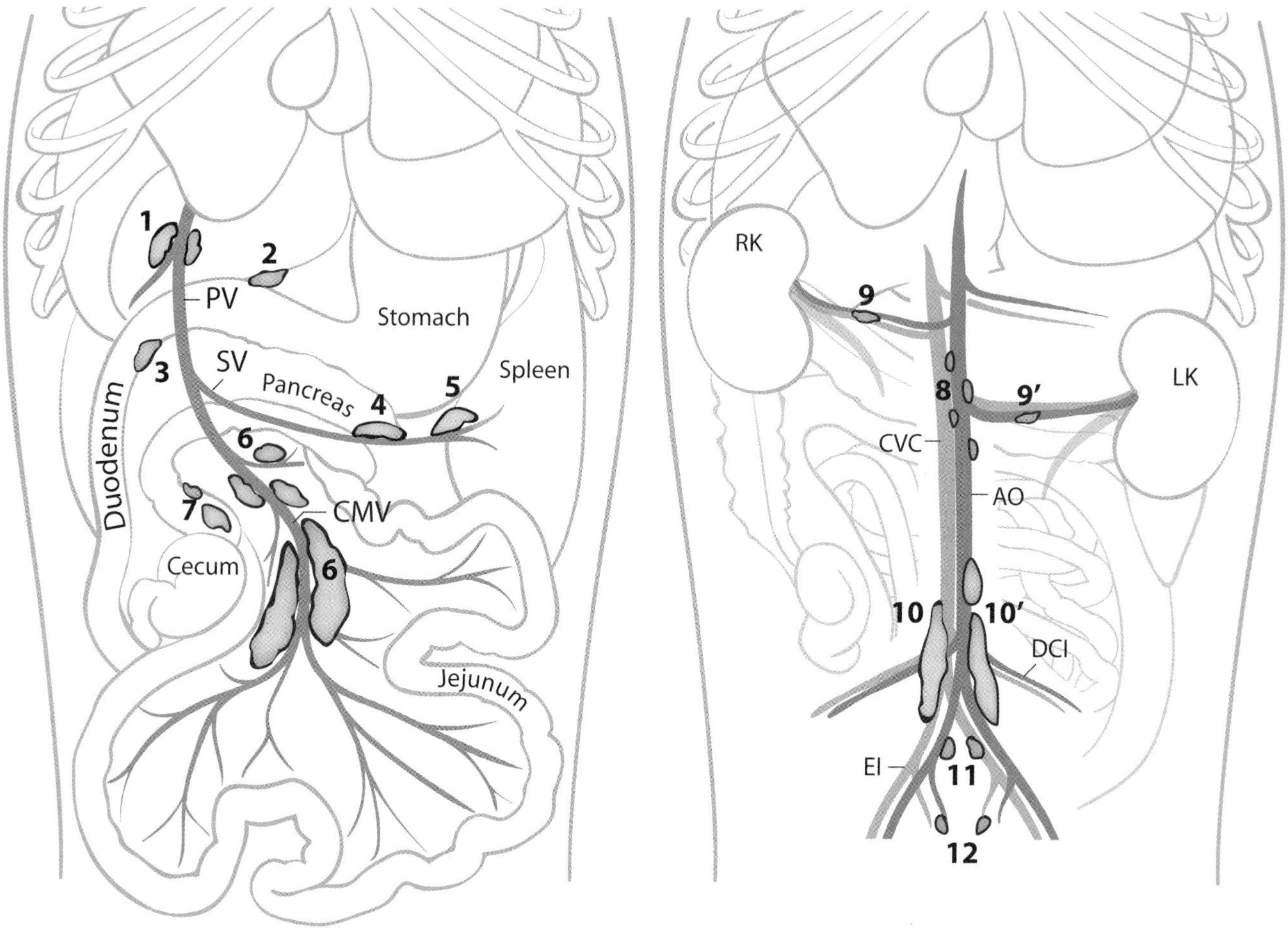

Figure 15.1. Schematic illustration of abdominal lymph nodes and major vessels. Note the intimate anatomical relationship between lymph nodes and vessels. **Lymph nodes:** 1, hepatic; 2, gastric; 3, pancreaticoduodenal; 4 and 5, splenic; 6, jejunal; 7, colic; 8, aortic; 9 and 9′, renal; 10 and 10′, medial iliac; 11, hypogastric; and 12, sacral. **Vessels:** AO, aorta; CMV, cranial mesenteric vein; CVC, caudal vena cava; DCI, deep circumflex iliac vessels; EI, external iliac vessels; PV, portal vein; and SV, splenic vein. **Other landmarks:** LK, left kidney; and RK, right kidney.

abdominal veins drain into the caudal vena cava (CVC). The CVC crosses the abdomen from caudal to cranial, remaining on the right of the midline. Visible veins with B-mode ultrasonography include, from cranial to caudal, hepatic veins, phrenicoabdominal veins, renal veins, and iliac veins (deep circumflex, common, external, and internal). The aorta is more dorsal than the CVC in the cranial abdomen and remains on the left side. Major abdominal branches of the aorta that can be localized ultrasonographically include, from cranial to caudal: celiac artery (left gastric, hepatic, and splenic arteries), cranial mesenteric and renal arteries. These vessels are useful landmarks for identifying abdominal lymph nodes. Lymph nodes are routinely evaluated in small animal patients, because the nodes drain several organs and structures. Table 15.1 lists the location and drainage of the abdominal lymph nodes in dogs and cats (Bezuidenhout 1993; Pugh 1994).

In dogs, several lymph nodes can be routinely identified (Spaulding 1997; Llabrés-Diaz 2004). Some can also be detected in cats. These lymph nodes are uniformly echogenic, relatively isoechoic or slightly hypoechoic to the adjacent fatty tissues, smooth, and fusiform to oval (Pugh 1994; Llabrés-Diaz 2004) (Figure 15.2). A thin hyperechoic capsule is often identified, and occasionally a normal hyperechoic central line can be seen crossing these nodes in the region of the nodal hilus. Although anatomical size references have been reported in dogs for normal lymph nodes (maximal 5-mm thickness) (Bezuidenhout 1993), reference ranges that can be reliably used with ultrasonography have not been reported for all sizes of dogs and cats. In the author's experience, lymph nodes can reach 7–8 mm

Table 15.1.
Location and drainage of abdominal lymph nodes

Lymph Node	Location	Drainage Areas
Hepatic	Along the portal vein, caudal to the *porta hepatis*	Liver, stomach, duodenum, and pancreas
Splenic	Along the splenic veins and the left pancreatic lobe	Liver, spleen, esophagus, stomach, pancreas, and omentum
Gastric	Near the pylorus	Diaphragm, liver, esophagus, stomach, duodenum, pancreas, and peritoneum
Pancreaticoduodenal	Near the cranial duodenal flexure, between the pylorus and the right pancreatic limb	Duodenum, pancreas, and omentum
Jejunal	Along the mesenteric vascular tree (cranial mesenteric artery and vein)	Jejunum, ileum, and pancreas
Colic	Near the ileocolic junction and mesocolon	Ileum, cecum, and colon
Lumbar aortic	Along aorta	Kidneys, adrenals, bladder, uterus, prostate, and gonads
Medial iliac, hypogastric, and sacral	At the caudal aortic trifurcation, between the deep circumflex and the external iliac arteries (medial), medial to the internal iliac arteries (hypogastric) and along the median sacral artery (sacral)	Ureters, bladder, uterus, prostate, gonads, peripelvic and pubic areas, abdominal skin, and muscles

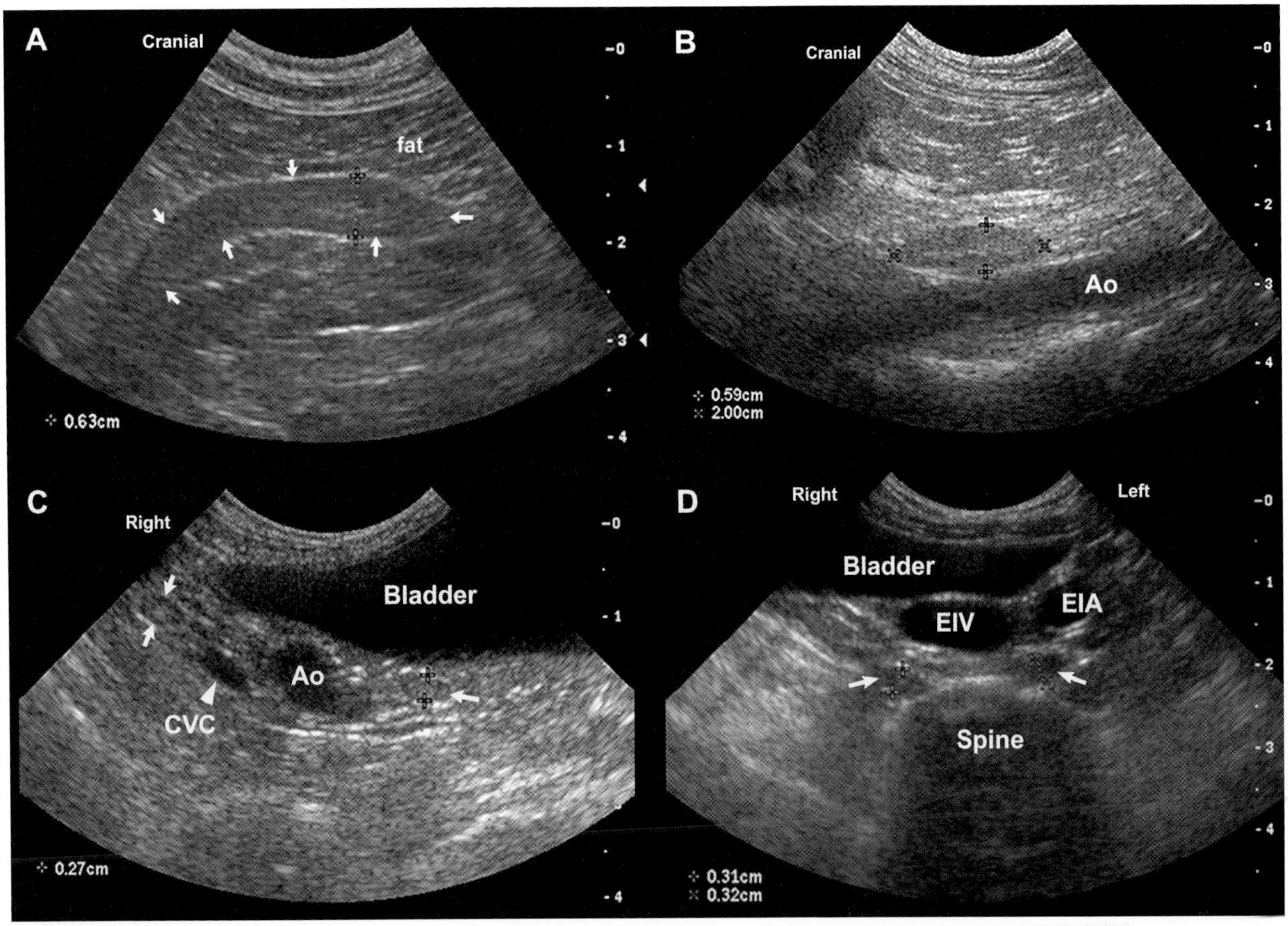

Figure 15.2. Normal lymph nodes. **A and B:** Longitudinal ultrasonographic images of normal mesenteric (**A**, arrows) and medial iliac (**B**, cursors) lymph nodes in two dogs. The nodes are fusiform, well defined, uniform, and mildly hypoechoic compared with the peripheral fat. The short-to-long axis ratio is less than 0.5. Ao, aorta. **C and D:** Transverse images of normal medial iliac (**C**, arrows) and hypogastric (**D**, arrows) lymph nodes in another dog. Note the proximity of these nodes to the urinary bladder and to the caudal vena cava (CVC) and aorta (Ao), as well as their branches (EIA and EIV: left external iliac artery and vein). The spine is located just dorsal to the hypogastric nodes and appears as a strongly shadowing interface.

thick in large normal dogs. The shape of these nodes may actually represent a more useful landmark. A ratio comparing the short and long axes should be less than 0.5 in normal nodes (Llabrés-Diaz 2004; Nyman et al. 2004).

Lymph nodes routinely identified include the jejunal (or mesenteric) and medial iliac lymph nodes. Jejunal nodes appear as a group of fusiform nodes aligned with the cranial mesenteric artery and vein and their branches within the omentum. Some of these nodes can be relatively long. The iliosacral lymphocenter is the group formed by the sublumbar lymph nodes, which are located along the caudal aortic trifurcation. The medial iliac lymph nodes, which are typically larger than the other nodes, may be more easily identified from a lateral flank approach rather than from the ventral abdomen, because the former allows placing the probe closer to the node and avoiding the descending colon (Llabrés-Diaz 2004).

Peritoneal Effusion

Peritoneal effusion can be detected with ultrasonography if the volume of free fluid exceeds approximately 2 mL/kg, which is half of what is needed for a radiographic diagnosis (Henley et al. 1989). Even smaller amounts of effusion are likely identified with more recent ultrasound systems. Peritoneal fluid distribution depends on its nature and on gravity. Free fluid moves with gravity, between abdominal organs, and locates itself according to the position of the animal. Free fluid is more likely to be detected when scanning the dependent portion of a dog that is in lateral recumbency (Boysen et al. 2004). Small volumes of free fluid can be identified at the left lateral margin of the spleen, between hepatic lobes or intestinal loops, or cranial to the apex of the bladder (Spaulding 1993), often as triangular foci that are anechoic or hypoechoic to the surrounding tissues (Figure 15.3). However, trapped or loculated fluids can remain in the nondependent portion of the abdomen. Trapped fluids are more commonly associated with chronic exudates. Care must be taken not to confuse free or trapped peritoneal fluid with fluid-filled structures, such as severe hydronephrosis, hydroureter, dilated bowel loops, or cysts (Figure 15.4A). Structures such as bowel loops or mesenteric folds are usually observed moving within the fluid, particularly if a large volume of peritoneal fluid is present (Figure 15.4B).

The echogenicity of the peritoneal fluid is usually proportional to its content in cells and other debris, which act as ultrasound reflectors (Spaulding 1993; Hanbidge et al. 2003). Low cellular fluids, such as pure or modified transudates, are typically anechoic to hypoechoic (Figures 15.4 and 15.5), in comparison with exudates, which are typically moderately echogenic

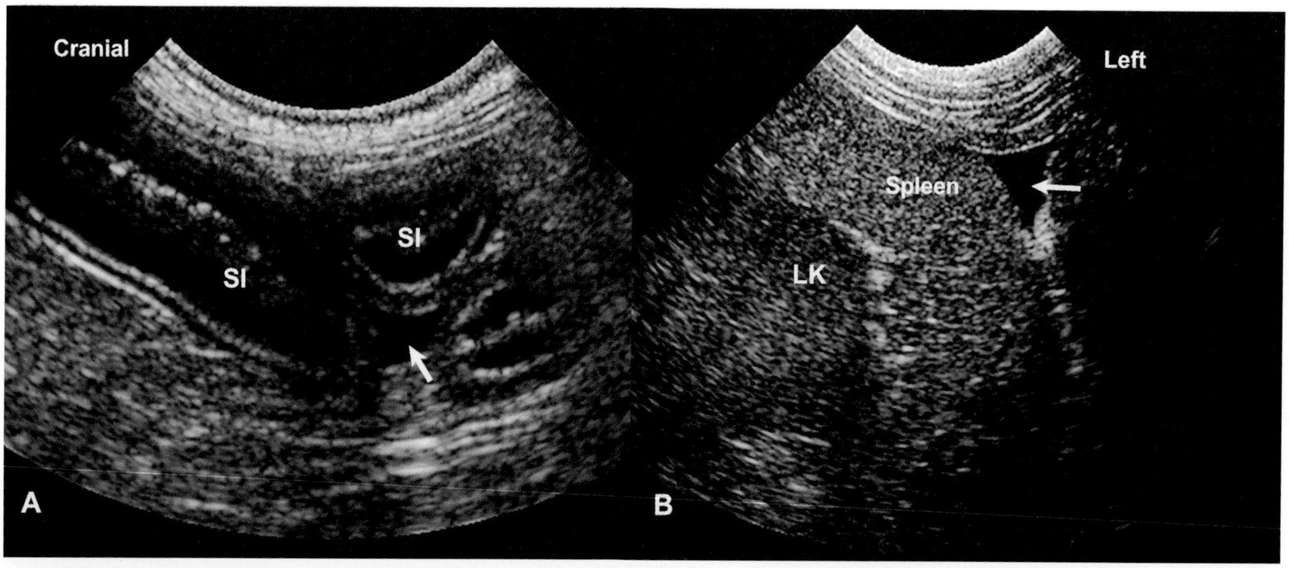

Figure 15.3. Mild peritoneal effusion. Longitudinal **(A)** and transverse **(B)** images obtained in a dog with hypoproteinemia in the midventral and left-lateral portions of the abdomen, respectively. Small triangular anechoic foci (arrows) are between small intestinal loops (SI) and lateral to the spleen, consistent with a low cellular fluid. A pure transudate was aspirated under ultrasound guidance. LK, left kidney.

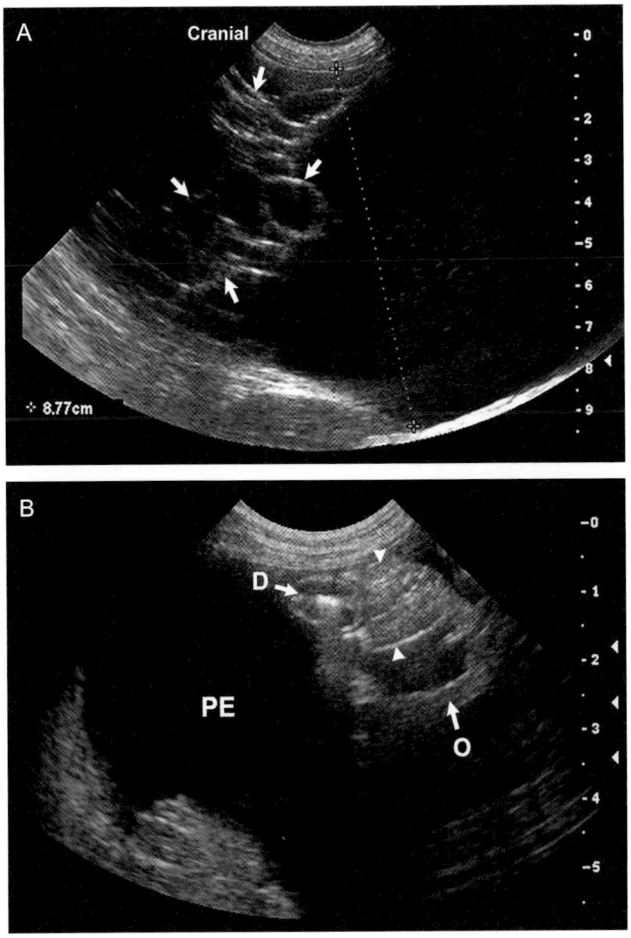

Figure 15.4. Loculated fluid compared with peritoneal effusion. **A:** Longitudinal image obtained in the right abdominal quadrant of a cat with a chronically distended abdomen. A large fluid-filled multiloculated cyst is identified, displacing all surrounding structures. Several septa (arrows) are seen throughout this benign cavitary structure that originated from the omentum. **B:** Transverse image obtained in the right cranial abdomen of a dog with cardiac tamponade. The peritoneal space is distended by a large volume of anechoic effusion (PE). The descending duodenum (D), pancreas (arrowheads), and omentum (O) are distinctly visualized within the contrasting anechoic fluid.

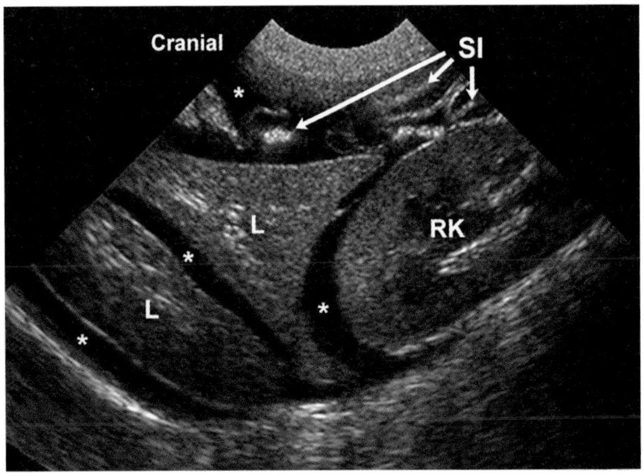

Figure 15.5. Modified transudate. Longitudinal image obtained in the right cranial abdomen of a dog with peritoneal effusion. Several structures, such as liver lobes (L), right kidney (RK), and small intestinal loops (SI) are separated by anechoic areas (*). The appearance of this effusion is suggestive of a pure or modified transudate rather than an exudate.

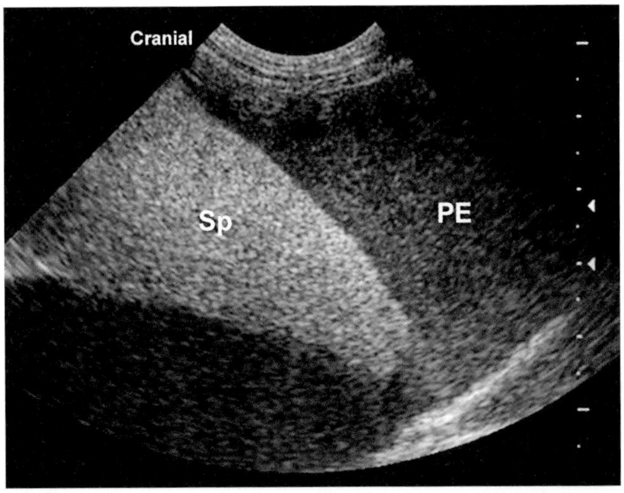

Figure 15.6. Echogenic peritoneal effusion. Longitudinal image of a dog with abdominal distension and pain. A large volume of particulate, echogenic, peritoneal effusion (PE) is seen around the spleen (Sp). These features are suggestive of a cellular effusion, such as exudate or hemorrhage. A diagnosis of septic peritonitis was made based on fluid aspiration.

(Figure 15.6). Highly cellular and homogeneous purulent exudates can actually appear isoechoic to soft-tissue organs, such as the spleen, and sometimes be recognized only because of their visible motion and lack of vascularity. Exudates can also be septated because of fibrin strands that commonly develop with this type of effusion, particularly with purulent peritonitis (Spaulding 1993).

Peritoneal hemorrhage varies in appearance according to the interval between the onset of bleeding and the time of the ultrasonographic exam. Fresh peritoneal blood may appear anechoic or echogenic, with swirling of particles within the fluid (Hanbidge et al. 2003; Pintar et al. 2003). Hematomas can develop and initially appear as homogeneous echogenic masses. Lysis of the hematoma produces a more heterogeneous appearance, with the formation of cystic areas and

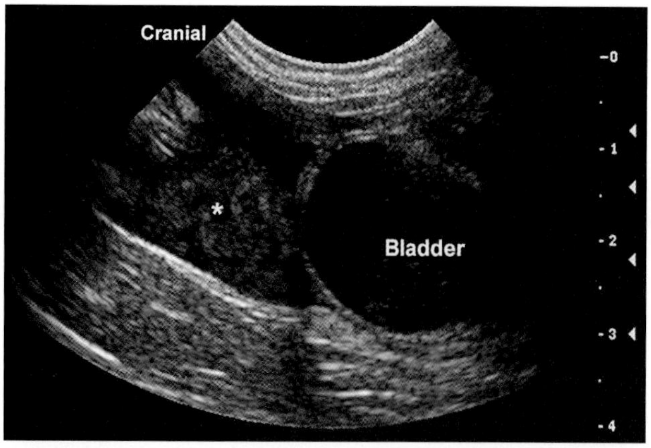

Figure 15.7. Hemoabdomen. Longitudinal image of the caudal abdomen of a cat diagnosed with multifocal biliary carcinomas. Floating, echogenic structures (*), not attached to any structure and consistent with blood clots, were identified cranial to the bladder.

Table 15.2.
Typical ultrasonographic appearance of peritoneal effusions

Ultrasonographic Appearance	Diagnostic Differential
Anechoic or hypoechoic fluid	Pure or modified transudate Serohemorrhagic fluid Urine leak Chylous effusion
Echogenic with mobile particles	Fresh hemorrhage Modified transudate Purulent exudate or loculated abscess Serosanguinous exudate Carcinomatosis Chylous effusion
Highly echogenic with fibrous strands	Purulent exudate
Mobile echogenic masses	Blood clots Masses or nodules attached to the mesentery, omentum or visceral serosa (carcinomatosis)

septa (Hanbidge et al. 2003) (Figure 15.7). In a previous study of dogs with nontraumatic hemoabdomen, a malignancy was identified in 80% and hemangiosarcoma in 70% of cases (Pintar et al. 2003).

However, it must be pointed out that some overlap exists in regard to the echogenic appearance of different types of fluids. Hence, modified transudates may look similar to exudates. Other ultrasonographic findings, such as the presence of nodules on the surface of the peritoneum in cases of carcinomatosis or with the presence of a large splenic mass, should be used to orient the diagnosis.

Table 15.2 describes the typical appearance of variable types of peritoneal effusion (Spaulding 1993; Hanbidge et al. 2003) in dogs and cats.

Peritonitis, Steatitis, and Pneumoperitoneum

A variable amount of effusion is observed with peritonitis in dogs and cats, usually with moderate to high echogenicity because of the high cellular content (Boysen et al. 2003). However, in some types of peritonitis, such as feline infectious peritonitis (FIP), the effusion can be less echogenic (Spaulding 1993) (Figure 15.8A). The peritoneum, omentum, and mesentery may also appear thickened, hyperechoic, and hyperattenuated, focally or more diffusely (Hanbidge et al. 2003). These features can significantly limit the penetration of the ultrasound beam and consequently the ability to visualize and assess deep organs. In these instances, the abdominal structures appear ill-defined, and their inner architecture cannot be well recognized. An area of mesenteric fat hyperechogenicity is suggestive of inflammation (steatitis) in dogs and cats, and should be thoroughly investigated for a possible nearby source of inflammation, such as intestinal perforation or pancreatitis (Boysen et al. 2003) (Figure 15.8B).

Idiopathic omental and mesenteric sterile steatitis has also been recognized in dogs, resembling the human disease called mesenteric panniculitis (Komori et al. 2002). Although the etiology of this condition is unknown, predisposing factors could include recent surgery, retained surgical material, prior abdominal trauma, ulcerative disease, autoimmune disease, or drugs. Sonographic features reported in people include a well-defined hyperechoic mass in the root of the mesentery, displacing intestinal loops (Roson et al. 2006) (Figure 15.9). Thickening and hyperechogenicity of the mesentery can also be associated with infarction or neoplastic invasion (Hanbidge et al. 2003).

Leakage or rupture of the gastrointestinal (GI) tract is one of the most common causes of septic peritonitis in dogs and cats. GI leakage may be caused by postsurgical intestinal dehiscence, GI perforation caused

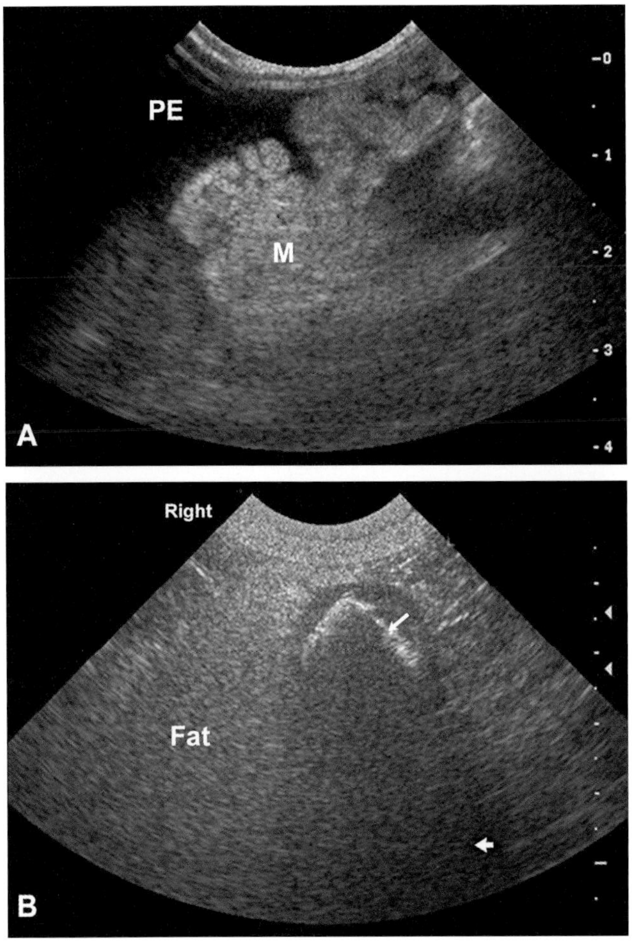

Figure 15.8. Peritonitis and steatitis. **A: Feline infectious peritonitis.** A large volume of hypoechoic peritoneal effusion (PE) is seen around a markedly thickened, irregular, hyperechoic mesentery (M). The changes to the mesentery were caused by pyogranulomatous vasculitis and steatitis (the same cat as in Figure 10.16). **B: Intestinal perforating foreign body.** Transverse image obtained in the right midabdomen of a dog with a history of acute vomiting and severe abdominal pain. A triangular hyperechoic interface (long arrow) is in a small intestinal loop, associated with far acoustic shadowing (short arrow), consistent with a foreign body. The peripheral mesenteric and omental fat is hyperechoic and hyperattenuating, and a mass effect was observed on other peripheral structures. These features are typical of steatitis caused by intestinal perforation.

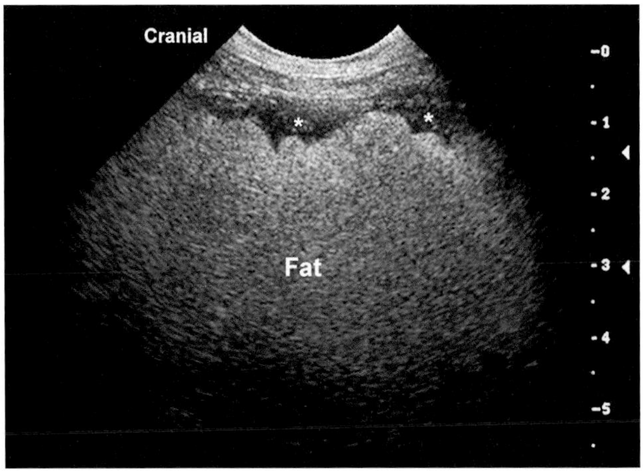

Figure 15.9. Omental steatitis. Longitudinal image of the right abdomen of a dog that had recent surgery for splenic torsion. An irregular, hyperechoic, hyperattenuating mass occupies a large portion of the right abdomen and is surrounded by hypoechoic peritoneal effusion (*). These changes were attributed to omental steatitis, possibly secondary to surgical manipulation. They eventually resolved. The ultrasonographic changes to the fat prevented any visualization of deep abdominal structures.

by a penetrating foreign body, GI ulcer (benign or malignant), gastric dilatation and volvulus, intestinal intussusception, intestinal infarction, penetrating abdominal trauma, or iatrogenic cause (Boysen et al. 2003). Inflamed perienteric fat often appears as a mass effect, displacing adjacent structures such as intestinal loops. In addition to the other aforementioned ultrasonographic changes, GI ileus with fluid accumulation is commonly observed (Boysen 2003). GI contents such as foreign material or free gas can sometimes be recognized in the peritoneal space. Free gas appears as echogenic foci or lines that are associated with reverberation artifacts such as comet tails. The lines collect between the nondependent abdominal wall and intra-abdominal structures such as the liver, omentum, stomach, or intestine (Boysen et al. 2003) (Figure 15.10). When peritoneal effusion is present, gas bubbles can appear as floating echogenic foci (Hanbidge et al. 2003). Free gas tends to shift in position with bowel or patient movement.

Spontaneous pneumoperitoneum can also be caused by abdominal wall trauma, bladder rupture, an extension of pneumothorax, splenic necrosis, clostridial peritonitis, or be idiopathic (Saunders and Tobias 2003). If a large volume of free air is in the peritoneal cavity, ultrasonographic visualization of deep structures may be significantly hampered by reverberation artifacts or shadowing. Because free air can persist several days before complete resorption, the significance of free air found in dogs or cats after surgery must be interpreted with caution, particularly if other signs of intestinal dehiscence are not present.

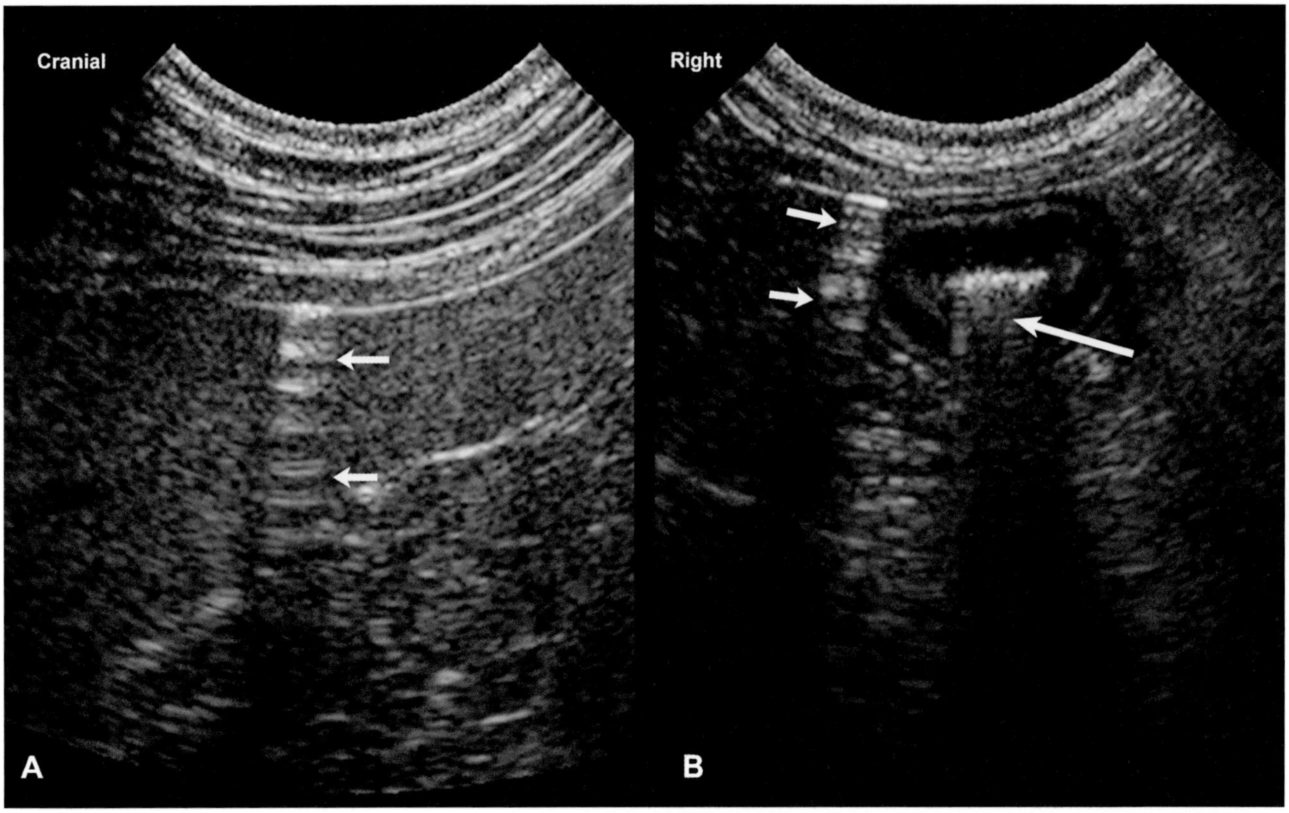

Figure 15.10. Free air in the peritoneal space. Longitudinal **(A)** and transverse **(B)** images obtained in the left cranial and mid-right abdomen of a dog that had surgery a few days earlier. Short, redundant, hyperechoic lines (short arrows), which appear as "comet tails" and are consistent with reverberation artifacts, are in the upper portion of the abdomen. These artifacts move during the exam along the inner surface of the abdominal wall, indicating free air. Air is also observed in an intestinal lumen (long arrow), associated with "dirty" acoustic shadowing.

Peritoneal Abscesses, Granulomas, and Pyogranulomas

Abscess formation can precede or follow the onset of peritonitis. Ultrasonographically, peritoneal abscesses often present as fluid pockets with particles, surrounded by an ill-defined hyperechoic wall and sometimes internal septa or gas foci (Konde et al. 1986; Hanbidge et al. 2003) (Figure 15.11). The cavitary portion of the abscess is often hypoechoic, and far acoustic enhancement may be recognized if the cell count is not too high. Conversely, caseous abscesses may be associated with some acoustic shadowing. The presence of gas in the central portion of a peritoneal mass, recognized as hyperechoic foci with reverberation artifacts, should be considered as a relatively specific sign of an abscess (Hanbidge et al. 2003).

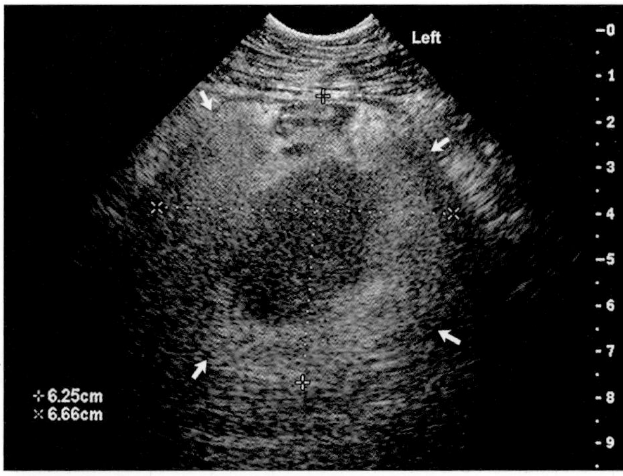

Figure 15.11. Peritoneal abscess. Transverse image of the left caudal abdomen of a dog with abdominal pain. An ill-defined hypoechoic area, surrounded by an ill-defined hyperechoic rim (arrows), is present without evidence of organ involvement. A sterile abscess, attached to the omentum and mesentery, was confirmed at surgery.

Peritoneal granulomas or pyogranulomas are rare in small animals. They can be found with feline infectious

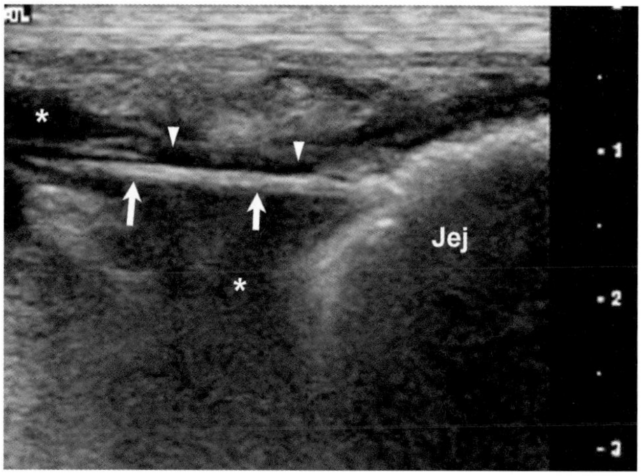

Figure 15.12. Wooden stick foreign body in a dog. A hyperechoic linear interface consistent with a stick (arrows) is noted, surrounded by a hypoechoic cast of inflammatory cells (arrowheads). The stick was impaling a segment of jejunum (Jej) and the left kidney (the same dog as in Figure 10.28A). A small amount of free fluid (*) is near the perforation site. Image courtesy of D. Penninck.

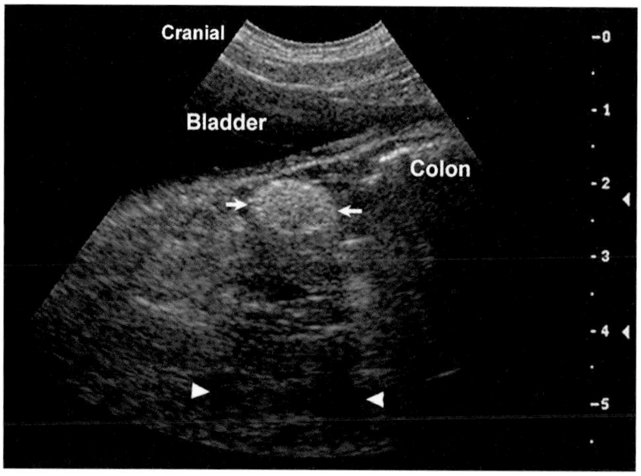

Figure 15.13. Fat nodular necrosis. Longitudinal image obtained in the caudal abdomen of a dog with chronic renal disease. A well-defined, oval, hyperechoic nodule (arrows) is dorsal to the bladder trigone. Partial acoustic shadowing is noted in the far field (arrowheads), indicating ultrasound-beam hyperattenuation in comparison with adjacent fat. These features are consistent with incidental fat nodular necrosis.

peritonitis or fungal diseases or be caused by foreign bodies, such as retained surgical sponges (Merlo and Lamb 2000). Fungal pyogranulomas, such as those caused by botryomycosis, are similar to bacterial abscesses on ultrasonographic exam (Share and Utroska 2002). Foreign bodies can produce a suppurative granulomatous or pyogranulomatous response of variable size. Some foreign bodies, such as wooden sticks or grass awns, can migrate through the abdominal wall or GI and create a sinus tract that can be recognized by their tubular, often tortuous, shape and their marked hypoechogenicity in comparison with the surrounding tissues that appear hyperechoic because of the inflammatory reaction and/or scar tissue (Penninck and Mitchell 2003; Staudte et al. 2004). The foreign body itself is not always ultrasonographically visible. Wooden sticks usually appear as linear hyperechoic interfaces, with acoustic shadowing in most cases (Figure 15.12). However, plant materials chronically imbedded in tissues can undergo a degradation that can render these objects less attenuating and therefore less likely to be associated with acoustic shadowing (Staudte et al. 2004). Grass awns appear as spindle-shaped, linear, hyperechoic interfaces measuring 3–4 cm long, with acoustic shadowing less commonly observed than with wood (Staudte et al. 2004; Gnudi et al. 2005). Retained surgical sponges typically appear as a hypoechoic mass with central hyperechoic foci and are associated with other variable signs of peritonitis (Merlo and Lamb 2000). Foreign bodies migrating into the abdominal cavity are not necessarily associated with signs of peritonitis (Penninck and Mitchell 2003).

Nodular Fat Necrosis

A benign and incidental finding in dogs and cats, this can appear as partially mineralized circular to oval soft-tissue masses in the abdominal fat. With ultrasound, these foci can be recognized as well-defined hyperechoic and hyperattenuating (acoustic shadow) nodules or masses in the abdominal fat, which can be multiple in the same patient (Schwarz et al. 2000) (Figure 15.13). A hypoechoic center may also be observed.

Peritoneal and Retroperitoneal Neoplasia

Primary peritoneal neoplastic processes, such as mesotheliomas, are extremely rare in dogs and cats (Morini et al. 2006). Peritoneal soft-tissue masses seen with ultrasonography are most often related to abdominal organs, such as the spleen, liver, pancreas, or intestine. Lipomas, infiltrative or not, may also be found within the omentum, mesentery, or other portions of the abdomen (Figure 15.14). These fatty masses are typically hyperechoic and hyperattenuating.

Other neoplastic processes, such as lymphoma, may infiltrate the omentum or mesentery, which can appear markedly heterogeneous (Figure 15.15).

Widespread dissemination of neoplasia throughout the peritoneum, a condition referred to as carcinomatosis, is more common than primary peritoneal tumors. The term carcinomatosis is used in veterinary medicine to include peritoneal invasion by epithelial, mesenchymal, or hematopoietic tumors (Monteiro and O'Brien 2004). In cats, the most common sites of primary carcinomas associated with carcinomatosis are the liver, pancreas, and intestine (Monteiro and O'Brien 2004). In dogs, peritoneal spread by ruptured hemangiosarcoma probably represents the most common type of carcinomatosis or sarcomatosis (Monteiro and O'Brien 2004). Free peritoneal effusion is expected in most cases of carcinomatosis (Figures 15.16 and 15.17). The volume and echogenicity of the fluid can vary and may be influenced by a high protein content, concurrent presence of sterile or septic peritonitis, or hemorrhage. Peritoneal effusion contributes to the visibility of nodules attached to the peritoneal surfaces or within the floating omentum or mesentery (Hanbidge et al. 2003) (Figures 15.16 and 15.17). Metastatic nodules tend to appear isoechoic to the abdominal wall or hypoechoic to adjacent fat (Monteiro and O'Brien 2004), although their echogenicity, as well as their size and shape, can vary (Figures 15.16–15.18). Infiltrated omentum or mesentery can appear focally or diffusely thickened, which has been described as "omental or mesenteric cakes" in people (Hanbidge et al. 2003). Additionally, mineral foci may be observed as hyperechoic foci casting an acoustic shadow.

Soft-tissue sarcomas, especially hemangiosarcoma, can be found in the retroperitoneal space, particularly in dogs. Ultrasonography can be useful in differentiating a retroperitoneal mass from retroperitoneal effusion, renomegaly, or renal mass suspected on radiographs. Retroperitoneal soft-tissue masses are often heterogeneous and ill-defined, and may invade major vessels such as the CVC, aorta, or renal vessels. However, it can be difficult to differentiate true large retroperitoneal masses from masses originating from the adrenal glands or urinary system. Alternate imaging such as computed tomography and magnetic resonance imaging may also help in better defining the origin and extent of retroperitoneal masses.

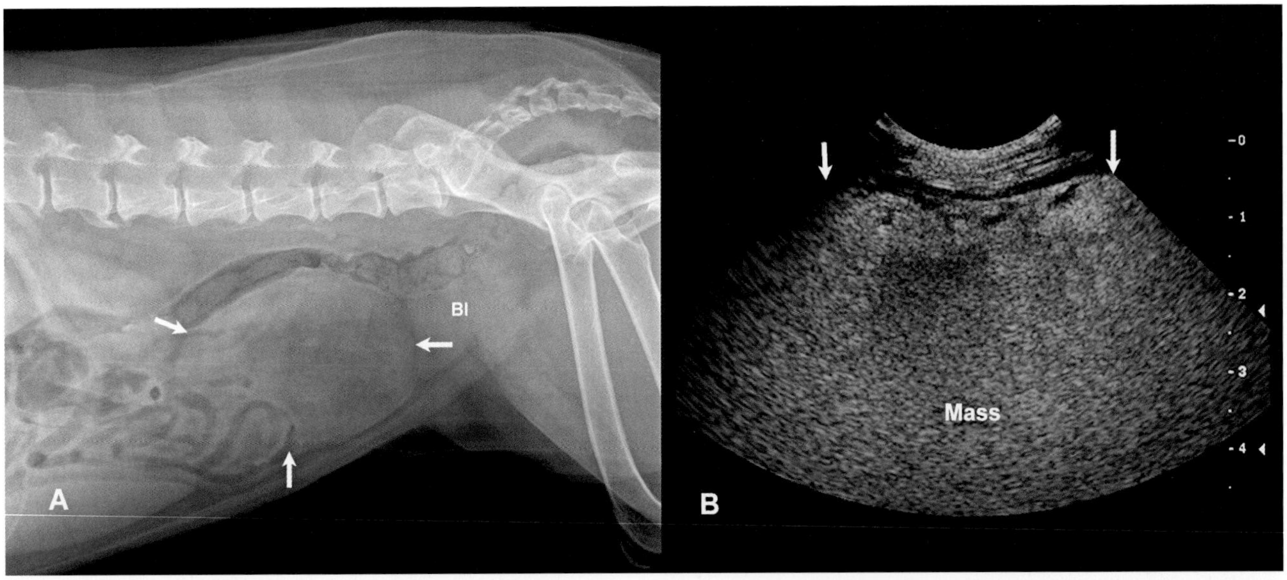

Figure 15.14. Mesenteric lipoma. **A:** Lateral abdominal radiograph of the abdomen of a large-breed dog with a palpable abdominal mass. A mildly inhomogeneous mass (arrows) in the caudal abdomen is deforming the descending colon and bladder (Bl). The mass is of intermediate opacity between fat and soft tissue. **B:** Longitudinal sonographic image of a portion of this mass that contacts the ventral abdominal wall (arrows) and extends beyond the limits of the scanned field of view. This mass is hyperechoic, hyperattenuating, and relatively uniform. A mesenteric lipoma was surgically confirmed.

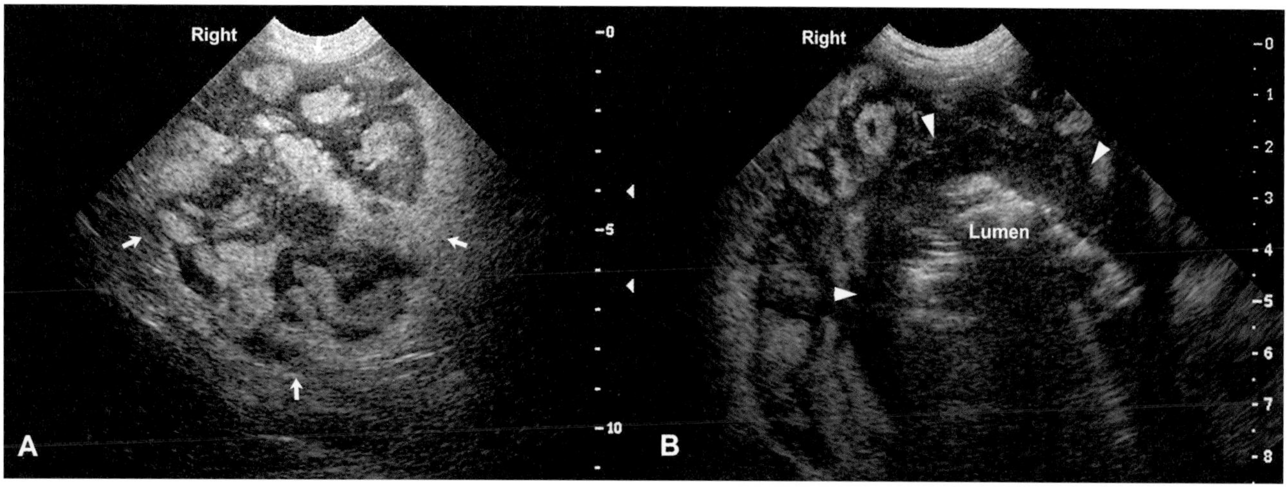

Figure 15.15. Mesenteric infiltrative mass. Transverse images obtained in the right caudal abdomen of a dog with intestinal lymphoma. **A:** A large ill-defined mass with mixed echogenicity is observed (arrows), surrounded with hyperechoic fat. **B:** In the central portion of this mass, a segment of small intestine is found with thickened and irregular hypoechoic walls (arrowheads). Mesenteric infiltration by the intestinal lymphoma was confirmed.

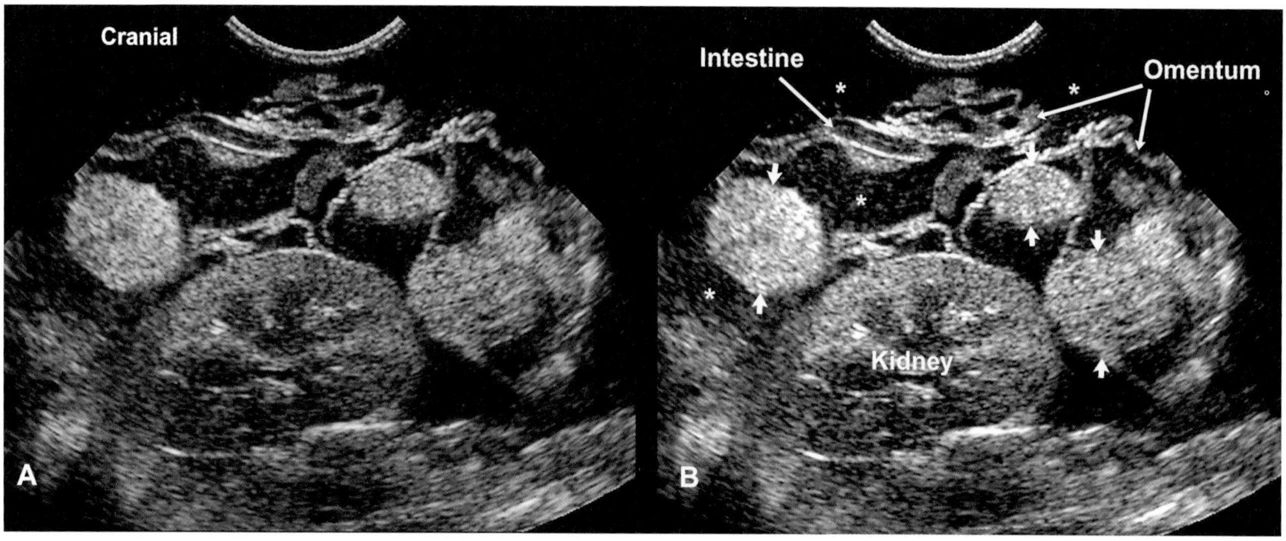

Figure 15.16. Sarcomatosis. Longitudinal sonographic **(A)** and schematic **(B)** images of the right portion of the abdomen of a cat with disseminated soft-tissue sarcoma. Multiple hyperechoic masses, consistent with metastases, are in the mesentery and omentum (arrows). Severe hypoechoic peritoneal effusion is also present (*), delineating abdominal structures.

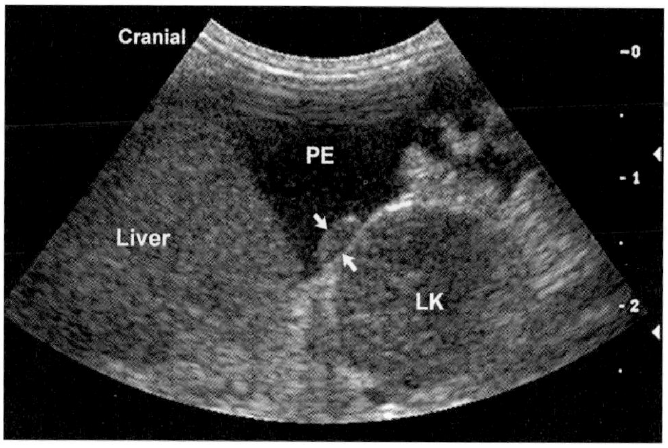

Figure 15.17. Carcinomatosis. Longitudinal image obtained in the left cranial abdomen of a cat with biliary carcinoma. An oval, mildly echogenic nodule (arrows) is on the surface of the peritoneum, at the level of the left kidney (LK). Several similar nodules were detected in the rest of the abdomen, consistent with carcinomatosis. A large volume of hypoechoic peritoneal effusion (PE) related to the metastatic disease is also present.

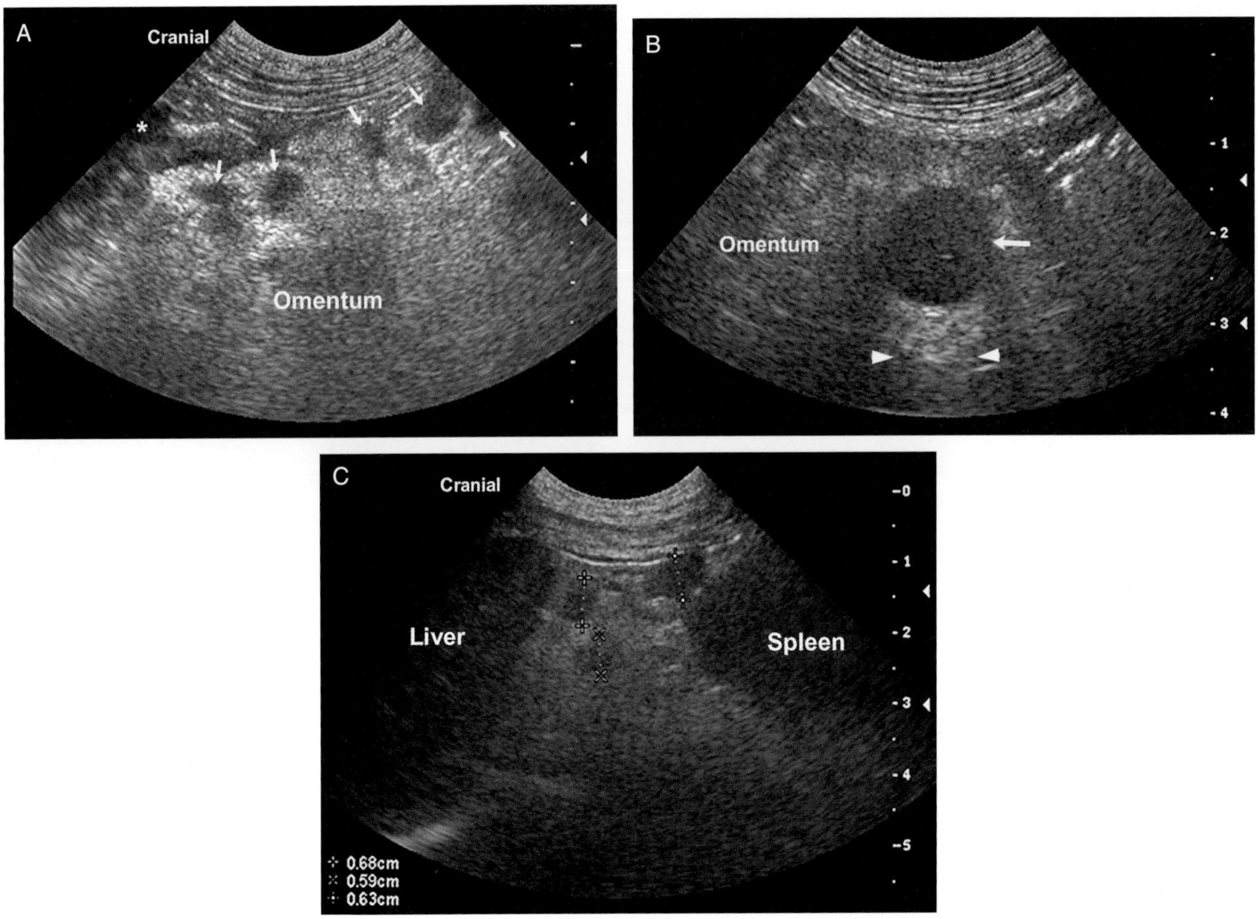

Figure 15.18. Omental carcinomatosis and sarcomatosis. **A:** Longitudinal image of the midabdomen of a cat diagnosed with pancreatic adenocarcinoma. The omentum is enlarged, hyperechoic, and filled with small hypoechoic nodules (arrows) consistent with metastases. **B:** Transverse image obtained in the right cranial abdomen, medial to the region of the pancreas, in a dog. A well-defined, circular, hypoechoic focus is in the omentum (arrow). The region dorsal to this focus is hyperechoic (arrowheads), consistent with acoustic enhancement. This hypoechoic focus contrasts with the surrounding hyperechoic and hyperattenuating omental fat. A necrotic metastatic focus was cytologically identified with fine-needle aspiration. Ileocecal adenocarcinoma was confirmed. **C:** Longitudinal image of the left cranial abdomen of a dog with a large splenic mass and peritoneal effusion (not shown). Three, small, ill-defined, hypoechoic foci (between the cursors) are in the omental fat between the liver and the spleen. Rupture splenic hemangiosarcoma with hepatic and omental metastases were identified in surgery.

Lymphadenopathy

Changes in size, shape, contour, and internal echogenicity and echotexture are important criteria that help to detect lymphadenopathies and differentiate benign from malignant processes. Enlarged lymph nodes typically become more rounded. Ratios comparing their short (S) and long (L) axes increase more significantly with neoplastic infiltration (Llabrés-Diaz 2004; Nyman et al. 2004). S/L axis ratios > 0.5 are usually predictive of neoplasia (Figure 15.19), as opposed to ratios < 0.5, which are usually calculated for normal or reactive lymph nodes (Figure 15.20). Internal nodal architecture tends to be more affected by neoplastic infiltration (Llabrés-Diaz 2004; Nyman et al. 2004). Reactive lymph nodes tend to present a hyperechoic hilus unlike with neoplastic infiltrations (Figure 15.20). Primary or metastatic neoplastic lymph nodes are commonly hypoechoic (Figures 15.19, 15.21, and 15.22), facilitating their identification, although areas of hyperechogenicity may be present if coagulative necrosis, hemorrhage, or mineralization is also present (Figure 15.23).

Massively infiltrated lymph nodes can become markedly enlarged and distorted (Figure 15.24). Hypoechoic or anechoic areas may also be seen as the result of liquefaction necrosis or cyst formation (Llabrés-Diaz 2004) (Figures 15.24 and 15.25). Cyst formation may also be seen in benign lymph nodes (Figure 15.25A). Malignant nodes may also be inflamed or abscessed and can therefore become markedly heterogeneous (Figure 15.25D).

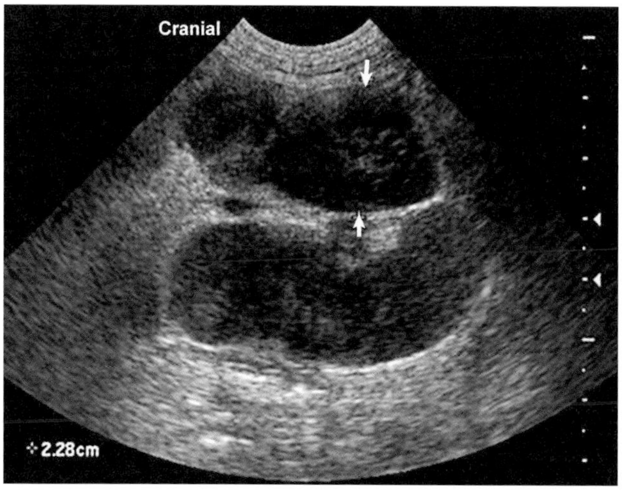

Figure 15.19. Malignant lymph nodes. Longitudinal image obtained in the midabdomen of a dog with peripheral lymphadenomegaly. Multiple oval to rounded, well-defined, hypoechoic masses are in the root of the mesentery, consistent with enlarged mesenteric lymph nodes (arrows). The ultrasonographic features of these nodes are highly suggestive of malignancy, particularly lymphoma.

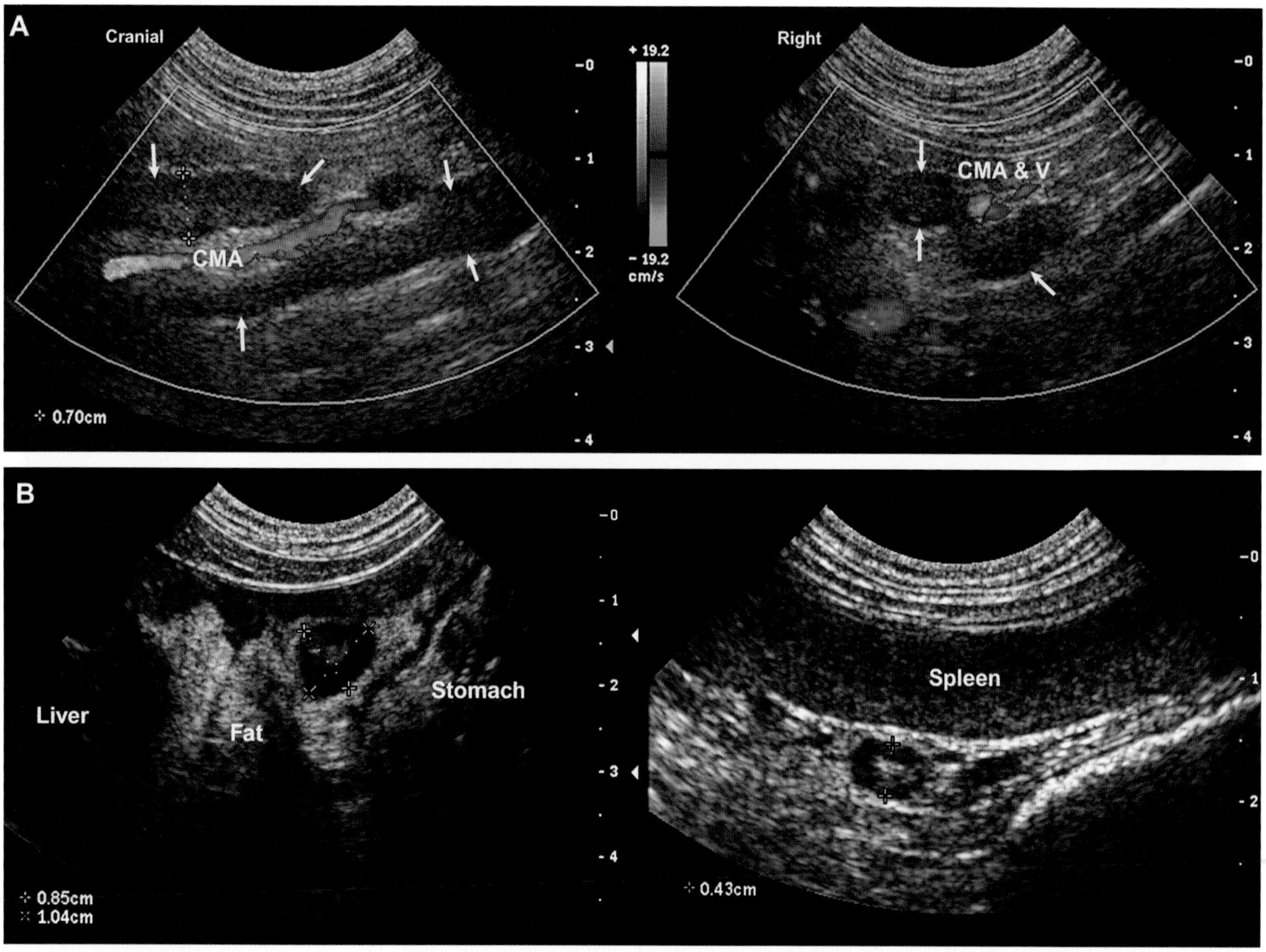

Figure 15.20. Reactive lymphadenopathy. **A:** Longitudinal image of the midabdomen of a dog with a history of inflammatory bowel disease. The mesenteric lymph nodes (arrows) are more prominent because of reduced echogenicity, particularly peripherally, as well as mild mesenteric fat hyperechogenicity. The cranial mesenteric artery and vein (CMA & V) are noted between these nodes, serving as a useful landmark for their identification. The orientation of the flow in the artery, which is directed toward the probe, is displayed as a red signal on color Doppler. **B:** Ultrasound images of mildly enlarged gastric (left) and splenic (right) lymph nodes in a cat with septic peritonitis. The fat around the gastric lymph node is hyperechoic, contrasting with the hypoechoic lymph node. The hilar portion of these nodes remains hyperechoic.

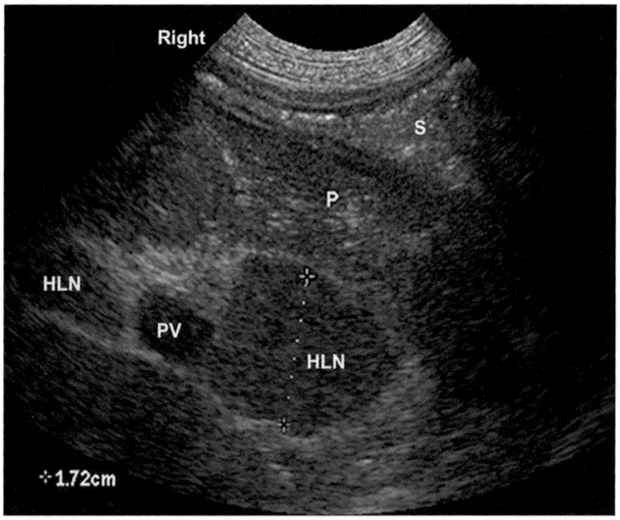

Figure 15.21. Neoplastic hepatic lymph nodes. Transverse sonographic image obtained at the porta hepatis in a dog with pulmonary histiocytic sarcoma. The hepatic lymph nodes (HLN) are identified adjacent to the portal vein (PV) and dorsal to the body of the pancreas (P) and stomach (S). These nodes are enlarged, irregular, and less echogenic than normal. They remain relatively uniform. Disseminated histiocytic sarcoma was identified in the liver and several abdominal lymph nodes.

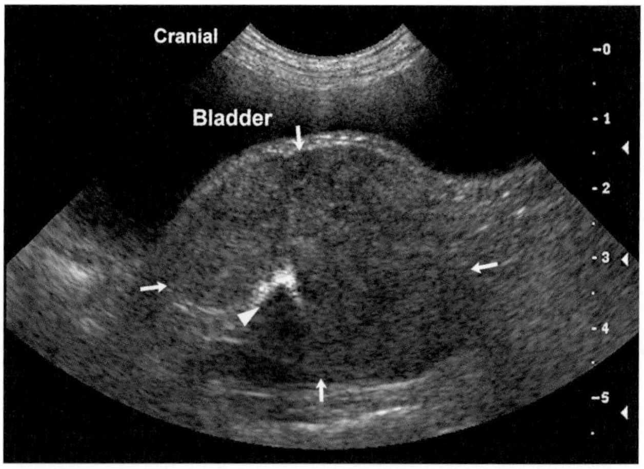

Figure 15.22. Anal sac gland lymphatic metastases. Longitudinal image obtained in the caudal abdomen of a dog with a perianal mass. A large heterogeneous mass (arrows) with well-defined contours is dorsal to the urinary bladder, in the region of the medial iliac lymph nodes. A hyperechoic focus (arrowhead) associated with acoustic shadowing, consistent with mineralization, is in the cranial portion of the mass. Metastatic anal sac carcinoma was diagnosed with cytology on fine-needle aspiration.

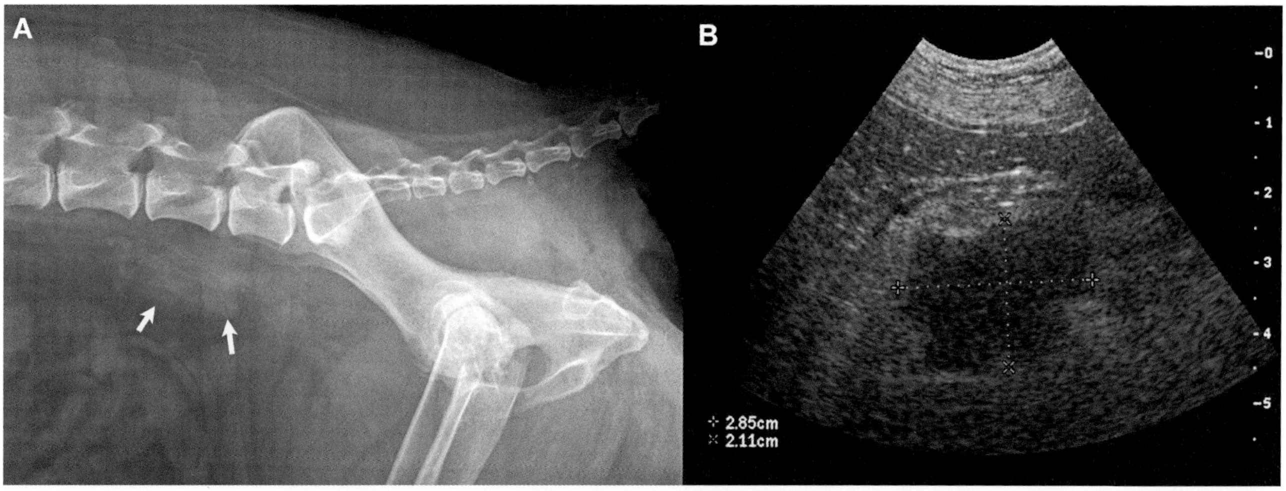

Figure 15.23. Sublumbar lymphadenopathy caused by metastatic carcinoma. **A:** Lateral abdominal radiograph of a medium-sized breed dog with metastatic carcinoma. An ill-defined, lobulated, soft-tissue opacity (arrows) is ventral to the sixth and seventh lumbar vertebrae. **B:** Longitudinal sonographic image obtained in the same region, lateral to the right iliac artery and vein (not shown). An irregular, hypoechoic mass with surrounding mildly hyperechoic fat, consistent with metastatic disease, is at the location of a medial iliac lymph node.

Figure 15.25. Cavitary lymph nodes. **A: Benign cystic node.** Multiple, irregular, well-defined anechoic cysts are incidentally found in the hepatic node of this dog with urinary calculi. HA, hepatic artery; and PV, portal vein. **B: Cystic node with lymphoma.** Longitudinal image of a mesenteric lymph node in a dog with multicentric lymphoma. A large, oval, anechoic, avascular area (arrows) is in the cranial region of the enlarged lymph node (arrowheads). Fine-needle aspiration confirmed the presence of a fluid-filled cavity or cyst within this portion of the node, and lymphoma was confirmed in the caudal solid portion. **C: Necrosis.** On this ultrasound image, two adjacent mesenteric lymph nodes are severely enlarged, nearly anechoic, and ill-defined. The surrounding fat is markedly hyperechoic. Fine-needle aspiration revealed the presence of metastatic carcinoma associated with necrosis and inflammation. **D: Abscessed malignant node.** Transverse image of a severely enlarged hepatic lymph node in a dog with multicentric lymphoma and suspected pancreatitis. Echogenic fluid is in the affected node, with a cellular sediment forming a line (arrow) parallel to the horizontal plane (probe placed obliquely). The adjacent pancreas (P) is hypoechoic and the peripheral fat is mildly hyperechoic. PV, portal vein.

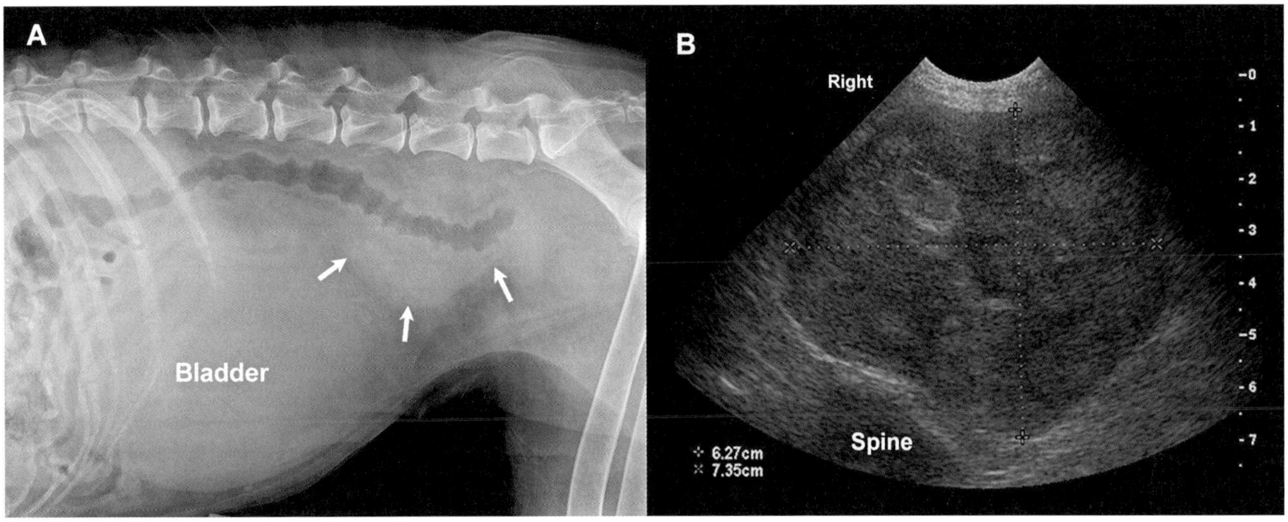

Figure 15.24. Sublumbar lymphadenopathy caused by metastatic sarcoma. **A:** Lateral abdominal radiograph of a large-breed dog with partial urinary obstruction and signs suggestive of colitis. A somewhat lobulated soft-tissue opacity is in the caudodorsal abdomen and displacing the descending colon ventrally and associated with marked bladder distension. The colon is corrugated. **B:** Transverse sonographic image obtained in the caudal abdomen. The mass suspected on radiographs is large and heterogeneous (between the cursors). Metastatic soft-tissue sarcoma to lymph nodes was highly suspected based on fine-needle aspiration.

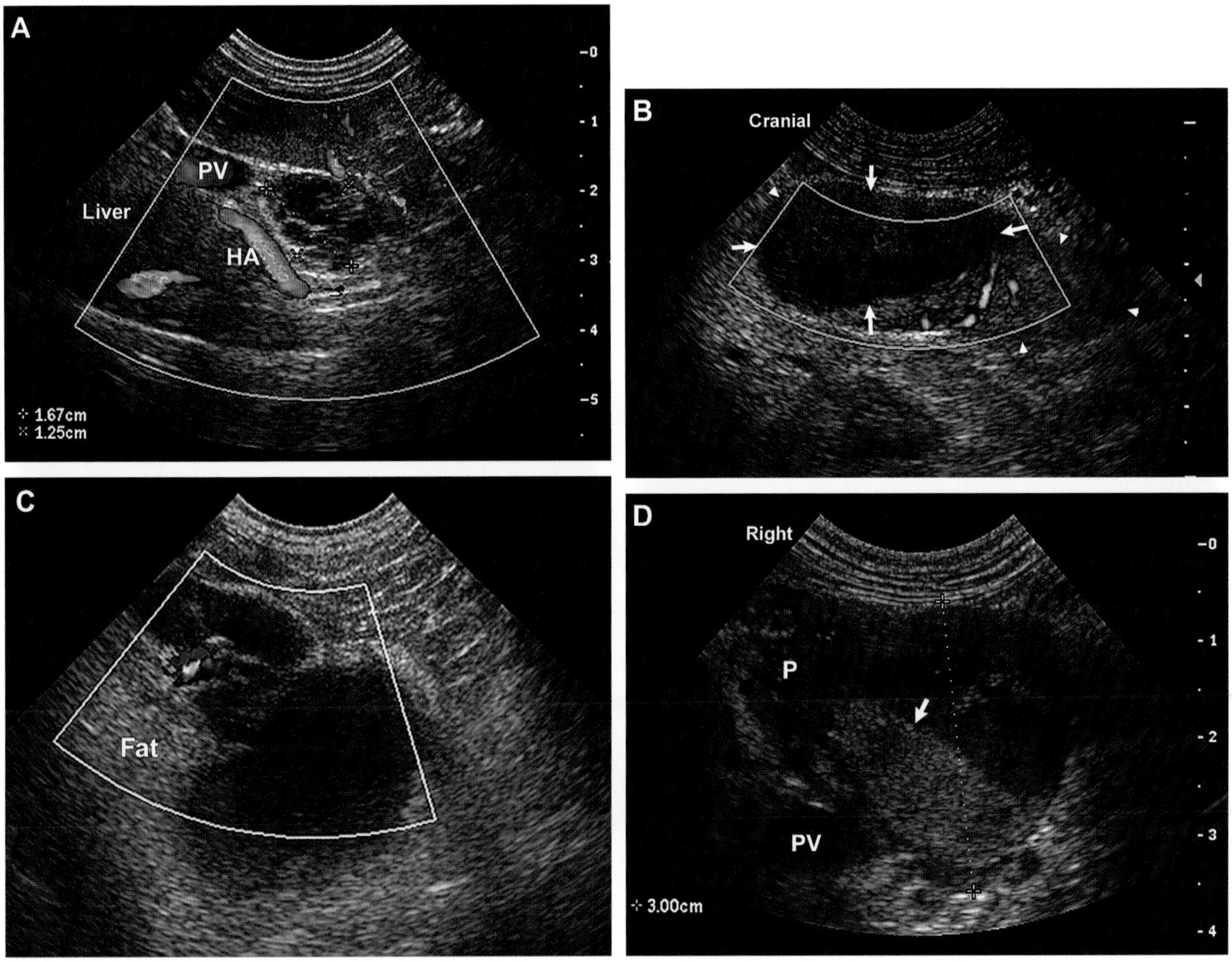

Figure 15.25.

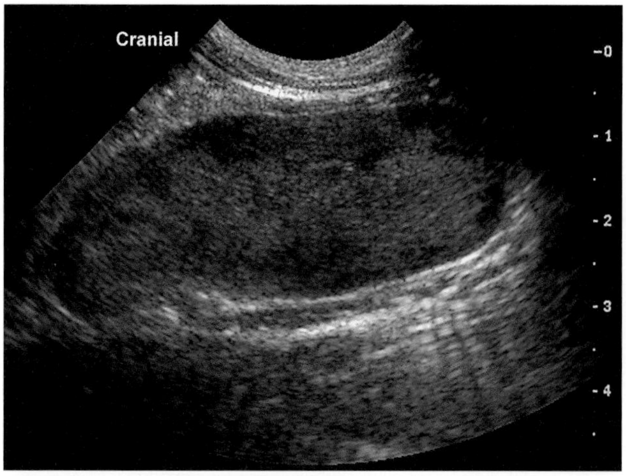

Figure 15.26. Granulomatous lymphadenopathy. Longitudinal image obtained in a dog diagnosed with an intestinal mass, on which a mesenteric lymph node appears moderately enlarged (2cm thick × 6cm long). This lymph node is not as hypoechoic as typically seen with lymphoma. Surgery confirmed the presence of severe granulomatous enteritis caused by pythiosis.

Inflammatory lymph nodes also tend to be ill-defined (Nyman et al. 2004). Noninflamed malignant nodes are usually sharper in contour and may be associated with acoustic enhancement. However, some overlap exists in the ultrasonographic appearance of benign and malignant lymph node pathologies. For example, granulomatous diseases, such as pythiosis, can mimic neoplasia (Figure 15.26).

In people, the use of color Doppler, power Doppler, or contrast ultrasonography increases the accuracy in differentiating benign from malignant nodes (Nyman et al. 2004). In benign nodes, the blood flow distribution is primarily hilar, whereas it tends to be more peripheral or mixed with malignancies. Resistive and pulsative indices are also higher in malignant nodes (Nyman et al. 2004).

Vascular Thrombosis and Other Anomalies

In addition to the portal system, thrombi and emboli involving the CVC, aorta, or iliac vessels can be detected with ultrasonography in dogs or cats. A thorough evaluation of all vascular branches, including femoral veins and arteries, is required when pelvic thromboembolic disease is suspected.

The appearance of thrombosis can vary in the acute and chronic phases. Initially, the thrombus may be poorly echogenic and more difficult to identify using standard B-mode. The lack of flow as evaluated with spectral Doppler, color Doppler, or power Doppler, as well as the lack of compressibility (applicable to distal CVC and peripheral veins), are useful signs in the identification of acute thrombosis (Linkins et al. 2006). With time, an echogenic area, usually attached to a portion of the vessel wall, is observed filling a portion of the vascular lumen. The thrombus can appear uniform or heterogeneous because of blood clot lysis and recanalization.

CVC thrombosis can be caused by the cranial extension of spontaneous femoral or iliac vein thrombosis, or by the invasion of malignant tumors involving adja-

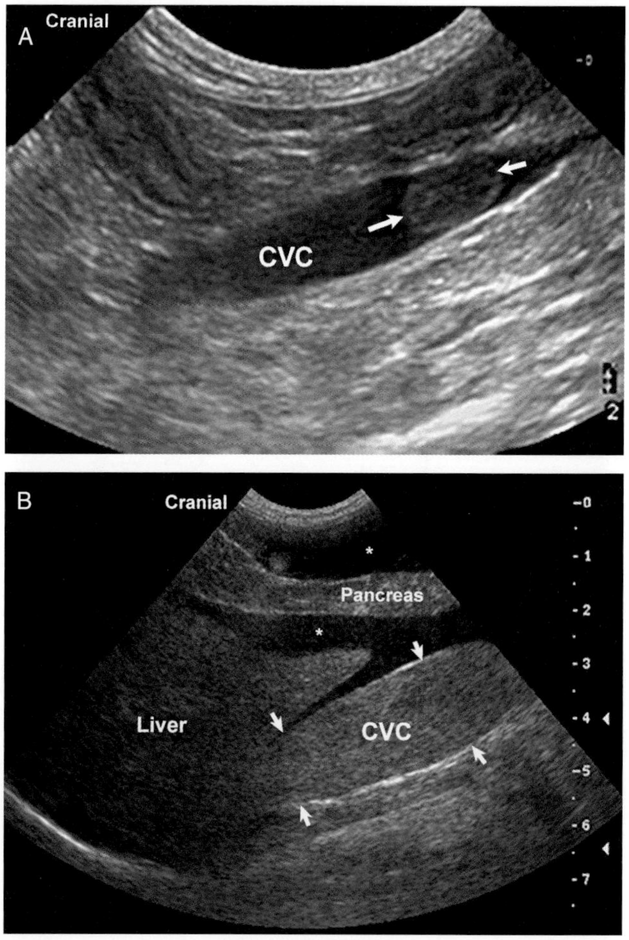

Figure 15.27. Thrombosis of the caudal vena cava. **A: Small thrombus.** Longitudinal image of the caudal portion of the caudal vena cava (CVC) of a cat on which a well-defined, oval, mildly echogenic thrombus is seen (arrows). This thrombus was partially obliterating the vessel lumen. Image courtesy of D. Penninck. **B: Massive thrombosis.** Longitudinal image obtained in the right cranial abdomen of a dog with severe ascites (*). The CVC is enlarged, and its lumen is diffusely and uniformly echogenic, consistent with thrombosis. There was no evidence of flow on color or power Doppler. A hepatic mass infiltrating the CVC was suspected.

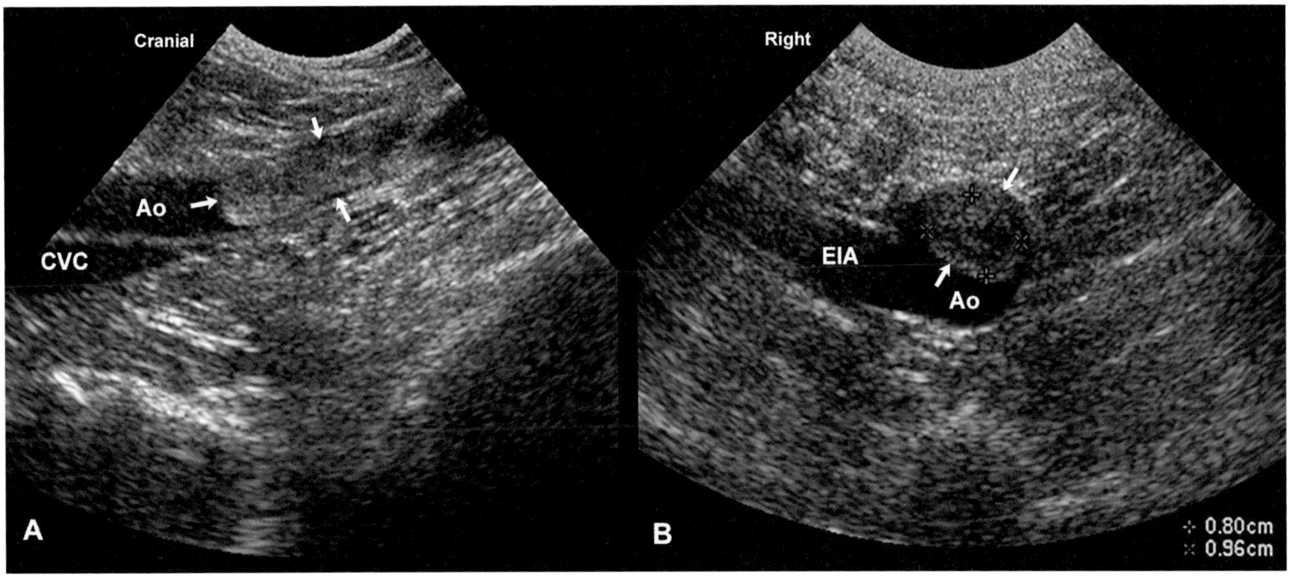

Figure 15.28. Aortic thromboembolism. Longitudinal **(A)** and transverse **(B)** images of the caudal portion of the abdominal aorta (Ao) in a dog with pelvic weakness. An echogenic, relatively well-defined, tubular structure in the aorta is occluding most of its lumen, consistent with a thromboembolus (arrows). The dog had hyperadrenocorticism, which was considered as the probable predisposing factor for thrombus formation. CVC, caudal vena cava; and EIA, external iliac artery.

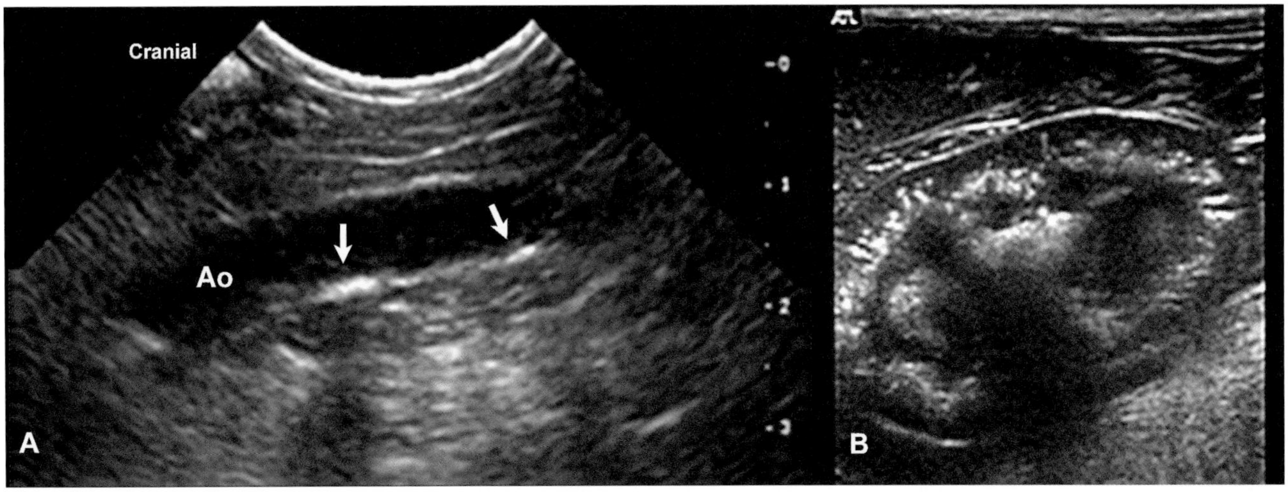

Figure 15.29. Aortic wall mineralization. **A:** Longitudinal sonographic image of the caudal abdominal aorta of a dog with chronic Cushing's disease. Linear hyperechoic foci (arrows) with acoustic shadowing are along the inner margin of the dorsal aortic (Ao) wall. **B:** Extensively distributed hyperechoic striations and dots are also found in the left kidney, particularly in the cortex, of this dog, which is consistent with nephrocalcinosis. Similar changes were present in the other kidney.

cent organs, such as the liver and adrenal glands, that produces endothelial damage (Finn-Bodner and Hudson 1998). External compression of the CVC may cause flow congestion, which represents a predisposing factor for thrombus formation (Figure 15.27). Peritoneal effusion may develop if venous flow is significantly reduced through the CVC. Additionally, thrombosis is favored by the presence of a hypercoagulable status.

Distal aortic and iliac thromboembolism represents an important complication associated with cardiomyopathies in cats. In dogs, aortic and iliac thromboembolism is usually present because of a disorder associated with a hypercoagulable state, cardiac disease or neoplasia (Boswood et al. 2000) (Figure 15.28).

Vascular wall mineralization, particularly involving the aorta, can sometimes be observed in dogs and is usually considered an incidental finding. Hyperechoic plaquelike lesions can be observed at the inner margin of the wall, with acoustic shadowing if large enough (Figure 15.29).

Abdominal vascular malformations other than portosystemic shunts are extremely rare in dogs and cats. The use of ultrasonography in the identification of segmental aplasia of the CVC with azygos continuation has been reported in dogs (Barthez et al. 1996).

Interventional Procedures

Fine-needle aspiration of peritoneal fluids is used routinely with ultrasonography in dogs and cats. With minimal practice, even small amount of fluids can be securely aspirated. Abdominal masses and lymph nodes can also be aspirated or biopsied. Cavitated masses, abscesses, or cysts can also be drained with ultrasound guidance.

References

Barthez PY, Siemens LM, Koblik PD (1996) Azygos continuation of the caudal vena cava in a dog: Radiographic and ultrasonographic diagnosis. Vet Radiol Ultrasound 37:354–356.

Bezuidenhout AJ (1993) The lymphatic system. In: Evans HE, ed. Miller's Anatomy of the Dog, 3rd edition. Philadelphia: WB Saunders, pp. 717–757.

Boysen SR, Rozanski EA, Tidwell AS, Holm JL, Shaw, SP, Rush JE (2004) Evaluation of a focused assessment with sonography for trauma protocol to detect free abdominal fluid in dogs involved in motor vehicle accidents. J Am Vet Med Assoc 225:1198–1204.

Boysen SR, Tidwell AS, Penninck D (2003) Ultrasonographic findings in dogs and cats with gastrointestinal perforation. Vet Radiol Ultrasound 44:556–564.

Boswood A, Lamb CR, White RN (2000) Aortic and iliac thrombosis in six dogs. J Small Anim Pract 41:109–114.

Evans HE (1993a) The Heart and Arteries & Chapter 12: Veins. In: Evans HE, ed. Miller's Anatomy of the Dog, 3rd edition. Philadelphia: WB Saunders, pp. 586–681.

Evans HE (1993b) Veins. In: Evans HE, Christensen GC, eds. Miller's Anatomy of the Dog, 3rd edition. Philadelphia: WB Saunders, pp. 682–716.

Finn-Bodner ST, Hudson JA (1998) Abdominal vascular sonography. Vet Clin North Am Small Anim Pract 28:887–943.

Gnudi G, Volta A, Bonazzi M, Gazzola M, Bertoni G (2005) Ultrasonographic features of grass awn migration in the dog. Vet Radiol Ultrasound 46:423–426.

Hanbidge AE, Lynch D, Wilson SR (2003) US of the peritoneum. Radiographics 23:663–684.

Henley RK, Hager DA, Ackerman N (1989) A comparison of two-dimensional ultrasonography and radiography for the detection of small amounts of free peritoneal fluid in the dog. Vet Radiol Ultrasound 30:121–124.

Komori S, Nakagaki K, Koyama H, Yamagami T (2002) Idiopathic mesenteric and omental steatitis in a dog. J Am Vet Med Assoc 221:1591–1593.

Konde LJ, Lebel JL, Park RD, Wrigley RH (1986) Sonographic application in the diagnosis of intraabdominal abscess in the dog. Vet Radiol Ultrasound 27:151–154.

Linkins LA, Stretton R, Probyn L, Kearon C (2006) Interobserver agreement on ultrasound measurements of residual vein diameter, thrombus echogenicity and Doppler venous flow in patients with previous venous thrombosis. Thromb Res 117:241–247.

Llabrés-Diaz FJ (2004) Ultrasonography of the medial lymph nodes in the dog. Vet Radiol Ultrasound 45:156–165.

Merlo M, Lamb CR (2000) Radiographic and ultrasonographic features of retained surgical sponge in eight dogs. Vet Radiol Ultrasound 41:279–283.

Monteiro CB, O'Brien RT (2004) A retrospective study on the sonographic findings of abdominal carcinomatosis in 14 cats. Vet Radiol Ultrasound 45:559–564.

Morini M, Bettini G, Morandi F, Burdisso R, Marcato PS (2006) Deciduoid peritoneal mesothelioma in a dog. Vet Pathol 43:198–201.

Nyman HT, Kristensen AT, Flagstad A, McEvoy FJ (2004) A review of the sonographic assessment of tumor metastases in liver and superficial lymph nodes. Vet Radiol Ultrasound 45:438–448.

Penninck D, Mitchell S (2003) Ultrasonographic detection of ingested and perforating wooden foreign bodies in four dogs. J Am Vet Med Assoc 223:206–209.

Pintar J, Breitschwerdt EB, Hardie EM, Spaulding KA (2003) Acute nontraumatic hemoabdomen in the dog: A retrospective analysis of 39 cases (1987–2001). J Am Anim Hosp Assoc 39:518–522.

Pugh CR (1994) Ultrasonographic examination of abdominal lymph nodes in the dog. Vet Radiol Ultrasound 35:110–115.

Roson N, Garriga V, Cuadrado M, et al. (2006) Sonographic findings of mesenteric panniculitis: Correlation with CT and literature review. J Clin Ultrasound 34:169–176.

Saunders WB, Tobias KM (2003) Pneumoperitoneum in dogs and cats: 39 cases (1983–2002). J Am Vet Med Assoc 223:462–468.

Schwarz T, Morandi F, Gnudi G, et al. (2000) Nodular fat necrosis in the feline and canine abdomen. Vet Radiol Ultrasound 41:335–339.

Share B, Utroska B (2002) Intra-abdominal botryomycosis in a dog. J Am Vet Med Assoc 220:1025–1027.

Spaulding KA (1993) Sonographic evaluation of peritoneal effusion in small animals. Vet Radiol Ultrasound 34:427–431.

Spaulding KA (1997) A review of sonographic identification of abdominal blood vessels and juxtavascular organs. Vet Radiol Ultrasound 38:4–23.

Staudte KL, Hopper BJ, Gibson NR, Read RA (2004) Use of ultrasonography to facilitate surgical removal of non-enteric foreign bodies in 17 dogs. J Small Anim Pract 45:395–400.

Szatmari V, Sotonyi P, Voros K (2001) Normal duplex Doppler waveforms of major abdominal blood vessels in dogs: A review. Vet Radiol Ultrasound 42:93–107.

CHAPTER SIXTEEN

MUSCULOSKELETAL SYSTEM

Martin Kramer and Marc-André d'Anjou

SHOULDER

Scanning Technique

Ultrasonography of the shoulder joint and the surrounding tissues is best performed with a linear transducer using frequencies greater than 10 MHz. Curvilinear probes may be used to facilitate the approach to deeper portions or areas with a curved surface, such as the axillary area. The hair around the joint is clipped. All tendons and muscles are scanned longitudinally and transversally (Figure 16.1).

The sonogram of the shoulder joint starts by scanning the supraspinatus and infraspinatus muscles down to their attachment sites at the major tubercle (Figure 16.2). Then the biceps muscle is examined, after maximal external rotation of the shoulder joint (Figures 16.1 and 16.2). Abducting the limb may also help gaining better access to the region. The scan begins at the muscle belly, along the craniomedial aspect of the humeral diaphysis. The probe is then gradually moved proximally along its proximal tendon, which lies within the intertubercular groove, at the medial aspect of the shoulder joint. The biceps tendon is then followed to its origin on the supraglenoid tubercle of the scapula. The most important standard scan plane is the cross section of the intertubercular groove between the major and minor tubercles. At that level, the tendon is encircled by a sheath filled with a small amount of synovial fluid that connects with the joint space proximally (Figure 16.2). The tendon and its sheath are contained in the intertubercular groove by a transverse ligament between the major and minor tubercles (Kramer and Gerwing 1994).

The intra-articular structures of the shoulder are imaged by positioning the transducer laterally in a craniocaudal orientation immediately distal to the acromion, which serves as a landmark (Figure 16.3). The joint is scanned by slowly adducting and simultaneously rotating the limb while the probe remains in the same position. As there is limited space, a second image—perpendicular to the first—is difficult to achieve, particularly with a linear transducer that has a long footprint. Scanning the cranial aspect of the shoulder joint is difficult because of the presence of the major tubercle, which allows only a small surface of probe contact. Medial imaging of the shoulder joint may be facilitated by the use of a curved or sector transducer because of the intimate relationship between the thoracic limb and the thoracic wall (Figure 16.4).

Normal Sonographic Anatomy of the Shoulder

Supraspinatus Muscle

The supraspinatus muscle originates on the supraspinatus fossa of the scapula and is scanned distally in longitudinal sections over the extensor side of the humerus to its insertion site on the major tubercle (Figures 16.2 and 16.5). The muscle is hypoechoic and loosely striated, and smoothly marginated. The major tubercle appears as a curvilinear hyperechoic interface, with irregular margins and acoustic shadowing, on which the supraspinatus muscles inserts (Figure 16.5). At that level, because of the orientation of the tendon fibers, this portion remains similar in appearance to the muscle belly, in comparison to the adjacent biceps tendon (Kramer and Gerwing 1994).

Infraspinatus Muscle

The infraspinatus muscle is scanned in longitudinal and transverse planes from its origin on the infraspinous fossa to its short tendon at the caudolateral margin of the major tubercle. The muscle belly is striated with thin hyperechoic bands that run obliquely connecting a central line to the periphery, giving a characteristic fish-bone pattern (Figure 16.6). The muscle belly becomes narrower distally, merging into a tendon beyond the joint. The tendinous tissue displays typical hyperechoic fibrils arranged in parallel lines, with a peripheral hyperechoic outline (peritendineum). The greater tubercle appears as a hyperechoic convex structure on which the tendon ends, laterally, while curving and tapering when scanned

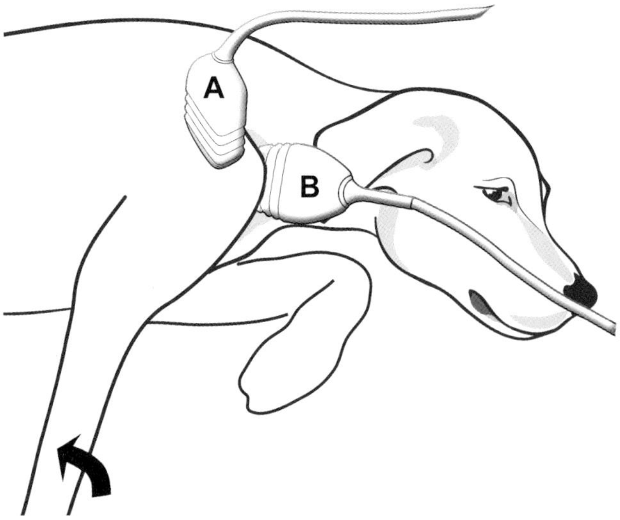

Figure 16.1. Scanning technique for the shoulder. Illustration showing the position of the dog and ultrasound probe to obtain longitudinal images of the supraspinatus and infraspinatus muscles (A) and biceps tendon (B). For the assessment of the biceps tendon, the leg must be pulled and externally rotated (curved arrow), facilitating the approach to the intertubercular groove, which is located in the medial portion of the shoulder.

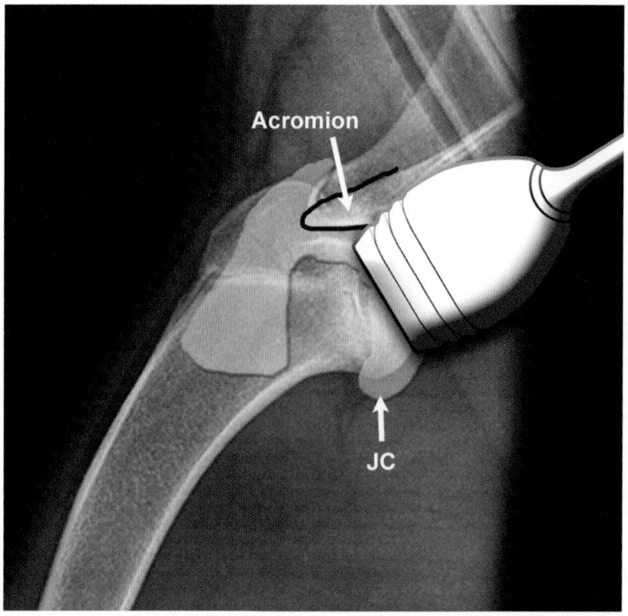

Figure 16.3. Sonographic approach to the shoulder joint. The caudolateral portion of the shoulder joint can be evaluated after placing the probe just caudal to the acromion, which can be easily palpated. The caudal extent of the joint space and capsule (JC) can be assessed. Illustration by M.A. d'Anjou.

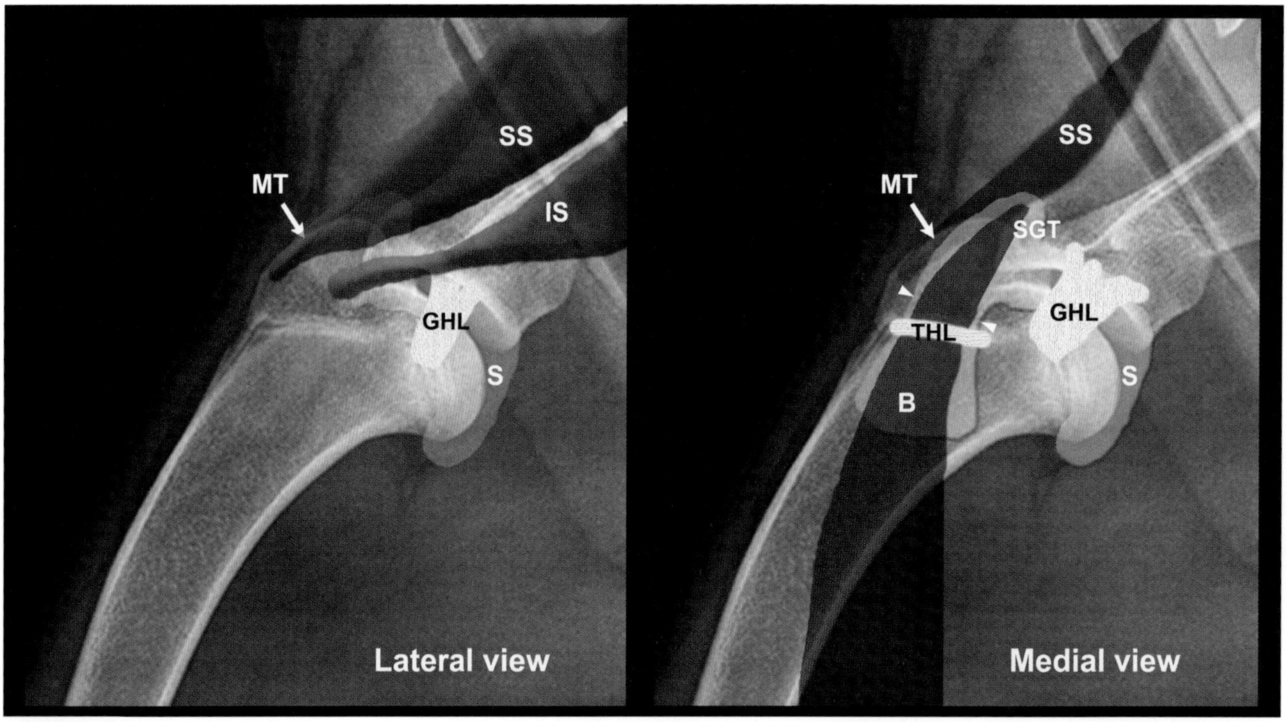

Figure 16.2. Schematic views of the normal shoulder anatomy in dogs. **Lateral view:** The supraspinatus (SS) and infraspinatus (IS) muscles and tendons are cranial and caudal to the scapular spine, respectively. The SS tendon inserts on the major tubercle (MT), just lateral to the bicipital groove. The IS inserts on the humeral head more laterally. The lateral glenohumeral ligament (GHL) is lateral to the joint capsule and synovial space (S). **Medial view:** The biceps (B) muscle and tendon course along the medial aspect of the humerus. The tendon of origin is in the intertubercular groove, just medial to the major tubercle (MT). It extends within a tendon sheath (arrowheads) that connects with the shoulder joint synovium (S) and is contained by the transverse humeral ligament (THL). The biceps tendon courses along the insertion site of the supraspinatus (SS) tendon, located craniolaterally, and originates on the supraglenoid tubercle (SGT). The medial glenohumeral ligament (GHL) is fan-shaped proximally. Illustrations by M.A. d'Anjou.

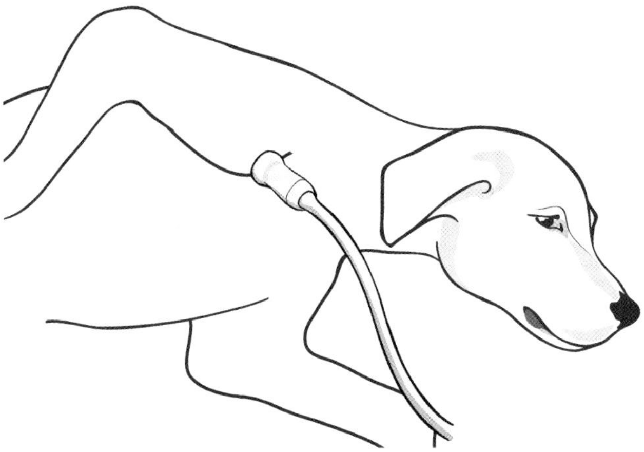

Figure 16.4. Scanning technique for the medial aspect of the shoulder joint. Illustration showing the position of the dog and ultrasound probe when scanning the medial aspect of the shoulder and axillary area. The leg must be abducted. The approach can also be facilitated by pulling (as shown) or extending the leg.

longitudinally (like a bird's beak). The infraspinatus muscle is covered by the deltoid muscle, which displays typical muscle echotexture (Figure 16.6). The fascias of both muscles can be distinguished sonographically (Kramer and Gerwing 1994) (Figure 16.6).

Biceps Brachii Muscle

In the longitudinal plane, the biceps muscle appears hypoechoic, with a hyperechoic line in the center representing the border between the two fused muscle bellies. Hyperechoic lines extend from this central line and run at a slightly oblique angle to the longitudinal axis (fish-bone pattern). In cross section, the shape of the muscle resembles a section of citrus fruit. The transducer is then positioned proximal to the muscle-tendon interface, which is ill-defined (Figure 16.7A). The proximal tendon runs within the humeral intertubercular groove, also called the bicipital groove, which

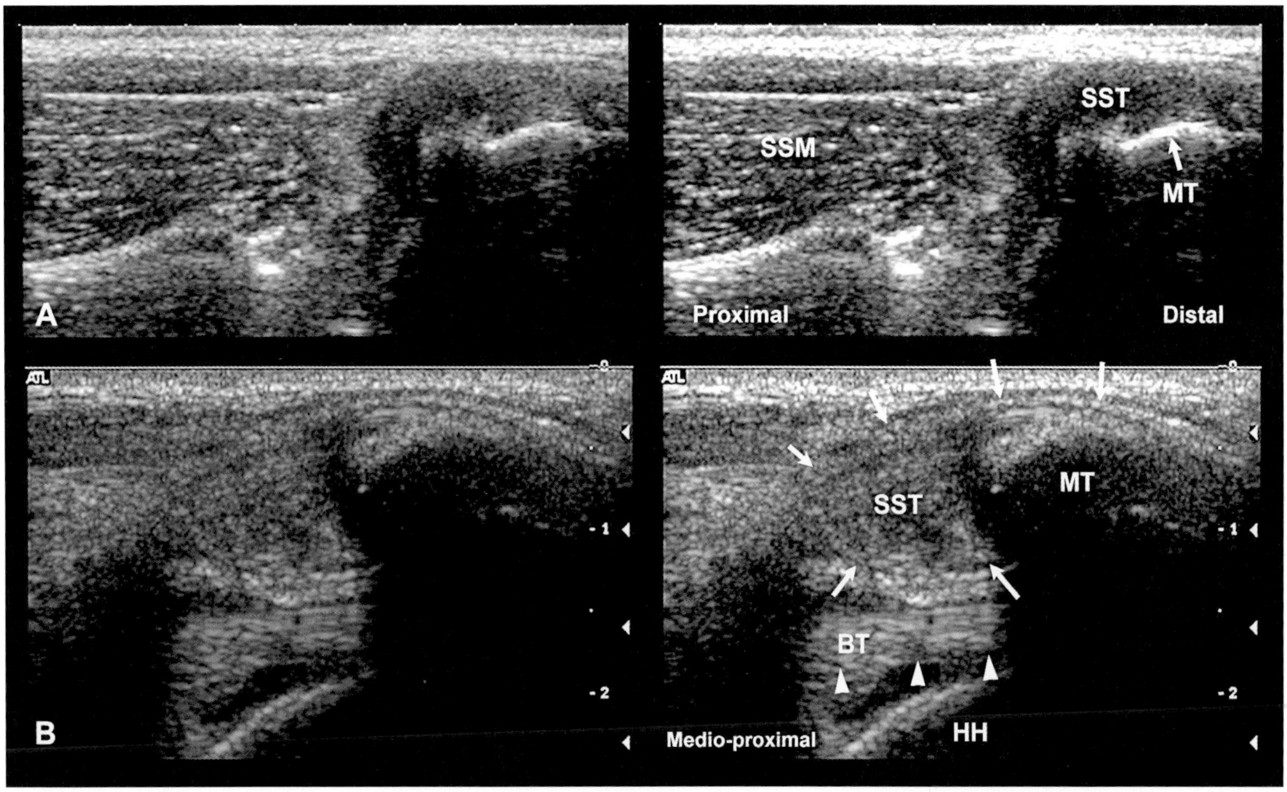

Figure 16.5. Normal sonographic anatomy of the supraspinatus muscle and tendon. Longitudinal **(A)** and transverse **(B)** sonographic and schematic images of the normal supraspinatus muscle (SSM) and supraspinatus tendon (SST) in a large breed dog. The characteristic hypoechoic echotexture with small hyperechoic dots and lines of the supraspinatus muscle is seen. Because of the orientation and distribution of the tendon fibers, this portion also appears hypoechoic. It fans (arrows) around the humeral major tubercle (MT) on which it inserts. The major tubercle and the surface of the humeral head (HH) appear as thin hyperechoic interfaces casting acoustic shadow. The biceps tendon (BT, arrowheads) and its sheath course caudally and medially, in proximity to the SST.

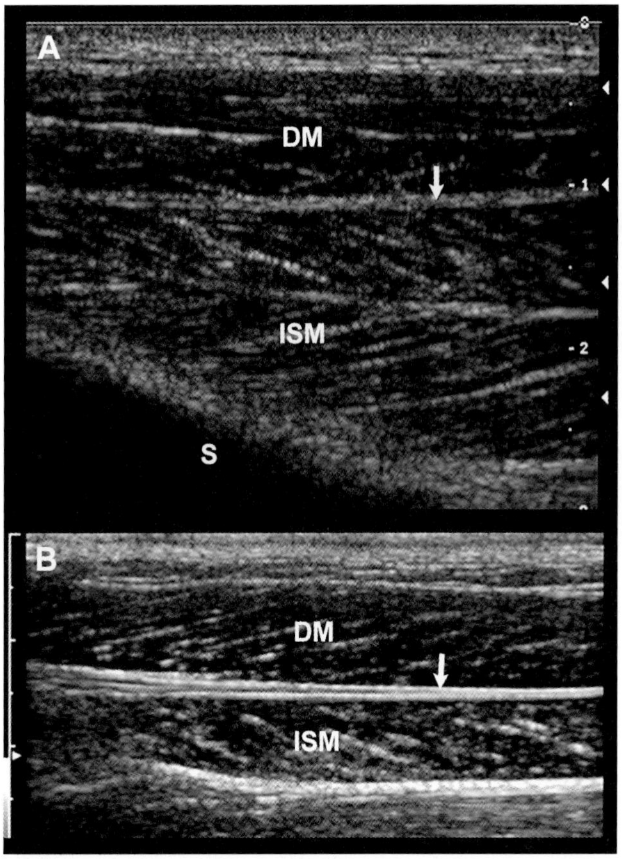

Figure 16.6. Normal sonographic anatomy of the infraspinatus muscle. **A and B:** Longitudinal sonographic images of the normal infraspinatus muscle (ISM) obtained at two different levels. The characteristic echotexture of the muscle is present. The deltoid muscle (DM) is in the near field, separated by a thin hyperechoic interface (arrow) that represents the intermuscular fascia. The shadowing hyperechoic surface of the scapula (S) is seen in the far field in **A**.

lies medial to the major tubercle, deep in the medial groove of the shoulder. At that level, transverse scans are preferred for assessing the tendinous texture, the tendon sheath, and the intertubercular groove. On a transverse plane, the tendon appears as an oval, uniformly hyperechoic structure measuring approximately 3 mm thick in medium-sized to large dogs (Figure 16.7C). The transducer must be placed carefully perpendicular to the tendon fiber to avoid a drop in tendon echogenicity (anisotropy) that could be confused for a lesion (Figure 16.7A and B). The tendon is surrounded by a thin hypoechoic halo, consistent with the tendon sheath, which is typically fusiform to oval on cross section (Figure 16.7C). Thin, linear, hyperechoic interfaces can be seen at the superficial and deep margins of the sheath at the interface level of the tendon sheath wall and humeral surface, respectively. The major tubercle appears as a hyperechoic convex line at the lateral aspect of the bicipital groove and tendon. It is more distinct than the minor tubercle medially, which is seen only as a small elevation of the reflective line on the surface of the bone. The intertubercular groove appears as a mildly concave hyperechoic line extending into the reflective lines of the tubercle (Figure 16.7C). The intertubercular ligament cannot be distinguished from the surrounding soft tissue. Distally, the distal outpouch of the synovial sheath can appear lobulated in some dogs.

The longitudinal examination is then performed by following the tendon across the joint to its origin on the supraglenoid tubercle. In the far field, the hyperechoic line of the humeral bone surface becomes visible. Proximal to this point of orientation, the hypoechoic to anechoic area of the joint space and dorsally the supraglenoid tubercle can be distinguished. The latter structure is visible as a slightly convex, hyperechoic interface associated with acoustic shadowing. In this region, the use of a cross-sectional plane does not provide additional information. Because of its curvature along the intertubercular groove, the tendon hyperechoic echotexture can be evaluated only when perpendicular to the probe (Figure 16.7B). At the level of the supraglenoid tubercle, the tendinous fibers curve and become hypoechoic as they enter the bone (Figure 16.7A). This region should not be confused for a lesion.

Finally, the tendon is dynamically examined by flexing, extending, abducting, and adducting the shoulder joint. During these manipulations, the fine fibrillar structure of the biceps tendon is visualized throughout its length. When the joint is flexed, the hypoechoic joint space enlarges to approximately twice its original size (Kramer et al. 2001b).

Shoulder Joint Space

Craniocaudal positioning of the transducer perpendicular to the joint space enables visualization of the surface of the humeral head as a semicircular, convex, hyperechoic line with distal acoustic shadowing. The line should appear smooth, distinct, and continuous. The humeral head is located at a depth of 1–3 cm and is covered by muscles. Because of the semicircular anatomy of the head, only a small section of the surface can be assessed. In these perpendicular views, the bone surface appears as a distinct, curvilinear, hyperechoic line, with a 0.5- to 0.7-mm anechoic central band that represents the cartilage. The caudal and cranial borders of the humeral head are scanned tangentially

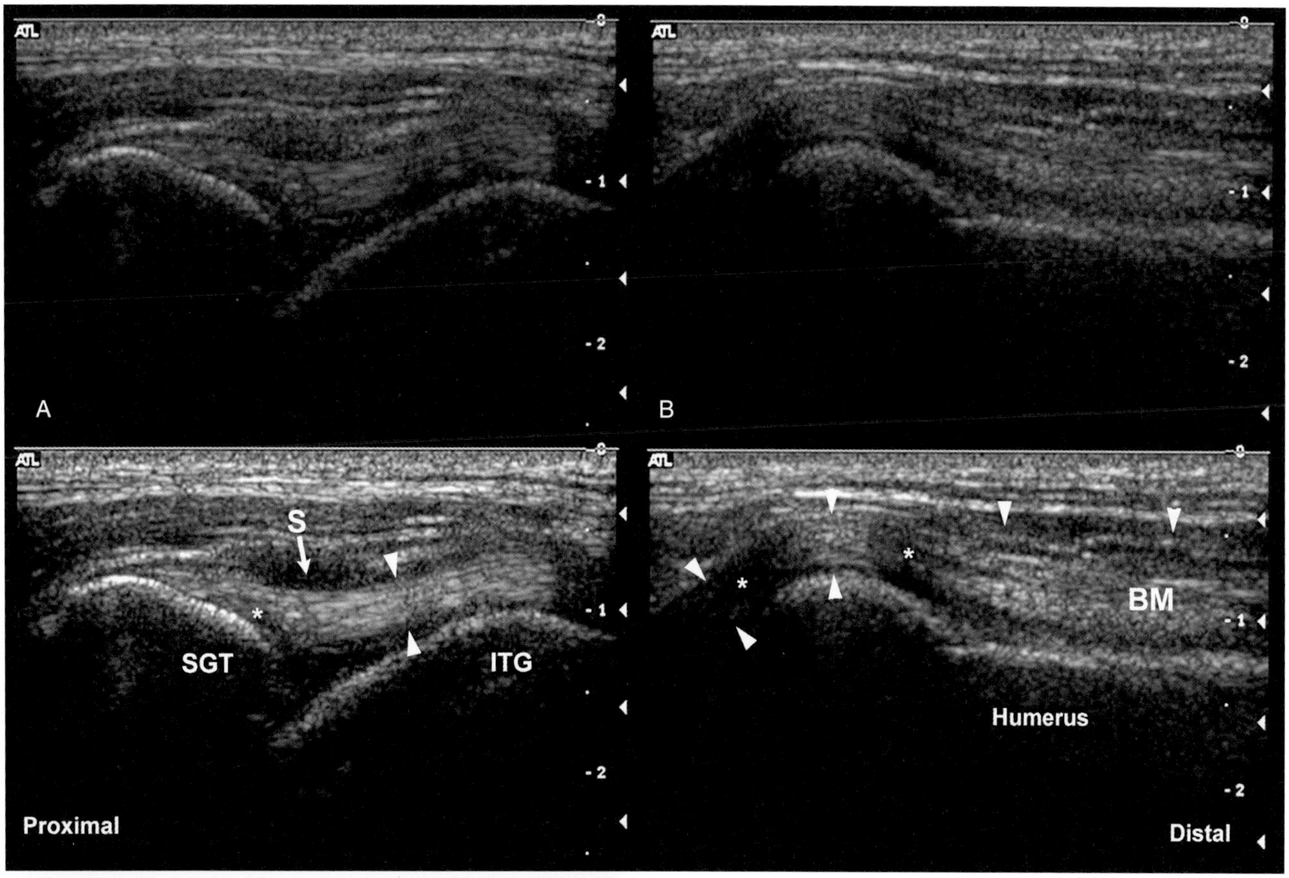

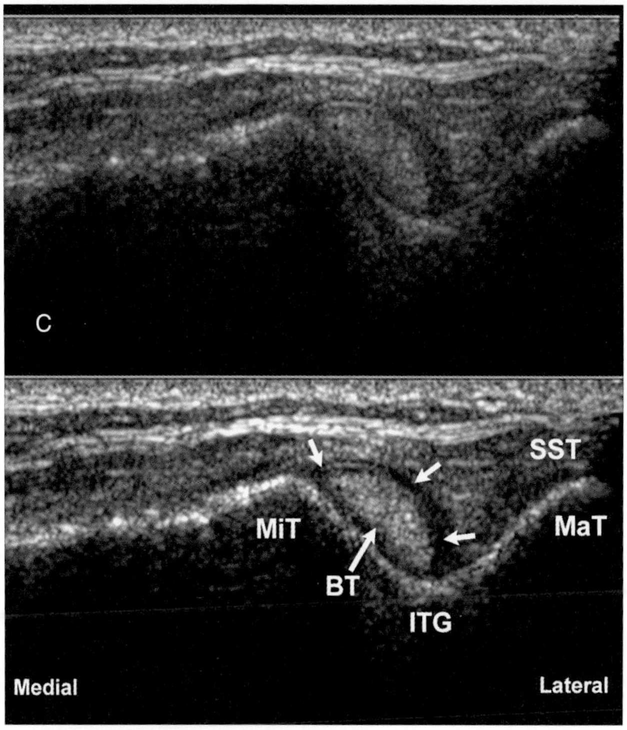

Figure 16.7. Normal sonographic anatomy of the biceps tendon in dogs. **A and B:** In these longitudinal sonographic and schematic images of the normal biceps tendon, the most proximal **(A)** and distal **(B)** portions of this tendon are seen (between the arrowheads) (see probe B on Figure 16.1). The characteristic hyperechoic echotexture of the tendon is well visualized when imaged perpendicularly. This tendon is hypoechoic (*) at the level of origin on the supraglenoid tubercle (SGT), as well as in curved portions more distally. Deep to the tendon, the intertubercular groove (ITG) appears as a curved, hyperechoic interface. The proximal portion of the biceps muscle (BM) is seen distal to the humeral head. **C:** Transverse sonographic and schematic images obtained at the level of the intertubercular groove (ITG). When imaged perpendicularly, the biceps tendon (BT) appears as a uniformly hyperechoic oval to flat structure surrounded by a thin hypoechoic rim (arrows) representing the tendon sheath with some fluid. The biceps tendon slides along the lateral aspect of the minor tubercle (MiT), medial to the major tubercle (MaT) and supraspinatus tendon of insertion (SST).

and appear indistinct, making them difficult to assess. In these planes, the synovium appears hypoechoic with small hyperechoic dots. The outer, curved line above the cartilage represents the joint capsule (Figure 16.8). This merges with the echotexture of the covering musculature. Accurate differentiation of these structures is usually not possible (Kramer and Gerwing 1994).

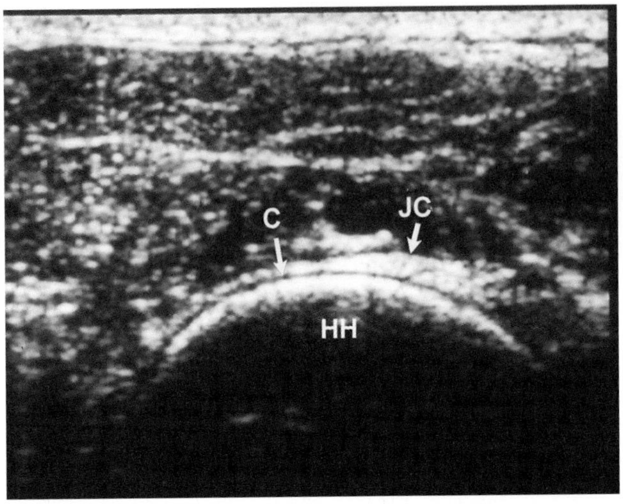

Figure 16.8. Normal sonographic anatomy of the shoulder joint. Longitudinal sonographic image obtained at the caudolateral aspect of the shoulder. The humeral head (HH) appears as a shadowing, hyperechoic, convex interface. The adjacent articular cartilage and small volume of synovial fluid appear as a thin hypoechoic band. The surrounding joint capsule (JC) is hyperechoic. C, thin layer of cartilage and synovial fluid.

Sonographic Features of Specific Shoulder Disorders

Supraspinatus Muscle

Supraspinatus Tendonitis and Mineralization Inflamed or degenerated supraspinatus tendons can be thickened and inhomogeneous because of fibrous disruption, hemorrhage, and/or fibrosis. Mineralization can also be found in the region of insertion on the major tubercle in the distal part of the tendon, although it may also be found in some clinically normal dogs. These mineral foci appear as small, hyperechoic, irregularly defined structures, with or without distal acoustic shadowing and with or without a surrounding hypoechoic to anechoic area (reaction tissue) (Gerwing and Kramer 1994; Long and Nyland 1999) (Figures 16.9 and 16.10).

Infraspinatus Muscle

Contracture of the Infraspinatus Muscle Distinct abnormalities in both echogenicity and echo pattern are seen in the affected muscle. The transition from muscle to tendon, and the tendon itself, are usually affected. These areas are highly inhomogeneous with hypoechoic and hyperechoic zones. The tendinous tissue appears edematous with irregular margins (Kramer et al. 1996; Siems et al. 1998).

Biceps Tendon

Tenosynovitis The ultrasonographic characteristics of bicipital tenosynovitis in dogs can be classified according to severity (Kramer et al. 2001b) (Table 16.1). The bicipital tendon appears mildly to severely thickened, losing its normal flat to oval shape to become rounded. Its normal fibrillar pattern can also be affected. Hypoechoic areas caused by partial tears and/or hemorrhage can be seen (Figure 16.11). The affected tendon may also appear significantly inhomogeneous.

Tendon sheath effusion, which is often observed, appears as an enlarged hypoechoic to anechoic halo surrounding the affected tendon. The effusion can range from mild to severe and is well visualized on transverse images over the intertubercular groove (Figures 16.11 and 16.12). In most cases, the thickened synovium cannot be easily distinguished from the synovial fluid. However, irregular synovial thickening or flocculent synovial fluid can be observed in some dogs (Long and Nyland 1999). Fibrous adhesions with

Table 16.1.
Bicipital tenosynovitis in dogs

Grade 1	Mild effusion of the tendon sheath (anechoic ring <2 mm thick) Normal tendon
Grade 2	Moderate effusion of the tendon sheath (anechoic ring 2–3 mm thick) Tendon mildly inhomogeneous
Grade 3	Severe effusion of the tendon sheath (anechoic ring >3 mm, extending further distally and medially in the tendon sheath) Tendon moderately to severely inhomogeneous and thickened or reduced to a stump
Grade 4	Maximal distension of the tendon sheath because of traumatic hemorrhage Tendon only mildly to moderately abnormal

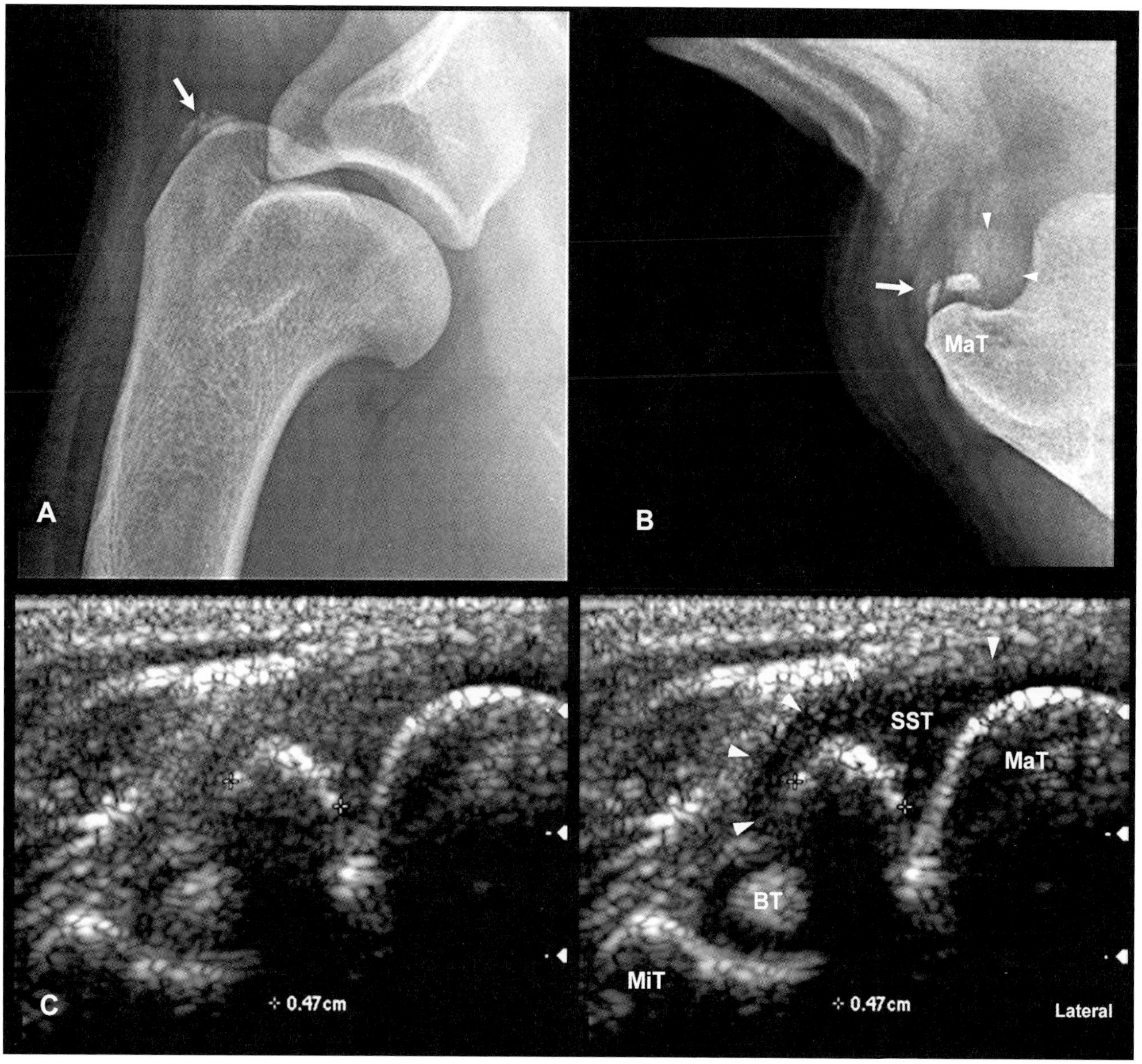

Figure 16.9. Calcifying supraspinatus tendinopathy. **A and B:** Mediolateral and tangential radiographs of the intertubercular groove in a large-breed dog with shoulder pain. Small mineral opacities (arrows) are observed in the region of insertion of the supraspinatus tendon, located just lateral to the intertubercular groove and biceps tendon (arrowheads). **C:** Transverse sonographic and schematic images of the intertubercular groove in the same dog. An irregular, hyperechoic, shadowing focus is in the distal supraspinatus tendon (SST), consistent with mineralization. This mineralization, as seen in the tangential radiographic projection, is adjacent to the biceps tendon (BT). Moderate distension of the biceps tendon sheath is observed, as the result of tenosynovitis, which was suspected to be secondary to the supraspinatus tendon lesion. MaT, major tubercle; and MiT, minor tubercle.

the tendon, particularly within the bicipital groove, can also be seen on dynamic sonograms. In severe cases, the tendon sheath develops a bulge in the direction of the minor tubercle. The wall of the tendon sheath is clearly visible as a hyperechoic line representing the border between the fluid and the surrounding musculature (Rivers et al. 1992; Kramer et al. 2001b; Esterline et al. 2005) (Figure 16.11E and F).

Exostoses (osteophytes) can form within the intertubercular groove as a result of chronic degenerative joint disease and/or bicipital tenosynovitis. The exostoses are attached to the tendon sheath and appear as

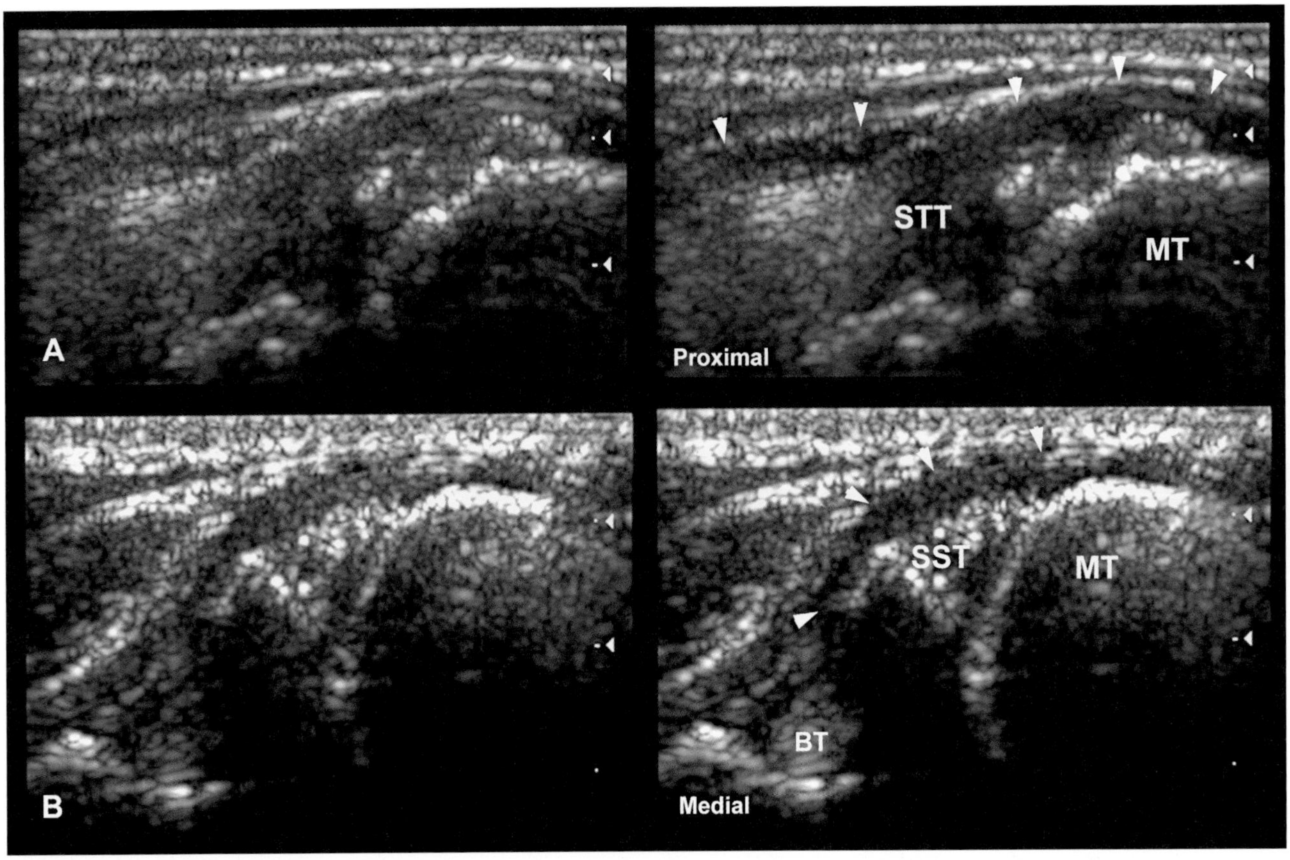

Figure 16.10. Calcifying supraspinatus tendinopathy. Longitudinal **(A)** and transverse **(B)** sonographic and schematic views of the supraspinatus tendon (SST) in a large-breed dog with shoulder pain. The supraspinatus tendon is inhomogeneous and presents several hyperechoic foci, some of which cause acoustic shadowing, consistent with fibrosis and mineralization. BT, biceps tendon; and MT, major tubercle.

hyperechoic, more or less concave, smooth, curved structures. Acoustic shadowing is usually present when these mineral deposits exceed 2–3 mm (Figure 16.12). In severe cases, the surrounding osteophytic formations may form a tunnel around the tendon, significantly hampering the visualization of the tendon (Figure 16.13). Mineralization of the bicipital tendon sheath cannot easily be distinguished from migrating calcified bodies, such as those related to osteochondritis dissecans.

Complete and Partial Tendon Ruptures With complete rupture, the homogeneous parallel, fibrillar structure of the tendon is destroyed. The gap between retracted tendon stumps is usually anechoic or hypoechoic, and moderate to severe tendon sheath effusion can be observed as the result of hemorrhage (Figure 16.14). The distal stump commonly is of mixed echogenicity and echotexture.

Most partial ruptures occur in the area of the supraglenoid tubercle. At this site, multiple, small, hyperechoic bone fragments with acoustic shadowing can be visible (Figure 16.15A). The proximal part of the tendon tissue appears hypoechoic and mildly to moderately inhomogeneous. In contrast to a complete rupture, areas of tendon tissue displaying a normal fibrillar echotexture can be found in a transverse image. A hypoechoic to anechoic region, also called *core lesion*, can be found in the central portion of the affected tendon, at the level of fibrillar disruption and hematoma formation, associated with tendon enlargement (Figures 16.11 and 16.15B) A cleft can also be observed in some partially ruptured tendons (Figure 16.13B). Tendon sheath effusion develops around the tendon (Kramer et al. 2001b).

Fractures of the Supraglenoid Tubercle The fractured supraglenoid tubercle is visualized at the proximal extent of the biceps tendon as a hyperechoic, more or less convex structure with smooth margins and acoustic shadowing. The fragment can be seen moving with the tendon during dynamic flexion and extension

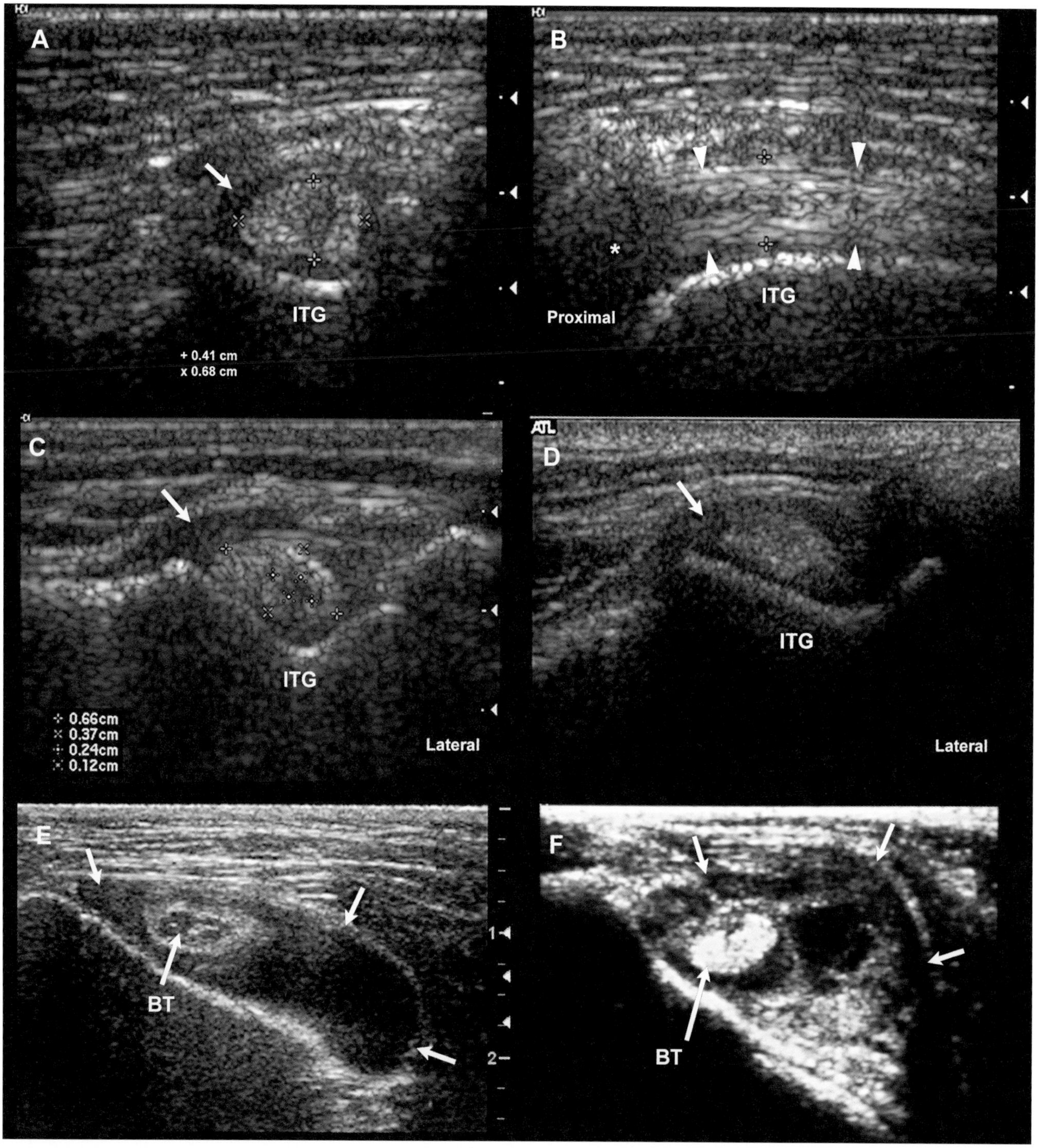

Figure 16.11. Bicipital tenosynovitis. **A and B:** Transverse **(A)** and longitudinal **(B)** sonograms of the biceps tendon (arrowheads) of a Labrador retriever scanned at the level of the intertubercular groove (ITG). The tendon is enlarged and rounded. A hypoechoic core lesion is in the center of the tendon, consistent with tendonitis with probable partial rupture. The tendon sheath (arrow) is mildly distended. **C–E:** Variable levels of tendon sheath distension (arrows) in several dogs with tenosynovitis. Hypoechoic lesions are in the central portion of the biceps tendon (BT) **(E)**. **F:** Distension of the tendon sheath in another dog with bicipital rupture and hemorrhage. The tendon sheath (arrows) is filled with inhomogeneously echogenic hematomas that encircle the biceps tendon (BT).

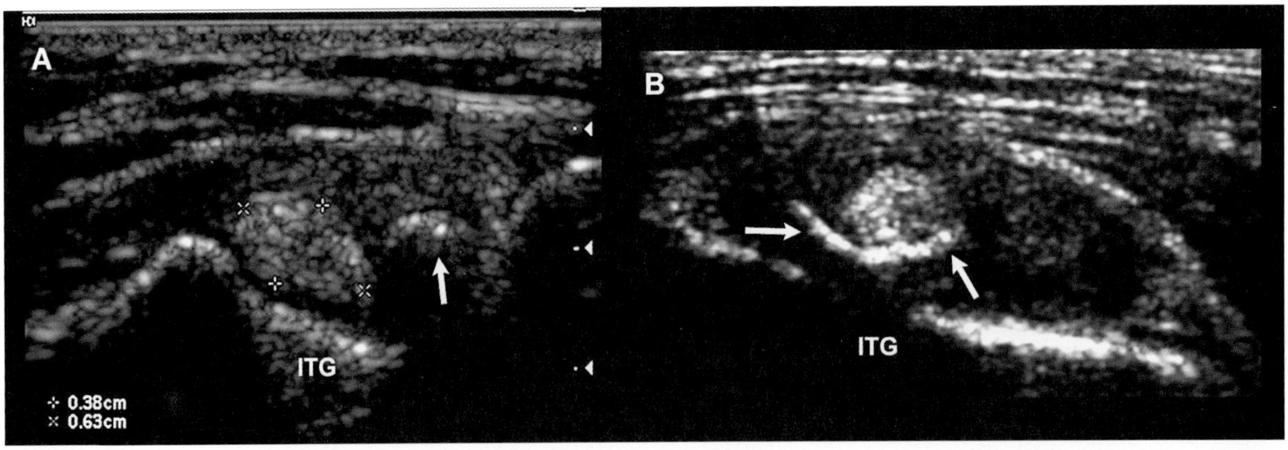

Figure 16.12. Chronic bicipital tenosynovitis with mineralization. Transverse sonographic images obtained in two dogs at the level of the intertubercular groove (ITG). **A:** A hyperechoic, shadowing mineral focus (arrow) is present at the lateral aspect of the bicipital tendon sheath. The adjacent tendon (between the cursors) is mildly thickened. **B:** Tendon sheath wall mineralization can appear as a hyperechoic semicircular groove (arrows) that may partially or completely encircle the biceps tendon.

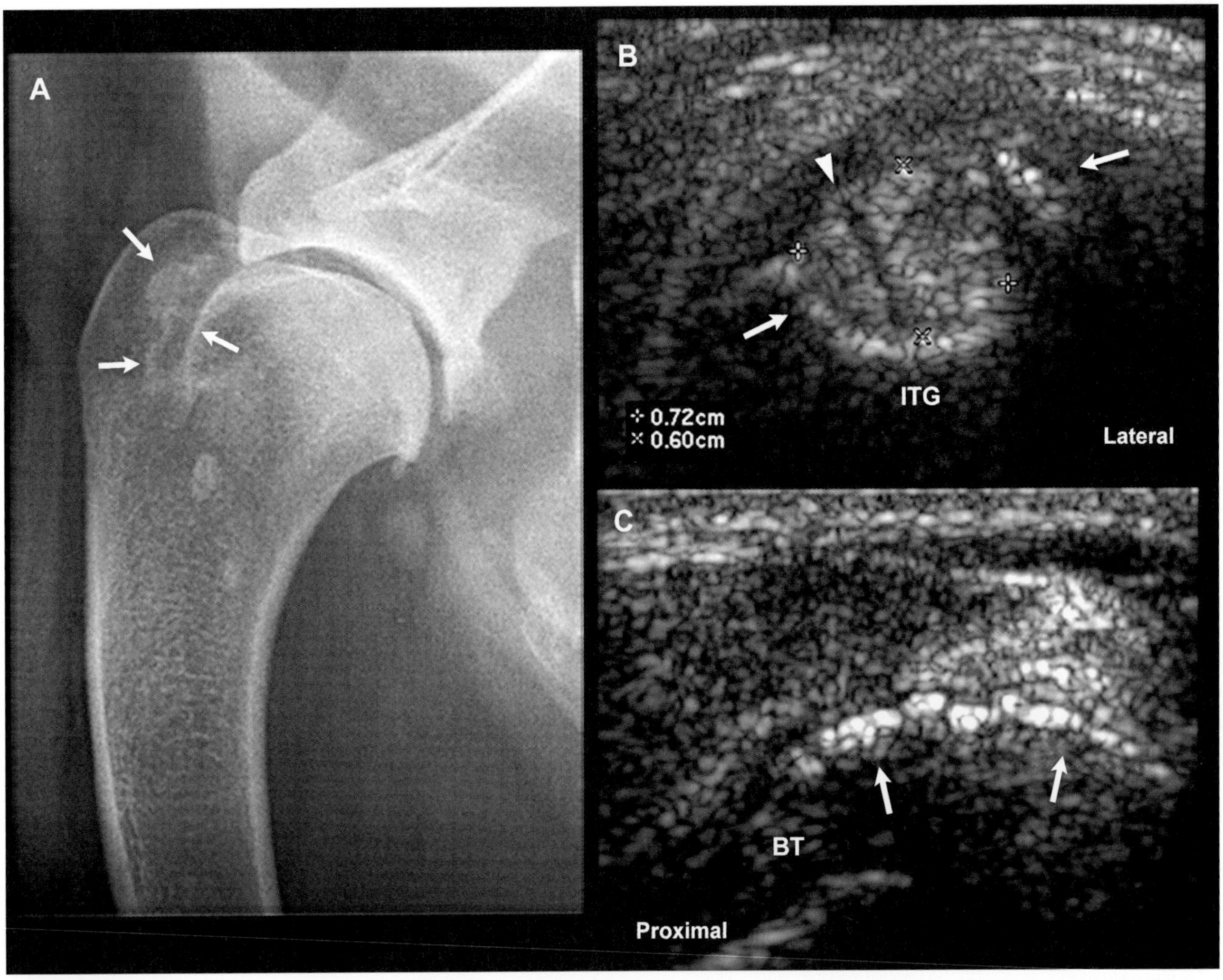

Figure 16.13. Chronic bicipital tenosynovitis with mineralization. **A:** Mediolateral radiographic view of the shoulder of a 4-year-old Rottweiler with chronic shoulder pain and lameness. Mineralization is found along the intertubercular groove (arrows), as well as in the distal region of the tendon sheath. Periarticular new bone formation is also present at the caudal aspect of the shoulder, consistent with degenerative joint disease. **B and C:** Transverse **(B)** and longitudinal **(C)** sonographic images of the intertubercular groove (ITG) on which an irregular and hyperechoic mineral cast partially encircles the biceps tendon (arrows). The tendon (between the cursors) is enlarged and presents a hypoechoic line (arrowhead) consistent with a tear.

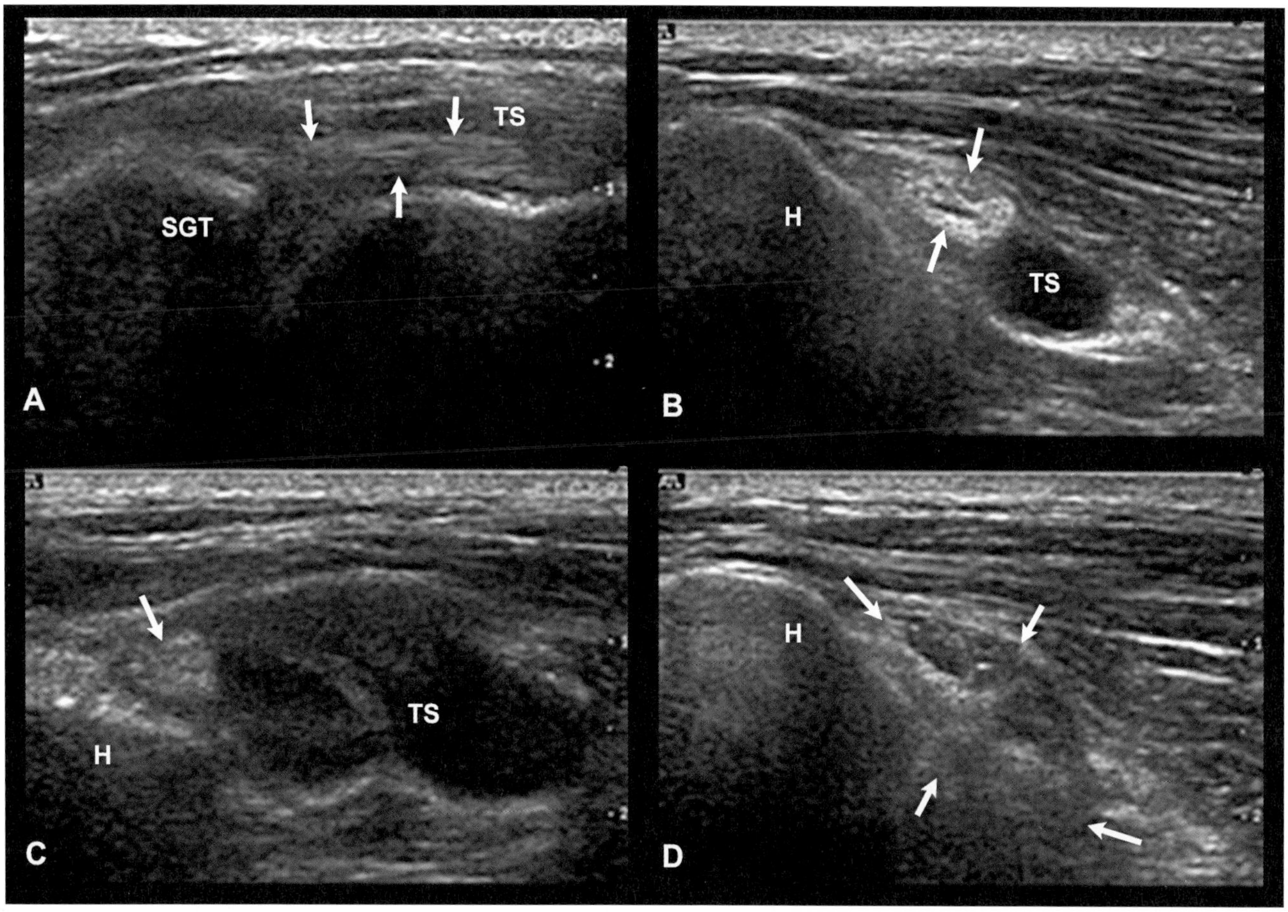

Figure 16.14. Complete bicipital tendon rupture. Longitudinal **(A)** and transverse **(B–D)** sonographic images of the biceps tendon and muscle in a dog with non–weight-bearing lameness. Significant distension of the tendon sheath (TS) is recognized. Hyperechoic and inhomogeneous retracted ends of the biceps tendon (arrows in **B** and **C**) are noted. Mildly echogenic regions, consistent with hemorrhage, are in the synovial sheath **(C)**. The proximal portion of the biceps tendon (**A**, arrows) and muscle (**D**, arrows) is inhomogeneous. Chronic bicipital tenosynovitis with rupture was diagnosed. H, humerus; and SGT, supraglenoid tubercle. Images courtesy of D. Penninck.

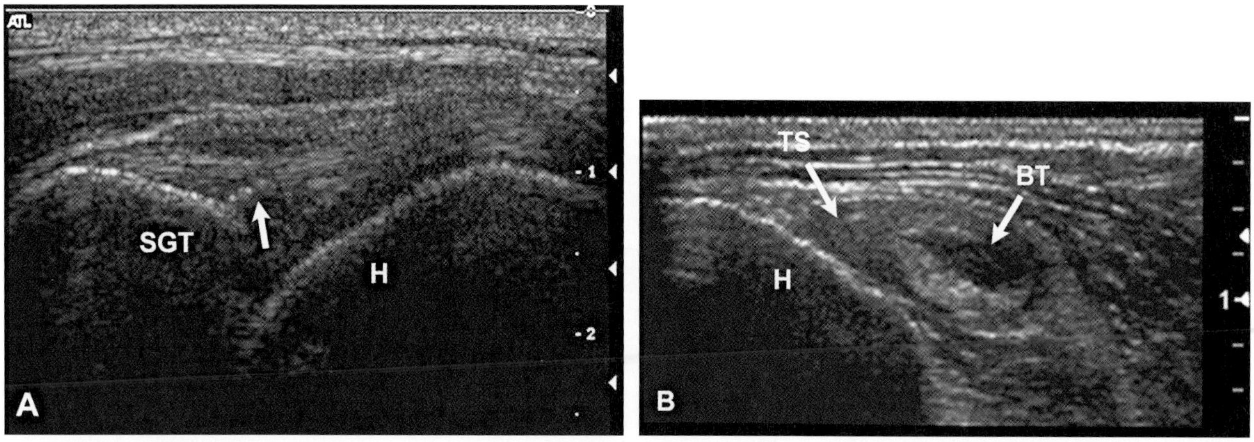

Figure 16.15. Partial bicipital tendon rupture. **A:** Longitudinal sonogram of the proximal portion of the biceps tendon in a dog with partial biceps tendon avulsion. An inhomogeneous, hypoechoic area (arrow) with small hyperechoic dots consistent with mineral fragments is just distal to the region of insertion on the supraglenoid tubercle (SGT). H, humerus. **B:** Transverse sonogram in another dog with partial tendon rupture. An oval anechoic area is in the central portion of the biceps tendon (BT), which is also enlarged. The tendon sheath (TS) has excessive fluid accumulation. H, humerus. Image B courtesy of D. Penninck.

of the shoulder, in association with moderate tendon sheath effusion (Gerwing and Kramer 1994). The surface of the tubercle appears irregular, and a bone defect can be observed. In cases of partial avulsion fracture, small bone fragments can be identified adjacent to the supraglenoid tubercle. Hyperechoic foci are observed in the proximal tendon and may be associated with acoustic shadowing (Kramer et al. 2001b) (Figure 16.15A).

Calcified Bodies in the Tendon Sheath Free bodies in the tendon sheath and caudal to the humeral head are usually caused by osteochondritis dissecans (OCD). Depending on their size, these are chips (>2 mm), microchips (1–2 mm), or stipples (<1 mm). Ultrasonographically, these bodies appear as hyperechoic, rounded or flat structures of different sizes that may cast acoustic shadows. They can be located anywhere around the tendon within the synovial sheath, which is usually distended (Kramer et al. 2001b) (Figure 16.16). These migrated bodies may adhere to the synovium and be difficult to differentiate from osteophytic formations, osteochondromas (Figure 16.17), or even primary bone tumors.

Tendon Luxation Rupture of the transverse ligament causes medial luxation of the tendon over the minor tubercle, which then cannot be demonstrated in the intertubercular groove. Instead, a moderate effusion of the tendon sheath is seen. The oval tendon with its typical fibrillar echotexture can be found in the region of the minor tubercle (Figure 16.18). During dynamic examination, the tendon slides back into the groove intermittently. The ruptured ligament cannot be visualized sonographically (Gerwing and Kramer 1994; Kramer et al. 2001b).

Joint

Osteochondritis Dissecans The subchondral defect on the caudal part of the humeral head can be visualized as an irregularity in the hyperechoic convex bone surface. The defect appears hypoechoic, with or without hyperechoic dots or lines, because of disturbed endochondral ossification and osteochondral fissures or fragments (Figure 16.19). The length of the defect can be measured (0.5–20 mm) via a craniocaudal scan. "Joint mice" might be present within the bicipital tendon sheath along with effusion of both the joint space and tendon sheath (Tacke et al. 1999; Vandevelde et al. 2006) (Figure 16.16).

Osteoarthritis In chronic osteoarthritis, the joint space of the shoulder appears distended and hypoechoic. The joint capsule is visible as a hyperechoic, thickened line (Figure 16.20). The cartilage can be thickened and, depending on the duration of the disease, becomes increasingly echogenic and inhomogeneous (Gerwing and Kramer 1994). Irregularities of the bone surface at the periphery of the joint are recognized when periarticular osteophytes develop.

Instability Shoulder joint instabilities can be determined by performing a dynamic scan of the joint to see

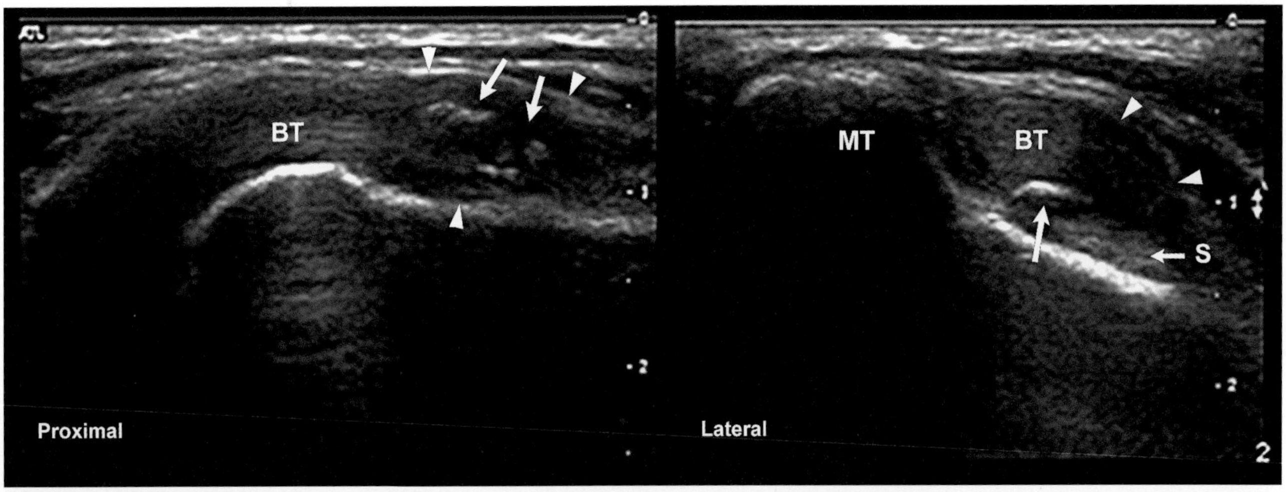

Figure 16.16. Migrating osteochondral fragments. Longitudinal and transverse sonograms of the distal tendon sheath in a dog with osteochondritis dissecans of the humeral head. Numerous hyperechoic foci (arrows) are in the distended tendon sheath (arrowheads), around the bicipital tendon (BT). Thickening of the synovial lining (S), consistent with synovitis, is also apparent on the surface of the humerus. MT, major tubercle. Images courtesy of D. Penninck.

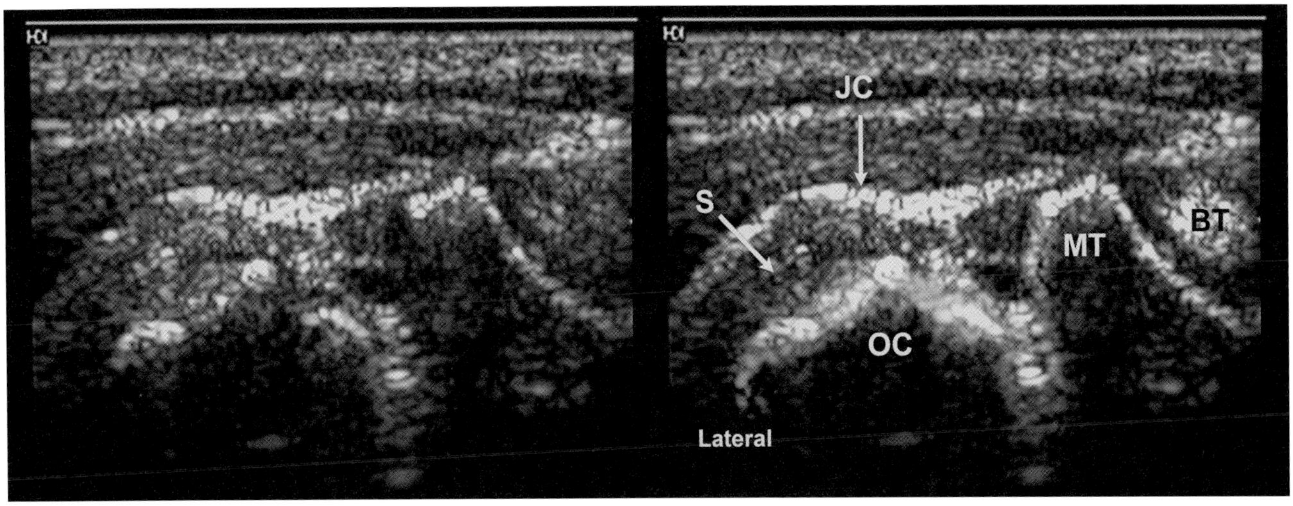

Figure 16.17. Osteochondromatosis. Transverse sonographic and schematic images obtained at the proximolateral aspect of the shoulder in a large-breed dog with chronic shoulder pain. An irregular, hyperechoic, strongly shadowing interface is lateral to the major tubercle (MT) and biceps tendon (BT), associated with thickening of the synovium (S) and joint capsule (JC). Calcified bodies attached to the joint capsule, in association with chronic synovitis, were identified at surgery. OC, osteochondroma.

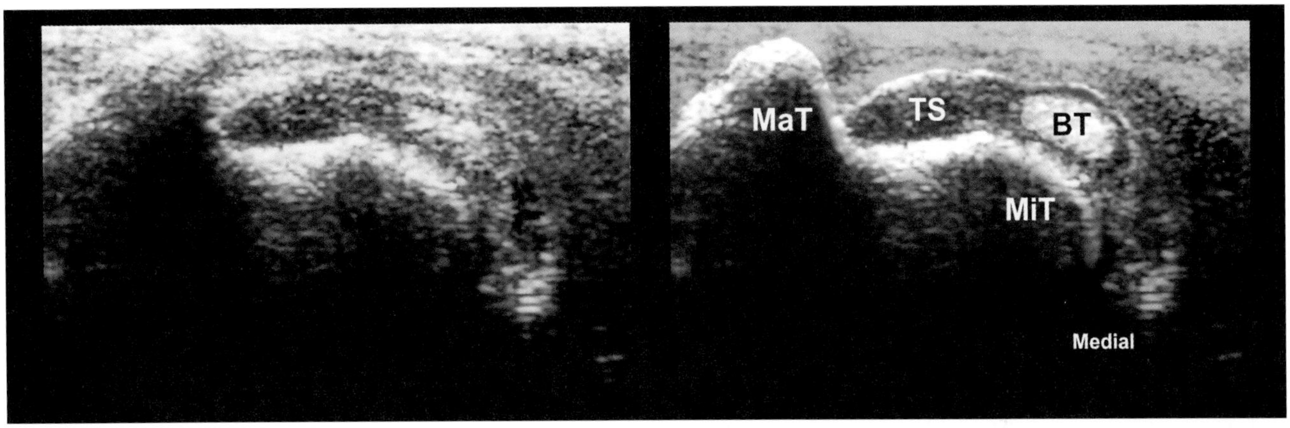

Figure 16.18. Biceps tendon luxation. In these transverse sonographic and schematic images of the intertubercular groove of a dog, the biceps tendon (BT) appears displaced medially over the minor tubercle (MiT). The tendon sheath is filled with fluid at the level of the bicipital groove. MaT, major tubercle; and TS, tendon sheath.

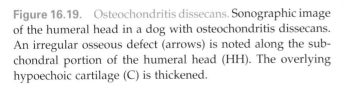

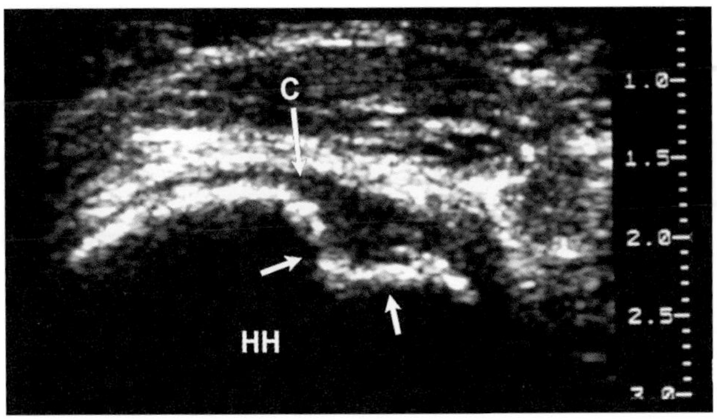

Figure 16.19. Osteochondritis dissecans. Sonographic image of the humeral head in a dog with osteochondritis dissecans. An irregular osseous defect (arrows) is noted along the subchondral portion of the humeral head (HH). The overlying hypoechoic cartilage (C) is thickened.

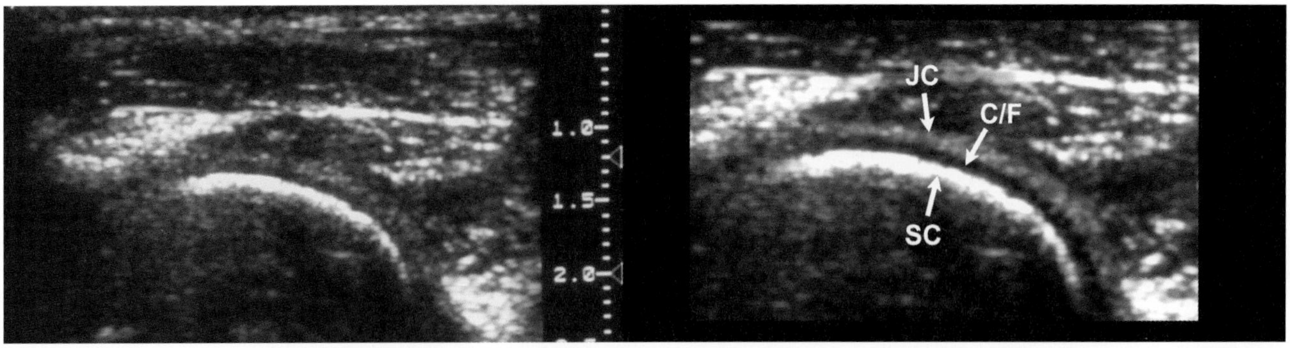

Figure 16.20. Osteoarthritis. Sonographic and close-up schematic images of the shoulder joint in a dog with degenerative joint disease. The thickened synovium and joint capsule (JC) appear as a hyperechoic band adjacent to the hypoechoic articular cartilage and fluid (C/F). SC, subchondral bone of the humeral head.

the abnormal gliding of the humeral head. However, this evaluation is subjective and often requires a comparison with the contralateral shoulder.

Elbow

Although radiography, computed tomography, and magnetic resonance imaging are most commonly used to image the elbow, ultrasonography can represent a useful tool in practice, particularly in the assessment of soft-tissue structures. The approach to the normal canine elbow has been well described (Knox et al. 2003; Lamb and Wong 2005).

Scanning Technique and Normal Ultrasonographic Anatomy

A linear, high-frequency (>10 MHz) ultrasound transducer is preferred for assessing all portions of the elbow. This joint can usually be examined without sedation. The hair around the elbow is clipped, and the patient initially is placed in lateral recumbency with the elbow of interest up. After the lateral aspect of the joint has been evaluated, the patient is turned over to assess the medial structures more easily (Figure 16.21).

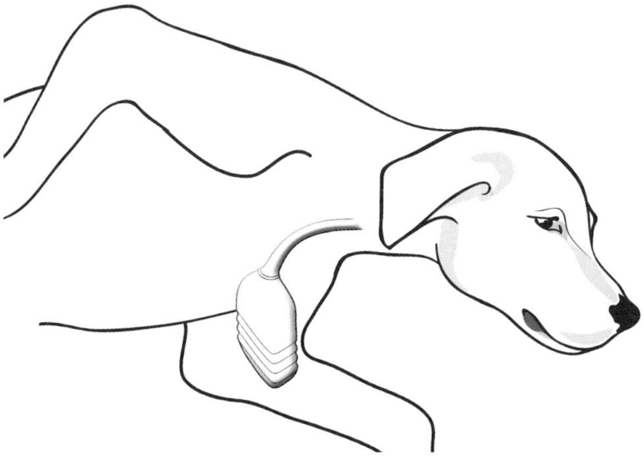

Figure 16.21. Scanning technique for the medial aspect of the elbow. Illustration showing the position of the dog and ultrasound probe when scanning the medial aspect of the elbow.

Lateral Aspect: Muscles and Lateral Collateral Ligament

The humerus and the brachialis muscle on the proximal craniolateral aspect of the joint are examined. During flexion and extension of the elbow, the hypoechoic brachialis muscle can be shown to slide against the smooth, linear, hyperechoic interface of the humerus. The distal portion of the triceps muscle can be seen caudolaterally inserting onto the olecranon.

Distally, the lateral region of the elbow is initially scanned in cross section to better identify all muscles and tendons. Each muscle and tendon is then scanned longitudinally. The most conspicuous muscle is the extensor carpi radialis located on the craniolateral aspect of the forearm. Caudal to this region, the common and lateral digital extensor tendons, as well as the extensor carpi ulnaris, are visualized.

The lateral collateral ligament is very thin and more easily assessed proximally because it displays multiple, fine, hyperechoic parallel lines that attach to the lateral humeral epicondyle. The distal aspect of the ligament is typically hypoechoic because the sound beam cannot be directed perpendicular to its longitudinal axis.

Caudal Aspect: Triceps, Olecranon, and Anconeal Process

The elbow joint is flexed, and the ultrasound probe is initially placed cranially on the olecranon. When a sagittal, perpendicular plane is used, the distal portion of the triceps muscle appears as a hyperechoic structure with multiple fine parallel lines, representing the collagen fibers, which insert onto the olecranon. Two distinct protuberances are recognized on the proximal aspect of the olecranon: the craniolateral and craniomedial tuberosities, which are located proximal to the anconeal process. The transducer is then slightly rotated laterally, enabling visualization of the outline of the anconeal process. This process is examined as the transducer is moved medially from the most lateral edge of the olecranon. The normal anconeal process appears as a curved, hyperechoic interface. Artifactual pseudoindentations are a common finding on the surface of the bone. The caudal joint capsule is usually not visible. The caudal structures of the joint are scanned in flexion and extension of the elbow by placing the probe on the lateral epicondyle.

Cranial Aspect: Joint Space, Muscles, Vessels, and Nerves

This region is examined after the elbow joint has been extended. Proximally, both the brachialis and biceps brachii muscles (Figure 16.22A) can be distinguished; distally, the extensor carpi radialis muscle is visible. In addition, vessels and nerves embedded within the adipose tissue can be visualized. The cranial portion of the humeroradial joint space appears as a thin, hypoechoic cleft between the smooth, hyperechoic contours of the humeral condyles and radial head. The normal joint capsule and synovium cannot differentiated.

Medial Aspect: Medial Collateral Ligament and Medial Coronoid Process

In the proximal caudomedial region of the elbow, the two heads of the triceps brachii muscle can be differentiated. The medial epicondyle is initially assessed in a longitudinal plane and appears as curved, slightly irregular, hyperechoic interface on the distomedial aspect of the humerus. The medial collateral ligament, which merges from the medial epicondyle, appears proximally as a thin, linear, hyperechoic structure that is densely packed with fine, parallel echoes (Figure 16.22B). The ligament fibers spread caudally to the ulna and become slightly thicker near the radius. Because of the oblique course of the medial collateral ligament, it is often not possible to identify the fibrillar pattern in the distal portion (Lamb and Wong 2005). The biceps brachii tendon can be visualized on the cranial aspect of the distal humerus and followed to its insertion sites on the ulnar and radial tuberosities, just adjacent to the medial coronoid process (Lamb and Wong 2005) (Figure 16.22A). This tendon shows a typical echotexture with hyperechoic lines. When the probe is moved proximally during a transverse scan, the surface of the medial coronoid process (MCP) comes into view as an angular process on the medial aspect of the ulna (Figure 16.22). The MCP is located deep to the medial collateral ligament and biceps tendon (Lamb and Wong 2005). A 90° flexion of the elbow and rotation of the forearm around its longitudinal axis may facilitate the identification of this structure.

Sonographic Features of Specific Elbow Disorders

Osteoarthritis and Septic Arthritis

Even minor effusions of the elbow joint can be visualized. Anechoic fluid in a recess of the joint can always be interpreted as a sign of a pathological process and is most commonly related to elbow dysplasia. With chronic degenerative joint disease (DJD), the joint capsule is visible as a hyperechoic, thick line between the synovium and the surrounding musculature. Periarticular new bone formations, caused by osteoarthritis, appear as irregularly circumscribed protuberances on the bony surfaces (Michele et al. 1998) (Figure 16.24). However, it must be pointed out that similar findings may be found with septic arthritis. Rapidly progressive, echogenic joint effusion is more suggestive of a septic process or hemorrhage (Figure 16.23).

Osteochondritis Dissecans

Osteochondrosis or OCD, which typically affects the medial articular portion of the humeral condyle, is difficult to assess sonographically because of the localization of the defect (Michele et al. 1998). Displaced osteochondral fragments may be visible.

Fragmented Medial Coronoid Process

A completely detached coronoid bone fragment can sometimes be identified as a very hyperechoic

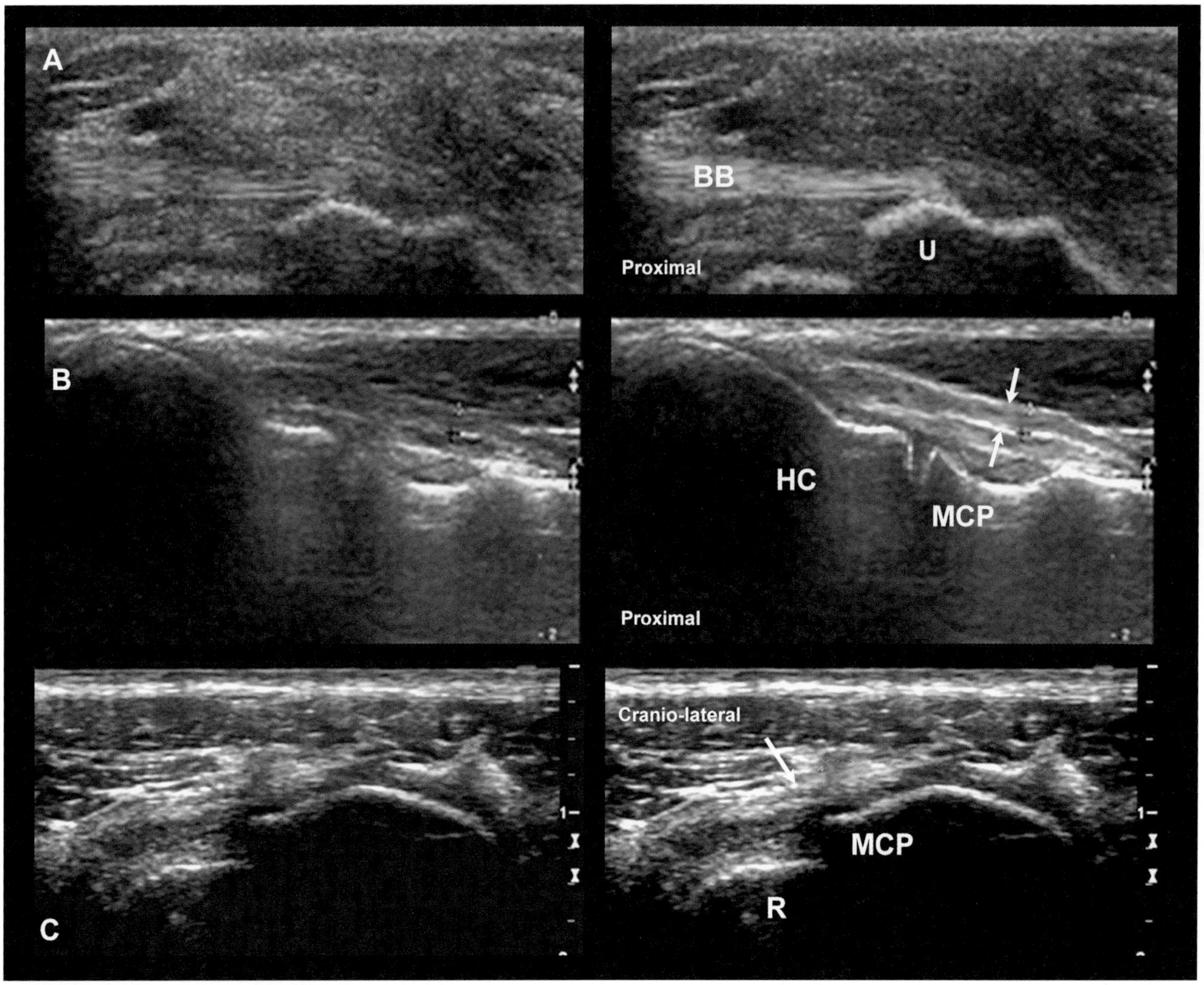

Figure 16.22. Normal sonographic anatomy of the canine elbow. **A:** Longitudinal sonographic and schematic images of the craniomedial aspect of the elbow. A portion of the distal biceps brachii (BB) appears as a hyperechoic fusiform structure with dense hyperechoic lines inserting on the craniomedioproximal surface of the ulna (U). **B:** Longitudinal sonographic and schematic images obtained just medial to **A**. The medial collateral ligament (arrows) is just medial to the medial coronoid process (MCP) and humeral condyle (HC). **C:** Transverse-oblique sonographic and schematic images of the craniomedial aspect of the elbow. The hyperechoic interface of the medial coronoid process (MCP) is well visualized adjacent to the head of the radius (R). The joint capsule is a hyperechoic band (arrow) that cannot be consistently distinguished from collateral ligaments.

structure with acoustic shadowing, cranial or medial to its anatomically correct position (Figure 16.24). The presence of new bone formation on the medial coronoid process, as the result of DJD, may be confused for fragmentation of the MCP. In general, fissures of the MCP cannot be displayed sonographically. Performing a dynamic examination with flexion and extension of the joint may lead to movement of the fragment, thereby confirming the diagnosis (Schleich et al. 1992).

Ununited Anconeal Process

Ununited anconeal process is recognized as an interruption of the hyperechoic outline of the protuberance (Figure 16.25). In some cases, movement of the fragment can be demonstrated with a dynamic sonogram. In chronic disease, an anechoic moderate effusion, hyperechoic thickening of the joint capsule, and/or irregularly circumscribed, hyperechoic, arthritic new

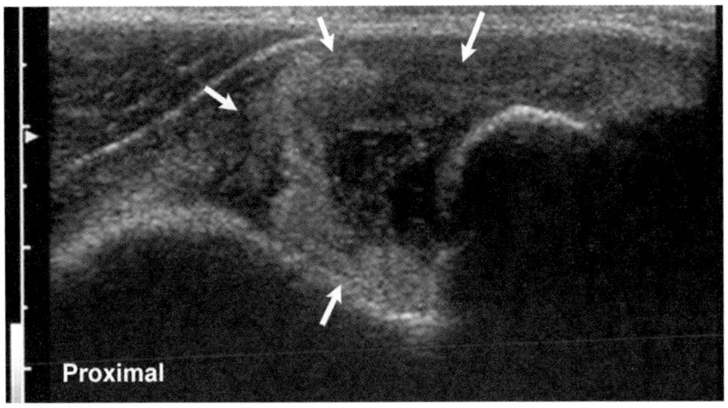

Figure 16.23. Septic arthritis. Longitudinal sonogram of the caudolateral aspect of the elbow of a dog with septic arthritis. A focal accumulation of inhomogeneous, echogenic fluid (arrows) is present, consistent with pus.

bone formations may be observed (Michele et al. 1998).

Fragmentation or Avulsion of the Medical Humeral Epicondyle and Metaplasia of the Deep Digital Flexor Muscle

Mineralization associated with the carpal and digital flexor muscles, which originate on the medial humeral epicondyle, are sometimes seen in dogs. These may relate to avulsion fractures, fragmentation, and/or dystrophic mineralization (Figure 16.26). These may also relate to muscular metaplasia (Michele and Gerwing 1999) (Figure 16.27). Adhesions to the joint capsule can be present, although this feature cannot be

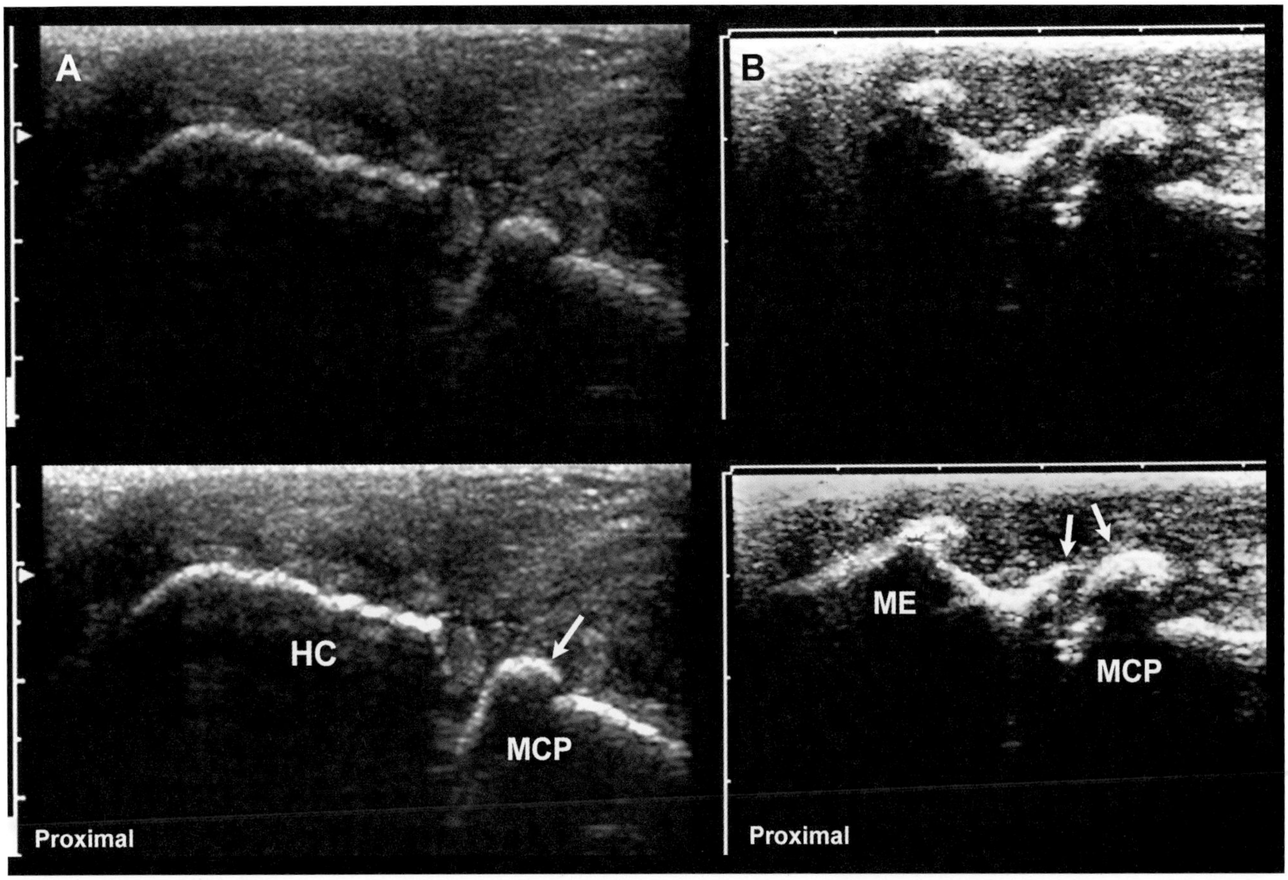

Figure 16.24. Fragmentation of the medial coronoid process. **A and B:** Longitudinal sonographic and schematic images obtained in two dogs in the region of the medial coronoid process (MCP). An irregular discontinuity of the craniomedial surface of these processes is noted, as well as suspected displaced fragments (arrows). Periarticular new bone formation consistent with degenerative joint disease has caused an irregularity in the medial surface of the humeral condyle (HC). ME, medial humeral epicondyle.

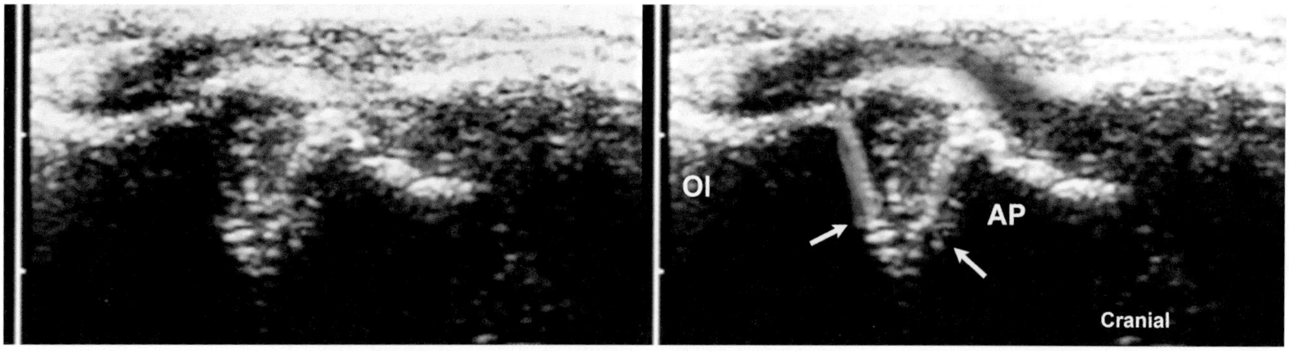

Figure 16.25. Ununited anconeal process. Longitudinal sonographic and schematic images obtained at the level of the anconeal process (AP) in a dog with suspected elbow dysplasia. The probe is placed on the dorsal (cranioproximal) surface of this process. A V-shaped cleft (arrows) is noted cranial to the olecranum (Ol), consistent with an ununited anconeum. Hyperechoic dots consistent with partial mineralization are noted within the cleft.

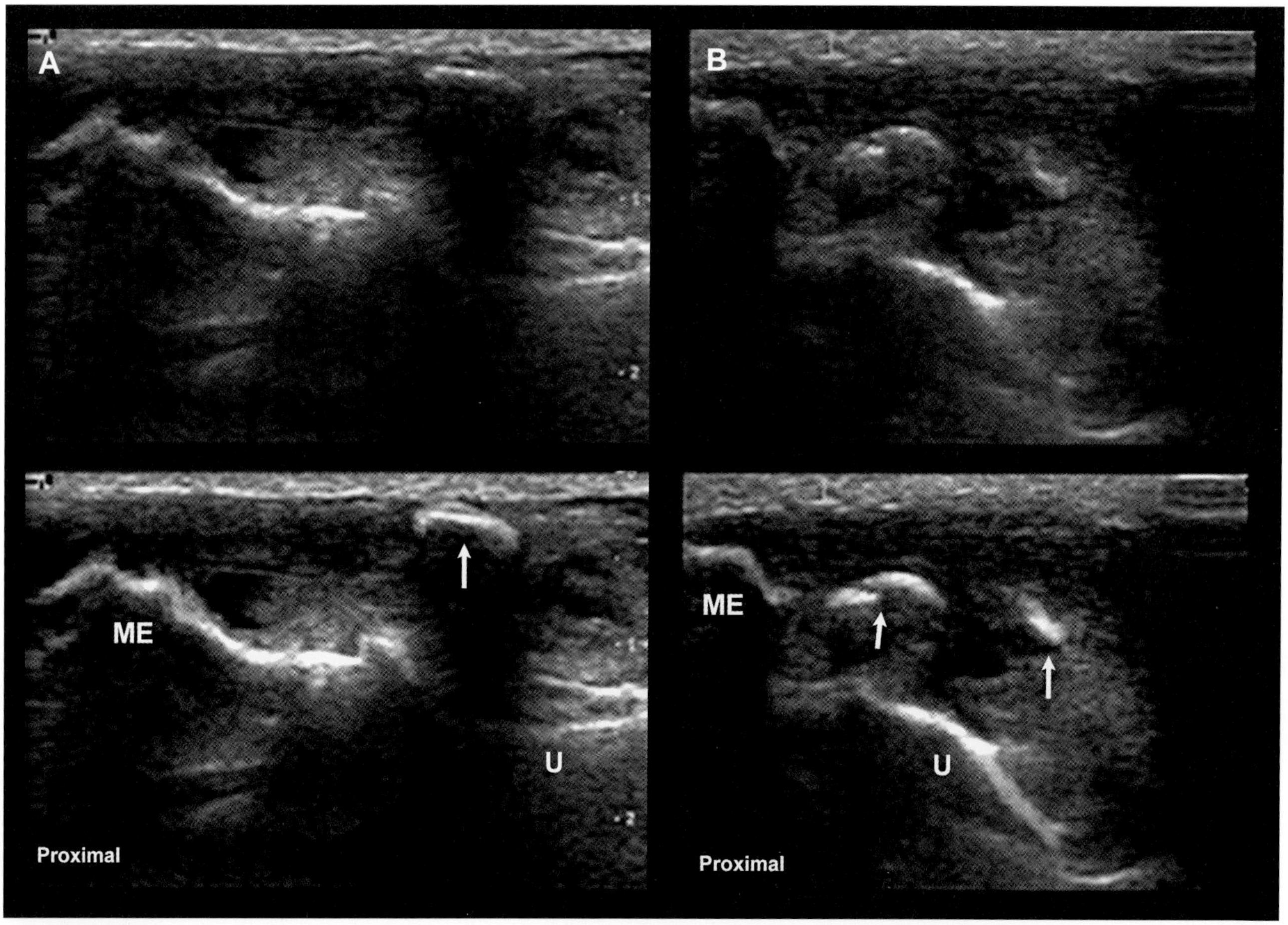

Figure 16.26. Fragmentation of the medial humeral epicondyle. **A and B:** Longitudinal sonographic and schematic images obtained at the caudomedial aspect of the medial humeral epicondyle (ME) in a dog. Numerous oval hyperechoic structures (arrows) consistent with calcified bodies are present at the medial aspect of the cubital joint and proximal ulna (U). The adjacent soft tissues are inhomogeneous and enlarged. The medial epicondyle surface is also irregular. Images courtesy of D. Penninck.

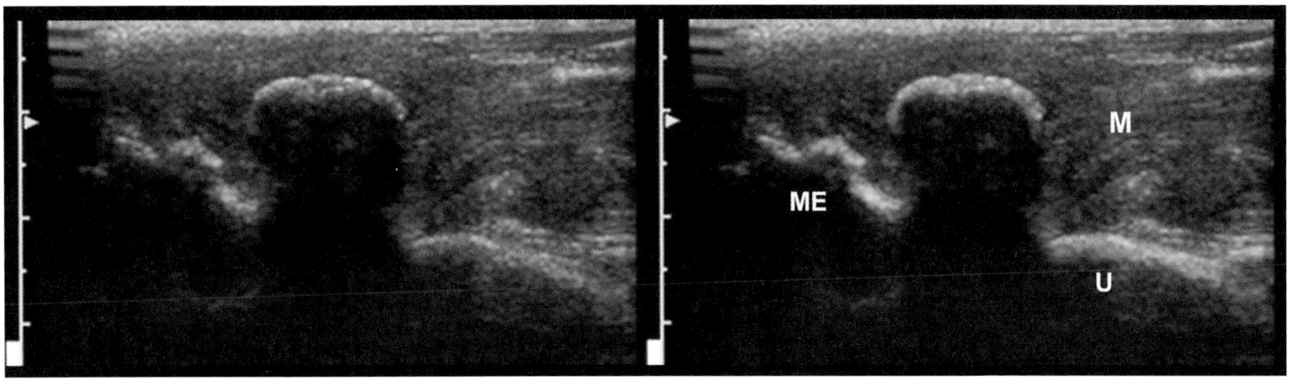

Figure 16.27. Metaplasia of the deep digital flexor muscle. Longitudinal sonographic and schematic images obtained at the caudomedial aspect of the medial humeral epicondyle (ME) in another dog. A well-defined, hyperechoic oval structure with strong acoustic shadowing is noted that is consistent with a calcified body. The adjacent muscles (M) are enlarged and inhomogeneous. Osseous metaplasia of the deep digital flexor tendon was diagnosed. U, ulna.

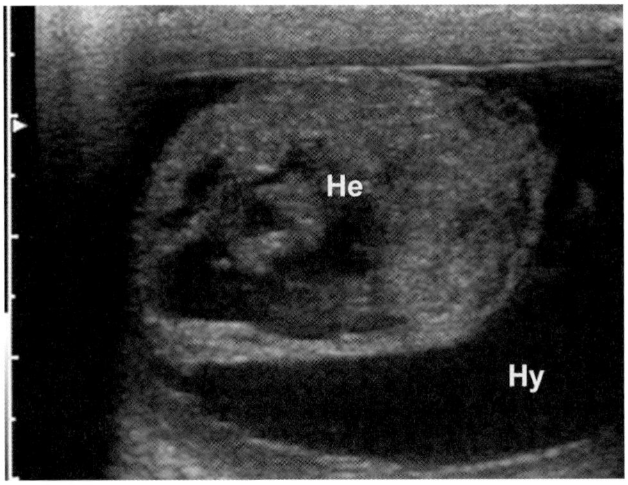

Figure 16.28. Hemorrhagic hygroma. The olecranon bursa is markedly distended and filled with an anechoic fluid consistent with hygroma (Hy). Additionally, a large inhomogeneous structure is found in the distended bursa indicative of a chronic hematoma (He).

easily seen ultrasonographically. Concurrent elbow dysplasia is common.

Hygroma

In large, heavy dogs, the olecranian bursa, which is located under the insertion of the triceps muscle, can become distended and/or inflamed. The bursa can be filled with variable fluid (blood, pus, or some other) of variable echogenicity. The capsule is hyperechoic and can be thickened (Michele et al. 1998) (Figure 16.28).

Stifle

Scanning Technique and Normal Sonographic Anatomy

A high-frequency linear transducer (>10 MHz) is usually preferred for assessing all structures of the knee. The hair must be clipped from the distal third of the femur to just below the tibial tuberosity. Initially, the dog is placed in lateral recumbency with the affected limb up (Figure 16.29A). The final dynamic examination requires flexion and extension of the joint, as well as inward and outward rotation of the knee in the area of the menisci (Engelke et al. 1997a; Kramer et al. 1999).

The stifle joint is examined from proximally to distally. After scanning the cranial, caudal, and lateral aspects of the joint, the dog is turned over so that the affected limb faces downward, allowing assessment of the medial region (Figure 16.29B). The stifle can be divided into five regions: suprapatellar, infrapatellar, lateral, caudal, and medial (Kramer et al. 1999).

Suprapatellar Region: Quadriceps Tendon, Femoral Trochlea, and Proximal Joint Recess

The suprapatellar region is proximal to the tendon of the quadriceps femoris muscle. The knee is flexed to 45°, and both longitudinal and transverse views are assessed, focusing on the distal femur, the patella, the joint capsule, the suprapatellar recess, as well as the quadriceps femoris muscle and tendon (Figure 16.29A). The hyperechoic convex surface of the patella can be used as a landmark. The suprapatellar indentation of the femoropatellar joint sac directly proximal to the

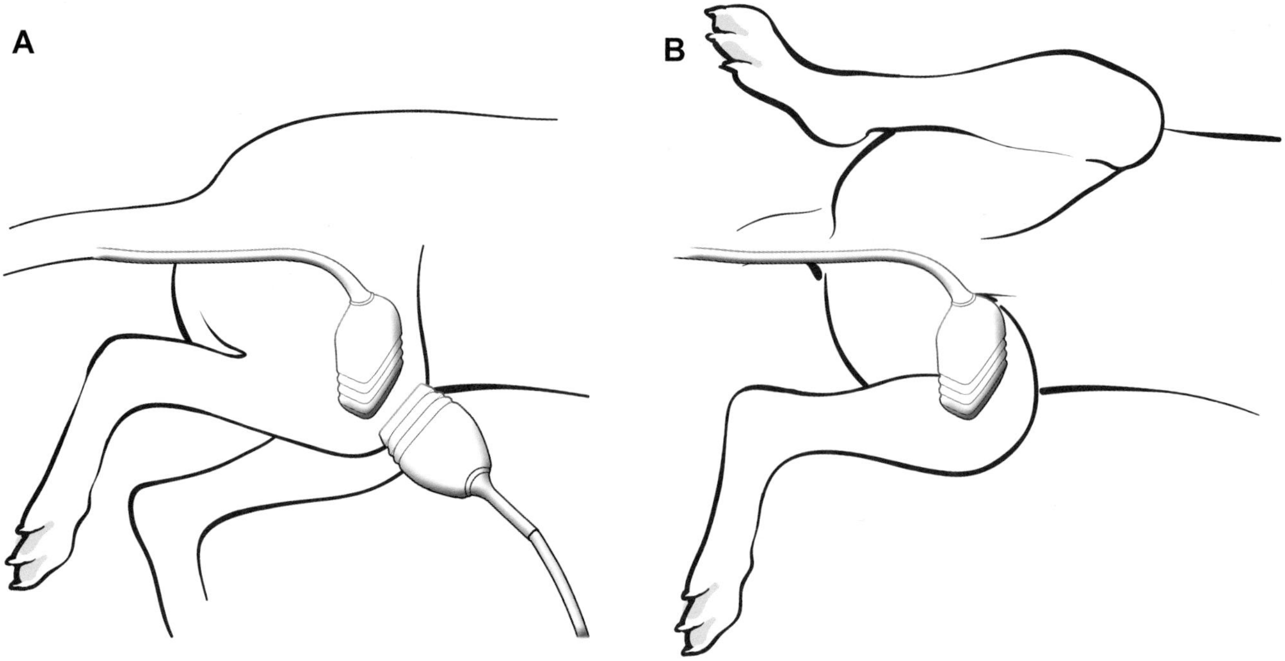

Figure 16.29. Scanning technique for the stifle. The position of the dog and ultrasound probe when using longitudinal planes to scan the lateral and cranial aspects of the stifle **(A)** and medial **(B)** regions. Longitudinal and transverse planes must be used in all regions.

patella is of particular interest. In a normal knee, the suprapatellar recess is a 1- to 2-mm-thick or smaller, anechoic, more or less inhomogeneous structure located above the hyperechoic shaft of the femur (Figure 16.30). On the femoral side, the joint capsule cannot be differentiated from the surrounding structures. However, in the region of the quadriceps femoris muscle, part of the joint capsule can be seen as a hyperechoic line. In most dogs, the fascia of the quadriceps muscle cannot be clearly differentiated from the surrounding structures.

The distal tendon of the quadriceps femoris muscle and the femoral condyles, trochlea, and covering cartilage become clearly visible by means of a dynamic scan. The articular cartilage is a 1- to 2-mm-thick anechoic band located directly above the curvilinear, hyperechoic subchondral surface of the femur. The depth and surface continuity of this cartilage must be examined (Figure 16.31).

The area above the patella can easily be evaluated in a transverse scan with the stifle maximally flexed. This position enables the assessment of the cartilage, as well as the shape and depth of the femoral trochlea. At this point, a dynamic examination (subsequent flexion and extension) enables the assessment of the sliding movement of the patella into the trochlear groove.

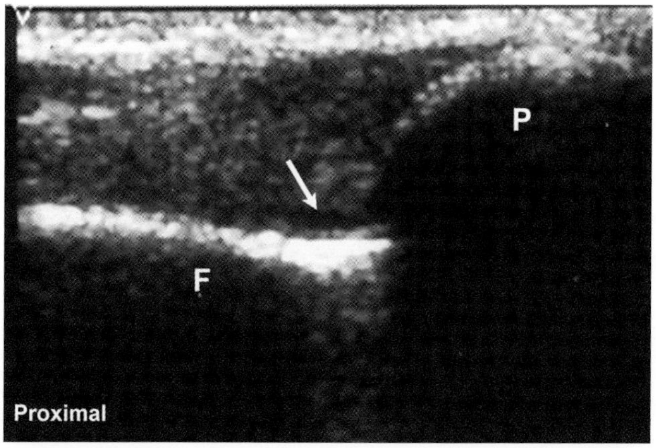

Figure 16.30. Normal suprapatellar region. Longitudinal sonogram of the suprapatellar region. The suprapatellar recess is seen as a small anechoic focus (arrow) at the proximal aspect of the femoral trochlea, just proximal to the patella (P). Only the convex, hyperechoic surface of the patella can be seen. This structure limits the visualization of the femoral trochlea. F, femur.

Infrapatellar Region: Patella and Patellar Ligament, Femoral Condyles, Infrapatellar Fat Body, and Cruciate Ligaments

Because of the convexity of the femoral condyles, only a few areas of the joint surface can be assessed. Multiple

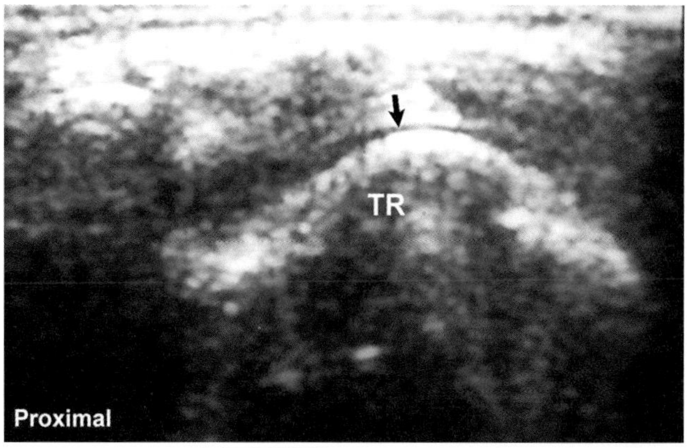

Figure 16.31. Normal trochlear ridge and cartilage. Longitudinal sonogram of one of the ridges of the trochlea in a normal dog. The osseous portion of the ridge appears as a smooth, convex, hyperechoic line and is covered by a thin hypoechoic band (arrow) that represents the cartilage and synovial fluid. These latter components cannot be distinguished. TR, trochlear ridge.

imaging planes of each condyle are necessary. When the stifle is extended, the patella slides proximally on the trochlea, and the medial and lateral femoral condyles can be more fully examined. The joint cartilage is anechoic and smoothly marginated (Figure 16.32). All planes must be used to ensure the identification of defects, as well as to rule out artifactual pseudodefects.

As the knee is 90° flexed, the transducer is moved over the patellar ligament and patella (Figure 16.29A). The patella, which appears as a hyperechoic, convex line with strong acoustic shadowing, is partially embedded in the patellar ligament, which presents a characteristic hyperechoic band with a fibrillar echotexture (Figure 16.32). A thin, echogenic, periligamentous sheath is also seen (Mattern et al. 2006). The distal margin of the patellar ligament appears slightly thicker and the insertion site is less echogenic than the rest of the structure. When viewed transversally, the curved margins of the ligament are not visible because of edge-shadowing artifacts.

Beneath the patellar ligament, the infrapatellar fat body is a triangular, poorly demarcated structure of mixed echotexture, but primarily hypoechoic, located cranial to the joint space (Figure 16.32). Within the infrapatellar fat body, vessels are often visible as hyperechoic thin, double-lined, tubular structures with an anechoic center. With the stifle still flexed, lateral rotation of the transducer by 20° enables visualization of the hypoechoic to anechoic cranial cruciate ligament, which extends from the cranial margin of the tibia to the region between the femoral condyles. The caudal cruciate ligament, which can be observed when the knee is maximally extended, appears as a hypoechoic, more or less ovoid structure. In small dogs, the ligament cannot be visualized because of limited space between the condyles that causes superimposition and artifacts. The space between the femur and tibia is filled with homogeneous tissue of medium echogenicity. Differentiation between the infrapatellar fat body and the meniscus is usually not possible from a cranial approach (Reed et al. 1995; Engelke et al. 1997a; Kramer et al. 1999).

Lateral Aspect: Fabella, Lateral Collateral Ligament, Long Digital Extensor Tendon, Lateral Meniscus, Joint Capsule, and Synovium

The surface of the lateral fabella is located immediately above the surface of the condyle. When a longitudinal plane is used, the head of the gastrocnemius muscle comes into view next to the caudolateral outline of the condyle and the fabella. The muscle is identified by the presence of the fabella within its tendon. The transverse parts of the biceps femoris muscle and the superficial digital extensor tendon run across the tibia.

By means of a longitudinal plane centered on the lateral joint space, the lateral femoral and tibial condyles are visualized proximally and distally, respectively (Figures 16.29A and 16.33). Static and dynamic sonograms are obtained with stifle flexion and extension, as well as internal and external rotations. The joint capsule, the collateral ligaments, and the lateral meniscus can all be assessed on a longitudinal plane (Figure 16.33).

The long digital extensor tendon, which demonstrates a typical fibrillar echotexture, runs between the lateral meniscus and the joint capsule, cranial to the collateral ligament. The origin of the tendon can be traced across the joint to the extensor fossa, a focal depression in the craniolateral margin of the lateral femoral condyle. The tendon, which is surrounded by its sheath, runs through the tibialis cranialis muscle. The tendon sheath is formed by an indentation of the joint sac and cannot be identified (Mueller et al. 2002).

The meniscus appears as a triangle structure of uniform, medium echogenicity located between the femoral condyle and the tibial plateau (Mueller and Kramer 2003) (Figure 16.33). The abaxial surface of the lateral meniscus should be linear and perfectly aligned with the surface of the adjacent femoral and tibial condyles. Additionally, a fine hypoechoic line may be seen on the femoral and tibial surfaces of the meniscus,

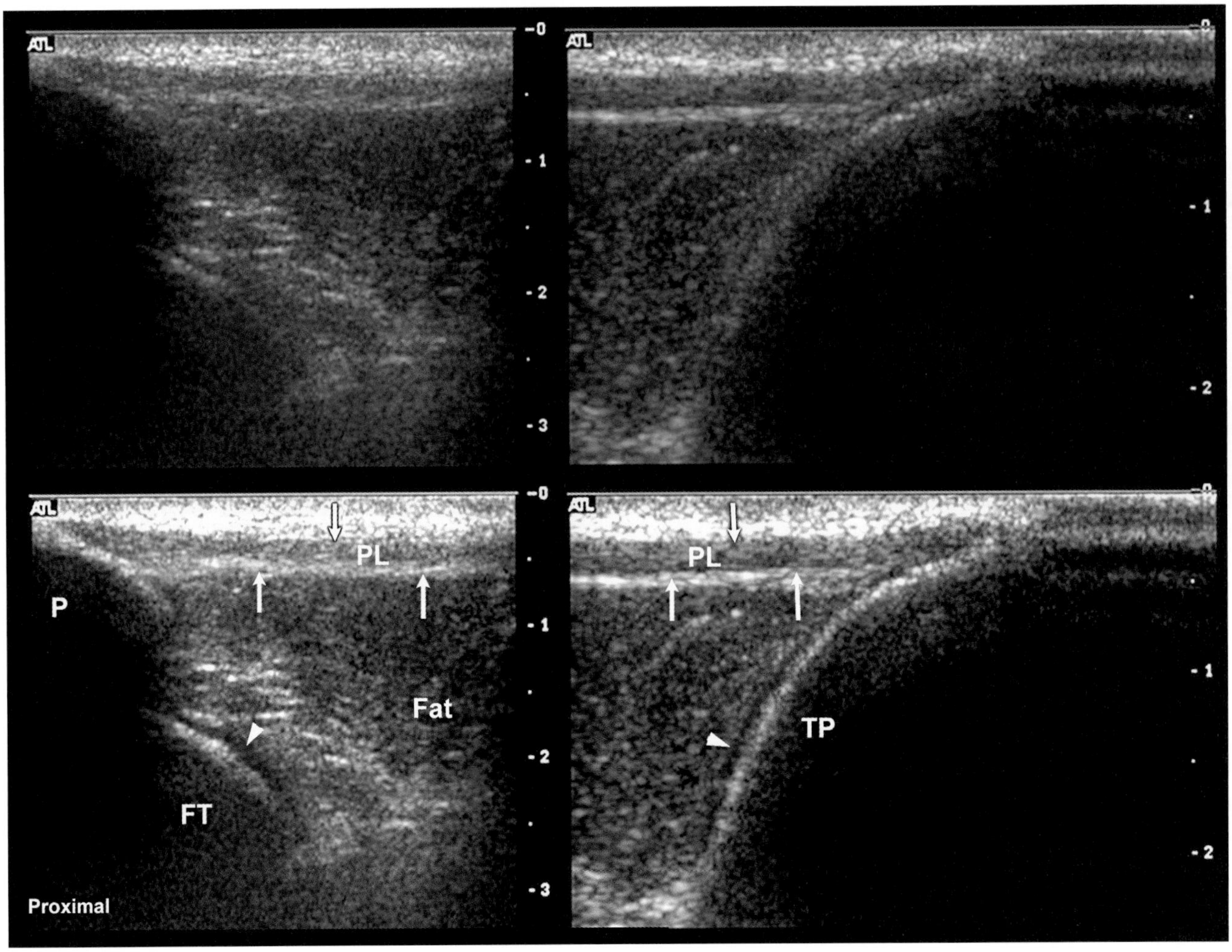

Figure 16.32. Normal infrapatellar region. Longitudinal sonographic and schematic images obtained of the proximal and distal portions of the infrapatellar region of a normal dog. The patellar ligament (PL and arrows) appears as a moderately echogenic, linear band connecting the patella (P) and the tibial crest. The infrapatellar fat pad located caudal to the patellar ligament is relatively hypoechoic and granular in echotexture. Small vessels located within this fat body appear as hyperechoic dots and lines. A thin hypoechoic band (arrowheads) consistent with cartilage and synovial fluid is noted on the surface of the femoral trochlea (FT) and tibial plateau (TP).

consistent with articular cartilage and synovial fluid (Mahn et al. 2005) (Figure 16.33). When the collateral ligament is used as a landmark, three different regions can be examined: cranial horn, middle portion, and caudal horn (Mahn et al. 2005).

Caudal Aspect: Popliteal Lymph Node

The caudal region of the stifle is examined in longitudinal and transverse scans with the joint in a slightly flexed position. As opposed to the approach in human knees, this approach provides fairly low visibility of intra-articular structures in dogs. The popliteal artery and lymph node can be found caudal to the stile joint, and portions of the caudal muscles of the thigh, as well as the popliteus and gastrocnemius muscles, are visible. The caudal horn of the meniscus appears sometimes between the condyles of the femur and tibia (Kramer et al. 1999).

Medial Aspect: Fabella, Medial Collateral Ligament, Medial Meniscus, Joint Capsule, and Synovium

With the stifle subsequently extended and flexed, the medial region is scanned from cranial to caudal, encompassing the medial femoral condyle. A longitudinal plane is most useful, and the medial femoral condyle, tibial plateau, medial collateral ligament, medial meniscus, joint capsule, and synovium are

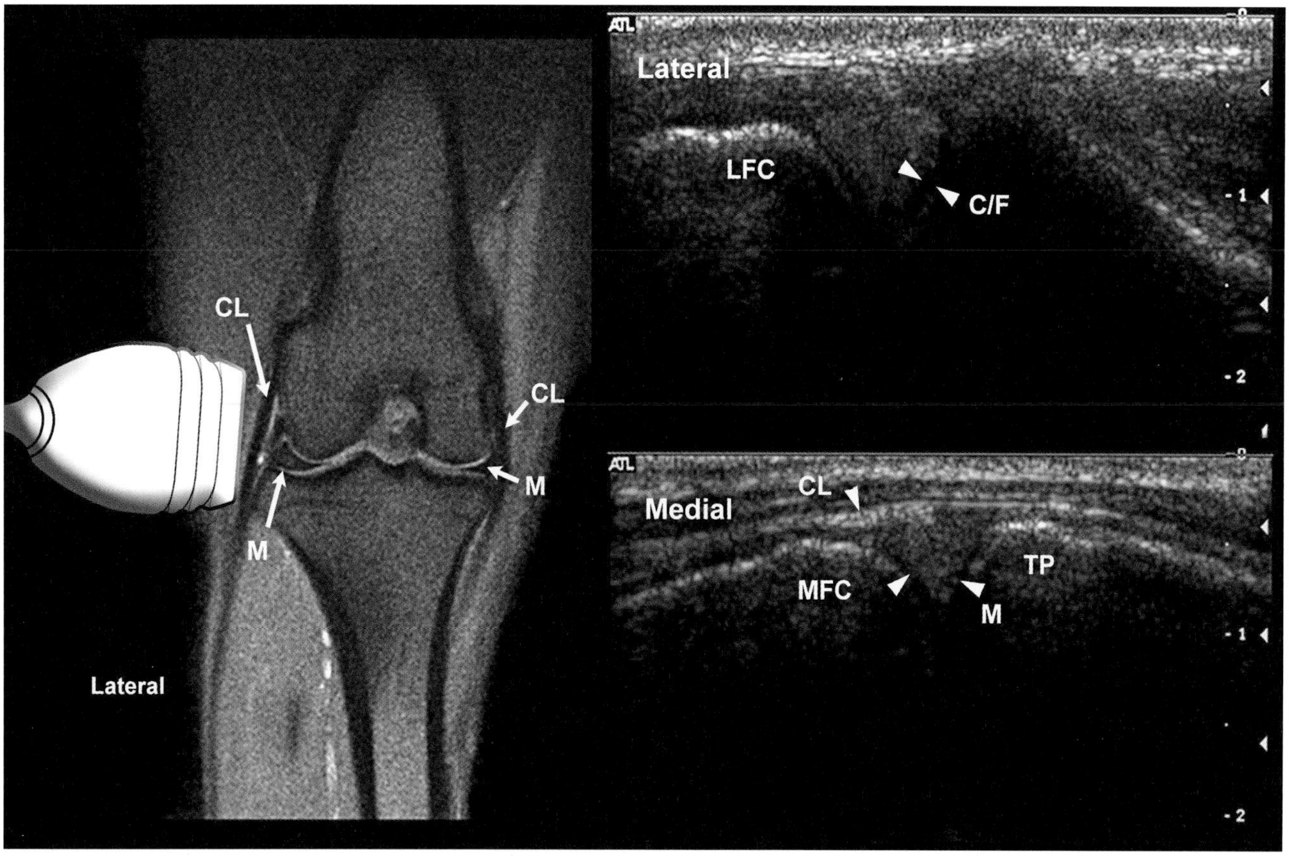

Figure 16.33. Femoral menisci: sonographic approach and normal anatomy. When scanned using a longitudinal plane, the menisci appear as moderately echogenic, triangular structures (M and arrowheads on the medial side) located between each femoral condyle and the opposite tibial plateau (TP). Thin hypoechoic layers consistent with articular cartilage and fluid (C/F and arrowheads) are observed on each side of the menisci. Collateral ligaments (CL) can also be seen crossing the medial and lateral aspects of the joint. LFC, lateral femoral condyle; and MFC, medial femoral condyle.

examined similarly as on the lateral side (Kramer et al. 1999; Mueller et al. 2002) (Figures 16.29B and 16.33).

Sonographic Features of Specific Stifle Disorders

Joint Effusion

In dogs with moderate to severe stifle effusion, dilatation of the suprapatellar recess is visible as an anechoic, tubelike structure surrounded by a hyperechoic line (joint capsule) (Figure 16.34A and B). Joint effusion also causes cranial displacement and compression of the infrapatellar fat body, which becomes outlined by the anechoic to hypoechoic fluid (Figure 16.35C). Distally, the distended synovial sheath that wraps around the tendon of the long digital extensor becomes clearly visible as an anechoic to hypoechoic tubular structure displacing the tibialis cranialis (Figure 16.34D).

In comparison to degenerative effusions, septic effusions appear more echogenic, and floating particles can be observed. Hemorrhagic effusions can range in echogenicity, depending on their chronicity.

Osteoarthritis

When osteoarthritic periarticular new bone formations develop, the contours of the patella, femoral trochlea ridges, condyles, and epicondyles, as well as the tibial plateau, become irregular (Figure 16.35). Joint effusion is typically observed, and the infrapatellar fat body appears inhomogeneous and more echogenic. Occasionally, small fluid-filled areas (cysts) can be seen within this fat body (Kramer et al. 1999). In addition, the joint capsule appears thickened (a hyperechoic band), and redundant synovial thickening can be visualized, particularly if associated with significant joint effusion.

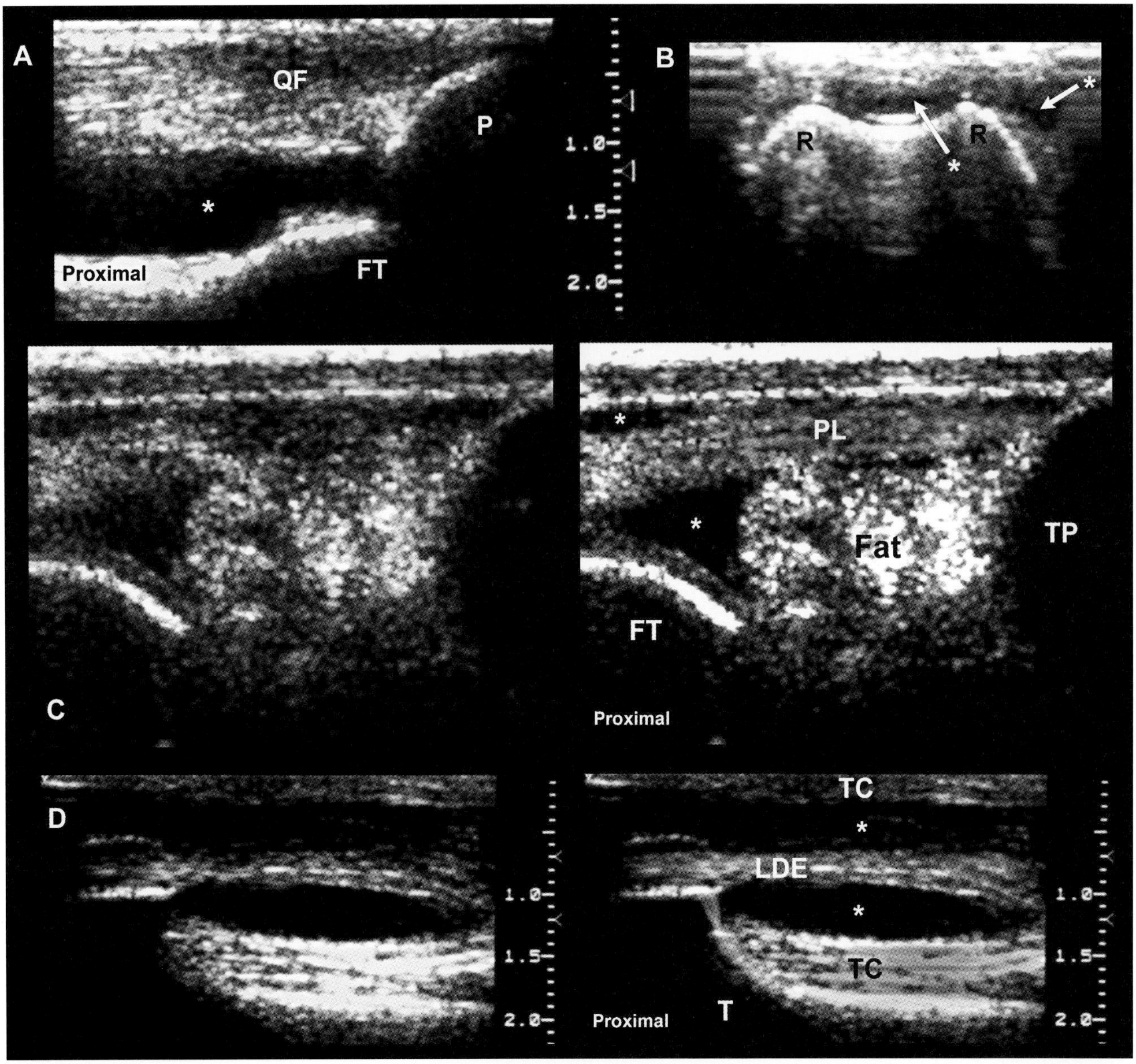

Figure 16.34. Stifle joint effusion. **A and B:** Longitudinal **(A)** and transverse **(B)** sonographic images in a dog with distension of the suprapatellar recess (*) along the femoral trochlea (FT) and ridges (R). P, patella; and QF, quadriceps femoris. **C:** Longitudinal sonographic and schematic images of the infrapatellar area with the infrapatellar fat body being displaced and heterogeneous. Anechoic effusion (*) is noted, delineating the degenerated articular cartilage that appears more echogenic along the femoral trochlea (FT). PL, patellar ligament; and TP, tibial plateau. **D:** Longitudinal sonographic and schematic images of the distal joint sulcus, which is distended with anechoic synovial fluid (*) and encircling the long digital extensor tendon (LDE) and displacing the tibialis cranialis (TC) muscle cranially. T, tibia.

Patellar Luxation

By using a transverse plane with the transducer placed at the level of the femoral trochlea, a luxated patella can be seen as an oval, hyperechoic structure with acoustic shadow located medially or laterally to the trochlea ridges. The trochlear groove is typically shallow. With subsequent extension and flexion of the stifle joint, the trochlear cartilage and groove depth can be assessed and measured.

Patellar Fractures and Desmopathies

A fracture of the patella is seen as an interruption of the outline of the smooth bone surface (Kramer et al. 1999) and is often associated with damage to the

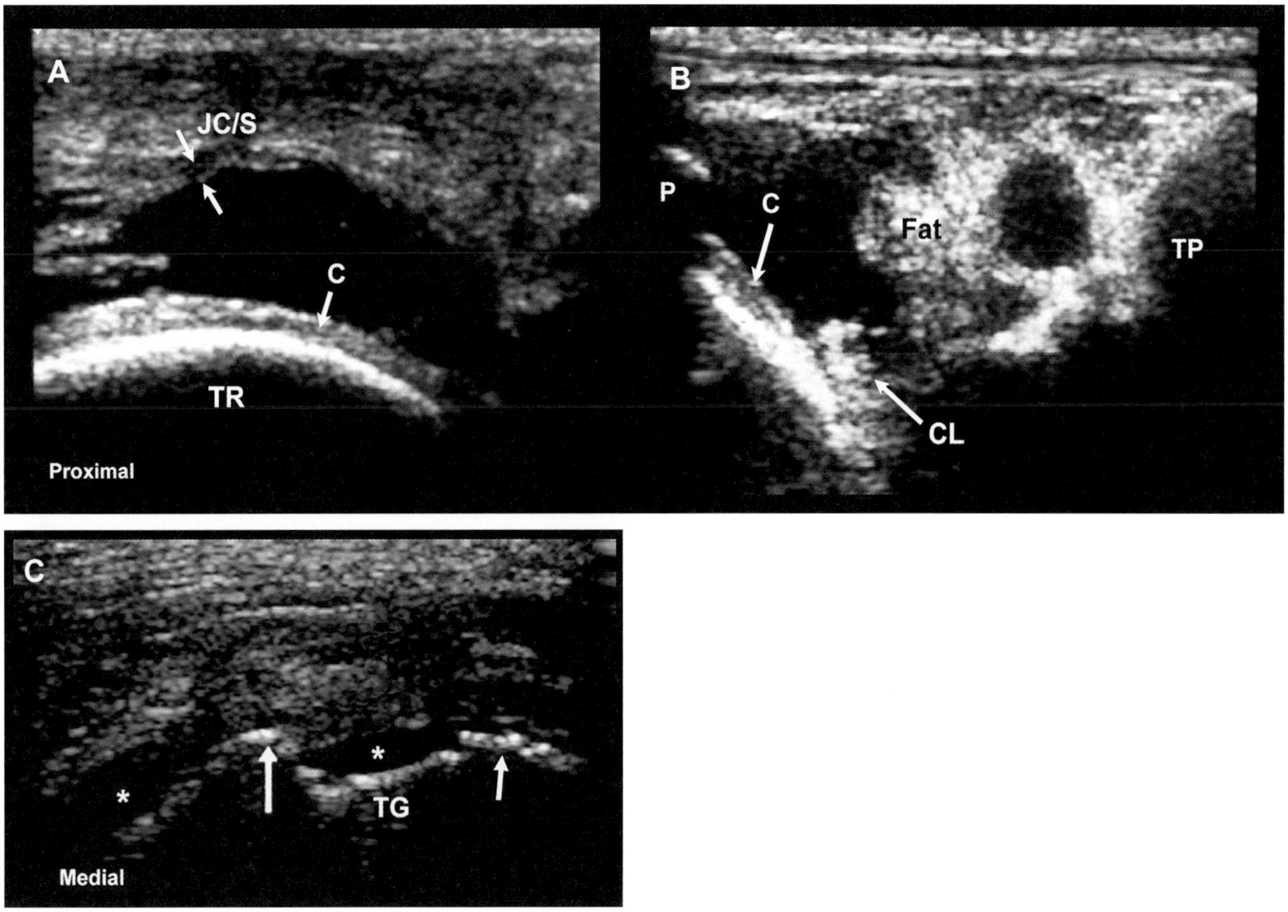

Figure 16.35. Stifle osteoarthritis. **A and B:** Longitudinal sonograms of the proximal joint recess **(A)** and infrapatellar region **(B)** in a dog with chronic stifle degenerative joint disease. Anechoic joint effusion is present, and the joint capsule and synovium (JC/S, arrows) are thickened. The cartilage (C) along the trochlea is hyperechoic and heterogeneous. The infrapatellar fat body is heterogeneous, and an irregular, hyperechoic structure is in the midportion of the joint, consistent with a degenerated and ruptured cranial cruciate ligament (CL). P, patella; TP, tibial plateau; and TR, trochlear ridge. **C:** Transverse sonographic image of the femoral trochlea in another dog with degenerative joint disease. The cranial surfaces of the trochlear ridges (arrows) are irregular because of osteophytosis. The proximal joint recesses at the medial aspect of the trochlea and over the trochlear groove (TG) are filled with anechoic fluid (*).

quadriceps tendon (proximally) or patellar ligament (distally).

Ruptures of the patellar ligament can be partial or complete. In both cases, the ligament appears edematous and hypoechoic to hyperechoic with irregular margins at the site of rupture. With avulsion fracture, small hyperechoic bone fragments are visible at the extremity of the ligament and associated with acoustic shadowing if more than 2–3 mm wide (Figure 16.36). When a longitudinal plane is used, a separation of the ruptured ends can be observed as the knee is flexed. During therapy, this view enables the evaluation and documentation of the healing and consolidation process. Initially, the area of insult becomes thicker and inhomogeneous with a mixed echotexture. Both ends of the ligament are clearly visible. Approximately 6–7 weeks later, the fibers are oriented longitudinally, resulting in decreased thickness of the tendon. The healing ligament appears more homogeneous, and its echogenicity resembles that of a normal ligament. However, some inhomogeneous areas may remain for months (Kramer et al. 1999).

Patellar thickening is also recognized following tibial plateau-leveling osteotomy (TPLO), particularly in large dogs (Mattern et al. 2006). Postoperative changes noted at 1 month also include hypoechoic to anechoic central lesions with partially disrupted ligaments. These changes have been significantly linked to the degree of tibial plateau rotation during the procedure, supporting the role for increased stress in the

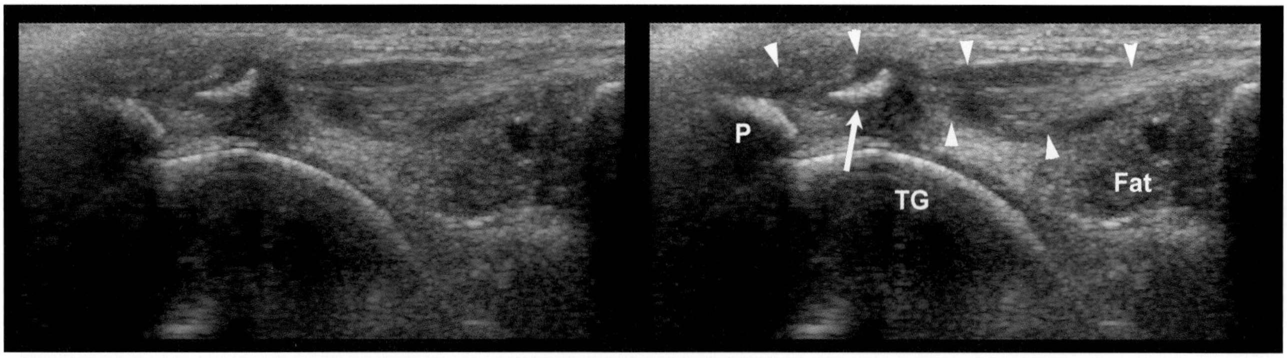

Figure 16.36. Avulsion fracture of the patella. Longitudinal sonographic and schematic images of the infrapatellar region in a dog with acute stifle pain and swelling. The patellar ligament (arrowheads) is irregularly thickened and heterogeneous. A hyperechoic, partially shadowing bony fragment (arrow) is just distal to the patella (P), consistent with fracture of the apex. The distal margin of the patella is abnormally flat, and the patella is displaced proximally. TG, trochlear groove.

development of patellar ligament desmitis (Mattern et al. 2006). However, these changes may be clinically insignificant in most dogs.

Avulsion fracture of the tibial tuberosity can also be visualized in the infrapatellar region. During a dynamic ultrasound exam, the acutely avulsed bony structure can move during flexion of the knee, confirming the diagnosis. However, this motion can be limited, particularly if a fibrous callous is already present.

Osteochondritis Dissecans

OCD appears as an irregular defect on the contour of the subchondral bone, typically at the lateral condyle. The abnormal cartilage can vary in thickness and echogenicity but often appears hyperechoic and heterogeneous. Detached pieces of cartilage are seen as hyperechoic structures of variable size. Other free bodies may also be visible, and their location can be determined (Kramer et al. 1999) (Figure 16.37). Joint effusion is typically observed in association with OCD, and periarticular osteophytes develop in the chronic phase.

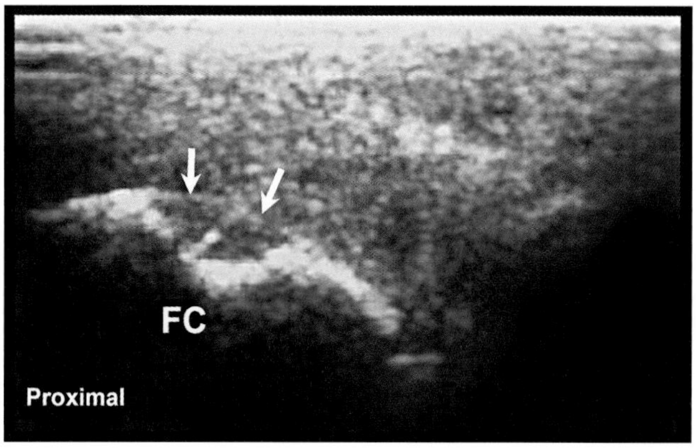

Figure 16.37. Osteochondritis dissecans. Longitudinal sonographic image of the lateral femoral condyle (FC) in a young dog. A concave defect (arrows) is filled with mildly echogenic and partially mineralized cartilage.

Cranial Cruciate Ligament Rupture

To assess the presence of cranial cruciate ligamentous damage, a cranial, longitudinal approach is used, and the stifle must be completely flexed, which may be difficult to accomplish in painful, unsedated dogs. An acutely ruptured cranial cruciate ligament cannot be identified in most cases (Gnudi and Bertoni 2001). However, in the region of the cranial cruciate ligament, an irregular, anechoic area (hematoma) can sometimes be identified (Kramer et al. 1999; Gnudi and Bertoni 2001). If the rupture has been present for a longer period (chronic rupture), the irregularly demarcated and hyperechoic stumps of the ligament can be seen (Figure 16.38). The stump close to the ligament insertion on the tibia can be more easily visualized, whereas the other stump, near the origin on the femur, is less often visualized (Engelke et al. 1997b; Kramer et al. 1999). The visibility of the cranial cruciate ligament is limited if a large volume of effusion is present, because this structure appears hypoechoic when scanned at an angle (Kramer et al. 1999; Gnudi and Bertoni 2001). Avulsion fragments may also be recognized as more or less shadowing hyperechoic foci in the central portion of the joint. Chronic ruptures are commonly associated with fibrous tissue proliferation in the region just cranial to the intercondylar groove, which appears as an irregular, hyperechoic structure (Gnudi and Bertoni 2001) (Figure 16.35B).

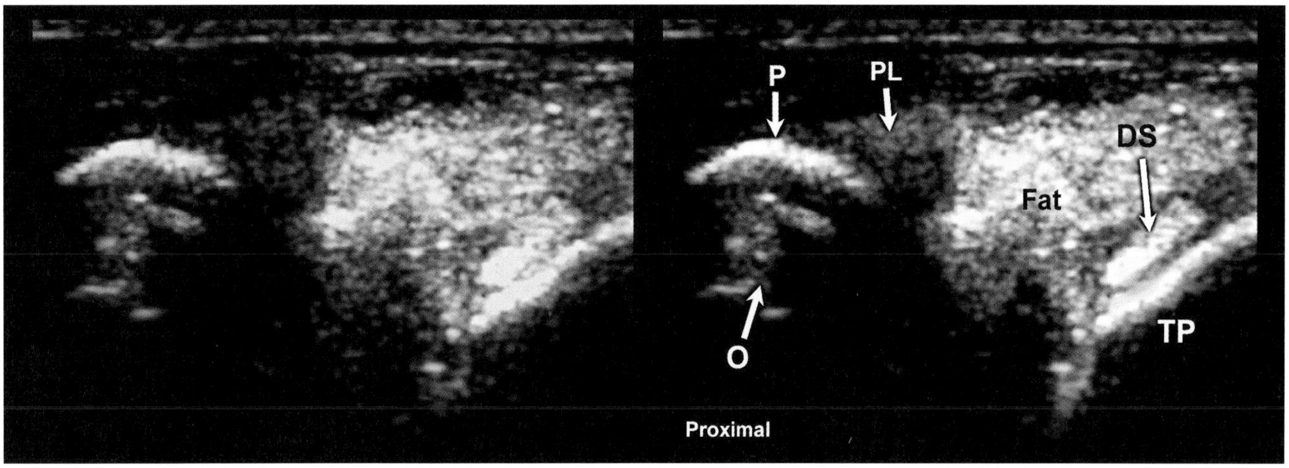

Figure 16.38. Cranial cruciate ligament rupture. Longitudinal sonographic and schematic images of the infrapatellar region in which the distal stump (DS) of the ruptured ligament appears as a hyperechoic band proximal to the tibial plateau (TP). O, osteophytosis over the femoral trochlea; P, patella; and PL, patellar ligament.

Meniscal Tears and Degeneration

Meniscal tears and degenerative changes are more commonly observed medially and secondary to stifle instability caused by cranial cruciate rupture. Isolated meniscal damage is rare in dogs and may affect more commonly the lateral meniscus (Mahn et al. 2005). Most tears appear to present a bucket-handle configuration. However, because of the difficulty in visualizing the internal portion of the menisci, partial and complete tears can be difficult to visualize.

Chronic meniscal degeneration has a characteristic appearance that can be more easily recognized. The involved meniscus appears edematous, and the echotexture is distinctly inhomogeneous with hyperechoic and hypoechoic areas (Figure 16.39A).

A decrease in the visibility of a meniscus may be due to its displacement. However, it must be pointed out that this sign does not necessarily indicate the presence of meniscal disease. Ultrasonographic assessment of the menisci can be limited by several factors, including severe fibrosis of the soft tissues along the medial aspect of the joint, marked osteophytosis caused by severe DJD, and previous surgery (Mahn et al. 2005). The size of the dog may also represent a limiting factor because thinner menisci (small patients) or deeper menisci (very large or obese dogs) can be more difficult to visualize well (Mueller and Kramer 2003).

Another sign of meniscal disease is the presence of hyperechoic lines, double lines, and stipples within a meniscus (Figure 16.39B). If these foci are widely distributed and numerous, large lesions within the meniscus are likely. However, a smaller size or number does not necessarily correlate with less severe lesions. Both minor and major lesions may be present. A hyperechoic double line is usually indicative of meniscal tear (Mueller and Kramer 2003).

Joint effusion can be observed at the periphery of the affected meniscus, as well as a change in meniscal shape or position (Mahn et al. 2005). Affected menisci may bulge axially (medial meniscus) or abaxially (lateral meniscus) or show an irregular contour (Figure 16.39A). Effusion or replacement tissue may also be found in the region of the meniscus after surgical excision (Figure 16.39C).

Collateral Ligament Rupture

In cases of severe and acute rupture of the medial or lateral collateral ligaments, a discontinuity of the affected ligament may be identified. Typically, hematomas are found at the level of the tear, seen as hypoechoic to anechoic, homogeneous to mildly inhomogeneous areas. When a longitudinal medial or lateral approach is used, a dynamic examination of the joint space while stressing its opening medially and laterally may confirm joint instability. Joint effusion rapidly develops and appears as bulging medial and/or lateral synovial recesses. Capsular tear may also be present, and fluid may have accumulated in the periarticular soft tissues.

Avulsion of the Long Digital Extensor Tendon

In cases of avulsion fracture of the origin of the long digital extensor tendon, shadowing hyperechoic foci consistent with bone fragments can be found just distal

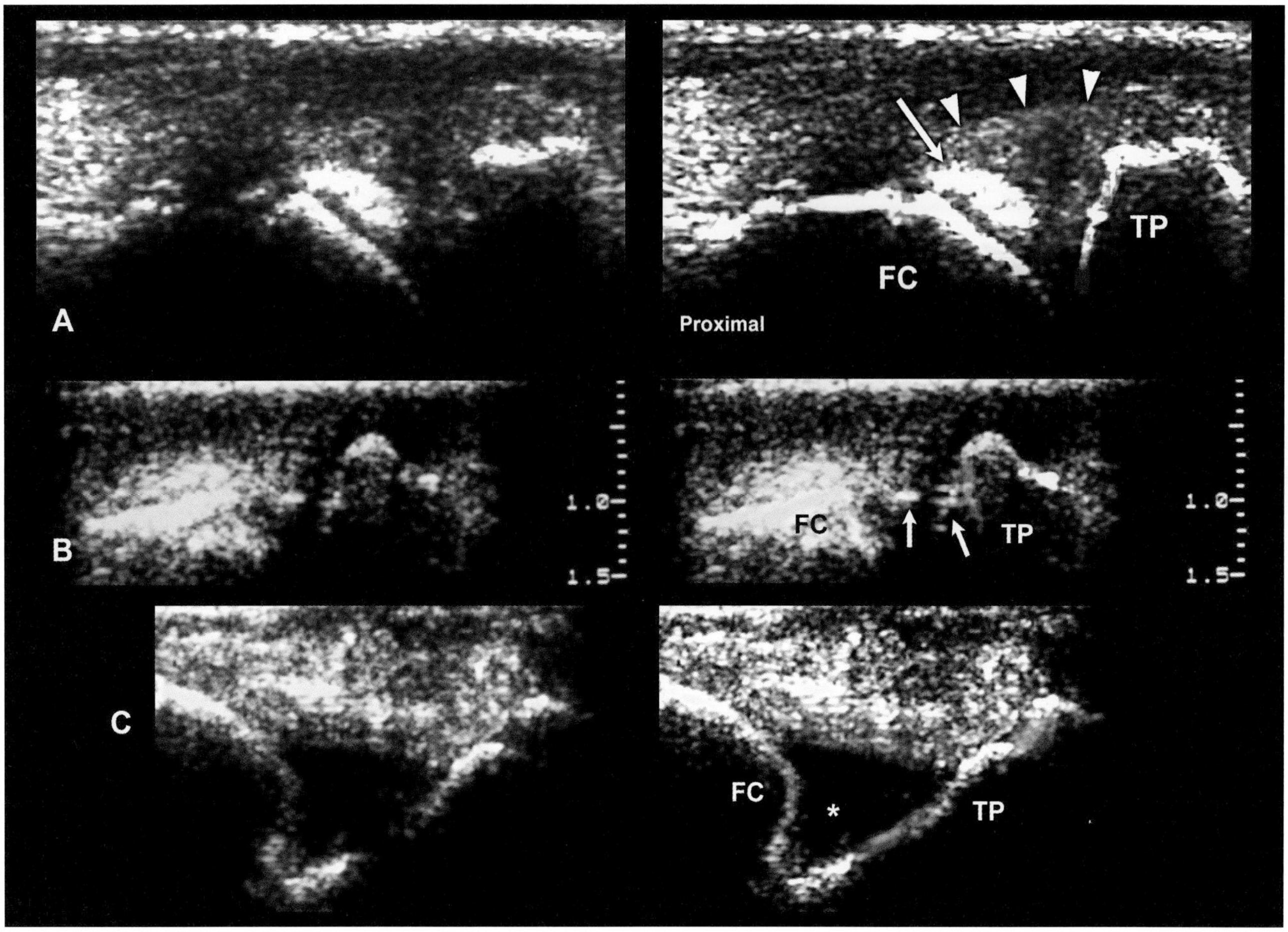

Figure 16.39. Meniscal degeneration and luxation. **A–C:** Longitudinal sonographic and corresponding schematic images of degenerated menisci in dogs. In all dogs, the medial margins of the tibial plateau (TP) and medial femoral condyle (FC) are irregular because of periarticular new bone formation. **A:** The medial meniscus is bulging medially (arrowheads) and presents a hyperechoic band (arrow). **B:** Hyperechoic stripes (arrows) are found in the meniscus of this other dog. **C:** The region of the medial meniscus is filled with synovial fluid (*) because of meniscal luxation.

to the level of the extensor fossa at the lateral femoral condyle (Kramer et al. 1999).

Hip

Scanning Technique and Normal Sonographic Anatomy

Animals are placed in lateral recumbency with the limb of interest up, and their hair is clipped around the hip. Although it can be useful in some patients, sedation or anesthesia is usually unnecessary (Greshake and Ackerman 1992; Floeck et al. 2003). A high-resolution (>8–10 MHz) linear transducer is recommended.

Longitudinal and transverse images are obtained by positioning the probe on the lateral aspect of the hip, dorsal to the greater trochanter (Figure 16.40). With slight movements of the probe in cranial and caudal directions, the joint capsule can be identified. The femoral head appears as a convex hyperechoic interface with acoustic shadowing. The shadowing caused by the femoral head represents a significant limiting factor in assessing the coxofemoral joint space and acetabulum, particularly when a transverse plane is used (Greshake and Ackerman 1992).

The articular cartilage appears a smooth hypoechoic layer around the femoral head. The joint capsule appears as a hyperechoic line at the periphery of the head and connected to the acetabular margins (Figure 16.41).

Hips can be evaluated in puppies that are up to 7–8 weeks of age (Greshake and Ackerman 1992). Each hip is evaluated preferably by using a longitudinal plane and dynamically examined while dorsolateral subluxation is forced (distraction) (Figure 16.42). The

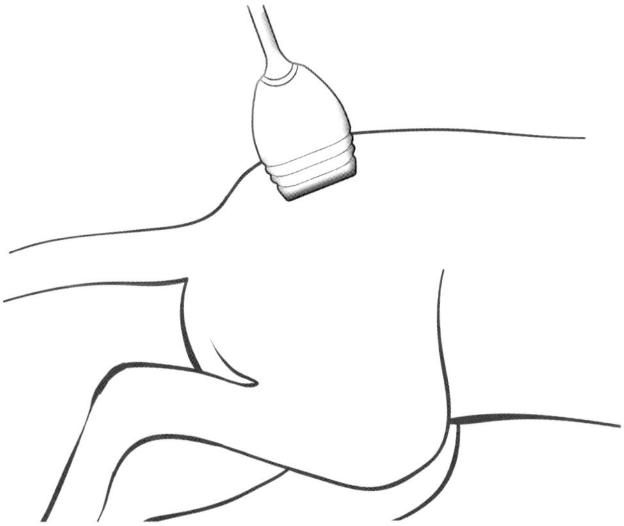

Figure 16.40. Scanning technique for the hip. The position of the dog and ultrasound probe when scanning the hip on a longitudinal plane. A dynamic exam is also performed while flexing, extending, abducting, and adducting the leg. Coxofemoral joint passive laxity can also be evaluated by forcing the femur laterally.

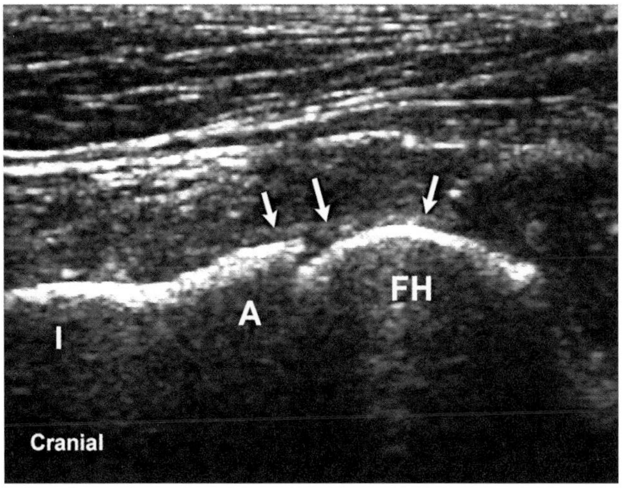

Figure 16.41. Normal hip joint in an adult dog. Longitudinal image of the coxofemoral joint in a normal, mature, large-breed dog. The dorsal surface of the femoral head (FH) appears as a convex hyperechoic line, and the craniodorsal acetabular rim (A) is seen as a triangular projection that is congruent with the femoral head. The joint capsule is a superficial, thin, and moderately echogenic band (arrows). The surface of the ilium (I) is seen cranially.

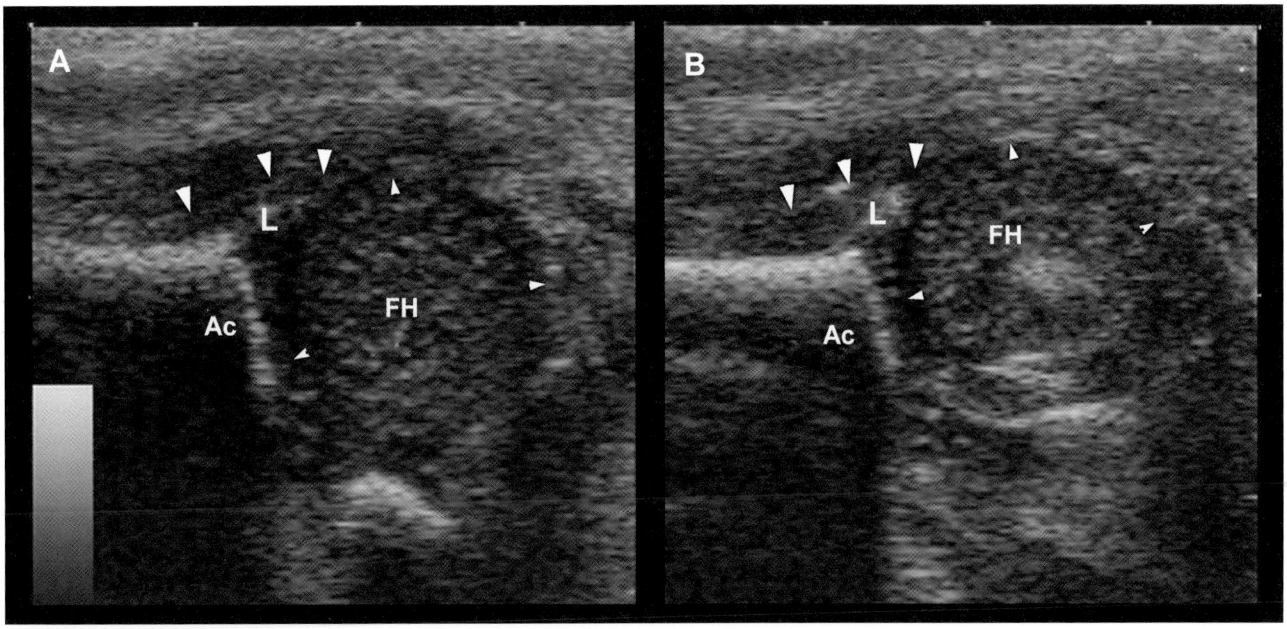

Figure 16.42. Normal hip joint in a young puppy: neutral and dynamic examination. **A:** In neutral position, the nonossified femoral head (FH and small arrowheads) is well visualized and appears in contact with the acetabular (Ac) fossa. **B:** Because of some normal degree of passive laxity, the femoral head (FH) can be moved dorsolaterally in relation to the incompletely ossified labrum (L and large arrowheads) of the acetabulum (Ac). The degree of passive laxity can be evaluated dynamically.

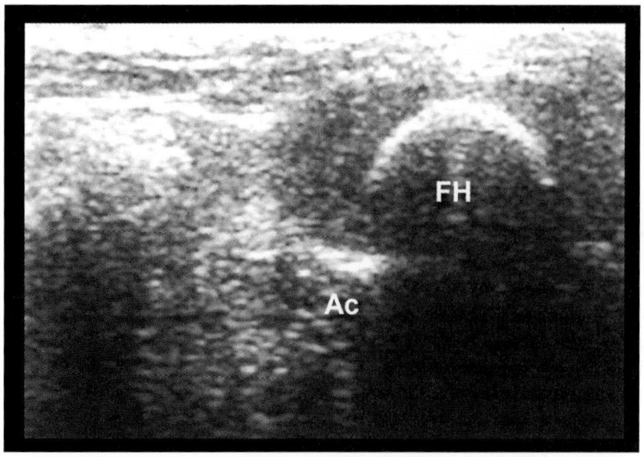

Figure 16.43. Hip luxation. Longitudinal image of the coxofemoral joint region in a traumatized dog. The femoral head (FH) appears dorsally displaced in relation to the acetabulum (Ac). Hypoechoic soft-tissue swelling is noted around the femoral head.

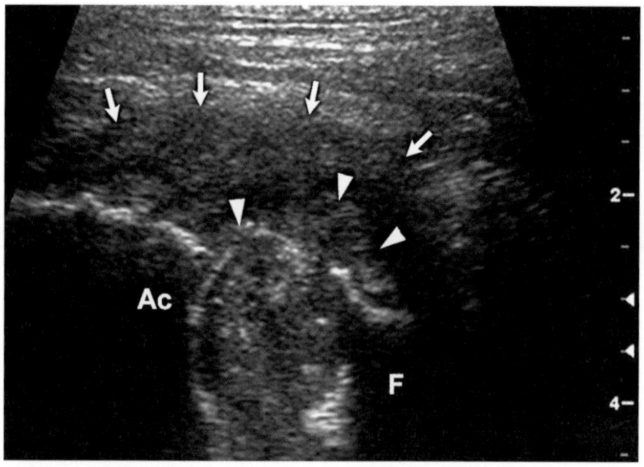

Figure 16.44. Femoral head and neck ostectomy. Longitudinal image of the coxofemoral joint region in a dog after femoral head and neck ostectomy. Hypoechoic soft-tissue swelling is noted around the joint (arrows). The joint space is filled with echogenic material consistent with hemorrhage and/or scar tissue. The dorsal margin of the acetabulum (Ac) is irregular because of periarticular new bone formation. F, proximal femur.

cartilage is thick at that time, and the subchondral bone is partially mineralized and irregular. The shadowing bony structures hamper complete assessment of these joints.

Hip Dysplasia and Osteoarthritis

The use of ultrasound in the diagnosis of hip dysplasia has been investigated in young puppies. Although dynamic measurements can predict the onset of osteoarthritis in some dogs such as Labrador retriever–golden retriever mix puppies (Adams et al. 2000), it is not currently recognized as a reliable clinical tool in the early diagnosis of hip dysplasia in dogs.

Joint effusion and capsular thickening related to osteoarthritis are of the same sonographic appearance as described in previous chapters.

Coxofemoral Joint Luxation

Coxofemoral joint luxation typically causes craniodorsal displacement of the femoral head (Figure 16.43). If present, secondary articular changes can be seen and the content of the acetabulum evaluated. Fibrin in the joint capsule appears as an accumulation of irregular material ranging from hyperechoic to hypoechoic.

After femoral head ostectomy, the acetabulum and surrounding tissue can be easily examined. The area around the joint can vary in echogenicity and homogeneity because of hemorrhage, edema, muscular contracture, and/or scar tissue (Figure 16.44).

Avascular Necrosis of the Femoral Head

With avascular necrosis (Legg-Calvé-Perthes disease), the femoral head and neck typically become irregular and lytic, with gaps noted at the osseous margins. The joint capsule can be thickened, and a moderate joint effusion can be evident.

Calcaneal Tendon (Achilles Tendon)

Injuries to the calcaneal tendon (Achilles tendon) are uncommon in small animals and are usually produced by direct trauma (Lamb and Duvernois 2005). The calcaneal tendon consists of all structures that attach to the calcaneal tuberosity. The gastrocnemius and the superficial digital flexor tendons represent the two main components. Tendons of the biceps femoris, semitendinosus, and gracilis muscles form another conjoined component, also called the *common calcaneal tendon* (CCT). The medial and lateral gastrocnemius muscles fuse at their distal aspect, becoming one tendon that runs within the deep portion of the calcaneal tendon and inserts on the calcaneal tuberosity. The superficial digital flexor tendon inserts both laterally and medially on this tuberosity, forming a caplike structure. The common calcaneal tendon is the deepest portion of the calcaneal tendon and inserts on the dorsal aspect of the calcaneal tuberosity (Hermanson and Evans 1993).

Scanning Technique

Ultrasonography of the calcaneal tendon is performed in a standardized fashion: The tarsocrural joint is slightly flexed, stretching the tendon that can be more easily imaged (Figure 16.45). Initially, a longitudinal scan is performed by placing the probe over the calcaneal tuberosity at the tendon insertion. The transducer is then moved proximally to examine the whole structure, as well as the musculotendinous junctions and muscles. Transverse views are then used to visualize individual portions of the tendon, from the level of their muscular origin to the level of the calcaneal tuberosity. Finally, a dynamic examination is performed (flexion and extension of the hock) (Kramer et al. 2001a; Lamb and Duvernois 2005).

Normal Sonographic Anatomy

A longitudinal image directly above the tuber calcanei shows the surface of the calcaneus as a convex hyperechoic line with distal acoustic shadowing (Figure 16.45A). Immediately proximal to this bony protuberance that serves as an important landmark is a 5 × 5-mm, hypoechoic, ill-defined area representing the calcaneal bursa with its surrounding connective tissue (Figure 16.45A). The CCT is a moderately echogenic, homogeneous structure with parallel hyperechoic lines (fibrillar echotexture) inserting on the tuberosity

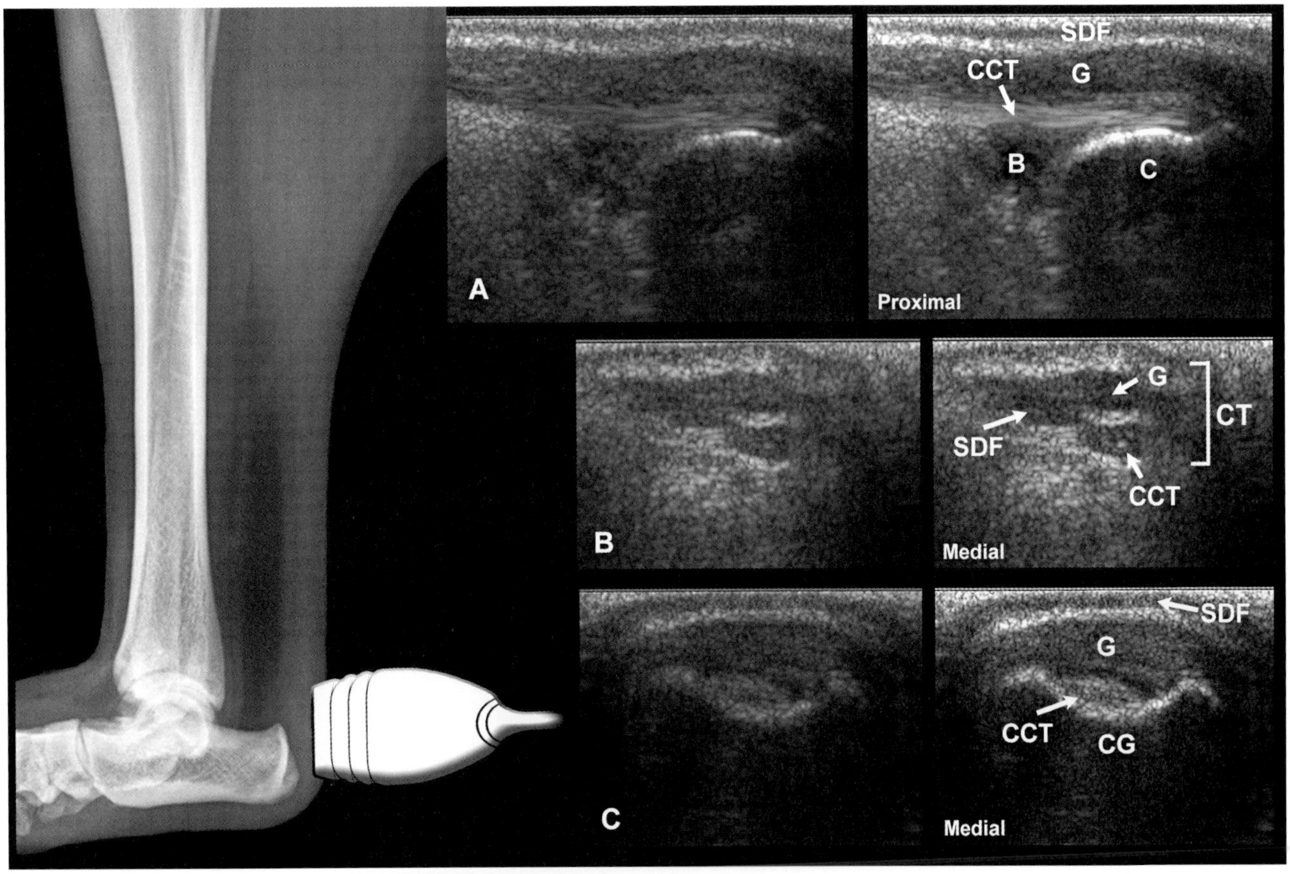

Figure 16.45. Normal sonographic anatomy of the calcaneal (Achilles) tendon. Sonographic and schematic images. **A: Longitudinal sonogram.** The common calcaneal tendon (CCT), which is the deepest component of the calcaneal tendon, has a characteristic hyperechoic, linear echotexture when scanned perpendicularly. The other components of the calcaneal tendon, i.e. the gastrocnemius (G) and superficial digital flexor (SDF) tendons, are seen more superficially. The calcaneal bursa (B) appears as a small, triangular anechoic area just proximal to the calcaneal tuberosity (C). **B and C: Transverse sonograms.** These images are obtained at the midlevel **(B)** and distal level **(C)** of the calcaneal tendon (CT). The superficial digital flexor (SDF), gastrocnemius (G), and common calcaneal (CCT) tendons can be seen distinctly. The superficial digital flexor tendon, which appears as a caplike, superficial structure around the calcaneal tuberosity, contains the gastrocnemius and common calcaneal tendons. (CG) calcaneal groove.

(Figure 16.45A). The peritendineum is a smooth hyperechoic band at the periphery of the tendon. Further proximally, the muscles display their typical echotexture (see section on Musculature). On transverse images, the CCT is a moderately echogenic, round structure with multiple small hyperechoic dots, that inserts deeply on the dorsoproximal margin of the calcaneal tuberosity (Figure 16.45B and C). The peritendineum surrounding the tendon is visible as a hyperechoic line. However, the presence of edge shadowing prevents a clear visualization of its curved axial and abaxial borders (Rivers et al. 1997; Kramer et al. 2001a; Lamb and Duvernois 2005).

Disorders of the Common Calcaneal Tendon

Partial and Complete Rupture and Healing Process In complete rupture, the echotexture of the CCT is completely interrupted, and a hypoechoic and inhomogeneous area (hematoma) is observed between the retracted ends of the tendon. The proximal and distal stumps of the tendon appear drumsticklike and inhomogeneous with a mixed echotexture. During dynamic examination, the movement of the ruptured ends is clearly visible.

With partial tendon rupture, the affected portion (deep or superficial) appears inhomogeneous and hypoechoic to anechoic with poorly demarcated areas (Figure 16.46). In contrast, the part of the tendon that is intact displays a normal fibrillar echotexture. Occasionally, a small anechoic fluid borderline is visible between the tendon and the peritendineum.

In chronic partial ruptures, images of the affected part of the tendon can vary from highly inhomogeneous to homogeneous and from hypoechoic to moderately hyperechoic. The surface of the calcaneal tuberosity is usually irregular and ill-defined because of new bone formation. Avulsed fragments and/or dystrophic mineralization can be recognized within the affected tendon as dispersed hyperechoic foci that can exhibit acoustic shadowing if their size exceeds 2–3 mm (Rivers et al. 1997; Swiderski et al. 2005).

By using ultrasonography, the healing process of the CCT with or without surgical intervention can be evaluated (Kramer et al. 2001a). Within the first day after trauma, the hematoma between the ends of the tendon stumps appears hypoechoic to anechoic. Organization of the hematoma during the first and second week leads to a more inhomogeneous image with echogenic areas. From weeks 2–6, the diameter and the inhomogeneity of the injured area increase. After 8 weeks, replacement tissue begins to grow in a longitudinal direction, and both diameter and inhomogeneity decrease. The decrease in diameter is accompanied by the reappearance of the characteristic tendinous fibrillar echotexture. This healing process is completed by 10–12 weeks after trauma. However, the injured CCT remains much less homogeneous in comparison to the unaffected tendon for a long period (up to years).

Tears of the Gastrocnemius Muscles Tears can be identified by visualizing an interruption of the normal echotexture. The accompanying hematomas are visible as inhomogeneous, hypoechoic to anechoic, and poorly demarcated areas at the site of injury (see section on Musculature) (Swiderski et al. 2005).

Displacement of the Superficial Digital Flexor Tendon Medial or lateral luxation of the superficial

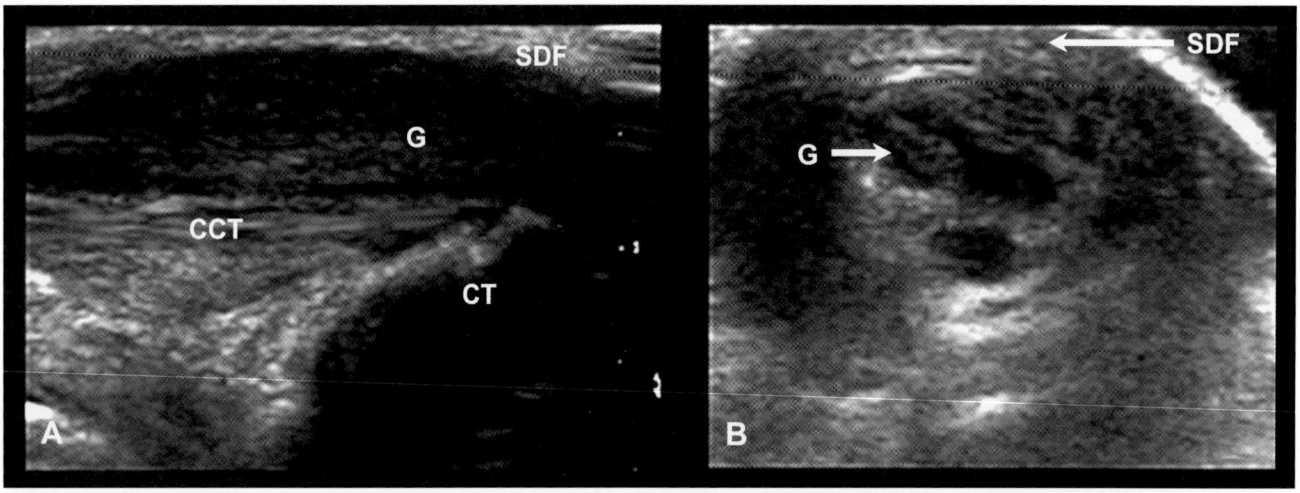

Figure 16.46. Partial rupture of the gastrocnemius tendon. Longitudinal **(A)** and transverse **(B)** sonograms of the calcaneal tendon in a dog with acute trauma. The gastrocnemius tendon (G) is markedly enlarged and hypoechoic. The superficial digital flexor tendon (SDF) is displaced caudally but appears intact. The common calcaneal tendon (CCT) is mildly inhomogeneous, which may also be because of partial rupture. Images courtesy of D. Penninck.

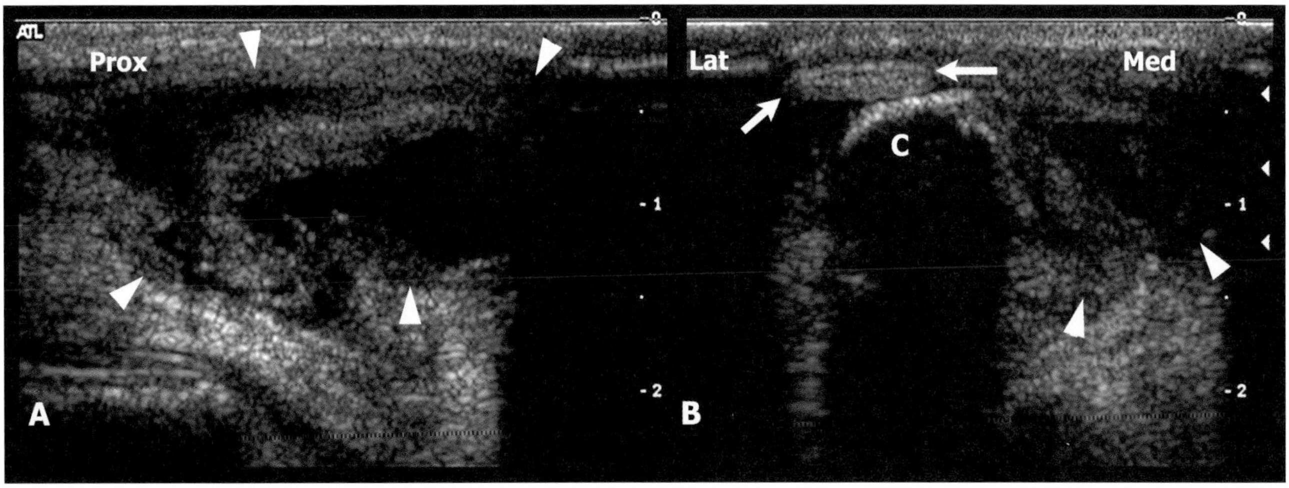

Figure 16.47. Chronic luxation of the superficial digital flexor tendon in large dog. **A:** In this longitudinal sonogram obtained medial to the calcaneum, an inhomogeneous mass (arrowheads) with anechoic fluid cavities is noted that is consistent with chronic hematoma and fibrous tissue. Prox, proximal. **B:** Transverse sonogram obtained at the plantaromedial aspect of the calcaneum (C), distal to the calcaneal tuberosity. The superficial digital flexor tendon (arrows) is displaced laterally. The changes caused by chronic hematoma and fibrous tissue thickening are noted medially (arrowheads) in the region of avulsion of tendon insertion. Lat, lateral; and Med, medial.

digital flexor tendon can be visualized by obtaining a transverse image above the calcaneal tuberosity. Adjacent to this convex, hyperechoic, shadowing structure, the medially or laterally displaced crescent-shaped to oval tendon comes into view. The luxated tendon can be enlarged and inhomogeneous, and a heterogeneous hematoma can also be observed at the level of fibrous avulsion on the medial or lateral aspect of the calcaneum.

Miscellaneous Musculoskeletal Disorders

Musculature

Scanning Technique

Muscles that are located laterally, cranially, or caudally are examined by placing the patient in lateral recumbency with the limb of interest up. Medially located muscles are assessed with the affected limb facing down while abducting the upper limb. Individual muscles are scanned between their origin and insertion by using both longitudinal and transverse planes.

The examination begins with images of the muscle belly, proceeds to the transition site of the muscle to its tendon, and finishes with the attachment and insertion sites, respectively (Kramer et al. 1997).

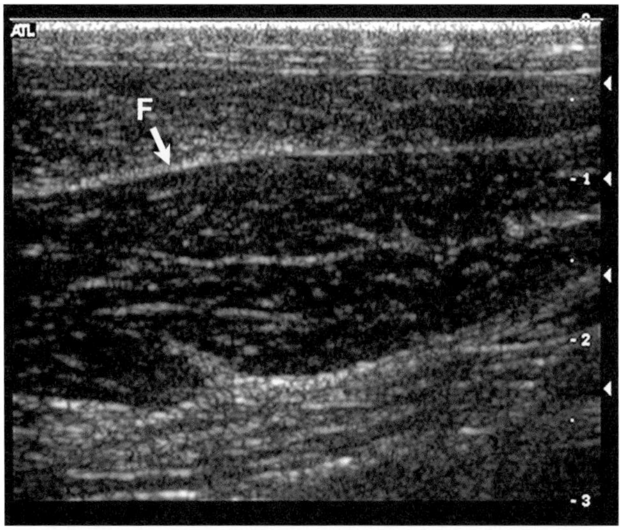

Figure 16.48. Normal muscle sonographic anatomy in a dog. Longitudinal sonographic image of a normal muscle showing the characteristic hypoechoic echotexture with fine hyperechoic dots and lines. Intermuscular fascias (F) appear as thin, hyperechoic planes between muscle bellies.

Normal Muscle Sonographic Anatomy

On longitudinal images, the structure of normal muscles appears hypoechoic with fine, oblique, hyperechoic striations. The fascias appear as smooth, continuous, hyperechoic lines, particularly when scanned perpendicularly (Figures 16.6 and 16.48). On transverse views, the background is hypoechoic with echoic dots representing the muscle septa, giving a coarse echotexture to the muscle belly. Tangential muscle boundaries are more difficult to image because of edge shadowing (Kramer et al. 1997). Subcutaneous and intramuscular fat planes are usually slightly hyperechoic to muscle bellies, although their appearance can vary.

Miscellaneous Disorders of Muscles and Tendons

Muscle Injuries The appearance of muscular trauma varies with the severity and onset of the injury. *Strain injuries*, which may or may not be secondary to a known traumatic event, likely represent an underestimated source of hind lameness in dogs (Breur and Blevins 1997; Nielsen and Pluhar 2004). Hip adductor, pectineus, and particularly iliopsoas muscles appear predisposed to strain injuries. In the acute phase, muscle swelling associated with hypoechoic areas is typically observed (Breur and Pluhar 1997) (Figure 16.49A–C). If the muscle is partially ruptured, the normal muscular echotexture is partially lost (Kramer et al. 1997).

Following muscular trauma, the healing process can be evaluated sonographically. In the chronic phase, a hyperechoic and variably inhomogeneous area (with or without acoustic shadowing) at the level of the previous trauma is indicative of scar formation (Breur and Pluhar 1997). The diameter of the muscle may be normal or smaller in the traumatized region.

A *fascial tear* appears as an interruption of the hyperechoic line enrobing the muscle belly, with protrusion of this muscle through the defect.

In *complete muscle rupture*, the typical echotexture of the muscle structure at the site of trauma is no longer visible. Because of acute hemorrhage, the area appears anechoic or hypoechoic (Figure 16.49B). In chronic rupture, the region appears highly inhomogeneous and has a mixed echotexture and echogenicity (organization of the hematoma) (Figure 16.50). The muscle stump can be described as a coblike, thickened, inhomogeneous structure that is more echogenic than the surrounding tissue. During a dynamic examination with flexion and extension of the limb, the separation of the muscle ends becomes evident (Kramer et al. 1997).

Muscular Contracture and Amyotrophy Muscular contracture affecting any muscle, but particularly the gracilis, infraspinatus, or quadriceps muscles, results in abnormal muscle echotexture and echogenicity.

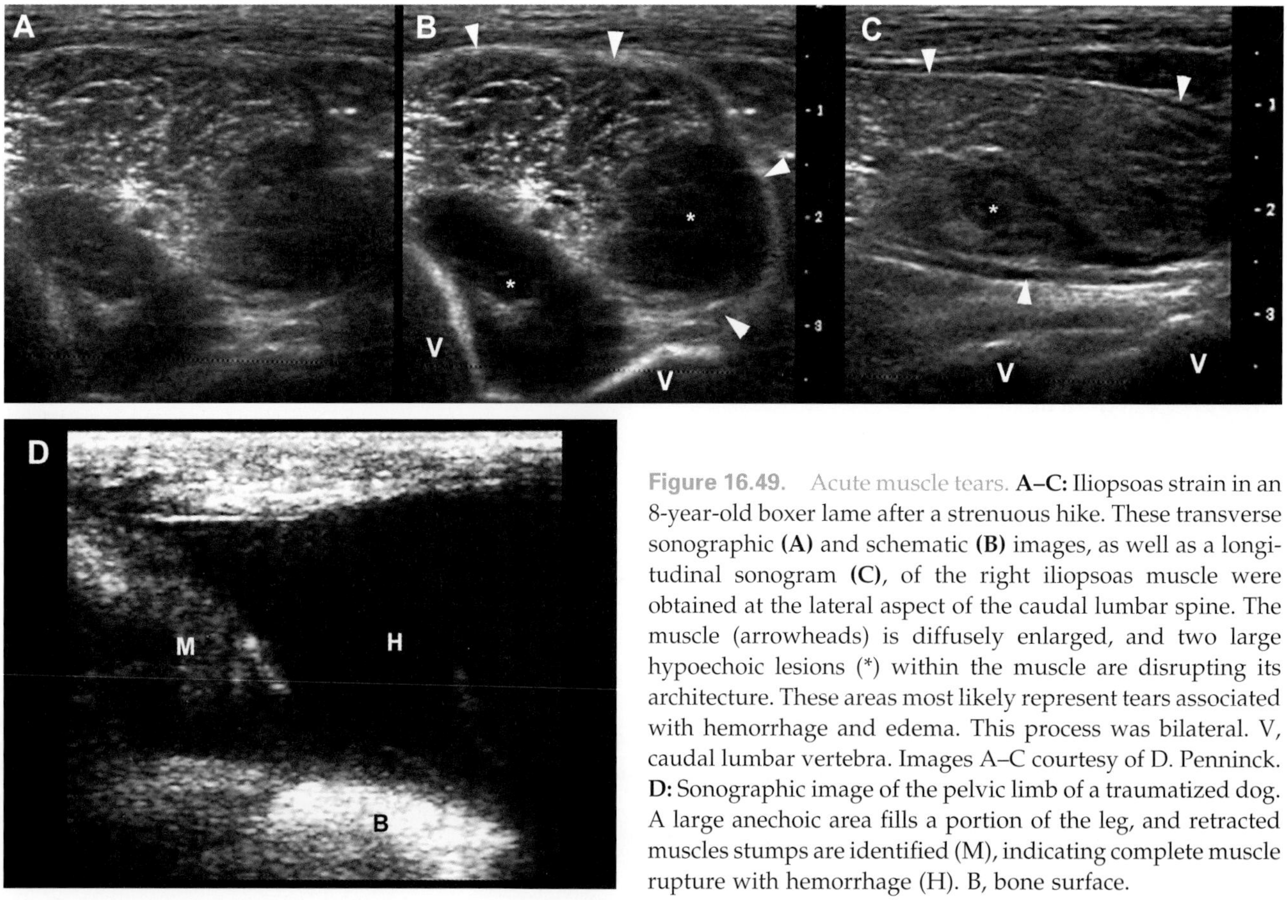

Figure 16.49. Acute muscle tears. **A–C:** Iliopsoas strain in an 8-year-old boxer lame after a strenuous hike. These transverse sonographic **(A)** and schematic **(B)** images, as well as a longitudinal sonogram **(C)**, of the right iliopsoas muscle were obtained at the lateral aspect of the caudal lumbar spine. The muscle (arrowheads) is diffusely enlarged, and two large hypoechoic lesions (*) within the muscle are disrupting its architecture. These areas most likely represent tears associated with hemorrhage and edema. This process was bilateral. V, caudal lumbar vertebra. Images A–C courtesy of D. Penninck. **D:** Sonographic image of the pelvic limb of a traumatized dog. A large anechoic area fills a portion of the leg, and retracted muscles stumps are identified (M), indicating complete muscle rupture with hemorrhage (H). B, bone surface.

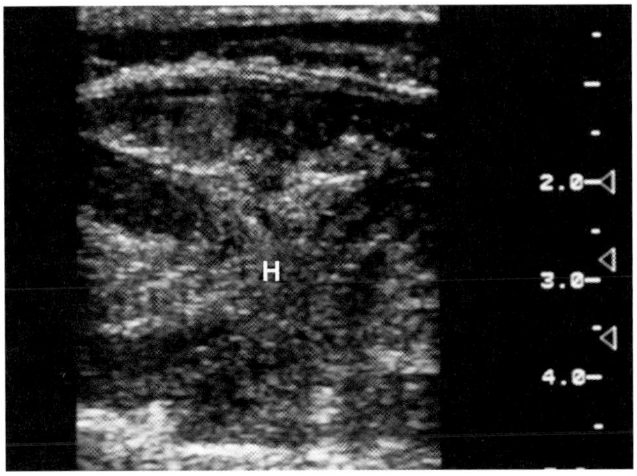

Figure 16.50. Muscle tear with hemorrhage. Sonographic image of a pelvic limb muscle in another dog with previous trauma. A large, inhomogeneous, intramuscular mass is noted that is consistent with an organizing hematoma (H). Note the difference in echotexture when compared with the normal muscle shown in Figure 16.48.

Hyperechoic and variably inhomogeneous regions are observed in the affected muscle, primarily because of fibrosis. The fascia is usually difficult to differentiate from the surrounding tissue. The appearance of the muscle begins to resemble a tendon, and the muscle fibers become indistinct. These changes often involve the entire muscle (Kramer et al. 1996).

Muscle atrophy caused by chronic disuse or neuropathy is associated with only minimal echotexture changes. The echogenicity of the affected muscle tends to be slightly increased but remains homogeneous.

Fibrosing and Calcifying Myopathies and Tendinopathies

Fibrosing and calcifying myopathies and tendinopathies, which may or may not be traumatic in origin, are occasionally seen in dogs. The muscular and/or tendinous part of the supraspinatus, iliopsoas, gluteal, biceps brachii, and abductor pollicis longus are more commonly affected (Figures 16.51 and 16.52). The calcium deposits are visible as hyperechoic, irregular structures that display acoustic shadowing. The affected tendon or muscle can also become enlarged, with an altered, inhomogeneous echotexture.

Ligaments

Scanning Technique and Normal Sonographic Anatomy

The ligaments of dogs and cats are usually very small and frequently close to uneven bony surfaces, making sonographic assessment difficult. The use of high-frequency (ideally >12 MHz), linear transducers directed perfectly perpendicular to the ligament is essential.

In longitudinal scans, linear ligaments appear as hyperechoic structures with a fibrillar echotexture (Figure 16.22). Most ligaments are too small to be consistently identified, particularly in cross-sectional planes, because they cannot be distinguished from the surrounding structures (capsule and muscle fascia). Ligaments with fanning fibers are oriented obliquely (e.g., cruciate ligaments) and are usually hypoechoic.

Sonographic Features of Ligament Disorders

Because of their small size, acutely ruptured ligaments cannot be easily visualized with ultrasound. A small anechoic or hypoechoic hematoma in the area of rupture may be seen in the initial phase. If the injury is associated with a bone avulsion fracture, the fragment is visible as a hyperechoic structure with acoustic shadowing within the reactive tissue. Ruptured ligament stumps can become hyperechoic and thickened, particularly in the chronic phase. Ligament rupture may cause joint instability, which may be evidenced by means of a dynamic examination. Over time, capsular thickening develops.

Cellulitis, Abscesses, and Foreign Bodies

Cellulitis is an inflammatory process involving the connective tissue and typically appears as alternating anechoic and hyperechoic bands in the subcutaneous planes, often resulting in increased ultrasound-beam attenuation that limits the assessment of deep structures (Figure 16.54B). Inflamed tissue can become enlarged. *Phlegmon* is a suppurative inflammation of the connective tissue that typically leads to accumulation of hypoechoic fluid pockets in the subcutaneous tissues (Figures 16.53 and 16.54).

More confined *abscesses* may also develop and appear as cavitary masses containing particulate fluid. A hyperechoic wall of variable thickness is often recognized in the chronic phase (Figures 16.54C and 16.56). Internal septa may also form. Thus, abscesses can be complex in ultrasonographic appearance and resemble neoplastic processes. An abscess can be identified as either intramuscular or intermuscular, subfascial, or subcutaneous. Ultrasound-guided fine-needle aspiration or drainage may assist in the diagnosis and treatment of the suppurative process (Figure 16.53B).

Inflammatory processes may be secondary to the presence of *foreign bodies* (FBs), such as wooden sticks,

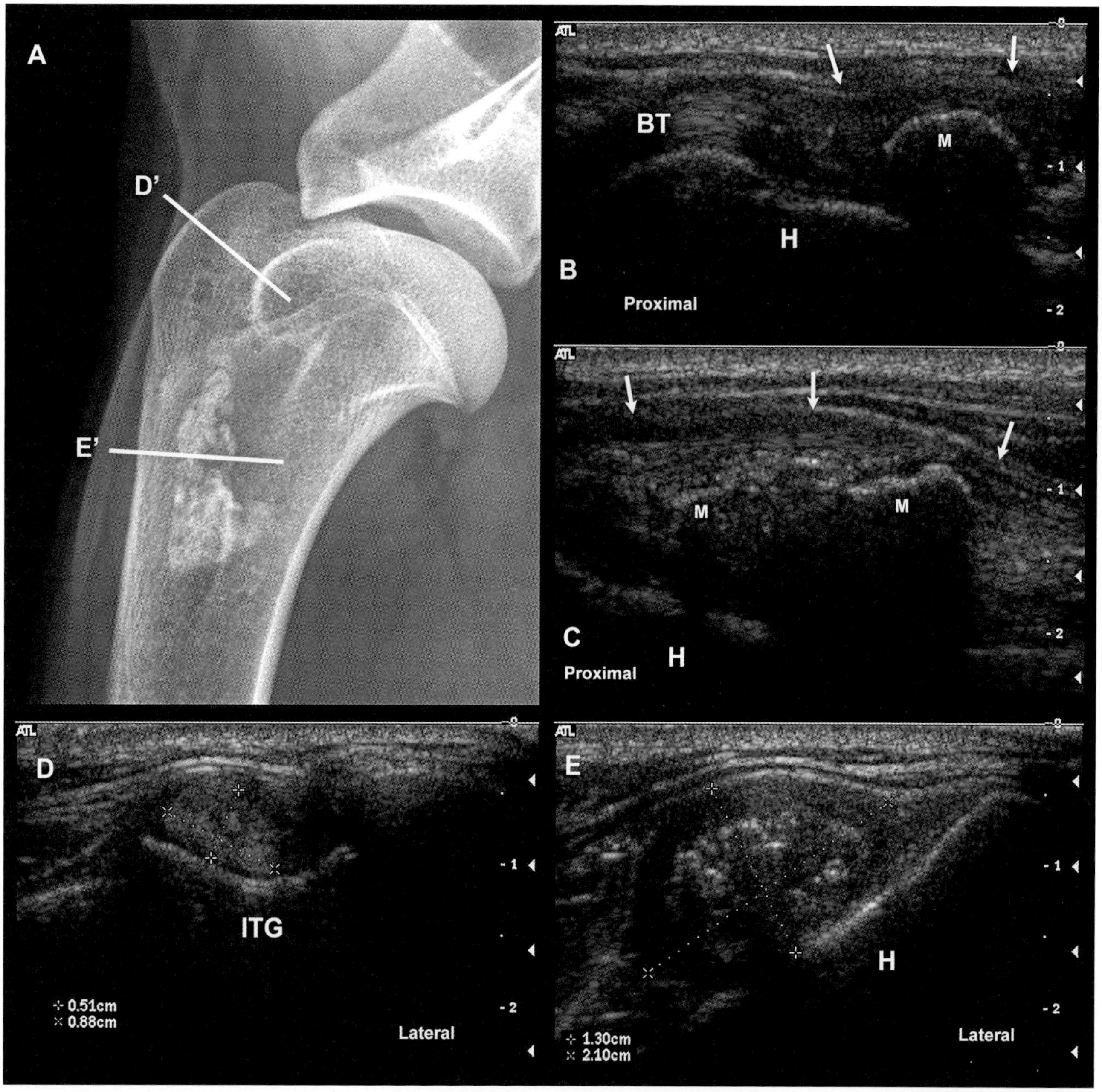

Figure 16.51. Bicipital calcifying myopathy. **A:** Mediolateral radiograph of the shoulder region of a 2-year-old large-breed dog with chronic thoracic lameness. An irregular mineral opacity is noted superimposed over the proximal humeral metaphysis in the region of the biceps muscle. **B and C:** Longitudinal sonograms obtained at the proximal aspect of the biceps muscle. This portion of the muscle is enlarged (arrows), heterogeneous, and contains irregular hyperechoic areas with acoustic shadowing, consistent with mineralization (M). **D and E:** Transverse sonograms The biceps tendon (BT) (cursors) is also mildly enlarged on this transverse image **(D)** obtained at the level of the intertubercular groove (ITG) (plane D′ in **A**). Just distal to the intertubercular groove (plane E′), the biceps muscle (between the cursors in **E**) is thickened and presents hyperechoic foci, some of which are associated with acoustic shadowing, consistent with mineralization and fibrosis. H, humerus.

porcupine quills, grass awns, glass, or plastic or metal objects (Figures 16.55–16.57). The accuracy of ultrasonography in detecting FBs, particularly if superficial, in people is high (Boyse et al. 2001). Although most FBs are hyperechoic to normal soft tissues, their echogenicity can vary, depending on their physical and acoustic characteristics (Boyse et al. 2001; Armbrust et al. 2003). Acoustic shadowing is expected; however, it may only be partial or be masked by the presence of a bony structure in the far field or by the ultrasono-

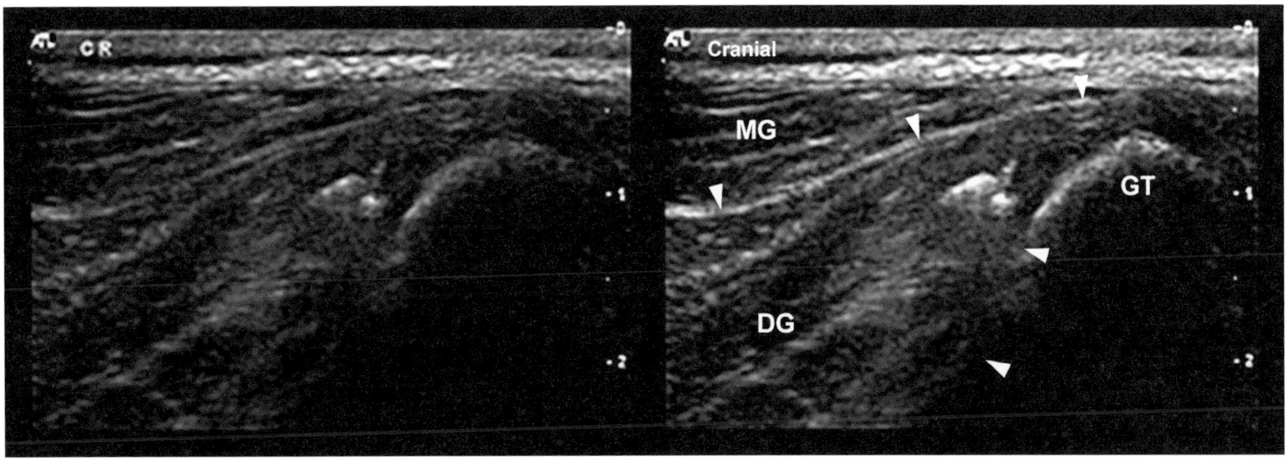

Figure 16.52. Gluteal calcifying myopathy. Longitudinal sonographic and schematic images of the distal portion of the middle gluteal (MG) and deep gluteal (DG) muscles. The deep gluteal muscle (arrowheads) is heterogeneous and presents hyperechoic foci near its insertion site on the greater trochanter (GT), consistent with mineralization. Image courtesy of D. Penninck.

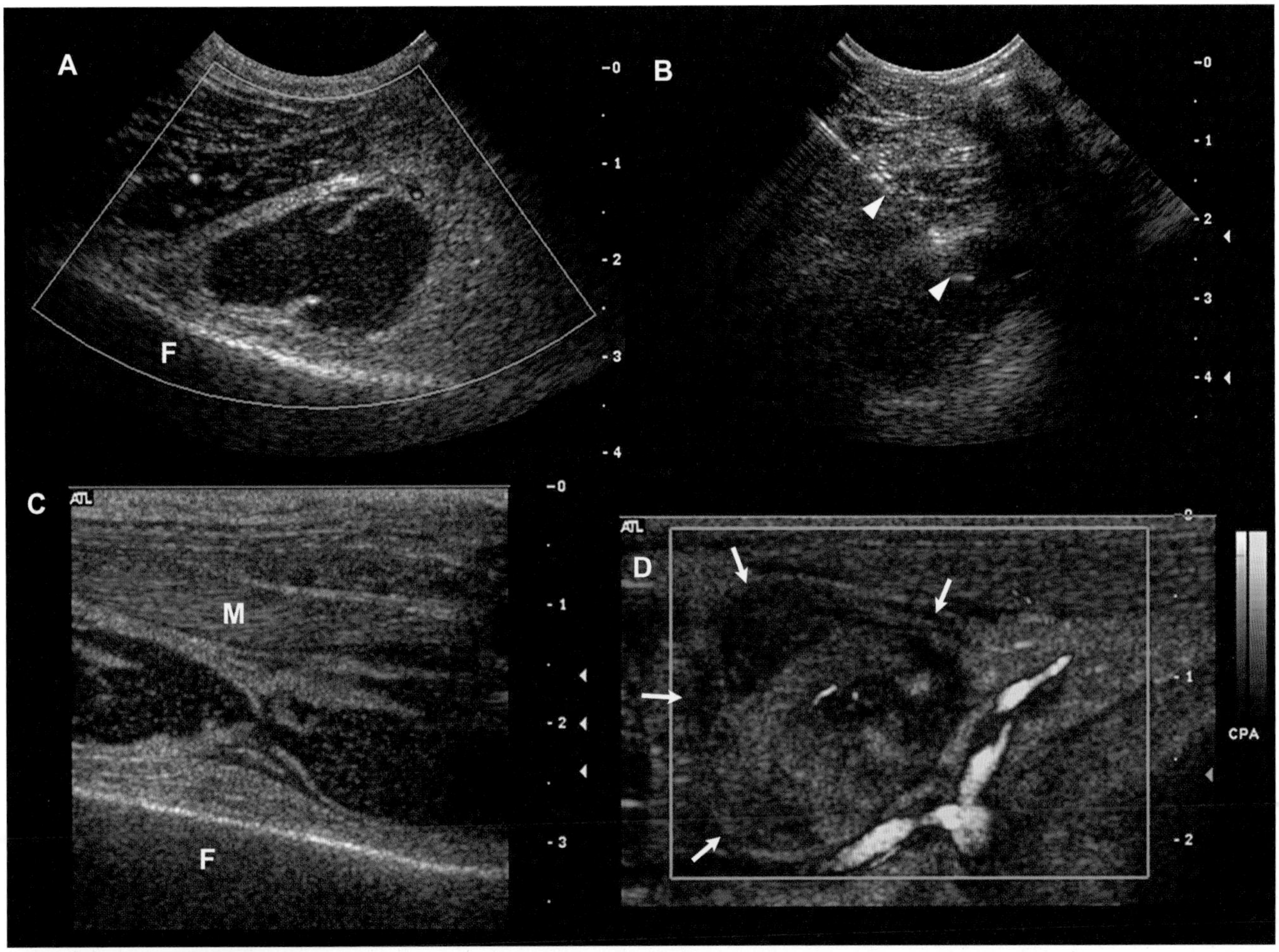

Figure 16.53. Intermuscular abscess and myositis in a cat. Transverse **(A)** and longitudinal **(C)** sonographic images obtained at the caudal aspect of the femur (F) in a cat with pelvic limb swelling and fever. An irregular accumulation of echogenic fluid is found between one of the muscles (M) and the femur. **B:** This cavitary lesion was aspirated using ultrasound guidance, which led to a diagnosis of a septic abscess. **D:** A nearby inhomogeneous mass (arrows) was found adjacent to large vessels. Fine-needle aspiration confirmed the presence of septic and necrotic myositis.

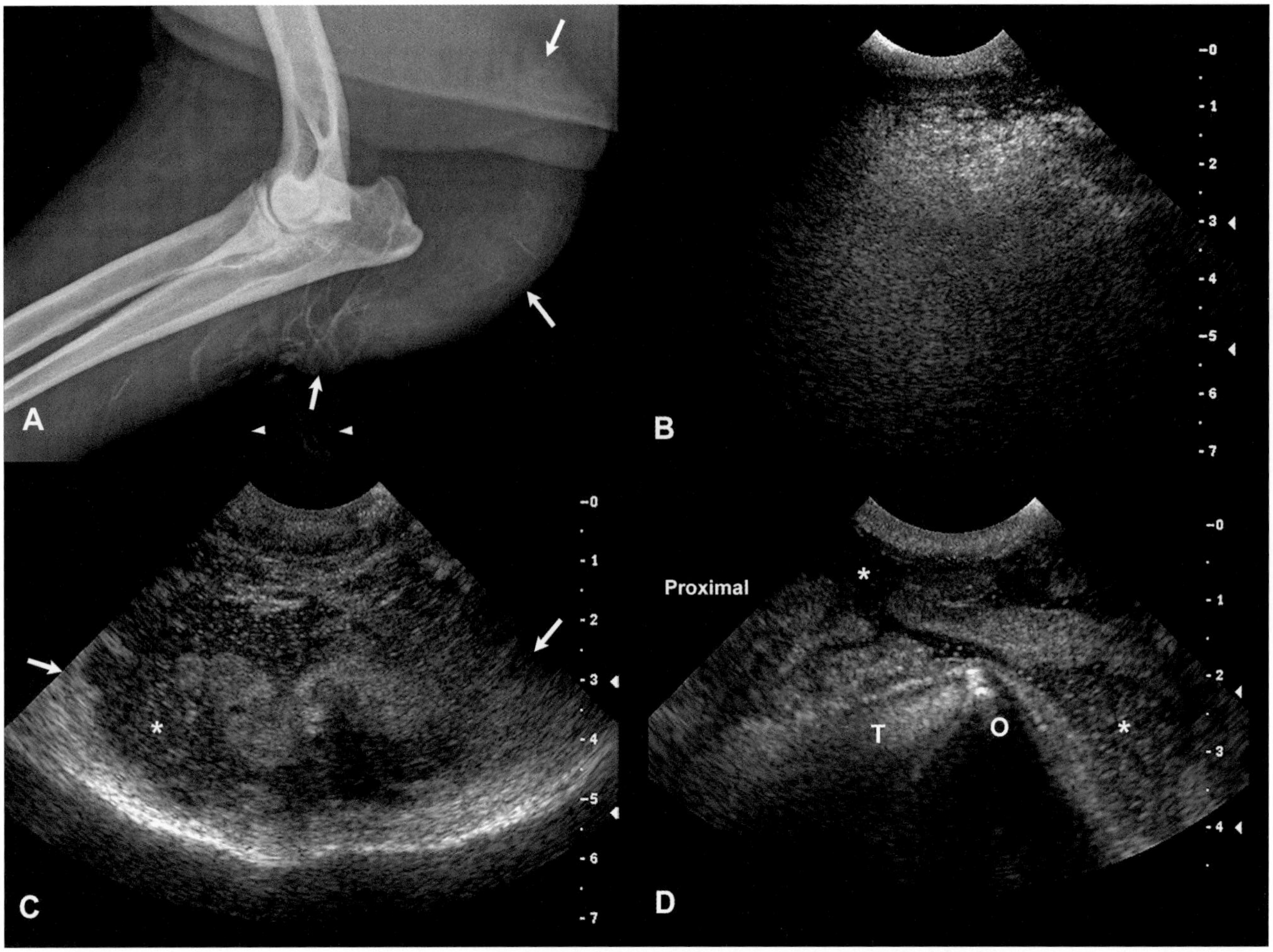

Figure 16.54. Septic abscess in the elbow region of a dog. **A:** Mediolateral radiograph of the elbow region of a 5-year-old large-breed dog with progressive, painful swelling caudal to the elbow. Soft-tissue swelling (arrows) is present without evidence of bone involvement or a radiopaque foreign body. This radiograph was obtained after the ultrasound exam, which explains the presence of artifacts caused by wet hair (arrowheads) caused by the presence of acoustic gel. **B:** In the proximal region of the limb, the subcutaneous tissue appears hyperechoic and hyperattenuating as the result of cellulitis. **C and D:** A large cavitary mass lesion (arrows) containing echogenic fluid (*) and mobile echogenic septa is caudal to the olecranon (O) and triceps tendon (T). An irregular, moderately echogenic capsule is noted proximally (arrow to the left in **C**).

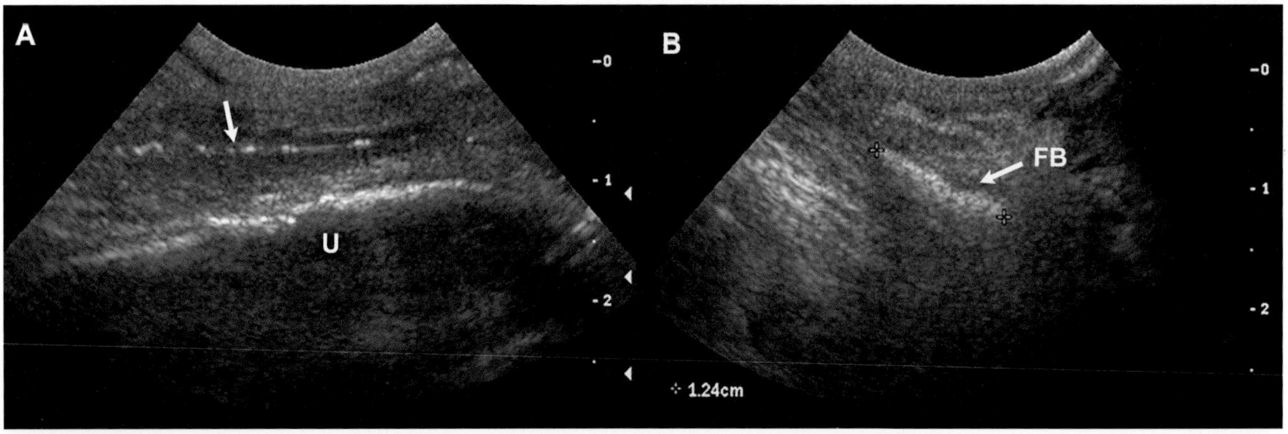

Figure 16.55. Fistular tract and foreign body. **A:** Longitudinal image of the region caudal to the proximal ulna (U) in a dog with a chronic draining tract. An interrupted hyperechoic line (arrow), consistent with gas, is seen within a hypoechoic cast of fibrous tissue. The caudal surface of the ulna is irregular because of periostitis. **B:** More distally, a 1.2-cm-long hyperechoic interface with dirty shadowing is found, which indicated a foreign body (FB).

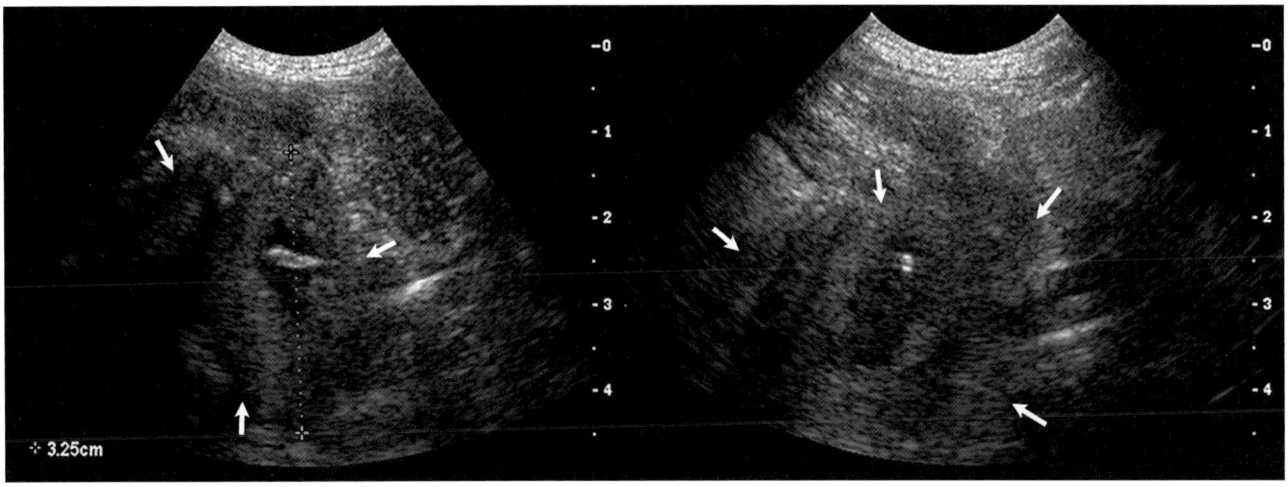

Figure 16.56. Porcupine quill migration and abscess. A 3.25-cm, moderately echogenic mass (arrows) is shown with a central fluid-filled cavity as well as a short, fusiform, double-lined hyperechoic structure when seen longitudinally and circular when seen transversally.

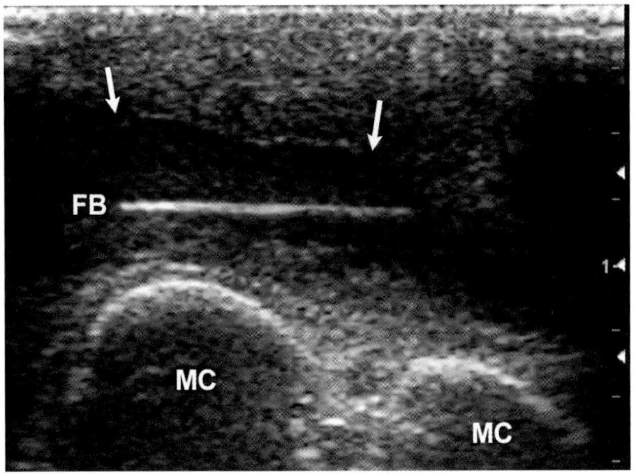

Figure 16.57. Wooden stick foreign body. Transverse sonographic image obtained at the dorsal aspect of the metacarpal bones (MC) of a dog. A thin, straight, hyperechoic foreign body (FB) is surrounded by mildly echogenic inflammatory tissue (arrows). A wooden stick was identified at surgery.

graphic complexity of the associated soft-tissue reaction. Wooden sticks often are of medium echogenicity that can be confounded by the surrounding tissue changes. A hypoechoic rim, consistent with an inflammatory cast or fistular tract, commonly develops around an FB, helping its identification (Shah et al. 1992; Kramer et al. 1997; Gnudi et al. 2005) (Figure 16.55). Also, in some instances, the artifacts associated with the FBs are more clearly visible than the body itself. The characteristics of the artifacts present deeper to the objects appear to be related to the surface shape of the FBs rather than to its composition (Boyse et al. 2001). Metal objects are typically associated with reverberation artifacts (comet tails), which may be confused with air bubbles. Metal objects of any size can easily be identifiable on standard radiographs. Glass is typically hyperechoic and may be recognized on radiographs. Porcupine quills appear as double-banded, fusiform, hyperechoic structures (Figure 16.56).

Small FBs may remain undetected if smaller than 2–3 mm or if deeply embedded in tissues. Furthermore, the presence of nearby mineral or aerated structures, such as in the region of the distal extremities (e.g., sesamoid bones) or the larynx and hyoid apparatus, may limit the identification of FBs.

Ultrasound may also be useful in the surgical planning or intraoperatively, assisting in the localization of a FB (Brisson et al. 2004) by placing a fine needle under ultrasound guidance to the level of the FB.

Benign and Malignant Tumors

Soft-tissue tumors can usually be identified by using ultrasonography and are classified as solid, cystic, or mixed lesions. Tumors often show mixed echogenicity, and their echotexture ranges from homogeneous to highly inhomogeneous and from anechoic to highly hyperechoic (Figures 16.58–16.60). The tumor margins may or may not be clearly visible. When color Doppler is used, malignant tumors can appear hypervascular with tortuous and randomly distributed vessels (Figure 16.59). However, malignant tumors may also be poorly perfused and/or necrotic (Figure 16.60). Ultrasonography cannot accurately differentiate malignant and benign diseases such as hemorrhage (Thiel et al. 2003) (Figure 16.61). Ultrasound-guided or surgical aspiration or biopsy is required in all cases.

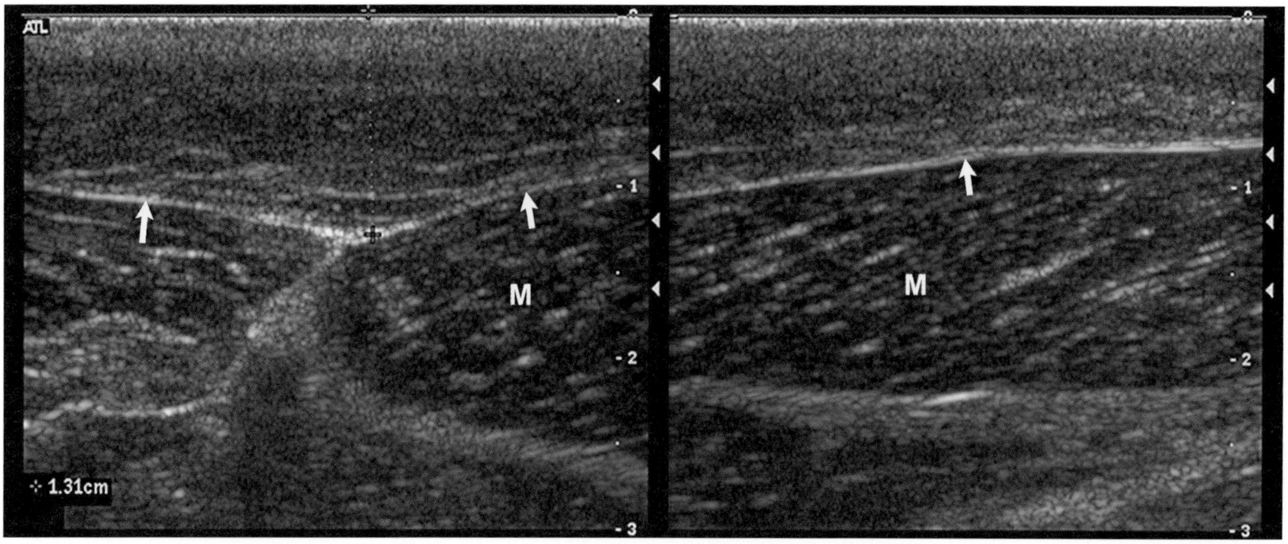

Figure 16.58. Subcutaneous lymphoma in a cat. In these sonographic images obtained at the lateral aspect of the pelvic limb, a moderately echogenic band in the near field is silhouetting with the dermis. Muscle bellies (M) are displaced, but not invaded by the neoplastic process. The muscle fascias (arrows) remain well defined.

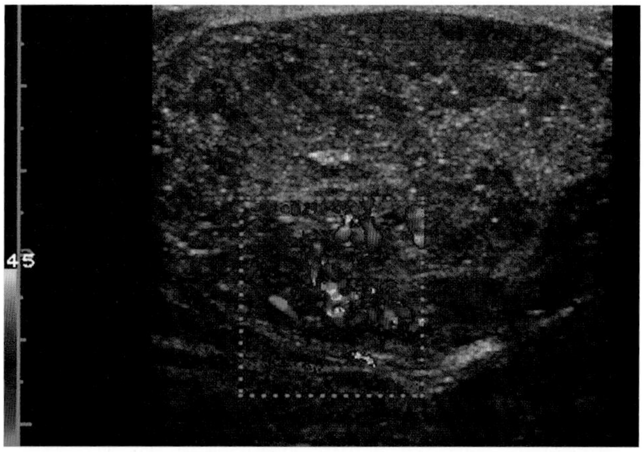

Figure 16.59. Muscular fibrosarcoma in a dog. Sonographic image a large soft-tissue mass involving the limb of a dog. The mass is relatively hyperechoic and well vascularized, as evidenced by using color Doppler in the deep portion of the mass.

Lipomas appear as mildly echogenic masses with diffuse hyperechoic dots and striations (Volta et al. 2006) (Figure 16.62). Lipomas can be located in the subcutaneous or intermuscular planes or within muscles (intramuscular). They are usually well encapsulated, although they can be ill-defined and invasive. The distinction between invasive or noninvasive lipomas cannot be made with accuracy by means of ultrasonography.

Ultrasound can also be very useful in the identification of *soft-tissue joint tumors* such as synovial cell sarcoma or histiocytic sarcoma. These tumors can vary in echotexture and echogenicity but typically appear as an irregular soft-tissue thickening that crosses the joint space, invades the osteochondral junctions, and protrudes into the synovial space (Figure 16.63). The bone surface at the periphery of the joint becomes irregular, and soft-tissue nodules or masses can be seen to extend within the metaphyseal cortex and medulla. These changes may also resemble severe DJD or other arthropathies, which justifies fine-needle aspiration or biopsy.

Bones

Scanning Technique and Sonographic Anatomy

Although radiography remains the principal modality in the investigation of bone diseases, ultrasonography can provide additional information, particularly in regard to the soft-tissue component of these processes. Linear transducers are preferred over convex or sectorial probes, because linear transducers provide a better image quality (higher resolution and less distortion). The exam is performed similarly as for muscles and tendons, with the patient in lateral recumbency.

The surface of a long bone is examined by slowly moving the probe along the long axis of the bone, usually with a longitudinal plane that enables visualizing a larger portion of the bone surface. This way, the area of interest can be compared with adjacent normal portions of the bone (e.g., tumor or fracture). A transverse view only rarely provides additional information (Risselada et al. 2003).

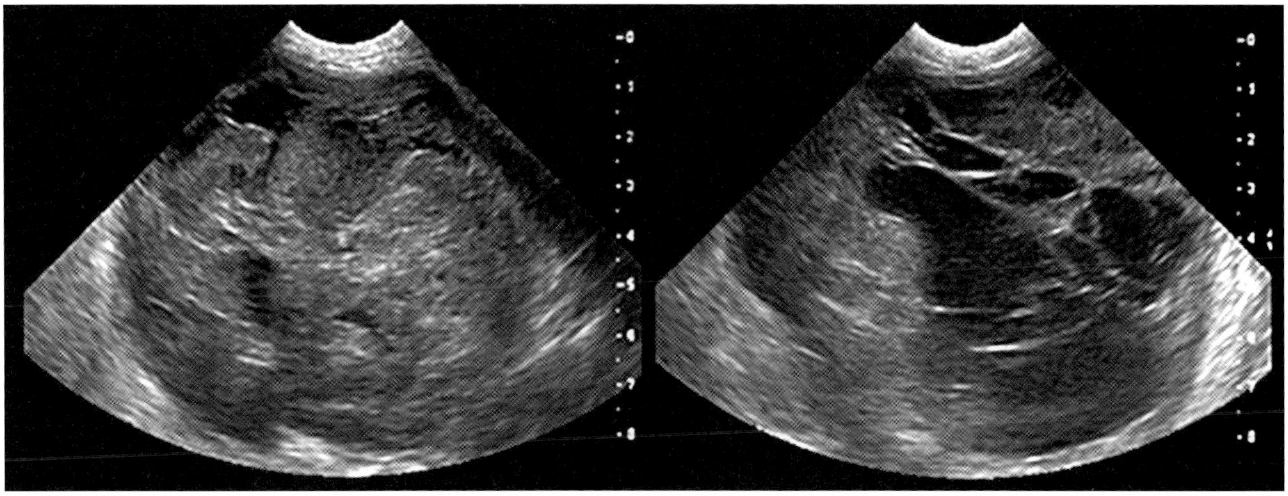

Figure 16.60. Fibrosarcoma. Sonographic images of a large soft-tissue mass involving the pelvic limb of a dog. This mass is solid and moderately echogenic in most areas, but also presents anechoic, fluid-filled necrotic and hemorrhagic cavities. Images courtesy of D. Penninck.

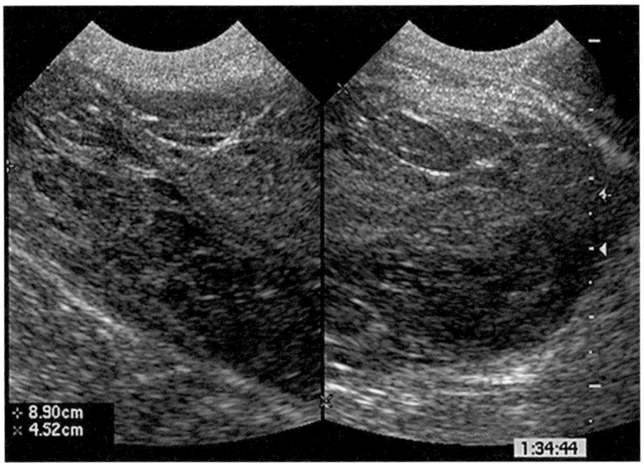

Figure 16.61. Muscular hemorrhage. Sonographic images of the pelvic limb of a dog with rapidly progressive swelling. A hypoechoic, inhomogeneous mass measuring more than 9 cm is noted involving the musculature. Hemorrhage was found on fine-needle aspiration. This mass resolved with time and was presumed to represent a benign spontaneous hematoma of uncertain origin.

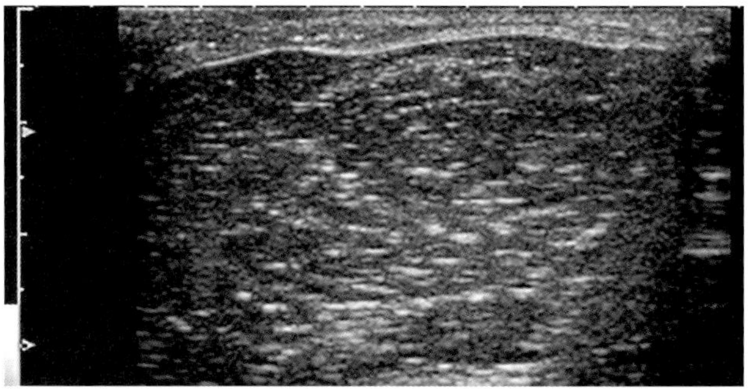

Figure 16.62. Lipoma. Sonographic image of a subcutaneous mass with features characteristic of a lipoma. The mass is moderately echogenic and has uniformly distributed hyperechoic dots and short lines.

Because of the reflection and absorption of the sound waves, the bone surface appears as a smooth, hyperechoic, continuous line with strong acoustic shadowing. This surface is more irregular at the sites of origin and insertion of tendons and ligaments. Superficial to the bony surface, the typical echotexture of soft-tissue structures, i.e., muscles and tendons, comes into view. In the near field, the image of the skin-transducer interface can be seen as a hyperechoic zone (Risselada et al. 2003).

Sonographic Features of Bone Disorders

Osteomyelitis and Bone Tumors Osteomyelitis can vary in ultrasonographic appearance. An ill-defined, irregular hyperechoic surface can be seen superficial to the bone cortex because of periosteal new bone formation. Peripheral, inflamed soft tissues appear swollen, hypoechoic, and inhomogeneous. The lytic cortical surface can be uneven, with multiple indentations (Kramer et al. 1997).

Primary and metastatic bone tumors associated with cortical lysis can be assessed sonographically, particularly if they extend into the surrounding soft tissue. They can vary in echogenicity and uniformity (Figures 16.64 and 16.65). Occasionally, periosteal elevation (Codman's triangle) is seen. If sufficient cortical lysis is present, the deeper bone tissue can be visualized.

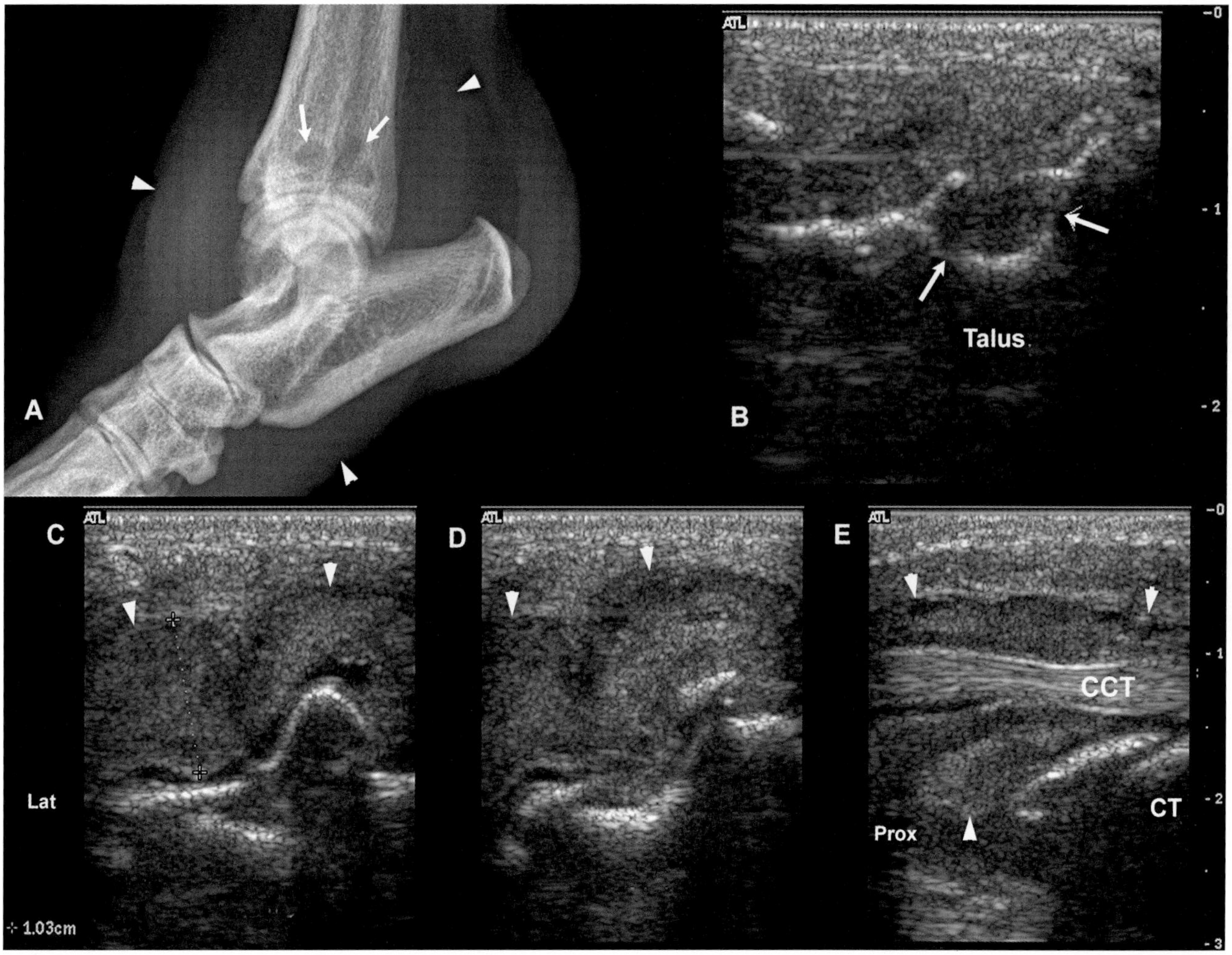

Figure 16.63. Synovial cell sarcoma. **A:** Mediolateral radiograph of the tarsus of a 6-year-old large-breed dog with chronic lameness. Soft-tissue swelling (arrowheads) is noted at the periphery of the tarsus, as well as lytic foci in the distal tibial metaphysis (arrows). **B–D:** Longitudinal **(B)** and transverse **(C and D)** sonograms of the dorsal aspect of the talus that show an irregular layer of echogenic tissue in the near field (arrowheads), as well as irregular bone defects (arrows). Lat, lateral. **E:** Longitudinal sonogram obtained at the plantar aspect. The soft-tissue thickening (arrowheads) is noted at the periphery of the common calcaneal tendon (CCT), reaching the level of the calcaneal tuberosity (CT). These features are typical of synovial cell sarcoma or synovial histiocytic sarcoma. Prox, proximal.

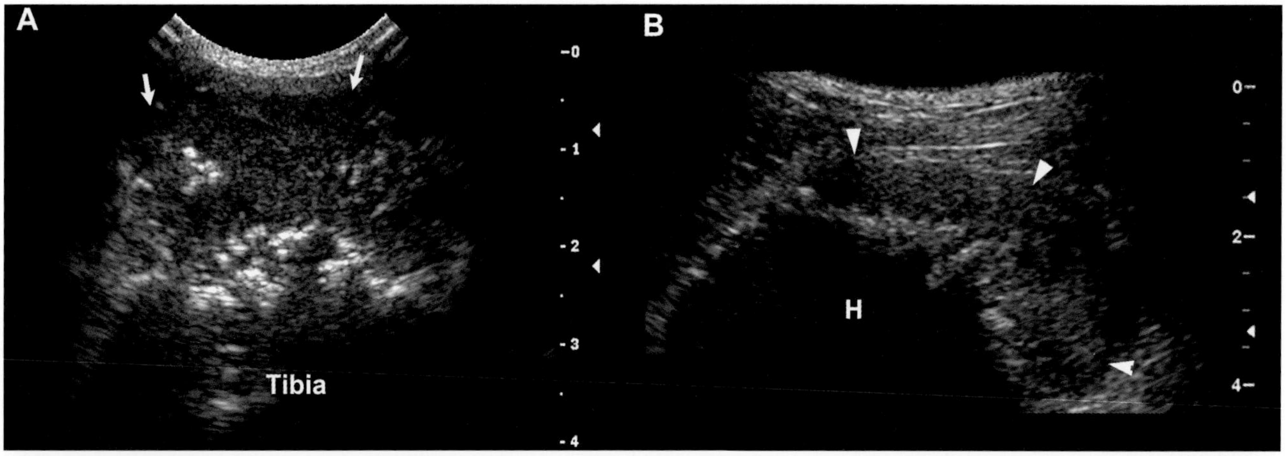

Figure 16.64. Osteosarcoma. Sonographic images of aggressive tibial **(A)** and humeral **(B)** mass lesions in two dogs. **A:** An ill-defined, hypoechoic mass (arrows) has hyperechoic foci, some of which are associated with acoustic shadowing, consistent with mineralization. The underlying bone cortex is no longer visible because of the extensive lysis. **B:** A well-defined, mildly echogenic mass (arrowheads) involves the humerus (H). The surface of the humerus is markedly irregular because of aggressive new bone formation and lysis.

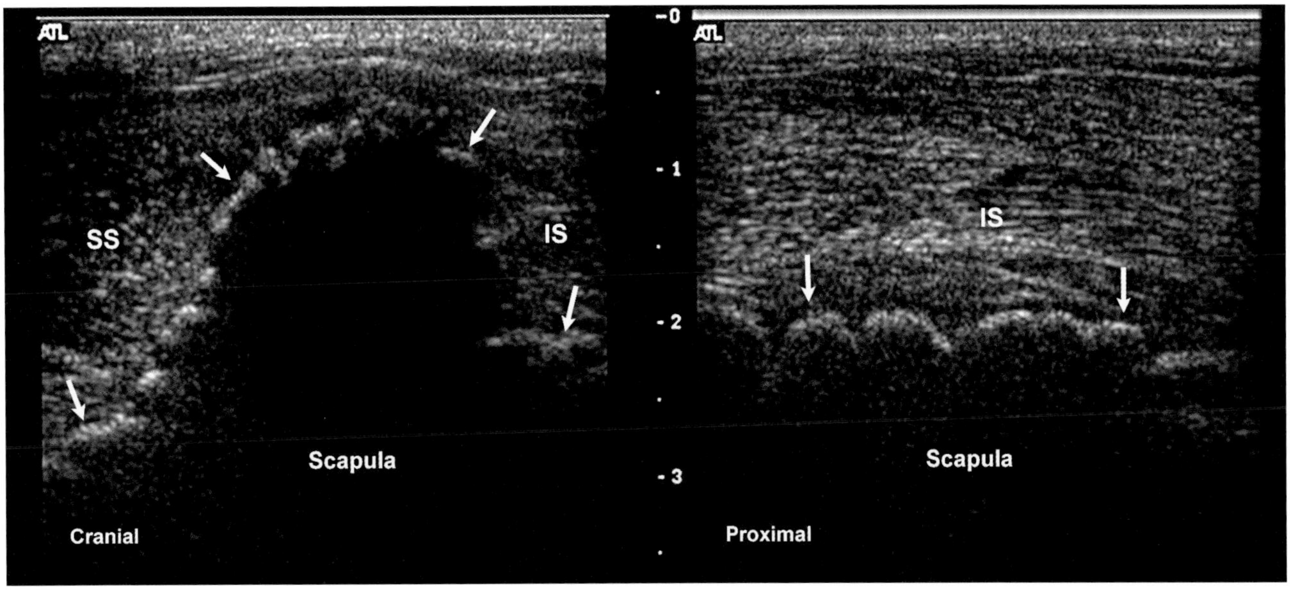

Figure 16.65. Metastatic carcinoma to the scapula. Transverse **(left)** and longitudinal **(right)** sonograms of the scapular spine in a dog with a transitional cell carcinoma and metastatic disease. Irregular new bone formation (arrows) is present at the level of the scapula. Adjacent supraspinatus (SS) and infraspinatus (IS) muscles are reduced in thickness and hyperechoic because of atrophy. Several similar lesions were identified in other bones, and metastatic carcinoma was confirmed.

Ultrasound can also assist in fine-needle aspiration or biopsy of bone lesions, avoiding the need for surgical biopsy in some patients (Samii et al. 1999).

Fractures Fractures of long bones and their healing process, as well as the associated soft-tissue damage (muscle rupture or hematoma), can be assessed ultrasonographically. Because there are no points of orientation, the exact relationship between the fractured ends is difficult to determine. To standardize the documentation of fracture healing of long bones, multiple and repeatable images must be obtained. The recommended transducer positions for the assessment of long bones are craniolateral (distal humerus, radius, ulna, and tibia) and caudolateral (proximal humerus cranial, femur medial, and fibula) (Risselada et al. 2003).

Ultrasonography can be used to evaluate secondary fracture healing in biologically treated fractures (Risselada et al. 2005). In comparison to radiography, the completion of fracture healing can be determined earlier. Secondary fracture healing can be divided into five stages.

Stage I (0–7 days after trauma): The area surrounding the fracture is homogeneous and hypoechoic to anechoic because of hematoma formation. The fracture site appears as a discontinuity (step) of the bone surface, which may be associated with the presence of several, separate hyperechoic interfaces indicating multiple fragments (Figure 16.66A). If the fracture gap is wide enough, the medulla region can be visualized. Surgical implants can be seen as hyperechoic, reverberating structures within or surrounding the bone.

Stage II (8–14 days after trauma): The tissue within the fracture gap appears hypoechoic to anechoic and more heterogeneous (resorption of the hematoma) (Figure 16.66B).

Stage IIIa (15–21 days after trauma): Fracture margins become irregular and blunted because of bone resorption. The early ossifying callus appears as an irregular or undulating hyperechoic surface. The surrounding tissue representing the maturing hematoma and the nonossified callus is inhomogeneous with a hypoechoic to isoechoic echotexture (compared with overlying muscles).

Stage IIIb (22–28 days after trauma): The nonossified callus becomes progressively more echogenic (Figure 16.66C).

Stage IV (29–42 days after trauma): The echogenicity of the callus increases and appears heterogeneous, consistent with incomplete ossification. Hyperechoic mineral foci, which may display acoustic shadowing, are noted in the callus (Figure 16.66D).

Stage V (more than 43 days after trauma): The fracture has healed completely. The cortex is seen as a continuous, smooth, or slightly irregular, hyperechoic line (Figure 16.66E). The surrounding soft-tissue thickening is reduced or resolved. Intramedullary implants

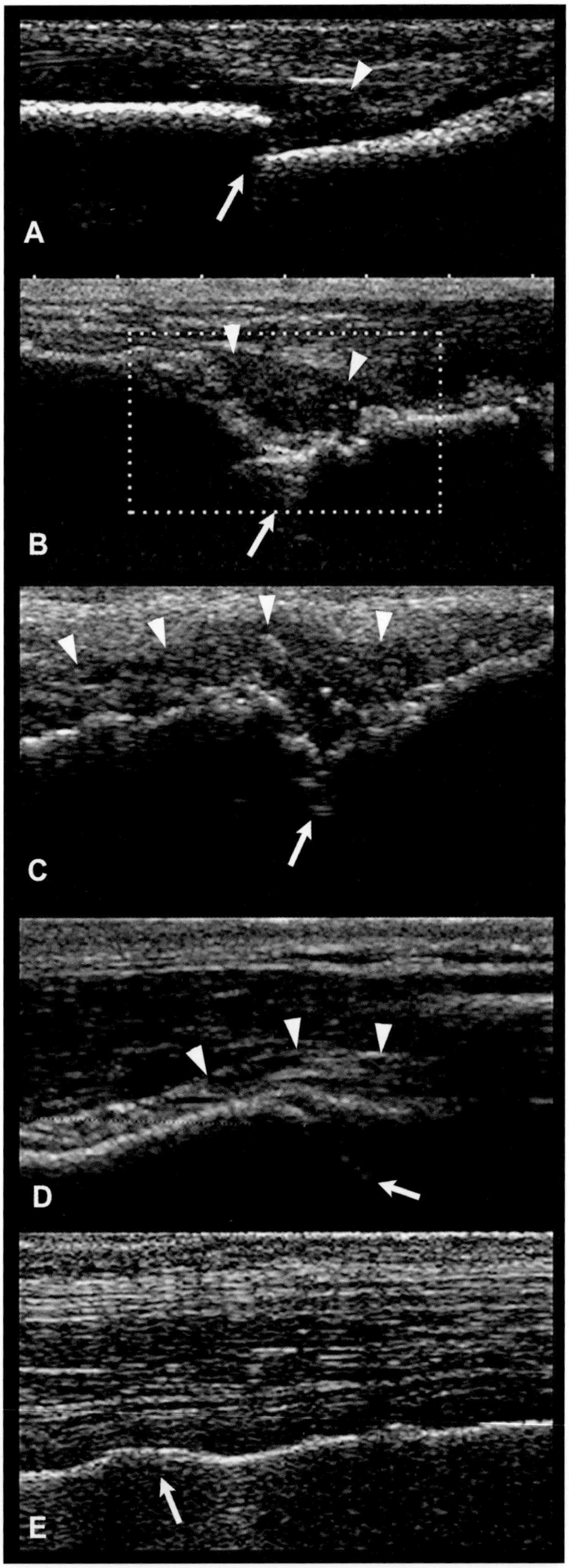

are no longer visible because the cortical integrity has been reestablished (Risselada et al. 2005).

During normal fracture healing, the newly developing tissues require more nutrients and have a higher metabolic rate. This requires the development of new vessels (neovascularization) at the fracture site and can be visualized using power Doppler ultrasound. A Doppler signal can be obtained as of day 10 after trauma, reaching a maximum between days 11 and 30, before gradually decreasing. Signals can be detected in and close to the callus (Risselada et al. 2006).

References

Adams WM, Dueland RT, Daniels R, Fialkowski JP, Nordheim EV (2000) Comparison of two palpation, four radiographic and three ultrasound methods for early detection of mild to moderate canine hip dysplasia. Vet Radiol Ultrasound 41:484–490.

Armbrust LJ, Biller DS, Radlinsky MG, Hoskinsons JJ (2003) Ultrasonographic diagnosis of foreign bodies associated with chronic draining tracts and abscesses in dogs. Vet Radiol Ultrasound 44:66–70.

Breur GJ, Blevins WE (1997) Traumatic injury of the iliopsoas muscle in three dogs. J Am Vet Med Assoc 210:1631–1634.

Brisson BA, Bersenas A, Etue SM (2004) Ultrasonographic diagnosis of septic arthritis secondary to porcupine quill migration in a dog. J Am Vet Med Assoc 9:1467–1470.

Boyse TD, Fessell DP, Jacobson JA, Lin J, van Holsbeeck MT, Hayes CW (2001) US of soft-tissue foreign bodies and associated complications with surgical correlation. Radiographics 12:1251–1256.

Engelke A, Meyer-Lindenberg A, Nolte I (1997a) Die Ultraschalluntersuchung des Kniegelenkes des Hundes [The ultrasonographic examination of the stifle joint in dogs]. Berl Munch Tierarztl Wochenschr 110:24–29.

Figure 16.66. Bone fracture: healing process. Sequential sonograms showing progressive bone healing. **A: Stage I (days 0–7).** A discontinuity of the bone cortex is identified that is associated with sharp ends (arrow). Hypoechoic soft-tissue swelling is noted at the fracture site (arrowhead). **B: Stage III (days 15–21).** The bone defect (arrow) is progressively remodeled. A nonossified callus (arrowheads) is present. **C: Stage IV (days 22–28).** The nonossified callus is progressively more echogenic (arrowheads), and the fracture gap (arrow) is progressively narrower. **D: Stage V (days 29–42).** The fracture gap is nearly completely filled with new bone and poorly seen (arrow). The peripheral callus is reduced in volume (arrowheads). **E: Stage VI (more than 43 days).** The fracture is healed. The surface of the bone remains mildly irregular (arrow).

Engelke A, Meyer-Lindenberg A, Nolte I (1997b). Die Ultraschalluntersuchung des inneren Kniegelenkes bei Hunden mit Kreuzbandriss [The ultrasonographic examination of the inner structures of the stifle joint in dogs with ruptured cranial cruciate ligament]. Dtsch Tierarztl Wochenschr 104:114–117.

Esterline ML, Armbrust L, Roush JK (2005) A comparison of palpation guided and ultrasound guided percutaneous biceps brachii tenotomy in dogs. Vet Comp Orthop Traumatol 18:135–139.

Floeck A, Kramer M, Tellhelm B, Schimke E (2003) Die sonographische Untersuchung des Hueftgelenks beim Deutschen-Schaeferhund-Welpen [Ultrasonographic examination of the hip joint of the German shepherd]. Tierarztl Prax 31:82–91.

Gerwing M, Kramer M (1994) Die Sononographie des Schultergelenkes und seiner umgebenden Weichteile beim Hund. Teil B: Sonographische Diagnostik von Erkrankungen im Bereich des Schultergelenkes [Ultrasonography of the shoulder joint and the surrounding soft tissue. Part B: Ultrasonographic diagnosis of diseases in the region of the shoulder joint]. Kleintierpraxis 39:141–156.

Gnudi G, Bertoni G (2001) Echographic examination of the stifle joint affected by cranial cruciate ligament rupture in the dog. Vet Radiol Ultrasound 42:266–270.

Gnudi G, Volta A, Bonazzi M, Gazzola M, Bretoni G (2005) Ultrasonographic features of grass awn migration in the dog. Vet Radiol Ultrasound 46:423–426.

Greshake RJ, Ackerman N (1992) Ultrasound of the coxofemoral joints of the canine neonate. Vet Radiol Ultrasound 33:99–104.

Hermanson JW, Evans HE (1993) Chapter 6: The Muscoloskeletal System. In: Evans HE, Christensen GC, eds. Miller's Anatomy of the Dog, 3rd edition. Philadelphia: WB Saunders, pp 258–384

Knox VW IV, Sehgal CM, Wood AK (2003) Correlation of ultrasonographic observations with anatomic features and radiography of the elbow joint in dogs. Am J Vet Res 64:721–726.

Kramer M, Gerwing M (1994) Die Sononographie des Schultergelenkes und seiner umgebenden Weichteile beim Hund. Teil A: Die sonographische Anatomie des Schultergelenkes und seiner Weichteile [Ultrasonography of the shoulder joint and the surrounding soft tissue. Part A: Ultrasonographic anatomy of the shoulder joint]. Kleintierpraxis 39:71–80.

Kramer M, Gerwing M, Hach V, Schimke E (1997) Sonography of the musculoskeletal system in dogs and cats. Vet Radiol Ultrasound 38:139–149.

Kramer M, Gerwing M, Michele U, Schimke E, Kindler S (2001a) Ultrasonographic examination of injuries to the Achilles tendon in dogs and cats. J Small Anim Pract 42:531–535.

Kramer M, Gerwing M, Sheppard C, Schimke E (2001b) Ultrasonography for the diagnosis of diseases of the tendon and tendon sheath of the biceps brachii muscle. Vet Surg 30:64–71.

Kramer M, Stengel H, Gerwing M, Schimke E, Sheppard C (1999) Sonography of the canine stifle. Vet Radiol Ultrasound 40:282–293.

Kramer M, Schimke E, Schachenmayr W, Gerwing M (1996) Diagnosis and therapy of special tendon and muscle diseases in the dog. Part I: Contracture of the gracilis and infraspinatus muscle [in German]. Kleintierpraxis 41:889–896.

Lamb C, Duvernois A (2005) Ultrasonographic anatomy of the normal canine calcaneal tendon. Vet Radiol Ultrasound 46:326–330.

Lamb C, Wong K (2005) Ultrasonographic anatomy of the canine elbow. Vet Radiol Ultrasound 46:319–325.

Long C, Nyland TG (1999) Ultrasonographic evaluation of the canine shoulder. Vet Radiol Ultrasound 40:372–379.

Mahn MM, Cook JL, Cook CR, Balke MT (2005) Arthroscopic verification of ultrasonographic diagnosis of meniscal pathology in dogs. Vet Surg 34:318–323.

Mattern KL, Berry RB, Peck JN, de Haan JJ (2006) Radiographic and ultrasonographic evaluation of the patellar ligament following tibial plateau leveling osteotomy. Vet Radiol Ultrasound 47:185–191.

Michele U, Gerwing M (1999) Sonographie bei Metaplasien im Ursprung des M. flexor digitalis profundus des Hundes [Ultrasonographic findings of metaplasias in the origin of the flexor digitals profundus muscle in dogs]. Ultraschall Med 20:76.

Michele U, Gerwing M, Kramer M, Schimke E (1998) Sonographische Möglichkeiten am Ellbogengelenk des Hundes: Anatomische Grundlagen und pathologische Befunde [Ultrasonographic possibilities in the elbow of the dog: Anatomical structures and pathological findings]. In: Jahrestagung der DVG-FG Kleintierkrankheiten 19.-22.11.1998 Stuttgart, Kongr.ber. [Annual Conference of the DVG-FG on Small Animal Illnesses, November 19–22, 1998, Stuttgart]. Proceedings 44:385–388.

Mueller S, Kramer M (2003) Die Eignung der Sonographie für die Diagnostik von Meniskusläsionen des Hundes [Usefulness of ultrasonography in the diagnosis of meniscal lesions in the dog]. Tierarztl Prax 31:10–15.

Mueller S, Kramer M, Tellhelm B, Schimke E (2002) Rupture of the origin of the long digital extensor muscle in a border collie [in German]. Prakt Tierarzt 83:416–421.

Nielsen C, Pluhar GE (2004) Diagnosis and treatment of hind limb muscle strain injuries in 22 dogs. Vet Comp Orthop Traumatol 18:247–253.

O'Brien RT, Dueland RT, Adams WC, Meinen J (1997) Dynamic ultrasonographic measurement of passive coxofemoral joint laxity in puppies. J Am Anim Hosp Assoc 33:275–281.

Reed AL, Payne JT, Constaninescu GM (1995) Ultrasonographic anatomy of the normal canine stifle. Vet Radiol Ultrasound 36:315–321.

Risselada M, Kramer M, de Rooster H, Taeymans O, Verleyen P, van Bree H (2005) Ultrasonographic and radiographic assessment of uncomplicated secondary fracture healing of long bones in dogs and cats. Vet Surg 34:99–107.

Risselada M, Kramer M, van Bree H (2003) Approaches for ultrasonographic evaluation of long bones in the dog. Vet Radiol Ultrasound 44:214–220.

Risselada M, Kramer M, van Bree H, Taeymans O, Verleyen P (2006) Power Doppler assessment of the neovascularization during uncomplicated fracture healing of long bones in dogs and cats. Vet Radiol Ultrasound 47:301–306.

Rivers B, Wallace L, Johnston GR (1992) Biceps tenosynovitis in the dog: Radiographic and sonographic findings. Vet Comp Orthop Traumatol 5:51–57.

Rivers BJ, Walter PA, Kramek B, Wallace L (1997) Sonographic findings in canine common calcaneal tendon injury. Vet Comp Orthop Traumatol 10:45–53.

Samii VF, Nyland TG, Werner LL, Baker TW (1999) Ultrasound-guided fine-needle aspiration biopsy of bone lesions: A preliminary report. Vet Radiol Ultrasound 40: 82–86.

Schleich S, Tellhelm B, Schimke E, Gerwing M, Kramer M (1992) Korrelation zwischen klinischen, röntgenologischen, sonographischen und Operationsbefunden bei fragmentiertem Processus coronoideus des Hundes [Correlation between clinical, radiographic, ultrasonographic, and surgical findings in fractured coronoid process in the dog]. In: Jahrestagung der DVG-FG Kleintierkrankheiten 06.-08.11.1992 Bonn, Kong.ber. [Annual Conference of the DVG-FG on Small Animal Illnesses, November 6–8, 1992, Bonn]. Proceedings 38:406–420.

Shah ZR, Crass JR, Dubravka CO, Bellon EM (1992) Ultrasonographic detection of foreign bodies in soft tissues using turkey muscle as a model. Vet Radiol Ultrasound 33:94–100.

Siems JJ, Breur GJ, Blevins WE, Cornell KK (1998) Use of two-dimensional real-time ultrasonography for diagnosing contracture and strain of the infraspinatus muscle in a dog. J Am Vet Medic Assoc 212:77–80.

Swiderski J, Fitch RB, Staatz A, Lowery J (2005) Sonographic assisted diagnosis and treatment of bilateral gastrocnemius tendon rupture in a Labrador retriever repaired with fascia lata and polypropylene mesh. Vet Comp Orthop Traumatol 18:258–263.

Tacke S, Kramer M, Schimke E, et al. (1999) Osteochondrosis dissecans (OCD) am Schultergelenk des Hundes [Osteochondritis dissecans in the shoulder joint of the dog]. Tierarztl Prax 27:81–90.

Thiel C, Kramer M, Schimke E (2003) The ultrasonographic examination of skin tumors (B-mode, color Doppler, power Doppler) and their differential diagnosis in dogs and cats [in German]. Kleintierpraxis 48:253–260.

Vandevelde B, Saunders JH, Kramer M, Van Ryssen B, van Bree H (2006) Comparison of the ultrasonographic appearance of osteochondrosis lesions in the canine shoulder with radiography, arthrography and arthroscopy. Vet Radiol Ultrasound 47:174–184.

Volta A, Bonazzi M, Gnudi G, Gazzola M, Bertoni G (2006) Ultrasonographic features of canine lipomas. Vet Radiol Ultrasound 47:589–591.

INDEX